Oxford Medical Publications

Soft Tissue Rheumatology

Oxford Medical Publications
Soft Tissue Rheumatology

Edited by

Brian Hazleman

Rheumatology Research Unit
Addenbrooke's Hospital
Hills Road
Cambridge

Graham Riley

Rheumatology Research Unit
Addenbrooke's Hospital
Hills Road
Cambridge

Cathy Speed

Rheumatology Research Unit
Addenbrooke's Hospital
Hills Road
Cambridge

OXFORD
UNIVERSITY PRESS

UNIVERSITY PRESS

Great Clarendon Street, Oxford OX2 6DP

Oxford University Press is a department of the University of Oxford.
It furthers the University's objective of excellence in research, scholarship,
and education by publishing worldwide in

Oxford New York

Auckland Bangkok Buenos Aires Cape Town Chennai
Dar es Salaam Delhi Hong Kong Istanbul Karachi Kolkata
Kuala Lumpur Madrid Melbourne Mexico City Mumbai Nairobi
São Paulo Shanghai Taipei Tokyo Toronto

Oxford is a registered trade mark of Oxford University Press
in the UK and in certain other countries

Published in the United States
by Oxford University Press Inc., New York

A catalogue record for this title is available from the British Library

Library of Congress Cataloging in Publication Data
(Data available)

ISBN 019 263093 8

10 9 8 7 6 5 4 3 2 1

Typeset by Newgen Imaging Systems (P) Ltd., Chennai, India
Printed in Italy
on acid-free paper by LegoPrint s.r.1

Preface

Rheumatology is a broad medical speciality, encompassing a wide range of musculoskeletal and connective tissue disorders. In the last decade, great strides have been made toward understanding the inflammatory process and its role in arthritis. However, many of the musculoskeletal conditions seen by rheumatologists and general practitioners are not primarily problems of the hard tissues of the joint, and are not associated with overt inflammation. Much of the rheumatologist's caseload comprises multifarious disorders of the musculoskeletal soft connective tissues including tendon, ligament, sheath, capsule, bursa, intervertebral disc and meniscus. These rather disparate conditions are grouped together as problems of 'soft tissue rheumatology'.

One of the major difficulties encountered when attempting to estimate the true burden of soft tissue rheumatology has been variation in definition and diagnostic criteria for specific disorders. The diagnostic challenge that many conditions present may be one explanation for the apparent lack of effect of current conventional management approaches. The majority of cases are regional disorders for which there are no clear guidelines for investigation and management, nor indications for referral to secondary care. Although many soft tissue disorders eventually resolve without intervention, a substantial proportion are chronic and resistant to treatment. Despite the prevalence of these conditions, less is known about the pathology compared to those primarily affecting bone and cartilage.

Fortunately, interest in soft tissue rheumatology is increasing, and this has led to an improvement in our understanding of these complex disorders. Despite this, relatively few medical texts devote much attention to the musculoskeletal soft connective tissues. As a consequence the editors felt compelled to compile this textbook of soft tissue rheumatology.

The authors hold a strong belief that a scientific approach is fundamental, and for that reason this book begins with a section on the basic science of the soft connective tissues. Written by researchers active in the field, these chapters provide a comprehensive update on the structure, organisation and molecular composition of the major soft connective tissues in both health and disease. The focus is on tendon, ligament, intervertebral disc and meniscus, since these tissues are commonly implicated in soft tissue rheumatology. Other connective tissues such as cartilage and muscle have been extensively reviewed elsewhere. This section should provide the reader with a broad grasp of the fundamentals of soft tissue pathology from the laboratory perspective.

A scientific and evidence-based approach is maintained where possible throughout the rest of the book. We have strived to bring coherence to the nomenclature and diagnostic criteria applied to disorders of the musculoskeletal soft connective tissues. Since pain is the common denominator of all soft tissue disorders, it is appropriate to review the recent advances in our understanding of pain mechanisms. It is also important to include a review of joint biomechanics and locomotion analysis, scientific disciplines having significant implications for the aetiology of specific disorders. General principles of the diagnosis and management are followed by discussion of specific disorders.

We trust that this book will provide a comprehensive and up-to-date resource for anyone interested in these diverse medical conditions, whether they are scientists, medical students, general practitioners or specialists in musculoskeletal medicine.

Brian Hazleman
Graham Riley
Cathy Speed

Acknowledgements

We would like to acknowledge the help received from the many contributors to this book. They have spent considerable amounts of their precious time providing us with accurate, up-to-date chapters, which has been essential to complete a project of this nature.

The work would never have reached the publishers without the extraordinary patience of Mrs Sheila Smith who has been heavily involved in the secretarial work of the editors. We would like to thank Phil Ball and Greg Harding, Medical Illustration Department at Addenbrooke's Hospital, and a financial contribution to the Artwork from Merck Sharpe and Dohme. Our thanks also go to Steve and Dan who acted as models. We would particularly like to acknowledge the financial support of Abbott Laboratories and Pharmacia for contributing towards the costs of the colour illustrations. Finally we would like to thank the staff of Oxford University Press for their help and support.

Contents

Part 6 Specific soft tissue disorders

Contributors

Mark Abrahams Fellow in Pain Management, Boyle Department of Anaesthesia, St Bartholomew's Hospital, West Smithfield, London EC1A 7BE

Rachel Batteson Tutor, School of Health and Community Studies, University of Derby, The Cedars, 138 Whitaker Road, Derby DE23 6AP

Michael Bayliss Professor (retired), Department of Veterinary Basic Sciences, Royal Veterinary College, Royal College Street, London NW1 0TU

Philip Bearcroft Consultant Radiologist, Department of Radiology, Addenbrooke's Hospital, Cambridge CB2 2QQ

Michael Benjamin Professor, Connective Tissue Biology Laboratories, Cardiff School of Biosciences, Biomedical Building, Museum Avenue, PO Box 911, Cardiff CF10 3US

Howard Bird Professor of Pharmacological Rheumatology, and Consultant Rheumatologist, Clinical Pharmacology Unit, Chapel Allerton Hospital, Chapeltown Road, Leeds LS7 4SA

Simon Boniface Consultant Neurophysiologist, Department of Clinical Neurophysiology, Addenbrooke's Hospital, Cambridge CB2 2QQ

Richard Brand, Professor, Department of Orthopaedic Surgery, University of Iowa Hospital, 200 Hawkins Drive, Iowa City, Iowa 52242, USA

Carol Chong Consultant in Anaesthesia and Pain Management, St Bartholomew's and Homerton Hospitals, London

Cyrus Cooper Professor of Rheumatology MRC Environmental Epidemiology Unit (University of Southampton), Southampton General Hospital, Southampton SO16 6YD

Adrian Crisp Consultant Rheumatologist, Department of Rheumatology, Addenbrooke's Hospital, Cambridge CB2 2QQ

Mike Cummings Medical Director of British Medical Acupuncture Society, British Medical Acupuncture Society, Royal London Homeopathic Hospital, Greenwell Street, London W1W 5BP

Seamus Dalton Consultant in Rehabilitation & Sports Medicine, North Sydney Orthopaedic & Sports Medicine Center, 272 Pacific Highway, Crows Nest, Sydney, New South Wales 2065, Australia

Victor Duance Professor, Connective Tissue Biology Laboratories, Cardiff School of Biosciences, Biomedical Building, Museum Avenue, PO Box 911, Cardiff CF10 3US

Jayesh Dudhia Senior Research Fellow, Department of Veterinary Basic Sciences, Royal Veterinary College, Royal College Street, London NW1 0TU

Jane Dutton Consultant in Nuclear Medicine, Department of Nuclear Medicine, Addenbrooke's Hospital, Cambridge CB2 2QQ

Jeremy Fairbank Consultant Orthopaedic Surgeon, Nuffield Orthopaedic Centre, Headington, Oxford OX3 7LD

Ignac Fogelnan Professor of Nuclear Medicine, Department of Nuclear Medicine, Guy's Hospital, London SE1 9RT

Roger Hackney Consultant Orthopaedic Surgeon, Leeds General Infirmary, Great George Street, Leeds LS1 3EX

Alison Hammond Senior Research Therapist, Rheumatology Department, Derby Royal Infirmary, London Road, Derby DE1 2QY

Brian Hazleman Consultant Rheumatologist, Rheumatology Research Unit, Addenbrooke's Hospital, Cambridge CB2 2QQ

Philip Helliwell Senior Lecturer in Rheumatology, The Rheumatology and Rehabilitation Unit, University of Leeds, 36 Clarendon Road, Leeds, West Yorkshire LS2 9NZ

Alison Hammond Senior Research Therapist, Rheumatology Department, Derby Royal Infirmary, London Road, Derby DE1 2QY

Graham Holloway Consultant Orthopaedic Surgeon, London Bridge Hospital, London Bridge, London

Glen Hunter Principal Lecturer, School of Allied Health Professions, Faculty of Health and Social Care, University of West of England, Glenside Campus, Blackberry Hill, Stapleton

Stephen Kirker Consultant in Rehabilitation Medicine, Lewin Stroke and Rehabilitation Unit, Addenbrooke's Hospital, Cambridge CB2 2QQ

Tarnya Marshall Consultant Rheumatologist, Norfolk & Norwich Hospital, Colney Lane, Norwich NR4 7UY

Audrey McAlinden Research Fellow, Department of Orthopaedics, Washington University School of Medicine, St Louis MO 63110, USA

Brian McNamara Consultant Neurophysiologist, Department of Clinical Neurophysiology, Cork University Hospital, Wilton, Cork, Ireland

Paula Muir Research Associate, Department of Veterinary Basic Sciences, Royal Veterinary College, Royal College Street, London NW1 0TU

Rajesh Munglani Consultant in Pain Management, West Suffolk Hospital, Bury St. Edmunds, Suffolk, IP33 2QZ

Donncha O'Gradaigh Specialist Registrar in Rheumatology, Rheumatology Department, Addenbrooke's Hospital, Cambridge CB2 2QQ

Andrew Östör Clinical Research Fellow, Rheumatology Research Unit, Addenbrooke's Hospital, Cambridge CB2 2QQ

David Perry Consultant Rheumatologist, Bart's and The London NHS Trust, Royal London Hospital (Mile End), Bancroft Road, London E1 4DG

Trevor Prior Consultant Podiatrist, Homerton University Hospital, Homerton Row, London E9 6SR

Julian Ray Consultant Neurophysiologist, Department of Clinical Neurophysiology, Addenbrooke's Hospital, Cambridge CB2 2QQ

Graham Riley Head of Soft Tissue Injury and Repair Group, Rheumatology Research Unit, Addenbrooke's Hospital, Cambridge CB2 2QQ

Sally Roberts Director of Research, Centre for Spinal Studies, The Institute of Orthopædics, The Robert Jones and Agnes Hunt Orthopædic and District Hospital NHS Trust, Oswestry, Shropshire, SY10 7AG

Andrew Robinson Consultant Orthopaedic Surgeon, Addenbrooke's Hospital, Cambridge CB2 2QQ

Cathy Speed Honorary Consultant Rheumatologist, Rheumatology Research Unit, Addenbrooke's Hospital, Cambridge CB2 2QQ

Karen Walker-Bone Senior Lecturer in Rheumatology, Brighton and Sussex Medical School, Falmer, Brighton BN1 9PX

Derek Yull GP Principal, Priors Field Surgery, 24 High Street, Sutton, Ely, Cambs CB6 2RB

Amy Zavatsky Lecturer, Department of Engineering Science, University of Oxford, Parks Road, Oxford OX1 3PJ

1

The science of soft tissue disorders

1.1 Soft connective tissues—normal structure, function, and physiology

Michael Benjamin

Introduction

The term 'soft connective tissue' is used here to include all connective tissues (CTs) except cartilage and bone. It is also called 'connective tissue proper' or 'ordinary connective tissue' and its subtypes are listed in Table 1. The purpose of this chapter is to introduce the reader to these tissues in a rheumatological and sports-related context.

Connective tissue is one of the four basic tissues that serve as 'building blocks' for organs—the others are epithelium, muscle, and nerve. In addition to its independent status as a 'pure basic tissue', CT is also an essential part of muscle and nerve—which can therefore be viewed as 'composite basic tissues'. In its most typical form, CT has large quantities of extracellular matrix (ECM) and relatively few cells. This contrasts vividly with a typical epithelium—which it invariably supports and underlies and from which it is separated by a basement membrane. However, some CTs are more cellular, for example, adipose tissue and reticular CT in the lamina propria of the gut. It is the ECM of CTs that allows them to act as binding and wrapping materials in the body, thus providing the body with vital physical support and promoting its mechanical integration. That CT (e.g. adipose tissue) can act as a packing material reflects its status as the predominant bulk component in the body.[1] The importance of CTs in determining three-dimensional form is evident from the start of embryonic development. Three-dimensional form and the organization of other tissues are controlled by proteoglycan (PG) and glycoprotein secretion at precise times. These molecules regulate cell proliferation, differentiation, and migration rates, as well as the development of collagen and elastic fibres in the ECM.

However, the importance of CTs extends far beyond the purely physical, for they:

1. contain the blood vessels that supply epithelia, muscle, and nerve;

2. provide the arena in which the body fights infection or where infection can spread from one region to another;

3. influence cell motility and proliferation in other tissues.

Proteoglycans in CTs can promote cell motility by blocking binding sites on cell membranes or on glycosaminoglycans (GAGs). The degradation of the ECM that occurs in inflammation or CT remodelling may 'unlock' growth factors capable of stimulating cell proliferation.[1] Tissue fluid accumulates within CTs and its dispersion is one of the benefits that is frequently suggested for massage therapy, which is now commonplace in sport.[2] The presence of CT implies functions geared towards structural support and the physiological integration of cells into tissues, tissues to organs, and of organs to the body as a whole (1).

There are essentially three types of CTs: loose CT; dense CT; and adipose tissue. Each will be considered separately below.

Loose connective tissue

This is named according to the loosely packed collagen and elastic fibres in the ECM that are interwoven together in a network. Several subtypes are recognized.

Areolar connective tissue

This is the most widespread of the subtypes and is regarded as synonymous with loose CT by some histologists.[3] Its name is now of historical interest only and derives from the observations of the early gross anatomists that the tissue traps bubbles of air within it as it is teased apart during dissection.[4] The artefactual space occupied by the air is an *areola* (diminutive of *area* (Latin), an open space).[5] Because the tissue frequently forms thin films, its general character is seen better in a spread preparation mounted on a slide with needles, rather than in a section cut with a microtome knife (Fig. 1(a)). In such spreads, the collagen fibres are grouped together into bundles—the larger the bundle, the more collagen fibres within it. Collagen fibres are readily distinguished from elastic fibres that appear as thin dark pencil lines in suitably stained spreads (Fig. 1(a)). Although individual collagen fibres do not branch, fibres within one bundle can be followed to neighbouring bundles. This contributes to a network formation. By contrast, elastic fibres do branch and thus the network created by them is rather different.

Functions of areolar connective tissue

Typically, areolar CT forms thin films of tissue that have the following functions.

1. They provide a plane of movement, for example, the superficial fascia that allows the skin to move over the structures beneath it or the loose CT that separates muscles, surrounds their fibres or lies between tendon fascicles (Fig. 1(a), (b)). In all skeletal muscles, the endomysium within fascicles and the perimysium that surrounds them are both relatively loose tissues so that fibres and fascicles can move freely over one another.[6] In many muscles, the epimysium (which envelops the whole muscle) is also a loose CT that in practice functions as a bursa, facilitating free movement of one muscle relative to another, or allowing the muscle to

Table 1 A classification of the soft connective tissues considered in the present chapter

Type	Distribution—examples
Loose connective tissue	
Areolar	Superficial fascia
	Within neurovascular bundles
	Forming the endomysia, perimysia, and some epimysia of skeletal muscles
	Supporting epithelial membranes (e.g. papillary layer of dermis)
	In association with glands (e.g. forming the connective tissue septa between the lobules of large exocrine glands such as the salivary glands or pancreas)
	Subendothelial connective tissue in the tunica intima of blood vessels
	Adventitia and serosa of gut
Reticular	Lymph nodes
	Spleen
	Lamina propria of small and large gut
Dense connective tissue (often classed as regular and irregular though distinction is often unclear)	Tendons and ligaments
	Dermis
	Joint capsules
	Aponeuroses
	Deep fascia
	Intermuscular septa
	Interosseous membranes
	Retinacula
	Fibrous digital sheaths and their associated annular and cruciform pulleys
	Fibrous tendon sheaths—e.g. paratenon of the Achilles tendon
	Investing fasciae of neurovascular bundles (e.g. carotid, femoral, and axillary sheaths)
	Dura mater
	Tunica adventitia of blood vessels
	Submucosa of gut (*NB*: this can be mixed with adipose tissue as well)
	Fibrous layer of the pericardium
	Epimysium of some muscles
	Thoracolumbar fascia
Adipose tissue	
White	Superficial fascia
	Palms and soles (where it is mixed with dense CT).
	Retroperitoneal locations—omenta, mesenteries, around kidneys
	Orbit, Ischiorectal fossa
	Appendices epiploicae of large gut serosa
Brown	Neck and axilla in newborn children—highly localized distribution

bulge prominently in a concentric contraction (e.g. in biceps brachii).[6] It is the loose nature of an epimysium that allows tissue fluid, blood, or inflammatory products to track down the muscle in injury or disease.[6] Thus, the sheath around psoas major can allow an exudate originating from a diseased lumbar vertebra to move into the thigh.[6] Yet, in other muscles, the epimysium is a dense CT that serves for the attachment of the muscle fibres (see below).

2. They support epithelial membranes and the epithelial cells of glands—epithelia are largely cellular and thus must receive additional physical support (Fig. 1(c)). Furthermore, by virtue of their exposed position facing the external environment, epithelia are necessarily avascular and must receive nutrients from blood vessels in the underlying CT.

3. They wrap up blood vessels and nerves into neurovascular bundles (Fig. 1(b)).

4. They form an integral part of some synovial membranes, notably those that are required to move freely over an adjacent joint capsule.[4]

Cell populations of areolar connective tissue

The cells of areolar CT fit broadly into two categories. First, a population of 'native cells' that differentiates *in situ* from mesenchymal cells that occupied the same site in the embryo during early development. Second, a variable number of 'immigrant cells' that have migrated into the CT from the bloodstream in response to the short-term demands associated with infection and/or injury. Bloom and Fawcett [3] refer to these cells as fixed and wandering cells, respectively. The native cells include fibroblasts, fat cells, and mast cells.

Fibroblasts are responsible for the production and maintenance of the ECM, fat cells store lipid, and mast cells (Fig. 1(g)) secrete histamine and other vasoactive compounds. The appearance of fibroblasts depends on whether they are actively synthesizing ECM. Active fibroblasts have an abundance of basophilic cytoplasm and a pale-staining ovoid nucleus. Inactive fibroblasts (i.e. most fibroblasts in adult CTs) have a barely recognizable cytoplasm and a dark, elongate nucleus (Fig. 1(c), (e)). In paraffin sections, fat cells appear as pale ghosts (Fig. 1(b), (d), (f)), for their large, central fat droplet is normally leached out by the alcohols and clearing agents routinely used for histology processing. The nucleus is dark-staining, flattened, and pushed to the edge of the cell by the fat droplet; the cytoplasm is reduced to a thin, peripheral rim (Fig. 1(f)).

The immigrant cells are all white blood cells that either remain in the CT unmodified (polymorphonuclear (PMN) leucocytes and T lymphocytes) or that differentiate further on leaving the blood (monocytes differentiate into macrophages, and B lymphocytes into plasma cells). The white blood cells merely use the bloodstream as a convenient mode of transport from their site of production (the bone marrow) to their site of function in the CTs. The PMN leucocytes are named according to their staining reactions and include neutrophils (the most common white blood cell; Fig. 1(k)), eosinophils, and basophils (the rarest of the white blood cells). Whole armies of neutrophils can be seen adhering to the capillary endothelial cells in an areolar CT at the site of an infection and large numbers of them die to contribute to the formation of pus.

The process of endothelial cell adhesion is called margination and is triggered by a chemotactic response to, for example, bacterial products or to substances produced by platelets or other neutrophils. Margination is a prelude to the entry of neutrophils into a loose CT by diapedesis. Neutrophils are avid phagocytes that are characterized by their multilobed nucleus (typically two to five lobes; Fig. 1(k)) and, at the ultrastructural level, by their numerous, pale-staining, cytoplasmic granules. These contain a broad range of highly cytotoxic proteins and include 'primary' granules that are packed with lysosomal enzymes

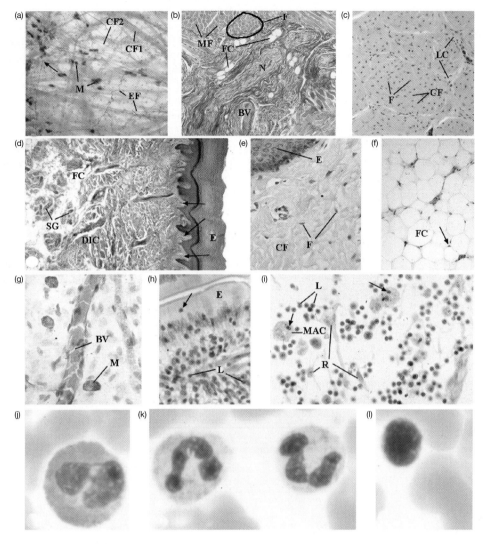

Fig. 1 The histological appearance of connective tissues. (a) An areolar connective tissue 'spread' (i.e. not a section) from the superficial fascia. The collagen fibres are grouped into bundles of different sizes (CF1 and CF2) and form a loose meshwork in conjunction with the thinner and more darkly stained elastic fibres (EF). Although the collagen fibres do not branch, the elastic fibres do (arrow). The majority of the nuclei probably belong to fibroblasts, but a few large and strongly staining mast cells (M) are prominent. (b) Areolar connective tissue in the tongue, serving as a conduit for nerves (N) and blood vessels (BV), and wrapping muscle fibres (MF) together into fascicles (F). Note the occasional fat cells (FC) within it. (c) Dense regular connective tissue as seen in a transverse section of a tendon. The tissue is characterized by abundant ECM that is dominated by large numbers of regularly arranged collagen fibres (CF) and by relatively small numbers of fibroblasts (F) identifiable only by their dark-staining nuclei. Thin films of loose, areolar connective tissue (LC) are present between the tendon fascicles. (d) Three connective tissues merging imperceptibly with each other in a piece of thick skin from the sole of the foot. Immediately beneath the epidermis (E), there is a thin film of areolar connective tissue that constitutes the papillary layer of the dermis (arrows). Deep to that is a more substantial layer of dense irregular connective tissue (DIC; the reticular layer of the dermis) and, finally, beneath the skin but blending with it there is a layer of adipose tissue. The adipose tissue is identified by its fat cells (FC) and contains the coiled portions of sweat glands (SG). (e) The typical appearance of fibroblasts (F) scattered among collagen fibres (CF) in a routine histology section of a connective tissue. This particular section shows the dense irregular connective tissue of the dermis, but the appearance is similar in most other connective tissues. Only fibroblast nuclei are clearly visible; they are darkly staining and irregular in shape. The cytoplasm is drawn out into such thin processes that they cannot be resolved in this photograph. E, epidermis. (f) White adipose tissue contains many large fat cells (FC). Each of these has a single fat droplet that dominates the cell and a small rim of peripheral cytoplasm in which the nucleus is located (arrow). Note the polygonal appearance of the closely packed cells—a consequence of mutual pressure. (g) Mast cells (M) packed with large, metachromatic granules are often located near blood vessels (BV) in spreads of areolar connective tissue. (h) The reticular connective tissue lying beneath the epidermis (E) of the small gut constitutes a mucosal-associated lymphoid tissue that is characterized by large numbers of lymphocytes (L). It is typical of this tissue that these cells can migrate into the overlying epithelium by squeezing between the lateral cell membranes of the absorptive cells. (i) Reticular connective tissue in the subcapsular sinus of a lymph node. As there are fewer lymphocytes (L) here than elsewhere in the node, the stellate-shaped reticular cells (R) are clearly visible. Several macrophages (MAC) can also be seen—some of which contain phagocytosed material (arrows). (j). A monocyte from a blood smear. This is a large cell with a deeply indented nucleus that differentiates into a macrophage when it migrates into a loose connective tissue. (k) Two neutrophils in a blood smear. Whole armies of these cells migrate into areolar connective tissues at the site of an infection. They are identified by their multilobed nucleus. (l) A lymphocyte within a blood smear. Note the rounded and darkly staining nucleus—the cytoplasm is restricted to a thin, peripheral rim.

and specific 'secondary' granules that contain lactoferrin in addition to lysozyme. The contents of both granules are released into phagosomes that contain and isolate micro-organisms that are ingested by phagocytosis. In addition, however, granule release can occur extracellularly.

Eosinophils normally have a bilobed nucleus and granules with a highly characteristic central, crystalloid structure. Although eosinophils are also phagocytic, their principal function is to combat parasitic infections by releasing their granule contents extracellularly. They are also known to produce aryl sulfatase and histaminase, which, when released into the ECM, can inactivate mast cell products and thus reduce the level of an inflammatory response.

Basophils are the rarest of the PMN leucocytes and are often difficult to distinguish from mast cells. They are packed with strongly staining, coarse granules that are also released in attacks upon parasites. The macrophages that differentiate from monocytes are large cells with abundant cytoplasm that are difficult to identify in routine histology sections unless they contain phagocytosed material (Fig. 1(i)). However, they can be strikingly visualized by immuno- or enzyme-histochemistry or by their ability to ingest Indian ink.

Reticular connective tissue

This forms the supporting framework of secondary lymphoid organs and tissues (lymph nodes, the spleen, and mucosal-associated lymphoid tissue; Fig. 1(h)). It forms a 'three-dimensional cobweb' of reticular cells and fibres, in the interstices of which are held enormous numbers of lymphocytes and related cells of the immune system. Lymphocytes are rounded cells that are dominated by their large, darkly staining nucleus (Fig. 1(h), (i), (l)) and, when present in large numbers, they make reticular cells difficult to identify. Reticular cells are thus easiest to visualize in the sinuses of lymph nodes where only small numbers of lymphocytes are present (Fig. 1(i)). Reticular fibres are highlighted by the traditional reticulin stains of the histologist, but are now known to contain laminin and type III or IV collagen.

Dense connective tissue

This is named according to the densely packed fibres in the ECM. They are usually collagen, but there are significant numbers of elastic fibres in the ligamentum nuchae and ligamenta flava. The fibres are either interwoven together in an irregular network (*dense irregular CT*) as in joint capsules, the dermis (Fig. 1(d)), or much of the deep fascia of the limbs, or arranged parallel to each other along the direction in which the principal tensile forces are acting (*dense regular CT*), as in tendons (Fig. 1(c)), ligaments, and some aponeuroses.

The most important functional property of a dense CT is its high tensile strength, that is, its resistance to stretch. It is this that allows tendons to transfer muscle pull to bone and ligaments to guide and limit joint movements. However, dense CT is also a major factor limiting muscle flexibility. The scar tissue that forms after a strain or tear can limit the contraction of a muscle and reduce joint range of motion. Appropriate physiotherapy and/or massage intervention can help by breaking down the CT physically.

Functions of dense connective tissues

Dense CTs provide for muscle attachment—particularly in the lower limb where movements are less precise than in the upper. Thus, both gluteus maximus and tensor fascia lata insert into a broad band of dense CT called the iliotibial (IT) tract, and tibialis anterior (a muscle implicated in shin splints) arises in part from the deep fascia that covers its anterior surface. Dense CTs also act as sheaths and restraining bands for tendons or as elastic cuffs for muscles.[6] They can compartmentalize blood vessels and nerves, for example, the carotid and femoral sheaths.[6] Dense CT is not a prominent feature of the lower abdominal wall, for its presence here would interfere with diaphragmatic breathing and make it difficult for the gut to distend after a heavy meal.

The range of dense connective tissues

Many of the named dense CTs in the body are listed in Table 1. Several are widely implicated in rheumatological conditions or sports injuries (Table 2).

The flexor retinaculum, which prevents the flexor tendons from 'bowstringing' in a flexed wrist, is directly involved in carpal tunnel syndrome. This is a compression neuropathy of the median nerve that can result from a swelling of tendon sheaths developing as a repetitive strain injury, or from osteophytes or anomalous muscle bellies that reduce the size of the carpal tunnel.

Rupture or subluxation injuries to analogous dense CTs that serve elsewhere as restraining bands for tendons are common in sport. The pulleys that restrain the digital flexor tendons have been known to fail under the extreme duress of rock climbing,[7] and subluxation of the peroneal tendons is often reported in athletes.[8]

The IT tract, a lateral thickening of the fascia lata that forms a stocking around the muscles of the thigh, is widely implicated in 'runner's knee'. This is an overuse injury common in distance runners, where the tract rubs against the lateral femoral epicondyle.[9]

Finally, dense CT formation is characteristic of many diseases, including neoplasias and scleroderma. The latter is an autoimmune disease characterized by a widespread increase in the amount of dense CT in the skin (particularly that of the hands and face), oesophagus, kidneys, and lung.[10]

'Fascia' is a rather vague term, widely applied in medicine to any collection of CTs that is large enough to be seen with the naked eye. Many fascias are dense CTs and several are implicated in rheumatological and/or sports injury conditions discussed elsewhere in this book (Table 2). They include the palmar and plantar fasciae that serve to protect blood vessels and nerves from the pressure associated with gripping or weight bearing. The palmar fascia is affected by Dupuytren's contracture and the plantar fascia by plantar fasciitis—a condition often linked with abnormal stresses on the foot where there is unusual torsion or tension in the fascia.[11] Such forces are magnified in patients with flat feet or a high medial longitudinal arch.

There are prominent intermuscular fascial septa in the limbs that separate muscles into their different compartments (e.g. flexor, extensor, adductor, etc.). 'Compartment syndromes' are well-documented sporting injuries that are associated with these dense CTs. They are particularly common in the lower leg (because the influence of gravity on venous and lymphatic drainage is most pronounced here) and are associated with an increase in compartmental, intramuscular pressure.[12]

Table 2 Examples of rheumatological conditions or sports injuries in which dense CTs are implicated

Rheumatological conditions and/or sports injuries	Description and brief comment on involvement of dense connective tissue
Dupuytren's contracture	Thickening and contraction of palmar fascia—a dense CT
Carpal tunnel syndrome	Narrowing of the carpal tunnel, creating pressure on median nerve—can be treated surgically by cutting through the flexor retinaculum (a dense CT)
Compartment syndromes (entrapment neuropathies)	Common sports injury involving increased pressure resisted by the dense CT of the deep fascia—the anterior compartment of the leg is the most commonly affected
de Quervain's tenosynovitis	Repetitive strain injury (RSI) of wrist tendons that involves thickening and stenosis of the tendon sheaths near the extensor retinaculum—both of these are dense CTs
Iliotibial band friction syndrome (runner's knee)	RSI where iliotibial tract (a dense CT) rubs on the lower end of the femur
Plantar fasciitis	Common RSI that gives rise to heel pain. Probably involves tearing and stretching of the dense CT that forms the plantar fascia
Autoimmune rheumatoid connective tissue diseases, e.g. scleroderma, systemic lupus erythematosus (SLE)	Scleroderma affects CT in the skin and/or other organs such as the lungs, kidneys, and oesophagus. SLE involves fibrous thickening in the walls of arterioles in skin, kidney, joints, and gut serosa

This pressure is in turn resisted by an overlying deep fascia with little ability to stretch. It is significant to note that during and after exercise, muscle volume may increase by as much as 20 per cent as a result of enhanced blood flow and the formation of tissue fluid within muscle CTs.[12] Conservative treatments for compartment syndromes involve stretching, strengthening, and icing programmes but, if these fail, the surgery involves a simple fasciotomy—as in carpal tunnel syndrome. Fascial hernias (where a more deeply located structure atypically protrudes through a weakening or a hole in a dense connective fascia) are well documented in patients suffering from compartment syndromes.[13] Such hernias are known to entrap the superficial peroneal nerve as it pierces the deep fascia in the lower leg.

Dense CT is almost invariably associated with thin films of loose CT, for example, the endotenon that separates tendon fascicles (Fig. 1(c)) or the papillary layer of the dermis (Fig. 1(d)). This loose CT both provides for motility and carries blood vessels that supply the cells of the dense CT. These are typically sparse and mainly fibroblasts (Fig. 1(c)). In tendons and ligaments, the cells are arranged in longitudinal rows and communicate with each other via gap junctions.[14] They also have elaborate, sheet-like, lateral cell processes that allow cells in neighbouring rows to maintain gap-junctional contact throughout a matrix dominated by collagen fibres—the cell processes create tunnels through which the collagen fibres run.

Adipose tissue

Distribution of adipose tissue

Adipose tissue (fat) is characterized by large numbers of fat cells (adipocytes) and is described as either 'white' or 'brown'. White adipose tissue is by far the most common. It is typically found beneath the skin, though the quantity varies with age and sex—subcutaneous fat is most widely distributed in young children.[6] Women typically have 8–10 per cent more body fat than men and there are characteristic regional differences in the distribution of the fat.[15] In women, fat is most typical of the breasts, buttocks, hips, and thighs, whereas in men it characteristically accumulates in the lower abdominal wall, nape of the neck, back, and buttocks.[6] Abdominal obesity is more associated with general health problems such as cardiovascular disease and hypertension.

In both sexes, yellow marrow is adipose tissue that is protected within the confines of bone. Only a few regions of the body are consistently devoid of fat—notably the eyelids and the scrotum.[3]

Brown adipose tissue is rare in man, but common in hibernating animals. In man, it is most prominent in the newborn where it is believed to play a role in temperature regulation. Brown fat is a highly vascular tissue with multilocular fat cells (i.e. with many small fat droplets rather than a single large one) that contrast vividly with the appearance of white adipocytes.

Functions of adipose tissue

White adipose tissue is often mixed with strands of dense fibrous CT (as in the palms and heels). The two together form an effective 'pressure pad', for the fat in the adipocytes is liquid at body temperature and thus incompressible. It has been estimated that 20–25 per cent of the contact force associated with the heel strike phase of the gait cycle is absorbed by the fat pad in the heel.[16] The strands of fibrous tissue serve to hold groups of fat cells together and prevent them from being pushed apart under compressive load. Thus, the functional interplay that exists at a gross level between fat cells (adapted to withstanding pressure) and strands of fibrous tissue (which resist tension) is analogous to that that exists at a molecular level between aggrecan and type II collagen in articular cartilage—the best documented pressure-tolerant tissue. 'Fat-pad syndrome', otherwise known as 'bruised heel', is a recognized sporting injury that occurs when the natural shock absorbing capacity of the heel pad is pushed beyond its tolerance limits.[16] It is a painful condition, for the fat pad is rich in free nerve endings and Pacinian corpuscles.

White fat has a number of important roles beyond that of pressure tolerance. Perhaps the most obvious and best documented are heat insulation and lipid storage. The superficial fascia is frequently fatty and thus provides an important layer of insulation just beneath the skin. The lipid content of the fat cells can be readily mobilized, and it thus provides a convenient temporary storage depot for fuel.[3] Fat cells synthesize lipid from carbohydrate and respond to both nervous and hormonal stimulation. Lipid is more suitable as a stored fuel than either carbohydrate or protein, for it weighs less and occupies less space per calorie of chemical energy.[3] The intracellular lipid of adipose tissue also provides a depot for the storage of fat-soluble vitamins (A, D, E, and K). Unfortunately, it is also where fat-soluble pesticides can accumulate.[1] Finally, white fat provides a plane of movement (e.g. behind the eyeball) or acts as a variable space filler (e.g. in the ischiorectal fossae), for the lipid content of the cells is liquid at body temperatures.

The cells of white adipose tissue

The cells (called 'adipocytes') in white adipose tissue have a single, large fat droplet and are thus identical to the occasional fat cells found in areolar CT (see above). The mutual pressure of neighbouring cells of equal size distorts the otherwise rounded fat cells into a hexagonal shape (Fig. 1(f)). In this way, the greatest number of cells can be packed into a finite volume, with a minimum of 'dead' space between them.[17]

References

1. **Pritzker, K.P.H.** (1997). Connective tissue. In *Encyclopaedia of Human Biology* (ed. R. Dulbecco), Vol. 3, pp. 11–20. Academic Press, San Diego.

2. **Hollis, M.** (1998). *Massage for therapists*, 2nd edn. Blackwell Science, Oxford.

3. **Bloom, W. and Fawcett, D.W.** (1975). *A Textbook of Histology*, 10th edn. Saunders, Philadelphia.

4. **Cormack, D.H.** (1987). *Ham's Histology*, 9th edn. Lippincott, London.

5. **Field, E.J. and Harrison, R.J.** (1968). *Anatomical Terms: Their Origin and Derivation*, 3rd edn. Heffers, Cambridge.

6. **Hamilton, W.J. and Yoffey, J.M.** (1977). Introduction. In *Textbook of Human Anatomy*, 2nd edn. (ed. W.J. Hamilton), pp. 1–17. Macmillan, London.

7. **Bollen, S.R. and Gunson, C.K.** (1990). Hand injuries in competition climbers. *Br. J. Sports Med.* **24**, 16–18.

8. **Kirk, K.L., Kuklo, T., and Klemme, W.** (2000). Iliotibial band friction syndrome. *Orthopedics* **23**(11), 1209–1214.

9. **Niemi, W.J., Savidakis, J. Jr, and DeJesus, J.M.** (1997). Peroneal subluxation: a comprehensive review of the literature with case presentations. *J. Foot and Ankle Surg.* **36**, 141–145.

10. **Smolle, J.** (1997). Skin disease. In *Pathology* (ed. I.A. Cree), pp. 415–477. Chapman & Hall, London.

11. **Lester, D.K. and Buchanan, J.R.** (1984). Surgical treatment of plantar fasciitis. *Clin. Orthop.* **186**, 202–204.

12. **Taunton, J., Smith, C., and Magee, D.J.** (1996). Leg, foot, and ankle injuries. In A*thletic injuries and rehabilitation* (eds J.E. Zachazewski, D.J. Magee, and W.S. Quillen), pp. 729–755. Saunders, Philadelphia.

13. **Pedowitz, R.A., Hargens, A.R., Mubarak, S.J., and Gershuni, D.H.** (1990). Modified criteria for the objective diagnosis of chronic compartment syndrome of the leg. *Am. J. Sports Med.* **18**, 35–40.

14. **McNeilly, C.M., Banes, A.J., Benjamin, M., and Ralphs, J.R.** (1996). Tendon cells *in vivo* form a three dimensional network of cell processes linked by gap junctions. *J. Anat.* **189**, 593–600.

15. **Lebrun, C.** (1998). The female athlete. In *The Oxford Textbook of Sports Medicine*, 2nd edn. (eds M. Harries, C. Williams, W.D. Stanish, and L.J. Micheli), pp. 743–779. Oxford University Press, Oxford.

16. **Karr, S.D.** (1994). Subcalcaneal heel pain. *Orthop. Clin. N. Am.* **25**, 161–175.

17. **Thompson, D'. A.W.** (1942). *On growth and form*. Cambridge University Press, Cambridge.

1.2 The structure and function of tendons

Michael Benjamin

General principles of tendon design and function

A tendon is generally a dense fibrous connective tissue that links a muscle to a bone and thus extends from its myotendinous junction to its enthesis (i.e. the bony attachment site). However, some tendons (e.g. the intermediate tendons of omohyoid and digastric and the tendinous intersections of rectus abdominis) simply link one muscle belly to another. Depending on the fibre arrangements in the muscle, tendons can extend into the muscle belly as tendinous septa. Such an arrangement is generally characteristic of the more powerful, multi-pennate muscles (e.g. deltoid) that have a short range of action. In such a muscle, the muscle fibres meet the tendon obliquely, and thus not all the force they generate is available to act along the long axis of the whole muscle. This restricts the range of motion of pennate muscles compared with parallel-fibred ones, but means that they are more powerful, as they contain a greater number of muscle fibres.[1] The shape of tendons varies greatly. They can be rounded, oval, or flattened—flat tendons are generally called 'aponeuroses'.

Biomechanics and tensile properties of tendon

The fundamental role of tendons is to transmit tensile force ('load') generated by muscle bellies to bone. In doing so, they form part of a continuum of connective tissue that extends from the endomysial harness of loose connective tissue that surrounds individual muscle fibres to the bone itself. Good elementary accounts of the biomechanical principles of tendon function are given by Moore[2] and Oakes.[3] Briefly, the tensile load on a tendon is expressed as *stress* (force per unit area) and the ensuing elongation as *strain* (percentage change in length). The changing relationship between stress and strain is depicted in a *stress–strain curve* (Fig. 1).

Tendons will initially elongate slightly with relatively little applied stress—that is, in the 'toe' region of the curve. This corresponds to the normal physiological range of a tendon or its *elastic limit* (typically 3–4 per cent elongation). Strain in the toe region is thought to be associated with the disappearance of collagen crimp,[3] but further elongation damages the tendon. In the initial stages of the damage, intermolecular collagen cross-links are broken, but eventually there is macroscopic tearing of fibrils, fibres, fascicles, and ultimately the whole tendon. If a tendon is loaded and unloaded repeatedly at the same rate but below its elastic limit, the stress–strain curves should be identical and the tendon does not experience any permanent deformation.[2] However, if the elastic limit in one loading cycle is exceeded,

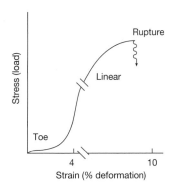

Fig. 1 A typical stress–strain curve for a tendon. The tendon elongates relatively easily and without damage in the 'toe' region of the curve, but continued elongation in the 'linear' region is accompanied by damage and eventually the tendon reaches its point of rupture. (Modified after reference 3, p. 495.)

the slope of the stress–strain curve changes and the tendon weakens because it has been permanently deformed. Tendons can withstand larger forces when these are applied quickly and exhibit the phenomena of *stress relaxation* (where the tensile load on a tendon diminishes as the load is held at a given level until the elongation equilibrates), *creep* (the elongation occurring during stress relaxation), and *hysteresis* (the different stress–strain curve that is followed by a tendon recovering from a load compared with that when receiving it).

Other functions of tendons

Tendons can have other functions as well. As they are smaller than muscles, they can allow them to pull through narrow, confined spaces—notably the carpal tunnel. This means that the more powerful movements of the hand can be governed remotely, that is, by muscles within the forearm. The same applies to the foot. Tendons also allow muscles to alter their angle of pull, for they can be bent around bony or fibrous pulleys (Fig. 2). They can withstand the associated compression and shear better than muscles because they are less vascular. Indeed, where the levels of compression demand it, tendons can be completely avascular—this requires that they be fibrocartilaginous.[4] As an extension of this general principle, it is worth noting that tendinous patches are present in muscles wherever they are subject to compression/friction, even if no change in muscle pull is involved.

The viscoelasticity of tendons can prevent or reduce muscle injury in high-velocity work when a force is suddenly applied and has subtle effects on the control and precision of movement. This is well illustrated

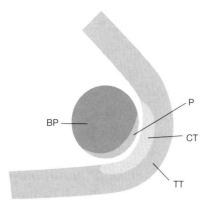

Fig. 2 Tendons can enable muscles to alter their angle of pull for, in contrast to fleshy muscle bellies, they can be wrapped around bony or fibrous pulleys. This highly diagrammatic representation of a wrap-around tendon curving around a bony pulley (BP) shows that the side of the tendon facing the pulley is subject to compression (CT) while the side facing away from it is under tension (TT). The bony pulley too is compressed by the tendon and its periosteum (P) in this region is frequently fibrocartilaginous.

by the work of Rack and Ross[5] on the tendon of flexor pollicis longus that helps to control the movements of the thumb. The compliancy of such a long tendon means that the effects of muscle contraction are dampened and that it is easier to control the forces acting on the thumb than its position. As the principal functional significance of the thumb relates to its oppositional movements (i.e. where the soft pad of its distal phalanx is opposed to that of one of the other fingers), the muscle–tendon unit is well adapted to its task. Rack and Ross[5] have also made the intriguing point that tendons are most compliant at low forces and that this promotes delicacy of touch in the fingers. However, where it becomes particularly important to maintain a constant position of a finger, we do this automatically by contracting simultaneously the flexor and extensor muscles so as to increase tendon rigidity.

Tendons eliminate the need for an unnecessary length of muscle belly between the origin and insertion of a muscle.[6] One of the consequences of the sliding filament mechanism of muscle action is that force can only be generated when actin and myosin filaments overlap. This automatically limits the change in length of each sarcomere (and thus the muscle as a whole) to about one-third. Thus, if there are enough sarcomeres along the length of the muscle to allow a given joint to be moved through its maximum range of motion, the rest of the muscle–tendon unit is constructed of tendon rather than muscle, for the former is metabolically less expensive than the latter. This reciprocal relationship between muscle belly and tendon length is well illustrated by the experiments of Crawford.[7] He re-routed the tendons of tibialis anterior in young rabbits so as to increase the distance by which the muscle belly needed to shorten in order to dorsiflex the foot. By maturity, the muscle belly was relatively longer and the tendon relatively shorter, compared with controls.

The functional interplay between a muscle and its tendon is thus complex and it can be difficult to predict the combined function of a muscle–tendon unit from a consideration of either structure alone.[8] Lower-limb tendons in particular can act as springs in locomotion, economizing on muscular effort.[9] Skeletal muscles are stretched prior to their subsequent shortening, and this enhances their performance

because of the elastic energy stored in the tendon.[10] This is exploited in the plyometric training methods that are now widely used in sport—particularly in sprinting and jumping. Fukashiro et al.[10] estimate that the percentage of elastic energy stored in the Achilles tendon during hopping movements amounts to 34 per cent of the total work performed by the calf muscles themselves. The storage of elastic energy in tendons means that their thickness becomes of critical importance.[11] If the tendon were too thin, it would be too extensible and this would mean that muscle mass would have to be increased substantially for the mechanical role of the tendon to be adequate. If the tendon were too thick, it would become too heavy. An inadequate thickness of a tendon would also increase the risk of its rupture for, clearly, tendons must have a suitable safety margin between the maximum stress applied to them by their muscle belly and their breaking point. The right compromise generally seems to be reached with tendons of intermediate thickness.[11] However, Ker et al.[11] have made the interesting point that the Achilles tendon has a thickness that places it fairly close to the safety limit—hence it is so vulnerable to rupture. The advantage accrued by such a 'risky' construction is that the tendon can efficiently store elastic energy.

Muscles, of course, can attach to bone without any tendons at all, and are then described as having 'fleshy attachments' to the skeleton. It is rare, however, for them to have fleshy attachments at both ends. Tendons are always present where muscle action changes the angle between two bones at a joint.[12] Wherever tendons are present, their site of attachment can generally be recognized on the skeleton by well defined (i.e. circumscribed) markings, for example, tubercles, tuberosities, or ridges. This highlights the well documented role of tendons in concentrating or focusing the site of muscle action.[12] Equally though, it creates the potential for dissipating muscle action to several sites simultaneously. This principle is well illustrated by the flexor and extensor tendons of the fingers and toes, where the action of the muscle belly can be spread across four digits.

Structure of tendons

For much of their course (in their mid-substance, tensional regions), tendons are dominated by type I collagen fibres and the predominant cell type is a fibroblast (sometimes called a 'tenocyte'). The molecular composition of the extracellular matrix (ECM) in such regions is considered in Chapter 1.3. However, where tendons also experience compression and/or shear—next to bony and sometimes fibrous pulleys and at many bony insertion sites (entheses), they are fibrocartilaginous.

Mid-substance, tensional regions

Many tendons have a fascicular structure (Fig. 3) and where this is very pronounced, for example, in the rat tail tendon, primary, secondary, and tertiary fascicles may be distinguished.[13] Frequently, the fascicles are arranged in a loose spiral, for example, in the Achilles tendon and in the flexor tendons of the fingers.[14, 15] Thin films of loose connective tissue separate them and serve as passageways for small blood vessels and as planes of movement between one bundle of collagen fibres and another. The loose connective tissue is often called 'endotenon' in contrast to the epitenon that surrounds the tendon as a whole. In some tendons (e.g. the Achilles) the fascicles spiral along

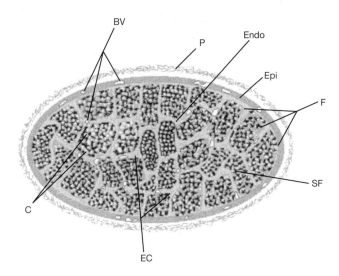

Fig. 3 Diagrammatic representation of the structure of the extrasynovial part of a tendon as seen in transverse section. The tendon contains numerous fascicles (F) that represent collections of bundles of collagen fibres (C) and the stellate fibroblasts (SF) that form them. Between the fascicles are thin films of loose connective tissue—the endotenon (Endo). Its thickness has been exaggerated in order to show the cells (EC) and blood vessels (BV) within it. The blood vessels enter via the epitenon (Epi) that surrounds the whole tendon. The paratenon (P) is a false tendon sheath, entirely separate from the tendon itself, that represents a condensation of the surrounding connective tissue.

their length and are interconnected as a plexus. Fascicle formation is probably important as a way of reducing the risk of catastrophic tendon failure, that is, even if one or more fascicles fail, there are still others to bear the load. Thus, the principle of protection against failure through the duplication of a structure operates at a number of hierarchical levels in tendons, from the molecular to the macroscopic. At the molecular level, the triple helical form adopted by the collagen fibrils parallels the spiralling, multifascicular nature of the fascicles that serves a similar purpose at a gross level. However, the ability of a tendon to withstand load can also be associated with the characteristic cross-linking that occurs between collagen molecules.[16]

Tendon 'crimp'

A conspicuous feature of tendons that has been reported by many investigators is crimp—a wavy or planar zigzag morphology.[13] Its significance is unclear, though according to some authors it accounts for the toe region of a typical stress–strain curve, where a tendon is stretched within its normal physiological range under load (Fig. 1). The slack it provides may act as a dampening buffer for the effects of muscle contraction at the myotendinous junction and/or the enthesis.[3] According to Oakes,[3] crimp is maintained by inter- and intramolecular cross-links between the collagen molecules as well as by the position of associated elastic fibres.

Cells of tendon

Far less attention has been paid to the cell biology of tendons, because of the obvious mechanical significance of collagen fibrils and because the cells in tendons are relatively inconspicuous. Typically, the cells lie in longitudinal rows separated by parallel collagen fibres and the only

evidence of them in a routine haematoxylin and eosin (H&E) section is their elongate, darkly staining nuclei. Recently, however, McNeilly et al.[17] have used confocal laser scanning microscopy to demonstrate that tendon cells have elaborate sheet-like processes that create tunnels through which the collagen fibrils pass. These cell processes enable the tendon cells to maintain direct cell–cell contact over a large three-dimensional domain, despite the dominance of the collagen. Furthermore, the tendon cells communicate with each other both within and between the longitudinal rows via gap junctions.[17] These findings provide an important basis for understanding how a co-ordinated cell response to changing mechanical load might occur. Furthermore, the presence of longitudinally orientated, actin stress fibres within tendon cell processes that are linked to adherens junctions opens the possibility that they could either be involved in initiating the signalling cascades that occur in response to mechanical signals and/or promoting the active recovery of tendon cells under stretch.[18]

Wrap-around regions

A 'wrap-around tendon' is one that bends around a bony or fibrous pulley so that the direction of muscle pull becomes altered. When the muscle fibres contract, the side of the tendon facing away from the pulley is placed under tension, but the side nearest the pulley becomes compressed (Fig. 2). As an adaptation to resisting this compression, the side near the pulley is fibrocartilaginous rather than purely fibrous, and the ECM commonly contains type II collagen and aggrecan.[19] These are molecules more often associated with the compression-tolerance properties of articular cartilage. The high charge density created by the glycosaminoglycans (GAGs) in aggrecan allows a tissue to imbibe large quantities of water by capillarity—and water of course is incompressible.[20] The associated, small-diameter collagen fibres could serve to prevent the tendon from splaying apart under compression and to control the swelling of aggrecan (see reference 4 for a review). The fibrocartilage cells are large, oval, or rounded and resemble cells in articular cartilage more than they resemble fibroblasts in the tensional region of the tendon. They are frequently characterized by large numbers of intermediate filaments—predominantly vimentin—but there can be a range of cytokeratins as well.[21] The fibrocartilage can be present throughout the tendon substance in the compressed region, or be restricted to the endotenon and/or epitenon.[22]

Well known wrap-around tendons that are fibrocartilaginous in man include several that pass behind the malleoli—fibularis (peroneus) longus and brevis, tibialis posterior, and flexor hallucis longus[22]—and also the extensor tendons of the fingers and toes over the metacarpophalangeal and interphalangeal joints (Fig. 4; references 23, 24). However, much important work on wrap-around tendons has centred around other species—notably the rabbit[21, 25] and cow.[26, 27] Experimental studies on the flexor digitorum profundus (FDP) tendons of these animals, both in vivo and in vitro, have established that the fibrocartilage is a dynamic tissue that responds to changes in mechanical load. Thus, when rabbit deep flexor tendons were surgically translocated to the extensor aspect of the limb so that they no longer experienced compression, large quantities of GAGs were lost from the tendon.[25] Comparable results have also been obtained with explants taken from the wrap-around region of bovine deep flexor tendons cultured in the presence or absence of compressive load.[28] Cells from explants subjected to cyclic uniaxial compression maintained their

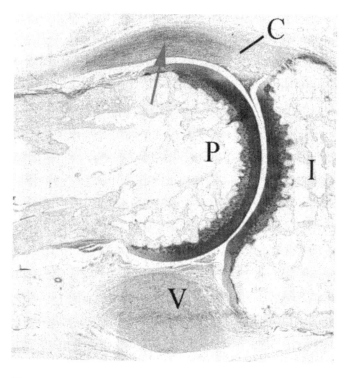

Fig. 4 A longitudinal section through the proximal interphalangeal joint of a finger, stained with toluidine blue to show the position of the sesamoid fibrocartilage (arrow) in the central slip (C) of the extensor tendon as it wraps around the head of the proximal phalanx (P). The sesamoid fibrocartilage is highlighted by its metachromasia, which is comparable to that of the articular cartilages and the volar plate (V). Note that the central slip inserts via a fibrocartilaginous enthesis into the base of the intermediate phalanx (I).

ability to synthesize large proteoglycan (probably aggrecan), whereas cells from unloaded explants synthesized predominantly small proteoglycans.

Wrap-around tendons are generally avascular for the same reason that articular cartilage is—because the blood vessels would be occluded by compression. The intermittent pressure experienced by wrap-around tendons is often accompanied by shear as the tendons slide longitudinally in response to muscle contraction. This means that the tensile load on a tendon is lower at a point distal, rather than proximal, to a pulley. This has been quantified for the digital flexor tendons either side of the flexor retinaculum.[29] When the wrist is flexed or extended to 65°, the distal strain is reduced by 40 per cent. The presence of compression and shear in addition to tension also means that pulley regions are common sites for wear and tear and this can be characterized by an increase in the amount of fibrocartilage—a condition sometimes known as mucoid degeneration.[30] Degenerative changes are also well documented in the conditions of posterior tibial tendinitis that particularly affects middle-aged women[31] and bicipital tendinitis that involves the distal tendon of biceps brachii in the region where it wraps around the radial tuberosity during pronation of the forearm.[32] Unfortunately, the absence of blood vessels in wrap-around tendon regions makes them difficult to heal. Histopathological changes have been reported in flexor hallucis longus where the tendon grooves the posterior surface of the talus and include fragmentation and partial delamination of tendon fibrocartilage.[22]

Just as wrap-around tendons are subject to compression, equally the tendons themselves exert compressive forces on the pulleys around which they pass (Fig. 2). Thus, the presence of fibrocartilage in a tendon is often correlated with the finding of a secondary cartilaginous/fibrocartilaginous periosteum on the surface of the adjacent bone instead of a fibrous periosteum, for example, on the lateral malleolus and cuboid where these are grooved by the tendon of peroneus longus.[22, 33] In marked contrast, however, the retinacula that hold wrap-around tendons in place against their bony pulleys are rarely fibrocartilaginous, though the inferior peroneal retinaculum and the annular and cruciform pulleys asociated with the flexor tendons of the fingers are notable exceptions.[22, 34]

Myotendinous junctions

The myotendinous junction (MTJ) is the region where the muscle belly meets the tendon. It may be relatively discrete, as in biceps brachii, or extend over a broad area, as in semimembranosus. It is a site of muscle growth, a target for muscle diseases,[35–38] and a region where force is transferred between muscle and tendon. It is important to recognize however, that the MTJ is not the exclusive site of force transfer, for this occurs wherever muscle cells meet connective tissue, that is, throughout the entire endomysial compartment of the muscle belly.[39]

In order to facilitate force transfer at the MTJ, the terminal muscle fibres have deep infoldings that dramatically increase the surface area of contact with tendon ECM (see references 40 and 41 for reviews). This not only decreases the stress concentration, but also affects the pattern of loading, for tensile stresses on the terminal sarcolemma are largely experienced as shear stresses. This makes the junctional region stronger. Intriguingly, the surface area is greater in slow than in fast twitch fibres, perhaps because the deformation of the terminal sarcolemma depends not only on the magnitude of the force applied, but also on its duration.[42] It is of further significance to note that the interface is a dynamic region and that its surface area decreases following periods of disuse.[43] This has obvious implications for the athlete returning to sport after an injury or an end-of-season break. MTJs fail more readily following a period of muscle disuse.[43] All professional athletes and coaches know from experience that a resumption of activity after enforced or voluntary rest should be gradual, and the above comments serve to give scientific credence to such common sense advice. Force transfer from muscle cell to tendon ECM is also enhanced by a modification of the terminal sarcolemma. There is a whole array of complex proteins here that is associated with the cytoskeleton and that allow force to be transmitted across the cell membrane (reference 41; reviewed in references 44 and 45). There are striking similarities at the molecular level between MTJs and focal adhesion sites in cultured cells. Recent evidence suggests that mechanical loading can regulate the synthesis of proteins involved in force transmission, for the quantities of talin, vinculin, and their mRNA are dramatically increased after rat hindlimb muscles are reloaded following a period of rest.[46]

The MTJ is of considerable significance in sports medicine, for it is the most common site of muscle pulls or tears.[40] It is also where most Golgi tendon organs (GTOs)[47] and other sensory receptors, including Ruffini and Vater–Pacinian corpuscles, are located.[48] GTOs are encapsulated mechanoreceptors that are innervated by large, fast-conducting Ib afferent nerve fibres and have long been implicated in the inverse stretch reflex, which is well known in sports science. The inverse stretch reflex occurs when the resistance a muscle offers to slow, continuous stretch diminishes so that the muscle lengthens and remains at its new length after the stretching force has been removed. The long-term benefits of enhanced flexibility that this mode of stretching conveys, compared with ballistic or dynamic stretching (i.e. that which is performed in a bouncy fashion), are well recognized by practising athletes. However, Jami[47] points out that the lengthening response of a muscle to stretch has been widely assumed to occur at the point where muscle tension reaches the *high* threshold of GTOs, whereas he argues that GTOs have a low threshold for contractile force. The functional significance of GTOs is thus more complex and exactly how they interact with sensory information that comes from other sources, for example, skin and joints, to control muscle contraction remains unclear.

Entheses

The enthesis is the junction between a tendon, ligament, or joint capsule and bone. It is of considerable importance in both rheumatology and sports medicine, for it is the site of tennis and golfer's elbow, jumper's knee, Osgood–Schatter's disease, Sever's disease, and the spondyloarthropathies (SpA). It is characteristic of the SpA that enthesitis affects several sites including the Achilles tendon, plantar aponeurosis, and several tendons that attach to the trochanters of the femur, to the knee, and the pelvis.[49]

Types of enthesis

Two fundamentally distinct types of enthesis have long been recognized histologically—fibrous and fibrocartilaginous (see references 41, 50, and 51 for reviews). They are also known as periosteo-diaphyseal and chondroapophyseal attachments[52, 53] or as indirect and direct insertions, respectively.[54] Fibrocartilaginous entheses are more common and are typical of the ends of long bones, but fibrous entheses are found on the metaphyses and diaphyses (Fig. 5). In fibrous entheses, the tendons attach either directly to the bone by fibrous tissue with no fibrocartilage cells being present, or indirectly to it via the periosteum. In marked contrast, fibrocartilaginous entheses have fibrocartilage cells present near the interface region so that four zones of tissue can be recognized: pure dense fibrous connective tissue (similar to that which characterizes the mid-substance of the tendon); uncalcified fibrocartilage; calcified fibrocartilage; and subchondral bone (Figs 6 and 7). These zones were originally described in the cat patellar tendon by Dolgo-Saburoff,[55] and his work was brought to the attention of a wider audience by the later studies of Cooper and Misol.[56] The zones of calcified and uncalcified fibrocartilage are separated from each other by a sharply defined calcification front called the tidemark (or 'cement line', though this term is now less commonly used). The tidemark is where the soft tissues fall away from the bone on maceration.[57] Although it is relatively straight (hence the markings left on dried bones by fibrocartilaginous entheses are smooth and resemble those of adjacent articular surfaces), the junction between the calcified fibrocartilage and the underlying subchondral bone can be highly irregular, with numerous finger-like interdigitations of the two tissues. It seems likely that the complexity of this interface contributes substantially to the strength of union of the tendon to the bone.[58]

Functions of entheses

According to Schneider[59] fibrocartilaginous entheses provide for a two-tier protection mechanism at the bony interface. The sinuosity of

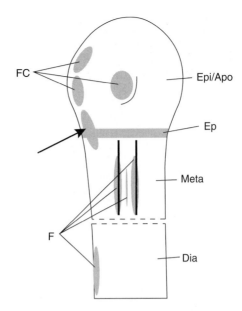

Fig. 5 A diagrammatic representation of the distribution of fibrous (F) and fibrocartilaginous (FC) entheses in a long bone. Fibrous entheses are typical of the metaphysis (Meta) and diaphysis (Dia), while fibrocartilaginous entheses are found on epiphyses or apophyses (Epi/Apo) towards the end of the long bone, above the level of the epiphyseal plate (EP). Note that it is possible for an enthesis (e.g. that of teres minor) to be partly above and partly below an epiphyseal plate (arrow).

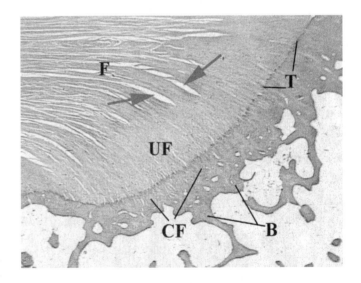

Fig. 6 The four zones of tissue that characterize the fibrocartilaginous enthesis at the insertion of the tendon of supraspinatus as seen in a section stained with haematoxylin and eosin (H&E): pure fibrous tissue (F); uncalcified fibrocartilage (UF); calcified fibrocartilage (CF); and bone (B). The two fibrocartilage zones are separated by a basophilic line called the tidemark (T). In a routine section such as this, artefactual shrinkage spaces (arrows) are prominent in the zone of fibrous tissue, but are not present in the zone of uncalcified fibrocartilage.

the calcified fibrocartilage–subchondral bone junction protects the site against shear, while the uncalcified fibrocartilage protects the tendon from undue bending at the hard tissue interface where stress concentration occurs. Schneider[59] has drawn a useful analogy between

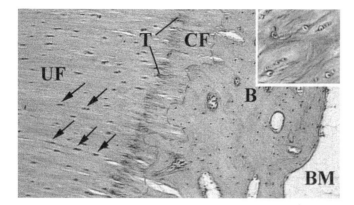

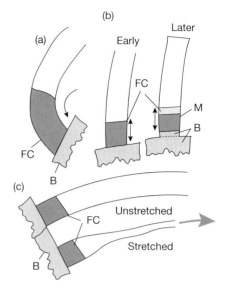

Fig. 7 High power view of the region of a fibrocartilaginous enthesis (supraspinatus insertion) either side of the tidemark (T) in a section stained with H&E. Note the rows of fibrocartilage cells (arrows) in the zone of uncalcified fibrocartilage and the highly irregular interface (broken line) between the calcified fibrocartilage (CF) and the subchondral bone (B). This sinuous junction contrasts markedly with the much straighter tidemark. Beneath the thin layer of subchondral bone is the fatty bone marrow (BM). The inset shows fibrocartilage cells in the zone of uncalcified fibrocartilage in a section of the same enthesis stained with toluidine blue.

Fig. 8 A schematic representation of the functional significance of uncalcified enthesis fibrocartilage (FC) in a tendon attaching to a bone (B). (a) Dissipating the bending of collagen fibres at the hard tissue interface. (b) Acting as a mini 'growth plate' that promotes the growth of the tendon into the bone. Note how, in the later stage of growth, bone has grown into the tendon by replacing fibrocartilage, but the thickness of the fibrocartilage zone is maintained (double-headed arrows) by the metaplasia (M) of tendon cells into fibrocartilage cells. (c) Preventing a stretched tendon from narrowing at its bony interface.

the role of uncalcified enthesis fibrocartilage in a tendon and that of a grommet on an electrical lead. Both dissipate the bending away from the hard interface (Fig. 8). Evans *et al.*[60] and Benjamin *et al.*[61] have shown that there is a correlation between the quantity of uncalcified enthesis fibrocartilage and the extent to which the insertional angle changes with joint movement. The greater the range of movement, the more fibrocartilage is present. It is intriguing therefore to note that fibrocartilage is increased in amount in patients with jumper's knee.[62]

Further functions that have been suggested for enthesis fibrocartilage are that it acts as a 'stretching brake' that prevents a stretched tendon from narrowing at its insertion site and that it provides for the growth of the underlying bone (Fig. 8).[53] The growth-promoting role of enthesis fibrocartilage has recently been supported by the developmental studies of Gao *et al.*[63] Although this work focused on the medial collateral ligament of the knee joint, the principles that emerge from it are also generally applicable to tendons. During the growing period, bone grows into a tendon/ligament by endochondral ossification (but where bone replaces a *fibrocartilaginous* rather than a *hyaline* cartilage template), but the enthesis fibrocartilage remains at the insertion site because neighbouring fibroblasts in the tendon metaplase into fibrocartilage cells. The stimulus is unknown, but is likely to be mechanical. The metaplastic origin of the enthesis fibrocartilage explains why the tissue can reappear after the surgical translocation of a tendon to a new bony insertion site.[64] It also suggests that the challenge facing surgeons trying to improve the quality of reconstructed entheses is to look for ways of encouraging the bone to grow into the tendon or ligament rather than vice versa. Bony spurs (enthesophytes) can grow into tendons as an extension of this normal mechanism of enthesis development, when bone is deposited in the walls of the tunnels created by the vascular invasion that occurs along the rows of enthesis fibrocartilage cells.[41] The invading blood vessels come from the underlying bone marrow. The mechanism has obvious parallels with the changes that occur in an epiphyseal growth plate

during the growth in length of a long bone. However, in an epiphyseal plate, the continued existence of the columns of chondrocytes is ensured by cell division, whereas in the enthesial fibrocartilage 'growth plate', the columns of fibrocartilage cells are maintained by fibroblastic metaplasia. Although bony spurs can result from inflammatory changes occurring in the underlying bone marrow, our work[41] does suggest that inflammation is not always a prerequisite for spur formation—though vascular invasion may be.

Pathology at the enthesis

Among the degenerative changes that can occur at entheses, attention is drawn to the presence of horizontal and vertical fissures in the uncalcified fibrocartilage or at its junction with the calcified tissue.[65] The vertical fissures are particularly significant because of the parallels they evoke with early changes that occur in articular cartilage during osteoarthritis. In both tissues, the fissures are bordered by clusters of cartilage cells. Radiological evidence, however, suggests that the metachromatic contents of the tendon fissures are calcified,[65] in contrast to the fissures in early osteoarthritic cartilage that are devoid of contents—possibly because they open into the synovial joint cavity itself. Horizontal tears seem fundamentally different as they do not invoke a cartilage cell response. Those reported by Rufai *et al.*[65] were located adjacent to the tidemark and associated with a fatty infiltrate.

The concept of an enthesis can be usefully extended beyond that of just the interface region itself, for there can be other closely related structures that help to dissipate stress concentration at the site where the tendon meets the bone. Collectively these constitute what Benjamin and McGonagle (2001)[66] have called an 'enthesis organ'.

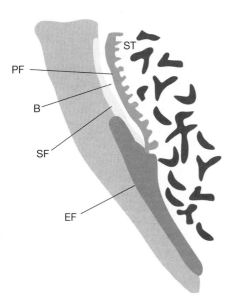

Fig. 9 A diagrammatic representation of the 'enthesis organ' of the Achilles tendon to show the location of its three fibrocartilages. The enthesis fibrocartilage (EF) lies at the tendon–bone junction and the sesamoid (SF) and periosteal (PF) fibrocartilages lie either side of the retrocalcaneal bursa (B). The latter two fibrocartilages are most prominent when the superior tuberosity (ST) of the calcaneus is large.

This is most clearly defined at the attachment of the Achilles tendon to the calcaneus and comprises periosteal and sesamoid fibrocartilages, an intervening synovial bursa and a fat pad (Fig. 9).[65] The sesamoid fibrocartilage is a specialization at the deep surface of the tendon next to the retrocalcaneal bursa that protects this part of the tendon from the pressure exerted on it by the bone when the foot is dorsiflexed (Fig. 9). Equally, the opposing surface of the bone is protected by a fibrocartilaginous periosteum and the relative movement between tendon and bone is promoted by the intervening bursa. This bursa is a well known source of much heel pain (retrocalcaneal bursitis) and the term 'bursitis' implies that it becomes inflamed—which is often the case. What our work[65] shows, however, is that fibrocartilages rather than synovial membrane line the distal end of the bursa and that degenerative changes in these fibrocartilages may contribute to the problem recognized as bursitis—or even be its underlying cause.

It is important to appreciate that any fibrous enthesis attached to the metaphysis or diaphysis of a long bone is always attached to the periosteum of the bone during the growing period and not directly to the bone itself (see Benjamin and Ralphs (2000) for a review).[67] It is only by this means that it can maintain the same relative position along the length of the bone during the growing period (Fig. 10). If a metaphyseal tendon/ligament were anchored directly to bone prior to the cessation of bone growth, it would eventually become a diaphyseal one. However, as the periosteum is capable of interstitial growth, the tendon/ligament can migrate as the bone lengthens and thus maintain a metaphyseal position.

Many entheses that are of particular interest to rheumatologists are fibrocartilaginous, for example, those of the rotator cuff and Achilles tendons, and contain aggrecan and type II collagen.[68] This molecular composition is often regarded as significant in understanding the link between the range of sites affected in spondyloarthropathies.[49] Targeted tissues are all regions where common

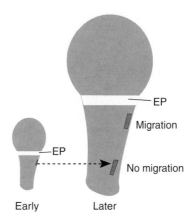

Fig. 10 A tendon (or ligament) that is attached to a metaphysis, just beneath the epiphyseal plate (EP) must migrate during development in order to maintain the same relative position of its enthesis. It does so by attaching indirectly to the periosteum during the growing period and not directly to the bone itself. If no migration occurred (e.g. because the immature tendon attached directly to bone—which is incapable of interstitial growth), the insertional site would eventually become diaphyseal.

autoantigens such as type II collagen or aggrecan are expressed. Fibrocartilaginous entheses are also common sites of sporting injuries, though the damage frequently occurs in the subchondral bone rather than in the fibrocartilage itself, for example, the avulsion injuries that occur in Osgood–Schlatter's and Sever's diseases.

Tendon sheaths

In order to facilitate the movement of a tendon when its muscle belly contracts, many tendons are surrounded by sheaths. Typically, these are true synovial sheaths, for example, those associated with tendons at the wrist, though these same tendons can have a 'false' sheath or paratenon as they cross the palm.[14] A paratenon is also well known in the Achilles tendon, for it is a common site of inflammatory changes that are associated with Achilles tendon pain in athletes. A paratenon is generally a condensation of the connective tissue surrounding a tendon that develops in response to movement. In contrast, true synovial sheaths are flattened sacs applied to a length of the tendon surface that contain a small quantity of synovial fluid and have distinct visceral and parietal layers. The visceral layer is applied directly to the tendon and is often represented by the epitenon. It is connected to the parietal layer by a sheet-like mesotenon, which in tendons with a significant longitudinal excursion can be reduced to a few thread-like vinculi (Figs 11 and 12). This is the case, for example, in the FDP tendons, where the excursion at the wrist can amount to 7 cm.[70] A persistent problem associated with tendon surgery is that adhesions frequently develop postoperatively between the tendon and its sheath that can severely limit tendon movement and compromise its normal function. There is thus great interest in any therapeutic approach that can reduce the risk of scar tissue in the tendon—for example, by applying neutralizing antibody to transforming growth factor beta 1 (TGF-β1) during the operation.[71]

Regions of tendons that are surrounded by true synovial sheaths are typically found in association with fibrous retinacula or pulleys that prevent the tendons from bowstringing as they cross synovial joints. The length of a tendon surrounded by a synovial sheath is generally

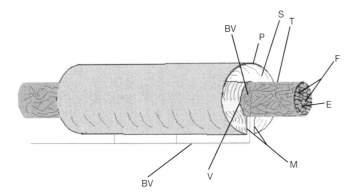

Fig. 11 Diagrammatic representation of the structure of a synovial sheath. The visceral layer (V) of the sheath is fused with the tendon (T) and represents its epitenon. It is separated from the parietal layer (P) by a synovial space (S) that contains a thin film of synovial fluid. Blood vessels (BV) enter the tendon and ramify throughout its epitenon via the mesotenon (M) that joins the visceral and parietal layer of the sheath. From the epitenon, blood vessels pass into the endotenon (E) that separates the tendon fascicles (F). (Redrawn and modified after Fig. 32 in Basmajian, J. V. Grant's Method of Anatomy, 1975, Williams & Wilkins, Baltimore.)

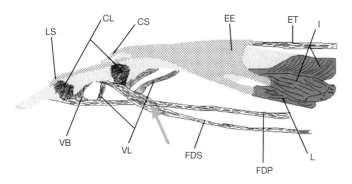

Fig. 12 A diagrammatic representation of the specialization of tendons in the middle finger. In the region of the metacarpophalangeal joint, the extensor tendon (ET) flattens into a dorsal digital expansion that surrounds the base of the finger as a hood and receives the attachment of the interosseous (I) and lumbrical (L) muscles. The central slip of the extensor tendon (CS) inserts into the base of the intermediate phalanx and two lateral slips (LS) insert into the base of the terminal phalanx. The flexor digitorum superficialis (FDS) tendon splits (arrow) to allow the tendon of flexor digitorum profundus (FDP) to pass through it on its way to its insertion at the base of the terminal phalanx. The FDS tendon inserts into the sides of the intermediate phalanx. The mesotenon of these tendons is reduced to strand-like vinculi breve (VB) near the enthesis and vinculi longi (VL) further away. CL, Collateral ligaments. (Modified from reference 69, plate 433.)

greater than the length of the retinaculum or pulley beneath which it passes. This allows the tendon to slide longitudinally on muscle contraction. Synovial sheaths can become inflamed (tenosynovitis) and accumulate a fibrin exudate in a variety of circumstances, notably in rheumatoid arthritis and as a result of repetitive motion injuries.[72, 73] Overuse injuries involving tendon sheaths are common in tennis, volleyball, and basketball players.[73] Injuries to retinacula or pulleys are also well documented, for example, tears of the pulleys associated with the digital tendons in rock climbers[74] or subluxations of the retinacula associated with the peroneal tendons. Fibrous pulleys may

become thickened and restrict the free movement of the tendon(s) within them. Such a condition is known as *stenosing tenosynovitis* and is exemplified by de Quervain's syndrome, where there is restricted movement of the tendons of abductor pollicis longus and extensor pollicis brevis in the region of the radial styloid process,[75] and trigger finger, where there is a painful locking of a digital flexor tendon in a finger or in the thumb.[76] Adhesions between the visceral and parietal layers of a synovial tendon sheath can occur following injury or surgery and can severely restrict the mobility of the tendons. Proliferative changes in the sheaths and subsequent infiltration of synovial cells into the tendon are widely implicated in the tendon ruptures that occur in rheumatoid patients.[77]

The presence of a synovial sheath alters the nutritive pathways available for the tendon cells. Digital flexor tendons are primarily nourished by diffusion from synovial fluid and their blood supply is less important than it is in extrasynovial regions.[78] Extensor tendons too rely significantly on synovial diffusion, though studies with radioactive tracers suggest that only 58 per cent of the nutrients come from this source in these tendons, compared with 90 per cent for the flexor tendons.[78, 79] This difference between flexor and extensor tendons probably relates at least in part to the more extensive mesotenon of the extensor tendons compared with the vincular attachments associated with the flexor tendons.[79] It may well be reflected in differences in healing rate and adhesion formation.[79] Predictably, tendons with a paratenon rather than a true synovial sheath rely totally upon vascular perfusion.[80]

Blood supply of tendons

Compared with skeletal muscle, tendons have a relatively poor blood supply that reflects the dominance of the ECM over the cells. This is why they appear white on gross inspection and why they were originally regarded as purely passive mechanical devices that are metabolically inert. Nevertheless, they *do* have more blood vessels than is commonly recognized, and this is highly significant to the functioning of the cells. The early literature on tendon vasculature has been briefly summarized by Elliott.[81] Blood vessels may enter at the MTJ, the paratenon, or the mesotenon/vinculae of true synovial sheaths and generally run longitudinally in the epitenon and endotenon (Fig. 3). The vessels may be rather tortuous where the longitudinal excursion of the tendons is marked so that the movement is accommodated.[14] Whether blood vessels cross the tendon–bone junction depends on the type of enthesis. At fibrocartilaginous entheses (which are the most common) no blood vessels pass across a healthy insertion site between the bone marrow and the tendon, because the fibrocartilage is avascular.[57, 82] However, at fibrous entheses, intratendinous vessels can anastomose directly with those of the bone.[83]

Avascularity and tendon pathology

The blood supply of the tendons of tibialis anterior was investigated by Gebbert *et al.*[84] in an attempt to see whether the common site of tendon rupture could be related to the pattern of blood supply. The tendon is supplied by two sets of arteries that enter it proximally and distally via branches of the anterior tibial and medial tarsal arteries respectively. Further vessels between these two sets enter the tendon separately from its synovial sheath. Gebbert *et al.*[84] showed that the entire tendon was adequately vascularized and that there was no hypovascular zone near the inferior extensor retinaculum, that is, where the ruptures most commonly occur. This is in line with the findings of Benjamin et al.[22] that the tendon is purely fibrous in this region, despite the presence of the pulley. Other tendons that are fibrocartilaginous near their fulcra are generally avascular or hypovascular,[22, 85, 86] as discussed briefly above. However, it does not necessarily follow that all avascular regions of tendons are fibrocartilaginous. One of the best known, poorly vascularized regions of a tendon is that in the Achilles tendon, approximately 2–6 cm above the calcaneus.[87] This is the region where ruptures most commonly occur—though it does not necessarily follow that the tears are related to the paucity of blood vessels.

The blood supply of the long, intrasynovial segments of the digital flexor tendons is precarious.[70] Both the FDP and flexor digitorum superficialis (FDS) tendons rely on two sets of blood vessels that enter via their vinculi and have avascular zones associated with the digital pulleys. Each tendon has a short vinculum near the end of its sheath and thus an independent supply at this level, but the long vinculum, which lies at the level of the proximal interphalangeal joint, is common to both tendons. Consequently, the surgical resection of the FDS tendon at this level deprives the FDP tendon of its blood supply.

Development and growth of tendons

Much of our knowledge of the early development of tendons has come from the study of the chick limb and was comprehensively reviewed by Benjamin and Ralphs.[41] A brief update on only some of the significant subsequent work is included here. Tendons develop from the lateral plate mesoderm as highly cellular condensations in which the cells soon become arranged into longitudinal rows in an organization that mirrors and controls the future organization of collagen fibres and fascicles. In chick limbs, the tendon cells condense on a tenascin-rich sheet of ECM called the 'mesenchyme lamina', though Gaunt[88] has recently suggested that this is a peculiarity of the chick and cannot be considered as a fundamental general feature of early tendon development in all species.

The initial formation of tendons is autonomous, but their later development involves a close interaction with the developing muscle belly (see reference 41 for a more extensive review). D'Souza and Patel[89] have further shown that tendon development is also closely coordinated with that of the cartilaginous skeletal elements. They found that two genes (Follistatin and Eph-A4) are expressed in the regions of avian limb buds where tendons develop and that the induction of cartilage formation by the application of TGFβ1 or the removal of foot-plate ectoderm, induces their expression. Whether one tissue controls the development of the other, or whether tendon and cartilage development is coordinated by a common signalling mechanism is unclear, though D'Souza and Patel[89] suggest the latter. They propose that the common signalling pathway involves TGFβ (which is expressed in both developing tendon and cartilage), a family of Gdf genes that are known to be involved in tendon development,[90] and Follistatin, which acts as an antagonist for the Gdfs. The expression profiles of Follistatin and Eph-A4 differ in developing tendons.[89] Eph-A4 is expressed in their core and Follistatin at their edge. As with Eya1 and Eya2, Follistatin and Eph-A4 are expressed in flexor tendons first, and extensor tendons later. Thus, there is a steadily increasing number of genes that are now known to be expressed in relation to tendon development.

References

1. Williams, P.L., Warwick, R., Dyson, M., et al. (1995). Gray's anatomy, 37th edn. Churchill Livingstone, Edinburgh.

2. Moore, J.S. (1992). Function, structure, and responses of components of the muscle–tendon unit. Occup. Med. 7, 713–740.

3. Oakes, B.W. (1994). Tendon–ligament basic science. In Oxford textbook of sports medicine (ed. M. Harries, C. Williams, W.D. Stanish, and L.J. Micheli), pp. 493–511. Oxford University Press, Oxford.

4. Benjamin, M. and Ralphs, J.R. (1998). Fibrocartilage in tendons and ligaments—an adaptation to compressive load. J. Anat. 193, 481–494.

5. Rack, P.M.H. and Ross, H.F. (1984). The tendon of flexor pollicis longus: its effects on the muscular control of force and position at the human thumb. J. Physiol. 351, 99–110.

6. Le Gros Clark, W.E. (1958). Tissues of the body, 4th edn. Oxford University Press, Oxford.

7. Crawford, G.N.C. (1954). An experimental study of muscle growth in the rabbit. J. Bone Joint Surg. 36B, 294–303.

8. Loren, G.J. and Lieber, R.L. (1995). Tendon biomechanical properties enhance human wrist muscle specialization. J. Biomech. 28, 791–799.

9. Alexander, R.McN. (1984). Elastic energy stores in running vertebrates. Am. Zool. 24, 85–94.

10. Fukashiro, S., Komi, P.V., Järvinen, M., and Miyashita, M. (1995). In vivo Achilles tendon loading during jumping in humans. Eur. J. Appl. Physiol. 71, 453–458.

11. Ker, R.F., Alexander, R.McN., and Bennett, M.B. (1988). Why are mammalian tendons so thick? J. Zool. (Lond.) 216, 309–324.

12. Jones, F.W. (1941). The principles of anatomy as seen in the hand. Baillière, Tindall and Cox, London.

13. Kastelic, J., Galeski, A., and Baer, E. (1978). The multicomposite structure of tendon. Connect. Tissue Res. 6, 11–23.

14. Semple, C. (1980). The design of tendons and their sheaths. In Scientific foundations of orthopaedics and traumatology (ed. R. Owen, J. Goodfellow, P. Bullough), pp. 74–78. Heinemann, London.

15. O'Brien, M. (1992). Functional anatomy and physiology of tendons. Clin. Sports Med. 11, 505–520.

16. Bailey, A.J., Robins, S.P., and Balian, G. (1974). Biological significance of the intermolecular crosslinks of collagen. Nature 251, 105–109.

17. McNeilly, C.M., Banes, A.J., Benjamin, M., and Ralphs, J.R. (1996). Tendon cells in vivo form a three dimensional network of cell processes linked by gap junctions. J. Anat. 189, 593–600.

18. Ralphs, J.R., Banes, A.J., and Benjamin, M. (1998). Tendon cells in vivo contain prominent longitudinal actin stress fibres, linked cell to cell via anchoring junctions. Trans. Orthop. Res. Soc. 23, 630.

19. Vogel, K.G., Evanko, S.P., and Robbins, J.R. (1999). What proteoglycan content says about the mechanical history of tendon. In Biology of the synovial joint (ed. C.W. Archer, B. Caterson, M. Benjamin, and J.R. Ralphs), pp. 301–313. Harwood Academic Publishers, Amsterdam.

20. Heinegård, D. and Oldberg, A. (1993). Glycosylated matrix proteins. In Connective tissue and its heritable disorders (ed. P.M. Royce and B. Steinmann), pp. 189–189. Wiley-Liss, New York.

21. Merrilees, M.J. and Flint, M.H. (1980). Ultrastructural study of tension and pressure zones in a rabbit flexor tendon. Am. J. Anat. 157, 87–106.

22. Benjamin, M., Qin, S., and Ralphs, J.R. (1995). Fibrocartilage associated with human tendons and their pulleys. J. Anat. 187, 625–633.

23. Milz, S., McNeilly, C., Putz, R., Ralphs, J.R., and Benjamin, M. (1998). Fibrocartilages in the extensor tendons of the interphalangeal joints of human toes. Anat. Rec. 252, 264–270.

24. Milz, S., Putz, R., Ralphs, J.R., and Benjamin, M. (1999). Fibrocartilage in the extensor tendons of the human metacarpophalangeal joints. Anat. Rec. 256, 139–145.

25. Gillard, G.C., Reilly, H.C., Bell-Booth, P.G., *et al.* (1979). The influence of mechanical forces on the glycosaminoglycan content of rabbit flexor digitorum profundus. *Connect. Tissue Res.* **7**, 37–46.

26. Vogel, K.G. and Koob, T.J. (1989). Structural specialization in tendons under compression. *Int. Rev. Cytol.* **115**, 267–293.

27. Vogel, K.G., Sandy, J.D., Pogany, D.L., and Robbins, J.R. (1994). Aggrecan in bovine tendon. *Matrix Biol.* **14**, 171–179.

28. Koob, T.J., Clark, P.E., Hernandez, D.J., Thurmond, F.A., and Vogel, K.G. (1992). Compression loading *in vitro* regulates proteoglycan synthesis by tendon fibrocartilage. *Arch. Biochem. Biophys.* **298**, 503–512.

29. Goldstein, S.A., Armstrong, T.J., Chaffin, D.B., *et al.* (1987). Analysis of cumulative strain in tendon and tendon sheaths. *J. Biomech.* **20**, 1–6.

30. Khan, K.M., Cook, J.L., Bonar, F., Harcourt, P., and Astrom, M. (1999). Histopathology of common tendinopathies. Update and implications for clinical management. *Sports Med.* **27**, 393–408.

31. Brandser, E.A., El-Khoury, G.Y., and Saltzman, C.L. (1995). Tendon injuries: application of magnetic resonance imaging. *Can. Assoc. Radiol. J.* **46**, 9–18.

32. Koch, S. and Tillmann, B. (1995). The distal tendon of the biceps brachii. Structure and clinical correlations. *Ann. Anat.* **177**, 467–474.

33. Stilwell, D.L. and Gray, D.J. (1954). The structures of bony surfaces in contact with tendons. *Anat. Rec.* **118**, 358–359.

34. Katzman, B.M., Klein, D.M., Garven, T.C., Claigiuri, D.A., and Kung, J. (1999). Comparative histology of the annular and cruciform pulleys. *J. Hand Surg. (Br.)* **24**, 272–274.

35. Williams, P.E. and Goldspink, G. (1971). Longitudinal growth of striated muscle fibres. *J. Cell Sci.* **9**, 751–767.

36. Law, D.J., Allen, D.L., and Tidball, J.G. (1994). Talin, vinculin and DRP (utrophin) concentrations are increased at *mdx* myotendinous junctions following onset of necrosis. *J. Cell Sci.* **107**, 1477–1483.

37. Law, D.J., Caputo, A., and Tidball, J.G. (1995). Site and mechanics of failure in normal and dystrophin-deficient skeletal muscle. *Muscle Nerve* **18**, 216–223.

38. Ridge, J.C., Tidball, J.G., Ahl, K., Law, D.J., and Rickoll, W.L. (1994). Modifications in myotendinous junction surface morphology in dystrophin-deficient mouse muscle. *Exp. Mol. Pathol.* **61**, 58–68.

39. Huijing, P.A. (1999). Muscle as a collagen fiber reinforced composite: a review of force transmission in muscle and whole limb. *J. Biomech.* **32**, 329–345.

40. Noonan, T.J., and Garrett, W.E. (1992). Injuries at the myotendinous junction. *Clin. Sports Med.* **11**, 783–806.

41. Benjamin, M. and Ralphs, J.R. (2000). The cell and developmental biology of tendons and ligaments. *Int. Rev. Cytol.* **196**, 85–130.

42. Tidball, J.G. and Daniel, L. (1986). Myotendinous junctions of tonic muscle cells: structure and loading. *Cell. Tissue. Res.* **245**, 315–322.

43. Tidball, J.G. (1984). Myotendinous junction: morphological changes and mechanical failure associated with muscle atrophy. *Exp. Mol. Pathol.* **40**, 1–12.

44. Tidball, J.G. (1991). Force transmission across muscle cell membranes. *J. Biomech.* **24**, (suppl.), 43–52.

45. Carlsson, L., Li, Z., Paulin, D., and Thornell, L-E. (1999). Nestin is expressed during development and in myotendinous and neuromuscular junctions in wild type and desmin knock-out mice. *Exp. Cell Res.* **251**, 213–223.

46. Frenette, J. and Tidball, J.G. (1998). Mechanical loading regulates expression of talin and its mRNA, which are concentrated at myotendinous junctions. *Am. J. Physiol.—Cell Physiol.* **275**, C818–C825.

47. Jami, L. (1992). Golgi tendon organs in mammalian skeletal muscle: functional properties and central actions. *Physiol. Rev.* **72**, 623–658.

48. Jozsa, L., Balint, J.B., Kannus, P., Järvinen, M., and Lehto, M. (1993). Mechanoreceptors in human myotendinous junction. *Muscle Nerve* **16**, 453–457.

49. McGonagle, D., Khan, M.A., Marzo-Ortega, H., O'Connor, P.O., Gibbon, W., and Emery, P. (1999). Enthesitis in spondyloarthropathy. *Curr. Opin. Rheumatol.* **11**, 244–250.

50. Benjamin, M. and Ralphs, J.R. (1995). Functional and developmental anatomy of tendons and ligaments. In *Repetitive motion disorders of the upper extremity* (ed. S.L. Gordon S.J. Blair, L.J. Fine), pp. 185–203. American Academy of Orthopaedic Surgeons, Rosemont.

51. Benjamin, M. and Ralphs, J.R. (1999). The attachment of tendons and ligaments to bone. In *Biology of the synovial joint* (ed. C.W. Archer, B. Caterson, M. Benjamin, and J. R. Ralphs), pp. 361–371. Harwood Academic Publishers, Amsterdam.

52. Biermann, H. (1957). Die Knochenbildung im bereich Periostaler-Diapysärer Sehnen- und Bandansätze. *Z. Zellforsch.* **46**, 635–671.

53. Knese, K-H. and Biermann, H. (1958). Die Knochenbildung an Sehnen- und Bandsätzen im Bereich ursprünglich chondraler Apophysen. *Z. Zellforsch.* **49**, 142–187.

54. Woo, S., Maynard, J., Butler, D., *et al.* (1988). Ligament, tendon, and joint capsule insertions to bone. In *Injury and repair of the musculoskeletal soft tissues* (ed. S.L.-Y. Woo), pp. 129–166. American Academy of Orthopaedic Surgeons, Park Ridge, Illinois.

55. Dolgo-Saburoff, B. (1929). Über Ursprung und Insertion der Skeletmuskeln. *Anat. Anz.* **68**, 80–87.

56. Cooper, R.R. and Misol, S. (1970). Tendon and ligament insertion. A light and electron microscopic study. *J. Bone Joint Surg.* **52A**, 1–20.

57. Benjamin, M., Evans, E.J., and Copp, L. (1986). The histology of tendon attachments to bone in man. *J. Anat.* **149**, 89–100.

58. Milz, S., Rufai, A., Buettner, A., Putz, R., and Benjamin, M. (2002). Three dimensional reconstructions of the Achilles tendon enthesis in man. *J. Anat.* **200**, 145–152.

59. Schneider, H. (1956). Zur Struktur der Sehnenansatzzonen. *Z. Anat. Entwick.* **119**, 431–456.

60. Evans, E.J., Benjamin, M., and Pemberton, D.J. (1990). Fibrocartilage in the attachment zones of the quadriceps tendon and patellar ligament of man. *J. Anat.* **171**, 155–162.

61. Benjamin, M., Evans, E.J., Donthineni Rao, R., Findlay, J.A., and Pemberton, D.J. (1991). Quantitative differences in the histology of the attachment zones of the meniscal horns in the knee joint of man. *J. Anat.* **177**, 127–134.

62. Ferreti, A., Ippolito, E., Mariani, P., and Puddu, G. (1983). Jumper's knee. *Am. J. Sports Med.* **11**, 58–62.

63. Gao, J., Messner, K., Ralphs, J.R., and Benjamin, M. (1996). An immuno-histochemical study of enthesis development in the medial collateral ligament of the rat knee joint. *Anat. Embryol.* **194**, 399–406.

64. Jones, J.R., Smibert, J.G., McCullough, C.J., Price, A.B., and Hutton, W.C. (1987). Tendon implantation into bone: an experimental study. *J. Hand Surg.* **12B**, 306–312.

65. Rufai, A., Ralphs, J.R., and Benjamin, M. (1995). Structure and histopathology of the insertional region of the human Achilles tendon. *J. Orthop. Res.* **13**, 585–593.

66. Benjamin, M. and McGonagle, D. (2001). The anatomical basis for disease localisation in seronegative spondyloarthropathy at entheses and related sites. *J. Anat.* **199**, 503–526.

67. Benjamin, M. and Ralphs, J.R. (2000). The cell and developmental biology of tendons and ligaments. *Int. Rev. Cytol.* **196**, 85–130.

68. Waggett, A., Kwan, A., Woodnutt, D., Ralphs, J., and Benjamin, M. (1998). Characterisation of collagens and proteoglycans at the insertion of the human Achilles tendon. *Matrix Biol.* **16**, 457–470.

69. Netter, F.H. (1997). *Atlas of human anatomy*, 2nd edn. Novartis, East Hanover.

70. Tubiana, R. and Beveridge, J. (1986). Flexor tendon injuries of the hand. *Curr. Orthop.* **1**, 91–99.

71. Chang, J., Thunder, R., Most, D., Longaker, M.T., and Lineweaver, W.C. (2000). Studies in flexor tendon wound healing: neutralizing antibody to TGF-beta1 increases postoperative range of motion. *Plast. Reconstr. Surg.* **105**, 148–155.

72. Järvinen, M., Józsa, L., Kannus, P., Järvinen T.L.N., Kvist, M., and Leadbetter, W. (1997). Histopathological findings in chronic tendon disorders. *Scand. J. Med. Sci. Sports* **7**, 86–95.

73. Kannus, P. (1997). Etiology and pathophysiology of chronic tendon disorders in sports. *Scand. J. Med. Sci. Sports* **7**, 78–85.

74. Bollen, S.R. and Gunson, C.K. (1990). Hand injuries in competition climbers. *Br. J. Sports Med.* **24**, 16–18.

75. Amadio, P.C. (1995). De Quervain's disease and tenosynovitis. In *Repetitive motion disorders of the upper extremity* (ed. S.L. Gordon, S.J. Blair, and L.J.Fine), pp. 435–438. American Academy of Orthopaedic Surgeons, Rosemont, Illinois.

76. Sampson, S.P., Badalamente, M.A., Hurst, L.C., *et al.* (1991). Pathobiology of the human A1 pulley in trigger finger. *J. Hand Surg.* **16A**, 714–721.

77. Williamson, S.C. and Feldon, P. (1995). Extensor tendon ruptures in rheumatoid arthritis. *Hand Clin.* **11**, 449–459.

78. Manske, P.R. and Lesker, P.A. (1983). Comparative nutrient pathways to the flexor profundus tendons in zone II of various experimental animals. *J. Surg. Res.* **34**, 83–93.

79. Manske, P.R. and Lesker, P.A. (1983). Nutrient pathways to extensor tendons within the extensor retinacular compartments. *Clin. Orthop.* **181**, 234–237.

80. Smith, J.W. (1965). Blood supply of tendons. *Am. J. Surg.* **109**, 272.

81. Elliott, D.H. (1965). Structure and function of mammalian tendon. *Biol. Rev.* **40**, 392–421.

82. Dörfl, J. (1969). Vessels in the region of tendinous insertions. I. Chondroapophyseal insertions. *Folia Morph.* **17**, 74–78.

83. Dörfl, J. (1969). Vessels in the region of tendinous insertions. II. Diaphysoperiosteal insertions. *Folia Morph.* **17**, 79–82.

84. Gebbert, M.J., Sobel, M., and Hannafin, J.A. (1993). Microvasculature of the tibialis anterior tendon. *Foot Ankle* **14**, 261–264.

85. Kolts, I., Tillmann, B., and Lüllmann-Rauch. (1994). The structure and vascularization of the biceps brachii long head tendon. *Ann. Anat.* **176**, 75–80.

86. Berenson, M.C., Blevins, F.T., Plaas, A.H.K., and Vogel, K.G. (1996). Proteoglycans of human rotator cuff tendons. *J. Orthop. Res.* **14**, 518–525.

87. Lagergren, C. and Lindholm, Å. (1958). Vascular distribution in the Achilles tendon: an angiographic and microangiographic study. *Acta Orthop. Scand.* **50**, 1–14.

88. Gaunt, M.K. (2000). Mammalian (mouse) and anuran amphibian (*Xenopus*) phalangeal tendon differentiation: a comparative immunohistochemical analysis. PhD Thesis, University College of Wales, Aberystwyth.

89. D'Souza, D. and Patel, K. (1999). Involvement of long- and short-range signalling during early tendon development. *Anat. Embryol.* **200**, 367–375.

90. Wolfman, N.M., Hattersley, G., Cox, K., *et al.* (1997). Ectopic induction of tendon and ligament in rats by growth and differentiation factors 5,6, and 7, members of the TGF-beta gene family. *J. Clin. Invest.* **100**, 321–330.

1.3 Tendon and ligament biochemistry and pathology

Graham Riley

Introduction

Tendon and ligament pathologies are often seen by general practitioners, rheumatologists, and specialists in musculoskeletal medicine. Increased participation in recreational exercise and sport, although beneficial for general health and well-being, has led to a substantial rise in their incidence. However, only belatedly are these conditions receiving the attention they deserve from the research community.

Tendons and ligaments are dense fibrous connective tissues, important for joint movement and stabilization, respectively. They have a similar composition and structure and are metabolically active and capable of responding to extrinsic factors such as mechanical load, exercise, and immobilization. Tendon and ligament are grouped together in this chapter so as to avoid repetition of common principles, although it is important to note that there are differences in the range of pathology affecting these tissues. Despite superficial similarities, there are differences in structure, composition, and function between tendon and ligament that make it unwise to extrapolate from one tissue to another.

The purpose of this chapter is to review what is known about the biochemistry and pathology of tendons and ligaments, focusing on conditions that are relevant to the practising rheumatologist and specialist in musculoskeletal medicine. Dr Benjamin has reviewed many aspects of the structure and function of tendon and their relevance to pathology in Chapter 1.2. This chapter begins with an overview of tendon and ligament biochemistry, which is fundamental to an understanding of the disease process.

Extracellular matrix components of tendon and ligament

Like all connective tissues, tendon and ligament are composite materials consisting of collagens, proteoglycans, and a variety of other non-collagenous proteins. Although the extracellular matrix (ECM) is predominantly collagen, many other components contribute to the strength, elasticity, and physiology of the tissue (Fig. 1). The relatively few cells in the mature tissue are responsible for the synthesis and organization of the ECM. These cells are also responsible for the degradation and replacement of ECM, an activity that is particularly important in tissue development, injury, and pathology. Degradation of the ECM is mediated largely by the resident fibroblasts and macrophages, either by phagocytosis or extracellular proteolysis. The maintenance of the normal tendon and ligament architecture is the result of a delicate balance between the synthesis and degradation of

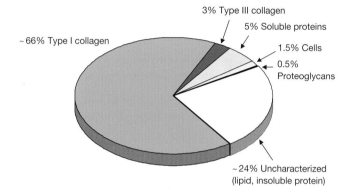

Fig. 1 Matrix (ECM) composition of tendon. Pie chart showing the approximate proportions of ECM components in a typical flexor tendon as a percentage of the tendon dry weight. The bulk of the tendon is collagen, predominantly type I with a small amount (up to 5 per cent) of type III collagen. The proportion of proteoglycan varies in different tendons and in different sites, representing 0.5–3.5 per cent of the matrix dry weight. A large proportion of the matrix is uncharacterized, thought to be insoluble protein and lipids. The composition of ligament is similar, although the proportion of type III collagen is greater—usually around 10 per cent but up to 40 per cent in some ligaments.

ECM. Disruption of this balance leads to a loss of ECM organization and will ultimately lead to pathology.

Collagens

The collagen family of glycoproteins has been extensively reviewed elsewhere.[1, 2] Collagen has a unique triple helix structure that, once secreted into the ECM, spontaneously associates with other collagen molecules to form characteristic banded fibrils (Fig. 2). Since early descriptions of collagen as a single entity, it is now known that there are at least 27 different collagen types, each with a different structure, function, and tissue distribution (Tables 1 and 2). However, it is increasingly apparent that collagens, once thought to be restricted to specific tissues, are in fact distributed more widely, albeit as minor constituents of the ECM though no doubt important for the tissue structure and function.

Tendon and ligament are predominantly type I collagen, organized into fibril bundles and orientated with the long axis of the tissue. Collagen comprises between 50 and 85 per cent of the tendon dry weight depending on the tendon, species, and location.[5] In studies of human tendon, collagen comprised on average 56 per cent of the dry weight in both the supraspinatus and the biceps brachii tendon,

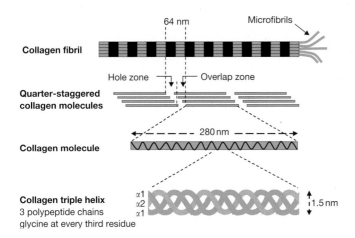

Fig. 2 Schematic representation of the prototypic collagen molecule. The collagen (type I) molecule consists of three polypeptide chains (designated α1 and α2), wound in a tight triple helix. This is made possible by the unusual amino acid content, with a high proportion of glycine, proline, and hydroxyproline in repeating triplets. Once secreted, each collagen molecule spontaneously associates end-to-end with other molecules, forming a quarter-staggered array. The 'hole zone' takes up electron-dense stains, which accounts for the striated appearance of the fibril under electron microscopy. (Reproduced (modified) from reference 3, fig. 1, p. 130, © 1998 with permission fron Elsevier Science.)

although there was considerable variation within each sample group.[6]

In the tendon mid-substance, approximately 95 per cent of the collagen is type I, with the remainder consisting of types III, IV, V, VI, XII, and XIV. Type V collagen is thought to form the core of the collagen fibril and may comprise around 2 per cent of the total collagen.[7] Type III collagen is thought to represent up to 5 per cent of the total collagen,[7] although in studies of normal human supraspinatus tendon we found an average of just over 2 per cent type III collagen.[6] Type III collagen is generally restricted to the endotenon or epitenon, the thin layers of connective tissue that surround the collagen fibre bundles.[8] However many older supraspinatus tendons show distribution of type III collagen throughout the matrix, consistent with the formation of heterotypic fibre bundles (reference 9 and Riley, G.P., unpublished observations). A similar distribution has been found in skin, with type I and type III collagens cross-linked together and found within the same fibrils.[10] This interaction appears to have a role in conditioning the collagen fibre organization and ultimate fibre diameter. Type III collagen tends to form smaller diameter fibrils, and changes in the ratio of type III to type I collagen are correlated with the average fibril diameter.[11] The resulting tissue may be more compliant and less resistant to mechanical strain. Although there have been suggestions that changes in the proportion of collagen types may be a consequence of ageing,[9] this is not a feature of all tendons, which suggests that other factors such as mechanical strain and injury are implicated. In the supraspinatus tendon the increase in type III collagen is thought likely to represent a history of previous injury and matrix remodelling events in the tissue. Changes in the proportion of collagen types I and III have been reported in other ruptured tendons,[12] consistent with some underlying process that weakens and predisposes the tendon to rupture. This is discussed in more detail below.

Type IV collagen is present in the basement membranes of tendon blood vessels, and type V collagen is encapsulated within the type I collagen fibrils.[13] Type VI collagen is found distributed throughout the matrix,[14] and collagen types XII and XIV are associated with the collagen (type I) fibril surface.[13, 15] The precise roles of these so-called 'minor' collagens are uncertain, but they are thought to be important for both cell and matrix interactions.

Ligaments are essentially similar in collagen composition to tendon, although the proportion of type III collagen is generally higher, with reported values from 12 per cent to greater than 40 per cent in some ligaments.[16, 17] The amount of type III collagen is thought to account for the elasticity of the tissue, with higher levels in intrinsic ligaments of the wrist (41 per cent) compared to extrinsic ligaments (19 per cent), and these correlated with the strain to failure.[17] Type III collagen is relatively abundant in the epiligament, the equivalent of the epitenon, that surrounds the ligament fibre bundles.[16] Type VI collagen in ligament is found in microfilaments stretching between the collagen fibrils in a network of electron-dense seams.[14]

Site-specific variations in collagen composition

The collagen composition and organization varies at different sites within tendons and ligaments—they are not homogeneous tissues. At the insertion of bovine knee ligaments and Achilles tendons there are found collagen types II, IX, X, and XI in addition to collagen type I.[18, 19] Type XIV collagen is more abundant at the insertion than elsewhere in the tendon/ligament.[7] Type X collagen is found at the Achilles insertion in the rodent, associated with the region of transition between calcified and non-calcified fibrocartilage.[20] In the human Achilles at the bone insertion there are found collagen types I, II, III, V, and VI.[21] A higher concentration of type III is reported in the rotator cuff tendon at or near the insertion where it might contribute to the high incidence of tear at this site.[6, 9, 22] Type II collagen is also found at regions of tendon fibrocartilage where tendon is compressed as it wraps around bone or passes through fibrous pulleys.[23, 24] In these regions the collagen has a different organization with a meshwork structure reminiscent of that of cartilage.[25] The cells in these regions are rounded and chondrocyte-like, and express proteoglycans once thought to be restricted to cartilage (see below). Type VI collagen, which is normally associated with microfibrillar networks between adjacent collagen fibres in the tendon mid-substance, is cell-associated in fibrocartilage, similar to the distribution seen in articular cartilage. Levels of matrix gene expression in the fibrocartilaginous regions of bovine tendon are higher than in the tension-bearing regions of the same tendon, demonstrating increased matrix turnover at these sites.[26]

Collagen fibril organization and structure

The hierarchical structure of a typical tendon was described by Kastelic et al.[27] as consisting of collagen molecules laid down into fibrils, bundles of fibrils forming fibres, and fibre bundles surrounded by endotenon to form fascicles (Fig. 3). A similar structure is found in ligament.

The smallest basic structural unit is the collagen fibril, with diameters ranging from 10 to 500 nm depending on the age, location, and species from which the tendon/ligament is sampled.[28] There is not a continuous spectrum of fibril sizes, but usually two or three distinct populations are present within a specific tendon or ligament.[28–30] In the young animal, fibrils are predominantly of small average diameter,

Table 1 Molecular composition and tissue distribution of collagens[a]

Collagen type	Molecular composition	Mature chain size[b] $Mr \times 10^{-3}$	Tissue distribution
Fibril-forming collagens			
I	$[\alpha 1(I)_2 \alpha 2(I)]$	95	Most connective tissues
II	$[\alpha 1(II)_3]$	95	Cartilage, vitreous
III	$[\alpha 1(III)_3]$	95	Synovium, skin, tendon, ligament
V/XI	$[\alpha 1(V)_2 \alpha 2(V)]$ $[\alpha 1(V)\alpha 2(V)\alpha 3(V)]$ $[\alpha 1(XI)\alpha 2(XI)\alpha 3(XI)]$ mixed molecules of V and XI	120–145	Heterotypic fibrils of type V with type I collagen, type XI with type II collagen, but mixed molecules possible
Network collagens			
IV	$[\alpha 1(IV)_2 \alpha 2(IV)]$ also unknown combinations of $\alpha 3(IV)$, $\alpha 4(IV)$, $\alpha 5(IV)$, $\alpha 6(IV)$	150	Basement membrane
VIII	$[\alpha 1(VIII)_2 \alpha 2(VIII)]$	70	Descemets membrane
X	$[\alpha 1(X)_3]$	59	Growth plate
Filamentous collagen			
VI	$[\alpha 1(VI)\alpha 2(VI)\alpha 3(VI)]$	$\alpha 1/\alpha 2 = 140$, $\alpha 3 = 200$–280	Skin, cartilage, tendon, blood vessels
Fibril-associated collagens (FACITs)			
IX	$[\alpha 1(IX)\alpha 2(IX)\alpha 3(IX)]$	$\alpha 1 = 66$ (short form) or 84 (long form) $\alpha 2 = 66$ (non-glycanated) or 66–115 (glycanated) $\alpha 3 = 72$	Cartilage, vitreous
XII	$[\alpha 1(XII)_3]$	220 (short form) 340 (long form) (long form can be glycanated)	Fetal tendon, skin
XIV	$[\alpha 1(XIV)_3]$	220 (can be glycanated)	Fetal tendon, skin
XVI	$[\alpha 1(XVI)_3]$	160	Fibroblasts, keratinocytes
XIX	$[\alpha 1(XIX)_3]$	115	Rhabdosarcoma
Multiplexins			
XV	$[\alpha 1(XV)_3]$	140	Fibroblasts
XVIII	$[\alpha 1(XVIII)_3]$	130	Liver, lung
Orphans			
VII	$[\alpha 1(VII)_3]$	270	Epithelial basement membrane
XIII	$[\alpha 1(XIII)_3]$	60	Many connective tissues
XVII	$[\alpha 1(XVII)_3]$	140	Epithelial hemidesmosomes

[a] Modified with permission from reference 4, table 1, p. 254 © 1998, Springer-Verlag.

[b] Mr, Relative molecular mass.

whilst in the adult there is a bimodal distribution, with large- and small-diameter fibrils.[30, 31] In adult human tendons, for example, there were two distinct populations with average diameters of 60 and 170 nm, respectively.[32] Since large-diameter fibrils are associated with greater tensile strength,[31] the factors that control the ultimate diameter of developing fibrils are important in both development and injury. An important contribution is thought to be provided by the glycosaminoglycan/proteoglycan content of the tissue, with different molecular species exerting differential effects on the formation of collagen fibres, at least *in vitro*.[33–35]

Fibre bundles (fascicles) exhibit a planar zigzag or 'crimp', and the stretching out of crimped fibrils is thought to account for the 'toe' region of the tendon/ligament stress–strain curve, as described in Chapter 1.2 and outlined in more detail below.[36] The angle of crimp can vary in different tendons and at different sites and has implications for the mechanical properties of tendon: collagen fibrils with smaller crimp angles will fail at a given strain before those with a larger crimp angle.[37]

Bundles of fascicles are bound together and surrounded by the epitenon. The number of fibre bundles in a fascicle and the number of fascicles varies between tendons, and often within the same tendon.[32] Fibre bundles are predominantly aligned with the long axis of the tendon and responsible for the mechanical strength of the tissue. However, not all fibres run parallel along the course of the tendon. A proportion of fibres run transversely, and there are more complex fibre arrangements including spirals and even a plait-like formation.[32, 38] This complex ultrastructure is thought to provide resistance against transverse shear, and rotational force.

Many tendons also exhibit a complex macrostructure, with a spiralling rotation of the fibre bundles in some tendons and a multidirectional orientation with interdigitation of fibres in others. In the Achilles, for example, fibre bundles may spiral up to 90° laterally, with a wide variation between individuals depending on the site of the fusion between the gastrocnemius and soleus fibre bundles.[32] The concentration of stress where the two tendons join, between 2 and 5 cm from the calcaneus insertion, has been associated with the high frequency of pathology at

Table 2 Schematic representation of the collagen superfamily[a]

Collagen type	Structure
I, II, III, V, XI	
IV	
VI	
VII	
VIII	
XII	
XV	
XVII	

[a] Each collagen contains at least some triple-helix structure (green) and variable amounts of globular (non-helical) domains (yellow). Some collagens form long rods (types I, II, III, V, and XI) with small globular domains at the ends. Other collagens have interrupted or short triple-helical regions resulting in a variety of different structures. (Modified with permission from reference 4, Fig. 1, p. 255 © 1998, Springer-Verlag.)

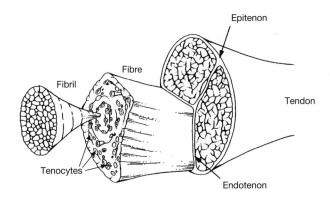

Fig. 3 Structural hierarchy of tendon and ligament. Collagen fibrils are arranged into fibres, and fibres are surrounded by a thin layer known as the endotenon. Bundles of fibres may form into fascicles, and the whole tendon is enveloped with a thin surface layer known as the epitenon. Fibroblasts (tenocytes) are dispersed throughout the fibre. The endotenon and epitenon contain a variety of different cell types and carry blood vessels, lymphatics, and nerves. The tendon is surrounded by paratenon, which at some sites is further specialized to form a sheath. (Reproduced from reference 27. Copyright 1978 from *Connective Tissue Research* by Kastelic J, Galeski A, and Baer E. Reproduced by permission of Taylor & Francis, Inc., http://www.routledge-ny.com.)

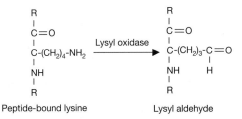

Fig. 4 Lysyl oxidase activity. The oxidative deamination of specific lysines (and hydroxylysines) is mediated by lysyl oxidase, forming aldehydes. Adjacent aldehydes then form reducible, covalent cross-links. Lysyl oxidase is the only enzyme required for cross-link formation in the matrix.

this site. Further demonstration of the complexity of organization in some tendons is provided by the multilayered organization of the supraspinatus tendon, which was shown to comprise at least five distinct layers, each with a different orientation and organization of fibres.[39] This structure has presumably developed to cope with the complex demands placed upon the supraspinatus in its role as a dynamic stabilizer of the shoulder joint. Pathology may be associated with the unequal distribution of load across the tendon, resulting in separation of adjacent layers within the tendon substance.[40]

The size of the fibre bundles is proportional to the macroscopic size of the tendon, with small fascicles generally found in digital tendons and large bundles in big, weight-bearing tendons such as the Achilles.[32] The fascicular structure provides a fail-safe mechanism, so that failure of one or a few collagen fibre bundles does not compromise the strength of the whole tendon. Tendons are normally immensely strong under tension, able to withstand loads of up to $100\ \mathrm{N\ m^{-2}}$, thought to be many times the functional requirements under normal conditions of loading.[5] However, the physical properties of tendon can be severely compromised by repeated strain, resulting in fatigue failure of the fibres and deterioration in tendon quality.[41, 42] This is the theoretical basis for tendon 'overuse injury' as discussed in more detail below.

Collagen cross-linking

Once synthesized and secreted into the matrix, collagen molecules associate together and these macromolecular assemblies are stabilized by the formation of stable cross-links.[43, 44] Cross-linking of collagen can occur by two different processes: (1) an enzyme-mediated process; (2) a non-enzymic reaction with plasma sugars known as glycation.

Cross-linking increases the stiffness of the collagen fibrils and is important for the mechanical properties of connective tissues. However, the process of glycation has deleterious effects on tissues, a problem particularly in diabetics as a result of elevated blood sugar levels.

Enzyme-mediated cross-linking

Enzyme-mediated cross-linking is initiated in the ECM by the action of lysyl oxidase, generating aldehydes from specific lysine or hydroxylysine residues (see Fig. 4).[43, 44] Lysyl oxidase is the only enzyme known to be involved in the process and all ensuing reactions are spontaneous. Immature aldimine and ketoimine cross-links form via the condensation of an aldehyde with an adjacent lysine or hydroxylysine residue (Fig. 5). In fibrillar collagens, aldehydes in the globular 'telopeptides' at each end of the molecule interact with lysines or hydroxylysines within the helical region of adjacent molecules. These di-functional cross-links are reducible, decrease in number with age, and are absent by the time of skeletal maturity. They are gradually replaced by tri-functional cross-links due to further reaction with adjacent aldehydes (Fig. 6). Although not all of the mature cross-links have been identified, the best characterized are hydroxylysylpyridinoline (HP, otherwise known as pyridinoline), derived from three

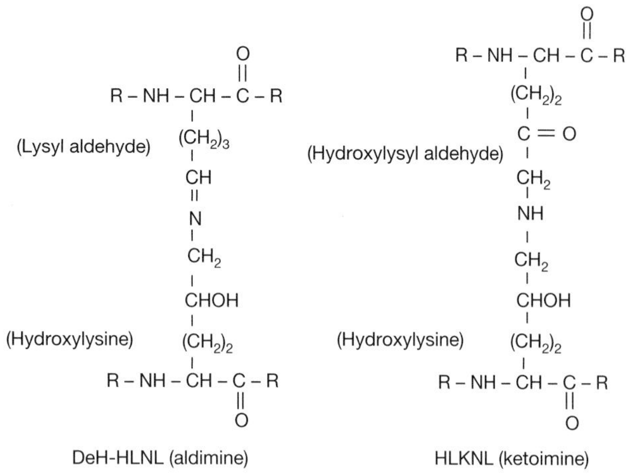

Fig. 5 Immature collagen cross-links. The initial products of cross-linking, such as dehydro-hydroxylysino-norleucine (deH-HLNL) and hydroxylysino-5-ketonorleucine (HLKNL), are between two adjacent amino acids. deH-HLNL, an aldimine, is derived from a lysyl-aldehyde in the non-helical domain of one collagen molecule and a hydroxylysine in the triple helix of an adjacent molecule. HLKNL, a ketoimine, is derived from a hydroxylysyl aldehyde in the non-helical domain of one collagen molecule and a hydroxylysine in the triple helix of an adjacent molecule. Aldimine cross-links, deH-HLNL in particular, are predominant in skin and tendon. They are readily cleaved at acid pH and by hot water, accounting for the high solubility of collagen in immature skin and tendon. Ketoimines are more abundant in bone and cartilage and, since they are stable to heat and acid pH, account for the insolubility of collagen from immature tissues.

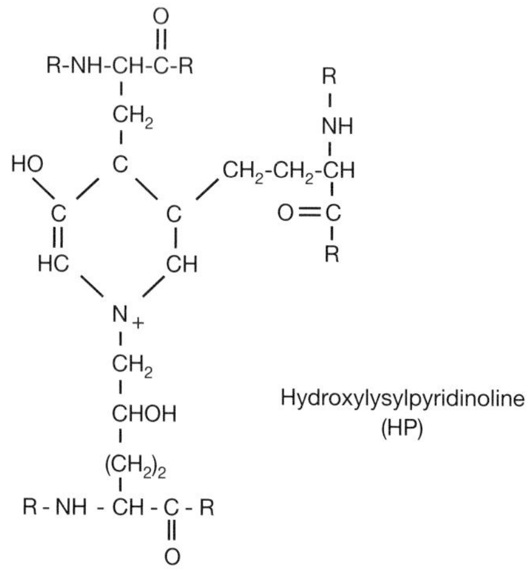

hydroxylysine residues, and lysylpyridinoline (LP, otherwise known as deoxypyridinoline), derived from two hydroxylysines and one lysine residue. LP is essentially restricted to bone and present only in small quantities in soft connective tissues.

The amount of HP in a given connective tissue is related to its mechanical function.[45] The highest concentration is reported in hyaline cartilage and intervertebral disc, with approximately two residues of HP per collagen molecule.[43] Flexor tendons have a high HP density compared to other type I collagen-containing tissues, although there are substantial variations between different tendons. Short head of biceps brachii tendons contained on average 0.25 residues of HP per collagen molecule compared to 0.8 residues of HP per collagen molecule in the supraspinatus.[46] These differences presumably reflect the different functional demands placed on these tendons, with the supraspinatus experiencing substantial shear and compressive loads as a consequence of its anatomical position in the shoulder joint. A high HP content was also reported in the compressed region of the bovine flexor digitorum profundus, compared to regions of the tendon experiencing purely tensile loads.[25] However since the levels of the HP cross-link do not change significantly with age post-maturity, they do not appear to contribute to the altered physicochemical properties with increasing age, such as the reduction in elasticity and decrease in solubility of the matrix.

Non-enzymic glycation of collagen

The second type of collagen cross-linking occurs by non-enzymic glycation.[47–49] Glycation reactions are a major cause of tissue dysfunction in the elderly due to cross-linking, which stiffens the tissues and alters normal cell–matrix interactions. Reducing sugars (e.g. pentoses) in the plasma react with matrix proteins resulting in the formation of advanced glycation end products (AGEs) (Fig. 7).

Fig. 6 Hydroxylysyl-pyridinoline (HP)—a mature collagen cross-link. Further condensation of the immature, di-functional cross-links with a third adjacent hydroxylysine residue results in the formation of mature, tri-functional cross-links such as hydroxylysyl-pyridinoline (HP). HP is the most abundant collagen cross-link in adult tendon and ligament.

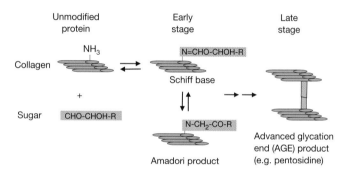

Fig. 7 Non-enzymatic glycation. Sugars accumulate on long-lived proteins such as collagen in a non-enzymatic and irreversible process known as glycation. Following a process of Amadori rearrangement, adjacent sugars become cross-linked to form various AGE cross-links such as pentosidine.

Over time, these sugars form irreversible cross-links with adjacent molecules as a result of Amadori rearrangement, producing Maillard browning products that alter the physical and chemical characteristics of tissues.[47, 49] These effects include a decrease in elasticity and a substantial decrease in solubility, even with chemical agents such as cyanogen bromide, making it difficult to assess the biochemical composition of ageing human tendon.[6] Although there are a variety of AGEs, the best characterized is the naturally fluorescent cross-link pentosidine.[50] Since the turnover of collagen in mature connective tissues is generally very low, it has been shown that AGEs such as pentosidine accumulate with age. Therefore pentosidine content serves as a marker of the age of the collagen network. We have found that pentosidine accumulates in a linear fashion with age in the human short head of biceps brachii tendon, consistent with very low levels of collagen turnover in this tissue (Fig. 8(a)).[46] However, pentosidine content was not correlated with age in the supraspinatus, consistent with significantly increased matrix (collagen) turnover at this site (Fig. 8(b)).[46] This turnover may have a number of implications for tendon pathology as discussed in more detail below.

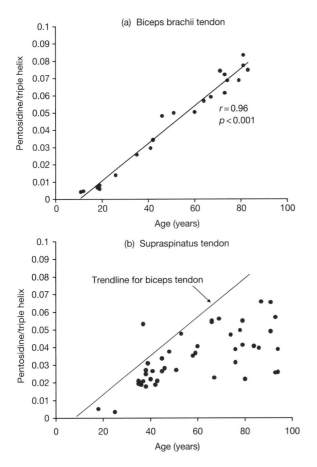

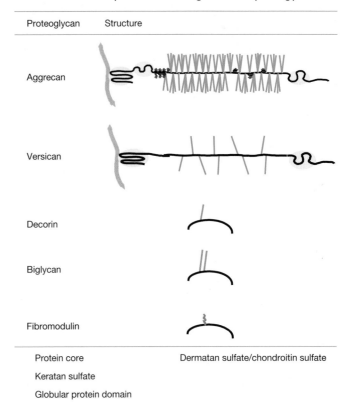

Table 3 Schematic representation of large and small proteoglycans[a]

Proteoglycan	Structure
Aggrecan	
Versican	
Decorin	
Biglycan	
Fibromodulin	

Protein core	Dermatan sulfate/chondroitin sulfate
Keratan sulfate	
Globular protein domain	

[a] Proteoglycans are a heterogeneous group of molecules with a wide range of sizes and functions, although all possess at least one chain of glycosaminoglycan (GAG). The large proteoglycans, aggrecan and versican, are rich in chondroitin sulfate, although only aggrecan has keratan sulfate chains. Decorin carries a single chain of GAG, which is predominantly dermatan sulfate in tendon and ligament. Biglycan has two GAG chains, either chondroitin sulfate or dermatan sulfate. Fibromodulin has a single keratan sulfate chain. (Modified from reference 51.)

Fig. 8 Pentosidine accumulation in human tendon. Pentosidine content was measured by reversed-phase high-performance liquid chromatography (HPLC) and expressed relative to the collagen content. (a) Pentosidine accumulated in a linear fashion with age in a sample of biceps brachii tendons, demonstrating minimal collagen turnover over lifetime. (b) In supraspinatus tendons the pentosidine content did not increase in a linear fashion with age, consistent with relatively high levels of collagen turnover, presumably as a consequence of repeated injury and matrix remodelling. (Modified from reference 46. Reproduced with permission from the BMJ publishing group.)

Proteoglycans

Proteoglycan nomenclature, structure, and function have been extensively reviewed elsewhere[51, 52] and are also covered in Chapters 1.4 and 1.5 on the intervertebral disc and meniscus, respectively. Briefly, proteoglycans are an extremely heterogeneous group of molecules, characterized by the presence of at least one chain of glycosaminoglycan (GAG) attached to the protein core (Table 3). There are five major classes of GAGs, each consisting of repeating disaccharides of hexosamine and a uronic acid, and those that bind to the proteoglycan core protein are sulfated. Their sulfate moiety and high uronic acid content mean that GAGs are highly anionic and therefore hydrophilic, in large part responsible for holding water within the tissues. The non-sulfated GAG hyaluronan forms huge multimolecular aggregates with large proteoglycans such as aggrecan, the major proteoglycan in articular cartilage. It has a core protein size of around 250 kDa, with three globular domains (G1, G2, and G3) and contains many GAG chains (chondroitin sulfate and keratan sulfate) attached to specific sites throughout its length.[51, 53] Versican is a large proteoglycan identified in soft connective tissues, with a similar structure to aggrecan although lacking the G2 domain and containing less GAG.[54]

Small proteoglycans are found in most connective tissues. Decorin has a core protein of 45 kDa and one GAG chain, which may be chondroitin sulfate (in muscle and bone) or dermatan sulfate (in tendon and articular cartilage).[55] It is found attached to collagen fibres at specific sites and is thought to modulate collagen fibril formation.[56] Fibromodulin has a closely related core structure and carries a single keratan sulfate GAG chain. As its name implies, it is thought to influence the development and ultimate diameter of collagen fibres. Biglycan contains two GAG chains, either chondroitin sulfate or dermatan sulfate, and although it is widely distributed its function is unknown. However, like other small proteoglycans, it binds to growth factors such as transforming growth factor β (TGFβ) and may act to sequester cytokines within the ECM and modulate their activity on the resident cell population.[57]

Proteoglycans in tendon and ligament

In the tension-bearing regions of a bovine flexor tendon, proteoglycans comprise between 0.2 and 0.5 per cent of the tendon dry weight. The most abundant is the small proteoglycan decorin carrying dermatan sulfate GAG side chains, in addition to small amounts of biglycan.[58] Small proteoglycans represent 88 per cent of the total and the remainder is large proteoglycan, thought to be a processed form of aggrecan rather than versican.[59]

In weight-bearing and compressed regions of bovine tendons, the proteoglycan content is around 3.5 per cent of the tendon dry weight, with a high content of aggrecan and biglycan.[25, 60] A similar proteoglycan composition has been described in fibrocartilaginous regions of rabbit and dog tendons.[61, 62] The accumulation of aggrecan at these sites occurs following weight bearing in the neonate, and the maintenance of synthesis is dependent on compressive load.[63] The presence of fibrocartilage at these sites is a protective adaptation, with the aggrecan functioning to hold water within the tissue and resist shear and compression as it does in articular cartilage.[25]

Regional differences in tendon morphology and composition have also been identified in human tendons.[21, 64–66] In Achilles tendons, decorin, biglycan, lumican, and fibromodulin have all been identified in both fibrocartilage and tension-bearing regions, at both the mRNA and protein level.[21] Versican was identified as the major large proteoglycan in the tendon mid-substance, with lesser amounts of aggrecan. In contrast, the fibrocartilage of the Achilles insertion contained mainly aggrecan with lesser amounts of versican. Site-specific variations in proteoglycan content are related to the mechanical history and function of the tendon. Short heads of biceps brachii tendons contain around 0.2 per cent proteoglycan, with the majority carrying dermatan sulfate GAG side chains (80 per cent) and the remainder chondroitin sulfate, consistent with a predominance of decorin in flexor tendons that experience mainly tensile loads.[64] Substantially higher levels of proteoglycan are found in supraspinatus tendons, mainly chondroitin sulfate with lesser amounts of dermatan sulfate and keratan sulfate.[64] These proteoglycans have since been characterized, confirming that aggrecan is the major large proteoglycan in the supraspinatus, in addition to significant amounts of biglycan.[67] This fibrocartilaginous composition is thought to be a result of adaptive metaplasia to the compressive load experienced by the tendon in the rotator cuff, which wraps around the head of humerus and may experience some impingement from the overlying bone and ligament. Similar fibrocartilaginous regions have also been described in human peroneus, tibialis, and extensor digitorum tendons.[65, 66]

In normal ligaments, 80 per cent of the proteoglycan is decorin, with the remainder biglycan and a large proteoglycan thought to be similar or related to versican.[68, 69] Ligaments also have fibrocartilaginous regions and the proteoglycan distribution is generally similar to that found in tendon,[66, 70] although there are differences between ligaments. In the collateral ligaments of the knee, for example, biglycan and decorin are found mainly between the collagen fibre bundles, whereas in cruciate ligaments these proteoglycans are largely cell-associated. Aggrecan is the major large proteoglycan in ligament fibrocartilage where the tissue is subject to compression, and versican is thought to be more characteristic of the fibrous, tensile-load-bearing regions.

Pathological significance of tendon and ligament fibrocartilage

The pathological significance of tendon (and ligament) fibrocartilage at insertions and other sites remains to be established. Fibrocartilage has an altered collagen composition and organization as well as an altered proteoglycan content.[25] The region is generally less vascularized, or even avascular, and therefore may be vulnerable if damaged and less capable of repair. Some studies have suggested that there is indeed a differential repair potential, although whether this is linked to biochemical, cellular, or vascular differences is unclear.[71] A lower elastic modulus was measured in the fibrocartilaginous region of the dog flexor digitorum profundus compared to the tensional region.[72] Pathology is frequently located in the fibrocartilaginous regions of tendons such as the supraspinatus, tibialis anterior, and tibialis posterior.

There may be a causal relationship between the relative avascularity and the development of fibrocartilage. However, other common sites of tendon pathology, such as the Achilles tendon mid-substance, that are thought to be relatively avascular (although this is questioned by some studies) are not fibrocartilaginous. Consequently, the development of fibrocartilage does not necessarily represent a pathological process, although fibrocartilaginous change may represent a precursor of tendon pathology induced by excessive compression or shear forces.

Non-collagen components of tendon and ligament

The other non-collagen components of the tendon/ligament ECM have not been extensively investigated. In biochemical studies we found that around that 20–25 per cent of the tendon dry mass was not accounted for by the collagen and proteoglycan component (Fig. 1).[6, 64] Apart from the cellular content, which is only 1–3 per cent of the dry weight,[32] the remaining mass consists of lipids, inorganic components, and non-collagen proteins such as elastin and various glycoproteins.

Elastin

Only a small proportion of the tendon ECM is elastin, with estimates in the literature of approximately 2 per cent of the tendon dry weight.[5] Elastin is a very stable and extremely insoluble protein composed mainly of hydrophobic amino acids, with a high proportion of glycine and proline.[73] Unlike collagen, it contains little hydroxyproline and no hydroxylysine and is rich in two unusual amino acids, desmosine and isodesmosine, that form covalent cross-links between the polypeptide chains.[43, 73] Elastin is a major component of elastic fibres, which consist of a central core and microfilaments that are found distributed throughout the ECM. Elastic fibres are found in young and old tendons, at the insertion as well as the mid-substance, and may be increased in some pathological conditions such as Ehlers–Danlos syndrome and chronic uraemia.[32, 74] The function of elastic fibres in tendon is unclear, but they may contribute to the recovery of the crimp in the collagen fibres after tendon is stretched.[36]

Fibronectin

Fibronectin is a high molecular weight extracellular protein important in mediating interactions between the cell and the surrounding matrix.[75] It is a multidomain protein, with specific domains involved in interactions with cells and molecules such as fibrin, actin, hyaluronan, collagen, heparin, and coagulation factors. It has a range of functions including cell adhesion, cell migration, control of differentiation, haemostasis, phagocytosis, and chemotaxis. Fibronectin has been detected in the matrix of tendons and ligaments, although there are site-specific variations, with a higher concentration in intrasynovial anterior cruciate ligaments (ACL) compared to extrasynovial medial collateral ligaments (MCL) and patellar tendon.[76, 77] It is not greatly abundant in normal tissues, comprising just 0.2 per cent of the ACL dry weight and less than 0.1 per cent of that of the patellar tendon.[76, 77] Fibronectin was primarily associated with synovial-like cells in the epitenon, which produce fibronectin in culture unlike cells from the centre of the tendon.[78] However, in human Achilles tendons fibronectin was not detected in the normal tendon mid-substance or paratenon, but was restricted to the vascular walls and myotendinous junction.[76, 79] After tendon rupture, fibronectin was massively increased and found associated with tenocytes and collagen fibres in the vicinity of the rupture, in addition to cells in macroscopically normal regions of the tendon.[79] It is not known whether the increase in fibronectin expression precedes tendon rupture, although it is an important part of the early tendon response to injury, implicated in fibroblast adhesion, migration, and differentiation at the wound site.[80, 81]

Tenascin-C

Tenascin-C is a disulfide-linked hexameric protein with subunits of between 200 and 300 kDa in the human, created by alternative splicing of a signal gene transcript.[82, 83] Tenascin-C was identified as a component of developing chick tendon, where it was particularly associated with the myotendinous junction, and consequently first described as myotendinous antigen.[82] Its distribution in mature tendon suggests at least two functional roles. In normal fibrous tendon, tenascin is associated with the collagen fibres, consistent with a role in collagen fibril organization, perhaps maintaining the interface between fibrils and adjacent structures.[84] The greatest concentration is at the myotendinous junction and bone insertion, suggesting a role in the transmission of tensile loads.[85] In fibrocartilaginous regions of tendon, tenascin-C was found to be predominantly cell-associated, and its expression may be implicated in the development of fibrocartilage and the altered cell activity in response to compressive load.[84, 86] An increase in tenascin-C expression was also associated with tendon and soft connective tissue injuries, where it has a restricted pattern of expression and a major role in the control of cell activities.[87, 88] Tenascin is a poor adhesive substratum for cells, and its effects on cell behaviour may be mediated by effects on cell shape, such as cell rounding and the development of a chondrocytic phenotype.[89] It is also strongly associated with connective tissue remodelling in development and disease, with increased expression in osteoarthritic cartilage.[90] We have shown that the there is an increase in tenascin-C expression in degenerate tendon pathology, with a change from predominantly the 200 kDa isoform to a mixed expression of 200 and 300 kDa isoforms.[84] Biochemical studies also showed evidence of enzymic degradation of tenascin-C in degenerate tendons, with the presence of multiple degradation products consistent with matrix metalloproteinase enzyme activity.[84, 91] It is not known whether changes in tenascin-C expression and structure occur before or after tendon rupture, although it is interesting to note that tenascin may have a direct stimulatory effect on matrix metalloproteinase (MMP) enzyme expression.[92]

Cartilage oligomeric matrix protein (COMP)

Despite its name COMP is not restricted to cartilage, but is found in other connective tissues and is a major component of tendon and ligament, representing up to 3 per cent of the tendon dry weight.[93, 94] A member of the thrombospondin gene family, it is now also referred to as thrombospondin 5.[95] COMP is a large (524 kDa) oligomer, composed of five subunits connected by disulfide bonds.[95] Its function is unclear, although its association with collagen fibre bundles suggests both a structural role and an interactive role with the cell population. There is a strong relationship with the loading pattern of tissues, with increased levels of COMP in flexor tendons compared to extensor tendons and ligaments, and it may function to signal cellular responses to mechanical load.[94] The structural importance of COMP is demonstrated by the discovery that a mutation in the COMP gene is responsible for pseudoachondroplasia, a rare genetic disorder characterized by short stature, lax joints, and early-onset osteoarthritis.[96] COMP levels increase as a function of age up to skeletal maturity in a variety of tissues, although only in weight-bearing tendons.[94] It also increases after injury as part of the healing response, possibly driven by mechanical forces across the granulation tissue. After skeletal maturity, levels of COMP in equine tendon decline, possibly by a combination of increased enzymic degradation and a decrease in the synthetic activity of mature tenocytes.[94] Thus it has been suggested that, in adult animals, strenuous exercise has deleterious effects on the biochemical composition of the tendon matrix, and that there is a window of opportunity for adaptive responses to exercise only in the immature animal.[97] Fragments of COMP released into the synovial fluid and bloodstream may be useful indicators of tendon injury, assuming that COMP fragments derived from tendon can be differentiated from those derived from cartilage and other tissues.[97]

Other matrix glycoproteins

Apart from serum proteins such as albumin, other glycoproteins in tendon/ligament include laminin, which is found as a major constituent of the blood vessel basement membranes, and link protein, which stabilizes large proteoglycan–hyaluronan interactions.[32, 51, 98] Other multidomain adhesive glycoproteins include members of the thrombospondin family, which like COMP, tenascin, and fibronectin mediate cell–matrix interactions in normal tissues as well as in repair and pathology.[99–101] Amongst other as yet unidentified proteins there are soluble proteins of 52, 54, and 55 kDa, respectively, that vary in distribution throughout the length of a tendon.[102]

Lipids

Cholesterol esters, thought to be derived from circulating plasma low-density lipoprotein, accumulate in tendons and fascia with increasing age.[103] There are also variable amounts of triglyceride, which are generally found between the collagen fibre bundles. Most lipid deposits are closely associated with GAGs, which act to entrap low-density lipoprotein similar to atherosclerotic plaques in arteries.[103] The GAG-rich tendon fibrocartilage is reported to contain more lipid deposits than normal tensile regions of tendon, and this may help the tissue withstand compression.[25] The precise contribution of lipids to tendon pathology is unknown, although increased lipid deposits are found relatively frequently in ruptured and degenerate tendons where they have been described as 'tendolipomatosis'.[104, 105]

Amyloid

Amyloid deposits are derived from normally soluble proteins, which can form insoluble aggregates in a number of connective tissues including cartilage, fibrocartilage, meniscus, and joint capsule. Deposition of amyloid is age-related and in osteoarthritic cartilage is associated with degenerative changes in the matrix attributable to the change in GAG composition.[106] Amyloid deposits were frequently found in ruptured supraspinatus tendons, localized to degenerate areas of the tendon where there was a high concentration of GAG.[107] Once deposited, amyloid is insoluble and resistant to proteolytic degradation, and may contribute to the structural and functional failure of the tissue. However, the incidence of amyloid deposition in normal tendon is not known; consequently the pathological significance is uncertain.

Inorganic components

A variety of inorganic constituents have been identified in tendon, with sodium, potassium, calcium, phosphorus, and magnesium most abundant among the different elements represented.[108] Most are primarily associated with soluble proteins, although the most abundant element, calcium, is also present as insoluble mineral deposits in tendon.[108, 109] The concentration of calcium was found to be similar in different tendons, accounting for around 0.1 per cent of the tendon dry weight in human supraspinatus and biceps brachii tendons.[109] There was a small but significant increase in calcium with age, and this was accompanied by an increase in phosphorus content, consistent with the accumulation of mineral deposits in ageing organelles and necrotic cell debris. Although the age-related increase in calcium is unlikely on its own to have any significance for tendon pathology, a substantial increase in calcium salt deposition is a common pathological feature in some tendons, particular at insertion sites and especially in the supraspinatus.[110–112] The increased deposition of calcific deposits in tendon pathology may be either degenerative ('dystrophic calcification') or a self-limiting and resolving condition ('calcific tendinitis').[113] This is discussed in more detail below.

Cell activity and matrix metabolism of tendon and ligament

Embryonic and neonatal tendon is a relatively cellular tissue, and there is a rapid fall in cell density during development and a gradual decrease in cellularity with increasing age post-maturity.[29, 114] Although adult tendons and ligaments were once considered metabolically inactive structures,[115, 116] tenocytes do have a significant aerobic capacity, but substantially less than that of liver and skeletal muscle.[117]

Tendon and ligament cells contain enzymes for all three pathways of energy generation: aerobic; anaerobic; and pentose phosphate shunt pathways.[118, 119] The metabolic activity changes with age, with a decline in aerobic and pentose phosphate shunt activity, and predominantly anaerobic metabolism at skeletal maturity.[120] Glycolytic activity is present even in old tendons, with similar levels of activity in young and old tendons.[120] Hypoxia has been suggested as a possible cause of tendon degeneration, although tendon cells are more resistant to hypoxia than other cell types.[119, 121] Differences in lactate dehydrogenase activity, an indicator of anaerobic glycolysis, have been detected in tendons from different sites, although there was no apparent correlation with age, tendon size, and strength.[32, 122] Tendons normally have a relatively good vascular supply (see Chapter 1.2), although the diffusion of nutrients may be an important factor in tendon segments where the blood supply is limited or restricted.[123] Restriction of the tendon blood supply by compression, arterial occlusion, or in the face of high demand from the actively contracting muscle may be a significant factor in tendon pathology.[124]

The ECM is synthesized and maintained by the activity of the resident fibroblasts.[29] In general, synthetic activity is high during development and diminishes with age, although activity may change dramatically in some pathological conditions. Normal tissue homeostasis requires a balance between the processes of synthesis and breakdown.[125, 126] This balance can be modified in response to nutritional and hormonal stimuli as well as trauma and mechanical stress. Our own studies have shown that the collagen in some adult tendons, such as short head of biceps brachii, turns over very slowly if at all, as shown by the accumulation of pentosidine and the racemization of D-aspartate.[46, 127] In tendons exposed to high mechanical demands, however, such as the supraspinatus and Achilles, the rate of collagen turnover is much higher, consistent with either a history of repair or a constant maintenance function. This activity is mediated by a variety of enzymes including MMPs, as described in more detail below.

Cell populations

There are a number of different cell populations within tendon, with regional variations in cell morphology and activity.[78, 128, 129] Synovial-like cells from the endotenon and epitenon have a greater proliferative potential than the cells of the tendon mid-substance, which are predominantly synthesizing matrix.[81, 129, 130] Similar cell populations are present in the epiligament. Cells from the epitenon (and perhaps also the endotenon) are more active in repair after injury, migrating to the site of the lesion and being responsible for the synthesis of new matrix.[129, 131] Since most tendon cells are terminally differentiated and relatively quiescent, repair activity has been ascribed to a resident subpopulation of mesenchymal 'stem' cells resident in the epitenon. Alternatively, cells from the surrounding tissues or derived from a circulating population of 'fibrocytes' may be involved in tendon/ligament repair.[132] The relative contribution of intrinsic and extrinsic cell populations may depend on the nature, site, and extent of the initial injury.

Epitenon-derived cells have a different matrix synthetic activity, producing fibronectin and type III collagen in culture, unlike the internal fibroblasts.[78] However, studies comparing human tendon fibroblasts from internal and superficial regions have shown no difference in their proliferative response to serum, and no difference in their ability to respond to growth factors and synthesize matrix (reference 133 and Riley, G.P., unpublished observations). Rounded, chondrocyte-like cells are a feature of the fibrocartilage at the insertion sites and in regions subject to compression.[25, 74] These cells have a very different pattern of matrix synthesis compared to that of tension-bearing regions of tendon, with higher levels of gene expression for matrix components such as type II collagen and aggrecan. These cells are responsive to the application of compressive load, and require continued dynamic compression for the maintenance of this synthetic activity *in vitro*.[134] The cell populations at the myotendinous junction have not been characterized.

A number of studies have shown that tendon and ligament cells, either in explant culture or isolated cell populations, respond to exogenous agents and factors such as the application of mechanical strain.[135–138] These studies are useful for understanding basic cellular mechanisms, but may not have physiological or pathological relevance. Cellular activities in standard culture conditions do not remotely resemble the situation *in vivo* where cells are surrounded by matrix and other chemical and physical interactions that modify the cell response. Chapter 1.2, for example, described how tenocytes within the fibres of a normal tendon communicate via gap junctions and how these mediate the tendon response to mechanical load.[139] Although some studies have shown differences in collagen expression between culture-derived cell populations from normal and diseased tendon,[140] other studies have shown no significant difference (Riley, G.P., unpublished observations). Research into the cell biology of tendon and ligament is complicated by the absence of any cell-specific markers that can be used to discriminate between different fibroblast populations.

Matrix degradation

The remodelling of the matrix in tendon and ligament is important for maintaining the health of the tissue. Although some matrix turnover is probably taking place in normal adult flexor tendons, the process is extremely slow, as shown by studies of pentosidine content and D-aspartate accumulation in the biceps brachii tendon.[46, 127] Turnover is higher in tendons such as the supraspinatus and Achilles, and this is probably associated with the high levels of strain normally experienced by these tendons in every day use.[46, 127] Increased turnover is also found in compressed regions of tendon and ligament, presumably part of the adaptation process to protect the tissue from damage.[26] After tissue injury, repair involves the limited destruction of matrix to weave new collagen into the existing structure. Scar tissue is also extensively remodelled during the maturation phase of wound healing. Inappropriate or excessive matrix degradation is a likely cause of matrix weakening in degenerative diseases. A failure of the remodelling process, such as in the injured ACL, may also account for the poor quality of repair at this site.[141]

Collagen degradation

The collagen (type I) fibres of tendon and ligament are highly resistant to degradation by most proteases. Some collagen is probably degraded by a phagocytic route, with fibroblasts and macrophages engulfing collagen molecules, which are then digested by lysosomal enzymes.[142, 143] This is a major activity in the remodelling peridontal

ligament, although few studies have investigated the relative importance of this route in tendon and ligament.

Several studies have shown release of collagen-degrading enzymes by tendon tissues in explant culture.[144–146] We have shown that collagenase-1, a member of the MMP superfamily, is the main mediator of collagen degradation in tendon explant culture, since levels of collagenase-1 (MMP-1) activity are closely associated with the release of collagen degradation products.[147] MMP-1 is one of the few enzymes capable of cleaving the intact type I collagen molecule, doing so at a specific locus in the triple helix, leaving three- and one-quarter length fragments that are in turn susceptible to other proteinases.[148–151]

The MMPs are a family of related enzymes that are major mediators of connective tissue turnover in the extracellular environment. MMPs are active at neutral pH, contain a catalytic zinc ion, and require calcium for activity. There are at least 23 MMPs, which can be subdivided into collagenases, gelatinases, stromelysins, and membrane-type MMPs, based on their structures and substrate specificities (Table 4).[148, 151, 152] MMPs

Table 4 The MMP superfamily—diversity in size and substrate specificity

MMP number	Enzyme name	Molecular weight (kDa)		Known substrates
		Latent	Active	
MMP-1	Collagenase -1	55	45	Collagens I, II, III, VII, VIII, X; gelatin; aggrecan; versican; link protein; casein; alpha-1 proteinase inhibitor; alpha2 macroglobulin (α2M); pregnancy zone protein; ovostatin; nidogen; myelin basic protein (MBP); pro-TNF; L-selectin; MMP-2; MMP-9
MMP-2	72 kDa gelatinase	72	66	Collagens I, IV, V, VII, X, XI, XIV; gelatin; elastin; fibronectin; aggrecan; versican, link protein; MBP; alpha-1 proteinase inhibitor; pro-TNF; MMP-9; MMP-13
MMP-3	Stromelysin-1	57	45	Collagens III, IV, IX, X; gelatin; aggrecan; versican, perlecan; link protein; nidogen; fibronectin; laminin; elastin; casein; fibrinogen; antithrombin-III; α2M; ovostatin; alpha-1 proteinase inhibitor; MBP; pro-TNF; MMP-1; MMP-7; MMP-8; MMP-9; MMP-13
MMP-7	Matrilysin (PUMP-1)	28	19	Collagens IV, X; gelatin; aggrecan; link protein; fibronectin; laminin; entactin; elastin; casein; transferrin; alpha-1 proteinase inhibitor; MBP; pro-TNF; MMP-1; MMP-2; MMP-9
MMP-8	Neutrophil collagenase	75	58	Collagens I, II, III, V, VII, VIII, X; gelatin; aggrecan; alpha-1 proteinase inhibitor; alpha-2 antiplasmin; fibronectin
MMP-9	92 kDa gelatinase	92	86	Collagens IV, V, VII, X, XIV; gelatin; elastin; aggrecan; versican; link protein; fibronectin; nidogen; alpha-1 proteinase inhibitor; MBP; pro-TNF
MMP-10	Stromelysin-2	57	44	Collagens III, IV, V; gelatin; casein; aggrecan; elastin; link protein; fibronectin; MMP-1; MMP-8
MMP-11	Stromelysin-3	51	44	alpha-1 proteinase inhibitor
MMP-12	Macrophage metalloelastase	54	45 / 22	Collagen IV; gelatin; elastin; alpha-1 proteinase inhibitor; fibronectin; vitronectin; laminin; pro-TNF; MBP
MMP-13	Collagenase-3	60	48	Collagens I, II, III, IV; gelatin; plasminogen activator inhibitor 2; aggrecan; perlecan; tenascin
MMP-14	MT1-MMP	66	56	Collagens I, II, III; gelatin; casein; elastin; fibronectin; laminin B chain; vitronectin; aggrecan; dermatan sulphate proteoglycan; pro-TNF; MMP-2; MMP-13
MMP-15	MT2-MMP	72	60	MMP-2; gelatin; fibronectin; tenascin; nidogen; laminin
MMP-16	MT3-MMP	64	52	MMP-2
MMP-17	MT4-MMP	57	53	
MMP-18	*Xenopus* collagenase	55	22	
MMP-19		54	45	Aggrecan
MMP-20	Enamelysin	54	22	Amelogenin
MMP-21	XMMP	70	53	
MMP-22	CMMP	52	43	Gelatin; casein
MMP-23		?	?	
MMP-24	MT5-MMP	63	45	MMP-2

Table 5 Schematic representation of the domain structure of the MMP superfamily[a]

MMP type	Structure
Collagenase (MMP-1, MMP-8, MMP-13)	
Gelatinase (MMP-2, MMP-9)	
Stromelysin (MMP-3, MMP-10, MMP-11)	
Membrane-type (MMP-14, MMP-15, MMP-16, MMP-17, MMP-24)	
Matrilysin (PUMP) (MMP-7)	

○ = Signal peptide   ◖■ = Pro-peptide   ▭ = Catalytic domain

▣ = Gelatin-binding domain   ⬠ = Zinc-binding domain   ∿ = Hinge region

✛ = Hemopexin domain   ◆○ =Transmembrane domain

[a] MMPs share common domains: a signal peptide that is cleaved prior to synthesis; a pro-peptide that renders the enzyme inactive until removed by proteolysis; a catalytic domain with zinc-binding site. The hemopexin domain confers substrate specificity. Gelatinases have an additional, gelatin-binding domain. Membrane-type MMPs have an additional transmembrane domain. Matrilysin (MMP-7) lacks the hemopexin domain. (Reproduced from *Extracellular matrix proteases and proteins technical guide*, Vol. 2, January 2002, with permission of Calbiochem.)

have a common domain structure, and most are secreted in an inactive form with a propeptide that is removed upon activation (Table 5).

The activity of MMPs is tightly controlled *in vivo*, with the regulation of transcription, translation, activation, and inhibition by specific inhibitors known as tissue inhibitors of metalloproteinases (TIMPs).[148, 153, 154] There are four TIMPs that have been characterized, and these may be constitutively expressed (TIMP-2) or stimulated by growth factors such as TGFβ (TIMP-1, TIMP-3). Each TIMP will bind to active MMPs in a stoichiometric ratio (1:1), resulting in an inactive complex. In general, expression and activity of the MMPs is stimulated by pro-inflammatory cytokines such as interleukin-1 (IL-1) and tumour necrosis factor (TNF) and inhibited by growth factors such as TGFβ.

In normal flexor tendons such as the biceps brachii, the activity of MMPs is low, consistent with the low rate of collagen turnover in these tendons.[127] MMP activity, particularly that of MMP-1, MMP-2, and MMP-3, is higher in normal supraspinatus tendons (Fig. 9). Similarly, high levels of MMP-3 are found in normal Achilles, suggesting an important role for MMPs in the maintenance of the tendon structure in tendons exposed to high levels of strain or repeated injury.[127] Further evidence for the importance of MMPs in tendon physiology comes from the observation that a broad-spectrum matrix metalloproteinase

inhibitor can induce painful tendon lesions.[155] The cause of the tendon pain is still unknown, and may be related to inhibition of one or more MMPs, although related metalloproteinase enzymes such as the ADAMs (A disintegrin and metalloprotease) may also be implicated.

There are at least 40 ADAMs, the majority of which function as zinc binding proteases, although the natural substrates and inhibitors are known for relatively few, such as tumour necrosis factor (TNF) for ADAM17 (otherwise known as TNF-alpha converting enzyme or TACE).[156] Their diverse range of activities, from cytokine processing to the control of matrix assembly, has made members of this group of enzymes an attractive target for therapeutic intervention in various pathologies. Inhibition of one or more of these proteases could account for the onset of tendon pain induced by inhibitors of metalloproteinases. The potential role of enzymes in chronic tendinopathy is discussed in more detail below.

Proteoglycan degradation

Proteoglycans are turned over much more rapidly than the fibrillar collagens. Although some members of the MMP family such as MMP-3 (stromelysin) can degrade proteoglycans such as aggrecan, most activity *in vivo* is associated with a related but distinct group of enzymes known as 'aggrecanases' (Fig. 10).

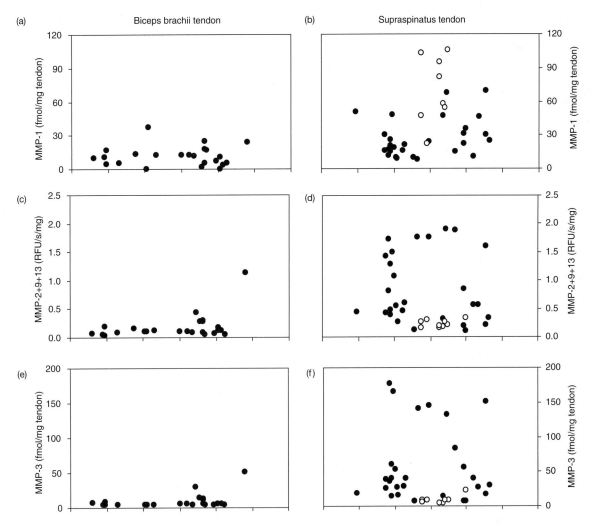

Fig. 9 MMP enzyme activities in tendon. MMPs were extracted from tendon and activities were measured using specific fluorogenic substrates. MMP-1 and MMP-3 activities were expressed as fentamoles per milligram tendon dry weight (fmol/mg tendon). Gelatinase activities (MMP-2, MMP-9, and MMP-13) were expressed as relative fluorescent units per second per milligram tendon dry weight (RFU/s/mg). Data for biceps brachii tendons are shown in (a), (c), and (e). Data for supraspinatus tendons are shown in (b), (d) and (f). Closed circles represent macroscopically normal 'control' tendons and open circles represent ruptured tendons. MMP-1, gelatinase (mostly MMP-2), and MMP-3 activities were significantly higher in control supraspinatus compared to biceps brachii tendons ($p < 0.01$ for each activity). Ruptured supraspinatus tendons had significantly higher levels of MMP-1 activity, but lower levels of gelatinase (mostly MMP-2) and MMP-3 compared to controls. (Data modified and reprinted from reference 127, © 2002 with permission from Elsevier Science.)

Aggrecanases, of which there are at least three members, were recently identified as members of the ADAM-TS family, a subgroup of ADAMs with thrombospondin (TS) type I motifs.[157] ADAM-TS4 (aggrecanase 1) and ADAM-TS5 (aggrecanase 2) both cleave aggrecan at a specific locus, between residues Glu[373] and Ala[374] in the interglobular domain of the core protein.[157–159] ADAM-TS1 can also degrade aggrecan at the same locus, at least *in vitro*.[160] ADAM-TS4 also has activity against the brain-specific proteoglycan brevican.[161] Little is known about the enzymes responsible for the degradation of other matrix proteoglycans.

Recent studies have demonstrated rapid catabolism and loss of proteoglycans from tendon and ligament explants maintained in culture.[138, 162] Antibodies to aggrecan, biglycan, and decorin showed that catabolites of these proteoglycans were present in both young and mature tendon, consistent with constitutively high levels of proteoglycan turnover.[138] Aggrecanase-generated fragments of aggrecan were found in both tensional and compressed regions, and the release of these fragments into the culture media was found both in control cultures and

in cultures stimulated by IL-1.[138] There was no evidence of MMP-mediated proteoglycan turnover, although aggrecan turnover did not correlate with the expression of mRNA for either ADAM-TS 1 or ADAM-TS2, at least in the compressed region of young tendon. Further work is required to determine which aggrecanases (and other proteoglycanases) are involved in tendon and ligament physiology and pathology.

Age-related changes of tendon and ligament matrix

Increasing age is associated with a number of significant changes in cell metabolism and in the structure, composition, and mechanical properties of the ECM. During development the cellularity decreases, collagen content increases, and there are changes in collagen fibre diameters and collagen cross-linking as described above. After maturity, there are additional changes including decreased solubility of the collagen and decreased GAG content.[6, 64, 163, 164] The total

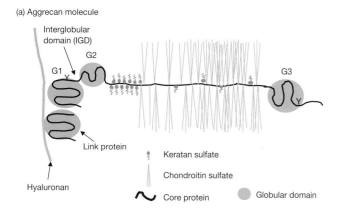

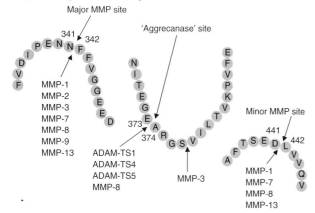

Fig. 10 Enzyme cleavage sites in aggrecan. (a) Aggrecan consists of three globular domains (G1 to G3) separated by linear core protein. The region between G2 and G3 is rich in sulfated glycosaminoglycans, which attract and hold water in the tissue. Aggrecan binds to hyaluronan via the G1 domain, stabilized by link protein, to form multimolecular aggregates. The interglobular domain (IGD) contains sequences susceptible to cleavage by several enzymes. (b) Although several MMPs can cleave aggrecan at multiple sites in the IGD, the predominant cleavage *in vivo* is made by aggrecanases, between specific glutamate and alanine residues (Glu[373] and Ala[374]). (Reproduced from reference 3, © 1998 with permission from Elsevier Science.)

collagen content in human tendon remains constant over a wide age range, from 12 to 96 years.[6] With ageing, however, collagen becomes stiffer, fibres shrink, and the tensile strength decreases.[165] The tensile modulus (stiffness) of canine tendons, calculated from the slope of the stress–strain curve, is not directly related to age, although it is positively correlated with the insoluble (cross-linked) collagen content.[166] The increase in tensile modulus with age in equine superficial digital flexor tendon (SDFT) was positively correlated with an increase in HP cross-link content and negatively correlated with the cross-sectional area of the central tendon fascicles, which decreased with age.[167] There was a corresponding increase in the number of fascicles with increasing age. There are changes in the average diameter of the collagen fibres, which in the equine SDFT increased to a peak of 170 nm at the age of 1.5 years and then declined gradually.[168] The angle of crimp and crimp length declined with age but reached a plateau in the mature animal. Mechanical properties such as hysteresis, the energy lost during stress-relaxation, decline considerably during maturation as a result of cross-link formation but change little as a result of ageing, at least in rat tail tendon.[169]

Age is strongly associated with the development of chronic tendon pathology, which tends to predominantly affect individuals in late middle-age. This is often thought to be associated with a lower cell activity and a reduction in tendon blood flow, implying a failure to repair or maintain the matrix. However, far from being senescent, tenocytes isolated from ageing individuals show proliferative potential similar to that of young tenocytes.[133] It is therefore important to distinguish the effects of ageing from pathological degenerative changes, such as lipid deposits, calcification, and mucoid degeneration, that may accumulate as a function of age.[170, 171] Although these are more frequently found in older tendons, they are not found in all tendons and are therefore likely to be an indirect consequence of ageing.[171] More work needs to be done to clarify the role of age in the tendon/ligament cell response to mechanical strain and injury.

Effect of exercise and immobilization on tendon and ligament

Tendons and ligaments are known to be capable of responding to changes in mechanical stresses and loading, although there are differences between tendons and more dramatic effects are seen in immature animals.[63, 118, 172, 173] Atrophy induced by immobilization is relatively slow compared to that in muscle, although there is a significant loss of water, GAGs, collagen, and tensile strength after a period of 8–9 weeks (Fig. 11).[117, 173–175] The reduction in strength was attributed to increased collagen degradation, although apparently not mediated by collagenase, which decreased in immobilized ligaments and tendons.[177] Collagen synthesis is also decreased and there is a reduction in both aerobic and anaerobic metabolism. Matrix properties return towards normal after the period of immobilization is ended, although there are site-specific variations, with a slower rate of recovery at the insertion compared to the tendon/ligament mid-substance.[178] Rehabilitation of immobilized tendons and ligaments takes much more time than that needed to cause the atrophy, and complete recovery of the original material properties of the ECM may never be reached.

Information on the functional adaptation of tendons/ligaments to exercise is limited and responses to training have been variable depending on anatomical site, species, and age. Exercise can produce an increase in collagen fibril size, ultimate strength, and stiffness, although the effects are small and more pronounced in (swine) extensor tendons compared to flexor tendons.[172, 173] Exercise can delay some of the changes with age such as the increase in maximum stress and stiffness.[179] Most studies have been conducted on immature animal tendons, however, and the effects of exercise on adult tendon may be minimal and possibly damaging. Exercise can have deleterious effects on equine tendons, for example, although this would appear to be highly dependent on the type and level of physical activity and the age of the animal. Tendons in trained horses were shown to have a reduced average fibril diameter, which was interpreted as the effect of microtrauma.[180] Since the average diameter of fibrils is correlated with tendon mechanical strength, this change represents a deterioration in the quality of the tendon matrix. The crimp angle was also reduced in the core of the tendon.[181] A hypothesis has been presented suggesting that improvement in tendon properties is only possible in immature animals and that exercise can only be damaging in older animals.[97] However, the flexor tendons of the equine athlete are operating close to their functional limits with very high levels of strain

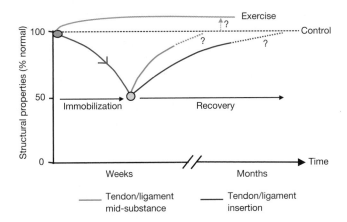

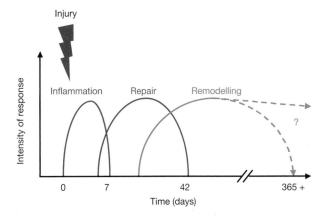

Fig. 11 Effects of immobilization and exercise on tendon and ligament. The structural properties of tendons and ligaments are considerably reduced following several weeks immobilization. There is a gradual recovery in the material properties after remobilization of the tissue, although it is questionable whether there is ever a full recovery. There are differences in the rate of recovery at different sites, with a more rapid rate in the mid-substance compared to the insertion. The effects of exercise on the structural properties are small (if any), greater in extensor tendons compared to flexors, and more pronounced in immature animals than in adults. (Modified and reproduced from reference 176, © 1988 with permission from the American Academy of Orthopaedic Surgeons.)

Fig. 12 The wound repair response. A schematic representation of the tissue response to injury, showing three overlapping phases of inflammation, repair (matrix synthesis), and remodelling. The time points shown are purely illustrative and vary according to tissue, site, age, etc. In tendons and ligaments the remodelling process may not be complete more than a year after injury.

and this theory may not be applicable to the human, particular the non-athletic population.

Tendon and ligament pathology

The range of pathology affecting tendons and ligaments is different. Both tissues may be subject to acute injury as a result of trauma, overload, or direct mechanical insult resulting from crushing blows or penetrating objects. The repair response is thought to follow the same general pattern, with the important proviso that some ligaments and tendons are apparently able to mount a more effective repair response than others. This has been linked to a number of factors, such as whether tendons are intrasynovial or extrasynovial, or whether ligaments are intraarticular or extraarticular. There is also evidence to suggest that the ability to repair is dependent on the quantity and quality of the vascular network at different sites. Repair may also be affected by the adaptive formation of fibrocartilage in response to compressive forces as described above.

Tendons are more prone to chronic, insidious forms of injury than ligaments. This pathology is often associated with repeated strain and repetitive microtrauma rather than a single traumatic episode. This form of soft tissue pathology, variously described as tendinitis, tendinosis, or tendinopathy, is commonly seen in rheumatology clinics and is one of the most difficult conditions to manage. Although more is now known about the biochemistry of this condition, there are still substantial gaps in our knowledge.

Acute tendon and ligament injuries

The cellular events occurring after traumatic injury to a tendon or ligament are thought to be broadly similar and common to all soft connective tissues.[129, 182] The response is usually divided into three or four phases, more for convenience as the phases merge imperceptibly

into each other and represent a continuum rather than discrete stages (Fig. 12). The timing of the different phases varies in different tissues and is influenced by nutrition, metabolic disorders (e.g. diabetes), age, and factors such as the location and extent of the tissue injury.

The first phase, occurring in the first 7 days after disruption of the tendon fibres, is characterized by inflammation. There is accumulation of serous fluid (oedema) and the infiltration of a variety of cell types attracted to the region by inflammatory mediators. Platelets and mast cells release histamine, a potent agent promoting vasodilatation and increasing blood vessel permeability. Serotonin, bradykinin, leukotrienes, and prostaglandins act together to recruit polymorphonuclear leucocytes and lymphocytes from the circulation. Growth factors released by platelets include platelet-derived growth factor (PDGF), TGFβ, and epidermal growth factor (EGF). Macrophages are present within 24 hours, phagocytosing tissue debris and releasing numerous inflammatory mediators and growth factors including basic fibroblast growth factor (bFGF), transforming growth factor alpha (TGFα), TGFβ, and PDGF. These growth factors are chemotactic for fibroblasts and other cells, and generally act to stimulate matrix synthesis. Angiogenic factors such as bFGF and vascular endothelial growth factor (VEGF) stimulate capillary ingrowth into the fibrous clot. Toward the end of the inflammatory phase, which may last several days, fibroblasts become the predominant cell type.

The second phase, lasting up to 6 weeks after injury, is characterized by cell proliferation and new matrix synthesis by fibroblasts. This new matrix is different in both quality and quantity from the normal matrix. Described as granulation tissue, it consists of a disorganized matrix with an elevated cell density that fills the tissue defect. The DNA content of the healing rabbit MCL reaches twice normal levels during this period.[182]

The third phase, occurring 3–6 weeks after injury and lasting for at least a year, is a prolonged period of remodelling and maturation in which the matrix components and tissue cellularity revert gradually toward normal. During this stage many cells in the scar are contractile myofibroblasts, specialized cells important for the organization of the wound tissue, approaching 10 per cent of the cells after 12 weeks of healing in the rabbit MCL.[183]

Cell response to injury

The cellular response of tendons to injury has been extensively studied in sheathed animal flexor tendons following a surgical laceration.[123, 184–188] Some investigators have suggested that lacerated tendons are incapable of healing without the involvement of cells from the surrounding connective tissues.[189] More recently, a number of studies have shown that the resident tenocytes have an intrinsic capacity to heal.[188, 190, 191] The first changes are observed in the epitenon, with cellular proliferation and migration of cells into the tendon and the site of the lesion by the seventh day after injury. However, it is likely that extrinsic cell proliferation and infiltration may overwhelm the intrinsic cell response and the contribution of each cell type may depend on the site and type of the tendon injury.[129] The cells from the outermost layers of the tendon (the epitenon) have been shown to synthesize both

collagen types I and III, whereas the innermost cells produced only type I collagen.[128] Some investigators have argued that the increase in type III collagen, observed in healing equine tendon, is a consequence of the activity of cells derived from the epitenon or peritendinous tissues.[192] The cells most active in tendon/ligament repair may be a subpopulation of mesenchymal 'stem' cells, possibly present as vascular pericytes in the epitenon, although some authors have suggested that circulating 'fibrocytes' may be involved in the soft tissue repair response.[132]

Growth factors

Growth factors are signalling peptides that regulate many cellular activities in connective tissues including proliferation, matrix synthesis, matrix degradation, differentiation, and death.[193, 194] A variety of growth factors have been associated with wound repair,[195] and some of these and their activities are summarized in Table 6. Growth factors are produced by most cell types and can act both locally and systemically. The expression and activity of growth factors can be

Table 6 Cytokines associated with wound repair and their effects[a]

Cytokine	Family	Action
PDGF-AB PDGF-BB	PDGF	Stimulates proliferation of most mesenchymal cells including fibroblasts and smooth muscle cells Stimulates chemotaxis Stimulates myofibroblast contraction
PDGF-AA	PDGF	Less potent than PDGF-AB: does not stimulate chemotaxis or myofibroblast contraction
VEGF	PDGF	Stimulates endothelial cell proliferation Increases vascular permeability
TGF-β1	TGF-β	Inhibits proliferation of most cells
TGF-β2		Stimulates fibroblast chemotaxis
TGF-β3		Stimulates matrix synthesis and protease inhibitor production
EGF	EGF	Stimulates proliferation of most epithelial cells, fibroblasts, and endothelial cells Stimulates keratinocyte migration
TGF-α	EGF	Similar to EGF, but more potent stimulator of angiogenesis
HB-EGF	EGF	Stimulates proliferation of keratinocytes, fibroblasts, and smooth muscle cells
Basic FGF	FGF	Stimulates proliferation of endothelial cells, keratinocytes, and fibroblasts Stimulates chemotaxis Stimulates protease synthesis
KGF	FGF	Stimulates epithelial cell proliferation Stimulates keratinocyte migration
IGF	Insulin	Stimulates proliferation of fibroblasts and endothelial cells Stimulates chemotaxis
IL-1	Interleukin	Stimulates fibroblast production of proteoglycans, collagen, and proteases (MMP-1, MMP-3, and others)
TNF-α	TNF	Stimulates macrophage production of proteases Increases vascular permeability Inhibits collagen synthesis
Endothelin		Stimulates contraction of smooth muscle cells and myofibroblasts
Scatter factor (HGF)		Stimulates motility and proliferation of epithelial and endothelial cells

[a] These cytokines have all been found in injured tissues and are thought to participate in wound healing on the basis of in vitro models and effects on cultured cells. Common acronyms are: PDGF, platelet-derived growth factor; VEGF, vascular endothelial growth factor (also known as VPF or vascular permeability factor); TGF, transforming growth factor; EGF, epidermal growth factor; HB-EGF, heparin-binding EGF-like growth factor; FGF, fibroblast growth factor; KGF, keratinocyte growth factor; IGF, insulin-like growth factor; IL-1, interleukin-1; TNF, tumour necrosis factor; HGF, hepatocyte growth factor. (Reproduced from reference 195, table 2, p. 719, © 1994, with permission from Elsevier Science.)

regulated at the level of transcription, translation, and secretion. Once secreted, activity is affected by specific and non-specific interactions with the surrounding matrix and other molecules. Activity is also influenced by other growth factors, forming a complex network of influences on the cell population. The activity of growth factors is mediated by specific receptors on the cell surface. Different cell types express different receptors, and levels of receptor expression can also be modulated, so that the responses of specific cell types are influenced by a complex array of factors.[195]

Despite the importance of growth factors as regulators of wound healing, relatively little is known about the timing of their expression in tendon and ligament injury. TGFβ, which directly or indirectly promotes cell recruitment, angiogenesis, and matrix synthesis and inhibits matrix breakdown, is found at low levels in normal tendon and is upregulated after injury.[196–198] Cells in the sheath and tendon mid-substance, including inflammatory cells infiltrating the lesion, showed increased levels of TGFβ1 expression just 1 day after injury, and these levels were maintained for up to 56 days.[196] bFGF, a growth factor that also stimulates angiogenesis, is not abundant in normal tendon.[199] After injury, bFGF is expressed in tenocytes concentrated along the epitenon and by infiltrating fibroblasts and inflammatory cells from the tendon sheath.[199] PDGF and EGF have also been shown to increase in injured digital flexor tendons.[197]

Slightly more is known about growth factors expressed after ligament injury. PDGF, bFGF, and TGFβ1 were elevated in the rabbit MCL 3–7 days after injury, and their levels began to decrease after 14 days.[200] The strong expression of PDGF, which has mitogenic and chemotactic properties, correlated with the increased cellularity of the tissue. In wounded ACL, expression of these growth factors was limited to the edge of the wound and levels were lower than in the MCL.[200] Expression of genes for endothelin-1 (ET-1), TGFβ1, insulin-like growth factor-1 (IGF-1), and IGF-2 was increased up to five times control levels 3 weeks after injury, returning close to normal at 14 weeks.[201] The importance of growth factor receptor expression was recognized in studies from Panossian et al. since these are essential for the transmission of growth factor effects after ligand binding at the cell surface.[202] These authors showed that bFGF and EGF receptors were strongly expressed during the early inflammatory phase after ligament injury, peaking at 7 days after injury.[202] Expression of the IGF-2 receptor rose and fell in parallel with the expression of IGF-2. Thus it is clear that, if the addition of exogenous growth factors is to be used to promote tendon/ligament repair, delivery must be timed to coincide with receptor expression, or additional factors provided to stimulate the expression of the appropriate receptors.

Biochemical changes in tendon and ligament injury

Collagen synthesis is seen during the first week after injury, with the initial deposition of a random, disorganized fibre network. A large proportion of the newly synthesized collagen is type III collagen.[80, 129, 192, 203] The concentration of immature, reducible cross-links is increased, the amount of mature tri-functional cross-links is low, and collagen is more readily extracted from the wound tissue. The collagen content increases through the next few weeks, with the gradual alignment of the collagen fibres with the long axis of the tendon/ligament. There is a slow transformation from loose fibrillar areas of types I and III collagen and pericellular type IV and V collagen to a dense network of parallel type I collagen fibre bundles.[203] Collagen maturation proceeds slowly but may not approach the normal composition, structure, and material properties even after many months.[80]

In the rabbit MCL injury model, collagen turnover was greatest 3–6 weeks after injury, with increased synthesis of type III collagen compared to type I collagen, and the rate returned toward the normal after 40 weeks.[181, 204] The collagen fibrils were initially a homogeneous population of small average diameter, and after 40 weeks there was a progressive increase in the proportion of slightly larger fibrils, but even at 2 years approximately 90 per cent of the fibrils were small.[205] Although the collagen concentration reached normal by 14 weeks, the mechanical strength of the ligament scar was 30 per cent of control values after 40 weeks, and there was a positive correlation with the HP cross-link density.[206] In gene expression studies, injured human ligaments (ACL) were shown to express much higher quantities of mRNA for types I and III collagen, biglycan, lumican, and TIMP-1 and lower levels of versican, and there was no change in decorin and fibromodulin mRNA compared to that of normal ligaments.[207, 208] Types I and III collagen, biglycan, and TIMP-1 mRNA levels were raised even 1 year after injury.[208] Thus, although the injured ACL demonstrates the ability to produce 'scar-like' molecules, healing is slow and there is a prolonged remodelling phase resulting in a low quality repair. Attempts to improve the repair of tendon and ligament must influence the cellular activity so as to promote the resolution of this extended remodelling phase and the restoration (as far as possible) of the normal matrix composition and organization.

Proteases in tendon and ligament injury

Proteolytic activity is an essential component of tissue repair, required to remove damaged matrix and remodel the resulting scar tissue so that it more closely resembles the normal tissue structure. Since most matrix proteolysis is thought to occur in the extracellular compartment, most importance is generally attributed to the MMP family described above. However, other proteinases such as the cathepsins may be implicated to some degree, and some matrix turnover may take place within the cell after phagocytosis, although there is relatively little research of these processes in tendon and ligament.

MMP-1 (interstitial collagenase) is stimulated by inflammatory mediators such as IL-1 during the inflammatory and proliferative phases of wound healing, declining in the later remodelling stages.[209] In slowly remodelling wounds, such as in the cornea, elevated levels of MMP-1 are found up to 9 months after injury.[210] Acute wounds contain MMP-2 (72 kDa gelatinase) and MMP-9 (92 kDa gelatinase), but levels are higher and remain elevated in chronic wounds such as leg ulcers.[211, 212] The factors that stimulate MMP expression and activity are not well characterized, although, in addition to inflammatory mediators and cytokines, proteolytic fragments of matrix molecules such as fibronectin and tenascin may directly stimulate proteolysis.[213]

Few studies have been conducted on protease expression in human tendon ruptures. A study of ruptured supraspinatus tendons showed co-localization of IL-1 and MMP-1 at the wound margin.[214] An analysis of MMPs extracted from ruptured supraspinatus has confirmed that there was an increase in the amount of active MMP-1 in the tendon (not just levels of MMP-1 protein) (Fig. 9).[127] There was also a decrease in MMP-2 and MMP-3 activities compared to those of control tendons. The increase in MMP-1 was associated with increased turnover of the matrix collagen as measured by pentosidine cross-link analysis and racemization of aspartate.[46, 127] The change in MMP activity may not represent an acute response, however, since ruptures of the supraspinatus are usually a consequence of a long-standing degenerative process. Thus it is not known if the change in matrix remodelling activity precedes or follows supraspinatus tendon rupture.

In contrast to the supraspinatus tendon, ruptured ACL showed an absence of MMP-1 and MMP-2 activity in the tissue remnant even 1 year after injury.[141] The lack of a matrix remodelling response could explain, at least in part, why the ACL (unlike the MCL) often fails to heal.[182]

Effects of exercise and mobilization on tendon and ligament repair

The use of controlled motion and exercise in the management of tendon and ligament injuries is now generally accepted. However, there is still considerable variation in the rehabilitation programme following tendon repair, despite objective evidence showing the benefits of early mobilization using techniques such as functional casting (for example) compared to rigid plaster casts.[215] Animal models have shown how non-repaired tendons rapidly lose a substantial proportion of their matrix, demonstrating the importance of early repair.[216] Prolonged immobilization after surgery has deleterious effects on the quality of repair, preventing the return to near-normal strength of transected rat Achilles tendon after 15 days immobilization.[217] There are a variety of other complications of an extended immobilization period following injury, including muscle atrophy, joint stiffness, cartilage deterioration, adhesions, and thrombosis.[215] Tension, applied cyclically or as a constant load, has a positive influence on the intrinsic fibroblast response and the strength of repair. It promotes cell proliferation and migration, facilitating the alignment of fibroblasts and the amount of synthesized collagen.[191, 218–221] Early passive mobilization of repaired tendons, using rubber bands or other devices to control or limit extension or flexion, results in better gliding function (reduced adhesions) and increased mechanical strength compared to immobilized tendons.[222, 223] Other data show the benefits of early active mobilization compared to passive mobilization, particularly in zone 2 flexor tendon repair, although care must be taken not to provoke re-rupture.[224, 225] Applied load has been shown to affect the orientation of fibroblasts, which become aligned with the direction of load.[226] It also has profound effects on the synthesis of matrix, with differences in the quantity, composition, and orientation of matrix depending on the direction (tension or compression) of the applied load as discussed above. There are also thought to be positive benefits as a result of improved nutrient provision, particularly for repair within the tendon sheath.[129] However more experimental work with controlled studies is required to define the optimum postoperative mobilization regime, designed to promote reorganization and remodelling of the repaired tendon/ligament so that higher strength and better function can be achieved.

Effects of exogenous agents on tendon/ligament repair

Growth factors

The application of exogenous, recombinant growth factors to damaged and healing ligaments and tendons has been attempted in a number of studies with variable levels of success. Bone morphogenetic protein 13 (BMP13, otherwise known as cartilage-derived morphogenetic protein 2 (CDMP-2) or growth differentiation factor 6 (GDF-6)), a member of the TGFβ superfamily of growth factors, improved the mechanical strength of repairing rat tendons by 39 per cent compared to controls,

8 days after injury.[227] GDF-5 (CDMP-1) also resulted in increased repair strength at 2 weeks, similarly to GDF-6.[228] BMP-2 has been used to enhance the healing of tendon to bone in the canine.[229] PDGF-BB increased the load to failure and stiffness of the healing MCL compared to untreated controls.[230, 231] Application of PDGF within 24 hours after injury was more effective compared to application after 48 hours.[230] The effect was dependent on dose, although structural properties never approached that of uninjured controls. Combinations of PDGF with a single additional growth factor (TGFβ, FGF, or IGF-1) did not result in significant improvement above PDGF alone.[231, 232] bFGF promoted neovascularization and the organization of collagen fibre bundles in defects of canine ACL between 6 and 24 weeks post-injury.[233] PDGF-AB and TGFβ2, applied separately, had no significant effect on the healing of rabbit MCL at 3 to 12 weeks after injury.[234]

Nonsteroidal anti-inflammatory drugs (NSAIDs)

NSAIDs are commonly used in the treatment of ligament and tendon injuries.[235–237] Their pharmacological target is cyclo-oxygenase (prostaglandin synthase), a key enzyme in the formation of prostaglandins that mediate the sensation of pain and inflammation in the tissues.[238] Studies of their effects on tendon healing have been inconclusive, with some studies showing deleterious effects on the repair quality and others showing no effect or even an increase in mechanical strength.[239–241] In vivo studies on both normal and healing tendons have shown an increase in the proportion of insoluble collagen, thought to be evidence of a decrease in collagen breakdown and an increase in cross-linked collagen.[242, 243] In vitro studies have shown that some NSAIDs (indomethacin, naproxen) may inhibit cell proliferation and matrix proteoglycan synthesis, while others (diclofenac, aceclofenac) have no effect and may even stimulate cell activity.[244] The significance of these finding to the in vivo situation is not known. Studies using a topical NSAID (ketoprofen) showed that levels of NSAID accumulate in the peritendinous tissues and reach levels many times higher than circulating plasma concentrations.[245] The rationale behind NSAID use in chronic tendon pain is uncertain, since inflammation is generally not a feature of these conditions and prostaglandin levels are not increased in the fluid surrounding painful tendons.[237, 246–248] There is also doubt about the effectiveness of NSAID treatment for ligament injuries.[235, 238]

Corticosteroids

There are many case reports describing rupture, often bilateral, of Achilles and other tendons after long-term oral corticosteroid therapy.[249–252] These ruptures are associated with a reduced collagen content and decreased mechanical strength as a result of decreased collagen synthesis over a long period of time. Local injections of steroid, sometimes given only once, have also been associated with tendon rupture, particularly in the Achilles.[253, 254] However, a review of the literature has shown that there are very few well controlled studies of the effects (and effectiveness) of corticosteroid injections on tendinopathy, particularly in the Achilles.[255] If there is a decrease in tendon strength it is in the first few weeks after injection, although there is no effect if the paratenon is injected rather than the tendon itself.[255] Other studies have suggested that it is the mode of delivery that is important.[256]

The results of animal studies are somewhat paradoxical and often contradictory. Short-term treatment with prednisolone, either orally or injected locally, has been shown to increase the strength of normal tendons, increasing both the total amount of collagen and the proportion of insoluble collagen.[257] Long-term treatment reduced the tendon dry weight but increased the stiffness, although the ultimate mechanical strength of the tissue was unchanged. These effects are similar to those of NSAIDs such as indomethacin, with inhibition of both collagen synthesis and collagen degradation, although the effects of corticosteroids are more rapid and dramatic.[242] Two different effects of corticosteroids are suggested to act on the tissue: (1) in the early period, a relatively fast increase in the stability of collagen; (2) over the long-term, a progressive reduction in collagen content caused by an inhibition of collagen synthesis.

In a rat model of Achilles tendon injury, multiple injections of hydrocortisone around the tendon were shown to have no deleterious effect on the repair quality up to 9 weeks post-injury.[258] In contrast, repeated injections of triamcinolone into the subacromial space of the rat shoulder resulted in focal inflammation, necrosis, and collagen fragmentation of the rotator cuff.[259] A single injection of dexamethasone had no effect on the healing of rat.[260] However, single injections of triamcinolone or betamethasone in rabbit MCL injury reduced the quality of repair.[261, 262] Thus the effects on tendons vary according to the species, timing, dosage, and type of corticosteroid preparation.

Anabolic androgenic steroids

The use and abuse of anabolic androgenic steroids (AAS) has been associated with tendon rupture. However, the literature is mostly case reports and far from conclusive.[263, 264] There is also a documented case of ligament rupture associated with the use of AAS, but this appears to be exceptional.[265] Some microscopic studies have shown ultrastructural changes in the tendon collagen,[266, 267] while clinical studies of ruptured tendon showed no significant changes.[268] Supraphysiological doses of AAS have been shown to stimulate the synthesis of collagen types I and III and decrease collagen degradation in athletes.[269] AAS are generally thought to promote muscle hypertrophy when combined with an exercise programme[263] and may also have some effect on immobilized and non-exercised muscle.[270] Although some studies have reported transitory inhibitory effects on collagen synthesis at very high doses,[271] the main reported effects on tendon are an increase in stiffness so that the tendon absorbs less energy.[267, 272] The altered mechanical properties are related to changes in the crimp morphology of the collagen fascicles.[273] There are reported to be no changes in fibril diameter, collagen type, or ultimate strength, and the change in mechanical properties is reversible.[272] The combination of increased muscle hypertrophy and a stiffer, less elastic tendon is thought to account for the incidence of rupture. The stimulation of collagen synthesis by AAS (such as norethandrolone) may result in an improved repair response post-injury. However, there is a lack of hard evidence, and even the effects of AAS on athletic performance are largely anecdotal.[274]

Miscellaneous factors and their effects on tendon and ligament repair

A variety of other factors and interventions are used in the treatment of tendon and ligament injuries, although few have shown clinical benefit in controlled trials. *In vitro* studies have shown benefit from the addition of vitamins (A, C, and E)[275] and exogenous electric currents.[276, 277] The sulfated GAG heparin, an anticoagulant and

stimulator of neovascularization, improved the collagen fibre organization of injured rabbit Achilles tendons.[278] Related compounds such as the synthetic polymer GAG polysulfate (GAGPS) have shown promise in the treatment of chronic tendinopathies, perhaps as a consequence of their inhibitory effects on proteolytic activities.[279] The addition of hyaluronan has been suggested to promote healing as well as inhibit adhesion formation, although the effect on tendon repair has been questioned.[280, 281] Protease inhibitors such as aprotinin and chemical agents such as 5-fluorouracil have also been used to inhibit tendon adhesions.[282, 283] Low-energy laser photostimulation stimulated the synthesis of collagen by 26 per cent in healing rabbit Achilles tendons, perhaps as a consequence of an effect on growth factor synthesis by the resident fibroblasts.[284] However, when combined with mechanical loading, there were no significant improvements in the tissue biomechanics[285] and there were only moderate improvements when combined with both ultrasound and mechanical loading.[286] Therapeutic ultrasound resulted in increased tensile strength and elasticity of healing chicken tendons, if applied during the early stages of healing.[287, 288] However no therapeutic effect of ultrasound was reported in a similar study of repaired cockerel tendon.[289] Extracorporeal shock wave therapy (ESWT) has recently been used in the treatment of tendon injuries and pathology such as rotator cuff tendinitis, plantar fasciitis, and calcific tendinitis.[290–292] Studies in animals have shown some benefit in the treatment of tendon injury, although the data presented were of a preliminary nature.[293] Some studies have shown negative effects such as necrosis, fibrosis, and inflammation if high-energy flux densities are used.[294] Systematic reviews of the literature have revealed the lack of controlled trials for ESWT and many of the commonly used modalities.[290, 295]

Chronic tendon pathology

Terminology

The terminology of chronic tendon pathology is both confused and confusing.[296] A variety of different classifications is present in the literature, and there is no consensus as to the best or most appropriate term to describe specific conditions. This confusion is due to the incomplete understanding of the pathological nature of the condition, primarily because diagnosis is imprecise and not based on an objective assessment. Terms such as tendinitis imply that there is inflammation, although there is little evidence of any inflammatory process in histological studies. Conditions are consequently best considered as either acute or chronic, whether caused by trauma, repeated microtrauma ('overuse'), or the result of an insidious process of clinically silent (pain-free) degeneration. Unless the presence of inflammation or degeneration has been unequivocally demonstrated, most tendon pain and dysfunction is best described as a 'tendinopathy'. A variety of chronic tendinopathies have been described, although basic entities commonly encountered are 'spontaneous' tendon rupture, painful tendinopathy, and calcific tendinitis. The histopathology and biochemistry of these conditions is considered below, preceded by an overview of their aetiology.

Aetiology of tendinopathy

The aetiology of most chronic tendinopathy is linked to multiple factors, both intrinsic and extrinsic (Table 7). These factors have been extensively reviewed elsewhere.[40, 295, 297–301] Salient points are discussed here and throughout this volume where appropriate. Many

Table 7 Factors implicated in the development of chronic tendinopathy

Intrinsic factors	Extrinsic factors
Age	Occupation
Vascular perfusion	Sport
Nutrition	Physical load
	Excessive force
Anatomical variants	Repetitive loading
Leg-length discrepancy	Abnormal/unusual movement
Malalignments (e.g. genu valgum)	
Bony impingement (e.g. acromiom)	Training errors
	Poor technique
Joint laxity	Fast progression
	High intensity
Muscle weakness/imbalance	Fatigue
Gender (?)	Shoes and equipment
Body weight	Environmental conditions
	Temperature
Systemic disease	Running surface

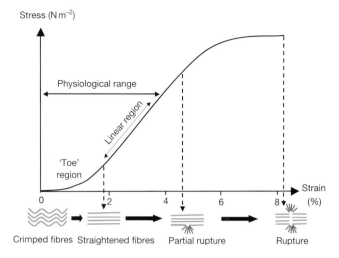

Fig. 13 The theoretical basis of tendon 'overuse' injury. The tendon stress–strain curve is used to illustrate the theoretical basis of tendon overuse injury. Strains of up to 4 per cent result in the stretching out of the crimped collagen fibres and do not damage the tendon. Strains above this level cause microscopic failure of fibrils within the tissue. If damage exceeds the ability of the tissue to repair, the tendon will rupture. (Reproduced from reference 308, © 2000 with permission from Oxford University Press.)

tendon lesions, whether spontaneous ruptures or painful tendinopathies, are commonly associated with a reduction in vascular perfusion, particularly at specific sites in the supraspinatus and the Achilles.[300, 302] However, this association and the importance of vascular perfusion has been questioned in other studies.[303–305] Since most tendon ruptures occur in the fifth decade, age-related changes are usually implicated, although ruptures of the Achilles are most common in a younger, physically active population with a mean age in the mid-thirties.[306] In most tendon ruptures there tends to be a preponderance of males to females, although it is uncertain whether this is directly associated with gender.[299] There is a strong association with particular sports and activities that result in high levels of stress being applied to specific sites. Genetic factors have been implicated, since a proportion of individuals tend to suffer from multiple types of soft tissue pathology such as Dupuytren's contracture, frozen shoulder, and various tendinopathies.[307] However, no genetic abnormality that is specifically implicated in tendinopathy has yet been identified. Leg-length discrepancies and other anatomical variants, such as the shape and slope of the acromion in the shoulder, are implicated in some individuals. Lifestyle factors are also likely to be important, and the combination of a more sedentary existence with increased leisure time, recreational sports, and a propensity to obesity may account for the greater incidence in the developed world.

'Overuse' pathology—a mechanical model of tendon injury

Most chronic tendinopathy is not associated with a single traumatic event, but is thought to be the consequence of repeated exposure to low-magnitude forces. Thus an overuse injury has been defined as a long-standing or recurring problem in the musculoskeletal system that arises during or soon after exertion due to repetitive microtrauma.[36, 297, 298] This concept now appears to be almost universally accepted and is usually explained with reference to the tendon stress–strain curve (Fig. 13).

Low levels of strain, up to a 2 per cent increase in the original length, are accommodated in normal tendon by the stretching out of the crimped collagen fibrils. This represents the 'toe' region of the stress–strain curve. Strains of up to 4 per cent are generally thought to represent the normal physiological range. Strains beyond this level result in fibril damage. Repeated stretching of the tendon results in accumulated damage that weakens the tendon. If the amount of damage exceeds the ability of the tendon cells to repair the matrix, the tendon will fail and rupture. The cellular response to mechanical strain is consequently a key factor in overuse pathology, and a failure of the cells to adapt to mechanical demands may precipitate the pathology.[309] The concept of tendon fatigue has been further developed by *in vitro* models that demonstrate that repeated loading at low levels of strain will result in tendon rupture.[42] Different tendons vary in their 'time-to rupture' and this correlates with the stresses experienced by the tendons *in vivo*. Thus specific tendons are thought to be 'engineered' to a minimum quality required for their normal function.

The ability of the tendon cell population to adapt, or to respond to tendon damage, is consequently thought to be a key factor in overuse tendinopathy.[309] Some researchers have questioned whether mature tendons are capable of adaptation, suggesting that exercise can only lead to deleterious effects on the adult (equine) tendon matrix.[97] In addition, exercise-induced hyperthermia, which can lead to an increase in temperature of several degrees in the core of the tendon, may be damaging to both tenocytes and matrix.[310] These factors depend on the levels and type of exercise, and may not be relevant to common clinical conditions, even in endurance athletes. Ageing, systemic diseases, nutritional factors, hormones, and drugs are all potentially able to have an impact on the tenocyte activities (see above). Reduced vascular perfusion, as a result of age or trauma, may also have a deleterious effect on the tenocytes. Thus the two major theories about the pathogenesis of tendinopathy, a mechanical theory and a vascular theory, are often linked and probably implicated to some degree in most tendinopathy. For example, damage to the vasculature as a result of microtrauma may increase intratendinous or intrasynovial pressure, obliterating vessels and beginning a vicious cycle of decreased blood flow, tissue hypoxia, and fibre degeneration.[309] The cell and blood vessel proliferation seen in painful tendinopathy and, less commonly, in spontaneous tendon rupture is assumed to represent a reparative response that is secondary to the initial lesion.

What is the cause of chronic tendon pain?

The model of overuse pathology presented above does not account for the onset of tendon pain. Damage to the vasculature and the cellular response to disrupted matrix has been suggested to precipitate an inflammatory response, resulting in oedema and pain. However, in the absence of any evidence of inflammation (see below), other causes of pain must be considered. The deterioration in material properties may result in the stimulation of stretch receptors in the tendon. Alternatively, receptors may be triggered by swelling in the tendon as a result of oedema, fibrosis, or (in some cases) calcific deposits. Very few studies have addressed the role of innervation in the perception of tendon pain, and it is not known whether the distribution of nociceptors is altered in tendinopathy. Some recent studies have identified nerve endings and neuropeptides (substance P and calcitonin gene-related peptide (CGRP)) at the site of the lesion in tendinopathies, although it was unclear whether this distribution was different from normal.[311] It is interesting to note that, in degenerative intervertebral disc, the in-growth of nerve endings accompanies the in-growth of blood vessels and is associated with the disc pathology (see Chapter 1.4).

Studies of fluids around painful tendons have led to new insights into the potential cause of pain in chronic tendinopathy. Using a microdialysis technique, Alfredson and co-workers found no difference in the amount of prostaglandin E_2 (PGE_2) around the patellar tendon in 'jumper's knee' compared to normal.[248] A similar result was found in Achilles tendinopathy and around the extensor carpi radialis brevis tendon in patients with tennis elbow, confirming the absence of 'classic' inflammation.[246, 247] However, the levels of the neurotransmitter glutamate were significantly increased in all three tendinopathies relative to controls.[246–248] Glutamate and glutamate N-methyl-D-aspartate receptor 1 (NMDAR1) have also been detected within Achilles tendons, located to nerve fibres, both in tendinopathy specimens and in controls.[312] Since glutamate is a potent mediator of pain in the central nervous system (CNS), it was suggested that glutamate NMDAR1 antagonists may be useful in the treatment of tendon pain. It has also been reported that substance P, another neuropeptide associated with the sensation of pain, is increased in the subacromial bursa in patients with rotator cuff tendinopathy.[313] The amount of substance P was shown to correlate with the degree of motion pain as assessed by a visual analogue scale. Whether this was due to an increase in the release of substance P or an increase in the number of nerve fibres was not clear, although immunohistochemistry showed more nerve fibres in bursal tissues of patients with a perforated rotator cuff.[313] Apart from the modulation of pain, substance P and other neuropeptides may have additional effects, regulating the local circulation and perhaps mediating neurogenic inflammation in and around the tendon.

Neurogenic inflammation and chronic tendinopathy

The pro-inflammatory role of neuropeptides such as substance P has been described with respect to the induction and progression of joint inflammation in other arthritides.[314, 315] More recently it has been proposed that the release of substance P and CGRP may be implicated in tendon (and ligament) pathology.[316, 317] Hart et al. have proposed

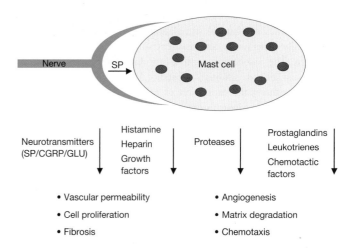

Fig. 14 Neurogenic inflammation. Schematic diagram illustrating the theoretical basis of neurogenic inflammation in tendon and ligament. Nerve endings in close proximity to mast cells release neuropeptides such as substance P (SP), calcitonin gene-related peptide (CGRP), and glutamate (GLU). Neuropeptides may have direct effects on the local cell population, but also stimulate mast cell degranulation, modulating a variety of different processes. (Modified and reproduced from reference 318, © 1995, with permission from the American Association of Orthopaedic Surgeons.)

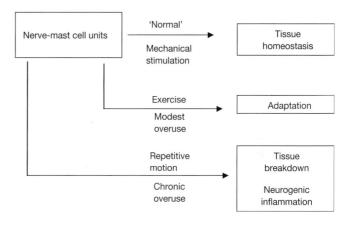

Fig. 15 Neurogenic control of tissue homeostasis. Nerve-mast cell units may function to modulate tissue homeostasis and the adaptive response to exercise. Excessive stimulation may result in negative effects on the tissue architecture. (Modified and reproduced from reference 318, © 1995, with permission from the American Association of Orthopaedic Surgeons.)

that regulatory units composed of nerve endings and mast cells reside in and around the tendon (Fig. 14). The release of neurotransmitters stimulates mast cell degranulation, releasing a variety of mediators (including growth factors) that influence oedema, angiogenesis, fibroblast proliferation, and many other aspects of cell activity. Biomechanical stimulation of these units may comprise part of the normal regulatory system, maintaining the tissue and also contributing to the adaptive response to increased load (Fig. 15). Excessive stimulation of these neural-mast cell 'units' may contribute to overuse pathology. Since the extent of innervation and vascularization probably varies between different tendons (and ligaments), the potential for the development of neurogenic dysfunction also varies. This theory potentially links mechanical stimulation of the paratenon, which is more richly innervated, and tissue changes in the tendon mid-substance. The association with tissue remodelling has not been conclusively proved, although substance P and CGRP can directly modulate (reduce) the expression of MMP-1 and MMP-3, at least *in vitro*.[316, 319] Thus innervation, and the stimulation of neuropeptide release by strain or friction at the tendon surface, are thought to be important for both normal tendon function and pathology.

Histopathology of tendinopathy

'Spontaneous' tendon rupture

The sudden rupture of tendons during low or moderate levels of activity, occurring without any preceding clinical symptoms such as pain or swelling, is often described as a spontaneous tendon rupture. However, the majority of ruptures are not truly spontaneous, since only rarely are they caused by excessive load acting on normal tendon. In most histopathological studies there is an absence of inflammatory cells and degeneration of the tendon matrix. Consequently this condition is attributed to 'tendinosis'.[320, 321] Very rarely, ruptures are associated with chronic systemic diseases such as rheumatoid arthritis, systemic lupus erythematosus (SLE), uraemia (haemodialysis), and diabetes, but these represented only 3 per cent of cases in one large study.[307] Other diseases directly affecting the tendon such as xanthoma and tendon tumours are very rare causes of rupture. Most ruptures of normal tendons as a result of excessive force tend to be avulsion injuries at the bone insertion, but these are also relatively rare.

The incidence of spontaneous tendon rupture has increased in recent years, and is more common in developed countries. Some tendons are more commonly affected than others, with the Achilles representing 45 per cent of all ruptures in one large study, followed by long head of biceps brachii (30 per cent), patellar (6 per cent), extensor pollicus longus (5 per cent), and quadriceps (4 per cent).[307] Rotator cuff pathology, usually affecting the supraspinatus, was not included in this particular study, although complete ruptures and partial thickness tears are also very common at this site.

Ruptures tend to be more commonly found at particular sites within tendons. In the supraspinatus, a site at or near the bone insertion is usually affected.[322, 323] In the patellar and quadriceps tendons, ruptures are also usually close to the bone insertion.[307, 324] In the Achilles, 83 per cent of ruptures occur in the tendon mid-substance, 3–6 cm from the calcaneus. In 12 per cent of cases, ruptures are found at the myotendinous junction and 5 per cent occur at the bone insertion.[307]

A number of features of matrix degeneration (tendinosis) have been described. In a heterogeneous group of 891 spontaneously ruptured human tendons, degenerative changes were found in the majority (97 per cent).[307] The most frequent observation was hypoxic cell changes (44 per cent), followed by 'mucoid degeneration' (GAG accumulation), often accompanied by cell rounding (21 per cent). 'Tendolipomatosis' (lipid accumulation) was seen in 73 tendons (8 per cent), with lipid deposits interspersed between the collagen fibres. Calcifying tendinopathy, with deposits of calcium on or between collagen fibres, was seen in 43 tendons. Similar degenerative changes were observed in non-ruptured cadaver tendons, but significantly less frequently, affecting 35 per cent of the sample. Other studies have shown an absence of degeneration in cadaver tendons from sites such as the biceps brachii (radius insertion) and Achilles (mid-substance), demonstrating that degeneration is not an inevitable consequence of ageing.[321, 325]

Chard *et al.* investigated degenerative changes in cadaver supraspinatus tendons and found that a significant proportion showed degenerative changes, the most common of which was GAG accumulation between the collagen fibrils (18 per cent), followed by a rounding up of the tendon cells to form regions with the appearance of fibrocartilage (8.5 per cent) (Fig. 16).[170, 321] Other observations included a reduction in cellularity, lipid deposits, calcification, and intimal hyperplasia of blood vessels. The severity of degeneration tended to increase with age, with the majority showing moderate to severe degeneration above the age of 60.[171] However, it was rare to find a normal supraspinatus tendon even in individuals under the age of 40, and less than 10 per cent of tendons in those over the age of 80 were considered normal. All specimens of ruptured supraspinatus tendons showed more severe degeneration, with the major change being a loss of cell number and disorganization of the matrix.[171]

Other studies have described a variety of features that can be interpreted as indicators of tendon matrix degeneration, including a reduction in the size of fascicles, microtears of fascicles, the presence of granulation tissue, disruption of the 'tide mark', dystrophic calcification, and bony spurs.[40, 323, 326] Degeneration was more prominent toward the articular side than the bursal side of the rotator cuff, and more severe degeneration was found in ruptured tendons.[326] Weakness of the tendon was correlated with the severity of degeneration at the insertion, not at the tendon mid-substance or 'critical zone'.[323] However, similar degenerative changes were found in all three rotator cuff tendons, demonstrating that additional factors must be involved in the pathogenesis of supraspinatus tendon pathology.[327]

Studies have differed over whether there is any evidence of repair (granulation tissue) in ruptured tendons. There have been observations of hypervascular areas with fibroblast proliferation in close proximity to avascular regions of limited cellularity. Cell and vessel proliferation, sometimes described as an angiofibroblastic response,[307] is thought to represent a repair process, although there was no evidence of repair activity at the proximal tendon stumps.[328] The cause of dysfunction in the supraspinatus has been linked to a combination of mechanical weakening and pain secondary to impingement caused by a swollen tendon.[40]

Painful tendinopathy

Similar histopathological features of degeneration have been identified in the mid-substance of tendons affected by chronic pain such as the Achilles, patellar, posterior tibialis, and common extensor tendons at the lateral epicondyle (tennis elbow) (Fig. 17).[321, 324, 329–331] Very few (if any) specimens show evidence of inflammation such as chronic inflammatory cells (macrophages). Typical observations in Achilles tendinopathy include abnormal fibre structure and arrangement, focal variations in cellularity (both increased and decreased), rounded nuclei, and an increased non-collagenous matrix.[331, 332] Increased vascularity was found in 65 per cent of pathological specimens and in 28 per cent of controls.[332] The amount of proteoglycan was increased, found interspersed between the fibrils, sometimes as vacuolated 'lakes'.[332]

In the Achilles, pain may be located at the insertion or in the tendon mid-substance.[329, 333] At the insertion, degenerative features include longitudinal fissures and transverse tears in the fibrocartilage, bony spurs, and granulation tissue.[333, 334] There is an association of calcification with mucoid degeneration (GAG infiltration), and the bony spurs form by a process of endochondral ossification following

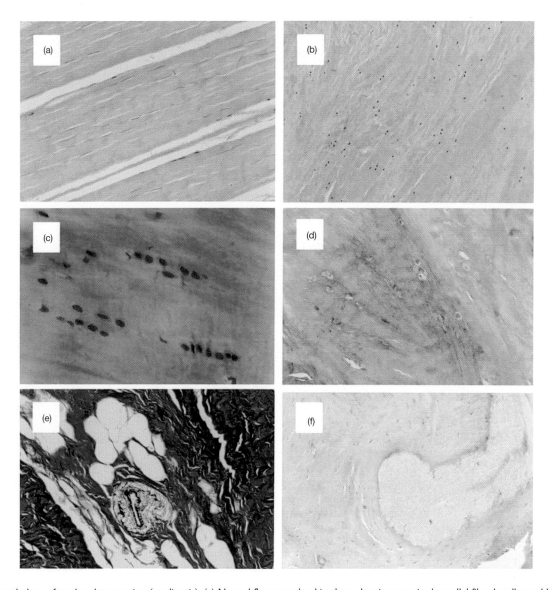

Fig. 16 Histopathology of tendon degeneration (tendinosis). (a) Normal flexor tendon histology, showing organized, parallel fibre bundles and long thin tenocytes dispersed throughout the matrix (H&E). (b) Ruptured supraspinatus tendon, showing hyaline (glassy) appearance, loss of matrix organization and rounded, shrunken nuclei (H&E). (c) Fibrocartilaginous change in supraspinatus tendon, showing rounded tenocytes in 'Indian file' (H&E). (d) Glycosaminoglycan (GAG) accumulation ('mucoid degeneration') in supraspinatus tendon, showing GAG (blue) surrounding rounded cells in the matrix (alcian blue/H&E). (e) Intimal hyperplasia of blood vessel and lipid droplets in the matrix (Elastin Ponceau S). (f) Calcium deposit in degenerate tendon, showing intense (blue) staining for GAG (Alcian Blue/H&E). (Reproduced from reference 321, © 1994, with permission from BMJ publishing group.)

vascular invasion of the fibrocartilage.[334, 335] In non-insertional Achilles tendon pain, the underlying tendinosis may or may not be associated with inflammation of the paratenon (paratenonitis).[329] Other studies have shown that inflammation of the paratenon is only rarely found in Achilles tendinopathy.[336]

Calcific tendinitis
Relatively few detailed histopathological studies of calcific tendinitis have been published. Two theories have dominated the literature regarding the possible pathogenesis of the condition. Some authors believe that mineralization results from necrotic, degenerative changes in the tendon.[110, 322] Indeed, calcific deposits are a common feature of degenerative tendinopathy, and found in many different tendons.[105, 109]

In contrast, others have postulated that calcification is the result of an endochondral transition, with mineral deposition occurring in a cartilaginous rudiment following chondrogenic metaplasia of the tenocytes.[113, 337] Studies of calcific tendinitis in supraspinatus tendons have not supported this hypothesis, showing an absence of type II collagen and alkaline phosphatase, both of which should be associated with chondrogenesis.[338] Uhthoff *et al.* recognized that there are two separate conditions associated with calcification of soft tissues.[339] One is degenerative and the other a cell-mediated process that is self-limiting and will eventually resolve. The nature and size of the deposit varies markedly, and a distinction must be made between mineralization and ossification (the formation of bone).[340] The formation of bone in tendon is normal in some tendons, particularly in the avian, and

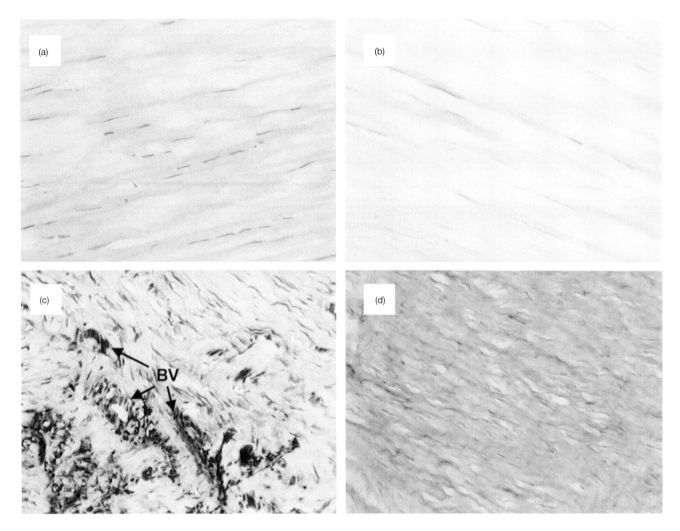

Fig. 17 Histopathology of painful tendinopathy. (a) Histology of normal Achilles tendon, showing organized, fibrous matrix with relatively few tenocytes (H&E). (b) Relative absence of glycosaminoglycan (GAG) in normal Achilles (toluidine blue). (c) 'Angiofibroblastic' activity in painful Achilles tendinopathy, showing increase in cell number and blood vessels (BV). (d) Increased GAG (blue) in painful tendinopathy, showing distribution throughout matrix (toluidine blue).

can also develop spontaneously in pathological conditions such as myositis ossificans, ankylosing spondylitis, and diffuse idiopathic skeletal hyperostosis (DISH).[340] Bone also develops following mid-point tenotomy of rodent Achilles tendons, with the formation of a cartilaginous intermediate in the regenerating granulation tissue.[341, 342] Osteogenic precursor cells were thought to derive from the tendon cells themselves, and not from circulating progenitors.[340, 342] We have recently demonstrated endochondral ossification in some Achilles and patellar tendinopathy specimens, resulting in discrete mineralized bony deposits.[343] These deposits showed a cartilaginous tissue consisting of type II collagen and the presence of both osteoblasts and osteoclasts within the bony nodule (Fig. 18). Tendons and ligaments appear to have an in-built capability to undergo cartilaginous and osteogenic transformation in certain pathological conditions and potentially as a result of trauma.[340]

Biochemistry and molecular pathology of chronic tendinopathy

There have been relatively few biochemical studies of chronic tendinopathy, and most have been of material collected at the end-stage of the condition after tendon rupture. Studies of ruptured supraspinatus tendons have found a small but significant decrease in total collagen content, and an increased proportion of type III collagen relative to type I collagen.[6] There was an increase in matrix proteoglycans and glycoproteins such as tenascin-C.[84] These changes in composition are generally consistent with wound repair as described above. This analysis supports the contention that accumulated micro-injuries result in a gradual deterioration in the quality of the tendon matrix. There is a transformation from a tendon consisting of predominantly organized type I collagen fibrils, to a tissue consisting of randomly organized, small-diameter fibrils of types I and III collagen. Similar changes are found in animal tendons, after both acute tendon injuries and in chronic tendinopathies, and these changes have been shown to persist, resulting in permanently altered mechanical properties of the tissue.[192, 203, 344]

Although some of the changes found in ruptured tendons are likely to be the result of the tendon rupture and not the cause, there are other reasons to suspect that a change in collagen turnover precedes and predisposes to tendon rupture. A study of the molecular age of the collagen network by an analysis of pentosidine content demonstrated that up to 50 per cent of the collagen in control (cadaver) supraspinatus

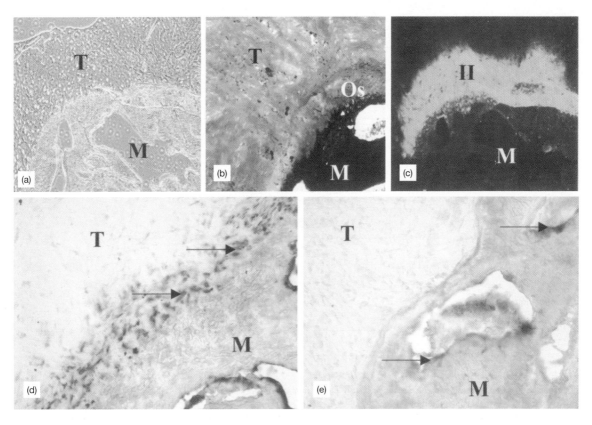

Fig. 18 Endochondral ossification in tendinopathy. A mineral deposit found in a specimen from patella tendinopathy was formed by a process similar or identical to endochondral ossification. Type II collagen was prominent in the matrix adjacent to the deposit, and markers of osteoblasts and osteoclasts were found in cells at the edge and within the deposit. (a) Phase contrast microscopy of mineral deposit. (b) Von Kossa staining of the calcific material (black). (c) Immunofluorescence staining of type II collagen (green). (d) Alkaline phosphatase activity, a marker of osteoblasts (red). (e) Tartrate-resistant acid phosphatase activity, a marker of osteoclasts (red). T, Tendon; M, Mineral deposit.

tendons had been replaced over the lifetime of the individual (Fig. 8).[46] An even greater proportion of collagen, up to 90 per cent of the total, was replaced in ruptured supraspinatus tendons.[46] These data have since been supported by an analysis of the racemization of the amino acid aspartate, another indicator of the molecular age of the protein network.[127] Since there were undetectable levels of immature collagen cross-links in these specimens, the data were consistent with increased remodelling of the collagen over a long time period—long enough to allow the maturation of the tri-functional HP cross-links.

Increased collagen turnover in supraspinatus tendons has been associated with several members of the MMP family. In control supraspinatus tendons, levels of MMP-1, MMP-2, and MMP-3 activity were significantly higher compared to those in normal biceps brachii tendons, which showed little or no collagen turnover (Fig. 9).[127] In ruptured supraspinatus tendons, there were increased levels of MMP-1 activity, reduced levels of MMP-2 and MMP-3, and increased collagen denaturation and turnover.[127] MMP-3 (stromelysin 1) is thought to be a key regulatory enzyme in the control of matrix turnover, and a decline in this enzyme activity may represent a failure in the control of the normal remodelling process. Thus tendinopathy may result from a failure to repair or maintain the tendon matrix in response to mechanical strain or microtrauma.

The key role of MMPs in chronic tendinopathy is further supported by the effect of a broad-spectrum inhibitor of metalloproteinases (Marimistat), which induces tendinopathy by an as yet unknown mechanism.[155] Detailed studies are required to determine which metalloproteinase activities are implicated, whether an MMP, ADAM, or ADAM-TS enzyme. Interestingly, other compounds such as fluoroquinolone antibiotics, which can induce tendinopathy in some patients, have recently been shown to modulate MMP activity *in vitro*. Studies on canine tenocytes showed a stimulation of a caseinase activity (possibly MMP-3) by canine tenocytes treated with ciprofloxacin.[345] We have shown no effect of ciprofloxacin on MMP-3 expression by human tenocytes, although pre-treatment with ciprofloxacin had a differential effect on the stimulation of MMPs by IL-1, increasing MMP-3 (protein) synthesis but not that of MMP-1.[346]

The importance of matrix remodelling activity in tendon was further emphasized in recent molecular studies of tendinopathy. Multiple changes in gene expression were detected in Achilles tendinopathy using cDNA arrays.[347] Of 265 genes that were analysed, 17 genes were upregulated and 23 were downregulated in degenerate tissue samples (Fig. 19). The absence of inflammation within the tendon was confirmed, and there were large increases in the expression of matrix genes such as collagen types I and III that were consistent with an attempt at repair. Proteoglycan mRNAs, such as versican, biglycan, and a cell-surface-associated heparan sulfate proteoglycan (HSPG2), were increased although there was no change in decorin mRNA. Matrix glycoproteins such as laminin, SPARC (secreted protein, acidic and rich in cysteine), and tenascin-C were also increased. In addition

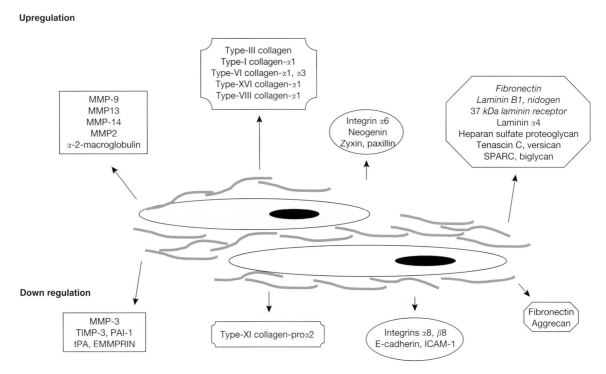

Fig. 19 Multiple changes in gene expression in chronic tendinopathy. Differential expression of genes for ECM and cell-adhesion molecules in degenerate Achilles tendon compared to normal, as identified by ATLAS™ cDNA arrays (Clontech, USA). Major changes, such as the increased expression of collagen type I and type III, and decreased expression of MMP-3 and TIMP-3, were confirmed by real-time reverse transcription polymerase chain reaction. (Reproduced (modified) from reference 346, © 2001, with permission from Elsevier Science.)

to matrix genes, there were also changes in MMP expression. The greatest difference between normal and pathological specimens was in the level of MMP-3 (stromelysin), which was present in normal Achilles and absent in tendinopathy specimens. This change was shown to be reflected in the level of MMP-3 protein and was similar to that reported in degenerate supraspinatus tendons (above). The data support the hypothesis that MMP-3 activity is required for normal tendon maintenance, at least in highly stressed tendons such as the supraspinatus and the Achilles.

Despite many elegant hypotheses, the factors that regulate matrix synthesis and degradation in chronic tendinopathy have not been characterized. Matrix interactions, insoluble deposits, mechanical strain, and neuropeptides (to name but a few factors) may have a direct effect on the cellular expression of matrix and enzyme activities. Very few studies have attempted to address the role of specific growth factors and cytokines in tendinopathy.

A study of TGFβ expression in the Achilles showed that one isoform (TGFβ2) was predominant in the fibrillar matrix of both normal and pathological tendons.[348] Although TGFβ2 was slightly increased in Achilles tendinopathy, an absence of one of the TGFβ signalling receptors (TGFβ-R1) suggested that TGFβ signalling was not actually taking place in the tendon. Consequently, a failure to control matrix degradation may result from a failure to upregulate TIMPs in response to TGFβ. This observation leads to the tentative hypothesis that the addition of growth factors such as TGFβ to facilitate tendon repair may be ineffective in chronic tendinopathy. It is also consistent with the hypothesis that the chronic nature of tendinopathy represents a

failure to appropriately regulate the cell activities during tendon repair and remodelling. Currently there are no therapies for tendinopathy that specifically address this problem.

Future directions

More work needs to be done to characterize the heterogeneous cell populations that populate tendons and ligaments and to determine how these cells respond to injury. We need to understand how ageing affects cell activities in different soft connective tissues, and how alterations in matrix structure and composition modulate the cell response to injury and stress. The mechanical environment plays a fundamental role in the regulation of cell activity, and future studies will increase our understanding of the signal transduction pathways involved in the response to different stresses and strains.

Presently much of our knowledge of soft tissue injury and repair is derived from studies of acute injuries in immature animals. There is a relative dearth of information about chronic pathology due to the absence of animal models that recreate the conditions seen in patients. These models may be developed once the pathology is better described in humans, allowing us to test new treatments. Little is known about early stages of the disease since most tissue samples reaching the laboratory come from the late or end-stage of the condition. Needle biopsies guided by ultrasound have recently been used to take small pieces of tendon from patients with chronic Achilles tendon pain, with no apparent ill effect.[349] The application of ultrasensitive techniques of molecular analysis to these biopsy specimens may allow us to identify changes in gene and protein expression at earlier stages, potentially identifying new targets for future research.

Diagnosis of soft tissue pathology is currently difficult due to the lack of biopsy material, and the absence of objective methods and criteria to assess the pathological process. Advances in imaging technologies such as magnetic resonance imaging (MRI) and ultrasound have already led to significant improvements in the diagnosis of soft tissue pathology, and these techniques are going to become more sensitive, more affordable, and more widely used in the objective assessment of individual conditions. In the future, early changes in protein structure and composition may be monitored by non-invasive techniques such as nuclear magnetic resonance (NMR) spectroscopic analysis. Already the biochemical analysis of protein degradation products released into the bloodstream or synovial fluid are being explored as potential markers for early tendon damage in horses, and a similar approach may be applied in human tendinopathies.

Based on the premise that much tendon and ligament pathology represents a failure by the resident cell population to adequately repair or maintain tissue after 'injury' (however caused), future treatment strategies may be targeted at improving the cellular activity in these tissues. Direct applications of recombinant growth factors such as TGFβ, PDGF, and IGF have been shown to have some possible benefit in animal models. However, application of these growth factors as proteins, given the proteolytic environment of many chronic wounds, may have little therapeutic use, particularly in the long term. There are problems of delivering these proteins and maintaining their concentration at the site of injury. An alternative strategy now being developed in animal models of tendon and ligament injury involves gene therapy. This can take a variety of forms, with one approach being to insert a gene encoding a particular growth factor into target cells at the wound site, increasing levels of expression and thus enhancing repair. Another approach is to apply small sequences of 'antisense' DNA, which bind to a specific gene and inhibit its expression, thus modulating some aspect of the wound healing response such as the formation of collagen fibrils. It is early days for these technologies, although the first clinical trials involving gene therapy on patients are now in progress.

Tissue repair requires a viable cell population that is able to respond to tissue injury and produce matrix of the correct composition and structure. All soft connective tissues are of mesenchymal origin, and contain a mixed population of cells. Some cells are less differentiated and specialized than others, and participate more actively in the repair response. Some of these cells may be derived from precursors known as 'stem cells', and enter tissues after injury or remain dormant in tissues as vascular 'pericytes'. Currently there is major research interest in developing ways to isolate and culture mesenchymal stem cells that may be used to repopulate sites of tendon injury and maintain the structure and composition of the tissue.[350]

Where tissues are extensively damaged, after cruciate ligament rupture, for example, there is currently no better option than to reconstruct the ligament, frequently using the central portion of the patient's own patellar tendon or hamstring. Alternative approaches with artificial materials such as carbon fibre have been disappointing. In the future, tissue engineering is likely to have a major impact on the reconstruction of soft tissues.[234] Techniques are being developed so as to create whole tissues in culture that replicate the structure and composition of the original tissue. Cartilage, skin, ligaments, and tendons have all been constructed from stem cells and supporting three-dimensional matrices, and it is surely only a matter of time before artificially grown ligaments and tendons are surgically transplanted into patients.

Summary

Ligaments and tendons are more complex and heterogeneous than commonly thought. They are metabolically active and responsive to changes in their mechanical and chemical environment. Injury results in substantial and often permanent changes in the quantity and quality of the ECM. There are regional differences in the response to injury that are related to the tissue cellularity, vascularity, composition, and organization. The repair tissue can be affected and modulated by physical and chemical factors, although the precise conditions required to optimize repair have not been defined scientifically. In tendon, most pathology is degenerative, resulting either in a 'spontaneous' tendon rupture or chronic (painful) tendinopathy, sometimes associated with calcification. Degeneration has been shown to be an active, cell-mediated process involving increased levels of matrix remodelling, with the increased synthesis and degradation of matrix components mediated by a variety of enzymes. The source of pain in chronic tendinopathy is uncertain, since inflammatory mediators may not be present in the tendon, although mediators of pain and inflammation may be increased in the surrounding peritendinous tissues or fluids. Current forms of treatment are based largely on empirical observations and their effectiveness is questionable. More clinical and experimental work remains to be done to develop a scientific approach to therapy.

Acknowledgements

The author gratefully acknowledges past and present members of the Rheumatology Research Unit who have all contributed in some part to the work presented in this chapter. Funding for the various research projects conducted at the Rheumatology Research Unit was provided by the Arthritis Research Campaign, The Isaac Newton Trust, REMEDI, The Wishbone Trust, The Sybil Eastwood Trust, and the Cambridge Arthritis Research Endeavour (CARE).

References

1. **Van der Rest, M. and Garrone, R.** (1990). Collagens as multidomain proteins. *Biochimie* **72**, 473–484.
2. **Prockop, D.J. and Kivirikko, K.I.** (1995). Collagens: molecular biology, diseases, and potentials for therapy. *Annu. Rev. Biochem.* **64**, 403–434.
3. **Cawston, T.E.** (1998). Matrix metallo proteinases and TIMPs: properties and implications for the rheumatic diseases. *Mol. Med. Today* **4**(3), 130–137.
4. **Aumailley, M. and Gayraud, B.** (1998). Structure and biological activity of the extracellular matrix. *J. Mol. Med.* **76**, 253–265.
5. **Elliott, D.H.** (1965). Structure and function of mammalian tendon. *Biol. Rev.* **40**, 392–421.
6. **Riley, G.P., Harrall, R.L., Constant, C.R., Chard, M.D., Cawston, T.E., and Hazleman, B.L.** (1994). Tendon degeneration and chronic shoulder pain: changes in the collagen composition of the human rotator cuff tendons in rotator cuff tendinitis. *Ann. Rheum. Dis.* **53**, 359–366.
7. **Niyibizi, C., Visconti, C.S., Kavalkovich, K., and Woo, S.L.-Y.** (1994). Collagens in an adult bovine medial collateral ligament: immunofluorescence localization by confocal microscopy reveals that type XIV collagen predominates at the ligament-bone junction. *Matrix Biol.* **14**, 743–751.

8. Duance, V.C., Restall, D.J., Beard, H., Bourne, F.J., and Bailey, A.J. (1977). The location of three collagen types in skeletal muscle. *FEBS Lett.* **79**, 248–252.

9. Kumagai, J., Sarkar, K., and Uhthoff, H.K. (1994). The collagen types in the attachment zone of rotator cuff tendons in the elderly: an immuno-histochemical study. *J. Rheumatol.* **21**, 2096–2100.

10. Lapiere, Ch.M., Nusgens, B., and Pierard, G.E. (1977). Interaction between collagen type I and type III in conditioning bundles organization. *Connect. Tissue Res.* **5**, 21–29.

11. Birk, D.E. and Mayne, R. (1997). Localization of collagen types I, III and V during tendon development. Changes in collagen types I and III are correlated with changes in fibril diameter. *Eur. J. Cell Biol.* **72**, 352–361.

12. Holz, U. (1980). [Achilles tendon rupture and achillodynia. The importance of tissue regeneration.] *Fortschr. Med.* **98**, 1517–1520.

13. von der Mark, K. (1981). Localization of collagen types in tissues. *Int. Rev. Connect. Tissue Res.* **9**, 265–324.

14. Bray, D.F., Bray, R.C., and Frank, C.B. (1993). Ultrastructural immunolo-calization of type-VI collagen and chondroitin sulphate in ligament. *J. Orthop. Res.* **11**, 677–685.

15. Shaw, L.M. and Olsen, B.R. (1991). FACIT collagens: diverse molecular bridges in extracellular matrices. *TIBS* **16**, 191–194.

16. Amiel, D., Frank, C., Harwood, F., Fronek, J., and Akeson, W.H. (1984). Tendons and ligaments: a morphological and biochemical comparison. *J. Orthop. Res.* **1**, 257–265.

17. Johnston, R.B., Seiler, J.G., Miller, E.J., and Drvaric, D.M. (1995). The intrinsic and extrinsic ligaments of the wrist. A correlation of collagen typing and histologic appearance. *J. Hand Surg. (Br.)* **20B**, 750–754.

18. Fukuta, S., Oyama, M., Kavalkovich, K., Fu, F.H., and Niyibizi, C. (1998). Identification of types II, IX and X collagens at the insertion site of the bovine Achilles tendon. *Matrix Biol.* **17**, 65–73.

19. Visconti, C.S., Kavalkovich, K., Wu, J.J., and Niyibizi, C. (1996). Biochemical analysis of collagens at the ligament–bone interface reveals presence of cartilage-specific collagens. *Arch. Biochem. Biophys.* **328**, 135–142.

20. Fujioka, H., Wang, G.J., Mizuno, K., Balian, G., and Hurwitz, S.R. (1997). Changes in the expression of type-X collagen in the fibrocartilage of rat Achilles tendon attachment during development. *J. Orthop. Res.* **15**, 675–681.

21. Waggett, A.D., Ralphs, J.R., Kwan, A.P.L., Woodnutt, D., and Benjamin, M. (1998). Characterization of collagens and proteoglycans at the insertion of the human Achilles tendon. *Matrix Biol.* **16**, 457–470.

22. Fan, L., Sarkar, K., Franks, D.J., and Uhthoff, H.K. (1997). Estimation of total collagen and types I and III collagen in canine rotator cuff tendons. *Calcif. Tissue Int.* **61**, 223–229.

23. Ralphs, J.R., Benjamin, M., and Thornett, A. (1991). Cell and matrix biology of the suprapatella in the rat: a structural and immunocyto-chemical study of fibrocartilage in a tendon subject to compression. *Anat. Rec.* **231**, 167–177.

24. Kumagai, J., Sarkar, K., Uhthoff, H.K., Okawara, Y., and Ooshima, A. (1994). Immunohistochemical distribution of type I, II and III collagens in the rabbit supraspinatus tendon insertion. *J. Anat.* **185**, 279–284.

25. Vogel, K.G. and Koob, T.J. (1989). Structural specialisation in tendons under compression. *Int. Rev. Cytol.* **115**, 267–293.

26. Perez-Castro, A.V. and Vogel, K.G. (1999). *In situ* expression of collagen and proteoglycan genes during development of fibrocartilage in bovine deep flexor tendon. *J. Orthop. Res.* **17**, 139–148.

27. Kastelic, J., Galeski, A., and Baer, E. (1978). The multicomposite structure of tendon. *Connect. Tissue Res.* **6**, 11–23.

28. Dyer, R.F. and Enna, C.D. (1976). Ultrastructural features of adult human tendon. *Cell Tissue Res.* **168**, 247–259.

29. Greenlee, T.K. and Ross, R. (1967). The development of the rat flexor digital tendon, a fine structure study. *J. Ultrastruct. Res.* **18**, 353–376.

30. Moore, M.J. and De Beaux, A. (1987). A quantitative ultrastructural study of rat tendon from birth to maturity. *J. Anat.* **153**, 163–169.

31. Parry, D.A., Barnes, G.R., and Craig, A.S. (1978). A comparison of the size distribution of collagen fibrils in connective tissues as a function of age and a possible relation between fibril size distribution and mechanical properties. *Proc. R. Soc. Lond B Biol. Sci.* **203**, 305–321.

32. Józsa, L. and Kannus, P. (1997). Structure and metabolism of normal tendons. In *Human tendons. Anatomy physiology and pathology* (ed. L. Józsa and P. Kannus), pp. 46–95. Human Kinetics, Champaign, Illinois.

33. Flint, M.H., Craig, A.S., Reilly, H.C., Gillard, G.C., and Parry, D.A.D. (1984). Collagen fibril diameters and glycosaminoglycan content of skins—indices of tissue maturity and function. *Connect. Tiss. Res.* **13**, 69–81.

34. Merrilees, M.J., Tiang, K.M., and Scott, L. (1987). Changes in collagen fibril diameters across artery walls including a correlation with glycosaminoglycan content. *Connect. Tissue Res.* **16**, 237–257.

35. Scott, J.E. (1990). Proteoglycan–collagen interactions and sub-fibrillar structure in collagen fibrils: implications in the development and remod-elling of connective tissues. *Biochem. Soc. Trans.* **18**, 489–490.

36. Butler, D.L., Grood, E.S., Noyes, F.R., and Zernicke, R.F. (1978). Biomechanics of ligaments and tendons. *Exer. Sport Sci. Rev.* **6**, 125–181.

37. Wilmink, J., Wilson, A.M., and Goodship, A.E. (1992). Functional signifi-cance of the morphology and micromechanics of collagen fibres in rela-tion to partial rupture of the superficial digital flexor tendon in racehorses. *Res. Vet. Sci.* **53**, 354–359.

38. Józsa, L., Kannus, P., Balint, J.B., and Reffy, A. (1991). Three-dimensional ultrastructure of human tendons. *Acta Anat. (Basel)* **142**, 306–312.

39. Clark, J.M. and Harryman, D.T. II (1992). Tendons, ligaments, and cap-sule of the rotator cuff. Gross and microscopic anatomy. *J. Bone Joint Surg. (Am.)* **74A**, 713–725.

40. Uhthoff, H.K. and Sano, H. (1997). Pathology of failure of the rotator cuff tendon. *Orthop. Clin. N. Am.* **28**, 31–41.

41. Schechtman, H. and Bader, D.L. (1997). *In vitro* fatigue of human tendons. *J. Biomech.* **30**, 829–835.

42. Ker, R.F., Wang, X.T., and Pike, A.V.L. (2000). Fatigue quality of mammalian tendons. *J. Exp. Biol.* **203**, 1317–1327.

43. Eyre, D.R., Paz, M.A., and Gallop, P.M. (1984). Cross-linking in collagen and elastin. *Ann. Rev. Biochem.* **53**, 717–748.

44. Bailey, A.J., Paul, R.G., and Knott, L. (1998). Mechanisms of maturation and ageing of collagen. *Mech. Ageing Dev.* **106**, 1–56.

45. Bailey, A.J., Robins, S.P., and Balian, G. (1974). Biological significance of the intermolecular crosslinks of collagen. *Nature* **251**, 105–109.

46. Bank, R.A., TeKoppele, J.M., Oostingh, G., Hazleman, B.L., and Riley, G.P. (1999). Lysylhydroxylation and non-reducible cross-linking of human supraspinatus tendon collagen: changes with age and in chronic rotator cuff tendinitis. *Ann. Rheum. Dis.* **58**, 35–41.

47. Sell, D.R. and Monnier V.M. (1989). Isolation, purification, and partial characterization of novel fluorophores from aging human insoluble collagen-rich tissue. *Connect. Tissue Res.* **19**, 77–92.

48. Reiser, K.M., Amigable, M., and Last, J.A. (1992). Nonenzymatic glyca-tion of type I collagen. The effects of aging on preferential glycation sites. *J. Biol. Chem.* **267**, 24207–24216.

49. Bailey, A.J., Sims, T.J., Avery, N.C., and Miles, C.A. (1993). Chemistry of collagen cross-links: glucose-mediated covalent cross-linking of type-IV collagen in lens capsules. *Biochem. J.* **296**, 489–496.

50. Sell, D.R. and Monnier, V.M. (1989). Structural elucidation of a senescence cross-link from human extra-cellular matrix. Implication of pentoses in the aging process. *J. Biol. Chem.* **264**, 21594–21602.

51. Hardingham, T.E. and Fosang, A.J. (1992). Proteoglycans: many forms and many functions. *FASEB J.* **6**, 861–870.

52. Iozzo, R.V. (1998). Matrix proteoglycans: from molecular design to cellular function. *Annu. Rev. Biochem.* **67**, 609–652.

53. Hardingham, T.E. and Fosang, A.J. (1995). The structure of aggrecan and its turnover in cartilage. *J. Rheumatol.* **22** (Suppl. 43), 86–90.

54. Margolis, R.U. and Margolis, R.K. (1994). Aggrecan–versican–neurocan family of proteoglycans. *Methods Enzymol.* **245**, 105–128.

55. Heinegård, D., Hedbom, E., Antonsson, P., and Oldberg, A. (1990). Structural variability of large and small chondroitin sulphate/dermatan sulphate proteoglycans. *Biochem. Soc. Trans.* **18**, 209–212.

56. Hedbom, E. and Heinegård, D. (1993). Binding of fibromodulin and decorin to separate sites on fibrillar collagens. *J. Biol. Chem* **268**, 27307–27312.

57. Hildebrand, A., Romarís, M., Rasmussen, L.M., Heinegård, D., Twardzik, D.R., Border, W.A., *et al.* (1994). Interaction of the small interstitial proteoglycans biglycan, and decorin and fibromodulin with transforming growth factor β. *Biochem. J.* **302**, 527–534.

58. Vogel, K.G. and Heinegard, D. (1985). Characterisation of proteoglycans from adult bovine tendon. *J. Biol. Chem.* **260**, 9298–9306.

59. Vogel, K.G., Sandy, J.D., Pogány, G., and Robbins, J.R. (1994). Aggrecan in bovine tendon. *Matrix* **14**, 171–179.

60. Koob, T.J. and Vogel, K.G. (1987). Site related variations in glycosaminoglycan content and swelling properties of bovine flexor tendon. *J. Orthop. Res.* **5**, 414–424.

61. Okuda, Y., Gorski, J.P., An, K.-N., and Amadio, P.C. (1987). Biochemical histological and biomechanical analyses of canine tendon. *J. Orthop. Res.* **5**, 60–68.

62. Merrilees, M.J. and Flint, M.H. (1980). Ultrastructural study of tension and pressure zones in a rabbit flexor tendon. *Am. J. Anat.* **157**, 87–106.

63. Gillard, G.C., Reilly, H.C., Bell-Booth, P.G., and Flint, M.H. (1979). The influence of mechanical forces on the glycosaminoglycan content of the rabbit flexor digitorum profundus tendon. *Connect. Tissue Res.* **7**, 37–46.

64. Riley, G.P., Harrall, R.L., Constant, C.R., Chard, M.D., Cawston, T.E., and Hazleman, B.L. (1994). Glycosaminoglycans of human rotator cuff tendons: changes with age and in chronic rotator cuff tendinitis. *Ann. Rheum. Dis.* **53**, 367–376.

65. Benjamin, M., Qin, S., and Ralphs, J.R. (1995). Fibrocartilage associated with human tendons and their pulleys. *J. Anat.* **187**, 625–633.

66. Vogel, K.G., Ördög, A., Pogány, G., and Oláh, J. (1993). Proteoglycans in the compressed region of human tibialis posterior tendon and in ligaments. *J. Orthop. Res.* **11**, 68–77.

67. Berenson, M.C., Blevins, F.T., Plaas, A.H.K., and Vogel, K.G. (1996). Proteoglycans of human rotator cuff tendons. *J. Orthop. Res.* **14**, 518–525.

68. Hey, N.J., Handley, C.J., Ng, C.K., and Oakes, B.W. (1990). Characterisation and synthesis of macromolecules by adult collateral ligament. *Biochim. Biophys. Acta* **1034**, 73–80.

69. Campbell, M.A., Tester, A.M., Handley, C.J., Checkley, G.J., Chow, G.L., Cant, A.E., *et al.* (1996). Characterization of a large chondroitin sulfate proteoglycan present in bovine collateral ligament. *Arch. Biochem. Biophys.* **329**, 181–190.

70. Benjamin, M. and Ralphs, J.R. (1998). Fibrocartilage in tendons and ligaments—an adaptation to compressive load. *J. Anat.* **193**, 481–494.

71. Nessler, J.P., Amadio, P.C., Berglund, L.J., and An, K.-N. (1992). Healing of canine tendon in zones subjected to different mechanical forces. *J. Hand Surg. (Br.)* **17B**, 561–568.

72. Amadio, P.C., Berglund, L.J., and An, K.-N. (1992). Biochemically discrete zones of canine flexor tendon: evaluation of properties with a new photographic method. *J. Orthop. Res.* **10**, 198–204.

73. Uitto, J. (1979). Biochemistry of the elastic fibers in normal connective tissues and its alterations in diseases. *J. Invest Dermatol.* **72**, 1–10.

74. Cooper, R.R. and Misol, S. (1970). Tendon and ligament insertion: a light and electron microscopic study. *J. Bone Joint Surg. (Am.)* **52A**, 1–20.

75. Labat-Robert, J., Bihari-Varga, M., and Robert, L. (1990). Extracellular matrix. *FEBS Lett.* **268**, 386–393.

76. Józsa, L., Lehto, M., Kannus, P., Kvist, M., Reffy, A., Vieno, T., *et al.* (1989). Fibronectin and laminin in Achilles tendon. *Acta Orthop. Scand.* **60**, 469–471.

77. Amiel, D., Foulk, R.A., Harwood, F.L., and Akeson, W.H. (1989). Quantitative assessment by competitive ELISA of fibronectin in tendons and ligaments. *Matrix* **9**, 421–427.

78. Banes, A.J., Link, G.W., Bevin, A.G., Peterson, H.D., Gillespie, Y., Bynum, D., *et al.* (1988). Tendon synovial cells secrete fibronectin *in vivo* and *in vitro*. *J. Orthop. Res.* **6**, 73–82.

79. Lehto, M., Józsa, L., Kvist, M., Jarvinen, M., Balint, B.J., and Reffy, A. (1990). Fibronectin in the ruptured human Achilles tendon and its paratenon. An immunoperoxidase study. *Ann. Chir. Gynaecol.* **79**, 72–77.

80. Williams, I.F., McCullagh, K.G., and Silver, I.A. (1984). The distribution of types I and III collagen and fibronectin in the healing equine tendon. *Connect. Tissue Res.* **12**, 211–222.

81. Gelberman, R.H., Steinberg, D., Amiel, D., and Akeson, W.H. (1991). Fibroblast chemotaxis after wound repair. *J. Hand Surg. (Am.)* **16A**, 686–693.

82. Chiquet, M. and Fambrough, D.M. (1984). Chick myotendinous antigen. II. A novel extracellular glycoprotein complex consisting of large disulfide-linked subunits. *J. Cell Biol.* **98**, 1937–1946.

83. Gulcher, J.R., Nies, D.E., Alexakos, M.J., Ravikant, N.A., Sturgill, M.E., Marton, L.S., *et al.* (1991). Structure of the human hexabrachion (tenascin) gene. *Proc. Natl Acad. Sci., USA* **88**, 9438–9442.

84. Riley, G.P., Harrall, R.L., Cawston, T.E., Hazleman, B.L., and Mackie, E.J. (1996). Tenascin-C and human tendon degeneration. *Am. J. Pathol.* **149**, 933–943.

85. Kannus, P., Józsa, L., Jarvinen, T.A., Jarvinen, T.L., Kvist, M., Natri, A., *et al.* (1998). Location and distribution of non-collagenous matrix proteins in musculoskeletal tissues of rat. *Histochem. J.* **30**, 799–810.

86. Mehr, D., Pardubsky, P.D., Martin, J.A., and Buckwalter, J.A. (2000). Tenascin-C in tendon regions subjected to compression. *J. Orthop. Res.* **18**, 537–545.

87. Mackie, E.J., Halfter, W., and Liverani, D. (1988). Induction of tenascin in healing wounds. *J. Cell Biol.* **107**, 2757–2767.

88. Whitby, D.J. and Ferguson, M.W.J. (1991). The extracellular matrix of lip wounds in fetal, and neonatal and adult mice. *Development* **112**, 651–668.

89. Mackie, E.J. (1994). Tenascin in connective tissue development and pathogenesis. *Perspect. Dev. Neurobiol.* **2**, 125–132.

90. Chevalier, X., Groult, N., Larget-Piet, B., Zardi, L., and Hornebeck, W. (1994). Tenascin distribution in articular cartilage from normal subjects and from patients with osteoarthritis and rheumatoid arthritis. *Arthritis Rheum.* **37**, 1013–1022.

91. Siri, A., Knäuper, V., Veirana, N., Caocci, F., Murphy, G., and Zardi, L. (1995). Different susceptibility of small and large human tenascin-C isoforms to degradation by matrix metalloproteinases. *J. Biol. Chem.* **270**, 8650–8654.

92. Tremble, P., Chiquet-Ehrismann, R., and Werb, Z. (1994). The extracellular matrix ligands fibronectin and tenascin collaborate in regulating collagenase gene expression in fibroblasts. *Mol. Biol. Cell* **5**, 439–453.

93. DiCesare, P., Hauser, N., Lehman, D., Pasumarti, S., and Paulsson, M. (1994). Cartilage oligomeric matrix protein (COMP) is an abundant component of tendon. *FEBS Lett.* **354**, 237–240.

94. Smith, R.K.W., Zunino, L., Webbon, P.M., and Heinegård, D. (1997). The distribution of cartilage oligomeric matrix protein (COMP) in tendon and its variation with tendon site, and age and load. *Matrix Biol.* **16**, 255–271.

95. Oldberg, A., Antonsson, P., Lindblom, K., and Heinegård, D. (1992). COMP (cartilage oligomeric matrix protein) is structurally related to the thrombospondins. *J. Biol. Chem.* **267**, 22346–22350.

96. Briggs, M.D., Hoffman, S.M., King, L.M., Olsen, A.S., Mohrenweiser, H., Leroy, J.G., *et al.* (1995). Pseudoachondroplasia and multiple epiphyseal dysplasia due to mutations in the cartilage oligomeric matrix protein gene. *Nat. Genet.* **10**, 330–336.

97. Smith, R.K., Birch, H., Patterson-Kane, J., Firth, E.C., Williams, L., Cherdchutham, W., *et al.* (1999). Should equine athletes commence training during skeletal development? Changes in tendon matrix associated with development, ageing, and function and exercise. *Equine Vet. J. Suppl.* **30**, 201–209.

98. Oldberg, A., Antonnsson, P., Hedbom, E., and Heinegård, D. (1991). Structure and function of extracellular matrix proteoglycans. *Biochem. Soc. Trans.* **18**, 789–792.

99. Sage, E.H. and Bornstein, P. (1991). Extracellular proteins that modulate cell–matrix interactions. SPARC, tenascin, and thrombospondin. *J. Biol. Chem.* **266**, 14831–14834.

100. Bornstein, P. (1992). Thrombospondins: structure and regulation of expression. *FASEB J.* **6**, 3290–3299.

101. Miller, R.R. and McDevitt, C.A. (1991). Thrombospondin in ligament, and meniscus and intervertebral disc. *Biochim. Biophys. Acta Gen. Subj.* **1115**, 85–88.

102. Jones, A.J. and Bee, J.A. (1990). Age and position related heterogeneity of equine tendon extracellullar matrix composition. *Res. Vet. Sci.* **48**, 357–364.

103. Adams, C.W.M. and Bayliss, O.B. (1973). Acid mucosubstances underlying lipid deposits in ageing tendons and atherosclerotic arteries. *Atherosclerosis* **18**, 191–195.

104. Józsa, L., Reffy, A., and Balint, B.J. (1984). The pathogenesis of tendolipomatosis—an electron microscope study. *Int Orthop SICOT* **7**, 251–255.

105. Jarvinen, M., Józsa, L., Kannus, P., Jarvinen, T.L.N., Kvist, M., and Leadbetter, W. (1997). Histopathological findings in chronic tendon disorders. *Scand. J. Med. Sci. Sports* **7**, 86–95.

106. Athanasou, N.A., West, L., Sallie, B., and Puddle, B. (1995). Localized amyloid deposition in cartilage is glycosaminoglycans-associated. *Histopathology* **26**, 267–272.

107. Cole, A.S., Cordiner-Lawrie, S., Carr, A.J., and Athanasou, N.A. (2001). Localised deposition of amyloid in tears of the rotator cuff. *J. Bone Joint Surg. (Br.)* **83B**, 561–564.

108. Ellis, E.H., Spadaro, J.A., and Becker, R.O. (1969). Trace elements in tendon collagen. *Clin. Orthop. Rel. Res.* **65**, 195–198.

109. Riley, G.P., Harrall, R.L., Constant, C.R., Cawston, T.E., and Hazleman, B.L. (1996). Prevalence and possible pathological significance of calcium phosphate salt accumulation in tendon matrix degeneration. *Ann. Rheum. Dis.* **55**, 109–115.

110. Urist, M.R., Moss, M.J., and Adams, J.M. (1964). Calcification of tendon. *Arch. Pathol.* **77**, 594–608.

111. Józsa, L., Balint, B.J., and Reffy, A. (1980). Calcifying tendinopathy. *Arch. Orthop. Trauma Surg.* **97**, 305–307.

112. Uhthoff, H.K. and Loehr, J.W. (1997). Calcific tendinopathy of the rotator cuff: pathogenesis, diagnosis, and management. *J. Am. Acad. Orthop. Surg.* **5**, 183–191.

113. Uhthoff, H.K. (1975). Calcifying tendinitis, an active cell-mediated calcification. *Virchows Arch. A* **366**, 51–58.

114. Squier, C.A. and Magnes, C. (1983). Spatial relationships between fibroblasts during the growth of rat-tail tendon. *Cell Tissue Res.* **234**, 17–29.

115. Neuberger, A., Perrone, J.C., and Slack, H.G.B. (1951). The relative metabolic inertia of tendon collagen in the rat. *Biochem. J.* **49**, 199–204.

116. Peacock, E. (1957). The vascular basis for tendon repair. *Surg. Forum* **8**, 65–86.

117. Vailas, A.C., Tipton, C.M., Laughlin, H.L., Tcheng, T.K., and Matthes, R.D. (1978). Physical activity and hypophysectomy on the aerobic capacity of ligaments and tendons. *J. Appl. Physiol.* **44**, 542–546.

118. Tipton, C.M., Matthes, R.D., Maynard, J.A., and Carey, R.A. (1975). The influence of physical activity on ligaments and tendons. *Med. Sci. Sports* **7**, 165–175.

119. Birch, H.L., Rutter, G.A., and Goodship, A.E. (1997). Oxidative energy metabolism in equine tendon cells. *Res. Vet. Sci.* **62**, 93–97.

120. Floridi, A., Ippolito, E., and Postacchini, F. (1981). Age-related changes in the metabolism of tendon cells. *Connect. Tissue Res.* **9**, 95–97.

121. Webster, D.F. and Burry, H.C. (1982). The effects of hypoxia on human skin, and lung and tendon cells *in vitro*. *Br. J. Exp. Pathol.* **63**, 50–55.

122. Vandor, E., Józsa, L., and Balint, B.J. (1982). The lactate dehydrogenase activity and isoenzyme pattern of normal and hypokinetic human tendons. *Eur. J. Appl. Physiol. Occup. Physiol.* **49**, 63–68.

123. Lundborg, G. and Rank, F. (1978). Experimental intrinsic healing of flexor tendons based upon synovial fluid nutrition. *J. Hand Surg.* **3**(1), 21–31.

124. MacNab, I. (1973). Rotator cuff tendinitis. *Ann. R. Coll. Surg. Engl.* **52**, 271–287.

125. Perez-Tamayo, R. (1982). Degradation of collagen: pathology. In *Collagen in health and disease* (ed. J.B. Weiss and M.I.V. Jayson), pp. 135–159. Churchill Livingstone, Edinburgh.

126. Stetler-Stevenson, W.G. (1996). Dynamics of matrix turnover during pathologic remodelling of the extracellular matrix. *Am. J. Pathol.* **148**, 1345–1350.

127. Riley, G.P., Curry, V., DeGroot, J., van El, B., Verzijl, N., TeKoppele, J.M., Hazleman, B.L., and Bank, R.A. (2002). Matrix metalloproteinase activities and their relationship with collagen remodelling in tendon pathology. *Matrix Biol.* **21**, 185–195.

128. Riederer-Henderson, M.A., Gauger, A., Olson, L., Robertson, C., and Greenlee, T.K. Jr. (1983). Attachment and extracellular matrix differences between tendon and synovial fibroblastic cells. *IN VITRO* **19**, 127–133.

129. Gelberman, R.H., Goldberg, V., An, K.-N., and Banes, A. (1988). Tendon. In *Injury and repair of the musculoskeletal soft tissues* (ed. S.L.-Y. Woo and J.A. Buckwalter), pp. 1–40. American Academy of Orthopaedic Surgeons, Park Ridge, Illinois.

130. Banes, A.J., Donlon, K., Link, G.W., Gillespie, Y., Bevin, A.G., Peterson, H.D., *et al.* (1988). Cell populations of tendon: a simplified method for isolation of synovial cells and internal fibroblasts. Confirmation of origin and biologic properties. *J. Orthop. Res.* **6**, 83–94.

131. Garner, W.L., McDonald, J.A., Koo, M., Kuhn, C., and Weeks, P.M. (1989). Identification of the collagen producing cells in healing flexor tendons. *Plast. Reconstr. Surg.* **83**(5), 875–878.

132. Chesney, J. and Bucala, R. (1997). Peripheral blood fibrocytes: novel fibroblast-like cells that present antigen and mediate tissue repair. *Biochem. Soc. Trans.* **25**, 520–524.

133. Chard, M.D., Wright, J.K., and Hazleman, B.L. (1987). Isolation and growth characteristics of adult human tendon fibroblasts. *Ann. Rheum. Dis.* **46**, 385–390.

134. Koob, T.J., Clark, P.E., Hernandez, D.J., Thurmond, F.A., and Vogel, K.G. (1992). Compression loading *in vitro* regulates proteoglycan synthesis by tendon fibrocartilage. *Arch. Biochem. Biophys.* **298**, 303–312.

135. Spindler, K.P., Nanney, L.B., and Davidson, J.M. (1995). Proliferative responses to platelet-derived growth factor in young and old rat patellar tendon. *Connect. Tissue Res.* **31**, 171–177.

136. Banes, A.J., Tsuzaki, M., Hu, P., Brigman, B., Brown, T., Almekinders, L., *et al.* (1995). PDGF-BB, and IGF-I and mechanical load stimulate DNA synthesis in avian tendon fibroblasts in vitro. *J. Biomech.* **28**, 1505–1513.

137. Schmidt, C.C., Georgescu, H.I., Kwoh, C.K., Blomstrom, G.L., Engle, C.P., Larkin, L.A., *et al.* (1995). Effect of growth factors on the proliferation of fibroblasts from the medial collateral and anterior cruciate ligaments. *J. Orthop. Res.* **13**, 184–190.

138. Rees, S.G., Flannery, C.R., Little, C.B., Hughes, C.E., Caterson, B., and Dent, C.M. (2000). Catabolism of aggrecan, and decorin and biglycan in tendon. *Biochem. J.* **350**(1), 181–188.

139. McNeilly, C.M., Banes, A.J., Benjamin, M., and Ralphs, J.R. (1996). Tendon cells *in vivo* form a three dimensional network of cell processes linked by gap junctions. *J. Anat.* **189**, 593–600.

140. Maffulli, N., Ewen S.W.B., Waterston, S.W., Reaper, J., and Barrass, V. (2000). Tenocytes from ruptured and tendinopathic Achilles tendons produce greater quantities of type III collagen than tenocytes from normal Achilles tendons—An *in vitro* model of human tendon heating. *Am. J. Sports Med.* **28**, 499–505.

141. Spindler, K.P., Clark, S.W., Nanney, L.B., and Davidson, J.M. (1996). Expression of collagen and matrix metalloproteinases in ruptured human anterior cruciate ligament: an *in situ* hybridization study. *J. Orthop. Res.* **14**, 857–861.

142. Everts, V., Van der Zee, E., Creemers, L., and Beertsen, W. (1996). Phagocytosis and intracellular digestion of collagen, and its role in turnover and remodelling. *Histochem. J.* **28**, 229–245.

143. Creemers, L.B., Jansen, I.D.C., Docherty, A.J.P., Reynolds, J.J., Beertsen, W., and Everts, V. (1998). Gelatinase A (MMP-2) and cysteine proteinases are essential for the degradation of collagen in soft connective tissue. *Matrix Biol.* **17**, 35–46.

144. Harper, J., Amiel, D., and Harper, E. (1988). Collagenase production by rabbit ligaments and tendon. *Connect. Tissue Res.* **17**, 253–259.

145. Piening, C. and Riederer-Henderson, M.A. (1989). Neutral metalloproteinase from tendons. *J. Orthop. Res.* **7**, 228–234.

146. Dalton, S.E., Cawston, T.E., Riley, G.P., Bayley, I.J.L., and Hazleman, B.L. (1995). Human tendon biopsy samples in organ culture produce procollagenase and tissue inhibitor of metalloproteinases. *Ann. Rheum. Dis.* **54**, 571–577.

147. Cawston, T.E., Curry, V.A., Summers, C.A., Clark, I.M., Riley, G.P., Life, P.F., *et al.* (1998). The role of oncostatin M in animal and human connective tissue collagen turnover and its localization within the rheumatoid joint. *Arthritis Rheum.* **41**, 1760–1771.

148. Cawston, T.E. (1995). Proteinases and inhibitors. *Br. Med. Bull.* **51**, 385–401.

149. Cawston, T.E. and Billington, C. (1996). Metalloproteinases in the rheumatic diseases. *J. Pathol.* **180**, 115–117.

150. Matrisian, L.M. (1990). Metalloproteinases and their inhibitors in matrix remodelling. *Trends Genet.* **6**, 121–125.

151. Matrisian, L.M. (1992). The matrix degrading metalloproteinases. *BioEssays* **14**, 455–463.

152. Nagase, H. (1994). Matrix metalloproteinases. A mini-review. *Contrib. Nephrol.* **107**, 85–93.

153. Murphy, G., Willenbrock, F., Crabbe, T., O'Shea, M., Ward, R., Atkinson, S., *et al.* (1994). Regulation of matrix metalloproteinase activity. *Ann. NY Acad. Sci.* **732**, 31–41.

154. Murphy, G. and Willenbrock, F. (1995). Tissue inhibitors of matrix metalloendopeptidases. *Methods Enzymol.* **248**, 496–510.

155. Millar, A.W., Brown, P.D., Moore, J., Galloway, W.A., Cornish, A.G., Lenehan, T.J., *et al.* (1998). Results of single and repeat dose studies of the oral matrix metalloproteinase inhibitor marimastat in healthy male volunteers. *Br. J. Clin. Pharmacol.* **45**, 21–26.

156. Schlondorff, J. and Blobel, C.P. (1999). Metalloprotease-disintegrins: modular proteins capable of promoting cell-cell interactions and triggering signals by protein-ectodomain shedding. *J. Cell Sci.* **112**, 3603–3617.

157. Kaushal, G.P. and Shah, S.V. (2000). The new kids on the block: ADAMTSs, and potentially multifunctional metalloproteinases of the ADAM family. *J. Clin. Invest.* **105**, 1335–1337.

158. Tortorella, M.D., Burn, T.C., Pratta, M.A., Abbaszade, I., Hollis, J.M., Liu, R., *et al.* (1999). Purification and cloning of aggrecanase-1: a member of the ADAMTS family of proteins. *Science* **284**, 1664–1666.

159. Abbaszade, I., Liu, R.Q., Yang, F., Rosenfeld, S.A., Ross, O.H., Link, J.R., *et al.* (1999). Cloning and characterization of ADAMTS11, and an aggrecanase from the ADAMTS family. *J. Biol. Chem.* **274**, 23443–23450.

160. Kuno, K., Okada, Y., Kawashima, H., Nakamura, H., Miyasaka, M., Ohno, H., *et al.* (2000). ADAMTS-1 cleaves a cartilage proteoglycan, and aggrecan. *FEBS Lett.* **478**, 241–245.

161. Nakamura, H., Fujii, Y., Inoki, I., Sugimoto, K., Tanzawa, K., Matsuki, H., *et al.* (2000). Brevican is degraded by matrix metalloproteinases and aggrecanase-1 (ADAMTS4) at different sites. *J. Biol. Chem.* **275**, 38885–38890.

162. Campbell, M.A., Winter, A.D., Ilic, M.Z., and Handley, C.J. (1996). Catabolism and loss of proteoglycans from cultures of bovine collateral ligament. *Arch. Biochem. Biophys.* **328**, 64–72.

163. Ippolito, E., Postacchini, F., and Ricciardi-Pollini, P.T. (1975). Biochemical variations in the matrix of human tendons in relation to age and pathological conoditions. *Ital. J. Orthop. Traum.* **1**, 133–139.

164. Ippolito, E., Natali, P.G., Postacchini, F., Accini, L., and de Martino, C. (1980). Morphological, immunological and biochemical study of rabbit achilles tendon at various ages. *J. Bone Joint Surg. (Am.)* **62A**, 583–598.

165. O'Brien, M. (1992). Functional anatomy and physiology of tendons. *Clin. Sports Med.* **11**, 505–520.

166. Haut, R.C., Lancaster, R.L., and DeCamp, C.E. (1992). Mechanical properties of the canine patellar tendon: Some correlations with age and the content of collagen. *J. Biomech.* **25**, 163–173.

167. Gillis, C., Pool, R.R., Meagher, D.M., Stover, S.M., Reiser, K., and Willits, N. (1997). Effect of maturation and aging on the histomorphometric and biochemical characteristics of equine superficial digital flexor tendon. *Am. J. Vet. Res.* **58**, 425–430.

168. Patterson-Kane, J.C., Parry, D.A., Birch, H.L., Goodship, A.E., and Firth, E.C. (1997). An age-related study of morphology and cross-link composition of collagen fibrils in the digital flexor tendons of young thoroughbred horses. *Connect. Tissue Res.* **36**, 253–26.

169. Vogel, H.G. (1983). Age dependence of mechanical properties of rat tail tendons (hysteresis experiments). *Akt. Gerontol.* **13**, 22–27.

170. Chard, M.D., Gresham, A., and Hazleman, B.L. (1989). Age related changes in the rotator cuff. *Br. J. Rheumàtal.* **28**, 19.

171. Riley, G.P., Goddard, M.J., and Hazleman BL. (2001). Histopathological assessment and pathological significance of matrix degeneration in supraspinatus tendons. *Rheumatology* **40**, 229–230.

172. Woo, S.L.-Y., Gomez, M.A., Amiel, D., Ritter, M.A., Gelberman, R.H., and Akeson, W.H. (1981). The effects of exercise on the biomechanical and biochemical properties of swine digital flexor tendons. *J. Biomech. Eng.* **103**, 51–56.

173. Woo, S.L., Gomez, M.A., Woo, Y.K., and Akeson, W.H. (1982). Mechanical properties of tendons and ligaments. II. The relationships of immobilization and exercise on tissue remodelling. *Biorheology* **19**, 397–408.

174. Akeson, W.H., Amiel, D., and La Violette, D. (1967). The connective tissue response to immobility: a study of the chondroitin 4 sulphate and 6-sulphate and dermatan sulphate changes in periarticular connective tissues of control and immobilized knees of dogs. *Clin. Orthop. Rel. Res.* **51**, 183–197.

175. Vailas, A.C., Pedrini, V.A., Pedrini-Mille, A., and Holloszy, J.O. (1985). Patellar tendon matrix changes associated with aging and voluntary exercise. *J. Appl. Physiol.* **58**, 1572–6.

176. Woo, S.L.-Y, Maynard, J., Butler, D., *et al.* (1988). Ligament, tendon and joint capsule insertions to bone. In *Injury and repair of the musculoskeletal soft tissues* (ed. S.L.-Y. Woo and J.A. Buckwalter), p. 156. American Academy of Orthopaedic Surgeons, Park Ridge, Illinois.

177. Harper, J., Amiel, D., and Harper E. (1992). Inhibitors of collagenase in ligaments and tendons of rabbits immobilized for 4 weeks. *Connect. Tissue Res.* **28**, 257–261.

178. Woo, S.L., Gomez, M.A., Sites, T.J., Newton, P.O., Orlando, C.A., and Akeson, W.H. (1987). The biomechanical and morphological changes in the medial collateral ligament of the rabbit after immobilization and remobilization. *J. Bone Joint Surg. (Am.)* **69A**, 1200–1211.

179. Nielsen, H.M., Skalicky, M., and Viidik, A. (1998). Influence of physical exercise on aging rats. III. Life-long exercise modifies the aging changes of the mechanical properties of limb muscle tendons. *Mech. Ageing Dev.* **100**, 243–260.

180. Patterson-Kane, J.C., Wilson, A.M., Firth, E.C., Parry, D.A.D., and Goodship, A.E. (1997). Comparison of collagen fibril populations in the superficial digital flexor tendons of exercised and nonexercised thoroughbreds. *Equine Vet. J.* **29**, 121–125.

181. Patterson-Kane, J.C., Wilson, A.M., Firth, E.C., Parry, D.A.D., and Goodship, A.E. (1998). Exercise-related alterations in crimp morphology in the central regions of superficial digital flexor tendons from young Thoroughbreds: a controlled study. *Equine Vet. J.* **30**, 61–64.

182. Andriacchi, T., Sabiston, P., DeHaven, K., Dahners, L., Woo, S.L.-Y., Frank, C., *et al.* (1988). Ligament: injury and repair. In *Injury and repair of the muskuloskeletal soft tissues* (ed. S.L.-Y. Woo and J.A. Buckwalter), pp. 103–128. American Academy of Orthopaedic Surgeons, Park Ridge, Illinois.

183. Faryniarz, D.A., Chaponnier, C., Gabbiani, G., Yannas, I.V., and Spector, M. (1996). Myofibroblasts in the healing lapine medial

collateral ligament: possible mechanisms of contraction. *J. Orthop. Res.* **14**, 228–237.

184. Postacchini, F., Accinni, L., Natali, P.G., Ippolito, E., and de Martino, C. (1978). Regeneration of rabbit calcaneal tendon. *Cell Tissue Res.* **195**, 81–97.

185. Postacchini, F. and de Martino, C. (1980). Regeneration of rabbit calcaneal tendon maturation of collagen and elastic fibers following partial tenotomy. *Connect. Tissue Res.* **8**, 41–47.

186. Goldin, B., Block, W.D., and Pearson, J.R. (1980). Wound healing of tendon—i. physical, and mechanical and metabolic changes. *J. Biomech.* **13**, 241–256.

187. Lundborg, G., Hansson, H.-A., Rank, F., and Rydevik, B. (1980). Superficial repair of severed flexor tendons in synovial environment. *J. Hand Surg.* **5**, 451–461.

188. Gelberman, R.H., Manske, P.R., Vande Berg, J.S., Lesker, P.A., and Akeson, W.H. (1984). Flexor tendon repair *in vitro*: a comparative histologic study of the rabbit, chicken, dog, and and monkey. *J. Orthop. Res.* **2**, 39–48.

189. Potenza, A.D. (1963). Critical evaluation of flexor-tendon healing and adhesion formation within artificial digital sheaths. *J. Bone Joint Surg. (Am.)* **45A**, 1217–1233.

190. Manske, P.R. and Lesker, P.A. (1984). Histologic evidence of intrinsic flexor tendon repair in various experimental animals. *Clin. Orthop. Rel. Res.* **182**, 297–304.

191. Graham, M.F., Becker, H., Cohen, I.K., Merritt, W., and Diegelmann, R.F. (1984). Intrinsic tendon fibroplasia: documentation by *in vitro* studies. *J. Orthop. Res.* **1**, 251–256.

192. Williams, I.F., Heaton, A., and McCullagh, K.G. (1980). Cell morphology and collagen types in equine tendon scar. *Res. Vet. Sci.* **28**, 302–310.

193. Dexter, T.M. and White, H. (1990). Growth factors: growth without inflation. *Nature* **344**, 380–381.

194. Haralson, M.A. (1993). Extracellular matrix and growth factors: an integrated interplay controlling tissue repair and progression to disease. *Lab. Invest.* **69**, 369–372.

195. Gailit, J. and Clark, R.A.F. (1994). Wound repair in the context of extracellular matrix. *Curr. Opin. Cell Biol.* **6**, 717–725.

196. Chang, J., Most, D., Stelnicki, E., Longaker, M., Silberstein, F.C., Lineaweaver, C., *et al.* (1998). Gene expression of transforming growth factor β-1 in rabbit zone II flexor tendon wound healing: evidence for dual mechanisms of repair. *Plast. Reconstr. Surg.* **100**, 937–44.

197. Duffy, F.J., Seiler, J.G., Gelberman, R.H., and Hergrueter, C.A. (1995). Growth factors and canine flexor tendon healing: initial studies in uninjured and repair models. *J. Hand Surg.* **20A**, 645–649.

198. Natsu-ume, T., Nakamura, N., Shino, K., Toritsuka, Y., Horibe, S., Ochi T. (1997). Temporal and spatial expression of transforming growth factor-β in the healing patellar ligament of the rat. *J. Orthop. Res.* **15**, 837–843.

199. Chang, J., Most, D., Thunder, R., Mehrara, B., Longaker, M.T., and Lineaweaver, W.C. (1998). Molecular studies in flexor tendon wound healing: the role of basic fibroblast growth factor gene expression. *J. Hand Surg. (Am.)* **23A**, 1052–1058.

200. Lee, J., Harwood, F.L., Akeson, W.H., and Amiel, D. (1998). Growth factor expression in healing rabbit medial collateral and anterior cruciate ligaments. *Iowa Orthop. J.* **18**, 19–25.

201. Sciore, P., Boykiw, R., and Hart, D.A. (1998). Semiquantitative reverse transcription-polymerase chain reaction analysis of mRNA for growth factors and growth factor receptors from normal and healing rabbit medial collateral ligament tissue. *J. Orthop. Res.* **16**, 429–437.

202. Panossian, V., Liu, S.H., Lane, J.M., and Finerman, G.A.M. (1997). Fibroblast growth factor and epidermal growth factor receptors in ligament healing. *Clin. Orthop.* **342**, 173–180.

203. Watkins, J.P., Auer, J.A., Gay, S., and Morgan, S.J. (1985). Healing of surgically created defects in the equine superficial digital flexor tendon: collagen-type transformation and tissue morphologic reorganization. *Am. J. Vet. Res.* **46**, 2091–2096.

204. Amiel, D., Frank, C.B., Harwood, F.L., Akeson, W.H., and Kleiner, J.B. (1987). Collagen alteration in medial collateral ligament healing in a rabbit model. *Connect. Tiss. Res.* **16**, 357–366.

205. Frank, C., McDonald, D., and Shrive, N. (1997). Collagen fibril diameters in the rabbit medial collateral ligament scar: A longer term assessment. *Connect. Tissue Res.* **36**, 261–269.

206. Frank, C., McDonald, D., Wilson, J., Eyre, D., and Shrive, N. (1995). Rabbit medial collateral ligament scar weakness is associated with decreased collagen pyridinoline crosslink density. *J. Orthop. Res.* **13**, 157–165.

207. Boykiw, R., Sciore, P., Reno, C., Marchuk, L., Frank, C.B., and Hart, D.A. (1998). Altered levels of extracellular matrix molecule mRNA in healing rabbit ligaments. *Matrix Biol.* **17**, 371–378.

208. Lo, I.K.Y., Marchuk, L.L., Hart, D.A., and Frank, C.B. (1998). Comparison of mRNA levels for matrix molecules in normal and disrupted human anterior cruciate ligaments using reverse transcription polymerase chain reaction. *J. Orthop. Res.* **16**, 421–428.

209. Ågren, M.S., Taplin, C.J., Woessner, J.F. Jr., Eaglstein, W.H., and Mertz, P.M. (1992). Collagenase in wound healing: Effect of wound age and type. *J. Invest. Dermatol.* **99**, 709–714.

210. Girard, M.T., Matsubara, M., Kublin, C., Tessier, M.J., Cintron, C., and Fini, M.E. (1993). Stromal fibroblasts synthesize collagenase and stromelysin during long-term tissue remodelling. *J. Cell Sci.* **104**, 1001–1011.

211. Salo, T., Mäkelä, M., Kylmäniemi, M., Autio-Harmainen, H., and Larjava, H. (1994). Expression of matrix metalloproteinase-2 and -9 during early human wound healing. *Lab. Invest.* **70**, 176–182.

212. Wysocki, A.B., Staiano-Coico, L., and Grinnell, F. (1993). Wound fluid from chronic leg ulcers contains elevated levels of metalloproteinases MMP-2 and MMP-9. *J. Invest. Dermatol.* **101**, 64–68.

213. Grinnell, F., Ho, C.H., and Wysocki, A. (1992). Degradation of fibronectin and vitronectin in chronic wound fluid: analysis by cell blotting, immunoblotting, and cell adhesion assays. *J. Invest. Dermatol.* **98**, 410–416.

214. Gotoh, M., Hamada, K., Yamakawa, H., Tomonaga, A., Inoue, A., and Fukuda, H.O. (1997). Significance of granulation tissue in torn supraspinatus insertions: an immunohistochemical study with antibodies against interleukin-1β, cathepsin, D., and matrix metalloprotease-1. *J. Orthop. Res.* **15**, 33–39.

215. Stehno-Bittel, L., Reddy, G.K., Gum, S., and Enwemeka, C.S. (1998). Biochemistry and biomechanics of healing tendon: Part I. Effects of rigid plaster casts and functional casts. *Med. Sci. Sports Exer.* **30**, 788–793.

216. Wiig, M., Hanff, G., Abrahamsson, S.-O., and Lohmander, L.S. (1997). Division of flexor tendons causes progressive degradation of tendon matrix in rabbits. *Acta Orthop. Scand.* **67**, 491–497.

217. Murrell, G.A.C. (1994). Effects of immobilization on Achilles tendon healing in a rat model. *J. Orthop. Res.* **12**, 582–591.

218. Slack, C., Flint, M.H., and Thompson, B.M. (1984). The effect of tensional load on isolated embryonic chick tendon cells in organ culture. *Connect. Tissue Res.* **12**, 229–247.

219. Mass, D.P., Tuel, R.J., Labarbera, M., and Greenwald, D.P. (1993). Effects of constant mechanical tension on the healing of rabbit flexor tendons. *Clin. Orthop.* **296**, 301–6.

220. Tanaka, H., Manske, P.R., Pruitt, D.L., and Larson, B.J. (1995). Effect of cyclic tension on lacerated flexor tendons *in vitro*. *J. Hand Surg. (Am.)* **20A**, 467–473.

221. Iwuagwu, F.C. and McGrouther, D.A. (1998). Early cellular response in tendon injury: the effect of loading. *Plast. Reconstr. Surg.* **102**, 2064–2071.

222. Woo, S.L., Gelberman, R.H., Cobb, N.G., Amiel, D., Lothringer, K., and Akeson W.H. (1981). The importance of controlled passive mobilization on flexor tendon healing. A biomechanical study. *Acta Orthop. Scand.* **52**, 615–622.

223. Gelberman, R.H., Woo, S.L., Lothringer, K., Akeson, W.H., and Amiel, D. (1982). Effects of early intermittent passive mobilization on healing canine flexor tendons. *J. Hand Surg. (Am.)* **7A**, 170–175.

224. Baktir, A., Türk, C.Y., Kabak, S., Sahin, V., and Kardas, Y. (1996). Flexor tendon repair in zone 2 followed by early active mobilization. *J. Hand Surg. (Br.)* **21B**, 624–628.

225. Bainbridge, L.C., Robertson, C., Gillies, D., and Elliot, D. (1994). A comparison of post-operative mobilization of flexor tendon repairs with 'passive flexion-active extension' and 'controlled active motion' techniques. *J. Hand Surg. (Br.)* **19B**, 517–521.

226. Eastwood, M., Mudera, V.C., McGrouther, D.A., and Brown, R.A. (1998). Effect of precise mechanical loading on fibroblast populated collagen lattices: morphological changes. *Cell Motil. Cytoskeleton* **40**, 13–21.

227. Forslund, C. and Aspenberg, P. (2001). Tendon healing stimulated by injected CDMP-2. *Med. Sci. Sports Exerc.* **33**, 685–687.

228. Aspenberg, P. and Forslund, C. (1999). Enhanced tendon healing with GDF 5 and 6. *Acta Orthop. Scand.* **70**, 51–54.

229. Rodeo, S.A., Suzuki, K., Deng, X.H., Wozney, J., and Warren RF. (1999). Use of recombinant human bone morphogenetic protein-2 to enhance tendon healing in a bone tunnel. *Am. J. Sports Med.* **27**, 476–488.

230. Batten, M.L., Hansen, J.C., and Dahners, L.E. (1996). Influence of dosage and timing of application of platelet-derived growth factor on early healing of the rat medial collateral ligament. *J. Orthop. Res.* **14**, 736–741.

231. Hildebrand, K.A., Woo, S.L., Smith, D.W., Allen, C.R., Deie, M., Taylor, B.J., *et al.* (1998). The effects of platelet-derived growth factor-BB on healing of the rabbit medial collateral ligament. An *in vivo* study. *Am. J. Sports Med.* **26**, 549–554.

232. Letson, A.K. and Dahners L.E. (1994). The effect of combinations of growth factors on ligament healing. *Clin. Orthop.* **308**, 207–212.

233. Kobayashi, D., Kurosaka, M., Yoshiya, S., and Mizuno, K. (1997). Effect of basic fibroblast growth factor on the healing of defects in the canine anterior cruciate ligament. *Knee Surg. Sports Traumatol. Arthrosc.* **5**, 189–194.

234. Woo, S.L., Hildebrand, K., Watanabe, N., Fenwick, J.A., Papageorgiou, C.D., and Wang, J.H. (1999). Tissue engineering of ligament and tendon healing. *Clin. Orthop.* S312–S323.

235. Almekinders L.C. (1990). The efficacy of nonsteroidal anti-inflammatory drugs in the treatment of ligament injuries. *Sports Med.* **9**, 137–142.

236. Almekinders, L.C. and Almekinders, S.V. (1994). Outcome in the treatment of chronic overuse sports injuries: a retrospective study. *J. Orthop. Sports Phys. Ther.* **19**, 157–161.

237. Almekinders, L.C. and Temple, J.D. (1998). Etiology, diagnosis, and treatment of tendonitis: an analysis of the literature. *Med. Sci. Sports Exerc.* **30**, 1183–1190.

238. Vane, J.R. (1971). Inhibition of prostaglandin synthesis as a mechanism of action for aspirin-like drugs. *Nature* **23**, 232–235.

239. Carlstedt, C.A. (1987). Mechanical and chemical factors in tendon healing. *Acta Orthop. Scand.* **58** (suppl. 224), 7–75.

240. Kulick, M.I., Smith, S., and Hadler, K. (1986). Oral ibuprofen: evaluation of its effect on peritendinous adhesions and the breaking strength of a tenorrhaphy. *J. Hand Surg. (Am.)* **11A**, 110–120.

241. Thomas, J.T., Taylor, D., Crowell, R., and Assor, D. (1991). The effect of indomethacin on Achilles tendon healing in rabbits. *Clin. Orthop. Rel. Res.* **272**, 308–311.

242. Vogel, H.G. (1977). Mechanical and chemical properties of various connective tissue organs in rats as influenced by non-steroidal antirheumatic drugs. *Connect. Tissue Res.* **5**, 91–95.

243. Carlstedt, C.A., Madsen, K., and Wredmark, T. (1986). The influence of indomethacin on collagen synthesis during tendon healing in the rabbit. *Prostaglandins* **32**, 353–358.

244. Riley, G.P., Cox, M., Harrall, R.L., Clements, S., and Hazleman, B.L. (2001). Inhibition of tendon cell proliferation and matrix glycosaminoglycan synthesis by non-steroidal anti-inflammatory drugs *in vitro*. *J. Hand Surg. (Br.)* **26B**, 224–228.

245. Rolf, C., Movin, T., Engstrom, B., Jacobs, L.D., Beauchard, C., and Le Liboux, A. (1997). An open, randomized study of ketoprofen in patients in surgery for Achilles or patellar tendinopathy. *J. Rheumatol.* **24**, 1595–1598.

246. Alfredson, H., Thorsen, K., and Lorentzon, R. (1999). *In situ* microdialysis in tendon tissue: high levels of glutamate, but not prostaglandin E2 in chronic Achilles tendon pain. *Knee Surg. Sports Traumatol. Arthrosc.* **7**, 378–381.

247. Alfredson, H., Ljung, B.O., Thorsen, K., and Lorentzon, R. (2000). *In vivo* investigation of ECRB tendons with microdialysis technique—no signs of inflammation but high amounts of glutamate in tennis elbow. *Acta Orthop. Scand.* **71**, 475–479.

248. Alfredson, H., Forsgren, S., Thorsen, K., and Lorentzon, R. (2001). *In vivo* microdialysis and immunohistochemical analyses of tendon tissue demonstrated high amounts of free glutamate and glutamate NMDAR1 receptors, but no signs of inflammation, in jumper's knee. *J. Orthop. Res.* **19**, 881–886.

249. Haines, J.F. (1983). Bilateral rupture of the Achilles tendon in patients on steroid therapy. *Ann. Rheum. Dis.* **42**, 652–654.

250. Potasman, I. and Bassan, H.M. (1984). Multiple tendon rupture in systemic lupus erythematosus: Case report and review of the literature. *Ann. Rheum. Dis.* **43**, 347–349.

251. Newnham, D.M., Douglas, J.G., Legge, J.S., and Friend, J.A. (1991). Achilles tendon rupture: an underrated complication of corticosteroid treatment. *Thorax* **46**, 853–854.

252. Kotnis, R.A., Halstead, J.C., and Hormbrey, P.J. (1999). Atraumatic bilateral Achilles tendon rupture: An association of systemic steroid treatment. *J. Accid. Emerg. Med.* **16**, 378–379.

253. Clark, S.C., Jones, M.W., Choudhury, R.R., and Smith, E. (1995). Bilateral patellar tendon rupture secondary to repeated local steroid injections. *J. Accid. Emerg. Med.* **12**, 300–301.

254. Smith, A.G., Kosygan, K., Williams, H., and Newman, R.J. (1999). Common extensor tendon rupture following corticosteroid injection for lateral tendinosis of the elbow. *Br. J. Sports Med.* **33**, 423–424.

255. Shrier, I., Matheson, G.O., and Kohl, H.W., III. (1996). Achilles tendonitis: are corticosteroid injections useful or harmful? *Clin. J. Sport Med.* **6**, 245–250.

256. Martin, D.F., Carlson, C.S., Berry, J., Reboussin, B.A., Gordon, E.S., and Smith, B.P. (1999). Effect of injected versus iontophoretic corticosteroid on the rabbit tendon. *South. Med. J.* **92**, 600–608.

257. Oxlund, H. (1984). Changes in connective tisssues during corticotrophin and corticosteroid treatment. *Dan. Med. Bull.* **31**, 187–206.

258. McWhorter, J.W., Francis, R.S., and Heckmann, R.A. (1991). Influence of local steroid injections on traumatized tendon properties. A biomechanical and histological study. *Am. J. Sports Med.* **19**, 435–439.

259. Tillander, B., Franzen, L.E., Karlsson, M.H., and Norlin, R. (1999). Effect of steroid injections on the rotator cuff: an experimental study in rats. *J. Shoulder. Elbow. Surg.* **8**, 271–274.

260. Campbell, R.B., Wiggins, M.E., Cannistra, L.M., Fadale, P.D., and Akelman, E. (1996). Influence of steroid injection on ligament healing in the rat. *Clin. Orthop.* 242–253.

261. Wiggins, M.E., Fadale, P.D., Barrach, H., Ehrlich, M.G., and Walsh, W.R. (1994). Healing characteristics of a type I collagenous structure treated with corticosteroids. *Am. J. Sports Med.* **22**, 279–288.

262. Wiggins, M.E., Fadale, P.D., Ehrlich, M.G., and Walsh, W.R. (1995). Effects of local injection of corticosteroids on the healing of ligaments. A follow-up report. *J. Bone Joint Surg. (Am.)* **77A**, 1682–1691.

263. Laseter, J.T. and Russell, J.A. (1991). Anabolic steroid-induced tendon pathology: a review of the literature. *Med. Sci. Sports Exerc.* **23**, 1–3.

264. Visuri, T. and Lindholm, H. (1994). Bilateral distal biceps tendon avulsions with use of anabolic steroids. *Med. Sci. Sports Exerc.* **26**, 941–944.

265. Freeman, B.J. and Rooker, G.D. (1995). Spontaneous rupture of the anterior cruciate ligament after anabolic steroids. *Br. J. Sports Med.* **29**, 274–275.

266. Michna, H. (1986). Organisation of collagen fibrils in tendon: changes induced by an anabolic steroid. I. Functional and ultrastructural studies. *Virchows Arch. B Cell Pathol. Incl. Mol. Pathol.* **52**, 75–86.

267. Miles, J.W., Grana, W.A., Egle, D., Min, K.-W., and Chitwood, J. (1992). The effect of anabolic steroids on the biomechanical and histological properties of rat tendon. *J. Bone Joint Surg. (Am.)* **74A**, 411–422.

268. Evans, N.A., Bowrey, D.J., and Newman, G.R. (1998). Ultrastructural analysis of ruptured tendon from anabolic steroid users. *Injury* **29**, 769–773.

269. Parssinen, M., Karila, T., Kovanen, V., and Seppala, T. (2000). The effect of supraphysiological doses of anabolic androgenic steroids on collagen metabolism. *Int. J. Sports Med.* **21**, 406–411.

270. Taylor, D.C., Brooks, D.E., and Ryan, J.B. (1999). Anabolic–androgenic steroid administration causes hypertrophy of immobilized and nonimmobilized skeletal muscle in a sedentary rabbit model. *Am. J. Sports Med.* **27**, 718–727.

271. Karpakka, J.A., Pesola, M.K., and Takala, T.E. (1992). The effects of anabolic steroids on collagen synthesis in rat skeletal muscle and tendon. A preliminary report. *Am. J. Sports Med.* **20**, 262–266.

272. Inhofe, P.D., Grana, W.A., Egle, D., Min, K.W., and Tomasek, J. (1995). The effects of anabolic steroids on rat tendon. An ultrastructural, biomechanical, and biochemical analysis. *Am. J. Sports Med.* **23**, 227–232.

273. Wood, T.O., Cooke, P.H., and Goodship, A.E. (1988). The effect of exercise and anabolic steroids on the mechanical properties and crimp morphology of the rat tendon. *Am. J. Sports Med.* **16**, 153–158.

274. Mottram, D.R. and George, A.J. (2000). Anabolic steroids. *Baillièr's Best. Pract. Res. Clin. Endocrinol. Metab.* **14**, 55–69.

275. Greenwald, D., Mass, D., Gottlieb, L., and Tuel, R. (1991). Biomechanical analysis of intrinsic tendon healing *in vitro* and the effects of vitamins A and E. *Plast. Reconstr. Surg.* **87**, 925–930.

276. Cleary, S.F., Li-Ming, L., Graham, R., and Diegelman, R.F. (1988). Modulation of tendon fibroplasia by exogenous currents. *Bioelectromagnetics* **9**, 183–194.

277. Fujita, M., Hukuda, S., and Doida, Y. (1992). The effect of constant direct electrical current on intrinsic healing in the flexor tendon *in vitro*. An ultrastructural study of differing attitudes in epitenon cells and tenocytes. *J. Hand Surg. (Br.)* **17B**, 94–98.

278. Williams, I.F., Nicholls, J.S., Goodship, A.E., and Silver, I.A. (1986). Experimental treatment of tendon injury with heparin. *Br. J. Plast. Surg.* **39**, 367–372.

279. Akermark, C., Crone, H., Elsasser, U., and Forsskahl, B. (1995). Glycosaminoglycan polysulfate injections in lateral humeral epicondylalgia: a placebo-controlled double-blind trial. *Int. J. Sports Med.* **16**, 196–200.

280. Wiig, M., Abrahamsson, S.O., and Lundborg, G. (1996). Effects of hyaluronan on cell proliferation and collagen synthesis: a study of rabbit flexor tendons *in vitro*. *J. Hand Surg. (Am.)* **21A**, 599–604.

281. Wiig, M., Abrahamsson, S.O., and Lundborg, G. (1997). Tendon repair—cellular activities in rabbit deep flexor tendons and surrounding synovial sheaths and the effects of hyaluronan: an experimental study *in vivo* and *in vitro*. *J. Hand Surg. (Am.)* **22A**, 818–825.

282. Komurcu, M., Akkus, O., Basbozkurt, M., Gur, E., and Akkas, N. (1997). Reduction of restrictive adhesions by local aprotinin application and primary sheath repair in surgically traumatized flexor tendons of the rabbit. *J. Hand Surg. (Am.)* **22A**, 826–832.

283. Akali, A., Khan, U., Khaw, P.T., and McGrouther, A.D. (1999). Decrease in adhesion formation by a single application of 5-fluorouracil after flexor tendon injury. *Plast. Reconstr. Surg.* **103**, 151–158.

284. Reddy, G.K., Stehno-Bittel, L., and Enwemeka, C.S. (1998). Laser photostimulation of collagen production in healing rabbit Achilles tendons. *Lasers Surg. Med.* **22**, 281–287.

285. Reddy, G.K., Gum, S., Stehno-Bittel, L., and Enwemeka, C.S. (1998). Biochemistry and biomechanics of healing tendon: Part II. Effects of combined laser therapy and electrical stimulation. *Med. Sci. Sports Exerc.* **30**, 794–800.

286. Gum, S.L., Reddy, G.K., Stehno-Bittel, L., and Enwemeka, C.S. (1997). Combined ultrasound, electrical stimulation, and laser promote collagen synthesis with moderate changes in tendon biomechanics. *Am. J. Phys. Med. Rehabil.* **76**, 288–296.

287. Enwemeka, C.S. (1989). The effects of therapeutic ultrasound on tendon healing. A biomechanical study. *Am. J. Phys. Med. Rehabil.* **68**, 283–287.

288. Stevenson, J.H., Pang, C.Y., Lindsay, W.K., and Zuker, R.M. (1986). Functional, mechanical, and biochemical assessment of ultrasound therapy on tendon healing in the chicken toe. *Plast. Reconstr. Surg.* **77**, 965–972.

289. Turner, S.M., Powell, E.S., and Ng, C.S. (1989). The effect of ultrasound on the healing of repaired cockerel tendon: is collagen cross-linkage a factor? *J. Hand Surg. (Br.)* **14B**, 428–433.

290. Fritze, J. (1998). [Extracorporeal shockwave therapy (ESWT) in orthopedic indications: a selective review.] *Versicherungsmedizin* **50**, 180–185.

291. Speed, C.A. and Hazleman, B.L. (1999). Calcific tendinitis of the shoulder. *New Engl. J. Med.* **340**, 1582–1584.

292. Haake, M., Sattler, A., Gross, M.W., Schmitt, J., Hildebrandt, R., and Muller, H.H. (2001). [Comparison of extracorporeal shockwave therapy (ESWT) with roentgen irradiation in supraspinatus tendon syndrome—a prospective randomized single-blind parallel group comparison.] *Z. Orthop. Ihre Grenzgeb.* **139**, 397–402.

293. Orhan, Z., Alper, M., Akman, Y., Yavuz, O., and Yalciner, A. (2001). An experimental study on the application of extracorporeal shock waves in the treatment of tendon injuries: preliminary report. *J. Orthop. Sci.* **6**, 566–570.

294. Rompe, J.D., Kirkpatrick, C.J., Kullmer, K., Schwitalle, M., and Krischek, O. (1998). Dose-related effects of shock waves on rabbit tendo Achillis. A sonographic and histological study. *J. Bone Joint Surg. (Br.)* **80B**, 546–552.

295. Huang, H.H., Qureshi, A.A., and Biundo, J.J., Jr. (2000). Sports and other soft tissue injuries, tendinitis, bursitis, and occupation-related syndromes. *Curr. Opin. Rheumatol.* **12**, 150–154.

296. Maffulli, N., Khan, K.M., and Puddu, G. (1998). Overuse tendon conditions: time to change a confusing terminology. *Arthroscopy* **14**, 840–843.

297. Kannus, P. (1997). Etiology and pathophysiology of chronic tendon disorders in sports. *Scand. J. Med. Sci. Sports* **7**, 78–85.

298. Józsa, L. and Kannus, P. (1997). Overuse injuries of tendons. *Human tendons: anatomy, physiology and pathology* (ed. L. Józsa and P. Kannus), pp. 164–253. Human Kinetics, Champaign, Illinois.

299. Józsa, L. and Kannus, P. (1997). Spontaneous rupture of tendons. In *Human tendons: anatomy, physiology and pathology* (ed. L. Józsa and P. Kannus), pp. 254–325. Human Kinetics, Champaign, Illinois.

300. Waterston, S.W., Maffulli, N., and Ewen, S.W.B. (1997). Subcutaneous rupture of the Achilles tendon: basic science and some aspects of clinical practice. *Br. J. Sports Med.* **31**, 285–298.

301. Teitz, C.C., Garrett, W.E., Miniaci, A., Lee, M.H., and Mann, R.A. (1997). Tendon problems in athletic individuals. *J. Bone Joint Surg. (Am.)* **79A**, 138–152.

302. Rathbun, J.B. and MacNab, I. (1970). The microvascular pattern of rotator cuff. *J. Bone Joint Surg. (Am.)* **52A**, 540–553.

303. Brooks, C.H., Revell, W.J., and Heatley, F.W. (1992). A quantitative histological study of the vascularity of the rotator cuff tendon. *J. Bone Joint Surg. (Br.)* **74B**, 151–153.

304. Ahmed, I.M., Lagopoulos, M., McConnell, P., Soames, R.W., and Sefton, G.K. (1998). Blood supply of the Achilles tendon. *J. Orthop. Res.* **16**, 591–596.

305. Astrom, M. and Westlin, N. (1994). Blood-flow in chronic Achilles tendinopathy. *Clin. Orthop. Rel. Res.* **308**, 166–172.

306. Kannus, P. and Józsa, L. (1991). Histopathological changes preceding spontaneous rupture of a tendon. *J. Bone Joint Surg. (Am.)* **73A**, 1507–1525.

307. Nirschl, R.P. and Pettrone, F.A. (1973). Tennis elbow. *J. Bone Joint Surg. (Am.)* **61A**, 832–839.

308. Stanish, W.O., Curwin, S., and Mandel, S. (2000). *Tendinitisi its etiology and treatment.* Oxford University Press, New York.

309. Leadbetter, W.B. (1992). Cell–matrix response in tendon injury. *Clin. Sports Med.* **11**, 533–578.

310. Wilson, A.M. and Goodship, A.E. (1994). Exercise-induced hyperthermia as a possible mechanism for tendon degeneration. *J. Biomech.* **27**, 899–905.

311. Sanchis-Alfonso, V., Rosello-Sastre, E., and Subias-Lopez, A. (2001). Neuroanatomic basis for pain in patellar tendinosis ('jumper's knee'): a neuroimmunohistochemical study. *Am. J. Knee Surg.* **14**, 174–177.

312. Alfredson, H., Forsgren, S., Thorsen, K., Fahlstrom, M., Johansson, H., and Lorentzon, R. (2001). Glutamate NMDAR1 receptors localised to nerves in human Achilles tendons. Implications for treatment? *Knee Surg. Sports Traumatol. Arthrosc.* **9**, 123–126.

313. Gotoh, M., Hamada, K., Yamakawa, H., Inoue, A., and Fukuda, H. (1998). Increased substance P in subacromial bursa and shoulder pain in rotator cuff diseases. *J. Orthop. Res.* **16**, 618–621.

314. O'Byrne, E.M., Blancuzzi, V., Wilson, D.E., Wong, M., and Jeng, A.Y. (1990). Elevated substance P and accelerated cartilage degradation in rabbit knees injected with interleukin-1 and tumor necrosis factor. *Arthritis Rheum.* **33**, 1023–1028.

315. Garrett, N.E., Mapp, P.I., Cruwys, S.C., Kidd, B.L., and Blake, D.R. (1992). Role of substance P in inflammatory arthritis. *Ann. Rheum. Dis.* **51**, 1014–1018.

316. Hart, D.A., Kydd, A., and Reno, C. (1999). Gender and pregnancy affect neuropeptide responses of the rabbit Achilles tendon. *Clin. Orthop.* **365**, 237–246.

317. Hart, D.A., Archambault, J.M., Kydd, A., Reno, C., Frank, C.B., and Herzog, W. (1998). Gender and neurogenic variables in tendon biology and repetitive motion disorders. *Clin. Orthop.* **351**, 44–56.

318. Hart, D.A., Frank, C.B., and Bray, R.C. (1995). Inflammatory processes in repetitive motion and overuse syndromes: potential role of neurogenic mechanisms in tendons and ligaments. In *Repetitive motion disorders of the upper extremity* (ed. S.L. Gordon, S.J. Blair, and L.J. Fine), pp. 247–262. American Association of Orthopaedic Surgeons, Rosemount, Illinois.

319. Hart, D.A. and Reno, C. (1998). Pregnancy alters the *in vitro* responsiveness of the rabbit medial collateral ligament to neuropeptides: effect on mRNA levels for growth factors, cytokines, iNOS, COX-2, metalloproteinases and TIMPs. *Biochim. Biophys. Acta Mol. Basis Dis.* **1408**, 35–43.

320. Khan, K.M., Cook, J.L., Bonar, F., Harcourt, P., and Astrom, M. (1999). Histopathology of common tendinopathies—Update and implications for clinical management. *Sports Med.* **27**, 393–408.

321. Chard, M.D., Cawston, T.E., Riley, G.P., Gresham, A., and Hazleman, B.L. (1994). Rotator cuff degeneration and lateral epicondylitis: a comparative histological study. *Ann. Rheum. Dis.* **53**, 30–34.

322. Codman, E.A. (1934). *The shoulder.* Todd Co., Boston, Massachusetts.

323. Sano, H., Uhthoff, H.K., Backman, D.S., Brunet, J.A., Trudel, G., Pham, B., *et al.* (1998). Structural disorders at the insertion of the supraspinatus tendon. Relation to tensile strength. *J. Bone Joint Surg. (Br.)* **80B**, 720–725.

324. King, J.B., Cook, J.L., Khan, K.M., and Maffulli, N. (2000). Patellar tendinopathy. *Sports Med. Arthrosc. Rev.* **8**, 86–95.

325. Maffulli, N., Barrass, V., and Ewen, S.W. (2000). Light microscopic histology of Achilles tendon ruptures. A comparison with unruptured tendons. *Am. J. Sports Med.* **28**, 857–863.

326. Sano, H., Ishii, H., Yeadon, A., Backman, D.S., Brunet, J.A., and Uhthoff, H.K. (1997). Degeneration at the insertion weakens the tensile strength of the supraspinatus tendon: a comparative mechanical and histologic study of the bone-tendon complex. *J. Orthop. Res.* **15**, 719–726.

327. Sano, H., Ishii, H., Trudel, G., and Uhthoff, H.K. (1999). Histologic evidence of degeneration at the insertion of 3 rotator cuff tendons: a comparative study with human cadaveric shoulders. *J. Shoulder Elbow Surg.* **8**, 574–579.

328. Fukuda, H., Hamada, K., and Yamanaka, K. (1990). Pathology and pathogenesis of bursal-side rotator cuff tears viewed from *en bloc* histologic sections. *Clin. Orthop.* **254**, 75–80.

329. Puddu, G., Ippolito, E., and Postacchini, F. (1976). A classification of Achilles tendon disease. *Am. J. Sports Med.* **4**, 145–150.

330. Mosier, S.M., Pomeroy, G., and Manoli, A. (1999). Pathoanatomy and etiology of posterior tibial tendon dysfunction. *Clin. Orthop. Rel. Res.* **365**, 12–22.

331. Tallon, C., Maffulli, N., and Ewen, S.W. (2001). Ruptured Achilles tendons are significantly more degenerated than tendinopathic tendons. *Med. Sci. Sports Exerc.* **33**, 1983–1990.

332. Movin, T., Gad, A., Reinholt, P., and Rolf, C. (1997). Tendon pathology in long-standing achillodynia—biopsy findings in 40 patients. *Acta Orthop. Scand.* **68**, 170–175.

333. Myerson, M.S. and McGarvey, W. (1998). Disorders of the insertion of the Achilles tendon and Achilles tendinitis. *J. Bone Joint Surg. (Am.)* **80A**, 1814–1824.

334. Rufai, A., Ralphs, J.R., and Benjamin, M. (1995). Structure and histopathology of the insertional region of the human achilles tendon. *J. Orthop. Res.* **13**, 585–593.

335. Benjamin, M., Rufai, A., and Ralphs, J.R. (2000). The mechanism of formation of bony spurs (enthesophytes) in the achilles tendon. *Arthritis Rheum.* **43**, 576–583.

336. Astrom, M. and Rausing, A. (1995). Chronic Achilles tendinopathy. A survey of surgical and histopathologic findings. *Clin. Orthop.* **316**, 151–164.

337. Uhthoff, H.K., Sarkar, K., and Maynard, J.A. (1976). Calcifying tendinitis. *Clin. Orthop. Rel. Res.* **118**, 164–168.

338. Archer, R.S., Bayley, J.I.L., Archer, C.W., and Ali, S.Y. (1993). Cell and matrix changes associated with pathological calcification of the human rotator cuff tendons. *J. Anat.* **182**, 1–12.

339. Uhthoff, H.K. and Sarkar, K. (1991). Classification and definition of tendinopathies. *Clin. Sports Med.* **10**, 707–720.

340. Rooney, P. (1994). Intratendinous ossification. In *Mechanisms of development and growth* (ed. B.K. Hall), pp. 47–84. CRC Press, Boca Raton, Florida.

341. Rooney, P., Grant, M.E., and McClure, J. (1992). Endochondral ossification and *de novo* collagen synthesis during repair of the rat achilles tendon. *Matrix* **12**, 274–281.

342. Rooney, P., Walker, D., Grant, M.E., and McClure, J. (1993). Cartilage and bone formation in repairing Achilles tendons within diffusion chambers: evidence for tendon–cartilage and cartilage–bone conversion *in vivo*. *J. Pathol.* **169**, 375–381.

343. Fenwick, S.A., Curry, V., Harrall, R.L., Hazleman, B.L., and Riley, G.P. (2002). Endochondral ossification in Achilles and patella tendinopathy. *Rheumatology*, in press.

344. Silver, I.A., Brown, P.N., Goodship, A.E., Lanyon, L.E., McCullagh, K.G., Perry, G.C., *et al.* (1983). A clinical and experimental study of tendon injury, healing and treatment in the horse. *Equine Vet. J.* (Suppl. 1), 1–24.

345. Williams, R.J., III, Attia, E., Wickiewicz, T.L., and Hannafin, J.A. (2000). The effect of ciprofloxacin on tendon, paratenon, and capsular fibroblast metabolism. *Am. J Sports Med.* **28**, 364–369.

346. Corps, A.N., Harrall, R.L., Curry, V., Hazleman, B.L., and Riley, G.P. (2002). Ciprofloxacin enhances the stimulation of matrix metalloproteinase-3 expression by interleukin-1β in human tendon derived cells. *Arthritis Rheum.* **46**(11), 3034–3040.

347. Ireland, D., Harrall, R.L., Holloway, G., Hackney, R., Hazleman, B., and Riley, G. (2001). Multiple changes in gene expression in chronic human Achilles tendinopathy. *Matrix Biol.* **20**, 159–169.

348. Fenwick, S.A., Curry, V., Harrall, R.L., Hazleman, B.L., Hackney, R., and Riley, G.P. (2001). Expression of transforming growth factor-beta isoforms and their receptors in chronic tendinosis. *J. Anat.* **199**, 231–240.

349. Movin, T., Guntner, P., Gad, A., and Rolf, C. (1997). Ultrasonography-guided percutaneous core biopsy in Achilles tendon disorder. *Scand. J. Med. Sci. Sports* **7**, 244–248.

350. Young, R.G., Butler, D.L., Weber, W., Caplan, A.I., Gordon, S.L., and Fink, D.J. (1998). Use of mesenchymal stem cells in a collagen matrix for Achilles tendon repair. *J. Orthop. Res.* **16**, 406–413.

1.4 The intervertebral disc—structure, composition, and pathology

Victor Duance and Sally Roberts

Introduction

The spine is a complex structure comprised of vertebrae, muscles and ligaments that combine to provide both strength and flexibility. To enable extension, flexion, lateral bending, and rotation each vertebral body is interposed with a soft deformable tissue, the intervertebral disc.[1] There are 24 intervertebral discs in the human spine, 7 in the cervical, 12 in the thoracic, and 5 in the lumbar regions (Fig. 1). The overall function of the intervertebral discs is to absorb and dissipate the high compressive and torsional forces experienced by the spine without compromising its flexibility.

In this chapter we will concentrate on the intervertebral disc, focusing on the recent advances to our knowledge of the structure and biochemical composition and how this changes in pathological conditions. Back pain remains one of the most prevalent disabling conditions in the Western world and is a significant public health and socio-economic issue.[3] In the United Kingdom alone, the total cost (including benefits, compensation, and lost production) is estimated at approximately 11 billion pounds per annum.[4]

Back pain encompasses many tissues associated with the spine[3] but degeneration of the intervertebral disc is thought to be directly or indirectly responsible in the majority of cases. Clearly a better understanding of intervertebral disc biology and its changes with age and disease is an important area of future research that could result in major benefits to society in the coming decades.

Structure of the intervertebral disc

The intervertebral disc can be divided into three anatomically distinct areas: the outer region that is the annulus fibrosus; the central nucleus pulposus; and the cartilaginous endplates on the superior and inferior surfaces (Fig. 2(a), (b)). The discs are attached to the adjacent vertebrae via both the annulus fibrosus and the cartilage endplates. Each region is described more fully below.

Annulus fibrosus

The annulus fibrosus can be considered as the outer shell of the disc. It is composed of 10–20 concentrically arranged lamellae of parallel bundles of collagen fibres (Fig. 2(c)).[5] X-ray diffraction studies have shown that each lamella is orientated at approximately 65° to the spinal axis with the inclination alternating in adjacent lamellae to the left and right of the axis (see Fig. 3).[8–10]

The collagen fibres in the periphery merge with the periosteum of the adjacent vertebrae and ligaments whereas centrally they intercalate with the cartilage endplate.[11, 12] The annulus fibrosus has been further subdivided into an inner and outer portion, which differ both

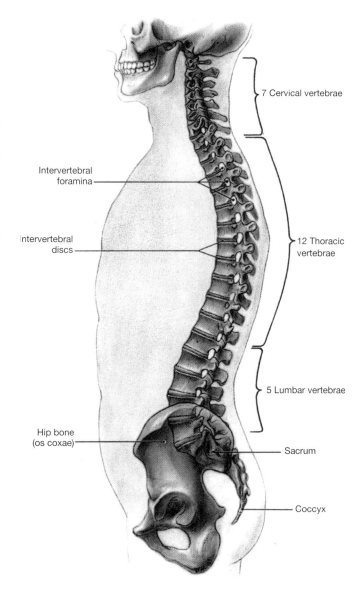

Fig. 1 Lateral view of the vertebral column showing the 24 vertebrae and the intervertebral discs. (Adapted from reference 2.)

morphologically and biochemically.[1] The outer annulus is more fibrous in nature and functions primarily to withstand tensional forces.[13, 14] The inner annulus is fibrocartilaginous and functions more to withstand compressive forces forming an interface with the central nucleus pulposus.[6]

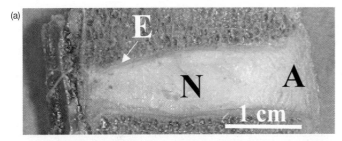

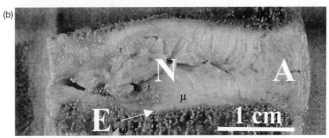

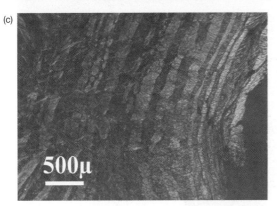

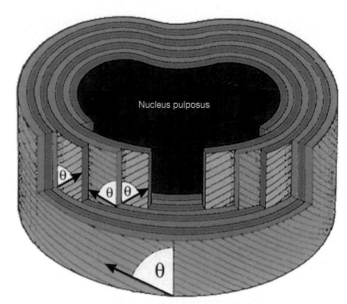

Fig. 3 Diagram showing the lamellae structure of collagen fibres in the annulus fibrosus. The lamellae are inclined to the long axis of the vertebral column by the angle θ. The inclination alternates to the left and right of the long axis in adjacent lamellae. (Adapted from reference 6 by A Hayes.[7])

Fig. 2 Intervertebral discs from the lumbar region of (a) a 17-year-old male and (b) an 82-year-old female cut in the sagittal plane to demonstrate the central nucleus pulposus (N) and outer annulus fibrosus (A) with the thin cartilage endplates (E) at the interface of the disc and vertebral body. (c) The organization of the collagen bundles within the annular lamellae can be visualized clearly with polarized light.

Nucleus pulposus

The nucleus pulposus is a highly hydrated gel-like structure being rich in proteoglycans and containing relatively few collagen fibres.[15] Although it exists as a discrete entity in the young, with age the interface with the inner annulus merges. The nucleus pulposus acts to dissipate compressive loads radially to the annulus fibrosus and axially to the cartilage endplates. Embryologically the nucleus pulposus is derived from the notochord but with age it becomes increasingly populated with chondrocytic cells resembling those of the inner annulus resulting in an increased collagen content and altered biomechanical properties.[16–19]

Cartilaginous endplates

The cartilage endplates are composed of hyaline cartilage and are located on the superior and inferior surfaces of the disc, merging peripherally with the annulus and thus essentially encapsulating the nucleus pulposus.[20] Although the endplates are derived from the vertebral body, they are usually considered as part of the disc because

of the strong attachments to the inner annulus and nucleus pulposus and because they act with the other components of the disc to dissipate loads.[15, 21] They are important shock absorbers protecting the vertebral body from axial loads and preventing the nucleus from bulging into the vertebral body. They are also important for disc nutrition. The disc is the largest avascular organ in the body and the major route of nutrition for the disc is through the cartilage endplates.[22, 23]

Extracellular matrix components of the intervertebral disc

Over the past 20 years there have been considerable advances in our knowledge of the extracellular matrix (ECM) of many tissues including the intervertebral disc.[24–31] The major constituents are collagen, proteoglycan, matrix glycoproteins, and water. The collagens and proteoglycans are the principal components conferring the mechanical properties to the tissue. The fibrous collagen network provides the necessary tensile component, whilst the proteoglycans retain the water necessary for the disc to withstand compressive forces. Less is known regarding the matrix glycoproteins of the disc but in other tissues they function as mediators of interactions between matrix components and connective tissue cells and are therefore important in matrix organization and integrity. Details of these individual constituents are given below.

Collagens of the intervertebral disc

Collagen is a major component of the intervertebral disc comprising over 50 per cent of the dry weight of the annulus fibrosus and 15–20 per cent of the nucleus pulposus.[32] It had been known for some time that the intervertebral disc is composed of more than a single collagen type when studies by Eyre and Muir[33, 34] revealed the presence of both collagen types I and II. Further studies showed that these two fibrillar collagen types are distributed radially in concentration gradients with type I collagen being the predominant collagen of the fibre bundles of the outer annulus while type II collagen is essentially the main collagen type of the random fibrillar network of the inner annulus and nucleus pulposus (Fig. 4).[33, 34] However, since these early studies it has been revealed that the collagenous composition of the intervertebral disc is significantly more complex with the discovery that the collagens are a large family of related proteins currently numbering 27 genetically distinct types. At least 10 of these have now been detected in the intervertebral disc (Table 1).

In a normal young intervertebral disc the annulus fibrosus is reported to contain collagen types I, II, III, V, VI, IX, X, XI, XII, and XIV, the nucleus pulposus types I, II, III, VI, IX, X, XI, and XII, and the endplate II, III, VI, IX, X, XI, and XII.[26, 31, 35, 38, 206] As with most connective tissues, the collagen fibrils can be considered as alloys, many fibrils being heterotypic, that is, containing more than one collagen type. Types I, II, III, V, and XI all belong to the fibrillar class of collagens

and a number of them are known to co-localize to the same fibril. The major fibrillar collagens in the disc are types I and II, and they are principally responsible for the mechanical properties of this tissue.[26]

Collagen cross-linking

The stability of the collagenous components and hence the mechanical integrity of connective tissues such as the disc is dependent on the degree and type of cross-links between the collagen molecules. Collagen initially undergoes enzyme-mediated cross-linking with the formation of divalent reducible cross-links, the aldimine dehydrohydroxylysinonorleucine and the keto-imine hydroxylysino-5-norleucine.[44] In mature tissues these reducible aldimine and keto-imine cross-links undergo spontaneous further reactions to form the non-reducible stable cross-links, histidinohydroxylysinonorleucine (HHL) and hydroxylysyl-pyridinoline (HL-Pyr), respectively.

The major cross-link present in the young disc is hydroxylysino-5-norleucine,[45] which disappears on maturation to give HL-Pyr.[46]

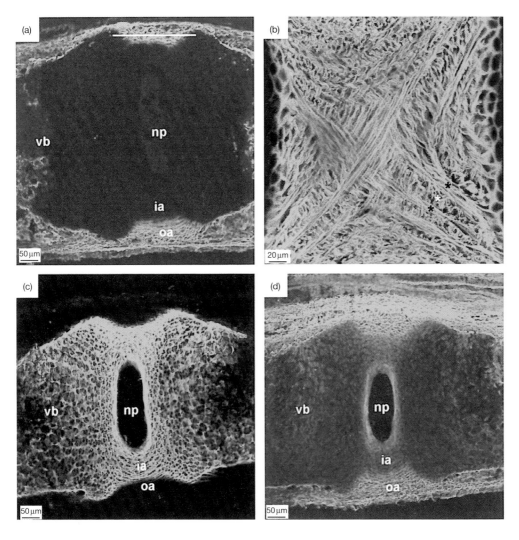

Fig. 4 Immunofluorescent localization of collagen types I, II and III in the neonate rat intervertebral disc. Strong immunolabelling (green) for collagen types I (a) and (d) III is seen in the outer annulus fibrosus (oa) but not the inner annulus (ia), nucleus pulposus (np), or the cartilaginous vertebral bodies (vb). Some labelling for type III is found surrounding the nucleus pulposus. (b) Three-dimensional reconstruction of the outer annulus from optical sections obtained by confocal laser scanning microscopy showing the alternately orientated lamellae of the type I collagen fibre bundles. (c) Immunolabelling for type II collagen showing strong staining in the inner annulus (ia) and vertebral bodies (vb) but little in the outer annulus (oa) and nucleus pulposus (np). (Reproduced from reference 7.)

Table 1 The genetically distinct collagen types of the intervertebral disc[a]

Type	Molecules	Macromolecular assembly	α chain Mr $\times 10^{-3}$	Distribution in the disc
I	$[\alpha1(I)]_2\alpha2(I)$	Fibril-forming	95	AF, NP
II	$[\alpha1(II)]_3$	Fibril-forming	95	AF, NP, EP
III	$[\alpha l(III)]_3$	Fibril-forming	95	AF, NP, EP
IV	$[\alpha1(IV)]–[\alpha6 (IV)]$ various molecular forms	Forms sheets	170–180	AF
V/XI	Combinations of $\alpha1(V)$ or $\alpha1(XI)$ with $\alpha2(V)$, $\alpha3(V)$, or $\alpha2(XI)$, $\alpha3(XI)$	Fibril-forming—often heterotypic fibrils	120–145	AF, NP, EP
VI	$[\alpha1(VI)\alpha2(VI)\alpha3(VI)]$	Beaded microfibrils (highly glycosylated)	140 340 ($\alpha3$)	AF, NP, EP
IX	$[\alpha1(IX)\alpha2(IX)\alpha3(IX)]$	FACIT collagen	64–84	AF, NP, EP
X	$[\alpha1(X)]_3$	Sheets form hexagonal lattices	59	AF, NP, EP
XII	$[\alpha1(XII)]_3$	FACIT collagen	220, 340	AF, NP, EP
XIV	$[\alpha1(XIV)]_3$	FACIT collagen	220	AF

Data taken from references 7, 26, and 31–43.

[a] Mr, Relative molecular mass; AF, annulus fibrosus; NP, nucleus pulposus; EP, cartilage endplate.

The intervertebral disc contains the highest level of HL-Pyr of any tissue, perhaps indicative of the high mechanical loads experienced by this tissue. However, there are regional variations in the levels, with the cartilage endplate having the highest levels of all.[47] The level of HL-Pyr is higher in the inner annulus and nucleus than in the outer annulus. The higher cross-link density of the nucleus may compensate for the much lower collagen content in this region of the disc.[47] However, the precise relationship between cross-link density and mechanical properties of tissues is currently unknown. In addition, collagen can become further cross-linked with increasing age by non-enzymic glycation.

'Minor' collagen components

The other fibrillar collagens, types III, V, and XI, are relatively minor components. However, these minor constituents play important roles in modifying the fibrillar architecture and fibril surface properties, thus influencing the structural and mechanical properties of the tissue. Type III collagen is often associated with type I collagen-containing tissues that require flexibility such as skin. Here it has been shown to be associated with type I collagen and may function to reduce the diameter of these fibrils.[48] It has been suggested that type III in the disc is also associated with type I collagen fibrils in the annulus fibrosus (see Fig. 4), although it also co-localizes to type II collagen fibrils in articular cartilage[49] and therefore could be associated more with type II in the disc. Type III collagen in the disc is predominantly associated with the cells. As in articular cartilage, the cells in both the adult annulus fibrosus and the nucleus pulposus are encapsulated in a fine fibrous capsule, the whole entity being termed a chondron. Type III collagen appears to be located at the periphery of the chondron and has been suggested to act as a link between the capsule and the surrounding interterritorial matrix.[35]

The fibrillar collagens types V and XI are homologous and it appears that hybrid molecules exist in some tissues such as the vitreous humour. Type V collagen is generally associated with type I collagen while type XI collagen is associated with type II collagen fibrils. Both type V and XI collagen retain a globular domain at the N-terminal end of the molecule, which is believed to be located on the fibril surface with the triple-helical domain buried within the typeI/II fibril.[50] In vitro fibrillogenesis studies have shown that these minor fibrillar collagens may function to regulate the diameter of the major fibrillar collagens and thus influence their mechanical properties. The localization of the N-terminal domain on the fibril surface also suggests they are involved in interactions with constituents of the interfibrillar space. Both type V and XI collagen genes undergo alternative splicing that alters the properties of these N-terminal domains and thus alters their interactions (reviewed in reference 50). At present the significance of these various forms and whether they are expressed in the intervertebral disc are unknown.

Type VI collagen

Type VI is an unusual collagen that aggregates to form beaded filaments. It has been found in the annulus fibrosus, nucleus pulposus, and the cartilage endplate. In the bovine disc it is a major collagenous constituent representing 20 per cent of the nucleus collagen and 5 per cent of the annulus fibrosus.[26, 39] In human discs it appears to be present at significantly lower levels by immohistochemistry but again is more prevalent in the nucleus pulposus. It is closely associated with the cells being found located near to the cell membrane and is a constituent of the chondron capsule (Fig. 5(a), (b)).[40] Since the disc is relatively acellular, the pericellular type VI collagen in the bovine nucleus pulposus must only represent a small proportion of the total type VI—the distribution for the most part must therefore be throughout the interterritorial matrix. Type VI is suggested to function as a link between the cell surface and the fibrillar ECM. Type VI collagen contains a number of RGD sequences, the amino acid motif recognized by many of the integrins, the cell surface receptors for ECM ligands.[51, 52]

Type VI is also composed of a number of domains with homology to von Willebrand factor that have been implicated in the interaction of type VI collagen with the fibrillar collagens. Thus type VI collagen appears to be important in linking the cell surface to the surrounding matrix.[51, 52] This pivotal link has important functions in maintaining tissue homeostasis and in cellular responses to tissue damage and degeneration by mechanotransduction via the cytoskeleton.

FACIT collagens

The remaining collagens, types IX, XII, and XIV, that have been found in the intervertebral disc all belong to the group termed FACIT collagens—fibril-associated collagens with an interrupted triple helix.[49, 52] These collagens are thought to decorate the surface of the collagen fibrils and restrict lateral associations, thus regulating fibril diameters. In addition, they all have a number of features that suggest they mediate interactions with other matrix components. They have non-triple helical domains that protrude away from the fibril surface and they can all be present in a glycanated form containing a chondroitin sulfate glycosaminoglycan (GAG) chain.[50, 53]

Type IX collagen is associated with the type II heterotypic fibrils in articular cartilage. In the intervertebral disc type IX collagen exists in both the long and short forms.[41, 206, 207] The short form lacks the globular NC4 domain of the alpha-1 chain that protrudes from the fibril surface and therefore would lack some of the putative interactive properties of the long form. There is more of the short form in the nucleus pulposus than in the annulus fibrosus—the significance of

this is unknown. As in articular cartilage, only the long form is present in the endplate. Both forms appear to be fully glycanated in the intervertebral disc.[41]

Type XII collagen has been located throughout both the annulus fibrosus and the nucleus pulposus of the intervertebral disc but is restricted to the territorial matrix of the chondrocytes in the endplate.[38] Type XII is usually associated with type I collagen fibrils but its localization in the nucleus pulposus of the disc implies it can also associate with type II collagen fibrils. The gene coding for type XII collagen contains a stress-response element in the promoter and therefore it may be an important collagen in responding to mechanically induced matrix degradation.[54] Type XIV collagen appears to co-localize with type XII in the annulus fibrosus but is not present in the nucleus pulposus or the cartilage endplate.[41] The precise function of all these minor collagenous components has yet to be elucidated.

Type X collagen

Type X collagen is a short-chain collagen that was originally thought to be restricted to the hypertrophic zone of growth plate cartilage and to contribute to the process of endochondral ossification (reviewed in reference 55). However, it has recently been found in small amounts in normal articular cartilage. Studies on the disc have resulted in conflicting reports as to whether it is a component of the normal disc. Lammi and co-workers[42] found that it was expressed in the cartilage endplate but not in the annulus fibrosus or nucleus pulposus, whereas others report that it is expressed in the developing/growing nucleus

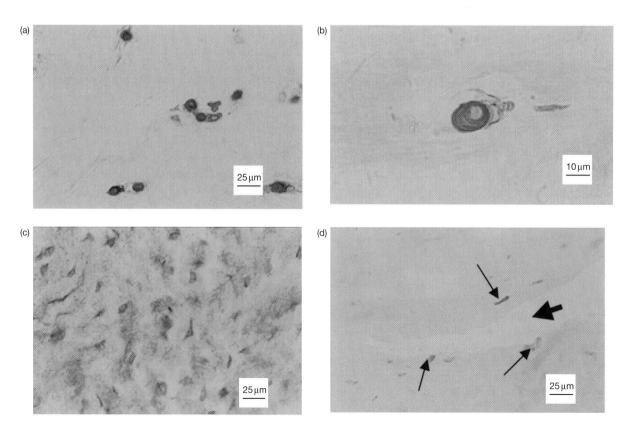

Fig. 5 Immunoperoxidase staining for type VI collagen is more prevalent in the (c) nucleus of bovine discs than (a), (b) in the nucleus of normal human disc where it is predominantly cell-associated. (d) There is more matrix staining in diseased human disc for type VI collagen and for type X collagen (as shown here) in localized areas of damage, for example, in cells (arrow) adjacent to a cleft in the tissue (arrowhead).

pulposus at <2 years of age, but is not present in the normal adult disc.[43] A number of reports have now reported type X in the degenerate disc (see Fig. 5(d)).

Proteoglycans of the intervertebral disc

Proteoglycans are a major constituent of the intervertebral disc representing around 10 per cent of the dry weight of the outer annulus with an increasing proportion towards the inner annulus and nucleus pulposus where they constitute approximately 50 per cent of the dry weight (Fig. 6).[56] Proteoglycans can be subdivided into large aggregating and small leucine-rich proteoglycans (SLRPs). Two members of the large aggregating proteoglycans have been found in the intervertebral disc, namely, aggrecan and versican (Fig. 7), while at least four members of the SLRPs have been identified, namely, decorin, biglycan, fibromodulin, and lumican.[57, 58] The large aggregating proteoglycans, when newly synthesized, associate with hyaluronan, a large non-sulfated GAG found in all connective tissues including the intervertebral disc and this association is stabilized by another glycoprotein, link protein.[59, 60] However, in the normal adult disc there is a significant proportion of the aggrecan and versican that is non-aggregating.

In comparison with human articular cartilage where 50–85 per cent of the large proteoglycans are aggregated, in the outer annulus 50 per cent are aggregated decreasing to 20 per cent in the nucleus pulposus.[24, 61] Hyaluronan is present throughout the disc but shows a higher concentration in the nucleus pulposus and inner annulus compared to that in the outer annulus.[62] The hyaluronan appears to have a higher proportion of associated aggrecan in the pericellular domain than in the interterritorial matrix. There is less hyaluronan in the outer annulus fibrosus, but it is abundant between the lamellae of collagen bundles and may be important for the plasticity of this structure.[62] It is also present throughout the cartilage endplate where there appears to be a high concentration of cell-associated hyaluronan.

Aggrecan

Aggrecan is the archetypal large aggregating proteoglycan. It contains a core protein with an approximate molecular weight of 230 kDa. It has three globular domains, G1, G2, and G3, and two GAG attachment regions: a keratan-sulfate-rich region and a chondroitin-sulfate-rich domain.[59] The G1 domain facilitates the aggregation of aggrecan to hyaluronan. The functions of the other globular domains are unclear. Aggrecan contains a number of keratan sulfate chains but the bulk of the attached GAGs are chondroitin sulfate chains that can be up to 150 in number.[59] The large aggregates of hyaluronan, aggrecan, and link protein produce a large negative charge and high osmotic pressure in the matrix of the disc, which are important for the maintenance of the high hydration state of the tissue and essential for withstanding the compressive forces experienced by the intervertebral disc. Both aggregating and non-aggregating forms of aggrecan have been isolated from discs, the latter being greater in older samples suggesting they represent a degradation product.[24, 61] Immunohistological studies have revealed variations in the staining intensity across the intervertebral disc with the highest levels in the nucleus pulposus, less in the annulus fibrosus, and the least in the cartilage endplate.[63] Versican, the other large aggregating proteoglycan found in the disc, has a core protein of 400 kDa with a hyaluronan-binding domain and a number of GAG attachment sites. It is subject to alternative splicing

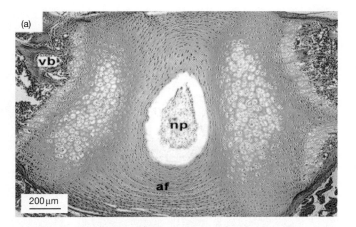

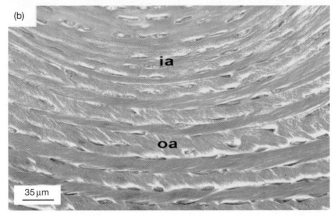

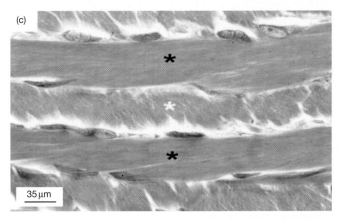

Fig. 6 Histochemical staining (Alcian blue and haematoxylin and eosin (H&E) of postnatal rat disc showing the high concentration of proteoglycans in the disc (blue) compared to that in the bone (red). (b), (c) Note the laminar appearance of both the inner (ia) and outer (oa) annulus fibrosus vb = vertebral, af = annulus fibrosus, np = nucleus pulposus. Individual lamallae are denoted by * (Reproduced from reference 7.)

and in the intervertebral disc both the shorter V1 and the larger V0 forms are expressed.[64] In other tissues it is expressed more highly in developing tissues and is often downregulated when aggrecan is upregulated. In the disc it is distributed in the anterior longitudinal ligament and matrix of the outer annulus, particularly in the young, with less towards inner annulus and nucleus, where it is mostly pericellular. In the cartilage endplate it is seen only in young specimens,

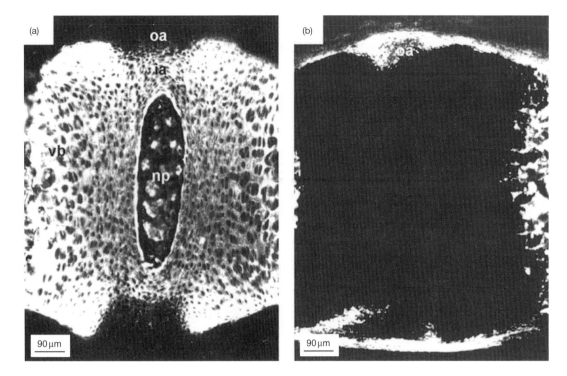

Fig. 7 Immunolabelling of neonatal rat disc showing the relative distribution of (a) aggrecan and (b) versican. Aggrecan is distributed throughout the disc except for the outer annulus (oa) whereas versican is present only in the outer annulus. Versican is evenly distributed in the posterior outer annulus (top) but restricted to the margins with the vertebral body (vb) in the anterior annulus. np, Nucleus pulposus. (Reproduced from reference 7.)

where it is weak in the matrix with some pericellular staining.[65, 66] The precise function of versican is not known.

Small leucine-rich proteoglycans (SLRPs)

The SLRPs are a family of non-aggregating proteoglycans with a small core protein that contains a leucine-rich domain and only one or two covalently linked GAG chains. Four members of this family have been identified so far as constituents of the intervertebral disc—decorin, biglycan, fibromodulin, and lumican.[58, 67] Decorin and biglycan both contain dermatan sulfate or chondroitin sulfate GAG side chains, whereas fibromodulin and lumican are keratan-sulfate-containing proteoglycans. The precise functions of these proteoglycans is not known but most interact with the fibrillar collagen network and appear to regulate its assembly and organization. For instance, decorin and fibromodulin inhibit collagen fibrillogenesis *in vitro* and are suggested to play some role in fibril formation.[68–70] Indeed, in the decorin knock-out mouse, the collagen network of the skin shows a disorganized and abnormal fibril morphology resulting in fragile skin.[71] Thus these proteoglycans can profoundly influence the mechanical properties of tissues. Decorin in articular cartilage has been located preferentially on the larger collagen fibrils, whereas type IX collagen predominates on the smaller fibrils.[72] In some way these two components appear to regulate the fibril morphology of the tissue. Lumican was first isolated from cornea and it has recently been shown to be important in maintaining the precise fibril spacing required in the cornea to retain transparency. It is assumed that lumican in other tissues also plays some role in fibril organization.[73]

The SLRPs are distributed throughout the different regions of the intervertebral disc but with some variations. Most information is available for decorin and biglycan, which have been found in high

content in the annulus fibrosus and cartilage endplate and to a lesser degree in the nucleus pulposus.[67] Decorin appears to be distributed in the interterritorial matrix, particularly in the nucleus pulposus and endplate, whereas biglycan is located more in the pericellular domain. Decorin and biglycan mainly contain dermatan sulfate GAG chains in the annulus fibrosus, whereas in the cartilage endplate they are mostly chondroitin sulfate. The significance of these differences is unknown.

Elastin and other matrix components of the intervertebral disc

Elastin is a highly insoluble protein that is very extensible and, as its name suggests, highly elastic. Elastin has been reported to occur in all intervertebral discs, estimates of its concentration ranging from 1 to 10 per cent of the total dry weight (references 74–76; Urban and Winlove, personal communication). Morphologically, elastin occurs in the annulus fibrosus in the form of uniform fibres aligned with the collagen fibrils, but in the nucleus pulposus it occurs as larger, more irregularly shaped fibres that are more randomly orientated than in the annulus fibrosus.[208, 209] The biochemical and amino acid analysis of this substance, however, is not identical to that of classical elastin extracted from the artery wall. The elastin-like material extracted from disc has a high methionine but lower valine content than artery elastin[76] and in some respects resembles lamprin, the glycoprotein found in the cartilage of lampreys.[77]

As in most connective tissues there are also present a number of large multidomain glycoproteins, although no thorough study has been carried out. Certainly, fibronectin, fibrillin, and laminin have been reported as being present but little information on their precise distribution has been published.[78, 210] The human intervertebral disc also contains a small amount of lipid in the form of cholesterol, triglyceride, and phospholipid. The lipid-derived pigment lipofuscin has also been reported particularly in older tissues.

Cells of the intervertebral disc

The intervertebral disc has a very low cell density in comparison to most tissues. Cells make up approximately 1–2 per cent of the tissue volume in disc whereas, for example, they make up approximately 80 per cent of the liver volume. Nonetheless, their metabolism and synthesis of extracellular molecules is obviously essential to the maintenance of a healthy, functioning intervertebral disc. Disc cells also have the capability to produce catabolic enzymes, which, whilst necessary for normal matrix turnover and remodelling, if produced in excess will have deleterious effects on the properties of the matrix.

The morphology of the cells varies in the different regions of the disc: in the cartilage endplate and outer annulus fibrosus they are thin elongated, fibroblast-like cells that are lying parallel to the collagen fibres. In young individuals these cells lie predominantly in sheets between the lamellar bundles, whereas in the mature human disc they are interspersed throughout the lamellar bundles, which themselves have become more irregular, with numerous bifurcations and interdigitations. This heterogeneity could arise in response to the loading history of the disc.

Towards the centre of the disc the cell density decreases to less than 50 per cent in the nucleus of that of the annulus,[79] and the cells take on a more rounded or oval appearance, often being described as chondrocyte-like. The exact origin of the cells in this region remains uncertain, though the most popular theory is that they have migrated inwards from the annulus when the previous population, the notochordal cells, receded. The lifespan of notochordal cells differs greatly between species. For example, in rodents, cats, rabbits, pigs, and non-chondrodystrophoid dogs, notochord cells remain into and throughout adult life in contrast to sheep, chondrodystrophoid dogs, and man where they do not. In man the number of notochord cells diminishes rapidly after birth until by the age of four very few, if any, remain. Indeed the disappearance of notochordal cells correlates with early degenerative changes in the disc, possibly due to a decrease in soluble factor(s) produced by notochordal cells that stimulate disc cells to synthesize proteoglycan molecules.[80]

Whilst cells in the centre of the disc may resemble cartilage chondrocytes in some respects, they differ in other ways, both functionally and morphologically.[211] Functionally, for example, cartilage chondrocytes exhibit a negative Pasteur effect, in common with most cell types, with a decreasing rate of glycolysis at low oxygen concentrations. Disc cells, in contrast, exhibit a strong positive Pasteur effect, with the glycolytic rate increasing steeply as the oxygen tension falls below 5 per cent O_2.[81] As far as morphology goes, disc cells have cell processes *in vivo* that are often long and extensive. The function of these processes is not certain, but it is suggested that they may be important for mechanotransduction within the cellular network.[82] Whatever their function in disc, no such processes were found in similar preparations of chondrocytes from articular cartilage in man, cow, pig, or rabbit.

Recent studies have focused on maintaining the phenotype of intervertebral disc cells *in vitro* in order to characterize better these cells.[83–86] Most studies have utilized alginate gels, which have been successfully used to culture chondrocytes from hyaline cartilages,[87] although in some cases matrix assembly appears aberrant in these cultures.[88] The limited studies to date have shown that the interverte- bral disc contains two distinct cell populations based on differences in phenotypic expression. The cells from the annulus fibrosus appear chondrocyte-like but also synthesize type I collagen, whereas the cells from the nucleus pulposus, although they phenotypically resemble articular cartilage chondrocytes, morphologically show features of notochordal cells.[82, 85, 211, 212] The use of *in vitro* systems for characterizing the cells of the intervertebral disc will aid our knowledge of the cell biology of this tissue. However, caution is necessary in the interpretation of this data as these systems provide an environment quite different from that experienced by the cells *in vivo*, such as, higher oxygen tension, greater nutritional availability, and an ECM different to that found in the disc.

Development of the intervertebral disc

The embryological origin of the intervertebral disc is the notochord that demarcates the midline of the developing embryo. The notochord derives from cells of Henson's node that, at gastrulation, migrate between the ectoderm and endoderm. The notochord induces the formation of a surrounding column of mesenchymal cells that become segmented, giving rise to the somites.[89] Cells in the ventromedial segment of each somite, the sclerotome, produce the vertebral column. The surrounding mesenchymal cells give rise to the ventral vertebral structures such as the vertebral body and the intervertebral disc. The mesenchymal cells giving rise to the vertebral body undergo differentiation to chondrocytes and the formation of the cartilaginous anlagen of the developing vertebrae whilst others form condensations that develop into the intervertebral mesenchyme (Fig. 8).[90, 91]

The development of this alternating segmental pattern of cartilage and intervertebral mesenchyme is under the control of a number of axial patterning genes, the most important being the Hox (homeobox-containing) and Pax (paired box) genes.[92, 93] These genes are regulated by various signalling molecules that are important in development such as retinoic acid, sonic hedgehog, and fibroblast growth factors.[94–96] The specific axial level is defined by the transcription of a unique combination of Hox genes.[97, 98] Pax genes are thought to mediate induction signals from the notochord for differentiation of the surrounding mesenchymal cells.[99–101] Loss of Pax 1 expression has been shown to result in abnormalities in sclerotome differentiation and the failure to form the vertebral body and intervertebral discs.[101]

The condensation of the intervertebral mesenchyme increases in density and becomes concentrically arranged around the notochord. Intervertebral disc differentiation begins with the rapid expansion of the notochord between the cartilaginous vertebral bodies giving rise to the primitive nucleus pulposus.[102] The mesenchymal cells closest to the notochord differentiate into chondrocytic cells to form the inner annulus. The outer fibroblastic cells organize into concentric sheets or laminae (Fig. 9(a), (b)).[36, 103] The orientation of these cells is associated with the formation of intercellular adherens junctions and intracellular longitudinal actin stress fibres (Fig. 9(c), (d)).[104] The stress fibres appear to direct the initial elongation of these fibroblastic cells and hence control the deposition of the oriented extracellular matrix. Once the template for the lamellar structure of the outer annulus fibrosus is established with an adequate ECM, the stress fibres disappear.[104]

During development, notochordal continuity between adjacent vertebrae is lost, with remnants of the notochord remaining only in the

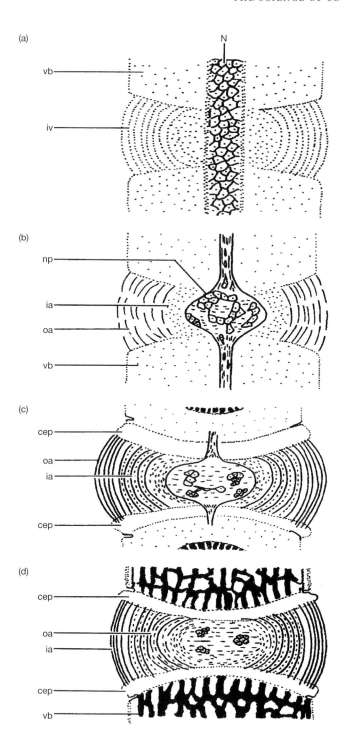

Fig. 8 Stages in the development of the intervertebral disc (based on reference 102). N, notochord; vb vertebral body; iv, intervertebral disc anlage; np, nucleus pulposus; ia, inner annulus fibrosus; oa, outer annulus fibrosus; cep, cartilage endplates.

intervertebral areas.[102] This loss of the notochord appears to be an essential step in the development of the intervertebral disc. Transgenic mice lacking expression of type II collagen retain a continuous notochord and fail to develop intervertebral discs. It is suggested that the type II collagen of the vertebral anlagen exerts mechanical pressure on

the notochord in this region of the developing vertebral column resulting in the decline of the notochord in these regions.[105, 106] Recent studies have shown that sox5 and sox6 are required for notochord and nucleus pulposus development.[213]

At parturition, the human intervertebral disc is fully formed with the lamellar annulus fibrosus and a large central nucleus pulposus that consists of clusters of notochordal cells embedded in a proteoglycan-rich matrix. The collagenous lamellae of the outer annulus fibrosus insert into the cartilaginous ends of the ossifying vertebral bodies, the cartilage endplate.[107] During skeletal growth the intervertebral disc continues to undergo development. The annulus fibrosus becomes increasingly fibrocartilaginous, whilst the nucleus pulposus becomes cartilaginous acquiring more chondrocytic cells, presumably from the inner annulus.[17, 36, 107, 108] The notochordal cells decline dramatically in number and are rarely present in the nucleus pulposus of the mature human intervertebral disc.[18, 19]

Immunohistochemical localization studies have revealed a differential expression and distribution of various ECM constituents. The cells of the nucleus pulposus and the inner annulus fibrosus generally exhibit a chondrogenic phenotype with expression of type II collagen and aggrecan and, initially, also versican.[7] Type II collagen is expressed as two forms, IIA and IIB. The type IIA variant is normally expressed only in pre-chondrogenic mesenchyme that, on differentiation to chondrocytes, switches to the alternatively spliced IIB form removing a 69 amino acid cysteine rich region of the N-terminal propeptide.[109, 214] However, in the intervertebral disc, the IIA form appears to persist in the cartilaginous vertebral body as well as in the notochord, especially in the notochordal sheath.[7, 110–112] The function of the IIA variant is unknown as the extra amino acid sequence occurs in the propeptide that is normally cleaved from the processed molecule. The high concentration of the proteoglycans in the notochord and notochordal sheath is thought to initiate the notochordal bulging giving rise to the nucleus pulposus and inner annulus fibrosus.[7]

As the fibroblastic cells of the outer annulus align, they express fibronectin and $\alpha 5\beta 1$ integrin, the fibronectin receptor. This appears to establish the template for the formation of the laminar matrix composed of types I, III, and IV collagen (see Fig. 4).[104] The latter collagen type is normally associated with basement membranes although there are reports of it occurring in non-basement membrane locations.[113, 114] In this instance it may be acting to orientate the fibroblasts of the outer annulus in order to lay down the laminar fibrillar network of types I and III collagen. Versican is progressively lost from the cartilaginous regions and becomes confined to the outer annulus and by the neonate stage is restricted to the posterior region of the outer annulus.[7] This differential expression in the posterior and not the anterior outer annulus raises intriguing questions as to the precise function of versican. Versican is known to inhibit mesenchymal chondrogenesis,[115] which may explain its loss from the nucleus pulposus and inner annulus. However, it may also influence cell proliferation and cell adhesion[116] and hence produce differential growth of the posterior versus the anterior outer annulus fibrosus.

Vascularization and nutrition of the intervertebral disc

The intervertebral disc is often referred to as the largest avascular tissue in the adult human. It does not begin life as such since in the

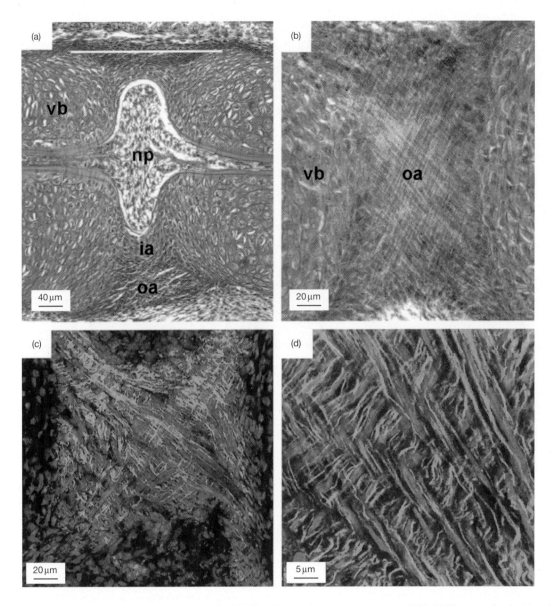

Fig. 9 (a), (b) Histological staining (alcian blue and H&E) of the developing rat disc at stage E 16. (a) The centrally placed nucleus pulposus (np) surrounded by an inner and outer annulus fibrosus (ia and oa, respectively). The nucleus pulposus contains notochordal cells in a sparse alcian blue positive matrix. The inner annulus is continuous with the cartilage of the vertebral bodies, while the outer annulus consists of sheets of fibroblasts that lack alcian blue staining. (b) A section through the outer annulus (white line in (a)) showing the lattice like arrangement of sheets of cells inclined to the long axis of the spine. (c), (d) Actin labelled with FITC–phalloidin (green) and the cell nuclei counterstained with propidium iodide (red). Actin label is prominent in the cell sheets of the outer annulus as a lattice-like pattern. (d) The higher power micrograph shows the obliquely running fibroblasts containing cables of actin. At least two layers of cells are present in this section producing the lattice-like pattern.[7, 104]

young individual blood vessels can be seen between the lamellae in the outer annulus. The adjoining hyaline cartilage endplates, lying superior and inferior to the disc, constitute more than 50 per cent of the intervertebral space in human neonates (Fig. 10). There are large vascular channels (Fig. 11(a), (b)) running through these that diminish and finally disapppear in the first few years of life. Simultaneously during skeletal development the cartilage endplate recedes and becomes thinner until in adulthood it is a totally avascular layer of hyaline cartilage approximately 1–3 mm in thickness.[117] Similarly, blood vessels in the outer annulus diminish.[118] Thus the cells of the intervertebral disc are dependent for their supply of nutrients on diffusion from the vasculature in adjoining tissues, that is, in the horizontal plane, from within the

longitudinal ligaments running anterior and posterior to the disc, and vertically from the vascular buds or marrow cavities and capillaries in the bony endplates of the vertebral bodies (Fig. 12(a), (b)). These are seen over the entire bone–cartilage interface, but are most dense in the central region adjacent to the nucleus pulposus.[119] These marrow spaces are believed to be very important to the nutritional pathway of the disc.[120, 121]

A gradient for solutes, whether of nutrients being lowest in the centre of the disc or of metabolites being greatest,[122] controls the rate of diffusion and flow of these solutes in and out of the disc. The gradients from the centre of the disc to the outer regions are steep and they are very important in determining nutrient supply and metabolite

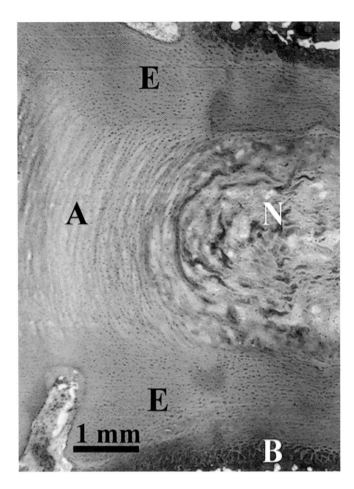

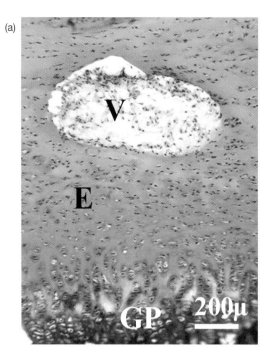

Fig. 10 In the neonate the cartilage endplates (E) constitute a much bigger proportion of the intervertebral space than later in life; see Fig. 2. B, Vertebral body; A, annulus fibrosus; N, nucleus pulposus.

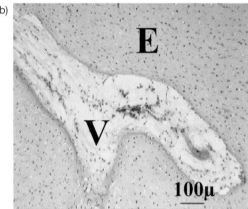

Fig. 11 In the human neonate there are large vascular channels (V) that recede in the first few years of life leaving a totally avascular but thinner cartilage endplate (E) in the skeletally mature human. GP, growth plate.

clearance. This in turn determines the cell density that can be supported in the disc.[123] Any factors that affect this gradient will influence the viability and vitality of the disc cells. The composition of the matrix through which the solutes must pass is also important: for example, if mineralization has occurred in the ECM of the cartilage endplate or disc, this will reduce the rate of transport.[124]

Other influencing factors include the area of exchange available, which in turn is influenced by the permeability of the vertebral bony endplate. Anything that decreases the contact area will disrupt transfer of solutes across the boundary with detrimental effects to the disc likely. Indeed, Nachemson *et al.*[120] found a significant correlation between the impermeability of the central portion of the vertebral endplate and the presence of degeneration in the adjacent disc. Cigarette smoking can also decrease the transport efficiency of solutes, such that smoking for 3 hours reduced the transport of oxygen by 50 per cent in dogs (Fig. 13).[125] Such a reduction is likely to alter cell physiology significantly. Since the nutritive status of the normal disc is precarious, any reduction in nutrition can be expected to have deleterious consequences for cell viability and functioning.[215]

In pathologically diseased discs, for example, those with degenerative disc disease, there is increased vascularization (Fig. 14). This may have complex influences on the disc. For example, whilst increasing the amounts of nutrients available, the increased vascularization may

also bring more cells with their own inevitable requirements for nutrients. In addition, vessels may introduce cytokines, growth factors, or enzymes, which are normally excluded from the ECM of the disc. The mixed results of increased vascularization may explain the poor correlation seen between oxygen and lactate concentrations in disc and the type and severity of disease.[122]

Innervation of the normal intervertebral disc

Nerves are found in all intervertebral discs but in the normal adult disc they are restricted to the outer annulus (Fig. 15(a)),[126] in vitro studies have shown that aggrecan inhibits nerve growth into the disc.[216] Nerve fibres are mostly thin and generally run parallel to the predominant collagen orientation in the annulus, particularly between the lamellae. These nerves pass into the annulus from the nerve plexi

(a)

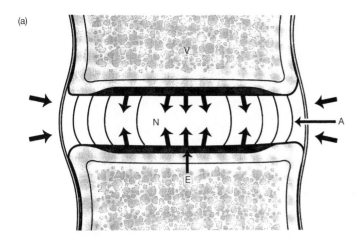

(b)

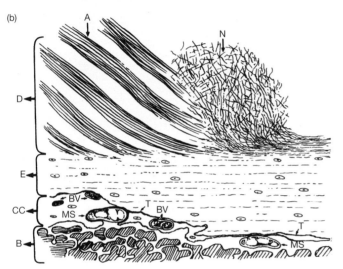

Fig. 12 (a) The adult disc is dependent on diffusion of nutrients and metabolites through the vasculature of either the anterior or posterior ligaments outside the annulus (A) or the vertebral body (V) and through the cartilage endplate (E). N, nucleus pulposus. (After reference 81.) (b) The marrow spaces (MS) and blood vessels (BV) in the calcified cartilage (CC) and bone (B) abutting the cartilage endplate (E) are important in supplying the nutrients to, and carrying the metabolites from, the cells of the disc (D) particularly those of the nucleus (N). A, annulus fibrosus; T, tidemark.

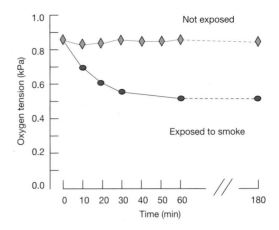

Fig. 13 The influence of cigarette smoking on the oxygen tension $p[O_2]$ in the intervertebral disc of dogs. Note the drop in $p[O_2]$ within the relatively short time frame of 30 minutes. (Adapted from reference 125.)

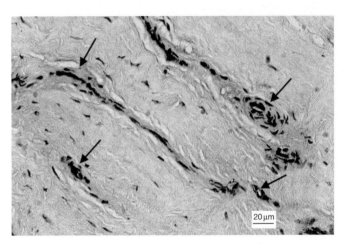

Fig. 14 Greater number of blood vessels (arrows) are found in degenerate human discs, such as are seen here immunostained with an endothelial marker, than in non-degenerate discs.

within the adjacent longitudinal ligaments lying anteriorly and posteriorly.[127] The nerve plexus overlying one individual disc receives innervation via the sinuvertebral nerve, not only from nerves derived from adjacent segments[128] but also those derived from several levels away.[129] Each sinuvertebral nerve arises from one or sometimes two rami communicantes close to the connection with the spinal nerve. Up to five sinuvertebral nerves have been observed in one intervertebral foramen, some being thick and others thin.

There appear to be both sympathetic and sensory components in the nerves of the disc. Immunohistochemical techniques have identified peptidergic nerves (represented by immunoreactivity to neuropeptide Y and vasoactive intestinal peptide (VIP)), noradrenergic nerves (reflected by tyrosine hydroxylase (TH) activity), and sensory, potentially nociceptive nerves (represented by substance-P and calcitonin gene-related peptide (CGRP) immunopositivity)(Fig. 15(b)).

Neuropeptide Y and TH positive nerves were predominantly found in the blood vessel walls whereas VIP and substance P stained nerves were mostly non-vascular.[130, 131] Neuropeptide Y and noradrenaline (also called norepinephrine) are both vasoconstrictive, implying that the function of these nerves in blood vessel walls is vasoregulatory.

Some of these nerves end in mechano- or proprioceptors, as demonstrated by immunohistochemical as well as traditional histological techniques.[123, 132, 133] These receptors provide the individual with the sensation of posture and movement and can even have a nociceptive role. Golgi tendon organs (GTO), Ruffini endings, and Pacinian corpuscles have all been reported in disc, GTO being found most frequently and Pacinian corpuscles least often (Fig. 16(a), (b)).[133] This relative incidence is likely to reflect their physiological function since GTO are slow-adapting, high-threshold receptors that are completely inactive in immobile joints. They are found commonly in ligamentous tissue elsewhere in the body and are thought to measure tension, only becoming active at extremes of their range of motion. The other receptor types, Ruffini endings and Pacinian corpuscles, are

(a)

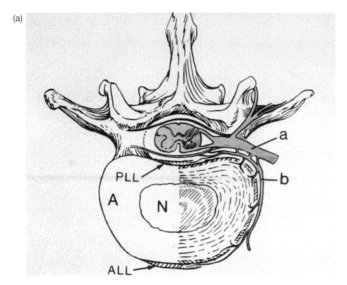

(b)

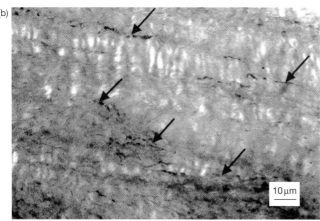

Fig. 15 (a) Schematic representation of the innervation of the normal adult intervertebral disc, restricted to the outer region of the annulus fibrosus, with nerves originating from branches (marked b) of the sinu-vertebral nerve (marked a) A, Annulus fibrosus; N, nucleus pulposus; ALL, anterior longitudinal ligament; PLL, posterior longitudinal ligament. (b) A section of the outer annulus immunostained for PGP 9.5 to demonstrate nerve fibres (arrows) lying predominantly parallel to the collagen bundles, viewed here under polarized light.

faster adapting and, in the case of Pacinian corpuscles, respond to sudden changes in stress. Their low frequency in the disc perhaps indicates that the stress levels do not normally change fast in the disc compared to other tissues.

The mechanoreceptors in the disc may play a role in influencing the activity of the spinal muscles. Certainly Indahl et al.[134] have shown that electrical stimulation of the disc innervation elicits reactions in the lumbar multifidus and longissimus paraspinal muscles.

Age changes of the intervertebral disc

There are a number of reported changes to the intervertebral disc that occur with age that may predispose to disc degeneration later in life. Ageing changes and degeneration can therefore be considered different

(a)

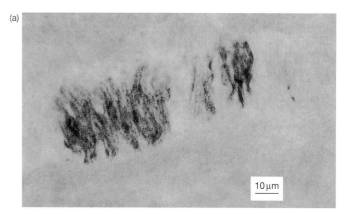

(b)

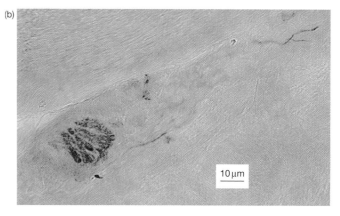

Fig. 16 Small numbers of mechanoreceptors are found in the outer extremities of the disc and longitudinal ligaments, most frequently resembling (a) Golgi tendon organs (b) and occasionally simple Pacinian corpuscles.

ends of the spectrum of the normal ageing process. During skeletal growth the intervertebral disc increases in volume considerably. The cells in the annulus fibrosus become increasingly fibrochondrocytic (Fig. 17(a)),[17] initially in the inner annulus, whilst the nucleus pulposus cells resemble chondrocytes (Fig. 17(b)).[7, 17, 106] The population of notochordal cells present at birth gradually becomes depleted (Fig. 17(c)).[18, 19] The inner annulus expands with age mainly at the expense of the nucleus pulposus such that they become less distinct tissue entities. There is a gradual loss of proteoglycans and water with an increase in non-collagenous proteins and age-related pigments such as lipofuscin and amyloid.[135, 136] Disc cells show a high incidence of apoptosis that is apparently higher in older people (Fig. 17(d)). Intervertebral disc cells, however, are not inactive, but it is suggested that the cells switch phenotype with age such that they accumulate an inappropriate matrix. These changes in composition and metabolism of the intervertebral disc are reflected in morphological changes.[137, 138, 217]

Collagens in the ageing intervertebral disc

Studies on the expression and turnover of the disc collagens reveal significant expression of types I and II collagen in the endplate of neonates and 2- to 5-year-old discs.[139] High levels of denatured type II collagen have also been detected in both the annulus fibrosus and the nucleus pulposus reflecting significant matrix turnover.[140, 141] With increasing age the level of turnover, defined by the level of denatured type II collagen,

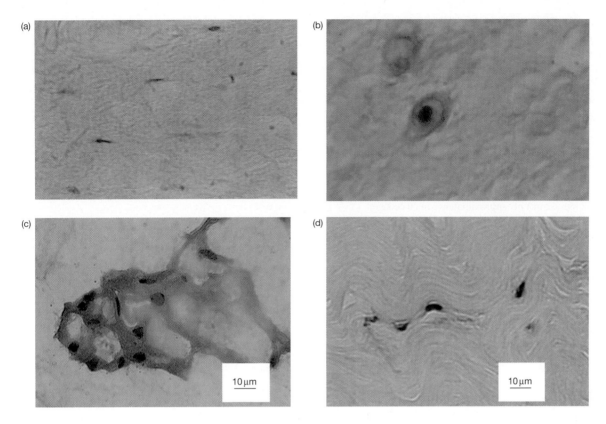

Fig. 17 In the annulus the cells resemble fibroblasts. Soon after birth (c) the notochordal cells in the nucleus are replaced by (b) chondrocyte-like nucleus cells. (d) With increasing age more and more cells become apoptotic, demonstrated here by TUNEL staining.

falls to low levels in the juvenile and young adult disc. In older discs the levels of denatured type II collagen epitope increase concomitant with a switch to greater type I collagen expression, suggesting changes consistent with disc degeneration. Such changes in expression result in an age-related increasing proportion of type I collagen in the nucleus pulposus and an increasing type II collagen concentration in the inner and outer annulus. Whether this reflects a change in the phenotypic expression of the resident cells or migration of the different cell populations is unknown.

Studies by Nerlich and co-workers[142] have shown there is an age-related accumulation of carboxymethyl lysine (CML), which is suggested to be an indicator of oxidative stress. CML was observed first in the nucleus pulposus in juvenile discs and found to increase significantly with age. In elderly people, both the nucleus pulposus and the annulus fibrosus showed extensive CML deposition. It is suggested this triggers an age-related change in the phenotypic expression of the cells in the annulus fibrosus but more particularly in the nucleus pulposus. Using immunohistochemical staining procedures, an initial increase in collagen types II, III, and VI followed by a loss of collagen type II, the occurrence of collagen type I, and the persistence of high levels of collagen types III and VI in the nucleus pulposus collagen have been observed.[143] These collagens also decrease as the disc becomes increasingly degenerate. In addition, a significant proportion of cells in the nucleus pulposus of adolescents and young adults positively stained for the basement membrane collagen type IV.[143] Interestingly, type IV collagen has been found throughout the rat disc during development with strongly positive immunolabelling in the outer annulus in the neonate but with lesser staining of the inner

annulus.[7] Many of the observed changes detailed above require confirmation by more quantitative biochemical methods. Type X collagen is not considered a component of the normal disc, although it has been reported to be a constituent of both the nucleus pulposus and annulus fibrosus of mature beagle dogs[55] and has also been reported in apparently normal human endplate, annulus fibrosus, and nucleus pulposus.[37, 42, 144] Type X has been found in degenerate discs (see below), and therefore it is unclear whether its presence reflects early stages of disc degeneration.

Collagen cross-linking

With increasing age, as well as changes in the types of collagen in the matrix, there are also changes in the collagen cross-linking that may compromise the biomechanical functions of the disc. The major cross-link present in the young disc is hydroxylysino-5-norleucine,[45] which disappears on maturation to give HL-Pyr.[46] The intervertebral disc contains the highest level of HL-Pyr of any tissue, perhaps indicative of the high mechanical loads experienced by this tissue. It has been suggested that HL-Pyr decreases with age in the mature disc.[145] However, most of the samples in this study were aged 40–80 years and the decrease may therefore represent changes indicative of disc degeneration.

In addition, collagen can become further cross-linked with increasing age by non-enzymic glycation. There are many so-called advanced glycation end-products (AGEs) but the only one characterized so far and shown to be a collagen cross-link is pentosidine.[146] Collagen of the intervertebral disc may be particularly susceptible to cross-linking in this way as low oxygen tension favours these reactions. Indeed, studies by Hormel and Eyre[147] and Yang et al.[148] show an age-related increase in collagen-associated fluorescence in the intervertebral disc, some of which is likely to be due to the presence of pentosidine. Indeed, studies recently carried out in our laboratory showed such an age-related increase specifically in pentosidine.[47] Pentosidine will accumulate at a slower rate in tissues with a faster turnover. The slightly lower level of pentosidine in the nucleus than in the outer annulus is therefore consistent with the higher level of reducible cross-links here, suggesting that the nucleus pulposus has a higher matrix turnover than the annulus fibrosus. The amount of pentosidine increases with age rising from 0.005 to 0.06 mol/mol collagen over the age range studied (Fig. 18). Although this is a 12-fold increase in this cross-link, it still represents only approximately 1 in 20 collagen molecules being cross-linked in the oldest tissue samples. It has been suggested that the age-related increase in these glycation products may cause an increase in tissue stiffness and decrease in elasticity and resilience to mechanical loads and thus contribute to eventual disc degeneration.[148] However, it is unclear if pentosidine directly influences tissue properties. There are other potential collagen cross-links, such as pyrroles and other glycation products, that may increase with age and which are thought to be present in more substantial amounts and therefore to have a greater influence on the properties of the tissues.[149–151]

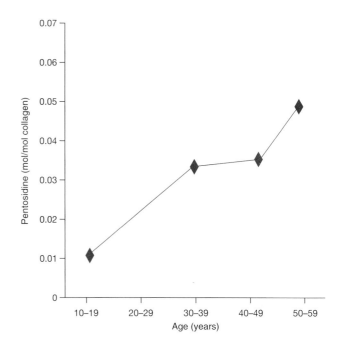

Fig. 18 Age-related changes in pentosidine in the nucleus pulposus. Pentosidine concentration is expressed as mol/mol collagen.

Proteoglycans in the ageing intervertebral disc

There are also age changes in the proteoglycans of the intervertebral disc. With age there is a steady increase in non-aggregating forms of aggrecan reflecting significant proteoglycan turnover or degradation.[24, 61] In addition, there is an accumulation of small fragments of link protein.[152] This accumulation of non-aggregating forms of aggrecan and degraded link protein may well contribute to further disc degeneration in the elderly. During growth of the immature disc, there is a high level of matrix metalloproteinase (MMP)-generated aggrecan degradation representing turnover during growth. Similarly, there is a significant amount of the aggrecanase-generated neoepitope in the annulus fibrosus but this declines in adulthood as turnover declines.[153, 154, 218] Based on the generation of these neo-epitopes, turnover in the nucleus pulposus declines to very low levels with age.

Changes also occur in the SLRPs. Both glycanated and non-glycanated forms of decorin and biglycan decrease with age after adolescence and fall to low levels in the nucleus pulposus. Fibromodulin is more abundant in the annulus fibrosus than the nucleus pulposus at all ages and shows a decline in the nucleus in the adult. In addition, fibromodulin without keratan sulfate chains becomes more prevalent with age.[58, 155] Lumican, which is more abundant in the nucleus pulposus than the annulus pulposus in young tissue, increases in the latter with age such that there are comparable levels in both in the adult.

Pathology of the intervertebral disc

Disc herniations

Prolapse or herniation of the intervertebral disc can occur to varying extents, resulting in protrusion or extrusion of the disc posteriorly or even sequestration, when a portion of the disc often migrates into the spinal canal breaking free from the disc itself (Fig. 19). Disc prolapse occurs most commonly in the lower spine at the L4–5 or L5–S1 discs

in physically active young or middle-aged adults. It presents as a clinical problem due, in part at least, to the pressure on the spinal nerves, the symptoms depending on the disc level and hence the tissues those spinal nerves supply and the extent of the 'bulge'. The sciatic nerve supplying the lower limb is often affected, leading to sciatica. In extreme cases a large midline bulge can cause paralysis of the bladder, requiring immediate surgical removal. In other cases, treatment ranges from conservative (analgesia or physiotherapy and manipulation) to surgical removal of the offending tissue. If surgery is not carried out it appears that the natural history of prolapsed disc tissue in many cases is for it to be resorbed.[156] Extruded and particularly sequestrated disc tissue becomes vascularized and demonstrates an increased presence of cytokines, proteases, etc. that are likely to be involved in degradation and diminution of the tissue. There are various theories as to what causes the herniation in the first place—is it increased load applied to the disc or diminished ability of the disc matrix to handle normal loads, due to perhaps increased enzyme activity leading to a 'weakening' of the matrix?

Posterior annular tears

Posterior annular tears are a further disorder of the posterior annulus fibrosus, when, as the name suggests, a fissure or rupture occurs through the annular lamellae.[157] It can be demonstrated by magnetic resonance imaging (MRI) (Fig. 19) or by injecting fluids into the disc when it reproduces the pain, and also, if radio-opaque, can be used to demonstrate the rupture. Unlike true disc herniation, annular tears are restricted to the outer region of the annulus, being either circumferential or radial tears. It is possible that they may develop into disc herniations with time if left untreated. Again, treatment can be conservative or surgical, when the offending part of the disc is removed.

Spinal deformities

Scoliosis or lateral curvature of the spine is the most common spinal deformity requiring surgical intervention. The curvature results from wedging of both intervertebral discs and vertebral bodies, often over several spinal levels (Fig. 20). It can develop secondarily to many diseases including muscular dystrophy, cerebral palsy, or several congenital connective tissue disorders such as Marfan's or Ehlers–Danlos syndrome. Alternatively, congenital abnormalities in the development of the vertebrae can lead to scoliosis, either through failure of the vertebrae to form symmetrically or through their failure to separate completely from each other.[158]

However, in the majority of patients there is no obvious cause, even though 'idiopathic scoliosis' has been researched for many years. This type most commonly affects adolescent girls with a thoracic curve to the right and a right-sided rib hump (a deformity seen when the patient leans forward), arising due to rotation of the spine.[159] If the curvature is seen to progress in adolescents, treatment again ranges from conservative bracing (the effectiveness remaining controversial) to surgery, when the deformity is corrected, the disc removed from the convex aspect of the curve, and fusion achieved, either anteriorly and/or posteriorly. Whilst there may be many causes of this disorder resulting in a similar symptom, genetic linkage studies have suggested a defect in fibrillin in at least a subgroup of patients.[160]

Kyphosis is curvature in the plane at 90° to that of scoliosis, resulting in a forward shift. It is less common than scoliosis and can be secondary to diseases such as Scheuermann's where there are many breaks and disorders of the cartilage endplate, or ankylosing spondylitis where calcification and fusion of the spine occurs spontaneously and progressively.

Spondylolisthesis

Spondylolisthesis is a 'forward slip' of one vertebra over another with the obvious distortion of the disc between. This often shows extensive remodelling, becoming much more ligamentous than usual. Spondylolistheses are graded ranging from I to IV depending on the level of overlap. The higher the grade, the more unstable it is and the more likely to require sugery. Spondylolisthesis can arise due to trauma, an ununited fracture of the pars interarticularis (the lamina between the facet joints), a dysplasia in the lamina allowing them to 'stretch' and the vertebrae to slide over one another, or even disc degeneration, especially at L4–5 in obese women in middle life.

Degenerative disc disease and spondylosis

Degenerative disc disease is identified radiologically as loss of disc space between the vertebrae. It is often accompanied by osteophyte formation at the vertebral rims and sclerosis of the bony endplate or rupture of the cartilage endplates. Whilst these are changes that occur more frequently with increasing age, they can occur earlier in some individuals, even in adolescence, when they are more likely to be associated with pain.[161, 219, 220] It is suggested that a genetic predisposition may result in this rapid advance of the normal degenerative process[221, 222] and recent studies indicate that gene polymorphisms of, for example, the vitamin D receptor[162] aggrecan[163] mmp3[223] or type IX callagen[206, 224, 225] could play a role in some patient groups.

Spinal stenosis

Disc degeneration later in life can contribute to spinal stenosis when either the central canal and/or the lateral recesses of the vertebrae are narrowed and result in neurogenic claudication. In addition to degenerate discs bulging increasingly and protruding into the canal, space in the spinal canal can be further diminished by increased sclerosis of the bony boundaries to the recess and canal. Thickening or even ossification of the ligamentum flavum can also further narrow the canal.[164] All will obviously diminish the space in the canals and increase the likelihood of compression of the cauda equina and spinal nerves. Symptoms will again depend on which nerves have pressure applied to them and the level of that pressure.

Animal models

Disc degeneration appears to occur spontaneously in certain animals, for example, the desert sand rat (*Psammomys obesus*). Approximately 50 per cent of these have significant disc disease by 18 months, with clear histological changes in 60 per cent of animals by the age of 30 months. Accompanying these changes in the disc, and perhaps even

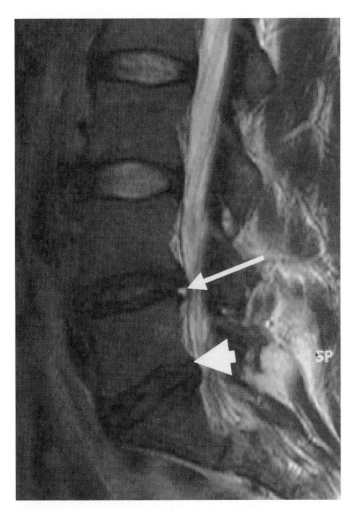

Fig. 19 Herniated disc (arrowhead) at L5–S1 level indicating compression on the cauda equina in the spinal canal as seen with magnetic resonance imaging (MRI). Note the increased signal at the disc level above this at L4–5 (arrow), demonstrating a posterior annular tear.

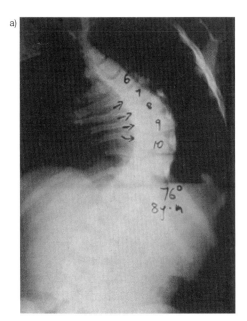
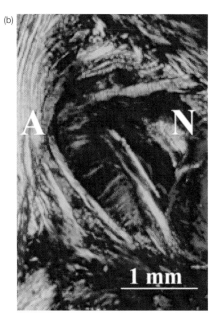
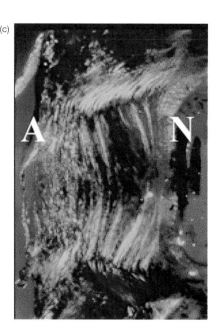

Fig. 20 (a) Lateral curvature of the spine occuring in scoliosis, with the primary curve being in the thoracic region with, in this case, the apex at T8–9. (b), (c) The discs here are wedged and the collagen bundles and annular lamellae disorganized and different at either side of the same disc. A, Annulus fibrosus; N, nucleus pulposus.

preceding them, are changes to the vertebral bone with subchondral bone sclerosis.[165] This provides evidence supporting one of the theories of a cause of disc degeneration—that of diminished nutrient pathways with calcification impeding the flow of nutrients into the intervertebral disc from the vertebrae. Another group of animals that suffers from disc degeneration is chondrodystrophoid dogs, such as beagles and dachshunds.[166] These animals frequently present with disc degeneration and herniations. Their discs resemble human discs in that notochord cells disappear during development, unlike in non-chondrodystrophoid dogs, where notochord cells remain into adulthood as in other species such as rabbit, pig, mouse, and cat.

Surgical disruption of the annulus in some animals including rabbits,[167] sheep,[168] and pigs[169] has been described as resulting in secondary degenerative changes in the central disc. A discrete cut in the outer annulus, made with a scalpel blade, results not only in remodelling of the outer lamellae but also biochemical and histological changes more centrally. However the changes do not mimic those seen in human spondylosis completely.

Various models of spinal deformities have also been developed, for example, by cutting ribs, muscles, ligaments, etc.[170] or actually applying asymmetrical loads across the disc.[171, 172] Whilst having all the usual problems associated with animal models and not replicating the disorder absolutely, animal models do at least provide an opportunity of studying an abnormality longitudinally, something that is technically very difficult in humans.

Extracellular matrix (ECM) changes in disc pathology

The degenerate intervertebral disc

The cause of disc degeneration is unknown but the disorder is considered to be a major cause of back pain and disability resulting in a significant drain on the economy and health services worldwide. In the

United Kingdom alone back pain affects 2–3 million people resulting in 14–15 million general practitioner (GP) consultations per annum.[173]

A number of potential causes of disc degeneration have been postulated. One likely cause is a deficiency in nutrition of the intervertebral disc leading to cell senescence and changes in cell phenotype and thus ultimately in the functional capabilities of the ECM. One of the major routes of nutrition for the intervertebral disc is through the cartilage endplate, which is known to calcify with increasing age.[124] Calcification would dramatically reduce the diffusion of essential nutrients into the disc as well as lowering the oxygen tension, giving rise to an altered cellular environment such as pH change through the increase in lactate concentration.[174] These changes might well result in changes in the cellular phenotype and consequent alterations in the ECM. It has been shown recently that nucleus pulposus chondrocytes synthezise significantly more proteoglycans when co-cultured with notochordal cells.[80] The age-related decline in the number of notochordal cells in the nucleus pulposus would therefore result in a deficiency in disc proteoglycans and a tissue less able to withstand compressive forces, one of its principal functions.

Collagens in the degenerate disc

Many of the age changes mentioned above are accentuated in the degenerate disc. For instance, there are changes in the collagenous constituents including an increase in the amount of denatured type II collagen and a loss of collagen types III and VI.[143] The low oxygen tension is thought to favour the formation of non-enzymic glycation of the collagens and it has been shown that glycanated type II collagen exhibits a reduced thermal stability, thus explaining the increase in the amount of denatured type II collagen present in the degenerate disc.[137, 145] Type X collagen has also been found in the degenerate disc closely associated with clusters of cells resembling hypertrophic chondrocytes. Type X collagen has been found in all regions of degenerate discs (Fig. 5(d)) and has been suggested to be an attempted repair response to altered loading.[37, 144] Type I collagen is also upregulated in the degenerate disc, resembling the response of articular cartilage to damage with the synthesis of a fibrocartilaginous tissue as an attempted repair process. As in cartilage, such tissue may be inadequate to withstand the mechanical loading imposed on these structures leading to a gradual degeneration and loss of function of the tissue.

Proteoglycans in the degenerate disc

There are also a number of changes that occur to the proteoglycan components of the disc. There is a loss of chondroitin-4-sulfate, particularly in the annulus fibrosus, that is most probably associated with aggrecan degradation. There is an increase in the carbohydrate epitopes 7D4 and 3B3(−) on the GAG chains of aggrecan, which, in cartilage, are normally only expressed during embryonic development and during attempted cartilage repair.[124, 175, 176] Their expression in the disc, however, did not correlate with disc degeneration. As stated above, the expression of fibromodulin decreases with age, but in the degenerate disc there is an upregulation of expression of fibromodulin throughout the disc and an increase in biglycan in the annulus fibrosus.[226] There is an increase in the non-glycanated forms of most of the proteoglycans. N-terminal sequence analysis has confirmed that these are indeed degradation products rather than alterations in the posttranscriptional events of proteoglycan biosynthesis.[58]

Genetic defects in matrix genes

Although the majority of the cases of disc degeneration may result from age-related nutritional deficiency, there are an increasing number of links with genetic defects in the genes coding for ECM components present in the disc and epidemiological evidence for genetic influence.[206, 221–225] Transgenic mice with a deletion mutation in the type II collagen gene revealed abnormalities to the vertebral column resulting in retarded removal of the notochord and abnormal shapes and sizes of the vertebral bodies and the intervertebral discs.[105, 106] Transgenic knock-out mice for the type II collagen gene revealed that, without type II collagen present during embryological development, notochordal bulging did not occur and intervertebral disc formation was prevented. Transgenic knock-out mice for the Col9a1 gene that codes for the alpha 1 chain of type IX collagen develop progressive joint degeneration with age as well as accelerated intervertebral disc degeneration.[177] A recent study has also shown linkage of intervertebral disc disease with a mutation in the COL9A2 gene that codes for the alpha 2 chain of type IX collagen.[178] A mutation altering a glutamic acid to a tryptophan residue was found in 6/157 patients. The mutation co-segregated with the disease giving a Lod score of 4.5. Disc degeneration has also been linked to the aggrecan gene. The cmd mouse, which lacks aggrecan, has severe skeletal malformations and dies shortly after birth. The heterozygote, however, appears to develop normally but with increasing age exhibits dwarfism and spinal misalignment.[179] It is suggested this could aid our search for mutations in humans that predispose to spinal degeneration. A recent study[163] has also linked a polymorphism associated with the aggrecan gene that predisposes to a high risk of multilevel disc degeneration. Those inheriting alleles with a shorter variable number tandem repeat exhibit this higher risk. Clearly, an increasing proportion of cases of disc degeneration will be found associated with mutations affecting disc ECM constituents. These mutations will lead to a tissue that lacks sufficient matrix integrity to withstand the mechanical loads that the spine is constantly subjected to, leading eventually to tissue failure.

Not all associations will necessarily be with ECM components. A recent study[162] has also revealed a vitamin D allelic polymorphism that is apparently linked to disc degeneration.

Matrix degradation and turnover in the degenerate disc

Whatever the underlying cause of the disease, the hallmark is the loss of matrix integrity of the intervertebral disc resulting in a tissue that is functionally inadequate. The common pathway is the imbalance of matrix degradation over matrix synthesis. A number of studies have investigated the role of proteinases in degenerative disc disease. ECM degradation is principally caused by the MMPs and the serine proteinases. A number of MMPs have been shown to be potentially involved in degradation of disc components including the collagenase MMP-1/13,[180] stromelysin MMP-3,[181, 182] and the gelatinases, MMPs 2 and 9.[183] MMP-3 has been found associated with inflammatory cells in herniated discs and is increased in expression/activation in degenerate discs.[180] There is also a reported decrease in TIMP-1 (tissue inhibitor of MMPs) altering the balance in favour of tissue degradation.[181] We studied the expression and activity of the gelatinases and showed a correlation between the grade of disc degeneration and the levels of both MMP-2 and 9 (Fig. 21(a)–(c)). Our related studies on the changes in the collagen cross-links with disc degeneration indicated that only in the severest grades was matrix degradation extensive, with a decrease in the age-related cross-link pentosidine (Fig. 22). No change was seen in the levels of HL-Pyr, indicating that the rate of tissue degradation was, in general, not rapid, consistent with the chronic progressive nature of the disease. However, changes in HL-Pyr have been observed by others in degenerative disc disease.

Innervation of the degenerate disc

Several studies have now identified degenerate intervertebral discs as having more extensive innervation than normal discs (Fig. 23).[184, 185] Physical probing of different regions of the spine has been carried out to try to identify the most likely tissue source responsible for back pain and sciatica.[186] This is obviously a very pertinent question to those involved in attempting to alleviate such clinical problems. Kuslich et al.[186] identified the outer annulus and vertebral endplate as the most common spinal tissue leading to pain production, second only to a compressed nerve root. The outer annulus in degenerative disc disease, having more innervation than the non-degenerate disc, would provide an explanation for the usefulness of discography, a diagnostic technique whereby a volume of radio-opaque material is injected that identifies the disc as the pain source when it reproduces the patient's pain syndrome.[187] Brown et al.[188] found proliferation of blood vessels and accompanying nerve fibres in the vertebral endplate and vertebral bodies of patients with disc degeneration and back pain compared to a control group. There were significantly more CGRP-positive sensory nerve fibres in low back pain patients compared to normal subjects.

Animal studies of disc degeneration provide mixed evidence regarding the disc and injury to it as a pain source. For example, a porcine model of disc degeneration caused by annular injury resulted in no increase in innervation in the wound area[189] whereas innervation was evident in a sheep model.[227] This is surprising in view of the fact that there was increased vascularity in the damaged disc, such that one would have expected sympathetic innervation for the control of this at least.

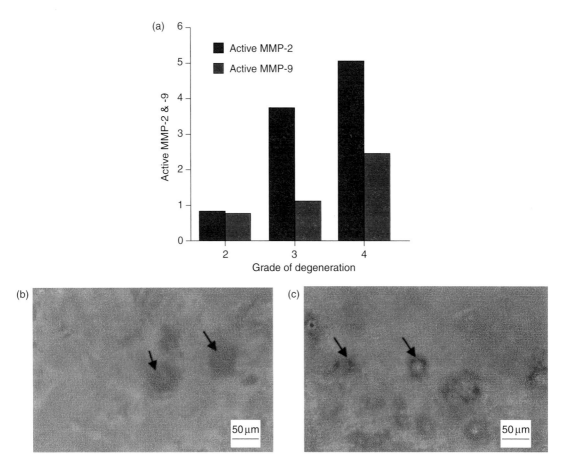

Fig. 21 (a) Active MMP-2 and -9 in the annulus fibrosus of the degenerate disc. Matrix metalloproteinases increase with grade of degeneration. Enzyme activity in a section of degenerate disc is demonstated by *in situ* zymography when there is loss of fluorescent signal around the cells (arrows) with a fluorescent-labelled substrate of (b) gelatin and (c) casein.

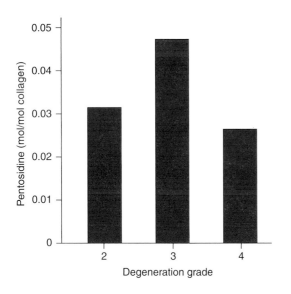

Fig. 22 Changes in pentosidine levels in disc degeneration. Pentosidine concentration is expressed as mol/mol collagen.

The presence of more innervation, with increased frequency, size, and penetration of nerves, into the degenerate human discs may, of course, be related to the sensation of pain in these patients. It may also have other physiological effects via the production of neuropeptides by the nerves. In addition to their role as neurotransmitters or modulators, many neuropeptides are known to have paracrine effects on connective tissue cells. For example, VIP stimulates bone resorption whilst CGRP inhibits it.[190, 191] Substance P has been shown to stimulate the release of cytokines[192] and enzymes (e.g. inteleukin-1(IL-1), tumour necrosis factor alpha (TNFα), collagenase) and also to increase proliferation in several connective tissue cells including disc cells.[193] Whether this is likely to be of relevance to the disc physiology remains unclear since the concentration used to produce these effects *in vitro* may be greater than is found in the disc *in vivo*.

The scoliotic disc and cartilage endplate

The primary cause of scoliosis is unknown but changes in the intervertebral disc and cartilage endplate will significantly contribute to the pathophysiology of the disease. The changes in composition and metabolism of the disc have been reviewed recently.[20, 194]

Proteoglycans in the scoliotic disc

The composition of the scoliotic disc and endplate differs from that of non-scoliotic discs of the same age, in having lower water and

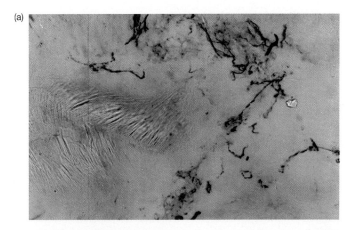

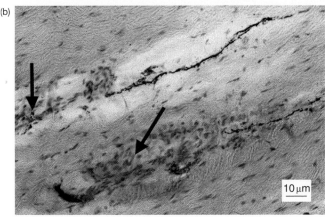

Fig. 23 (a) The density, size, and depth of penetration of nerves is greater in degenerate disc tissue, as shown here by PGP 9.5 immunostaining, than in non-degenerate disc (see Fig. 15(b)). (b) PGP 9.5 immunostaining and Mayer's haematoxylin. The nerves are sometimes, but not always, associated with blood vessels (arrows). Vascularization also increases with degeneration.

proteoglycan contents.[65, 195] The reduction tends to be greatest in the thinnest region of the disc, nearest the concavity of the scoliotic curve, with more difference being seen in the nucleus than in the annulus.[195] Other studies demonstrate no difference radially but the disc at the apex of scoliotic curve (the most deformed) have the highest water and proteoglycan content.[228] The structure of the proteoglycans also changes in scoliotic discs, with less aggregated and smaller proteoglycan monomers being found in the endplate nearer the convexity[196] and with scoliotic discs containing higher keratan sulfate concentrations than in normals.[197] If, as has been suggested, the production of keratan sulfate is favoured in areas of low oxygen concentration[198] such as have been found in scoliotic discs,[122] this could arise due to the calcification deposits in the endplate affecting nutrient flow.

Collagens in the scoliotic disc

In contrast to the proteoglycan and water contents, collagen content has been reported as being raised in the scoliotic nucleus[195] and in the concave side of the annulus.[199] It is not clear, however, if the amount of collagen actually increases or if its proportion changes as the result of loss of proteoglycan and other matrix components. The proportion of collagen types across the disc appears to alter in scoliosis. As stated previously, in the normal disc, the outer annulus is

predominantly type I collagen with type II collagen predominating towards the inner regions. In the scoliotic disc, however, there have been reports of a change in the proportion of these fibrillar collagens with a shift towards more type I collagen at the concavity.[199] The arrangement of the fibrillar collagen bundles and annular lamellae often differs in scoliotic discs compared to normals with severely crimped collagen bundles and changes in lamellar pattern seen contralaterally in the same scoliotic disc (Fig. 20(b), (c)).[65] Changes to the minor collagen population have also been reported. For example, more type III, VI, IX, and X collagen have been seen in the matrix of scoliotic discs than in normal discs.[31, 35, 37, 144] Similar changes have been reported in osteoarthritis, for example, type X collagen, the occurrence of which appears to correlate with remodelling in arthritic cartilage. Changes to the minor collagens can introduce subtle modifications in intermolecular interactions, which can in turn modulate the morphology of the matrix and the response of the embedded cells.[200]

Fibrillin

Other structural macromolecules besides collagen and proteoglycan may also be involved in scoliosis. For example, defects in the formation of fibrillin, a microfibrillar ECM component associated with elastin, have been identified in 17 per cent of patients with idiopathic scoliosis.[201]

Matrix degradation and turnover in the scoliotic disc

Altered composition of the ECM components in scoliosis may be the result of altered turnover in the disease, whether due to a change in loading, nutrition, genetics, or some other factor. For example, the levels of MMPs differ contralaterally in the scoliotic disc, being greater towards the convexity than the concavity (Fig. 24).[183] Although MMPs are involved in normal turnover and remodelling, aberration of the control mechanisms of their activity is thought to be responsible for degenerative changes in other connective tissues. Thus, increased MMP activity in arthritic cartilage appears to contribute to the breakdown and loss of matrix components such as proteoglycans. This raised activity can arise via an increase in synthesis of the enzymes, increased conversion from the latent to active form, or a decrease in the molecules that can bind to and render the enzyme inactive (TIMPs). More recently another enzyme, aggrecanase, has been identified as being responsible for proteoglycan degradation in osteoarthritis, particularly in the early stages. Aggrecanase has been identified in the intervertebral disc,[153, 154] but how it may be modulated in scoliosis remains to be investigated.

The collagen cross-link profile provides further evidence of matrix remodelling in the disc towards the convex side of the curve. Initially 'reducible' enzyme-mediated cross-links form, which, with time and maturity, undergo spontaneous further reactions to form the non-reducible, stable cross-links (see above). Levels of reducible cross-links are generally highest towards the convexity suggesting that the collagen population here is more recently synthesized than at the concavity.[47] As well as the indication of different rates of remodelling across the scoliotic disc, the collagen cross-link profile will also have implications for the integrity and mechanical properties of the matrix.

Calcification in the scoliotic disc

Deposits of calcium hydroxyapatite are frequently found in the cartilage endplates from scoliotic patients of all ages, sometimes making up as much as 47 per cent of the endplate's dry weight.[65] Since the

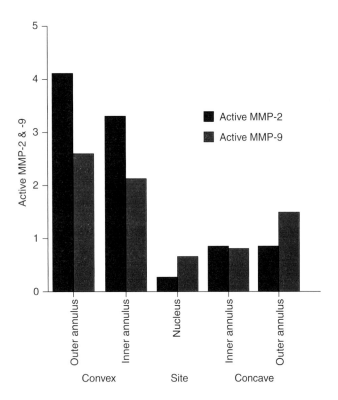

Fig. 24 Active MMP-2 and MMP-9 on the convex and concave sides of the intervertebral disc in scoliosis.

endplate contributes to the growth of the vertebrae, calcification here in young scoliotic patients is likely to affect this. Indeed premature closure of the growth plate at the concave side of the curve is reported by Pedrini-Mille *et al.*[196] Calcification in the body of the endplate is likely to have further additional consequences, since the disc relies primarily on diffusion of solutes to and from the vertebral body through the endplate for its clearance of waste products and nutrient supply, respectively.[202] Deposition of calcium salts can act as a barrier to transport, restricting the movement of even small molecules such as proline.[124] This could explain the findings of greatly reduced solute transport into scoliotic discs particularly at the apex where it is as low as 6% of that from unimpeded diffusion.[229]

Cell metabolism in the scoliotic disc

Levels of the metabolites, oxygen and lactate, have been measured across scoliotic discs.[122] Although variable, in general the oxygen concentration profile falls steeply (by as much as 80 per cent of the plasma levels) over the first 5 mm from the anterior surface before flattening out. Oxygen levels in some scoliotic discs were lower even than in degenerate discs from low back pain patients. In contrast, the lactate levels, as expected for a metabolite produced rather than consumed by cells, increased towards the centre of the disc and were greater than the concentration in the blood. The levels of these metabolites can have an influence on the metabolic activity of disc cells and affect matrix synthesis[173] with a decrease of either oxygen or pH reducing the ability of the disc cells to synthesize proteoglycans and proteins. The fall in pO_2 and rise in lactate in scoliotic discs would therefore reduce proteoglycan levels. Hence the change in metabolite levels may ultimately be responsible for the changes in composition seen in scoliotic discs.

Innervation of the scoliotic disc

There is some evidence that the nervous system could contribute to scoliosis. Experimental damage to the central nervous system at either the dorsal root or brainstem has been shown to produce scoliosis. Several studies have indicated abnormal neurological control of equilibrium and proprioception in scoliosis.[203, 204] The frequency of mechanoreceptors appears to differ in disc disorders. In spinal deformity patients, such as in scoliosis where there is lateral curvature of the spine and wedging of the discs, there is a lower frequency of receptors.[130] This may be important in the aetiology and presentation of the disorder in these patients, some at least of whom, it is suggested, have a central nervous system defect. Similarly, in an animal model of scoliosis in the chick, there appears to be reduced innervation and reduced proprioceptive receptors in the affected population (Raso and Bagnall, personal communication).

Future directions

Repair and even regeneration of intervertebral disc must be a target for the development of future therapies for disc disorders. Current treatments are either ineffectual in a significant number of patients and/or require the patient to undergo major surgical procedures. With the advent of tissue engineering, the physiology and functioning of disc cells or even other cell types may be harnessed and directed towards regenerating healthy disc matrix. Alternatively, synthetic but acellular artificial matrices with appropriate mechanical properties may be inserted into the disc space and suitably adhered to endogenous disc material. Such acellular approaches may be particularly pertinent for replacing a degenerate, non-functioning disc, where the mechanism of degeneration is largely unknown and where replacing cells, when it is not known what led to the death or malfunctioning of the original population, may be inappropriate. Alternatively, if our understanding of the breakdown of cell matrix functioning in disc diseases improves, we may be able to redress the situation by genetic engineering and insertion of appropriate genes, for example, perhaps for inhibition of MMPs or particular cytokines or growth factors. To date transfection of rabbit disc cells with transforming growth factor beta-1 (TGFβ1) gene has been performed by adenovirus-mediated transfer. This resulted in a subsequent 20-fold increase in active TGFβ1 production and 100 per cent increase in proteoglycan synthesis in the disc with transfected cells as compared to those in non-treated discs.[205] More recently sox9, the transcription factor that define the cartilaginous phenotype, has been used in studies to genetically modify intervertebral disc cells to aid regeneration.[220]

As our understanding of the aetiology and pathogenesis of disc diseases progresses, targets for the development of pharmacological agents will become obvious, for example specific enzymes or cytokines. By modulating the expression of particular factors it is to be hoped that such agents would have the potential for arresting or at least slowing down the degenerative cascade in the case of degenerative disc disease, or perhaps stimulating matrix synthesis at the narrowed, thinned region of the scoliotic disc.

Acknowledgements

We are indebted to Dr Tony Hayes, Cardiff University, for providing material from his doctoral thesis[7] for inclusion in this chapter.

References

1. Hukins, D.W.L. (1988). Disc structure and function. In *The biology of the intervertebral disc*, Vol. 1 (ed. P. Ghosh), pp. 1–37. CRC Press, Boca Raton, Florida.

2. Ager, A.M.R., Lee, M.J., and Grant, J.C. (eds.) (1999). *Grant's atlas of anatomy*, 10th edn. Lippin Cott Williams and Wilkins, Philadelphia.

3. Waddell, G. (1999). *The back pain revolution*. Churchill Livingston, London.

4. Maniadakis, N. and Gray, A. (2000). The economic burden of back pain in the U.K. *Pain* **84**, 95–103.

5. Taylor, J.R. (1990). The development and adult structure of lumbar intervertebral discs. *J. Man Med.* **5**, 43–47.

6. Bogduk, N. and Twomey, L.T. (1997). *Clinical anatomy of the lumbar spine and sacrum,* 3rd edn. Churchill Livingstone, London.

7. Hayes, A.J. (2000). The development of the annulus fibrosus of the intervertebral disc. PhD thesis, University of Wales, Cardiff.

8. Hickey, D.S. and Hukins, D.W.L. (1980). X-ray diffraction studies on the arrangement of collagenous fibres in human foetal intervertebral disc. *J. Anat.* **131**, 81–90.

9. Klein, J.A. and Hukins, D.W.L. (1982). Collagen fibre orientation in the annulus fibrosus of the intervertebral disc during bending and torsion measured by X-ray diffraction. *Biochim. Biophys. Acta* **717**, 61–64.

10. Klein, J.A. and Hukins, D.W.L. (1982). X-ray diffraction demonstrates reorientation of collagen fibres in the annulus fibrosus during compression of the intervertebral disc. *J. Biomech.* **16**, 211–217.

11. Inoue, H. and Takeda, T. (1975). Three-dimensional observation of collagen framework of lumbar intervertebral discs. *Acta. Orthop. Scand.* **46**, 949–956.

12. Inoue, H. (1981). Three dimensional architecture of lumbar intervertebral discs. *Spine* **6**, 138–146.

13. Taylor, J. and Twomey, L. (1988). The development of the human intervertebral disc. In *The biology of the intervertebral disc* (ed. P Ghosh), pp. 39–82. CRC Press, Boca Raton, Florida.

14. Klein, J.A., Hickey, D.S., and Hukins, D.W.L. (1983). Radial bulging of the annulus fibrosus during compression of the intervertebral disc. *J. Biomech.* **16**, 211–217.

15. Meachim, G. and Cornah, M.S. (1970). Fine structure of juvenile human nucleus pulposus. *J. Anat.* **107**, 337–350.

16. Bijlsma, F. and Peereboom, J.W. (1972). The ageing pattern of human intervertebral disc. *Gerontologia* **18**, 157–168.

17. Pritzker, K.P.H. (1997). Ageing and degeneration in the lumbar intervertebral discs. *Orthop. Clin. N. Am.* **8**, 65–77.

18. Trout, J.J., *et al.* (1982). Ultrastructure of the human intervertebral disc: I. Changes in notochordal cells with age. *Tissue Cell Res.* **14**, 359–369.

19. Trout, J.J., Buckwalter, J.A., and Moore, K.C. (1982). Ultrastructure of the human intervertebral disc: II. Cells of the nucleus pulposus. *Anat. Rec.* **204**, 307–314.

20. Roberts, S., *et al.* (2000). Structure and composition of the cartilage endplate and intervertebral disc in scoliosis. In Etiology of adolescent idiopathic scoliosis. *Spine* State of the art reviews (ed. R.G. Burwell, P.H. Dangerfield, T.G. Lowe, and J.Y. Margulies). *Spine* **14**, 371–381.

21. Humzah, M.D. and Soames, R.W. (1988). Human intervertebral disc: structure and function. *Anat. Rec.* **220**, 337–356.

22. Urban, J.P.G., *et al.* (1977). Nutrition of the intervertebral disc: an *in vivo* study of solute transport. *Clin. Orthop. Rel.* **129**, 101–114.

23. Crock, H.V. and Yoshizawa, H. (1976). The blood supply of the lumbar vertebral column. *Clin. Orthop.* **115**, 6–21.

24. Adams, P., Eyre, D.R., and Muir, H. (1977). Biochemical aspects of development and ageing of human lumbar intervertebral discs. *Rheumatol. Rehabil.* **16**, 22–29.

25. Bushell, G.R., Ghosh, P., Taylor, T.F.K., and Akeson, W.H. (1977). Proteoglycan chemistry of the intervertebral discs. *Clin. Orthop.* **129**, 115–123.

26. Eyre, D. (1988). Collagens of the disc. In *The biology of the intervertebral disc* (ed. P. Ghosh), Vol. 1, pp. 171–188. CRC Press, Boca Raton, Florida.

27. Ghosh, P. (ed.)(1988). *The biology of the intervertebral disc*, Vol. 1. CRC Press, Boca Raton, Florida.

28. Ghosh, P. (ed.)(1988). *The biology of the intervertebral disc*, Vol. 2. CRC Press, Boca Raton, Florida.

29. Ghosh, P., Bushell, G.R., Taylor, T.F.K., and Akeson, W.H. (1977). Collagens, elastin and noncollagenous protein of the intervertebral disc. *Clin. Orthop. Rel. Res.* **129**, 124–132.

30. Melrose, J. and Ghosh, P. (1988). The noncollagenous proteins of the intervertebral disc. In *The biology of the intervertebral disc*, Vol. 1 (ed. P. Ghosh), pp. 189–237. CRC Press, Boca Raton, Florida.

31. Roberts, S., Menage, J., Duance, V., and Wotton, S., and Ayad, S. (1991). Collagen types around the cells of the intervertebral disc and cartilage endplate: an immunolocalisation study. *Spine* **16**, 1030–1038.

32. Ayad, S. and Weiss, J.B. (1986). Biochemistry of the intervertebral disc. In *The lumbar spine and back pain* (ed. M.I.V. Jayson), pp. 100–137. Churchill Livingstone, London.

33. Eyre, D.R. and Muir, H. (1976). Types I and II collagens in human intervertebral disc. Interchanging radial distributions in annulus fibrosus. *Biochem. J.* **157**, 267–270.

34. Eyre, D.R. and Muir, H. (1977). Quantitative analysis of types I and II. collagens in human intervertebral disc at various ages. *Biochim. Biophys. Acta* **492**, 29–42.

35. Roberts, S., Menage, J., Duance, V., and Wotton, S.F. (1991). Type, III collagen in the intervertebral disc. *Histochem. J.* **23**, 503–508.

36. Rufai, A., Benjamin, M., and Ralphs, J.R. (1995). The development of fibrocartilage in the rat intervertebral disc. *Anat. Embryol.* **192**, 53–62.

37. Roberts, S., *et al.* (1998). Type X collagen in the intervertebral disc: an indication of repair or remodelling. *Histochem. J.* **30**, 89–95.

38. Newall, J.F., Morris, N.P., and Ayad, S. (1997). Immunolocalisation of collagens XII and XIV in the intervertebral disc. *Int. J. Exp. Pathol.* **78**, 24.

39. Wu, J.J., Eyre, D.R., and Slayter, H.S. (1987). Type VI collagen in the intervertebral disc: biochemical and electron-microscopic characterization of the native protein. *Biochem. J.* **248**, 373–381.

40. Roberts, S., Ayad, S., and Menage, P.J. (1991). Immunolocalization of type VI collagen in the intervertebral disc. *Ann. Rheum. Dis.* **50**, 787–791.

41. Newall, J.F. and Ayad, S. (1995). Collagen IX isoforms in the intervertebral disc. *Biochem. Soc. Trans.* **23**, 517.

42. Lammi, P., *et al.* (1998). Localization of type X collagen in the intervertebral disc of mature beagle dogs. *Matrix Biol.* **17**, 449–453.

43. Boos, N., Nerlich, A., Wiest, I., von der Mark, K., and Aebi, M. (1997). Immunolocalization of type X collagen in human lumbar intervertebral discs during ageing and degeneration. *Histochem. Cell. Biol.* **108** (6), 471–480.

44. Bailey, A.J. (1991). The eating quality of meat. *Chemi. Britain* **27**, 1013–1016.

45. Bailey, A.J., Herbert, C.M. and Jayson, M.I.V. (1976). In *The lumbar spine and back pain* (ed. M.I.V. Jayson). Sector Publishing Ltd., London.

46. Eyre, D.R. (1987). Collagen cross-linking amino acids. *Meth. Enzymol.* **44**, 115–139.

47. Duance, V.C., *et al.* (1998). Changes in collagen cross-linking in degenerative disc disease and scoliosis. *Spine* **23**, 2545–2551.

48. Fleischmajer, R., *et al.* (1990). Type I and type III collagen interactions during fibrillogenesis. *Ann. N.Y. Acad. Sci.* **580**, 161–175.

49. Young, R.D., *et al.* (2000). Immunolocalisation of collagen types II and III in single fibrils of human articular cartilage. *J. Histochem. Cytochem.* **48**, 423–432.

50. Duance, V.C., *et al.* (1999). Collagens of articular, growth plate and meniscal cartilages. In *Biology of the synovial joint* (ed. B. Caterson, C.W. Archer, M. Benjamin, and J. Ralphs), pp. 135–163. Harwood Academic Publishers, Amsterdam.

51. Timpl, R. and Engel, J. (1987). Type VI collagen. In *Structure and function of the collagen types* (ed. R.E. Mayne and R. Burgeson), pp. 105–143. Orlando, FL: Academic Press, Orlando, Florida.

52. Chu, M.L., *et al.* (1990). The structure of type VI collagen. *Ann. NY Acad. Sci.* **580**, 55–63.

53. Shaw, L.M. and Olsen, B.R. (1991). FACIT collagens—diverse molecular bridges in extracellular matrices. *Trends Biochem. Sci.* **16**, 191–194.

54. Trachslin, J. and Chiquet, M. (1998). Regulation of collagen, XII expression by mechanical stress. *FECTS* C21.

55. Kwan, A.P.L. (1999). Type X collagen. In *Biology of the synovial joint* (ed. B. Caterson, C.W. Archer, M. Benjamin, and J. Ralphs), pp. 165–176. Harwood Academic Publishers, Amsterdam.

56. Eyre, D.R. (1979). Biochemistry of the intervertebral disc. *Int. Rev. Connect. Tissue. Res.* **8**, 227–291.

57. Bayliss, M.T. and Johnstone, B. (1992). Biochemistry of the intervertebral disc. In *The lumbar spine and back pain*, 4th edn (ed. M.I.V. Jayson), pp. 111–131. Churchill Livingstone, London.

58. Johnstone, B., *et al.* (1993). Identification and characterization of glycanated and non-glycanated forms of biglycan and decorin in the human intervertebral disc. *Biochem. J.* **292**, 661–666.

59. Hardingham, T.E. and Fosang, A.J. (1992). Proteoglycans: many forms, many functions. *FASEB J.* **6**, 861–870.

60. Tengblad, A., Pearce, R.H., and Grimmer, B.J. (1984). Demonstration of link protein in proteoglycan aggregates from human intervertebral disc. *Biochem. J.* **222**, 85–92.

61. Johnstone, B. and Bayliss, M.T. (1995). The large proteoglycans of the human intervertebral disc: changes in their biosynthesis and structure with age, topography, and pathology. *Spine* **20**, 674–684.

62. Inkinen, R.I., *et al.* (1999). Hyaluronan distribution in the human and canine intervertebral disc and cartilage endplate. *Histochem. J.* **31**, 579–587.

63. Roberts, S., *et al.* (1994). Proteoglycan components of the intervertebral disc and cartilage end-plate—an immunolocalisation study of animal and human tissues. *Histochem. J.* **26**, 402–411.

64. Dours-Zimmerman, M.T. and Zimmerman, D.R. (1994). A novel glycosaminoglycan attachment domain identified in two alternative splice variants of human versican. *J. Biol. Chem.* **269**, 32992–32998.

65. Roberts, S., *et al.* (1994). Immunolocalisation of versican in the intervertebral disc. *Int. J. Exp. Pathol.* **75**, A30–31.

66. Johnstone, B., Roberts, S., and Menage, J. (1994). The occurrence of versican in the human intervertebral disc. *Trans. Orthop. Res. Soc.* **19**, 132.

67. Götz, W., *et al.* (1997). Immunohistochemical localization of the small proteoglycans decorin and biglycan in human intervertebral discs. *Cell. Tissue Res.* **289**, 185–190.

68. Hedbom, E. and Heinegård, D. (1993). Binding of fibromodulin and decorin to separate sites on fibrillar collagens. *J. Biol. Chem.* **268**, 27307–27312.

69. Sini, P., Denti, A., Tira, M.E., and Balduini, C. (1997). Role of decorin on *in vitro* fibrillogenesis of type I collagen. *Glycoconjugate J.* **14**, 871–874.

70. Svensson, L., *et al.* (1999). Fibromodulin-null mice have abnormal collagen fibrils, tissue organisation, and altered lumican deposition in tendon. *J. Biol. Chem.* **274**, 9636–9647.

71. Danielson, K.G., *et al.* (1997). Targeted disruption of decorin leads to abnormal collagen fibril morphology and skin fragility. *J. Cell. Biol.* **136**, 729–743.

72. Hagg, R., Bruckner, P., and Hedbom, E. (1998). Cartilage fibrils of mammals are biochemically heterogeneous: differential distribution of decorin and collagen, IX. *J. Cell. Biol.* **142**, 285–294.

73. Chakravarti, S., *et al.* (1998). Lumican regulates collagen fibril assembly: skin fragility and corneal opacity in the absence of lumican. *J. Cell. Biol.* **141**, 1277–1286.

74. Buckwalter, J.A., Cooper, R.R., and Maynard, J.A. (1976). Elastic fibers in human intervertebral discs. *J. Bone Joint Surg.* **58A**, 73–76.

75. Johnson, E.F., Chetty, K., Moore, I.M., Stewart, A., and Jones, W. (1982). The distribution and arrangement of elastic fibres in the intervertebral disc of the adult human. *J. Anat.* **135**, 301–309.

76. Mikawa, Y., Hamagami, H., Shikata, J., and Yamamuro, T. (1986). Elastin in the intervertebral disk. *Arch. Orthop. Traumat. Surg.* **105**, 343–349.

77. Robson, P., *et al.* (1993). Characterisation of lamprin, an unusual matrix protein from lamprey cartilage—implications for evolution, structure and assembly of elastin and other fibrillar proteins. *J. Biol. Chem.* **268**, 1440–1447.

78. Melrose, J. and Ghosh, P. (1988). The noncollagenous proteins of the intervertebral disc. In *The biology of the intervertebral disc* (ed. P. Ghosh), Vol. 1, pp. 189–237. CRC Press, Boca Raton, Florida.

79. Maroudas, A., Stockwell, R.A., Nachemson, A., and Urban, J. (1975). Factors involved in the nutrition of the human lumbar intervertebral disc: cellularity and diffusion of glucose *in vitro*. *J. Anat.* **120**, 113–130.

80. Aguiar, D.J., Johnson, S.L., and Oegema, T.R. (1999). Notochordal cells interact with nucleus pulposus cells: regulation of proteoglycan synthesis. *Exp. Cell Res.* **246**, 129–137.

81. Holm, S., *et al.* (1981). Nutrition of the intervertebral disc: solute transport and metabolism. *Connect. Tissue Res.* **8**, 101–119.

82. Errington, R.J., *et al.* (1998). Characterization of cytoplasm-filled processes in cells of the intervertebral disc. *J. Anat.* **192**, 369–378.

83. Chelberg, M.K., *et al.* (1995). Identification of heterogeneous cell populations in normal intervertebral disc. *J. Anat.* **186**, 43–53.

84. Gruber, H.E., *et al.* (1997). Human intervertebral disc cells from the annulus: three-dimensional culture in agarose or alginate and responsiveness to, TGFβ. *Exp. Cell Res.* **235**, 13–21.

85. Chiba, K., Andersson, G.B.J., Masuda, K., and Thonar, E.J.M.A. (1997). Metabolism of the extracellular matrix formed by intervertebral disc cells cultured in alginate. *Spine* **22**, 2885–2893.

86. Poiraudeau, S., *et al.* (1992). Phenotypic characteristics of rabbit intervertebral disc cells—comparison with cartilage cells from the same animals. *Spine* **24**, 837–844.

87. Buschmann, M., *et al.* (1992). Chondrocytes in agarose culture synthesise a mechanically functional extracellular matrix. *J. Orthop. Res.* **10**, 745–758.

88. Gregory, K.E., *et al.* (1999). Abnormal collagen assembly, though normal phenotype, in alginate bead cultures of chick embryo chondrocytes. *Exp. Cell. Res.* **246**, 98–107.

89. Pourquie, O., Coltey, M., Teillet, M.-A., Ordahl, C., and Le Douarin, N. (1993). Control of dorsoventral patterning of somitic derivatives by notochord and floor plate. *Proc. Natl Acad. Sci., USA* **90**, 5242–5246.

90. Verbout, A.J. (1985). The development of the vertebral column. *Adv. Anat. Embryol. Cell Biol.* **90**, 1–122.

91. Christ, B. and Wilting, J. (1992). From somites to vertebral column. *Ann. Anat.* **174**, 23–32.

92. Gilbert, S.F. (1997). *Developmental biology*, 5th edn. Sinauer Associates Inc, Sunderland, Massachusetts.

93. McGinnis, W. and Krumlauf, R. (1992). Homeobox genes and axial patterning. *Cell* **68**, 283–303.

94. Gospodarowicz, D. (1990). Fibroblast growth factor: chemical structure and biological function. *Clin. Orthop. Rel. Res.* **257**, 231–248.

95. Summerbell, D. and Maden, M. (1990). Retinoic acid, a developmental signalling molecule. *Trends Neurosci.* **13**, 142–147.

96. Weed, M., Mundlos, S., and Olsen, B.R. (1997). The role of sonic hedgehog in vertebrate development. *Matrix Biol.* **16**, 53–58.

97. Kessel, M. and Gruss, P. (1991). Homeotic transformations of murine vertebrae and concomitant alteration of Hox codes induced by retinoic acid. *Cell* **67**, 89–104.

98. Kessel, M., Balling, R., and Gruss, P. (1990). Variations of cervical vertebrae after expression of a Hox-1.1 transgene in mice. *Cell* **61**, 301–308.

99. Koseki, H., *et al.* (1993). A role for Pax-1 as a mediator of notochordal signals during the dorso-ventral specification of vertebrae. *Development* **119**, 649–660.

100. Ebensperger, C., *et al.* (1995). Pax-1, a regulator of sclerotome development is induced by notochord and floor plate signals in avian embryos. *Anat. Embryol.* **191**, 297–310.

101. Wallin, J., *et al.* (1994). The role of Pax-1 in axial skeleton development. *Development* **120**, 1109–1121.

102. Peacock, A. (1951). Observations on the pre-natal development of the intervertebral disc in man. *J. Anat.* **85**, 260–274.

103. Walmsley, R. (1953). The development and growth of the intervertebral disc. *Edinburgh Med. J.* **60**, 341–364.

104. Hayes, A.J., Benjamin, M., and Ralphs, J.R. (1999). Role of actin stress fibres in the development of the intervertebral disc: cytoskeletal control of extracellular matrix assembly. *Dev. Dyn.* **215**, 179–189.

105. Aszódi, A., *et al.* (1998). Collagen II is essential for the removal of the notochord and the formation of intervertebral discs. *J. Cell Biol.* **143**, 1399–1412.

106. Savantaus, M., Metsaranta, M., and Vuorio, E. (1997). Mutation in type II collagen gene disturbs spinal development and gene expression patterns in transgenic Dell mice. *Lab. Invest.* **77**, 591–600.

107. Peacock, A. (1951). Observations on the post-natal structure of the intervertebral disc in man. *J. Anat.* **86**, 162–179.

108. Benjamin, M. and Evans, E.J. (1990). Fibrocartilage. *J. Anat.* **171**, 1–15.

109. Ryan, M.C. and Sandell, L.J. (1990). Differential expression of a cysteine-rich domain in the amino-terminal propeptide of type II (cartilage) procollagen by alternative splicing of mRNA. *J. Biol. Chem.* **265**, 10334–10339.

110. Sandell, L.J. (1994). *In situ* expression of collagen and proteoglycan genes in notochord and during skeletal development and growth. *Microsc. Res. Tech.* **28**, 470–482.

111. Sandell, L.J., Morris, N., Robbins, J.R., and Golding, M.B. (1991). Alternatively spliced type II procollagen mRNAs define distinct populations of cells during vertebral development: differential expression of the amino-propeptide. *J. Cell Biol.* **14**, 1307–1319.

112. Oganesian, A., Zhu, Y., and Sandell, L.J. (1997). Type IIA procollagen amino propeptide is localised in human embryonic tissues. *J. Histochem. Cytochem.* **45**, 1469–1480.

113. Vinall, R.L. (1998). Identification and immunolocalisation of epithelial-like molecules within human articular cartilage. PhD thesis, University of Wales, Cardiff.

114. Durrant, L.A., Archer, C.W., Benjamin, M., and Ralphs, J.R. (1999). Organisation of the chondrocyte cytoskeleton and its response to changing mechanical conditions in organ culture. *J. Anat.* **194**, 343–353.

115. Zhang, Y., Cao, L., Kiani, C.G., Yang, B.L., and Yang, B.B. (1998). The G3 domain of versican inhibits mesenchymal chondrogenesis via the epidermal growth factor-like motifs. *J. Biol. Chem.* **273**, 33054–33063.

116. Zhang, Y., Cao, L., Kiani, C., Yang, B.L., Hu, W., and Yang, B.B. (1999). Promotion of chondrocyte proliferation by versican mediated G1 domain and, E.G.F.-like motifs. *J. Cell Biochem.* **73**, 445–447.

117. Roberts, S., Menage, J., and Urban, J.P.G. (1989). Biochemical and structural properties of the cartilage end-plate and its relation to the intervertebral disc. *Spine* **14**, 166–174.

118. Schmorl, G. (1971). Development, growth, anatomy and function of the spine. In *The human spine in health and disease*, 2nd edn (ed. E.F. Besemann), pp. 2–42. Grune and Stratton Inc, New York.

119. Yoshizawa, H., Ohiwa, T., Kubota, K., and Crock, H.V. (1986). Morphological study on the vertebral route for the nutrition of the intervertebral disc. *Neuro Orthopaedics* **1**, 17–32.

120. Nachemson, A., Lewin, T., Maroudas, A., and Freeman, M.A.R. (1970). *In vitro* diffusion of dye through the endplates and the annulus fibrosus of human intervertebral discs. *Acta Orthop. Scand.* **41**, 589–607.

121. Ogata, K. and Whiteside, L.A. (1981). Nutritional pathways of the intervertebral disc. An experimental study using hydrogen washout technique. *Spine* **6**, 211–215.

122. Bartels, E.M., Fairbank, J.C.T., Winlove, C.P., and Urban, J.P.G. (1998). Oxygen and lactate concentrations measured *in vivo* in the intervertebral discs of patients with scoliosis and back pain. *Spine* **23**, 1–8.

123. Stairmand, J.W., *et al.* (1991). Factors influencing oxygen concentration gradients in the intervertebral disc. *Spine* **16**, 444–449.

124. Roberts, S., Urban, J.P.G., Evans, H., and Eisenstein, S. (1996). Transport properties of the human cartilage endplate in relation to its composition and calcification. *Spine* **21**, 415–420.

125. Holm, S. and Nachemson, A. (1988). Nutrition of the intervertebral disc: acute effects of cigarette smoking. *Uppsala J. Med. Sci.* **93**, 91–99.

126. Jackson, H.C., Winkelmann, R.K., and Bickel, W.H. (1966). Nerve endings in the human lumbar spinal column and related structures. *J. Bone Joint Surg. Am.* **48** (7), 1272–1281.

127. Groen, G.J., Baljet, B., and Drukker, J. (1990). Nerves and nerve plexuses of the human vertebral column. *Am. J. Anat.* **188**, 282–296.

128. Bogduk, N., Tynan, W., and Wilson, A.S. (1981). The nerve supply to the human lumbar intervertebral discs. *J. Anat.* **132**, 39–56.

129. Suseki, K., *et al.* (1998). Sensory nerve fibres from lumbar intervetebral discs pass through rami communicantes. *J. Bone Joint Surg. Br.* **80**, 737–742.

130. Ahmed, M., *et al.* (1993). Neuropeptide Y, tyrosine hydroxylase and vasoactive intestinal polypeptide-immunoreactive nerve fibers in the vertebral bodies, discs, dura mater and spinal ligaments of the rat lumbar spine. *Spine* **18**, 268–273.

131. Ashton, I.K., *et al.* (1994). Neuropeptides in the human intervertebral disc. *J. Orthop. Res.* **12**, 186–192.

132. Malinsky, J. (1959). The ontogenetic development of nerve terminations in the intervertebral discs of man. *Acta Anat.* **38**, 96–113.

133. Roberts, S., *et al.* (1995). Mechanoreceptors in intervertebral discs. Morphology, distribution and neuropeptides. *Spine* **20**, 2645–2651.

134. Indahl, A., Kaigle, A.M., Reikeras, O., and Holm, S. (1997). Interaction between the porcine lumbar intervertebral disc, zygapophysial joints and paraspinal muscles. *Spine* **22**, 2834–2840.

135. Urban, J.P.G. and McMullin, J.F. (1988). Swelling pressure of the lumbar intervertebral discs—influence of age, spinal level, composition and degeneration. *Spine* **13**, 179–187.

136. Yasuma, T., *et al.* (1992). Age-related phenomena in the lumbar intervertebral discs: lipofuscin and amyloid deposition. *Spine* **17**, 1194–1197.

137. Postachinni, F., Bellocci, M., and Massobrio, M. (1984). Morphological changes in annulus fibrosus during ageing—an ultrastructural study in rats. *Spine* **9**, 596–603.

138. Hickey, D.S. and Hukins, D.W.L. (1982). Ageing changes in the macromolecular organisation of the intervertebral disc. An X-ray diffraction and electron microscopic study. *Spine* **7**, 234–242.

139. Antoniou, J., Goudsouzian, N.M., Heathfield, T.F., *et al.* (1996). The human lumbar endplate—evidence of changes in biosynthesis and denaturation of the extracellular matrix with growth, maturation, aging and degeneration. *Spine* **21**, 1153–1161.

140. Antoniou, J., *et al.* (1996). The human lumber intervertebral disc. Evidence for changes in the biosynthesis and denaturation of the extracellular matrix with growth, maturation, ageing and degeneration. *J. Clin. Invest.* **98**, 996–1003.

141. Hollander, A.P., *et al.* (1996). Enhanced denaturation of the α1(II) chains of type II collagen in normal adult human intervertebral discs compared with femoral articular cartilage. *J. Orthop. Res.* **14**, 61–66.

142. Nerlich, A.G., Schleider, E.D., and Boos, N. (1997). Immunohistologic markers for age-related changes of human lumbar intervertebral discs. *Spine* **22**, 2781–2795.

143. Nerlich, A.G., Boos, N., Wiest, I., and Aebi, M. (1998). Immunolocalisation of major interstitial collagen types in human lumbar intervertebral discs of various ages. *Virchows Arch.* **432**, 67–76.

144. Aigner, T., *et al.* (1998). Variation with age in the pattern of type X collagen expression in normal and scoliotic human intervertebral discs. *Calcif. Tissue Int.* **63**, 263–268.

145. Pokharna, H.K. and Phillips, F.M. (1998). Collagen crosslinks in human lumbar intervertebral disc aging. *Spine* **23**, 1645–1648.

146. Sell, D.R. and Monnier, V.M. (1989). Structure elucidation of a senescence cross-link from human extracellular matrix. Implication of pentoses in the aging process. *J. Biol. Chem.* **264**, 21597–21602.

147. Hormel, S.E. and Eyre, D.R. (1991). Collagen in the aging intervertebral disc: an increase in covalently bound fluorophores and chromophores. *Biochim. Biophys. Acta* **1078**, 243–250.

148. Yang, C., *et al.* (1994). Structural and functional implications of age-related abnormal modifications in collagen II from intervertebral disc. *Matrix Biol.* **14**, 643–651.

149. Hanson, D.A. and Eyre, D.R. (1996). Molecular site-specificity of pyridinoline and pyrrole cross-links in type-I collagen of human bone. *J. Biol. Chem.* **271**, 26508–26516.

150. Paul, R.G. and Bailey, A.J. (1996). Glycation of collagen: the basis of its central role in the late complications of ageing and diabetes. *Int. J. Biochem. Cell Biol.* **28**, 1297–1310.

151. Kuypers, R., *et al.* (1992). Identification of the loci of the collagen-associated Ehrlich chromogen in type-I collagen confirms its role as a trivalent cross-link *Biochem. J.* **283**, 129–136.

152. Pearce, R.H., *et al.* (1989). Effect of age on the abundance and fragmentation of link protein of the human intervertebral disc. *J. Orthop. Res.* **7**, 861–867.

153. Sztrolovics, R., *et al.* (1997). Aggrecan degradation in human intervertebral disc and articular cartilage. *Biochem. J.* **326**, 235–241.

154. Roberts, S., *et al.* (2000). Matrix metalloproteinases and aggrecanase: their role in disorders of the human intervertebral disc. *Spine* **25**, 3005–3013.

155. Sztrolovics, R., *et al.* (1999). Age-related changes in fibromodulin and lumican in human intervertebral discs. *Spine* **24**, 1765–1771.

156. Saal, J.A., Saal, J.S., and Herzog, R.J. (1990). The natural history of lumbar intervertebral disc extrusions treated nonoperatively. *Spine* **15**, 683–686.

157. Park, W.M., McCall, I.W., O'Brien, J.P., and Webb, J.K. (1979). Fissuring of the posterior annulus fibrosus in the lumbar spine. *Br. J. Radiol.* **52**, 382–387.

158. Eisenstein, S. and Jones, R. (1998). Spinal deformities. In *Orthopaedic physiotherapy* (ed. M. Tidswell), pp. 173–185. Mosby, London.

159. Lonstein, J.E. (1994). Adolescent idiopathic scoliosis. *Lancet* **344**, 1407–1412.

160. Miller, N.H., *et al.* (1996). Genetic analysis of structural elastic fiber and collagen genes in familial adolescent idiopathic scoliosis. *J. Orthop. Res.* **14**, 994–999.

161. Jaffray, D.C. (1998). Degeneration of the lumbar spine. In *Orthopaedic physiotherapy* (ed. M. Tidswell), pp. 165–171. Mosby, London.

162. Videman, T., Leppavuori, J., Kaprio, J., *et al.* (1998). Intragenic polymorphism of the vitamin D receptor gene associated with intervertebral disc degeneration. *Spine* **23**, 2477–2485.

163. Kawaguchi, Y., *et al.* (1999). Association between an aggrecan gene polymorphism and lumbar disc degeneration. *Spine* **24**, 2456–2460.

164. Porter, R.W. (1995). The pathophysiology of neurogenic claudication. In *Lumbar spine disorders. Current concepts* (ed. R.M. Aspden and R.W. Porter), pp. 120–131. World Scientific, Singapore.

165. Ziran, B.H., *et al.* (1994). Biomechanical, radiologic, and histopathologic correlations in the pathogenesis of experimental intervertebral disc disease. *Spine* **19**, 2159–2163.

166. Sether, L.A., Nguyen, C., Yu, S., *et al.* (1990). Canine intervertebral disks: correlation of anatomy and MR imaging. *Radiology* **175**, 207–211.

167. Lipson, S.J. and Muir, H. (1981). Proteoglycans in experimental intervertebral disc degeneration. *Spine* **6**, 194–210.

168. Osti, O.L., Vernon-Roberts, B., and Fraser, R.D. (1990). Annulus tears and intervertebral disc degeneration. An experimental study using an animal model. *Spine* **15**, 762–767.

169. Kaapa, E., *et al.* (1994). Neural elements in the normal and experimentally injured porcine intervertebral disc. *Eur. Spine J.* **3**, 137–142.

170. Michelsson, J.-E. (1965). The development of spinal deformity in experimental scoliosis. *Acta Orthop. Scand.* **81** (suppl.), 62–77.

171. Sarwark, J.F., Dabney, K.W., Salzman, S.K., *et al.* (1988). Experimental scoliosis in the rat. I. (1988). Methodology, anatomic features, and neurologic characterization. *Spine* **13**, 466–471.

172. Stokes, I.A.F., Aronsson, D.D., Spence, H., and Iatridis, J.C. (1998). Mechanical modulation of intervertebral disc thickness in growing rat tails. *J. Spinal Dis.* **11**, 261–265.

173. Oshima, H. and Urban, J.P.G. (1992). The effect of lactate and pH on proteoglycan synthesis rates in the intervertebral disc. *Spine* **17**, 1079–1082.

174. Clinical Standards Advisory Group (1994). *Epidemiological review: the epidemiology and cost of back pain.* HMSO, London.

175. Caterson, B., Mahmoodian, F., Sorrell, J.M., *et al.* (1990). Modulation of native chondroitin sulphate in tissue development and in disease. *J. Cell Sci.* **97**, 411–417.

176. Inkinen, R.I., Lammi, M.J., Lehmonen, S., Puustjarvi, K., Kääpä, E., and Tammi, M.I. (1998). Relative increase of biglycan and decorin and altered CS epitopes in the degenerating human intervertebral disc. *J. Rheumatol.* **25**, 506–514.

177. Kimura, T., Nakata, K., Tsumaki, N., *et al.* (1996). Progressive degeneration of articular cartilage and intervertebral discs—an experimental study in transgenic mice bearing a type IX collagen mutation. *Int. Orthop.* **20**, 177–181.

178. Annunen, S., Paassilta, P., Lohiniva, J., *et al.* (1999). An allele of, COL9A2 associated with intervertebral disc disease. *Science* **285**, 409–412.

179. Watanabe, H., Nakata, K., Kimata, K., Nakanishi, I., and Yamada, Y. (1997). Dwarfism and age-associated spinal degeneration of heterozygote cmd mice defective in aggrecan. *Proc. Natl Acad. Sci. USA* **94** (13), 6943–6947.

180. Matsui, Y., Maeda, M., Nakagami, W., and Iwata, H. (1998). The involvement of matrix metalloproteinases and inflammation in lumbar disc herniation. *Spine* **23**, 863–868.

181. Kanemoto, M., Hukuda, S., Komiya, Y., Katsuura, A., and Nishioka, J. (1996). Immunohistochemical study of matrix metalloproteinase 3 and tissue and tissue inhibitor of metalloproteinase 1 in human intervertebral discs. *Spine* **21**, 1–8.

182. Nemoto, O., Yamagishi, M., Yamada, H., Kikuchi, T., and Takaishi, H. (1997). Matrix metalloproteinase-3 production by human degenerate intervertebral disc. *J. Spinal Dis.* **10**, 493–498.

183. Crean, J.K.G., Roberts, S., Jaffray, D.C., Eisenstein, S.M., and Duance, V.C. (1997). Matrix metalloproteinases in the human intervertebral disc: role in disc degeneration and scoliosis. *Spine* **22**, 2877–2884.

184. Coppes, M.H., Marani, E., Tomeer, R.T.W.M., and Groen, G.J. (1997). Innervation of 'painful' lumbar discs. *Spine* **22**, 2342–2350.

185. Freemont, A.J., Peacock, T.E., Goupille, P., Hoyland, J.A., O'Brien, J., and Jayson, M.I.V. (1997). Nerve ingrowth into diseased intervertebral disc in chronic back pain. *Lancet* **350**, 178–181.

186. Kuslich, S.D., Ulstrom C.L., and Michael, C.J. (1991). The tissue origin of low back pain and sciatica. A report of pain response to tissue stimulation during operations on the lumbar spine using local anesthesia. *Orthop. Clin. N. Am.* **22**, 181–187.

187. Weinstein, J., Claverie, W., and Gibson, S. (1988). The pain of discography. *Spine* **13**, 1344–1348.

188. Brown, M.F., Hukkanen, M.V.J., McCarthy, I.D., Redfern, D.R., Batten, J.J., Crock H.V., Hughes, S.P., and Polak, J.M. (1997). Sensory and sympathetic innervation of the vertebral endplate in patients with degeneration. *J. Bone Joint Surg. Br.* **79**, 147–153.

189. Kääpä, E., Han, X., Holm, S., Peltonen, J., Takala, T., and Vanharanta, H. (1995). Collagen synthesis and types I, III, IV, and VI in an animal model of disc degeneration. *Spine* **20**, 59–67.

190. Hohmann, E.L., Levine, L., and Tashjian, A.H. (1983). Vasoactive intestinal peptide stimulates bone resorption via a cyclic adenosine 3′,5′-monophosphate-dependent mechanism. *Endocrinology* **112**, 1233–1239.

191. Zaidi, H., Fuller, K., Bevis, P.J.R., GainesDas, R.E., Chambers, T.J., and MacIntyre, I. (1987). Calcitonin gene-related peptide inhibits osteoclastic bone resorption: a comparative study. *Calcif. Tissue Int.* **40**, 149–154.

192. Lotz, M., Carson, D.A., and Vaughan, J.H. (1987). Substance P activation of rheumatoid synoviocytes; neural pathway in pathogenesis of arthritis. *Science* **235**, 893–895.

193. Ashton, I.K., Walsh, D.A., Polak, J.M., and Eisenstein, S.M. (1994). Substance P in intervertebral discs. Binding sites on vascular endothelium of the human annulus fibrosus. *Acta Orthop. Scand.* **65**, 635–639.

194. Taylor, T.K.F. and Melrose, J. (2000). The role of the intervertebral disc in adolescent idiopathic scoliosis. In *Spine: State of the art reviews on etiology of adolescent idiopathic scoliosis* (ed. R.G. Burwell, P.H. Dangerfield, T.G. Lowe, and J.Y. Margulies), pp. 359–369. Harley and Belfus Inc., Philadelphia.

195. Ponseti, I.V., Pedrini, V., Wynne-Davies, R., and Duval-Beaupere, G. (1976). Pathogenesis of scoliosis. *Clin. Orthop.* **120**, 268–280.

196. Pedrini-Mille, A., Pedrini, V.A., Tudisco, C., *et al.* (1993). Proteoglycans of human scoliotic intervertebral disc. *J. Bone Joint Surg. Am.* **65**, 815–823.

197. Melrose, J., Ghosh, P., and Taylor, T.K.F. (1994). Proteoglycan heterogeneity in the normal adult ovine intervertebral disc. *Matrix Biol.* **14**, 61–75.

198. Scott, J.E., Bosworth, T.R., Cribb, A.M., and Taylor, J.R. (1994). The chemical morphology of age-related changes in human intervertebral disc glycosaminoglycans from cervical, thoracic and lumbar nucleus pulposus and annulus fibrosus. *J. Anat.* **184**, 73–82.

199. Brinkley-Parsons, D. and Glimcher, M.J. (1984). Is the chemistry of collagen in the human intervertebral disc an expression of Wolff's law? *Spine* **9**, 148–163.

200. Reichberger, E. and Olsen, B.R. (1996). Collagens as organizers of the extracellular matrix during morphogenesis. *Semin. Cell Dev. Biol.* **7**, 631–638.

201. Hadley-Miller, N., Mims, B., and Milewicz, D.M. (1994). The potential of the elastic fibre system in adolescent idiopathic scoliosis. *J. Bone Joint Surg.* **76**, 1193–1206.

202. Urban, J.P.G., Holm, S., and Maroudas, A. (1978). Diffusion of small solutes into the intervertebral disc. *Biorheology* **15**, 203–223.

203. Yamada, K., Yamamoto, H., Nakagawa, Y., Tezuka, A., Tamura, T., and Kawata, S. (1984). Etiology of idiopathic scoliosis. *Clin. Orthop.* **184**, 50–57.

204. Geissele, A.E., Kransdorf, M.J., Geyer, C.A., Jelinek, J.S., and Van Dam, B.E. (1991). Magnetic resonance imaging of the brain stem in adolescent idiopathic scoliosis. *Spine* **16** (7), 761–763.

205. Nishida, K., Kang, J.D., Gilbertson, L.G., *et al.* (1999). Modulation of the biologic activity of the rabbit intervertebral disc by gene therapy of the human transforming growth factor β1 encoding gene. *Spine* **24**, 2419–2455.

206. Eyre, D.R., Matsui Y. and Wu, J-J. (2002). Collagen polymorphisms of the intervertebral disc. *Biochem. Soc. Trans.* **30**, 844–848.

207. Wu, J.-J. and Eyre, D.R. (2003). Intervertebral disc collagen. Usage of the short form of the alpha 1(IX) chain in bovine nucleus pulposus. *J. Biol. Chem.* 278, 24521–24525.

208. Yu, J., *et al.* (2002). Elastic fibre organization in the intervertebral discs of the bovine tail. *J. Anat.* **201**, 465–475.

209. Yu, J. (2002). Elastic tissues of the intervertebral disc. *Biochem. Soc. Trans.* **30**, 848–852.

210. Oegema, T.R., *et al.* (2000). Fibronectin and its fragments increase with degeneration in the human intervertebral disc. *Spine* **25**, 2742–2747.

211. Oegema, T.R. (2002). The role of disc cell heterogeneity in determining disc biochemistry: a speculation. *Biochem. Soc. Trans.* **30**, 839–843.

212. Thonar, E., An H. and Masuda, K. (2002). Compartmentalization of the matrix formed by nucleus pulposus and annulus fibrosus cells in alginate gels. *Biochem. Soc. Trans* **30**, 874–877.

213. Smits, P. and Lefebvre, V. (2003). Sox5 and Sox6 are required for notochord extracellular matrix sheath formation, notochord cell survival and development of the nucleus pulposus of intervertebral discs. *Development* **130**, 1135–1148.

214. McAlinden, A., Zhu, Y. and Sandell, L. (2002). Expression of type II procollagen during development of the human intervertebral disc. *Biochem. Soc. Trans.* **30**, 831–838.

215. Urban, J.P.G. (2002). The role of the physicochemical environment in determining disc cell behaviour. *Biochem. Soc. Trans.* **30**, 858–864.

216. Johnson, W.E., *et al.* (2002). Human intervertebral disc aggrecan inhibits nerve growth in vitro. *Arth & Rheum.* **46**, 2658–2664.

217. Boos, N., *et al.* (2002). Classification of age-related changes in lumbar intervertebral discs. Spine, 27, 2631–2644.

218. Roughley, P.J., *et al.* (2002). The role of proteoglycans in aging degeneration and repair of the intervertebral disc. *Biochem. Soc. Trans.* **30**, 869–874.

219. Fairbank, J. (2002). Clinical importance of the intervertebral disc, or back pain for biochemists. *Biochem. Soc. Trans.* **30**, 829–831.

220. Roberts, S. (2002). Disc morphology in health and disease. *Biochem. Soc. Trans.* 30, 864–869.

221. Battie, M.C., *et al.* (1995). Similarities in degenerative findings on magnetic resonance images of the lumbar spines of identical twins. *J. Bone & Joint Surg. (Am.)* 77, 1662–1670.

222. Sambrook, P.N., *et al.* (1999). Genetic influences on cervical and lumbar disc degeneration. *Arth. & Rheum.* **42**, 366–372.

223. Takahashi, M., *et al.* (2001). The association of degeneration of the intervertebral disc with 5a/6a polymorphism in the promoter of the human matrix metalloproteinase-3 gene. *J. Bone & Joint Surgery* (Br.) **83-B**, 491–495.

224. Paassilta, P., *et al.* (2001). Identification of a novel common genetic risk factor for lumbar disc disease. *JAMA* **285**, 1843–1849.

225. Solovieva, S., *et al.* (2002). COL9A3 gene polymorphism and obesity in intervertebral disc degeneration of the lumbar spine: evidence of gene-environment interaction. *Spine* 27, 2691–2696.

226. Cs-Szabo, G., *et al.* (2002). Changes in mRNA and protein levels of proteoglycans of the annulus fibrosus and nucleus pulposus during intervertebral disc degeneration. *Spine*, 27, 2212–2219.

227. Melrose, J., *et al.* (2002). Increased nerve and blood vessel ingrowth associated with proteoglycan depletion in an ovine anular lesion model of experimental disc degeneration. *Spine* 27, 1278–1285.

228. Urban, M.R., *et al.* (2001). Intervertebral disc composition in neuromuscular scoliosis. *Spine* **26**, 610–617.

229. Urban, M.R., *et al.* (2001). Electrochemical measurement of transport into scoliotic intervertebral discs in vivo using nitrous oxide as a tracer. *Spine* **26**, 984–990.

230. Paul, R., *et al.* (2003). Potential use of sox9 gene therapy for intervertebral degenerative disc disease. *Spine* **28**, 755–763.

1.5 The meniscus—structure, composition, and pathology

Jayesh Dudhia, Audrey McAlinden, Paula Muir, and Michael Bayliss

Introduction

The menisci of the human knee joint are two crescent-shaped fibrocartilaginous elements that play a critical role in the maintenance of normal synovial articulation. Once described as the functionless remains of leg muscle,[1] the menisci are now known to be integral components of the knee and to contribute significantly to its biomechanical properties.

The function, injury, and repair of the meniscus have long been topics of interest and discussion among orthopaedic surgeons. It is now generally accepted that the primary function of this tissue is to distribute load throughout the joint. The menisci have adapted to play this role and are composed predominantly of extracellular matrix (ECM). The cell (fibrochondrocyte) content is a very small proportion of the total volume of the tissue. The major component of the ECM is collagen, the majority of which is arranged circumferentially, that is, parallel to the periphery of the meniscus. Non-collagenous matrix components, such as proteoglycans and other glycoproteins, are either interspersed within, or bound to, the collagen network. Some of these matrix components are also present in articular cartilage, a tissue in close contact with the menisci. However, there are distinct differences in the ECMs of both tissues and these will be discussed in this chapter.

In marked contrast to articular cartilage, our knowledge of the biochemistry of collagens, proteoglycans (PGs), and non-collagenous proteins (NCPs) in the meniscus is poor. Limited studies have shown that the amounts of collagens, PGs, and NCPs vary with age and degeneration of the human meniscus.[2, 3] However, identification of the matrix components that are contributing to these age-related and pathological changes remains to be elucidated.

Anatomy of the knee joint

The human knee joint (Fig. 1(a)) is classified as a diarthrodial joint structure capable of flexion, extension, and rotation. These movements are complex and involve both rolling and gliding of the femur on the tibia. It is the largest of the human joints in terms of volume of its synovial cavity and the area of its articular cartilage. The human knee joint is an organ consisting of specialized tissues, the shapes and tensions of which contribute to its normal motion. Disruption in the structure of any of these tissues will ultimately lead to organ failure as exemplified in the degenerative clinical condition, osteoarthritis.

Major tissues of the knee joint

Fibrous capsule and ligaments aid in maintaining the integrity of the knee joint. These periarticular structures are fairly uniform in

histological appearance, chemical composition, and tissue organization. They are hyperhydrated with estimates of water ranging up to approximately 70 per cent. Like most connective tissues, they are composed predominantly of collagen fibres and relatively few cells (fibrocytes). Blood vessels and nerve fibres are interspersed within the collagen network. The dense fibrous tissue of the capsule occupies the entire joint and inserts into bones usually close to the articulating surface. This complex capsular structure is thickened in parts to form named ligaments, for example, the coronary and transverse ligaments (Fig. 1(b)).

Accessory ligaments include the anterior and posterior cruciates and the medial and lateral collateral ligaments. The cruciate ligaments are composed of bundles of fibres of different lengths that twist around a

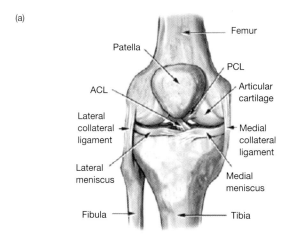
(a)

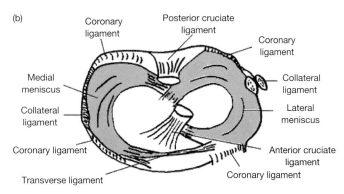
(b)

Fig. 1 (a) Anterior view of the human knee joint. ACL, Anterior cruciate ligament; PCL, posterior cruciate ligament. (b) Proximal view of a tibial plateau. The lateral and medial menisci (coloured) and associated capsular ligaments are shown.

main axis. This arrangement allows part of the ligament to be under tension in all positions of the joint. For example, the anterior cruciate ligament is described as being composed of two bands: an anteromedial, which is taut when the knee is flexed, and a posterolateral, which is taut when the knee is extended. Therefore, the capsule in association with the cruciate and collateral ligaments provides the joint with stability.

Synovium

Synovium is a vascular connective tissue, lining the inner surface of the capsule but not covering the articular cartilage.[4] The cells lining this tissue (synoviocytes) secrete synovial fluid. Normal synovial fluid is clear, pale yellow, and viscous. It is normally present in very small amounts (1–4 ml) in the human knee. The viscosity of the fluid is due to the presence of a large polyanionic molecule, hyaluronan and proteinaceous materials, which have considerable importance in lubrication. There is growing interest in the analysis of synovial fluid for molecular markers of disease and fragments of molecules derived from the surrounding connective tissues in the joint have been identified in this fluid.[5] Changes in the molecular composition of the fluid have been related to processes that may be occurring in the joint during degeneration.

Articular cartilage

Articular cartilage is a specialized connective tissue component found firmly attached to the underlying bones. It has been shown to vary in thickness depending on the site within the joint.[6] It is a dense, white tissue on gross inspection, which becomes yellow with age. Despite a high water content (up to 80 per cent), this avascular, anueral tissue is semisolid. Histological and ultrastructural examination of the cartilage demonstrates a predominance of ECM and only sparse cellularity. Distribution of these cells (chondrocytes), and matrix components synthesized by the chondrocytes, varies throughout the depth of the cartilage. Thus, four distinct zones—superficial, intermediate, deep, and calcified—have been described for this tissue.

The biomechanical function of articular cartilage is to withstand compressive forces within the joint. This property depends on the unique structural organization of the ECM. In particular, the collagen network is responsible for the tensile properties of the tissue and a high concentration of PGs endows the cartilage with important viscoelastic properties.[7] The balance between the tensile strength of the collagen fibres and the swelling pressure of the PGs gives cartilage its compressive stiffness and the ability to expand back to its original shape when load is removed.

The biochemical properties of this tissue have been the focus of attention for many years. These studies have enhanced our knowledge of the structure and turnover of components in the ECM in articular cartilage. More importantly, age-related and pathological changes in ECM composition have since been discovered. Aspects of these changes will be discussed and used as a comparison to the major joint tissue of interest in this chapter: the meniscus.

Anatomy and structure of the meniscus

The lateral and medial menisci of the human knee joint are two crescents of fibrocartilage, with a wedge-shaped cross-section, that fit into the space between the femoral condyles and the tibial plateau (Fig. 1(a)). These periarticular soft tissues are shaped to maximize their role as distributors of load within the joint: the proximal surface of the menisci in contact with the femoral condyles is concave, whereas the distal surface in contact with the tibial plateau is flat or slightly convex. Figure 1(b) shows the shape and attachments of the lateral and medial menisci on the tibial plateau. The lateral meniscus is of equal width throughout its length, whereas the posterior region of the medial meniscus is wider than its anterior end. Strong ligamentous horns attach the fibrocartilage to the tibial plateau. The tissue is further secured through various attachments to capsular components of the joint, for example, the collateral ligaments.

Microanatomy of the meniscus

The microanatomy of the meniscus is complex and age-dependent. The characteristic shapes of the lateral and medial menisci are attained early in prenatal development. At that time they are very cellular and highly vascularized throughout their substance.[8] Vascularity decreases postnatally, progressing from the central to the peripheral margin. After skeletal maturity, the peripheral portion constitutes from 10–30 per cent of the total structure. The most peripheral aspect of the meniscus is the meniscosynovial junction, which extends from the anterior to the posterior horns. This is a transitional zone with the deeper, collagenous tissue gradually shifting from meniscal tissue to capsular protein tissue. The blood supply originates from a network of vessels within the peripheral capsular and synovial attachments: the perimeniscal capillary plexus.[9] This arborizing network of vessels enters the meniscus through the fringe of the synovium and provides vascularity to the peripheral 25–33 per cent of the meniscus. The peripheral region also contains nerve endings[10] and probably provides the outermost part of the meniscus with oxygen and nutrients.[11] The remaining, more visceral portion of the meniscus is made up of an avascular, aneural, and alymphatic fibrocartilage consisting of an abundant ECM.

Biomechanical properties of the meniscus

The menisci serve several important biomechanical functions in the knee. They distribute stresses over a broad area of articular cartilage, absorb shocks during dynamic loading, and probably assist in joint lubrication. In addition, the menisci serve a secondary biomechanical function by providing stability to the injured knee when the cruciate ligaments or other primary stabilizers are deficient.[12]

The ability to perform these mechanical functions is based on the intrinsic material properties of the menisci as well as their gross anatomical structure and attachments.[13] The material properties of the menisci are determined by the organization and interactions of the major tissue constituents of the ECM: water; collagens; and PGs. These interactions render meniscal tissue a porous, permeable composite material similar to articular cartilage. The arrangement of collagen fibres in the meniscus allows the tissue to effectively distribute load throughout the joint. The most important mechanical properties of collagen fibres are their tensile stiffness and strength. They make their greatest contribution to tissue material properties when they are aligned along the direction of the load, as they are in tendons and ligaments. The majority of collagen fibres in the meniscus are arranged parallel to its periphery. These circumferential fibres maximize the ability of the tissue to function as a load-bearing structure.[14, 15]

Radially arranged fibres are also present in areas of the fibrocartilage.[16] It has been recently demonstrated that these radial fibres influence the tensile properties of the bovine medial meniscus. Meniscal tissue containing radial fibres were found to be significantly stronger and stiffer than specimens with no radial fibres.[17] In addition, there was regional variation in the tensile modulus, with the posterior meniscus being the stiffest portion. Such topographical variations in collagen arrangement emphasize the complexity of meniscus structure. The organization of meniscal components has probably been adapted to cope with a variety of load-bearing stresses applied on the tissue. These variations should be considered when analysing the structure and composition of the meniscus.

Partial or total removal of the meniscus (meniscectomy) dramatically alters the pattern of load transmission across the knee joint. Several investigators have noted greater stress concentrations[18, 19] and decreased shock-absorbing capability[20, 21] after total meniscectomy. Bourne and co-workers[22] concluded that both partial and total meniscectomy significantly alters the pattern of strain distribution across the tibial plateau. Therefore, it is likely that loss of the meniscus due to meniscectomy allows overloading of the articular cartilage and subsequent joint degeneration.

Extensive studies by Shrive[23] demonstrated that the menisci distribute approximately 40–60 per cent of the load acting on the knee. Fewer constraints operate on the movement of the lateral meniscus on the tibial plateau, making this tissue more efficient than the medial meniscus in distributing load. Movement of the medial meniscus on the tibia is approximately 2 mm compared to 10 mm for the lateral meniscus. Experiments carried out by Seedhom and co-workers[24] using cadaveric knees also showed that the menisci transmit a large portion of the load applied to the joint. Generally, it was found that the medial meniscus transmits 40–50 per cent and the lateral meniscus transmits 65–70 per cent of the load acting on the respective side. Thus, it is not surprising that injury to one or both menisci will affect their ability to carry out important biomechanical functions and lead to the disruption of normal knee joint articulation.

Extracellular matrix of the meniscus

The meniscus is a dense connective tissue in that it is composed of relatively few cells surrounded by an abundant ECM. The ECM is a system of insoluble fibrils and soluble polymers that has evolved to cope with load-bearing stresses of movement. This structurally stable material consists of water and four major classes of macromolecules: collagens, PGs, NCPs, and elastin. Together, these macromolecules contribute to the shape, strength, and resiliency of the tissue. The cells not only synthesize matrix components, but also continue to interact with the ECM products. Therefore, the metabolism, shape, and other properties of the cells are related to and are dependent on the composition and organization of the matrix.

ECM components in the meniscus are arranged so as to optimize the ability of the tissue to distribute load within the knee joint. The organization and composition of the ECM are therefore fundamental to the properties of the meniscus. Disruption of this organized structure as a result of tissue damage or osteoarthritis will ultimately lead to joint failure.

Water content of the meniscus

The meniscus consists of approximately 70 per cent water.[25] Meniscal tissues of young individuals are usually white, have a translucent

quality, and are supple on palpation. The menisci in older individuals lose their translucency, become thinner, more opaque, and yellow in colour, and feel less supple. It is likely that this thinning and lack of suppleness observed in different ages of tissue are due to loss of water.

There have been no studies reported on age-related or topographical changes in water content in the meniscus. However, in other connective tissues such as articular cartilage, water content was found to vary markedly through the depth of the tissue.[26, 27] Lower levels of water have been detected in areas of cartilage[27] and tendon[28] that have been subjected to loading. Dehydration was found to cause cell proliferation and inhibition of matrix synthesis in rabbit tendon.[29] Therefore, the presence of water in connective tissues is vital for maintaining both the structural characteristics of the tissue and the viability of the cells synthesizing the matrix.

Collagens

The collagens constitute a highly specialized family of glycoproteins.[30] Collagens are the major constituents of all ECMs and can be described as molecular ropes that transmit and resist tensile strain. Collagens are distinguished from other matrix components by the presence of a triple helix formed by the intertwining of three α-helical polypeptide chains. Glycine occupies every third residue and this is an absolute requirement, as glycine is the only residue with a small enough side-chain to fit into the centre of the triple helix without distorting it. Approximately 20–22 per cent of the remaining X and Y residues in the repeating triplet $[\text{Gly-X-Y}]_n$ are, respectively, the imino acids proline and hydroxyproline.

The α chains of the collagen molecules form the basis of their nomenclature. In addition, each collagen type has been designated by a roman numeral in the order in which they were discovered, for example, types I, II, III, etc. Therefore, the molecular composition of type I collagen, (a heterotrimer of two $\alpha 1(I)$ chains and one $\alpha 2(I)$ chain) is $[\alpha 1(I)]_2 \alpha 2(I)$. In contrast, type II collagen is a homotrimer of three identical chains designated $\alpha 1(II)$ giving a molecular composition of $[\alpha 1(II)]_3$.

The synthesis of collagen α chains follows the established pathway of other secretory proteins but involves several co- and posttranslational modifications. These include: (1) hydroxylation of proline and lysine; (2) glycosylation of hydroxylysine; (3) sulfation of tyrosine; (4) disulfide bond formation and chain association; and (5) the addition of complex carbohydrates and glycosaminoglycans (GAGs). The modified collagen chains are then secreted and deposited in the ECM. Additional modifications can occur in the ECM, which depend on the collagen type and specific supramolecular structure formed.

The superfamily of collagens[31] can be subdivided into several classes on the basis of the polymeric structures they form or related structural features. In most connective tissues, the majority of collagens in the ECM are organized into highly ordered thin filaments or fibrils that are subsequently aggregated into fibres or fibre bundles. These fibril-forming collagens or FFCs include types I, II, III, V, and XI. Collagen components that are located on the surface of collagen fibrils and regulate their aggregation are known as fibril-associated collagens with interrupted triple helix or FACITs. These include types IX, XII, XIV, XVI, and XIX.[32] Other classes of collagens include the network-forming collagens (the type IV family), short-chain collagens (types VIII and X), the collagen that forms beaded filaments (type VI), and collagens that have a transmembrane domain (types XIII and XVII).

Collagen types in the meniscus

Collagen constitutes 60–70 per cent of the dry weight of meniscal fibrocartilage. A seminal study by Eyre and Muir[33] established that the major type of collagen in porcine menisci was type I, an observation consistent with the fibrocartilaginous nature of the tissue. Like all FFCs, type I collagen is first synthesized as a large precursor procollagen molecule within the cell before secretion into the extracellular space. Pro-collagenases cleave the *N*- and *C*-terminal propeptides to form the triple-helix tropocollagen molecules that then self-aggregate to form fibrils. These fibrils are stabilized by intermolecular cross-links derived from specific lysine/hydroxylysine residues in both the non-helical (telopeptide) and helical domains.

Trace quantities of the FFCs, types III and V, have been demonstrated in the meniscus.[34] These collagens are generally present in type I collagen-containing tissues. Type III collagen has been found not only to co-polymerize with type I fibrils, but also to regulate the diameter of these fibrils.[35] In addition, heterotypic combinations of types I and III collagens have been identified in human skin[36] and tendon.[37] Similarly, assembly of types I and V collagens results in the formation of heterotypic collagen fibres.[38] The presence of type V fibres is thought to control the diameter size of collagen I fibrils. Types III and V collagen fibres generally result in a more compliant tissue. Therefore, although collagen interactions have not been studied in any great detail in the meniscus, it is likely that heterotypic I/III and I/V fibres exist to maximize the ability of the meniscus to distribute load.

A small but significant amount of type II collagen has been identified in the meniscus.[39, 40] This molecule is the major collagen type found in articular cartilage[41] and it has been found to assemble with type XI collagen[42] and type I collagen,[43] forming heterotypic fibre structures. Collagen type II is the product of a single gene (COL2A1), the mutation of which has been found to be associated with the early onset of primary generalized osteoarthitis.[44] Interestingly, increased levels of type II collagen have been identified in osteoarthitic menisci (Wardale, personal communication 1996), which may suggest that the matrices of these diseased menisci are of a more cartilaginous nature.

Type VI collagen constitutes approximately 2 per cent of the dry weight of the meniscus.[45] This ubiquitously expressed molecule is characterized by a relatively short, triple-helical domain that bears relatively large, globular glycoprotein domains at each extremity.[46] The function of type VI collagen is unknown but its role as an intermolecular adhesive protein has been postulated. In addition to type I collagen fibres, the small PG, decorin, has also been found to bind collagen type VI filaments.[47] Chung et al.[48] have analysed levels of type VI collagen in the medial posterior region of maturing and ageing sheep menisci. In this region of tissue, it was found that the concentration of type VI declined sharply at skeletal maturity and continued to decline during ageing. The enhanced type VI collagen levels during development of the sheep meniscus are consistent with a role for this protein in processes in which the assembly of a new matrix is required.

Arrangement and distribution of collagen fibres in the meniscus

Collagen fibres are orientated throughout the meniscus in such a way as to maximally resist the forces that are brought to bear on this tissue. Figure 2 shows that the majority of these fibres are circumferentially arranged, making the meniscus much stiffer in this direction than in the radial direction.[14, 15] Some investigators have suggested that the radial fibres, found deep within the tissue as well as on the femoral and tibial surfaces, act to resist both lateral spread of the tissue and longitudinal splitting that can lead to bucket handle tears.[16] Site-dependent variations in collagen composition in the meniscus were demonstrated by Eyre et al.[40] Comparison of articulating surfaces and deep

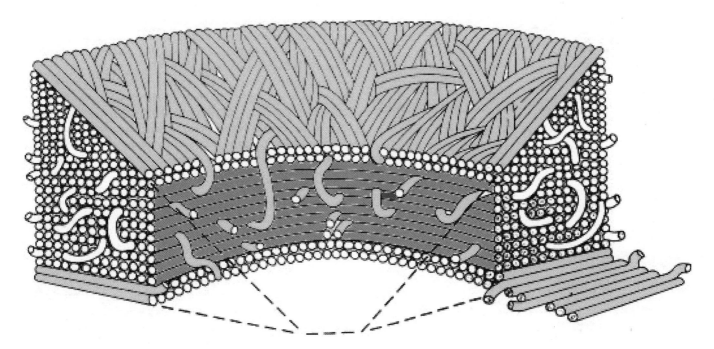

Fig. 2 Distribution of collagen type I fibres in the meniscus. The fibres are mostly circumferentially arranged (red), but radially arranged fibres are also present (yellow). The wedge of the meniscus is shown through the dashed lines.

zones of bovine menisci revealed three times as much type V collagen in the surface zone. Further variations in the distribution of collagen fibres were found between the outer two thirds and the inner third of bovine menisci.[39] The outer region was composed almost entirely of type I collagen with trace amounts of types III and V collagen. The inner region contained mainly types I and II collagen. This region has been shown to resemble articular hyaline cartilage both in gross appearance and histological examination.[49]

These observations highlight the heterogeneity of collagen composition in the meniscus. In addition, Table 1 displays the striking difference in collagen composition between menisci and articular cartilage. Even though these tissues have similar biomechanical functions in the knee joint, they are biochemically very different tissues. As will be discussed throughout this chapter, variations in other matrix components, such as PGs, also contribute to the differences in ECM composition between these tissues.

Proteoglycans

PGs are very complex macromolecules consisting of a central protein core with one or more negatively charged carbohydrate side-chain substituents, termed glycosaminoglycans (GAGs).[50] These ubiquitous molecules are found on cell surfaces, within intracellular vesicles, and in ECMs. Only PGs found in the ECM will be discussed in this chapter. PGs have no unifying features such as a collagen triple helix, and they display a great diversity of protein forms with regard to their protein core size as well as the amount and composition of GAG chain attachments.

The general features of the biosynthetic assembly of PGs[51] are as follows: (1) synthesis of the core protein; (2) xylosylation of specific serine moieties of the core protein; (3) addition of a galactose (Gal) residue to the xylose (Xyl), followed by a Gal and glucuronic acid (GlcUA) residue to complete the GlcUA-Gal-Gal-Xyl tetrasaccharide protein–GAG linkage moiety; (4) repeat addition of hexosamine residues alternating with GlcUA or Gal residues to form the large heteropolymer GAG chain; and (5) modification of these GAG chains by variable N-deacetylation/N-sulfation, and/or O-sulfation, and variable

epimerization of GlcUA to iduronic acid. In addition, glycoprotein-like N-linked or O-linked glycosylation takes place before or while the oligosaccharide linkage region and GAGs are being formed.

The assembly of the linkage region on the core protein followed by GAG polymerization, sulfation, and epimerization occurs completely isolated from the cytoplasm within the intracellular membrane system composed of the endoplasmic reticulum, transfer vesicles, Golgi apparatus, and secretory vesicles. Each step in the synthesis of PGs is controlled by specific enzymes, but how these enzymes are regulated to produce specific PGs has yet to be elucidated.

Glycosaminoglycans

GAGs are polyanionic chains of variable length constructed from repeating disaccharide units that contain a hexosamine and a uronic acid residue.[52] In mammalian tissues, there are five major classes of GAGs: hyaluronic acid; chondroitin sulfate; dermatan sulfate; keratan sulfate; and the heparan sulfate/heparin class. Figure 3 shows the repeating disaccharide structure of each GAG. GAGs dominate the physical properties of the protein to which they are attached. PGs in the ECM function physically as creators of a water-filled compartment. Their high fixed negative charge attracts counter-ions and the osmotic balance caused by a local high concentration of ions draws water from the surrounding area.[53] Therefore, the GAGs are responsible for the hydration of the ECM. A further physical property of the GAG chain is that they exclude other matrix macromolecules while retaining permeability to low molecular weight solutes. The PGs thus create a water compartment, only part of which is available to other matrix macromolecules, and, therefore, may increase reaction rates and promote all interactions that are concentration-dependent.

Hyaluronan (HA) consists of an alternating polymer of glucuronic acid and N-acetylglucosamine (GlcNAc), joined by a β1–3 linkage (Fig. 3). This GAG is unique since it functions in vivo as a free carbohydrate. The biosynthesis of HA is different from that of the PGs. It is not formed within or attached to intracellular membrane structures, but is synthesized at the inner surface of the plasma membrane by pathways quite distinct from those of PG GAG formation.[54] HA synthesis involves the transfer of UDP-glucuronate and UDP-N-acetylglucosamine to nascent HA by HA synthase.

A study has shown that HA synthase, identified in plasma membranes from a eukaryotic cell line, contains two subunits of 52 and 60 kDa that bind to the precursor UDP-glucuronate.[55] A single molecule of HA can have a molecular weight of up to 10 million. It assumes a randomly kinked, coil structure that endows solutions with high viscosity. The individual molecules can self-associate and form networks and a number of PGs can associate with HA, forming supramolecular aggregates in the ECM. Electron microscopic characterization of HA showed that the region bound to articular cartilage PG (aggrecan) monomers was condensed to approximately half of its original length.[56] This implies that HA adopts a defined spatial arrangement within the central filament of the aggregate, probably different from its secondary structure in solution.

HA has been suggested to be an important factor in various processes including transforming growth factor-β (TGF-β) binding[57] and regulation of PG synthesis.[58] Recently, it has been shown that HA may induce meniscal tissue remodelling after partial meniscectomy.[59]

Chondroitin sulfate (CS) is composed of repeating units of N-acetylgalactosamine (GalNAc) and glucuronic acid (GlcUA) joined

Table 1 Collagen types in the meniscus and articular cartilage

Collagen class and type	Formula	Total collagen (%) in	
		Meniscus	Articular cartilage
FFCs			
I	$[\alpha1(I)]_2\alpha2(I)$	95	—
II	$[\alpha1(II)]_3$	< 1	95
III	$[\alpha1(III)]_3$	1	—
V	$[\alpha1(V)]_2\alpha2(V)$	1	Variable
FACIT			
IX	$[\alpha1(IX)\alpha2(IX)\alpha3(IX)]$	—	1–2
XII	$[\alpha1(XII)]_3$	—	< 1
XIV	$[\alpha1(XIV)]_3$	—	< 1
Filamentous			
VI	$[\alpha1(VI)\alpha2(VI)\alpha3(VI)]$	2–3	0–1
Short-chain			
X	$[\alpha1(X)]_3$	—	1

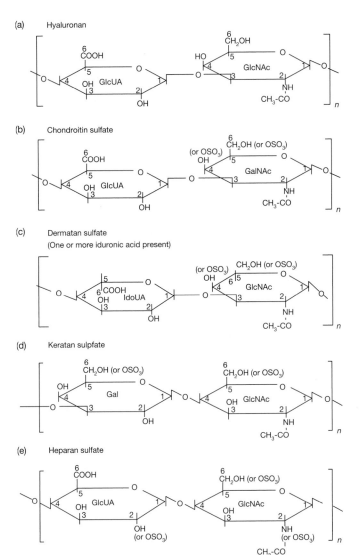

Fig. 3 The repeating disaccharide units of glycosaminoglycans.

by a β1–3 linkage (Fig. 3). There are three known sites of ester sulfation in the sugar moieties of the CS chain: the 2-hydroxyl of the glucuronic acid and the 4- and 6-hydroxyls of the GalNAc residue.[60] Monosulfated disaccharides, where the sulfate is located in either the 4- or 6-hydroxyls of GalNAc, are the most common forms of CS found in nature and the proportion of the two varies with growth and development. In addition, non-sulfated isomers of CS also occur, but these are often only in discrete domains within the CS GAG chain and are more frequently found in embryonic and young, developing tissues. The biological function and significance of these isomeric variations are not known at present.

Dermatan sulfate (DS) has a similar structure to that of CS except that one or more glucuronic acid residues are epimerized and converted to iduronic acid. Once formed, the iduronic acid residues may be sulfated in the 2 position. The glycosidic bond is also changed to α1–3. Variations in the distribution of DS have been noted, for example human articular cartilage,[61] bovine tendon,[62] and bovine skin[63] all contain DS proteoglycans whereas bovine bone[64] and porcine laryngeal cartilage[61] are devoid of iduronate.

Keratan sulfate (KS) consists of a repeating disaccharide sequence comprising galactose (Gal) and GlcNAc joined by a β1–3 linkage. Therefore, in contrast to the other GAGs listed above, KS does not contain uronic acid. Proteoglycan KS chains are normally sulfated on the 6-position of either or both sugar moieties. The degree of sulfation is variable, and oversulfation is common, with the extra sulfate ester group found at position 2 of the galactose residues.

High molecular weight, aggregating proteoglycans

Both aggrecan and versican are termed 'aggregating' due to their ability to bind to HA in the ECM.[65, 66] The interaction with HA is mediated by a common core protein element localized at the N-terminus of the PG molecules, thus forming large macromolecular complexes.

A matrix protein termed link protein or LP[67] stabilizes the aggrecan/HA aggregate[68] by binding to both components. It was demonstrated recently that the concentration of LP is an important factor influencing the stability of the PG aggregates.[69] In articular cartilage, LP exists in three forms (LP1, LP2, and LP3) differing in molecular weight (41–48 kDa) due to differential glycosylation and a loss of the N-terminal portion as a result of proteolytic cleavage.[70] LP in the versican/HA interaction has not yet been characterized.

Aggrecan is the major PG component in articular cartilage. The large number of GAG chains attached to aggrecan endows the tissue with important viscoelastic properties.[7] Figure 4 shows the domain structure of aggrecan including the attachment sites of the GAG chains. The intact core protein of aggrecan is 2316 amino acids long with a molecular weight of approximately 220 kDa.[65] The main globular domains of aggrecan are termed G1, G2, and G3.

The G1 domain, also referred to as HA binding region (HABR), is located at the N-terminus of aggrecan and has a molecular weight in the range 70–100 kDa. This region contains an immunoglobin (Ig) fold that shares sequence homology with members of the IgG superfamily of proteins.[71] Two PG tandem repeat (PTR) sequences are also present in the G1 domain and contain a sequence similar to that found in the lymphocyte homing receptor CD44, a glycoprotein that also binds to hyaluron.[72] The G2 domain (110 kDa) contains a tandem repeat structure similar to that found in the G1 domain and link protein. The function of this domain is unclear—the isolated domain does not interact with HA, LP, aggrecan monomers, or other major components of the ECM.[73] Although the exact function of it is still unknown, it appears to function by inhibiting aggrecan secretion.[74] It has been shown that both G1 and G2 work in concert with each other inhibiting secretion of aggrecan, whilst G3 and the chondroitin sulfate-glycosylated core protein region promote secretion. Therefore, G2 acts as a secretion retardant, ensuring that only fully glycosylated aggrecan monomer is secreted.[75]

Aggrecan is extensively modified with CS, KS, and other oligosaccharides. KS chains are covalently bound to aggrecan core protein and are concentrated near the G2 domain. CS chains are covalently linked to the central region of the core protein and there may be up to 150 chains per aggrecan monomer. Some KS chains are also present in this CS-dominant region.

At the C-terminal end of aggrecan are three types of subdomains that together form a globular structure, the G3 domain, for which no direct functional properties have been assigned. The G3 domain is readily cleaved from secreted aggrecan and there is a steady decline with advancing age in the number of aggrecan molecules in the ECM

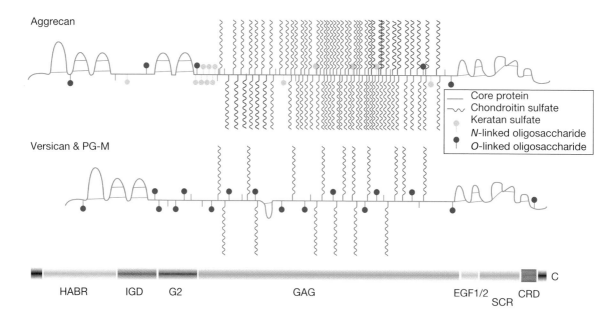

Fig. 4 Domain structures of the large aggregating proteoglycans, aggrecan and versican. HABR, Hyaluronan-binding region (G1 domain); IGD, interglobular domain; G2, G2 domain (which versican lacks); GAG, glycosaminoglycan attachment region; EFG1/2, epidermal fibroblast growth factor-like modules; CRD, carbohydrate recognition module; SCR, short complement recognition module. The EGF1/2, CRD, and the SCR modules together make up the G3 domain.

that contain this domain.[76] It is comprised of two epidermal growth factor-like domains (EGF1 and 2), a carbohydrate recognition domain (CRD) similar to the mammalian type C lectins, and a complement regulatory protein B component (short complement repeat, SCR). Each of these is encoded by separate exons,[77] which are alternatively spliced.[65, 78–80] Thus, both the EGF-like and the SCR modules can undergo alternative splicing independently, resulting in multiple variants of aggrecan mRNA of which the shortest transcript, lacking the EGF and SCR modules, is the most abundant.[78, 80] The CRD module is not known to be alternatively spliced and is always present on the mRNA. The G3 domain appears to provide the core protein with a correctly folded C-terminal cap that is essential for intracellular trafficking of aggrecan and preventing core protein degradation.[81–85] The domain is conserved amongst other members of the lectican PGs, and evidence suggests that the CRD module can bind to various carbohydrate moieties such as fucose and galactose[86, 87] and to tenascin-R core protein and the glycoprotein fibulin-1,[88, 89] suggesting a role in ECM adhesion. The EGF-like modules may provide growth-promoting activity during skeletal formation because the G3 domain of versican, and to a lesser extent that of aggrecan, can inhibit mesenchymal chondrogenesis and induce proliferation in cultured chicken limb bud cells.[90] The SCR module may function by promoting GAG chain attachment to the core protein[91] during aggrecan synthesis and both the G3 and CS-rich core protein are required for effective secretion of aggrecan.[75] A requirement for a heat shock protein of 25 kDa (HSP25) has also been implicated in G3-mediated aggrecan secretion.[83]

Versican[92, 93] is a large, aggregating CS PG,[66] the domain structure of which is shown in Fig. 4. The deduced 2409 amino acid polypeptide of human fibroblast versican has a molecular weight of approximately 265 kDa.

Versican is structurally similar to aggrecan except that it lacks a G2 domain and KS GAG chains. In addition, versican contains fewer CS chains than aggrecan. Recently, three different splice variants (V0, V1, and V2) of human versican were identified as a result of alternative splicing of two large exons.[94] Each of these exons encodes a GAG attachment domain termed GAG-α and GAG-β. Both of these domains are present in the largest (V0) isoform of versican. Versican V1 contains only the GAG-β domain and versican V2 only the GAG-α domain. A fourth versican isoform (V3) lacks both GAG attachment domains and thus appears to be devoid of GAG side-chains.[95] Thus, the calculated molecular weights of the core proteins of the four splice variants are approximately 370, 262, 180, and 72 kDa for the V0, V1, V2, and V3 isoforms, respectively. At present, only versican V0 and V1 have been identified on the protein level, whereas data for the V2 and V3 splice forms are solely based on reverse transcription-polymerase chain reaction (RT-PCR) experiments. On sodium dodecyl sulfate (SDS)-polyacrylamide gel electrophoresis (PAGE), the two largest and most prominent splice variants of versican, V0 and V1, migrate as a double band in the range above 400 kDa after chondroitinase ABC digestion.[94]

A PG similar to versican, termed PG-M, has been isolated from developing chicken limb buds.[96] Binding experiments suggests that PG-M interacts with collagen type I and fibronectin.[97] These molecules, therefore, are candidates for ligands of either the GAG chains or the various binding elements of versican core protein. Immunohistochemical studies using anti-PG-M antibodies have shown that versican is present in osteoarthritic cartilage.[98, 99] Here, PG-M was found to be expressed in the superficial zone of degenerative cartilage, and also in the intermediate and deep zones as the disease progressed.

A recent, detailed immunohistochemical study using antibodies recognizing the V0 and V1 versican variants showed widespread distribution in normal adult human tissues.[100] For example, versican was found in the loose connective tissues of various organs and was often associated with the elastic fibre network. This PG was also localized in most smooth muscle tissues, the central and peripheral nervous system, the basal layer of the epidermis, and the wall layers of veins and elastic arteries. In addition, versican was also analysed in fibrous and elastic cartilage: versican was completely absent from the ECM and cells of hyaline cartilage from rib and trachea. Some positive staining was noted in tendon and in the fibrous cartilage of the intervertebral disc. Versican gene expression has been noted in human articular cartilage[101] and a versican-like PG was shown to be present as an endogenous and newly synthesized PG in bovine collateral ligament.[102] The highly diversified distribution of versican in normal adult tissues may reflect the functional versatility of this large aggregating PG.

Non-aggregating, leucine-rich proteoglycans

Three PGs (decorin, biglycan, and fibromodulin) that have been characterized from connective tissues[50, 103] belong to this family of low-molecular-weight, leucine-rich proteins. The core proteins of decorin, biglycan, and fibromodulin are approximately 40–50 kDa and they contain a homologous region consisting of 10–14 repeats of a 23-residue leucine-rich sequence. Decorin (PG-SII) and biglycan (PG-SI) contain one or two CS/DS chains, respectively, which are situated close to the N-terminus of the protein. GAG chain sequence analysis has shown that decorin from bone and articular cartilage and biglycan from articular and nasal cartilage carry mostly CS chains and some DS chains. In addition, decorin and biglycan from articular cartilage were found to have similar glycan chains.[104]

Fibromodulin is different from decorin and biglycan in that it contains N-linked KS chains that are located within the leucine-rich repeat region of the core protein. These three PGs are commonly termed 'non-aggregating' molecules as it is generally held that they do not form complexes with hyaluronic acid. However, recent in vitro studies have shown that, when decorin, biglycan, and fibromodulin are mixed together, multimeric complexes are formed, either via core protein or GAG chain interactions. These complexes were shown by rotary shadowing microscopy to associate with hyaluron in solution.[105] Thus, a similar interaction could occur in vivo, where the binding of small PGs with hyaluron may have a functional significance in the maintenance of ECM homeostasis.

Interaction with the fibrillar collagens is also a common feature of decorin.[106, 107] Biglycan has been shown to bind to collagen type I in vitro.[108] There are at least two separate binding domains for the interaction between decorin core protein and type I collagen and binding is not necessarily correlated with an alteration of collagen fibrillogenesis. Decorin and fibromodulin have been shown to interact at defined sites along the collagen molecules,[109] but do not compete for the same sites.[110] It has been found that decorin and fibromodulin form bridges of anti-parallel GAG chains linked via their core protein to the fibrils. These proteoglycans are horseshoe-shaped, which enables them to bind to adjacent collagen fibrils.[111]

An additional function of decorin, biglycan, and fibromodulin is the ability to bind to transforming growth factor beta (TGFβ).[112] In turn, it has been shown that TGFβ downregulates decorin mRNA in fibroblasts. Decorin binds to TGFβ via the leucine-rich region of the protein core, thus preventing the growth factor from binding to cell surface receptors.[113] Thus, release of TGFβ from the growth factor complex enables the cytokine to carry out functions including selective stimulation of decorin and biglycan and modulation of GAG attachment. Many studies have analysed the decorin/growth factor interaction. One process by which TGFβ activities could be activated in vivo is by matrix metalloproteinase (MMP) activity. MMPs are key enzymes present during normal physiological remodelling and pathological degradation of ECMs.[114] MMP-2 (gelatinase A), MMP-3 (stromelysin 1), and MMP-7 (matrilysin) degrade decorin resulting in the release of TGFβ from the complex. Interestingly, removal of the GAG chain from decorin reduces the susceptibility of decorin to MMP-2 and MMP-3 activity, but not to that of MMP-7. This may be due to a conformational change of decorin core protein as a result of deglycosylation.

The small, non-aggregating PGs thus carry out a diverse range of functions within the ECM and are therefore important components in the control of matrix assembly, homeostasis, and remodelling. It is interesting that, in fibrous connective tissues, which are composed primarily of collagen type I, the small PGs predominate, representing as much as 95 per cent of all the interstitial PGs.[115]

Proteoglycans and glycosaminoglycans of the meniscus

Endogenous GAGs and PGs in the meniscus have been studied using standard biochemical techniques including density gradient centrifugation, gel electrophoresis, and ion-exchange chromatography. These analyses involved pooling tissue from humans or animals of similar age and, in some cases, lateral and medial menisci were not treated as separate entities. In addition, some studies analysed GAGs and PGs from the whole meniscus, whereas other studies analysed and compared the PG composition from specific regions of the meniscus. Canine menisci were found to contain 10 per cent less water and approximately eightfold less GAGs than articular cartilage from the same knee joint.[116] More 6-sulfated than 4-sulfated CS chains were also identified in these menisci. DS chains were also found, but at lower levels than CS chains. In addition, HA accounted for 6 per cent of the total uronic acid. In this study, anterior and posterior regions of lateral or medial menisci were pooled and compared to the composition of the central region (Fig. 5). Levels of GAGs were higher in the lateral menisci, but no significant differences were found between different regions of each meniscus. Later studies by Adams et al.[117] found two populations of high-molecular-weight PGs in canine menisci that were able to interact with HA. Lateral and medial menisci were pooled in these experiments. A joint study of GAG structure in canine and human menisci found major difference between the two tissues: human menisci contains more DS than canine tissue.[118]

Recently, Scott et al.[119] analysed GAGs and PGs from different regions of porcine menisci, in particular, the inner, middle, and outer regions (Fig. 5). Lateral and medial menisci were treated separately, but no statistically significant differences in PG composition were noted between the two tissues. The most abundant GAG was CS: lower levels of this GAG were found in the outer regions of the menisci compared to the inner regions. DS was the second most abundant GAG, the concentrations of which were higher in the outer zones. HA accounted for 4–5 per cent of total GAG content in the inner zones and 10 per cent in the outer zones. In addition, large CS- and KS-containing PGs and small DS-containing PGs (decorin and biglycan) were identified. Decorin and biglycan in the inner zones of porcine menisci were found to contain longer DS chains than PGs in the outer zones.

Further analyses[120] involving the isolation and characterization of these small PGs showed that biglycan was the major small PG and was more concentrated in the inner regions of porcine menisci. Decorin was also identified and was present at high concentrations in the outer regions of the porcine meniscus. Like biglycan, fibromodulin was concentrated in the inner regions. This PG distribution fits well

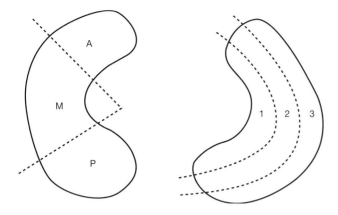

Fig. 5 Dissection of human menisci for biochemical analyses. Topographical variations in matrix composition have been compared between the anterior (A), middle (M), and posterior (P) regions and also between the inner (zone 1), centre (zone 2), and outer regions (zone 3) of menisci.

with the proposed functions of biglycan and decorin as a regulator of cellular activities and a modulator of collagen fibrillogenesis, respectively, because the inner regions of the meniscus contain more fibrochondrocytes, whereas the outer regions are composed mainly of collagen fibres, particularly type I collagen. However, fibromodulin also binds collagen fibres and its localization in the inner region of the meniscus suggests that, in comparison to decorin, it binds to different collagen fibres. Collectively, these results show that the ECM of knee meniscus varies continuously across its width, which may reflect regional adaptations to functional demands.

There have been fewer studies analysing GAGs and PGs in the *human* meniscus. The first investigation of intact PG characterization in the human meniscus[121] found PG molecules of similar size and GAG content (CS, KS, and no DS) to those present in articular cartilage. Further characterization[122] revealed that this 'cartilage-like' PG was able to bind to HA. In addition, these 'cartilage-like' PGs were similar, but not identical, to PGs present in an equivalent preparation from age-matched human articular cartilage. The meniscus PG contained more 4-sulfation and an increased abundance of CS relative to KS. Such parameters are more comparable with those PGs isolated from immature human articular cartilage. This study also revealed the presence of small, non-aggregating DS-containing PGs. The DS-containing PGs of adult human meniscus have recently been analysed in more detail.[123] In contrast to porcine meniscus, the major PG in human tissue was decorin and the DS chains contained three times as much 4- as 6-sulphation. The predominance of decorin in the adult meniscus and its ability to interact both with itself and collagen fibrils is compatible with a role in maintaining tissue integrity and strength.

In summary, similarities and differences in GAG and PG composition have been identified in various studies of the ECM of animal and human menisci. However, it is difficult to relate these studies because different regions and different ages of menisci were analysed. Studies on the porcine meniscus mentioned above showed topographical variations in the localization of PGs in the matrix. Age-related changes in matrix composition of the human meniscus have also been found. Thus, it is important to consider both the age and the region of the tissue when analysing the meniscus.

Non-collagenous matrix components of the meniscus

In addition to collagen and PGs, the ECM of connective tissues also contains a population of NCPs for which no functional role has yet been identified.[124] They appear to participate in the assembly of the matrix and/or to be involved in the regulation of tissue homeostasis. Some of these proteins have been identified and characterized from articular cartilage, but very little information is available on proteins present in the ECM of the meniscus.

The function of many of these matrix proteins is, at present, unclear. Some turn over relatively slowly, suggesting a structural role, whereas others turn over more rapidly. It is likely that the matrix proteins are as important as the collagens and PGs in maintaining tissue function and, as their abundance may vary between different sites, they may also be important in determining the different functional roles played by connective tissues. At present, only a few proteins have been identified in the meniscus, including LPs and a high-molecular-weight component that is probably a subunit of cartilage oligomeric matrix protein (COMP).[125] More attention needs to be focused on characterizing these proteins in the meniscus and other connective tissues.

Cells of the meniscus

Cells of the meniscus are referred to as fibrochondrocytes (FCs) because their appearance is chondrocytic, yet they synthesize a fibrocartilage matrix. Articular cartilage chondrocytes, in contrast, synthesize their own distinctive hyaline cartilage matrix. The FCs serve to maintain the biomechanical integrity and function of the meniscus through ongoing production of the constituents of the ECM.

Two populations of FCs can be discerned at both the light (Fig. 6) and electron-microscopic levels.[126] Unlike fibroblasts, FCs are either round or oval and are situated in well-formed lacunae. Cells of the superficial zone (closest to the articular surface) are generally oval with a few cell processes. Those in the deep zone, which constitutes the majority of the meniscal midsubstance, tend to be more rounded, with numerous and elaborate cell processes that project into an amorphous pericellular zone. Both cell types contain abundant endoplasmic reticulum and Golgi complex. Mitochondria are only occasionally visualized, suggesting that, as in articular chondrocytes,[127] the major pathway for energy production for the FCs in their avascular milieu is probably anaerobic glycolysis.

These two distinct cell populations probably carry out different functions in the meniscus depending on where they are situated. Those in the superficial zone may be more suited to respond to load applied on the tissue during extension and flexion of the knee joint. In addition, these superficial cells are likely to be the first to 'detect' and respond to meniscus injury or degeneration. As a result, these cells may 'communicate' with the cells of the deeper zone to then synthesize the components essential to induce a repair process. When complete tissue sections are stained (e.g. with safranin O) to reveal the presence of sulfated PGs, more intense staining is visualized in the central region of the deep zone. Therefore, the round, deep zone cells are probably more efficient than the other cell population in either synthesizing ECM components or retaining synthesized PGs in their pericellular coat. It would be interesting to study the effects of these two cell populations in culture to identify if their response to various cytokines and growth factors differ. Heterogeneity of cells in articular cartilage, however, has been studied in detail.[128] Chondrocytes in

(a)
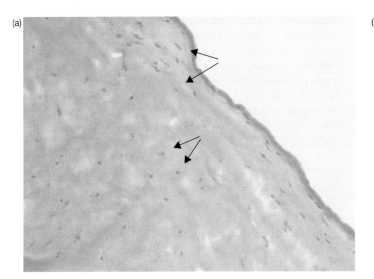

(b)
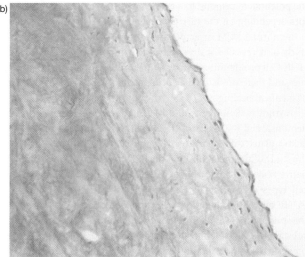

Fig. 6 Histochemistry of human meniscus. Tissue sections (10 μM thick) from the medial meniscus of a 34-year-old specimen stained with (a) haematoxylin and eosin (H&E) and (b) toluidine blue. There is a low density of fibrochondrocytes with cells on the periphery of the meniscus mostly having an oval (or flattened) appearance, while cells within the deep zone mostly appear more rounded in shape (arrows in (a)). The glycosaminoglycans visualized by toluidine blue are distributed throughout the tissue, but more concentrated in the deep zone. (40× magnification.)

cartilage display differences in terms of their morphology, metabolism, phenotypic stability, and responsiveness to interleukin-1α (IL-1α). Chondrocytes from the superficial layer (zone 1) of articular cartilage were found to display an irregular shape with numerous cell processes when cultured in agarose gel. In contrast, chondrocytes from the deep zone (zone III) retained a rounded shape and morphological features typical for chondrocytes.[129] This is analogous to the two populations of cells observed in meniscal tissue *in vitro*. Recent studies[130] have shown that cells in the superficial layer of human articular cartilage display greater sensitivity to the damaging effects of IL-1 than cells of the deeper layers. This suggests that, in intact articular cartilage, the chondrocytes that would be the most responsive to IL-1 *in vitro* are those that are closest to the surface of the tissue, and most likely to be exposed to IL-1 in synovial fluid.

In vitro culture of fibrochondrocytes

FCs from the meniscus were first cultured under monolayer conditions by Webber *et al.*[131] In this study, rabbit FCs were enzymatically released from the fibrocartilaginous mid-substance and, under the culture regimens employed, the cells proliferated vigorously. Morphologically, the FCs displayed the typical flattened appearance of cells in monolayer culture. However, two subpopulations of cells could be grown depending on the type of basal nutrient medium used for the primary culture. One cell type appeared more elongated and the other more polygonal in shape. It was suggested that these two cell subpopulations may represent the *in vitro* correlate of the superficial and deep zone FCs, respectively, as described in the electron-microscopic investigations of rabbit menisci by Ghadially and co-workers.[126]

Webber and co-workers[132] also found that the population doubling times (PDT) of the FCs were within the range (15–20 hours) previously described for hyaline articular chondrocytes.[133] However, the fibroblast-like cells were found to proliferate more than the chondrocyte-like cells. The proliferative rate of these meniscal cells could be increased in a dose-dependent manner by exposure to

mitogenic factors such as pituitary fibroblast growth factor (FGF) and platelet lysate. Human FCs grown under the same culture conditions were found to proliferate more slowly than rabbit, porcine, or canine FCs.[134] In addition, canine FCs have been shown to be capable of using the RGD (arginine–glycine–aspartate) peptide to enhance their attachment to artificial surfaces. The RGD peptide was first demonstrated by Pierschbacher *et al.*[134] to be the cell attachment site of fibronectin, the glycoprotein used *in vivo* by numerous mesenchymal cell types to attach to their physiological substrates such as collagen and fibrin during wound healing.

Using radiolabelling procedures, Webber *et al.*[131] also found that both subtypes of the monolayer rabbit FCs synthesize sulfated PGs. The 'fibroblastic' cells synthesized approximately three times more PGs than the 'chondrocytic' cells. The addition of FGF or ascorbate reduced the rate of PG synthesis by both subtypes. Furthermore, there was a higher level of retention of radiolabelled PGs in the pericellular coat of the deep zone cells compared to the superficial zone cells. The addition of ascorbate to the culture medium increased the retention of PGs in both cell types. This phenomenon has been demonstrated previously with rabbit[132] and human[135] articular chondrocytes. Thus, regardless of their differences, both types of FCs were shown to proliferate well in culture, synthesize sulfated PGs, and respond to ascorbate, FGF, and platelet lysate.

Natsu-Ume *et al.*[136] showed that hepatocyte growth factor (HGF) receptor upregulated mRNA expression in meniscal FCs. HGF was originally described as a potential mitogen for normal adult rat hepatocytes. Subsequent studies revealed HGF secretion by mesenchymal cells and that it promotes motility, morphogenesis, and proliferation of epithelia expressing the HGF receptor, c-proto-oncogene product.[137] Moreover, recent studies have shown that non-epithelial cells, in particular chondrocytes,[138] can be targets of HGF. However, contrary to results obtained from cultured FCs isolated from the surrounding matrix by enzymatic digestion, no expression of HGF receptor was detected in meniscal tissue. This suggests that meniscal cells may have the potential to respond to a whole range of cytokines and growth factors depending on the surrounding external environment, whether it is the normal ECM or artificial culture conditions. Results from this study also revealed a dose-dependent proliferative effect of FCs by HGF. Cell proliferation is an essential process in the healing of soft tissues and therefore HGF may be a potential candidate for the purpose of meniscal healing.

A study by Spindler et al.[139] using sheep meniscal organ cultures demonstrated that FCs are capable of responding to another growth factor, platelet-derived growth factor (PDGF). Organ cultures allow the study of the metabolism of the FC while it is still surrounded by its native fibrocartilaginous matrix but devoid of the influences of other cell types or other in vivo physiological parameters. The effect of PDGF on cell proliferation was compared between meniscal cells in the peripheral, vascular region and those in the avascular midsubstance. Results demonstrated that cells of the central region of the meniscus did not respond to doses of PDGF that were effective in the peripheral region.

Similarly, zonal variations in the response of bovine meniscal cells to various cytokines have been addressed.[140] The proliferation and migration of cells from the outer vascular region, the central region, and the inner area of the meniscus were compared. In particular, PDGF, bone morphogenic protein-2 (BMP-2), and HGF stimulated DNA synthesis in all distinctly localized fibrochondrocytes in a dose-dependent manner. However, insulin-like growth factor-1 (IGF-1) had no effect.

Migratory responses of meniscal cells to different cytokines varied: PDGF and HGF were found to stimulate migration of meniscal cells from all three zones, but IL-1 preferentially stimulated the migration of outer cells, while epidermal growth factor (EGF) stimulated the migration of inner and outer cells.

The in vitro culture analyses described above emphasize the heterogeneity that exists in the meniscus due to the presence of different cell populations. Variations in proliferation, migration, and PG synthesis in response to cytokines and growth factors have been demonstrated between: (1) cells of the superficial and deep zones of the meniscus; (2) cells of the peripheral, central, and inner regions of the meniscus; and (3) isolated FCs in culture and FCs from meniscal tissue. It is important to evaluate these differences in order to successfully treat injuries in particular regions of this fibrocartilaginous tissue. Thus, having the potential to respond to various cytokines and growth factors, FCs need only to be exposed to the proper stimuli to express their intrinsic repair capabilities, that is, proliferation and ECM synthesis.

Ageing and degenerative joint disease

Changes in ECM structure and composition of connective tissues in ageing and degenerative joint disease have been studied in great detail. Analysis of osteoarthritic tissue is important, but any changes in matrix structure observed in these tissue specimens generally corresponds to the end-point of the disease process. Therefore age-related studies of normal tissue are essential in order to interpret the findings described in disease, because some repair processes may involve the re-expression of juvenile genes.

Age-related changes in the meniscus

Data describing changes in the composition of the ECM in the meniscus during tissue development and ageing are lacking. One of the first studies analysing the composition of human menisci of different ages was carried out by Ingman and co-workers.[141] It was found that levels of total collagen increased in developing menisci and, thereafter, remained constant. No other age-related studies have been done with respect to human tissue, but, more recently, it has been shown that levels of collagen type VI in sheep menisci were higher in immature tissue compared to mature menisci.[48] This is consistent with a role for this protein in processes in which the assembly of a new matrix is required.

An early study that characterized PGs from the human meniscus[117] is the only study to date that has analysed PGs in menisci of different ages. The KS in the meniscus was found to increase with age as did the 6:4 ratios of CS isomers and this was later confirmed by Bayliss et al.[142]

In summary, changes affecting GAG chains in cartilage appear to be of synthetic origin and are presumably designed to meet the changing needs of the developing tissue. In contrast, many of the changes affecting PG core protein structure may be of degradative origin, and the products probably result from the accumulation of normal turnover processes occurring throughout life. It is likely that proteinases released by the chondrocytes themselves are responsible for much of these changes in clinically normal tissue.[143] It is difficult to suggest processes that may be occurring in the meniscus due to the lack of data on age-related trends in this tissue. In addition, more research in this area would advance our knowledge of changes that may occur in the meniscus prior to and during degeneration of the knee joint.

Pathology and repair of the meniscus

The menisci, because of their central anatomical and functional positions in the knee joint, are the targets of numerous forms of inflammatory, traumatic, metabolic, and degenerative disease.[144] Meniscal tears (Fig. 7) constitute the most important pathological condition of the tissue.

Diagnosis of a meniscal tear on clinical grounds is often difficult. Arthroscopy has been useful, but has fallen out of favour in recent

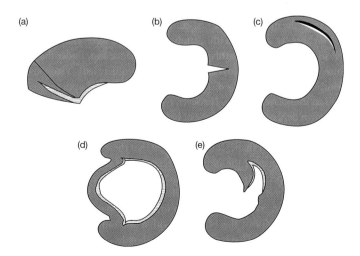

Fig. 7 Types of meniscal tears. Tears are shown in grey. (a) Horizontal; (b) vertical (radial); (c) vertical (longitudinal); (d) bucket handle; (e) flap.

years due to the availability of magnetic resonance imaging (MRI). MRI offers many advantages, including excellent resolution of soft tissue structures without pain or joint manipulation, with no ionizing radiation, and with non-invasive techniques.[145] It is hoped that MRI may be useful for decreasing the total treatment time by clarifying clinical findings initially and thus enabling appropriate treatment options from the onset of significant symptoms. This could theoretically decrease overall treatment time and in the long run be more cost-effective.[146] However, in order for MRI to be included in the routine evaluation of a knee injury in which meniscal damage is suspected, MRI accuracy rates need to surpass that of a well-performed physical examination in order to justify its routine use.

Healing of meniscal tears can occur through two general pathways: (1) an *intrinsic* ability of the meniscal cells to migrate, proliferate, and synthesize matrix provided they are given the proper stimuli; (2) *extrinsic* stimulation through neovascularization. The extrinsic pathway is activated when the meniscus is injured within the peripheral vascular region. A fibrin clot is formed that acts as a scaffold for proliferation of the capillary plexus, attracting undifferentiated mesenchymal cells from the outside along with nutrients necessary to accomplish healing.[147] This fibrovascular tissue seals the defect and promotes further neovascularization. Animal studies[148, 149] have confirmed that lesions in this vascular region of the meniscus do have the potential to heal.

The fibrin clot appears to possess the requisite ingredients to nurture the intrinsic meniscal healing pathway. Even cells from the avascular region of the meniscus have been shown to proliferate and synthesize matrix without a blood supply if they are provided with the proper environment. It is thought that the fibrin clot not only acts as a scaffold, but provides the chemotactic and mitogenic stimuli necessary to support the required cellular response. As well as affecting the cells in the meniscus, these factors probably entice synovial cells and migrating peripheral blood elements into the repair site.

The need to provide extra stimulation to the tear site is related to the inherent healing potential of any tear. There is an increased necessity for an adequate biological environment during healing if the tear is located more centrally, that is, further from the vascular periphery. This has been recognized by clinicians, who have based their decision to repair a particular meniscal lesion on where the tear is located.[150]

New approaches to repair of the meniscus

Studies of meniscal healing have demonstrated that, although partially or totally meniscectomized knees have regenerative capacity, the natural repair is usually incomplete and early degenerative arthritis is the end result of the incompetent meniscus remnant.[151, 152] Interest has been rekindled in the topic of meniscal repair and research efforts are under way to make meniscal replacement (either allograft, tendon autograft, or prosthetic) a clinically useful procedure.

Meniscus transplantation procedures have been attempted with some success in humans[153, 154] and dogs.[155] However, although some consider the meniscus to be an immunoprivileged tissue, there is concern about the immunogenicity of meniscal allografts.[156] Therefore, attempts have been made to replace the meniscus with autograft tissue. Successful autograft replacements have been reported in one study where part of the patellar tendon was used as a replacement meniscus because, histologically, the meniscus periphery is similar to tendon tissue.[157]

Collagen-based prostheses have attracted much interest as a method for meniscal regeneration. A prosthesis, or regenerated tissue, must account for the complete shape of the meniscus. Otherwise, it cannot be expected to accommodate the subtleties of force transmission or recreate normal joint stability. Preliminary studies revealed that collagen scaffolds could induce cellular adherence, migration, division, and matrix formation.[158] These regenerated templates were produced by cross-linking various combinations of GAGs found within the normal human meniscus to purified collagen from bovine Achilles tendon.

Recent studies have examined the effects of cell-based meniscus regeneration. Previously, it was suggested that bone marrow-derived mesenchymal stem cells recapitulate the embryonic lineage cascade in articular cartilage and tendon defect repair.[159] Therefore, Walsh and co-workers[160] used a collagen scaffold loaded with autologous bone marrow-derived mesenchymal stem cells to replace the partially meniscectomized medial meniscus in rabbits. These implants resulted in abundant repair tissue production that was grossly and histologically meniscus-like. In addition to stem cells, it was found that seeding meniscal cells on to synthetic biodegradable polymer scaffolds (polyglycolic acid (PGA)) and implanting them subcutaneously into nude mice produced tissue constructs resembling normal menisci.[161] Similar studies also revealed that these tissue constructs developed biomechanical compressive properties similar to those of the normal meniscus.[162] Ertl *et al.*[163] used a PGA/meniscal cell artificial construct, produced in tissue culture, to analyse meniscal repair in rabbits. This was the first reported evidence of successful repair and subsequent healing of avascular meniscal lesions utilizing tissue-engineered meniscal constructs.

Even though prosthetic methods are rapidly improving, no artificial material identified to date has matched the unique characteristics of the meniscus. None has been able to tolerate the 1 to 3 million load-bearing cycles per year at up to five times body weight that the normal meniscus encounters. Methods to induce natural healing of the meniscus, thus retaining the original tissue, would obviously be the best option. Difficulties in the production of suitable tissue constructs has led to a new area of meniscal healing research: gene transfer. Cytokines and growth factors have been shown to promote cell responses important in the repair process. However, in the avascular region of the meniscus, the cells are not exposed to these factors for prolonged periods of time. One solution to this problem is the transfer of the corresponding gene to the meniscal cells resulting in local secretion of the cytokine over predictable time periods. This therapeutic approach depends on vectors that enable the cellular uptake and expression of DNA. Preliminary studies have compared the efficiency of several viral vectors as candidates for gene transfer to ligaments and menisci.[164] It was demonstrated that all investigated cells from the rabbit knee joint were susceptible to viral infection. Therefore, the success of natural, cell-based regeneration procedures seems probable. Since cells are pivotal to the repair of meniscal tissue, detailed knowledge of these cells and their repair capacity, that is, response to stimuli such as cytokines and growth factors, is required for the progress of effective treatments for pathological conditions of the meniscus.

Structure and biochemistry of osteoarthritic menisci

Information on the biochemistry of osteoarthritic menisci is lacking. More interest has been focused on how the effects of meniscectomy or meniscus injury contribute to the development of osteoarthritis (OA). Structural and biochemical changes have been studied in great detail in articular cartilage with very little attention to what changes may be occurring in the meniscus. Radiographs reveal obvious changes in the structure of articular cartilage, but changes in the meniscus are not as apparent. However, examination of menisci from osteoarthritic joints show thinning and fibrillation. It is not known if the menisci, like cartilage, swell during the early stages of OA.

Three studies on osteoarthritic menisci have shown that changes in the composition of the ECM of the meniscus do occur. Adams et al.[165] analysed the menisci from beagles after OA was induced by sectioning the anterior cruciate ligament. One week after induction of OA, the water content of the tissue increased, whereas the GAG content decreased. In particular, like osteoarthritic cartilage, the content of KS decreased. However, as long as 15–18 months after induction, the GAG levels were elevated above normal, which suggests that the meniscus is capable of some regeneration. An earlier, unrelated study[166] analysed osteoarthritic menisci from several human patients. Basic biochemical techniques revealed a decrease in collagen and an increase in hexosamines and non-collagenous matrix proteins in degenerative areas. Recent, unpublished data has also shown that osteoarthritic menisci contain elevated levels of type II collagen compared to normal tissue (Wardale, personal communication).

It is evident that more experimental analyses on osteoarthritic menisci are required to determine the processes occurring in the diseased tissue. It is likely, however, that the meniscus, as well as other major joint tissues, will be affected by proteases resulting in the breakdown of matrix components and their release into the surrounding synovial fluid. There is growing interest in the use of diagnostic 'markers' of OA in synovial fluid to diagnose the disease at an earlier stage and perhaps assess the severity of the disease and its treatment.

Summary and future directions

This chapter described the complexity of the knee joint as an organ with an emphasis on the meniscus. Biomechanical and biochemical properties of the meniscus were discussed and it is apparent that there is a lack of knowledge of the structure and metabolism of the ECM of this tissue, especially from ageing and osteoarthritic knee joints. In addition, a basic understanding of the structure and organization of the meniscus will improve strategies for repairing pathological tears in the tissue, thus preventing the need for partial or total meniscectomies, which are known to predispose the knee joint to OA.

Acknowledgements

The authors would like to thank the Arthritis Research Campaign, UK, for their financial support.

References

1. Sutton, J.B. (1897). *Ligaments: their nature and morphology*, 2nd edn. H.K. Lewis and Co, London.
2. Ingman, A.M., Ghosh, P., and Taylor, T.K. (1974). Variation of collagenous and non-collagenous proteins of human knee joint menisci with age and degeneration. *Gerontologia* **20**, 212–213.
3. Ghosh, P., Ingman, A.M., and Taylor, T.K. (1975). Variations in collagen, non-collagenous proteins, and hexosamine in menisci derived from osteoarthritic and rheumatoid arthritic knee joints. *J. Rheumatol.* **2**, 100–107.
4. Edwards, J. (1994). Synovium. In *Rheumatology* (ed. J.H. Klippel and P.A. Dieppe), pp. 3.7.1–3.7.8. Mosby Year Book Europe Ltd, London.
5. Rørvik, A.M. and Grøndahl, A.M. (1995). Markers of osteoarthritis—a review of the literature. *Vet. Surg.* **24**, 255–262.
6. Heinegård, D. and Paulsson, M. (1987). Cartilage. *Methods Enzymol.* **145**, 336–363.
7. Hardingham, T.E.M., Muir, H., Kwan, M.K., Lai, W.M., and Mow, V.C. (1987). Viscoelastic properties of proteoglycan solutions with varying proportions present as aggregates. *J. Orthop. Res.* **5**, 36–46.
8. Clark, C.R. and Ogden, J.A. (1983). Development of the menisci of the human knee joint. *J. Bone Joint Surg.* **65A**, 538–547.
9. Arnoczky, S.P. and Warren, R.F. (1982). Microvasculature of the human meniscus. *Am. J. Sports Med.* **10**, 90–95.
10. Arnoczky, S.P., Adams, M., DeHaven, K., Eyre, D., and Mow, V. (1988). Meniscus. In *Injury and repair of the muscoskeletal soft tissues* (ed. S.L-Y. Woo and J. Buckwalter), pp. 487–548. American Academy of Orthopaedic Surgeons, Park Ridge, Illinois.
11. Arnoczky, S.P., Marshall, L.L., Joseph, A., Jarhe, C., and Yoshioka, M. (1980). Meniscal nutrition: an experimental study in the dog. *Orthop. Trans.* **5**, 127.
12. Shoemaker, S.C. and Markolf, K.L. (1986). The role of the meniscus in the anterior–posterior stability of the loaded anterior cruciate-deficient knee. Effects of partial versus total excision. *J. Bone Joint Surg. (Am.)* **68**, 71–79.
13. Fithian, D.C., Kelly, M.A., and Mow, V.C. (1990). Material properties and structure–function relationships in the menisci. *Clin. Orthop.* **252**, 19–31.
14. Aspden, R.M., Yarker, Y.E., and Hukins, D.W. (1985). Collagen orientations in the meniscus of the knee joint. *J. Anat.* **140**, 371–380.
15. Bullough, P.G., Munuera, L., Murphy, J., and Weinstein, A.M. (1970). The strength of the menisci of the knee as it relates to their fine structure. *J. Bone Joint Surg. (Br.)* **52**, 564–567.
16. Cameron, H.U. and MacNab, I. (1972). The structure of the meniscus of the human knee joint. *Clin. Orthop.* **89**, 215–219.
17. Skaggs, D.L., Warden, W.H., and Mow, V.C. (1994). Radial tie fibers influence the tensile properties of the bovine medial meniscus. *J. Orthop. Res.* **12**, 176–185.
18. Fukubayashi, T. and Kurosawa, H. (1980). The contact area and pressure distribution pattern of the knee. A study of normal and osteoarthrotic knee joints. *Acta Orthop. Scand.* **51**, 871–879.
19. Kurosawa, H., Fukubayashi, T., and Nakajima, H. (1980). Load-bearing mode of the knee joint: physical behavior of the knee joint with or without meniscus. *Clin. Orthop.* **149**, 283–290.
20. Seedhom, B.B. (1976). Loadbearing function of the menisci. *Physiotherapy* **62**, 223–226.
21. Voloshin, A.S. and Wosk, J. (1983). Shock absorption of meniscectomized and painful knees: a comparative *in vivo* study. *J. Biomed. Eng.* **5**, 157–161.
22. Bourne, R.B., Finlay, J.B., Papadopoulos, P., and Andreae, P. (1984). The effect of medial meniscectomy on strain distribution in the proximal part of the tibia. *J. Bone Joint Surg. (Am.)* **66**, 1431–1437.
23. Shrive, N. (1974). The weightbearing role of the menisci of the knee. *J. Bone Joint Surg.* **56B**, 381.
24. Seedhom, B.B., Dowson, D., and Wright, V. (1984). The load bearing function of the menisci: a preliminary study. In *The knee joint* (ed. O.S. Ingwersen, B. Van Linge, and T.J.G. Van Rens), pp. 37–42. American Elsevier, New York.
25. Atencia, L.J., McDevitt, C.A., Nile, W.B., and Sokoloff, L. (1989). Cartilage content of an immature dog. *Connect. Tissue Res.* **18**, 235.
26. Maroudas, A., Bayliss, M.T., and Venn, M.F. (1980). Further studies on the composition of human femoral head cartilage. *Ann. Rheum. Dis.* **39**, 514–523.

27. Thonar, E.J., Sweet, M.B., Immelman, A.R., and Lyons, G. (1978). Hyaluronate in articular cartilage: age-related changes. *Calcif. Tissue Res.* **26**, 19–21.

28. Hannafin, J.A. and Arnoczky, S.P. (1993). The effect of cyclic and static tensile loading on water content and solute diffusion in canine flexor tendon—an *in vitro* study. *Trans. Orthop. Res. Soc.* **18**, 367.

29. Abrahamsson, S.-O., Lundborg, G., and Lohmander, L.S. (1991). Dehydration inhibits matrix synthesis and cell proliferation. An *in vitro* study of rabbit flexor tendons. *Acta Orthop. Scand.* **62**, 159–162.

30. Prockop, D.J. and Kivirikko, K.I. (1995). Collagens: molecular biology, diseases, and potentials for therapy. *Annu. Rev. Biochem.* **64**, 403–434.

31. Hulmes, D.J. (1992). The collagen superfamily—diverse structures and assemblies. *Essays Biochem.* **27**, 49–67.

32. Gordon, M.K. and Olsen, B.R. (1990). The contribution of collagenous proteins to tissue-specific matrix assemblies. *Curr. Opin. Cell. Biol.* **2**, 833–838.

33. Eyre, D.R. and Muir, H. (1975). Characterisation of the major CnBr-derived peptides of porcine type II collagen. *Connect. Tissue Res.* **3**, 165–170.

34. Eyre, D.R. and Wu, J.J. (1983). Collagen of fibrocartilage: a distinctive molecular phenotype in bovine meniscus. *FEBS Lett.* **158**, 265–270.

35. Romanic, A.M., Adachi, E., Kadler, K.E., Hojima, Y., and Prockop, D.J. (1991). Copolymerization of pNcollagen III and collagen I. pNcollagen III decreases the rate of incorporation of collagen I into fibrils, the amount of collagen I incorporated, and the diameter of the fibrils formed. *J. Biol. Chem.* **266**, 12703–12709.

36. Keene, D.R., Sakai, L.Y., Bachinger, H.P., and Burgeson, R.E. (1987). Type III collagen can be present on banded collagen fibrils regardless of fibril diameter. *J. Cell Biol.* **105**, 2393–2402.

37. Fleischmajer, R., Perlish, J.S., Burgeson, R.E., Shaikh-Bahai, F., and Timpl, R. (1990). Type I and type III collagen interactions during fibrillogenesis. *Ann. NY Acad. Sci.* **580**, 161–175.

38. Linsenmayer, T.F., Fitch, J.M., Gross, J., and Mayne, R. (1985). Are collagen fibrils in the developing avian cornea composed of two different collagen types? Evidence from monoclonal antibody studies. *Ann. NY Acad. Sci.* **460**, 232–245.

39. Cheung, H.S. (1987). Distribution of type I, II, III and V in the pepsin solubilized collagens in bovine menisci. *Connect. Tissue Res.* **16**, 343–356.

40. Eyre, D.R., Koob, T.J., and Chun, L.E. (1983). Biochemistry of the meniscus: unique profile of collagen types and site-dependent variations in composition. *Trans. Orthop. Res. Soc.* **8**, 56.

41. Eyre, D.R. (1991). The collagens of articular cartilage. *Semin. Arthritis Rheum.* **21**, 2–11.

42. Mendler, M., Eich-Bender, S.G., Vaughan, L., Winterhalter, K.H., and Bruckner, P. (1989). Cartilage contains mixed fibrils of collagen types II, IX and XI. *J. Cell Biol.* **108**, 191–197.

43. Linsenmayer, T.F., Fitch, J.M., and Birk, D.E. (1990). Heterotypic collagen fibrils and stabilizing collagens. Controlling elements in corneal morphogenesis? *Ann. NY Acad. Sci.* **580**, 143–160.

44. Ala-Kokko, L., Baldwin, C.T., Moskowitz, R.W., and Prockop, D.J. (1990). Single base mutation in the type II procollagen gene COL2A1 as a cause of primary osteoarthritis associated with a mild chondrodysplasia. *Proc. Natl Acad. Sci. USA* **87**, 6565–6568.

45. Wu, J.J., Eyre, D.R., and Slayter, H.S. (1987). Type VI collagen of the intervertebral disc. Biochemical and electron-microscopic characterization of the native protein. *Biochem. J.* **248**, 373–381.

46. Engel, J., Furthmayr, H., Odermatt, E., von der Mark, H., Aumailley, M., Fleischmajer, R., and Timpl, R. (1985). Structure and macromolecular organization of type VI collagen. *Ann. NY Acad. Sci.* **460**, 25–37.

47. Bidanset, D.J., Guidry, C., Rosenberg, L.C., Choi, H.U., Timpl, R., and Hook, M. (1992). Binding of the proteoglycan decorin to collagen type VI. *J. Biol. Chem.* **267**, 5250–5256.

48. Chung, S.T., McDevitt, C.A., and Turner, A.S. (1997). The effect of maturation and aging on the concentration of type VI collagen in the sheep meniscus. *Trans. Orthop. Res. Soc.* **22**, 486.

49. McDevitt, C.A. and Webber, R.J. (1990). The ultrastructure and biochemistry of meniscal cartilage. *Clin. Orthop.* **252**, 8–18.

50. Hardingham, T.E. and Fosang, A.J. (1992). Proteoglycans: many forms and many functions. *FASEB J.* **6**, 861–870.

51. Silbert, J.E. and Sugumaran, G. (1995). Intracellular membranes in the synthesis, transport and metabolism of proteoglycans. *Biochim. Biophys. Acta—Rev. Biomembranes* **1241**, 371–384.

52. Kjellen, L. and Lindahl, U. (1991). Proteoglycans: structures and interactions. *Annu. Rev. Biochem.* **60**, 443–475.

53. Hardingham, T. and Bayliss, M.T. (1990). Proteoglycans of articular cartilage: changes in aging and in joint disease. *Semin. Arthritis Rheum.* **20**, 12–33.

54. Prehm, P. (1983). Synthesis of hyaluronate in differentiated teratocarcinoma cells. Mechanism of chain growth. *Biochem. J.* **211**, 191–198.

55. Klewes, L., Turley, E.A., and Prehm, P. (1993). The hyaluronate synthase from a eukaryotic cell-line. *Biochem. J.* **290**, 791–795.

56. Mörgelin, M., Paulsson, M., Heinegård, D., Aebi, U., and Engel, J. (1995). Evidence of a defined spatial arrangement of hyaluronate in the central filament of cartilage proteoglycan aggregates. *Biochem. J.* **307**, 595–601.

57. Locci, P., Marinucci, L., Lilli, C., Martinese, D., and Becchetti, E. (1995). Transforming growth factor β1-hyaluronic acid interaction. *Cell Tissue Res.* **281**, 317–324.

58. Bansal, M.K., Ward, H., and Mason, R.M. (1986). Proteoglycan synthesis in suspension cultures of Swarm rat chondrosarcoma chondrocytes and inhibition by exogenous hyaluronate. *Arch. Biochem. Biophys.* **246**, 602–610.

59. Sonoda, M., Harwood, F., Amiel, M., Wada, Y., Moriya, H., and Amiel, D. (1997). Characterization of tissue remodelling in menisci following partial meniscectomy: the effects of hyaluronan treatment. *Trans. Orthop. Res. Soc.* **22**, 420.

60. Caterson, B., Griffin, J., Mahmoodian, F., and Sorrell, J.M. (1990). Monoclonal antibodies against chondroitin sulphate isomers:their use as probes for investigating proteoglycan metabolism. *Biochem. Soc. Trans.* **18**, 820–823.

61. Sampaio, L.O., Bayliss, M.T., Hardingham, T.E., and Muir, H. (1988). Dermatan sulphate proteoglycans from human articular cartilage. Variation in its content with age and its structural comparison with a small chondroitin sulphate proteoglycan from pig laryngeal cartilage. *Biochem. J.* **254**, 757–764.

62. Vogel, K. and Heinegård, D. (1985). Characterization of proteoglycans from the adult bovine tendon. *J. Biol. Chem.* **260**, 9298–9306.

63. Pearson, C.H., Winterbottom, N., Fackre, D.S., Scott, P.G., and Carpenter, M.R. (1983). The NH_2-terminal amino acid sequence of bovine skin proteodermatan sulfate. *J. Biol. Chem.* **258**, 15101–15104.

64. Sato, S., Rahemtulla, F., Prince, C.W., Tomano, M., and Butler, W.T. (1985). Proteoglycans of adult bovine compact bone. *Connect. Tissue Res.* **14**, 65–76.

65. Doege, K.J., Sasaki, M., Kimura, T., and Yamada, Y. (1991). Complete coding sequence and deduced primary structure of the human cartilage large aggregating proteoglycan, aggrecan—human-specific repeats, and additional alternatively spliced forms. *J. Biol. Chem.* **266**, 894–902.

66. LeBaron, R.G., Zimmermann, D.R., and Ruoslahti, E. (1992). Hyaluronate binding-properties of versican. *J. Biol. Chem.* **267**, 10003–10010.

67. Doege, K., Hassell, J.R., Caterson, B., and Yamada, Y. (1986). Link protein cDNA sequence reveals a tandemly repeated protein-structure. *Proc. Natl Acad. Sci. USA* **83**, 3761–3765.

68. Mörgelin, M., Paulsson, M., Hardingham, T.E., Heinegård, D., and Engel, J. (1988). Cartilage proteoglycans—assembly with hyaluronate and link protein as studied by electron-microscopy. *Biochem. J.* **253**, 175–185.

69. Tang, L.H., Buckwalter, J.A., and Rosenberg, L.C. (1996). Effect of link protein-concentration on articular cartilage proteoglycan aggregation. *J. Orthop. Res.* **14**, 334–339.

70. Nguyen, Q., Liu, J., Roughley, P.J., and Mort, J.S. (1991). Link protein as a monitor *in situ* of endogenous proteolysis in adult human articular cartilage. *Biochem. J.* **278**, 143–147.

71. Perkins, S.J., Nealis, A.S., Dudhia, J., and Hardingham, T.E. (1989). Immunoglobulin fold and tandem repeat structures in proteoglycan N-terminal domains and link protein. *J. Mol. Biol.* **206**, 737–753.

72. Aruffo, A., Stamenkovic, I., Melnick, M., Underhill, C.B., and Seed, B. (1990). CD44 is the principal cell surface receptor for hyaluronate. *Cell* **61**, 1303–1313.

73. Fosang, A.J. and Hardingham, T.E. (1989). Isolation of the N-terminal globular protein domains from cartilage proteoglycans. Identification of G2 domain and its lack of interaction with hyaluranate and link protein. *Biochem. J.* **261**, 801–809.

74. Watanabe, H., Cheung, C.S., Itano, N., Kimata, K., and Yamada, Y. (1997). Identification of hyaluronan-binding domains of aggrecan. *J. Biol. Chem.* **272**, 28057–28065.

75. Kiani, C., Lee, V., Cao, L., Chen, L., Yaojiong, W., Zhang, Y., Adams, M.E., and Yang, B.B. (2001). Roles of aggrecan domains in biosynthesis, modification by glycosaminoglycans and product secretion. *Biochem. J.* **354**, 199–207.

76. Dudhia, J., Davidson, C.M., Wells, T., Vynos, D., Hardingham, T.E., and Bayliss, M.T. (1996). Age-related changes in the content of the C-terminal region of aggrecan in human articular cartilage. *Biochem. J.* **313**, 933–940.

77. Valhmu, W.B., Palmer, G.D., Rivers, P.A., Ebara, S., Cheng, J.-F., Fischer, S., and Ratcliffe, A. (1995). Structure of the human aggrecan gene:exon–intron organization and association with the protein domains. *Biochem. J.* **309**, 535–542.

78. Baldwin, C.T., Reginato, A.M., and Prockop, D.J. (1989). A new epidermal growth factor-like domain in the human core protein for the large cartilage-specific proteoglycan—evidence for alternative splicing of the domain. *J. Biol. Chem.* **264**, 15747–15750.

79. Fülöp, C., Walcz, E., Valyon, M., and Glant, T.T. (1993). Expression of alternatively spliced epidermal growth factor-like domains in aggrecans of different species. Evidence for a novel module. *J. Biol. Chem.* **268**, 17377–17383.

80. Dudhia, J., Flannelly, J.K., and Bayliss, M.T. (2000). Developmental regulation of the alternatively spliced EGF and CRP motifs of aggrecan. *Trans. Orthop. Res. Soc. USA* **24**, 17.

81. Vertel, B.M., Walters, L.M., Grier, B., Maine, N., and Goetinck, P.F. (1993). Nanomelic chondrocytes synthesize, but fail to translocate, a truncated aggrecan precursor. *J. Cell. Sci.* **104**, 939–948.

82. Li, H., Schwartz, N.B., and Vertel, B.M. (1993). cDNA cloning of chick cartilage chondroitin sulfate aggrecan core protein and identification of a stop codon in the aggrecan gene associated with the chondrodystrophy, nanomelia. *J. Biol. Chem.* **268**, 23504–23511.

83. Luo, W., Kuwada, T.S., Chandrasekaran, L., Zheng, J., and Tanzer, M. (1996). Divergent secretory behavior of the opposite ends of aggrecan. *J. Biol. Chem.* **271**, 16447–16450.

84. Day, J.M., Murdoch, A.D., and Hardingham, T.E. (1999). The folded protein modules of the C-terminal G3 domain of aggrecan can each facilitate the translocation and secretion of the extended chondroitin sulfate attachment sequence. *J. Biol. Chem.* **274**, 38107–38111.

85. Dudhia, J. and Bayliss, M.T. (1998). Deletion of the lectin-like motif of the G3 domain of aggrecan results in the secretory and glycosylation failure of the protein. *Trans. Orthop. Res. Soc. USA* **23**, 108.

86. Saleque, S., Ruiz, N., and Drickamer, K. (1993). Expression and characterization of a carbohydrate-binding fragment of rat aggrecan. *Glycobiology* **3**, 185–190.

87. Halberg, D.H., Proulx, G., Doege, K., Yamada, Y., and Drickamer, K. (1988). A segment of the cartilage proteoglycan core protein has lectin-like activity. *J. Biol. Chem.* **263**, 9486–9490.

88. Aspberg, A., Binker, C., and Ruolahti, E. (1995). The versican C-type lectin domain recognizes the adhesion protein tenascin-R. *Proc. Natl Acad. Sci. USA* **92**, 10590–10594.

89. Aspberg, A., Miura, R., Bourdoulous, S., Shimonaka, M., Heinegård, D., Schachner, M., Rouslahti, E., and Yamaguchi, Y. (1997). The C-type lectin domains of lecticans, a family of aggregating chondroitin sulfate proteoglycans, bind tenascin-R by protein–protein interactions independent of carbohydrate moiety. *Proc. Natl Acad. Sci. USA* **94**, 10116–10121.

90. Zhang, Y., Cao, L., Kiani, C.G., Yang, B.L., and Yang, B.B. (1998). The G3 domain of versican inhibits mesenchymal chondrogenesis via the epidermal growth factor-like motifs. *J. Biol. Chem.* **273**, 33054–33063.

91. Yang, B.L., Cao, L., Kianai, C., Lee, V., Zhang, Y., Adams, M.E., and Yang, B.B. (2000). Tandem repeats are involved in G1 domain inhibition of versican expression and secretion and the G3 domain enhances glycosaminoglycan modification and secretion via the complement-binding protein motif. *J. Biol. Chem.* **275**, 21255–21261.

92. Zimmermann, D.R. and Ruoslahti, E. (1989). Multiple domains of the large fibroblast proteoglycan, versican. *EMBO J.* **8**, 2975–2981.

93. Krusius, T., Gehlsen, K.R., and Ruoslahti, E. (1987). A fibroblast chondroitin sulfate proteoglycan core protein contains lectin-like and growth factor-like sequences. *J. Biol. Chem.* **262**, 13120–13125.

94. Dours-Zimmermann, M.T. and Zimmermann, D.R. (1994). A novel glycosaminoglycan attachment domain identified in 2 alternative splice variants of human versican. *J. Biol. Chem.* **269**, 32992–32998.

95. Zako, M., Shinomura, T., Ujita, M., Ito, K., and Kimata, K. (1995). Expression of PG-M V3, an alternative splice form of PG-M without a chondroitin sulfate attachment region in mouse and human tissues. *J. Biol. Chem.* **270**, 3914–3918.

96. Kimata, K., Oike, Y., Tani, K., Shinomura, T., Yamagata, M., Uritani, M., and Suzuki, S. (1986). A large chondroitin sulfate proteoglycan PG-M synthesized before chondrogenesis in the limb bud of chick-embryo. *J. Biol. Chem.* **261**, 3517–3525.

97. Yamagata, M., Yamada, K.M., Yoneda, M., Suzuki, S., and Kimata, K. (1986). Chondroitin sulfate proteoglycan PG-M-like proteoglycan is involved in the binding of hyaluronic acid to cellular fibronectin. *J. Biol. Chem.* **261**, 3526–3535.

98. Ito, K., Shinomura, T., Yamakawa, N., Usui, M., Ishii, S., and Kimata, K. (1995). Expression of a large chondroitin sulphate proteoglycan PG-M in degenerative articular cartilage. *Trans. Orthop. Res. Soc.* **20**, 411.

99. Nishida, K., Inoue, H., Toda, K., and Murakami, T. (1995). Localization of the glycosaminoglycans in the synovial tissues from osteoarthritic knees. *Acta Med. Okayama* **49**, 287–294.

100. Bode-Lesniewska, B., Dours-Zimmermann, M.T., Odermatt, B.F., Briner, J., Heitz, P.U., and Zimmermann, D.R. (1996). Distribution of the large aggregating proteoglycan versican in adult human tissues. *J. Histochem. Cytochem.* **44**, 303–312.

101. Grover, J. and Roughley, P.J. (1993). Versican gene-expression in human articular-cartilage and comparison of messenger-RNA splicing variation with aggrecan. *Biochem. J.* **291**, 361–367.

102. Campbell, M.A., Tester, A.M., Handley, C.J., Checkley, G.J., Chow, G.L., Cant, A.E., Winter, A.D., and Cain, W.E. (1996). Characterization of a large chondroitin sulfate proteoglycan present in bovine collateral ligament. *Arch. Biochem. Biophys.* **329**, 181–190.

103. Iozzo, R.V. (1997). The family of the small leucine-rich proteoglycans: key regulators of matrix assembly and cellular growth. *Crit. Rev. Biochem. Mol. Biol.* **32**, 141–174.

104. Cheng, F., Heinegård, D., Malmstrom, A., Schmidtchen, A., Yoshida, K., and Fransson, L.A. (1994). Patterns of uronosyl epimerization and 4-/6-O-sulfation in chondroitin/dermatan sulfate from decorin and biglycan of various bovine-tissues. *Glycobiology* **4**, 685–696.

105. Roughley, P.J., Rodriguez, E., and Lee, E.R. (1995). The interactions of non-aggregating proteoglycans. *Osteoarthritis Cartilage* **3**, 239–248.

106. Schonherr, E., Hausser, H., Beavan, L., and Kresse, H. (1995). Decorin-type-I collagen interaction—presence of separate core protein-binding domains. *J. Biol. Chem.* **270**, 8877–8883.

107. Svensson, L., Heinegård, D., and Oldberg, Å. (1995). Decorin-binding sites for collagen type I are mainly located in leucine-rich repeats 4–5. *J. Biol. Chem.* **270**, 20712–20716.

108. Schonherr, E., Witsch-Prehm, P., Harrach, B., Robenek, H., Rauterberg, J., and Kresse, H. (1995). Interaction of biglycan with type I collagen. *J. Biol. Chem.* **270**, 2776–2783.

109. Scott, J.E. (1992). Supramolecular organization of extracellular matrix glycosaminoglycans, *in vitro* and in the tissues. *FASEB J.* **6**, 2639–2645.

110. Hedbom, E. and Heinegård, D. (1993). Binding of fibromodulin and decorin to separate sites on fibrillar collagens. *J. Biol. Chem.* **268**, 27307–27312.

111. Scott, J.E. (1996). Proteodermatan and proteokeratan sulfate decorin, lumican/fibromodulin proteins are horseshoe shaped. Implications for their interactions with collagen. *Biochemistry* **35**, 8795–8799.

112. Hildebrand, A., Romaris, M., Rasmussen, L.M., Heinegård, D., Twardzik, D.R., Border, W.A., and Ruoslahti, E. (1994). Interaction of the small interstitial proteoglycans biglycan, decorin and fibromodulin with transforming growth factor beta. *Biochem. J.* **302**, 527–534.

113. Yamaguchi, Y., Mann, D.M., and Ruoslahti, E. (1990). Negative regulation of transforming growth factor-β by the proteoglycan decorin. *Nature* **346**, 281–284.

114. Birkedal-Hansen, H. (1995). Proteolytic remodeling of extracellular matrix. *Curr. Opin. Cell Biol.* **7**, 728–735.

115. Heinegård, D. and Sommarin, Y. (1987). Proteoglycans: an overview. In *Methods of immunology, structural and contractile proteins*, Part D: Extracellular matrix (ed. L.W. Cunningham), pp. 305–319. Academic Press, Orlando, Florida.

116. Adams, M.E. and Muir, H. (1981). The glycosaminoglycans of canine menisci. *Biochem. J.* **197**, 385–389.

117. Adams, M.E., McDevitt, C.A., Ho, A., and Muir, H. (1986). Isolation and characterization of high-buoyant-density proteoglycans from semilunar menisci. *J. Bone Joint Surg. Am.* **68**, 55–64.

118. Adams, M.E. and Ho, Y.A. (1987). Localization of glycosaminoglycans in human and canine menisci and their attachments. *Connect. Tissue Res.* **16**, 269–279.

119. Scott, P.G., Dodd, C.M., Tredget, E.E., Ghahary, A., and Rahemtulla, F. (1995). Immunohistochemical localization of the proteoglycans decorin, biglycan and versican and transforming growth factor-β in human postburn hypertrophic and mature scars. *Histopathology* **26**, 423–431.

120. Scott, P.G., Nakano, T., and Dodd, C.M. (1997). Isolation and characterization of small proteoglycans from different zones of the porcine knee meniscus. *Biochim. Biophys. Acta* **1336**, 254–262.

121. McNicol, D. and Roughley, P.J. (1980). Extraction and characterization of proteoglycan from human meniscus. *Biochem. J.* **185**, 705–713.

122. Roughley, P.J., McNicol, D., Santer, V., and Buckwalter, J. (1981). The presence of a cartilage-like proteoglycan in the adult human meniscus. *Biochem. J.* **197**, 77–83.

123. Roughley, P.J. and White, R.J. (1992). The dermatan sulfate proteoglycans of the adult human meniscus. *J. Orthop. Res.* **10**, 631–637.

124. Heinegård, D., Larsson, T., Sommarin, Y., Franzen, A., Paulsson, M., and Hedbom, E. (1986). Two novel matrix proteins isolated from articular cartilage show wide distributions among connective tissue. *J. Biol. Chem.* **261**, 13866–13872.

125. Fife, R.S. (1985). Identification of link proteins and a 116,000-Dalton matrix protein in canine meniscus. *Arch. Biochem. Biophys.* **240**, 682–688.

126. Ghadially, F.N., Thomas, I., Yong, N., and Lalonde, J.M. (1978). Ultrastructure of rabbit semilunar cartilages. *J. Anat.* **125**, 499–517.

127. Mankin, H.J. (1978). The metabolism of articular cartilage. In *The human joint in health and disease* (ed. W.H. Simon), p. 53. University of Pennsylvania Press, Philadelphia.

128. Aydelotte, M.B., Schumacher, B.L., and Kuettner, K.E. (1992). Heterogeneity of articular chondrocytes. In *Articular cartilage and osteoarthritis* (ed. K.E. Kuettner, R. Schleyerbach, J.G. Peyron, and V.C. Hascall), pp. 237–249. Raven Press Ltd, New York.

129. Aydelotte, M.B. and Kuettner, K.E. (1988). Differences between subpopulations of cultured bovine articular chondrocytes. I. Morphology and cartilage matrix production. *Connect. Tissue Res.* **18**, 205–222.

130. Hauselmann, H.J., Flechtenmacher, J., Michal, L., Thonar, E.J., Shinmei, M., Kuettner, K.E., and Aydelotte, M.B. (1996). The superficial layer of human articular cartilage is more susceptible to interleukin-1-induced damage than the deeper layers. *Arthritis Rheum.* **39**, 478–488.

131. Webber, R.J., Harris, M.G., and Hough, A.J. Jr (1985). Cell culture of rabbit meniscal fibrochondrocytes: proliferative and synthetic response to growth factors and ascorbate. *J. Orthop. Res.* **3**, 36–42.

132. Webber, R.J., Malemud, C.J., and Sokoloff, L. (1977). Species differences in cell culture of mammalian articular chondrocytes. *Calcif. Tissue Res.* **23**, 61–66.

133. Webber, R.J. (1990). *In vitro* culture of meniscal tissue. *Clin. Orthop.* **252**, 114–120.

134. Pierschbacher, M., Hayman, E.G., and Ruoslahti, E. (1983). Synthetic peptide with cell attachment activity of fibronectin. *Proc. Natl Acad. Sci. USA* **80**, 1224–1227.

135. Kilar, M., Goldberg, R., and Schwartz, E.R. (1984). Cell coat formation in normal and osteoarthritic chondrocyte cultures. *Trans. Orthop. Res. Soc.* **9**, 234.

136. Natsu-Ume, T., Nakamura, N., Shino, K., Hashimoto, N., Matsumoto, N., and Nakata, K. (1997). The effects of hepatocyte growth factor/scatter factor HGF/SF on meniscal fibrochondrocytes. *Trans. Othop. Res. Soc.* **22**, 421.

137. Matsumoto, K., Tajima, H., Okazaki, H., and Nakamura, T. (1992). Negative regulation of hepatocyte growth factor gene expression in human lung fibroblasts and leukemic cells by transforming growth factor-β1 and glucocorticoids. *J. Biol. Chem.* **267**, 24917–24920.

138. Takebayashi, T., Iwamoto, M., Jikko, A., and Matsumura, T. (1995). Hepatocyte growth factor/scatter factor modulates cell motility, proliferation, and proteoglycan synthesis of chondrocytes. *J. Cell. Biol.* **129**, 1411–1419.

139. Spindler, K.P., Mayes, C.E., Miller, R.R., Imro, A.K., and Davidson, J.M. (1995). Regional mitogenic response of the meniscus to platelet-derived growth factor PDGF-AB. *J. Orthop. Res.* **13**, 201–207.

140. Attia, E., Bhargava, M.M., Dolan, M., Murrell, G.A.C., Warren, R.F., and Hannafin, J.A. (1997). Effect of cytokines on proliferation and migration of bovine meniscal cells. *Trans. Orthop. Res. Soc.* **22**, 422.

141. Ingman, A.M., Ghosh, P., and Taylor, T.K. (1974). Variation of collagenous and non-collagenous proteins of human knee joint menisci with age and degeneration. *Gerontologia* **20**, 212–213.

142. Bayliss, M.T., Davidson, C., Woodhouse, S.M., and Osborne, D.J. (1995). Chondroitin sulphation in human joint tissues varies with age, zone and topography. *Acta Orthop. Scand.* **66**, 142–164.

143. Roughley, P.J. (1987). Structural changes in the proteoglycans of human articular cartilage during aging. *J. Rheumatol.* **14**, 14–15.

144. Hough, A.J. Jr and Webber, R.J. (1990). Pathology of the meniscus. *Clin. Orthop.* 32–40.

145. Fitzgerald, S.W. (1994). Magnetic resonance imaging of the meniscus. Advanced concepts. *Magn. Reson. Imaging Clin. N. Am.* **2**, 349–364.

146. Hutchinson, C.H. and Wojtys, E.M. (1995). MRI versus arthroscopy in evaluating knee meniscal pathology. *Am. J. Knee Surg.* **8**, 93–96.

147. Arnoczky, S.P., Warren, R.F., and Spivak, J.M. (1988). Meniscal repair using an exogenous fibrin clot. An experimental study in dogs. *J. Bone Joint Surg. Am.* **70**, 1209–1217.

148. Arnoczky, S.P. and Warren, R.F. (1983). The microvasculature of the meniscus and its response to injury: an experimental study in the dog. *Am. J. Sports Med.* **11**, 131–141.

149. Newman, A.P., Anderson, D.R., Daniels, A.U., and Dales, M.C. (1989). Mechanics of the healed meniscus in a canine model. *Am. J. Sports Med.* **17**, 164–175.

150. Newman, A.P., Daniels, A.U., and Burks, R.T. (1993). Principles and decision making in meniscal surgery. *Arthroscopy* **9**, 33–51.

151. Allen, P.R., Denham, R.A., and Swan, A.V. (1984). Late degenerative changes after meniscectomy. Factors affecting the knee after operation. *J. Bone Joint Surg. Br.* **66**, 666–671.

152. Jorgensen, U., Sonne-Holm, S., Lauridsen, F., and Rosenklint, A. (1987). Long-term follow-up of meniscectomy in athletes. A prospective longitudinal study. *J. Bone Joint Surg. Br.* **69**, 80–83.

153. Garrett, J.C., Steensen, R.N., and Steensen, R.N. (1991). Meniscal transplantation in the human knee: a preliminary report [published erratum appears in *Arthroscopy* (1991) **72**, 256.]. *Arthroscopy* **7**, 57–62.

154. van Arkel, E.R. and de Boer, H.H. (1995). Human meniscal transplantation. Preliminary results at 2 to 5-year follow-up. *J. Bone Joint Surg. Br.* **77**, 589–595.

155. Arnoczky, S.P., Warren, R.F., and McDevitt, C.A. (1990). Meniscal replacement using a cryopreserved allograft. An experimental study in the dog. *Clin. Orthop.* 121–128.

156. Khoury, M.A., Goldberg, V.M., and Stevenson, S. (1994). Demonstration of HLA and ABH antigens in fresh and frozen human menisci by immunohistochemistry. *J. Orthop. Res.* **12**, 751–757.

157. Kohn, D. (1993). Autograft meniscus replacement: experimental and clinical results. *Knee Surg. Sports Traumatol. Arthrosc.* **1**, 123–125.

158. Stone, K.R., Rodkey, W.G., Webber, R.J., McKinney, L., and Steadman, J.R. (1990). Future directions. Collagen-based prostheses for meniscal regeneration. *Clin. Orthop.* **252**, 129–135.

159. Wakitani, S., Goto, T., Pineda, S.J., Young, R.G., Mansour, J.M., Caplan, A.I., and Goldberg, V.M. (1994). Mesenchymal cell-based repair of large, full-thickness defects of articular cartilage. *J. Bone Joint Surg. Am.* **76**, 579–592.

160. Walsh, C.J., Goodman, D., Caplan, A.I., and Goldberg, V.M. (1996). Cell-based meniscus regeneration in a partial meniscectomy model. *Trans. Orthop. Res. Soc.* **21**, 100.

161. Ibarra, C., Hidaka, C., Hannafin, J.A., Torzilli, P.A., and Warren, R.F. (1998). Tissue engineered repair of canine meniscus explants *in vitro* and in a nude mice model. *Trans. Orthop. Res. Soc.* **23**, 148.

162. Ibarra, C., Ellisseff, J., Vacanti, J.P., Cao, Y., Kim, T.H., Upton, J., and Langer, R. (1997). Meniscal tissue engineered by subcutaneous implantation of fibrochondrocytes on polymer develops biomechanical compressive properties similar to the normal meniscus. *Trans. Orthop. Res. Soc.* **22**, 549.

163. Ertl, W., Paulino, C., Manji, R., and Grande, D. (1996). Successful meniscal repair utilizing meniscal tissue engineered constructs: one year results. *Trans. Orthop. Res. Soc.* **21**, 539.

164. Gerich, T.G., Kang, R., Georgescu, H.I., Nita, I.M., Fu, F., Robbins, P.D., and Evans, C.H. (1996). Comparison of viral vectors of potential use for gene transfer to ligaments and menisci. *Trans. Orthop. Res. Soc.* **21**, 285.

165. Adams, M.E., Billingham, M.E., and Muir, H. (1983). The glycosaminoglycans in menisci in experimental and natural osteoarthritis. *Arthritis Rheum.* **26**, 69–76.

166. Ghosh, P., Ingman, A.M., and Taylor, T.K. (1975). Variations in collagen, non-collagenous proteins, and hexosamine in menisci derived from osteoarthritic and rheumatoid arthritic knee joints. *J. Rheumatol.* **2**, 100–107.

2

The science of pain from theory to clinical practice

2.1 The science of chronic pain from theory to clinical practice

Derek Yull and Rajesh Munglani

The study and treatment of pain

There always seems to be a dichotomy between academic research into pain and practical treatment. There seems to be a sense of random choice as to whether, for example, one treats back pain with drugs, injections, psychotherapy, or physiotherapy or a combination of some or all of these. Any model of pain has to explain why such different therapies may achieve similar results—lip service is given to a biopsychosocial model, but the details of this model on a neurobiological level are still be elucidated. This chapter provides a brief overview of pain mechanisms and in a small way attempts to provide a rational basis for various modalities of treatment. Some of the treatments mentioned here will be covered in more detail in other chapters but it is important to provide a framework on which to add further knowledge.

The definition of pain endorsed by the International Association for the Study of Pain is as follows, 'Pain is an unpleasant sensory and emotional experience associated with actual or potential tissue damage, or described in terms of such damage.' Pain can be subdivided into four areas to help understand its nature:[1]

1. *Nociception* is the detection of tissue damage by the free nerve endings of Aδ and C fibres.

2. *Perception of pain* is highly subjective and is frequently triggered by noxious stimuli such as an injury or disease. It can also be generated by lesions in the peripheral or central nervous system (CNS), that is, there may be pain without nociception. With chronic pain, the intensity of pain perception often bears little or no relation to the extent of tissue injury.

3. *Suffering* is a negative response induced not only by pain but also by fear, anxiety, and stress.

4. *Pain behaviours* result from pain and suffering, and are what a person does or does not do in response to pain, for example, limping or seeking medical attention.

Pain can also be subdivided into three main types:[1]

1. *Transient pain* is elicited by the activation of nociceptors in the periphery in the absence of any tissue damage. It evolved to protect man from physical damage and is ubiquitous in everyday life.

2. *Acute pain* is the result of substantial injury of body tissue and nociceptor activation at the site of injury. The injury will alter the response characteristics of the nociceptors and their central connections. Examples occur after trauma, surgery, and some diseases, and most people will seek medical attention. The important features are that the injury does not overwhelm the body's response mechanisms and the report of pain stops long before

healing has been completed. The healing process usually takes a few days or weeks.

3. *Chronic pain.* Defining chronic pain in terms of the duration or existence of a pain is not useful. It is distinguished from acute pain in that it may exceed the body's capability for healing, and pain may persist when treatment or healing stops. Changes may occur within the pain pathways both peripherally and centrally to allow the persistence of a painful perception. Finally, because chronic pain is unrelenting, it is likely that stress, environmental, and affective factors may be superimposed and actually contribute to the intensity and persistence of the pain.

Summary of pathways from nociceptor to brain

The human response to acute pain is an entirely useful and important reaction to an acute noxious stimulus. It quite clearly is a protective mechanism as shown by the severe deformities in those with congenital insensitivity to pain.

Chronic pain is less easy to understand. Different pathophysiological processes occur following inflammation and nerve injury compared to those occurring in acute pain states. These will be discussed later, but first a summary of the pain pathways is required.

Primary afferent nociceptors

These are the initial structures involved in nociception and they are widespread in skin, muscle, connective tissues, blood vessels, and thoraco-abdominal viscera. They are activated by thermal, mechanical, or chemical stimuli that have the potential to cause damage.[2]

The nociceptors are pseudounipolar neurons with the cell body found in the dorsal root ganglion. Innervation of many tissues occurs where the nociceptors lose their perineural sheath from the peripheral processes. There is no specialized structure for detection of noxious stimuli—they are basically 'free' nerve endings. As well as detecting changes in mechanical, thermal, and chemical energy, these endings release peptides in response to injury such as substance P, calcitonin gene-related peptide (CGRP), and neurokinin A.[2]

The two main categories of nociceptor are C fibres and Aδ fibres, which are unmyelinated and thinly myelinated, respectively. Most nociceptors are C fibre polymodal, which means they respond to noxious chemical, thermal, and mechanical stimuli—the ratio of unmyelinated to myelinated fibres in cutaneous nerves is 4:1. Approximately 10 per cent of cutaneous myelinated fibres and 90 per cent of cutaneous unmyelinated fibres are nociceptive. The two fibre types differ in the type of sensation detected: Aδ fibres conduct 'fast' pain, which is perceived as short-lasting and pricking in nature. 'Slow' pain, which is dull, poorly localized, and burning, is conducted by C fibres.[2]

Cutaneous nociceptors on the head and face transmit pain via the three divisions of the trigeminal nerve to the trigeminal or Gasserian ganglion, which is analagous to the dorsal root ganglion of spinal nerves.[2]

Generally speaking, the increasing intensity of a peripheral stimulus is encoded by a primary afferent nociceptor as increasing frequency of discharge. In addition, the number of afferents stimulated provides information since the area of skin innervated by a single afferent fibre is less than 1 cm squared.[3]

Visceral afferents

Visceral pain is the most common form of pain in disease states and relatively little is known about it. It has been conventionally thought that visceral pain is simply a variant of somatic pain, although this is not now thought to be true. There are different neurological mechanisms involved in the transmission of visceral pain, and its perception and psychological processing is also distinct from those of somatic pain.[4]

Visceral pain is not evoked from all viscera and is not always linked to visceral injury. It is diffuse, can be referred to other locations, and is accompanied by motor and autonomic reflexes (e.g. nausea). It commonly results from distension of a hollow organ or prolonged contraction of the smooth muscle making up its wall.[4]

It is now thought that there are two distinct classes of nociceptive sensory receptors innervating internal organs: high-threshold nociceptors that are only activated by stimuli within the noxious range; and intensity-coding receptors that have a low threshold to natural stimuli and therefore respond to stimuli ranging from innocuous to noxious. Chronic visceral stimulation may result in the sensitization of high-threshold receptors such that they begin to respond to innocuous stimuli. This will lead to increased afferent input into the central nervous system.[4]

Visceral afferent inputs terminate on spinal cord laminae I and V, as do some somatic afferents—hence the ability to achieve referred pain.

Sympathetic nervous system

It is best to consider the sympathetic nervous system (SNS) as an efferent neuroeffector system modulating cardiovascular, bronchial, visceral, metabolic, and sudomotor function. Sympathetic preganglionic fibres leave the spinal cord through the ventral root of the thoracolumbar spinal nerves and end in a sympathetic ganglion. Here they synapse with postganglionic fibres that then leave the ganglion and connect to the effector tissues mentioned above. Preganglionic fibres are myelinated B fibres and postganglionic fibres are small, unmyelinated C fibres.[2]

Dorsal horn

Nearly all sensory afferents terminate in the dorsal horns of the medulla and spinal cord. Most of these sensory afferents enter via the dorsal root, although some unmyelinated ones enter via the ventral root. Light microscopic morphology is used to divide the spinal cord grey matter into 10 laminae according to Rexed's classification. The dorsal horn consists of six laminae (I–VI) with I being the most superficial. The ventral horn consists of four (VII–X) with X surrounding the central canal.[2]

Unmyelinated C-fibre nociceptors terminate in lamina II (the substantia gelatinosa) and some also ascend and descend in Lissauer's tract before terminating. Small, unmyelinated Aδ nociceptors terminate mainly in laminae I and V, and large fibre nociceptors (transmitting fine touch, proprioception, and vibration) terminate in III and IV or in the dorsal columns.[2]

The terminations of the primary afferent nociceptors transmit information to second-order neurons. Second-order neurons consist of two main classes:

1. nociceptive specific (high threshold);

2. wide dynamic range (convergent).

They have different responses to afferent inputs and are also found in different areas of the dorsal horn. Nociceptive-specific neurons are found superficially in the dorsal horn and only respond to noxious stimuli. Wide dynamic range neurons are found deeper in the dorsal horn and respond to noxious and non-noxious stimuli.[2]

Wide dynamic range neurons hence can accurately encode a range of afferent stimuli from light touch to intense pain. Their receptive fields are vast in comparison to those of primary afferent neurons since both primary nociceptor afferents and propriospinal tracts converge on them. Wide dynamic range neurons are recruited in the face of increasing nociceptive stimulation, and the field size is larger. They can generate long-lived responses in the face of only brief discharges in C and Aδ fibres.[3]

Neurotransmitters

Within the dorsal horn are many peptide and amino acid neurotransmitters released by the various primary nociceptor afferent, proprioceptive, and second-order neurons. The effects can be either excitatory or inhibitory depending upon which neurotransmitter is released and where. Neurotransmission within the dorsal horn includes:[2]

1. excitatory neurotransmitters released from primary afferent nociceptors;

2. excitatory transmission between neurons of the spinal cord;

3. inhibitory neurotransmitters released by interneurons within the spinal cord;

4. inhibitory neurotransmitters released from supraspinal sources.

It is clear that there is not a single neuron releasing a single neurotransmitter within the synaptic cleft in the dorsal horn. Two or more compounds are commonly released at the same time, which is called co-release. Neurotransmitters found in the dorsal horn include:

1. peptides—substance P, CGRP, somatostatin, neuropeptide Y, galanin, neurokinin A;

2. excitatory aminoacids—aspartate, glutamate;

3. inhibitory aminoacids—gamma amino butyric acid (GABA), glycine;

4. nitric oxide;

5. arachidonic acid metabolites;

6. endogenous opioids;

7. monoamines—serotonin, noradrenaline (also called norepinephrine).

Peptides

Substance P coexists in primary afferents with glutamate and it plays a modulatory role in nociception by modifying the gain of afferent transmission. The release of substance P as well as neurokinin A from primary afferent nociceptors is required to produce intense pain.[2]

Excitatory amino acids

Glutamate is the major neurotransmitter within the CNS and plays a major role in nociceptive transmission in the dorsal horn. It acts at α-amino-3-hydroxy-5-methyl-4-isoxazolepropionic acid (AMPA) receptors, N-methyl-D-aspartate (NMDA) receptors, kainate (KA), and metabotropic glutamate receptors. Variants of each glutamate receptor subtype are expressed throughout the CNS.

AMPA receptors are ligand-operated ion channels that permit Na^+ entry. They are activated by both non-nociceptive and nociceptive afferent inputs, and can also activate NMDA receptors. NMDA receptors are not activated by glutamate alone due to ion blockade by Mg^{2+}—activation of AMPA receptors will remove this blockade and allow Na^+ and Ca^{2+} ion flux through the NMDA receptor. Hence AMPA receptor activation is necessary in order to 'prime' the NMDA receptor such that it is ready for activation. Glutamate coexists with substance P in some nociceptive neurons and both may be released together after intense noxious stimulation. The significance is that substance P, as well as AMPA receptor activation, can lead to a reduction in the Mg^{2+} blockade of the NMDA receptor.[2, 3, 5]

Once activated, NMDA receptors cause a longlasting depolarization associated with Ca^{2+} mobilization in neurons that are already partly depolarized. What this does in effect is lower the threshold for other subsequent lower-intensity stimuli to generate postsynaptic action potentials. This is important, as will be discussed later, in the process of wind-up, long-term potentiation and also pain radiation.[2, 3]

Following the initial increase in intracellular Ca^{2+} there is activation of protein kinase C which has both pre- and postsynaptic effects. It increases glutamate and aspartate release and reduces the Mg^{2+} blockade on the NMDA receptor.[3]

Metabotropic glutamate receptors are G-protein-coupled and linked to the phosphoinositide and cyclic adenosine 3'-5'-phosphate (cAMP) second-messenger systems. Their role is unclear at present.[2]

Inhibitory amino acids

Both GABAergic and glycinergic interneurons are vital in the inhibition of the nociceptive stimulus. It is thought that $GABA_A$-receptor-mediated inhibition occurs mainly through postsynaptic mechanisms and that of $GABA_B$ via presynaptic mechanisms involving the suppression of excitatory amino acid release from primary afferent terminals. These inhibitory interneurons help to explain the gate theory whereby non-noxious input along large-diameter afferent nerves will primarily activate inhibitory interneurons and noxious input along small-diameter afferents will inhibit the inhibitory interneurons. A further component of the gate theory is inhibition of noxious inputs by descending pathways from the brain.[2]

Nitric oxide

Nitric oxide (NO), a small freely diffusible molecule, can act as an intracellular messenger that does not require synaptic contacts.

NMDA receptor activation is linked to NO production via the Ca^{2+} activated constitutive enzyme nitric oxide synthase (NOS). NO then activates guanylate cyclase to produce cyclic guanosine 5'-phosphate (cGMP). There seems to be upregulation of NOS in injured neurons leading to increased NO production, which may lead to neuropathic pain. NO may have pre- and postsynaptic neuronal sensitizing effects, including the release of sustance P and CGRP.[3]

Arachidonic acid metabolites

Following NMDA receptor activation there is an increase in intracellular Ca^{2+}, which is essential for a number of events. These include activation of phospholipase A2 and hence conversion of arachidonic acid into prostacyclins via cyclo-oxygenase. In inflammatory states, there is known to be prostaglandin production in spinal cord neurons and Schwann cells.[3]

Endogenous opioids

Opioid receptors modulate nociceptive input at spinal and supraspinal levels within the CNS. The different subtypes (μ, δ, κ or OP-1, OP-2, OP-3 plus the orphan opioid receptor ORL-1) are distributed throughout the CNS and are activated by the endogenous opioid ligands β-endorphin and endomorphin 1 and 2 (μ ligands), enkephalin (κ), and dynorphin (δ). An endogenous ligand for the ORL-1 receptor has been isolated called nociceptin. Opioid receptors are G-protein-linked and lead to a reduction in cAMP.[2]

At the spinal level, opioids act in the dorsal horn to inhibit glutamate and neurokinin release from primary afferent terminals pre- and postsynaptically to inhibit second-order neuron depolarization. The release of cholecystokinin in the dorsal horn modulates opioid analgesic mechanisms. There is a high density of opioid receptors supraspinally in the periaqueductal grey, nucleus raphe magnus, and locus ceruleus.[2]

Monoamines

Both noradrenaline (norepinephrine) and serotonin are important neurotransmitters in descending neuronal pathways within the spinal cord. Electrical stimulation of the nucleus raphe magnus and periaqueductal grey causes increased serotonin release in the spinal cord, and stimulation of the locus ceruleus causes noradrenaline release from noradrenaline-containing terminals in the upper laminae of the dorsal horn.[2]

Adenosine

The endogenous compound adenosine is present in all cells and may be released from cells directly or via degradation of adenosine triphosphate (ATP). Adenosine, along with ATP, adenosine monophosphate (AMP), and adenosine diphosphate (ADP), is a purine that acts at purine receptors P1 and P2. P1 receptors can be further subdivided into A1, A2a, A2b, and A3 receptors, the first three of which occur in the spinal cord. There is now evidence that adenosine can modulate nociception via A1 receptors, having an antinociceptive effect.[6]

Ascending spinal tracts

There is a multiplicity of pain pathways connecting the dorsal horns to the brain. These include the spinothalamic, spinoreticular, spinomesencephalic, spinolimbic, spinocervicothalamic, and the postsynaptic dorsal column pathways.[2]

Spinothalamic tract

This has a central role in pain perception and transmits information regarding pain, warmth, and touch. It originates within laminae I, IV, V, VII, and also X. Nociceptive afferents may ascend one or two segments from their point of entry to the spinal cord before decussating via the dorsal commissure and ascending to the contralateral thalamus. A few fibres do project to the ipsilateral thalamus. Spinothalamic neurons have restrictive receptive fields and there is somatotopic organization such that fibres arising caudally are more lateral than those entering more cranially.[2]

Spinoreticular tract

This pathway originates in the deep layers of the dorsal horn and laminae VII and VIII of the ventral horn. It projects largely non-somatotropically to the reticular formation of the brainstem. It appears that the pathway is involved in the basic autonomic, motor, and endogenous analgesic responses to nociceptive input.[2]

Spinomesencephalic tract

Originating in laminae I, IV, V, VI, and X, these neurons project somatotropically to midbrain nuclei such as the periaqueductal grey, cuneiform nucleus, superior colliculus, and Edinger–Westphal nucleus. Neurons in this tract have large and complex receptive fields and it is involved in more organized and integrated motor, autonomic, and antinociceptive responses.[2]

Spinolimbic pathway

The spinolimbic pathway involves projections from neurons in laminae I, VII, and X to the hypothalamus and from lamina X and the deep dorsal horn to the amygdala. These pathways may be responsible for the motivational or affective responses associated with pain perception.[2]

Spinocervicothalamic pathway

This pathway runs from lamina IV to the lateral cervical nucleus at C1 and C2, and then decussates and ascends with the medial lemniscus to end in the thalamus. It is primarily involved with light touch transmission rather than nociception.[2]

Postsynaptic dorsal column pathway

This pathway transmits information regarding fine touch, proprioception, and vibration. It is possible that stimulation of the medial aspect of the nucleus gracilis (part of the dorsal colum pathway) may cause pain. Cells in the gracile nucleus also respond to noxious stimulation of viscera. The pathway originates in laminae III and X.[2]

Supraspinal structures

Thalamus

Positron emission tomography (PET) studies have illustrated several subcortical structures involved in nociception transmission and pain perception including the thalamus, putamen, caudate nucleus, hypothalamus, amygdala, periaqueductal grey, hippocampus, and cerebellum. Studies have shown that acute painful stimuli result in increased thalamic activity, whereas chronic pain results in decreased thalamic activity.[2]

The thalamus is hence one of the key areas involved in pain transmission and it consists of separate areas. One group of the spinothalamic fibres terminates in the posterior thalamus (transmitting the sensory discriminative component of pain) and another terminates more medially, which then projects to the somatosensory cortex. The centromedian fibres project more diffusely, including to the limbic system (involved in the affective–motivational aspects of pain). The spinoreticular and spinomesencephalic tracts project to the medial thalamus, and the spinocervicothalamic and postsynaptic dorsal column pathways terminate in the posterior complex.[2]

Cortex

PET and functional magnetic resonance imaging (MRI) have helped ascertain which cortical regions are involved in pain processing. Painful stimuli may cause activation of somatosensory, motor, premotor, parietal, frontal, occipital, insular, and anterior cingulate regions of the cortex. It is suggested that the parietal regions evaluate the temporal and spatial features of pain, whereas the frontal cortex is responsible for the emotional response to pain.[2]

Neurosurgical lesions of cortical regions produce varying effects depending upon the region ablated. Lesions of the frontal and cingulate cortex leave pain perception intact, but with a reduced component of suffering. In contrast, lesions to the medial thalamus and hypothalamus give pain relief without demonstrable analgesia.[2]

Descending pathways

These inhibitory influences arising from the brain have already been mentioned. They descend in the spinal cord and can have powerful modulatory (inhibitory and also facilitatory) effects on spinal reflexes. The inhibitory pathways arise from the hypothalamus, periaqueductal grey, locus ceruleus, and nucleus raphe magnus. These areas in turn receive projections from the amygdala and the frontal and insular cortex. In addition, endorphins synthesized in the pituitary are released into the cerebrospinal fluid (CSF) and blood where they can exert inhibitory effects at these centres.[2, 6]

Electrical stimulation and microinjection of excitatory amino acids into these centres will inhibit nociception. Descending inhibition is activated by external factors such as stress or noxious input. There is also a background activity within the system to maintain a resting level of inhibitory function.[2]

Fibres from each of these centres descend either directly or indirectly within the dorsolateral and ventrolateral funiculi and terminate within the dorsal horn (e.g. within laminae I, II, and V). Within the dorsal horn, the terminals of the descending pathways interact with projection neurons that transmit information from spinal regions to the brain, local interneurons, and primary afferent endings. They allow inhibition either by presynaptically modulating neurotransmitter release or by postsynaptically exciting local inhibitory interneurons or inhibiting second-order projection neurons.[2]

What initiates chronic pain?

The next section looks at changes that may occur within the peripheral and central nervous systems to maintain a chronic pain. But what are the actual events that can trigger such potentially debilitating pain? There are three possible mechanisms:[7]

1. Ongoing nociceptive input is the simplest explanation of chronic pain and is typified by chronic inflammatory degenerative

conditions such as rheumatoid arthritis. There is ongoing activation of peripheral nociceptors leading to peripheral and central sensitization.

2. Persistence of pain after healing. Chronic pain persists long after the tissue damage that initially triggered its onset has resolved, for example, back pain in disc prolapse. Pain perception requires activity only in cortical and associated supraspinal regions many synapses distant from the peripheral nociceptor. Therefore, ongoing afferent input into the spinal cord is not a prerequisite for ongoing pain.

3. Chronic pain in the absence of any tissue injury, such as fibromyalgia, myofascial pain syndrome, or headache.

Neuropathic pain

Neuropathic pain is a pathological, maladaptive pain typically resulting from damage to the nervous system—the peripheral nerve, the dorsal root, or the CNS. It comprises a complex combination of negative symptoms or sensory deficits such as partial or complete loss of sensation, and positive symptoms that include dysaesthesia, paraesthesia, and pain.[5] Chronic pain may be neuropathic or non-neuropathic.

Fibromyalgia

Fibromyalgia is a non-articular form of rheumatism wherein patients complain of chronic generalized musculoskeletal aching and stiffness, sleep disturbances, fatigue, and exaggerated tenderness called 'tender points'. It is now thought to be a disturbance of endogenous pain control mechanisms leading to increased sensory perception. It is associated with irritable bladder syndrome, irritable bowel syndrome, and depression. More females than males suffer from fibromyalgia and, indeed, increased tenderness has been demonstrated in the postmenstrual phase of the cycle in normally cycling women. There is an association with other rheumatic and systemic illnesses and there may be a linkage of fibromyalgia to the HLA region. Laboratory tests on serum may show disturbances of hormonal function as well as altered peptide levels in the CSF. Treatment is difficult, but there is limited evidence that antidepressant, cognitive behavioural therapy, exercise therapy, and acupuncture are effective.[8, 9]

Myofascial pain syndrome

The generalized musculoskeletal aching and stiffness of fibromyalgia is different from the myofascial pain syndrome in that in the latter the pain is much more localized to distinct muscle groups. These muscle groups such as shoulder muscles have trigger points that produce predictable pain that varies from a slight discomfort to severe unrelenting pain and is either sharp or dull. The mechanism is thought to be that trauma, fatigue, or stress initiate a physiological response and a particular trigger point sends nociceptive signals to the CNS. Muscles of the trigger point become tense, then fatigued, and eventually ischaemic. Inflammatory mediators are released and there may be sympathetic activity leading to increased pain. Each muscle has a distinctive myofascial pain syndrome with its own referred pain pattern specific for the trigger points in that muscle. Travell and Simons have mapped these trigger points and their referred pain patterns. When examining the patient, the trigger point is felt as a taut band of fibres under the tip of the finger.[10]

Maintenance of chronic pain

This section will look at where the pain pathways described previously malfunction and how this can maintain a state of chronic pain. The persistence of pain may be a result of plastic changes within the nervous system both in the periphery and centrally within the spinal cord, with or without the persistence of the original stimulus.

Peripheral sensitization

Denervated peripheral tissue such as skin does not sit passively and await reinnervation, but actively responds to the lack of electrical and chemical communication by inducing and directing the regenerative efforts of injured and collateral axons to regain appropriate connectivity with the CNS (Colburn and Munglani, unpublished observations). The result of a chronic pain stimulus is peripheral sensitization such that there may be increased nociceptive input via the peripheral nervous system. This sensitization is brought about as follows.

Inflammatory 'soup'

When a stimulus is repeated, nociceptors exhibit sensitization such that there is a reduction in the threshold for activation, an increase in the response to a given stimulus, or the appearance of spontaneous activity. This is caused by the release of inflammatory mediators such as K^+, H^+, serotonin, bradykinin, substance P, histamine, cytokines, nitric oxide, leukotrienes, thromboxanes, and prostaglandins. These chemicals sensitize high-threshold nociceptors such that their threshold for response in lowered and a heightened response to noxious stimulation occurs. This produces a zone of 'primary hyperalgesia' surrounding the injury that is commonly observed following surgery or other forms of trauma.[2]

Silent nociceptors

This group of nociceptors cannot normally be activated and only become excitable under pathological conditions such as inflammation. They have been identified in joints, viscera, and cutaneous tissue.[2, 11]

Abnormal Na^+ channels

It is now known that dorsal root neurons express at least six types of Na^+ channel.[6] Nerve injury may cause the expression of abnormally excitable Na^+ channels at the site of injury and in the dorsal root ganglia. All normal sensory neurons have Na^+ channels that are sensitive to tetrodotoxin, a potent puffer fish toxin. There are tetrodotoxin-insensitive Na^+ channels found only on nociceptor sensory neurons that have much slower activation and inactivation kinetics. After nerve injury, both types of Na^+ channels accumulate in the axon and cell body of injured sensory neurons. Both injured and uninjured sensory neurons may then develop ectopic discharges, particularly the tetrodotoxin-insensitive Na^+ channels.[2, 5] It has also been predicted that K^+ channels may have a role to play, in that a reduction of K^+ channel density after nerve injury could contribute to sensory neuron hyperexcitability.[6]

Sympathetic nervous system

There is evidence that neurons of the sympathetic nervous system may release products of arachidonic acid metabolism after peripheral injury. This may provide a link between the peripheral sympathetic efferent and the peripheral nociceptor that is important in sympathetically mediated pain states such as chronic regional pain syndrome (CRPS).

In addition, injured and uninjured axons may begin to express α-adrenoreceptors, which renders them sensitive to catecholamines. There is evidence that the sensitivity of nociceptors can be increased by the release of catecholamines from the adrenal gland in response to sympathetic nervous system activity.[6]

Peripheral nerve lesions have another effect on the sympathetic nervous system in that they cause a massive sprouting response and invasion of the dorsal root ganglion by sympathetic fibres. There is build up of basket formations around cell bodies of dorsal root ganglion neurons, and it is thought that this is a basis for sympathetic–sensory coupling. More work is needed in this field, but it is clear that the baskets are usually found around large sensory neurons—what is not clear is whether the mechanism is actually responsible for excitatory responses in the dorsal root ganglion following low-frequency sympathetic stimulation.[6]

Nerve growth factor

Nerve growth factor (NGF) has recently been shown to have a central role in the aetiology of inflammatory pain. NGF belongs to the family of neurotropic peptides that specify the phenotypic development of central and peripheral neurons. NGF is expressed constitutively at low levels, and it may have a role in determining nociceptor phenotype. However, inflammation is associated with increased NGF expression and synthesis in peripheral tissues. There is rapid onset of hyperalgesia following subcutaneous administration of NGF and this strongly suggests a direct peripheral action mediating peripheral sensitization. It may also be possible that NGF mediates upregulation of various types of Na^+ channel including the tetrodotoxin-insensitive type mentioned earlier.[2]

Muscle

As discussed earlier, myofascial pain syndromes can lead to nociceptive inputs into the CNS and peripheral sensitization.

Central sensitization

Peripheral sensitization and primary hyperalgesia occur in the periphery following trauma. This sensitization only partly explains the overall changes that occur in the periphery—there is a centrally mediated component as well. Centrally mediated sensitization is associated with the following features.[5]

1. Enlargement of the receptive field size so that a spinal neuron responds to stimuli outside the region of cutaneous innervation that responds to nociceptive stimuli in the non-sensitized state.

2. There is an increase in the magnitude and duration of the response to stimuli that are above threshold in strength. This gives rise to 'secondary hyperalgesia', which is a heightened response to noxious stimulation that is centrally mediated.

3. There is a reduction in threshold such that stimuli that are non-noxious activate neurons that normally transmit nociceptive information. This gives rise to 'allodynia', which is the interpretation of previously innocuous sensation as if it were noxious.

There are various proposed mechanisms by which central sensitization occurs.

Wind up

Low-frequency (0.1 Hz) C fibre afferent input gives a constant response from the dorsal horn neurons. However, stimulation frequencies of 0.5 Hz or above cause a large increase in the response of the dorsal horn neuron. This frequency-dependent phenomenon is called 'wind up' and may play a role in some chronic pain conditions such as neuralgias. One problem, however, is that this increased responsiveness of dorsal horn neurons only persists for 5 minutes after the initial stimulus and therefore is not a long-term feature.[3]

Long-term potentiation (LTP) is a process in the brain that is involved in memory formation. It is the strengthening of the efficacy of synaptic transmission that occurs following activity across that synapse. LTP has been demonstrated in the dorsal horn neurons, and therefore 'memory traces' within the spinal cord are talked of. Whether LTP is of sufficient duration to maintain central sensitization independent of peripheral stimuli long enough to cause chronic pain is unclear.[2, 3]

Glutamate and the NMDA receptor

The glutamate/NMDA system is one of the key systems involved in central sensitization. The NMDA receptor can cause longlasting depolarizaton that lowers the threshold for other subsequent low-intensity stimuli, and it is thought that this is part of the mechanism responsible for wind up and LTP. NMDA receptor activation would also explain the expansion of the receptive fields of wide dynamic range (WDR) neurons, with the clinical consequence of pain radiation and temporal summation of pain.[3]

GABA

Small GABAergic inhibitory interneurons are particularly susceptible to neuronal and glial death for periods long after the initial injury. This may occur by programmed mechanisms involving protein synthesis (apoptosis). The result is a net loss of inhibitory tone within the dorsal horn after nerve injury.[2, 11]

Nitric oxide

As previously described, NO production is linked to NMDA receptor activation and as such can cause hyperalgesia. Other NMDA-mediated phenomena such as wind up have been shown to be critically dependent on NO production. NOS inhibition reduces the hyperalgesia seen in established pain states.[3]

Prostaglandins

Since NMDA receptors can activate phospholipase A_2, prostaglandins are produced in the spinal cord during inflammatory pain states. This has the effect of sensitizing nerve terminals to substances such as bradykinin.[11]

Neuropeptides

Nociception can cause substance P, neurokinin A, and CGRP release in the dorsal horn—these may be co-released with glutamate. All three neuropeptides may have presynaptic actions, causing increased glutamate release as well as perhaps acting as co-agonists on the NMDA receptor. CGRP has also been shown to inhibit substance P breakdown by endopeptidase, thereby synergistically enhancing the effect of substance P upon glutamate-induced depolarization. In inflammatory pain states, the increased levels of substance P and CGRP at both the peripheral and central terminals of primary afferent fibres may be controlled by the increased production of neurotrophins such as NGF. In contrast to the raised levels of substance P and CGRP in the dorsal horn in inflammatory pain states, there are decreases in levels of these peptides after nerve injury. Vasoactive intestinal peptide (VIP) levels, however, increase after nerve injury, and it has been suggested that VIP takes over the excitatory role of substance P in these situations. Other neuropeptides such as cholecystokinin, galanin, and neuropeptide Y (NPY) also rise in response to nerve injury, the latter two having an analgesic role.[3]

Neuronal sprouting and synaptic rewiring

When an injured sensory neuron sustains a lesion to its central axonal process (dorsal root), there is degeneration of the associated central axon and terminal connections. Associated spinal interneurons may also degenerate. The normal pattern of incoming electrical signals is replaced by either a barrage of signals, ectopic noise, or quiescence. These electrical changes coupled with glial cell activation provoke compensatory responses within the spinal dorsal horn, some of which may exacerbate the sensory malfunction (Colburn and Munglani, unpublished observations). There is sprouting of $A\beta$ fibres in lamina III of the dorsal horn into lamina II resulting in a reorganization of the normal synaptic architecture. This may give rise to the formation of inappropriate synapses that may allow the low-threshold afferent input to be interpreted as nociceptive input by the spinal cord. This will allow mechanical allodynia. Furthermore, there is a suggestion that there may be sprouting of neurons from the superficial layers to deeper ones, causing the loss of the $A\beta$ inhibitory control from the deeper layers[2, 3, 5].

A fibre phenotype switching

Substance P and CGRP are usually expressed by afferent C and $A\delta$ fibres. However, after peripheral nerve injury, the expression of these neuropeptides by these neurons is downregulated, only to be expressed by large $A\beta$ fibres instead. This phenotypic switching means that low-threshold stimuli cause release of substance P in the dorsal horn and therefore allow central sensitization.

Cytokines

CNS glial cells (microglia, astrocytes, and oligodendrocytes) were once thought of as merely a physical support system for neurons. They have more recently come to be appreciated as key neuromodulatory, neurotrophic, and neuroimmune elements in the CNS. When a neuron is injured, adjacent glial cells are stimulated to mount a dramatic neuroimmunological response, including glial cell hypertrophy, proliferation, and the release of inflammatory cytokines, adhesion molecules, chemokines, and factors from the complement cascade. The main cytokines involved are interleukin-1β (IL-1β), tumour necrosis factor-α (TNFα), and interleukin-6 (IL-6). TNFα has three main functions: it directly excites neurones through an ill-defined mechanism; it amplifies local inflammatory cascades resulting in the release of prostaglandins, bradykinin, histamine, and NGF; and it induces other cytokines such as IL-1β and IL-6. The end result is, once again, augmentation of neuronal excitability (Colburn and Munglani, unpublished observations).

Glia also provide neurotrophic support for regenerating neurons and play a critical role in the synaptic remodelling that occurs following neuronal loss (Colburn and Munglani, unpublished observations).

Opioid insensitivity

Nerve injury induces a number of changes that diminish the action of opioids. It causes a loss of opioid receptors, a reduction in sensitivity to opioids, and the *de novo* production of cholecystokinin, which antagonizes the actions of opioids. This reduction in opioid sensitivity may apply to both endogenously produced and exogenously administered opioids. It has been shown that activation of NMDA receptors causes tolerance to develop at the opioid receptor. Opioids do have some effect in chronic pain, but it is likely to be mediated in the brain rather than spinally.[2, 3, 11]

Descending pathway changes

It was mentioned earlier that the central descending pathways can be facilitatory as well as inhibitory, with a background inhibitory effect overall. After injury, both inhibitory and facilitatory pathways concurrently activate, and the interaction between these pathways will dictate the development of spinal hyperexcitability and hyperalgesia. The dynamic plasticity of descending pathways may sometimes render the system vulnerable and lead to pathological consequences.[6]

Immediate early genes

Immediate early genes were originally described as a class of genes rapidly and transiently expressed in cells stimulated with growth factors without the requirement for *de novo* protein synthesis. Examples such as c-*fos* and c-*jun* have been shown to be transcription factors and are expressed in the CNS following specific types of stimulation. The proteins Fos and Jun effect the transcription of other genes. It has been shown that Fos is expressed postsynaptically in dorsal horn neurons following noxious stimulation. The protein product appears within 1–2 hours poststimulation and then tends to decline rapidly. Fos-positive neurons are restricted to laminae I, II, and V, that is, the laminae that receive the nociceptive primary afferents. However, another peak of Fos expression occurs at 8–16 hours within the deep layers (V, VI, VII, and X) independently of any further inputs from the afferents. It has been shown that even if a peripheral nerve injury has resolved, the changes associated with it in the spinal cord in expression of c-*fos* may continue to persist. The amount of protein product of the c-*fos* gene in the spinal cord seems to correlate with the magnitude of the initial stimulus yet also mediates some of the adaptive responses of the spinal cord. These responses may include the activation of analgesic opioids such as dynorphin.[3, 11]

Treatment of chronic pain

It is now generally accepted that the management of chronic pain needs an interdisciplinary approach. The patient should receive comprehensive rehabilitation that includes multiple therapies provided in a coordinated manner. This section will therefore describe the various treatment modalities in turn, covering pharmacological and non-pharmacological therapies, interventional and implantable treatments, behavioural/cognitive treatments, and pre-emptive therapy. Where possible, the treatment will be related to the underlying neurobiological mechanism. Some of these will not be covered in detail as they are covered more thoroughly elsewhere in the book.

Pharmacological therapies

Nonsteroidal anti-inflammatory drugs (NSAIDS)

Most NSAIDS inhibit the synthesis of prostaglandins and thromboxane by inhibition of the enzymes cyclo-oxygenase (COX) 1 and 2.

COX 1 is the constitutive form that has a role in the normal homeostasis of renal and hepatic tissue, and COX 2 is induced in inflammatory states. Various new COX 2-specific inhibitors are available that may reduce the side-effects due to COX 1 inhibition, such as gastrointestinal irritation and ulceration, inhibition of platelet aggregation, renal dysfunction, and hepatic damage.[2, 3, 7, 12] NSAIDS clearly have a role in chronic pain systemically, and it has also been shown that intrathecal indomethacin and other NSAIDS suppress hyperalgesia in inflammatory pain states.[3, 6, 13, 14]

Opioids

Although controversial, regular use of low-dose, long-acting opioids can effectively control chronic pain in selected patients. Some generalities about opioid utility are known: for example, they seem to work better for inflammatory pain than for neuropathic pain.[15] Their side-effect profile can be a problem as well as tolerance and addiction, which need careful monitoring to avoid.[3] In some patients, there is a reduction in the efficacy of opioid drugs for reasons already discussed and therefore their use is quite limited. Animal studies have suggested that administration of an NMDA antagonist can prevent both development of tolerance to morphine and the withdrawal syndrome.[2, 3] The combination of opioid and NMDA antagonist has been shown to be synergistic in preventing wind up, and therefore the NMDA antagonist can reverse opioid insensitivity. The site of action of the NMDA antagonist has been shown to be the spinal cord rather than the brain.[3]

Antidepressants

Antidepressants are widely used to treat symptoms other than depression such as neuropathic pain, atypical facial pain, fibromyalgia, temperomandibular joint dysfunction, and irritable bowel syndrome. Even though no antidepressant is licensed for such use, trials have shown that tricyclic antidepressants (TCAs) are effective for several of these conditions. The median effective dose is 75 mg, which is lower than that for treating depression. They are used either instead of or in addition to conventional analgesics when the latter are unsuccessful or intolerable.[16] It has been thought that the TCAs work in the chronic pain setting by facilitating the descending inhibitory spinal pathways by blocking serotonin and noradrenaline reuptake. However, TCAs have also been shown to be potent Na^+ channel blockers, NMDA receptor blockers, and also sympatholytic agents. Newer non-TCA antidepressants have been less effective than TCAs at reducing chronic pain, possibly because of some of them being more specific inhibitors of serotonin reuptake. Clinical trials of newer non-TCAs that affect both serotonin and noradrenaline reuptake are needed.[6]

Anticonvulsants

Anticonvulsants have an established role in the treatment of chronic neuropathic pain, and there was a dogma that burning pain should be treated with antidepressants and shooting pain with anticonvulsants—this has been since disproved.[16] Anticonvulsants are a broad category of drugs tied together only by their ability to suppress epileptic seizures. They differ in their mechanism of action with some acting by blocking Na^+ channels, others directly or indirectly by inhibiting release of excitatory amino acids, some by blocking neuronal Ca^+ channels, and others by augmenting inhibitory CNS pathways by increasing GABAergic transmission.[6]

Carbamazepine, phenytoin, and lamotrigine work by suppressing the abnormal ectopic Na^+ channel activity described earlier, and they work at concentrations two to three orders of magnitude lower than those required to block normal impulse propagation.[6] Lamotrigine also inhibits excessive central release of glutamate and aspartate.[6, 12]

Gabapentin was developed to be an analogue of the neurotransmitter GABA, but has since been shown to not interact at either $GABA_A$ or $GABA_B$ receptors. Its mechanism is unclear, although postulated ideas include increasing GABA release from nerve terminals, enzyme effects, or decreased GABA breakdown. Gabapentin has quickly become popular with physicians, mainly because of reasonable efficacy, fewer interactions with other drugs, and fewer side-effects.[6, 12]

Valproate is structurally unrelated to any of the other anticonvulsants and is thought to act by increasing GABAergic neurotransmission, increasing brain GABA, and altering brain levels of excitatory amino acids.[6]

Antiarrhythmics

Intravenous administration of local anaesthetic agents such as lignocaine can result in a marked reduction in pain following peripheral nerve injury. Relatively low concentrations of local anaesthetic can reduce ectopic activity in specific populations of Na^+ channels in damaged nerves at concentrations below those required to produce conduction block at classical tetrodotoxin-sensitive Na^+ channels.[2] Whilst lignocaine has the ability to block primary afferent fibre discharge, it is also thought to have a central effect by some investigators.[6] Oral congeners of local anaesthetics such as mexilitine or flecainide are more commonly used for long-term analgesia in neuropathic pain, usually following an improvement in symptoms with an intravenous lignocaine infusion.[2]

NMDA antagonists

Controlled clinical trials in healthy volunteers show that NMDA receptor antagonists inhibit experimentally induced pain, including secondary hyperalgesia, allodynia, and temporal summation. Currently available examples include ketamine, dextromethorphan, and amantadine, all of which have side-effects, particularly ketamine with its psychic disturbances.[6] As mentioned above, NMDA antagonists act synergistically with opioids to reduce chronic pain.

Clonidine

The α_2 agonist clonidine is analgesic when administered epidurally or intrathecally in CRPS states that are opioid-insensitive. It inhibits primary afferent neurotransmitter release and second-order neuronal depolarization.[2]

GABA agonists

Baclofen is an agonist at the $GABA_B$ receptor and has been used in settings where the pain is due to muscle spasm.[17] Its antispastic effects are peripherally mediated. Attempts at producing centrally acting $GABA_A$ agonists have given mixed results, although gabapentin, albeit not a true GABA analogue, has been successful.

Guanethidine

This inhibits the release of noradrenaline from peripheral adrenergic neurons and therefore impairs the sympathetic response to stimulation.[17] It is used in sympathetically mediated pain states via Bier's block. Does it work by inhibiting catecholamine action on α_2 adrenoceptors expressed abnormally on primary afferent nociceptors?

Capsaicin

Capsaicin is found in hot pepper and can be administered as an ointment in postherpetic neuralgia and painful diabetic neuropathy. It acts by antagonizing the actions of neuropeptides involved with peripheral sensitization.[12] It causes a local burning sensation when applied topically that lasts for 3–4 weeks. This is probably due to substance P release.[6] Once the burning sensation has ceased, the efficacy of the treatment usually becomes evident.[12]

Transdermal fentanyl

Due to its high lipid solubility, fentanyl has been successfully used in the treatment of cancer pain. However, its use in non-malignant pain is controversial, although there are suggestions that it may be useful in patients with low back pain who are already taking oral morphine.[12]

Other drugs

Cannabinoids

The recent cloning of the CB1 cannabinoid receptor and its localization in central and peripheral tissues involved in nociceptive processing has suggested a probable role for endogenous cannabinoids in pain modulation. Cannabinoids in the brain, spinal cord, and peripheral tissues modulate the release of neurotransmitters such as acetylcholine, noradrenaline, dopamine, GABA, and aspartate. Animal models have shown anti-nociceptive activity in acute, inflammatory, and neuropathic pain. Developing clinical trials to assess the effects of cannabinoids is more difficult due to lack of standardized plant material and drug delivery systems.[6]

Adenosine

Human studies have shown a reduction in the area of dynamic tactile allodynia in patients with peripheral neuropathic pain following intravenous infusion of adenosine. There was also subjective global improvement of the clinical pain condition. As previously described, the anti-nociceptive effects of adenosine may be mediated primarily via adenosine A1 receptors in the dorsal horn.[6]

Substance P antagonists

Substance P, acting via neurokinin NK 1 receptors, plays an important role in pain transmission in animals. However, NK 1 receptor antagonists have been surprisingly poor in human studies at producing pain relief. This has raised concerns as to the general relevance of animal assays and their ability to predict clinical analgesic efficacy.[6]

Neuroimmune manipulation

Areas of interest include manipulating microglia, astrocytes, and the cytokines. Current research is examining ways of targeting microglia and astrocytes to prevent their activation. Functional antagonism of inflammatory cytokines has been achieved by either administering agents that bind them (for example TNF-bp) or applying neutralizing antibodies. Stimulating endogenous production of antibodies directed against inflammatory cytokines (IL-6) has been achieved using the superantigenic Sant-1 molecule. A further method is the enhancement of so-called anti-inflammatory cytokines such as interleukins-4 and -10, and transforming growth factor beta (TGF-β). These cytokines suppress the expression of TNFα and IL-1β, and can reduce the hyperalgesia associated with the latter's injection (Colburn and Munglani, unpublished observations).

Botulinum toxin

Botulinum toxin A is one of eight subtypes of a potent biological toxin produced by *Clostridium botulinum*. It weakens skeletal muscle by blocking calcium-mediated release of acetylcholine from motor nerve endings—the effect is mainly on α-motor neurons although it may also affect χ-motor neurons in the muscle spindles resulting in lower muscle resting tone. Botulinum toxin A has been shown to be effective in the treatment of blepharospasm, strabismus, hemifacial spasm, spasmodic torticollis, oromandibular dystonia, and spasmodic dysphonia.[18]

There is emerging evidence that botulinum toxin may relieve the pain associated with myofascial pain syndromes such as whiplash injuries. The basis for this action is speculative, although it is possible that by relaxing muscles in a spastic state the toxin may indirectly reduce peripheral stimuli into the CNS. This would alter neuropeptide and inflammatory modulator release and therefore reduce central sensitization of the spinal cord. The toxin is injected at the tender muscle trigger points.[18, 19]

Other areas

As the understanding of chronic pain mechanisms increases, the potential for further sites of interruption of the pathways increases. Thus areas that are being examined include: bradykinin B_1 and B_2 antagonists; NGF inhibitors; NOS inhibitors; selective Na^+ channel blockers; neuropeptide Y, galanin, and somatostatin analogues; VIP and cholecystokinin antagonists; antisense oligonucleotide to c-*fos*.[3, 11]

Interventional treatments

Central sensitization, once initiated, may be maintained by further input from the periphery. This input may be from damaged nerves or from surrounding undamaged nerves. It has been shown clinically that peripheral blocks could bring about general decreases in pain perception over large areas of the body. These findings suggest that peripheral nerve activity entering the spinal cord will continue to maintain central sensitization and they have implications as to why nerve denervation procedures may work in so many patients, regardless of whether the nerve traffic is abnormal or not. However, what is even more interesting is the prolonged action of these nerve blocks, outlasting the known action of the local anaesthetic. Nerve blockade, as performed in many chronic pain clinics, may play a helpful role by producing a global reduction in nerve traffic into the spinal cord, allowing the system to 'wind down' again. In addition, the administration of epidural steroids, NMDA antagonists, and α_2 agonists, for example, helps to antagonize the actions of upregulated spinal cord second messengers and therefore reduce central sensitization.[11]

Areas targeted include somatic nerves (facet and sacroiliac joints, dorsal roots), sympathetic nerves (stellate, lumbar, coeliac plexus), and axial blocks such as by epidural local anaesthetic. An alternative approach to the problem of intractable back pain is not to concentrate on the source of the pain but the consequences, such as muscle spasm. Intramuscular stimulation (IMS, a modified form of acupuncture) is said to desensitize muscles so that they tend not to go into spasm so easily. It has been shown to produce long-lasting reductions in pain scores in back pain patients and may be useful in treating whiplash-associated pain.[11, 20] Hence targeting these trigger points can reduce myofascial pain.

Implantable technologies

When other therapies have failed, the next step to consider is implantable treatments. These consists of two main areas—epidural and intrathecal drug delivery systems and dorsal column stimulators. Both methods require surgical implantation and therefore carry extra risks.[7]

Epidural and intrathecal drug delivery

This method has been effective in the treatment of both cancer and chronic pain. A pre-implantation trial should be carried out first to assess whether the patient will respond to the implanted device. The usual agent administered is morphine, although baclofen has also been used. The intrathecal/epidural catheter is tunnelled subcutaneously and connected to the pump which is usually sited anteriorly. The pump reservoir will require intermittent refilling which is done directly through the skin.[7, 17]

Spinal cord stimulation

Spinal cord stimulation is used widely throughout Europe for treating peripheral vascular disease and ischaemic pain. It is also used in neuropathic pain, sympathetically mediated pain, and radicular low back pain. Spinal cord stimulation is performed either percutaneously using a wire electrode threaded into the epidural space and fed cranially or by laminectomy to suture a plate electrode to the dura. A trial will show whether appropriate paraesthesia can be achieved in a particular patient and indicate the optimal placement. Though originally inspired by the gate theory of pain, and developed to block the propagation of painful nerve impulses, spinal cord stimulation is now linked to many other mechanisms. It activates GABAergic (and possibly adenosine) inhibitory pathways and may work at a cerebral level.[7, 12, 21]

Pre-emptive therapy

Pre-emptive analgesia is an anti-nociceptive treatment that prevents establishment of altered central processing of afferent input and therefore prevents postoperative hyperalgesia. There is evidence that severe postoperative pain may be a significant predictor of long-term pain and that steps that reduce or abolish noxious input to the spinal cord during surgery may reduce spinal cord changes and therefore chronic pain. However, what duration or degree of noxious input is required before these long-term changes occur remains unclear—central sensitization caused by noxious stimulation is a complex phenomenon. The sensitization may fade rapidly or very slowly, or even become permanent. Surgery-induced central sensitization has two phases: incisional and inflammatory. The former may be brief, whereas the latter could play the dominant role in central sensitization.[2, 6]

Much of the focus of pre-emptive analgesia has been on reducing acute pain in the early postoperative period, although it may also be important in reducing chronic pain. The study that generated most interest was the finding that preoperative epidural blockade of patients undergoing lower limb amputation resulted in a lower incidence of phantom limb pain at 6 and 12 months postsurgery. Unfortunately, this has not been replicated by subsequent studies, and other studies looking at pre-emptive analgesia in general have been both positive and negative. Research has examined the effects of local anaesthetics, opioids, and NSAIDS given locally, epidurally, intrathecally, or systemically on postoperative pain. Studies have also looked at the effects of pre-emptive anaesthetic agents such as isoflurane on central sensitization (for example by measuring immediate early gene expression such as that of c-*fos*): these suggest that noxious stimulation still enters the spinal cord during seemingly adequate anaesthesia and therefore it

is not surprising that clinical studies show such a small effect of pre-emptive analgesia. It has been demonstrated previously that radically different outcomes in terms of long-term pain behaviour and spinal cord changes can be produced experimentally with different adjuncts to isoflurane anaesthesia such as α_2 agonists, NMDA antagonists, and peripheral blocks with local anaesthetic.[6, 11, 14]

There are therefore two areas that need to be addressed in clinical trials to attempt to show unequivocal benefits of pre-emptive analgesia. The first concerns the misleading nature of the term pre-emptive analgesia. This implies that giving a therapy before incision reduces postoperative pain as compared to giving it after incision. However, emphasis should be placed not on the timing of treatment initiation but on the central sensitization it is trying to prevent. Expanding this further, one may wish to state whether there is prevention of central sensitization caused by incisional or inflammatory injuries. The second area is that 'pre-emptive' therapy should continue long enough to effectively suppress the afferent input and prevent the reappearance of central sensitization after some time.[6, 11]

Non-pharmacological therapies

It is becoming increasing obvious that the complementary–conventional boundaries are beginning to blur in actual clinical practice. What might have been considered an alternative treatment for pain in the past (e.g. psychotherapy, acupuncture, hypnotherapy) may now be considered part of informed, responsible practice. Other examples of non-pharmacological therapies include transcutaneous electrical nerve stimulation (TENS), dietary prescription, chiropractice, meditation, prayer, and spiritual direction, herbal/botanical medicine, t'ai chi, art therapy, homeopathy, and aromatherapy.[22] TENS produces analgesia in a wide range of medical conditions, but its usefulness is questioned by recent studies. It probably works by increasing inhibitory inputs into the spinal cord.[17]

Behavioural/cognitive therapies

The lifetime prevalence rates for any psychiatric condition are far greater for patients with one or more medical conditions than for those patients without medical conditions. Chronic pain patients consider themselves to suffer from a physical illness for which physicians cannot seem to develop a cure. This physical illness is associated with significant impairment and disability that has tremendous impact on the patient's life. Because often no apparent tissue damage can be found to explain the cause of chronic pain, physicians frequently attribute the chronic pain patient's pain to underlying psychiatric illness.[23]

Once pain is experienced by someone, the impact may be displayed externally in the form of pain behaviour and internally in terms of the subjective experience of suffering. Pain behaviours are overt expressions that communicate pain and distress to others. They include simple verbal or motor behaviours such as limping and grimacing, or they can be higher-order behavioural patterns such as taking medication or seeking medical help. Some patients acquire and maintain pain behaviours because of the environmental contingencies that provide reinforcement for such behaviours—for example, limping may elicit more attention from family members. Once such a contingency is established, pain is no longer needed to maintain limping behaviour. Suffering is where one perceives a threat or damage to the integrity of the self, and it can lead to a disparity between what one expects of one's self and what one actually achieves.[24, 25]

Patients with chronic pain are a heterogeneous group, differing in terms of pain severity, emotional distress, and disability. Physical, psychological, and social circumstances contribute to their pain to differing degrees. There are three unique subgroups of pain patients described: dysfunctional patients who report that their pain affects a broad range of functioning; interpersonally distressed patients who perceive their relatives/friends as unsupportive; and adaptive copers who deny significant negative effects of pain. Patients in the dysfunctional group report more pain, display more pain behaviours and medication consumption, spend more time in bed due to pain, demonstrate higher levels of pain-related anxiety, and are more likely to be unemployed compared to the other two subtypes.[26]

Cognitive–behavioural models of chronic pain emphasize the importance of pain-related cognitions and beliefs in chronic pain adjustment. It is possible that certain cognitions and beliefs may be adaptive and help patients cope with the experience of pain, although others may actually contribute to increased pain and affective distress. Cognitions are self-statements that are specific responses to an environmental event. Negative cognitions about pain have repeatedly been shown to predict pain, disability, and distress amongst chronic pain patients; they have also been associated with greater use of health care resources and medication consumption.[27] One other problem with chronic pain is actually assessing whether a treatment has been useful, particularly if a patient is having negative cognitions. It has been shown that verbal reports from the patient reflecting their views on the success of any previous treatments are poor indicators of true changes in chronic pain, partly due to distortions in pain memory. The suggestion is that assessment of treatment success should be based upon the patient's pain measured at the time of consultation or from pain diaries.[28]

In order to help patients cope more effectively with their chronic pain, pain management programmes have been set up. There are different types of programmes, although most use group cognitive behavioural therapy to change patients' attitudes, beliefs, and behaviour in relation to their pain.[12] Active psychological treatments based on the principle of cognitive behavioural therapy have been shown to be effective.[29]

The programme usually includes progressive muscular relaxation therapy, goal setting and pacing, group cognitive therapy, education about the physiology and pharmacology of pain, and progressive supervised physiotherapy exercises. Rather than measuring changes in pain, the groups look for improvements in mood, catastrophizing, physical performance, overall function, and use of drug treatment. In terms of patients returning to work after a pain management programme, the numbers vary between countries, with the United Kingdom having one of the lowest percentages of patients managing to work again. Pain management programmes have been set up and run successfully now in district hospitals and primary health care areas.[12]

References

1. Loeser, J.D. and Melzack, R. (1999). Pain: an overview. *Lancet* **353**, 1607–1609.

2. Siddall, P.J., Hudspith, M.J., and Munglani, R. (2000). Sensory systems and pain. In *Basic and applied science for ànesthesia* (ed. H.C. Hemmings Jr and P.M. Hopkins). Mosby International, London.

3. Munglani, R., Hunt, S.P., and Jones, J.G. (1996). The spinal cord and chronic pain. In *Anaesthesia Review 12* (ed. L. Kaufman and R. Ginsburg), pp. 53–76. Churchill Livingstone, New York.

4. Cervero, F. and Laird, J.M.A. (1999). Visceral pain. *Lancet* **353**, 2145–2148.

5. Woolf, C.J. and Mannion, R.J. (1999). Neuropathic pain: aetiology, symptoms, mechanisms, and management. *Lancet* **353**, 1959–1964.

6. Devor, M., Roubotham, M.C., and Wiesenfeld-Hallin, Z. (eds.) (2000). *Proceedings of the 9th World Congress on Pain, Progress in pain research and management*, Vol. 16. IASP Press, Seattle.

7. Ashburn, M.A. and Staats, P.S. (1999). Management of chronic pain. *Lancet* **353**, 1865–1869.

8. Buskila, D. (2000). Fibromyalgia, chronic fatigue syndrome, and myofascial pain syndrome. *Curr. Opin. Rheumatol.* **12** (2), 113–123.

9. Yunus, M.B., Inanici, F., Aldag, J.C., and Mangold, R.F. (2000). Fibromyalgia in men: comparison of clinical features with women. *J. Rheumatol.* **27** (2), 485–490.

10. Wall, P.D. and Melzack, R. (1984). *Textbook of pain.* Churchill Livingstone, Edinburgh.

11. Munglani, R. (1998). Advances in chronic pain therapy with special reference to low back pain. In *Anaesthesia review 14* (ed. L. Kaufman and R. Ginsburg), 153–174. Churchill Livingstone.

12. Nurmikko, T.J., Nash, T.P., and Wiles, J.R. (1998). Recent advances—control of chronic pain. *Br. Med. J.* **317**, 1438–1441.

13. Besson, J.M. (1999). The neurobiology of pain. *Lancet* **353**, 1610–1615.

14. Carr, D.B. and Leonidas, C.G. (1999). Acute pain. *Lancet* **353**, 2051–2058.

15. Loeser, J.D. (2000). Perils in the pursuit of mechanisms. *Pain* **86**, 1–2.

16. McQuay, H.J. and Moore, R.A. (1997). Antidepressants and chronic pain—effective analgesia in neuropathic pain and other syndromes. *Br. Med. J.* **314**, 763–764.

17. Prithvi Raj, P. (1996). *Pain medicine—a comprehensive review.* Mosby, St Louis.

18. Freund, B.J. and Schwartz, M. (2000). Treatment of whiplash associated with neck pain with Botulinum toxin A: a pilot study. *J. Rheumatol.* **27** (2), 481–484.

19. Diaz, J.H. and Gould, H.J. III. (1999). Management of post-thoracotomy pseudoangina and myofascial pain with botulinum toxin. *Anesthesiology* **91** (3), 877–879.

20. Munglani, R. (2000). Neurobiological mechanisms underlying chronic whiplash associated pain: the peripheral maintenance of central sensitization. *J. Musculoskeletal Pain* **8** (1/2), 169–178.

21. American Society of Anesthesiologists task force on pain management, chronic pain section (1997). Practice guidelines for chronic pain management. *Anesthesiology* **86**, 995–1004.

22. Berman, B.M. and Bausell, R.B. (2000). The use of non-pharmacological therapies by pain specialists. *Pain* **85**, 313–315.

23. Fishbain, D.A. (1999). Approaches to treatment decisions for psychiatric comorbidity in the management of the chronic pain patient. *Med. Clin. N. Am.* **83** (3), 737–760.

24. Turk, D.C. and Okifuji, A. (1999). Assessment of patients' reporting of pain: an integrated perspective. *Lancet* **353**, 1784–1788.

25. Chapman, C.R. and Gavrin, J. (1999). Suffering: the contributions of persistent pain. *Lancet* **353**, 2233–2237.

26. McCracken, L.M., Spertus, I.L., Janeck, A.S., Sinclair, D., and Wetzel, F.T. (1999). Behavioural dimensions of adjustment in persons with chronic pain: pain-related anxiety and acceptance. *Pain* **80**, 283–289.

27. Stroud, M.W., Thorn, B.E., Jensen, M.P., and Boothby, J.L. (2000). The relation between pain beliefs, negative thoughts, and psychosocial functioning in chronic pain patients. *Pain* **84**, 347–352.

28. Feine, J.S., Lavigne, G.J., Thuan Dao, T.T., Morin, C., and Lund, J.P. (1998). Memories of chronic pain and perceptions of relief. *Pain* **77**, 137–141.

29. Morley, S., Eccleston, C., and Williams, A. (1999). Systematic review and meta-analysis of randomized controlled trials of cognitive behaviour therapy and behaviour therapy for chronic pain in adults, excluding headache. *Pain* **80**, 1–13.

3

Biomechanics and locomotion

3.1 Biomechanics

Amy Zavatsky

Introduction

Biomechanics is the application of the principles of mechanics and the techniques of engineering to the study of biological systems, including the human body. From an early date, one of the major areas of biomechanical study has been the musculoskeletal system or locomotor system. Diagnosis and treatment of disorders and diseases of the musculoskeletal system are the main goals of orthopaedics. Practitioners in this field require an understanding of bone, muscle, connective tissue, and nerve. They need to understand how these tissues function and interact on all levels—from genetic and cellular levels to the macroscopic level of the joints and limbs.

There are many reasons why orthopaedic surgeons should make an effort to understand the basics of biomechanics. First, the musculoskeletal system is affected not only by genetic and metabolic factors, but also by mechanical factors.[1] This was recognized over a century ago by Wolff,[2] who studied the adaptation of bone to the forces applied to it. The idea that bone perceives and adapts to its functional demands is widely known today as Wolff's law.

Second, many orthopaedic surgical procedures are based on simple mechanical principles. For example, a 'closing osteotomy'—an operation that can be used to correct deformity or to reduce pain and disability at an arthritic joint—involves first cutting into two parts one of the bones that meets at the affected joint. A wedge of bone is then removed, followed by realignment and healing of the cut bone ends. The resulting redistribution of load at the joint depends critically on the size and shape of the bone removed, and this should be calculated based on mechanical principles before the procedure is attempted.

Third, the design and application of orthopaedic devices and prostheses and of rehabilitation regimes requires a knowledge of the magnitude and frequency of the forces likely to be transmitted by the bones, muscles, and joints during activities of daily living. This also requires an understanding of biomechanics.

Finally, many cases seen by an orthopaedic surgeon involve trauma. To understand the mechanisms of traumatic injury, to know how the tissues will react or ultimately fail, and to develop preventative measures requires the assessment of high-speed impact forces, another topic from the realm of mechanics. So, as shown by these examples, a knowledge of basic biomechanics can only be an asset to anyone involved in orthopaedics and traumatology.

To cover the range of biomechanical applications in orthopaedics would take an entire volume.[3–7] Similarly, to explain and illustrate the principles of engineering mechanics[8, 9] and the techniques of modern engineering would require much space. Indeed, this has been done successfully by others. Instead of duplicating their work, this chapter will explain how loads are transmitted by the bones, muscles, and other soft tissues. In doing so, some basic concepts useful for further study in biomechanics will be introduced.

Loads applied to the body

To find the forces acting in the bones, muscles, and soft tissues of the body, one could attempt to measure them *in vivo*. Direct measurement of forces and strains in living human tissues is not impossible,[10, 11] but it is difficult. In addition, ethical considerations mean that most such measurements are done either in animals or *in vitro*. Regardless of which approach is taken, a detailed understanding of the measurement process itself is needed and also a knowledge of the possible physical, biochemical, and physiological interactions of the measurement device with the tissue being measured.[12]

One alternative to direct measurement of forces is the creation and solution of a mathematical model of the system of interest. The particular body or mechanical system to be analysed is isolated and all the forces or loads that act on it are defined clearly and completely. This isolation of the body of interest is accomplished by means of a 'free-body diagram', which is a diagrammatic representation of the isolated body showing all the forces applied to it by mechanical contact and all body forces, such as those due to gravitational attraction. The construction of the free-body diagram is the single most important step in the solution of problems in mechanics.[8] Only when a clear free-body diagram has been completed should mathematical relationships between the force quantities be written and solved.

Consider the physical situation in Fig. 1(a), which shows a man carrying a briefcase climbing some stairs. The system of interest is the man, and so he is drawn separately as the first step in constructing a free-body diagram (Fig. 1(b)). Then it is necessary to draw as arrows all the forces acting on the man and to specify their magnitudes, directions, and points of application. In the language of mechanics, these forces are known as vectors. A vector is usually written in boldface type ($\mathbf{F}$) or with an arrow over it ($\vec{F}$).

Forces may be either concentrated or distributed. When the area over which the force is applied is small compared with the other dimensions of the body, the force may be considered to be concentrated at a point. These are the types of force acting on the man's

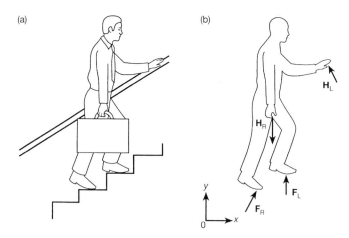

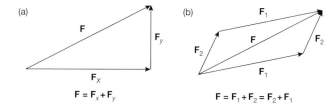

Fig. 3 The parallelogram law of vector addition. (a) perpendicular forces $\mathbf{F}_x$ and $\mathbf{F}_y$ add to give $\mathbf{F}$. (b) Forces $\mathbf{F}_1$ and $\mathbf{F}_2$ add to give $\mathbf{F}_3$. Note that the order of addition is not important: $\mathbf{F}_1 + \mathbf{F}_2 = \mathbf{F}_2 + \mathbf{F}_1 = \mathbf{F}_3$.

Fig. 1 (a) A man climbing stairs. (b) Free-body diagram of a man climbing stairs, excluding the force of body weight.

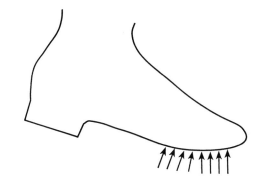

Fig. 2 Distributed forces on the left foot of the man in Fig. 1.

feet (labelled $\mathbf{F}_L$ and $\mathbf{F}_R$ and in Fig. 1(b)) and on the hand which he rests on the handrail (labelled $\mathbf{H}_L$ in Fig. 1(b)). These particular forces are a good example of Newton's third law of mechanics (sometimes known as 'action and reaction'). The man's foot pushes against the stair with a certain force, and the stair pushes back on the foot with a force of the same magnitude and line of action, but in the opposite direction. The forces $\mathbf{F}_L$, $\mathbf{F}_R$, and $\mathbf{H}_L$ all have units of newtons (N) in the SI system.

An arrow (labelled $\mathbf{H}_R$) indicating the downward force due to the weight of the briefcase that the man carries in his right hand must also be drawn on the free-body diagram. The force $\mathbf{H}_R = m_B \mathbf{g}$, where m_B is the mass of the briefcase in kilograms (kg) and $\mathbf{g}$ is the acceleration associated with the gravitational force of attraction (9.81 m/s^2). Note that 1 N = 1 kg m/s^2. Note also that the force $\mathbf{H}_R$ acts downward, towards the centre of the Earth.

Distributed forces are applied over an area, or they may be distributed over a volume. The weight of a body or body segment is the force of gravitational attraction distributed over its volume, but this is usually taken as a concentrated force acting through the centre of gravity of the body or the relevant body segment. The weight of the man (not included in Fig. 1(b)) is equal to the mass of the man m_M (in kg) times $\mathbf{g}$.

If, instead of the whole man, the bones, muscles, and joints of his feet were of interest, the non-uniform distributed forces (Fig. 2), rather than the concentrated forces $\mathbf{F}_L$ and $\mathbf{F}_R$ (Fig. 1(b)), would have to be considered. The distributed forces act over the area of contact

between the man's feet and the stairs. The parts of these forces perpendicular to the soles of the man's shoes can be thought of as pressures; they have units of force per unit area, namely N/m^2 or pascals (Pa). Instrumentation has been designed to measure plantar pressure using either shoe insole devices or special plates set in the floor,[13, 14] but the majority of these devices are limited in that they can only measure pressure in a direction perpendicular to the device itself.

In addition to the forces, pertinent dimensions may also be represented on the free-body diagram. Numerical values for average body segment lengths have been compiled in tables.[15] The study of such physical measurements of the human body is called anthropometry. In biomechanical studies, a wide variety of physical measurements are required, including not only body segment lengths and masses, centres of mass, and moments of inertia, but also locations of muscle origins and insertions, angles of pull of tendons, and lengths and cross-sectional areas of muscles. In the past, most of these measurements were made on cadavers, but now many subject-specific measurements can be made *in vivo* using plane radiography, computerized tomography (CT), or magnetic resonance imaging (MRI).

It is also usual to indicate a set of co-ordinate axes on the free-body diagram. For simplicity, only two dimensions will be considered in this example, and so in Fig. 1(b) the axes x and y have been added. The x-axis points to the right, and the y-axis points upward. If a z-axis were included, it would point out of the page. The origin O of this global co-ordinate system is fixed on the bottom stair.

Note that each force vector in Fig. 1(b) could instead be drawn as the sum of two perpendicular vectors, one parallel to the x-axis and one parallel to the y axis. An example is given in Fig. 3(a), in which $\mathbf{F} = \mathbf{F}_x + \mathbf{F}_y$. The absolute values of the two perpendicular vectors ($|\mathbf{F}_x| = F_x$ and $|\mathbf{F}_y| = F_y$) are known as the 'components' of the vector $\mathbf{F}$. The graphical construction in Fig. 3(a) is an example of the 'parallelogram law of vector addition', in which the resultant of two vectors is found by drawing each vector to scale and arranging them tip to tail. The resultant then connects the tail of the first vector drawn to the tip of the last vector drawn. The vectors to be added need not necessarily be parallel, nor does it matter in which order they are drawn (Fig. 3(b)).

External loads applied to the body can often be measured accurately using force transducers, which give an electrical signal proportional to the applied force. Excluding the gravitational force, the most common external force acting on the body is the ground reaction force ($\mathbf{F}_L$ or $\mathbf{F}_R$ in Fig. 1(b)) that acts on the foot during standing, walking, or running.[15] The device used to measure the ground reaction force is called a force plate or force platform and is an important tool in clinical gait analysis.[16] Most force plates are rectangular in shape, lie flush with the ground, and are supported below ground level at each

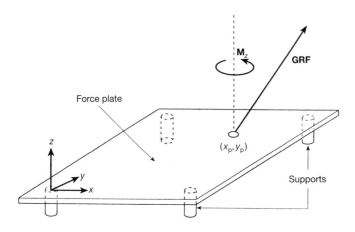

Fig. 4 The force plate. The ground reaction force (**GRF**), the free moment of rotation (**M**$_z$), and the centre of pressure (x_p, y_p) are shown. Note that the axis directions differ from those shown in Fig. 1.

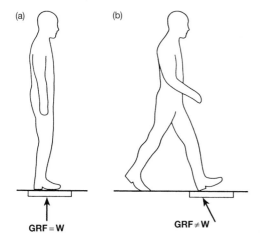

Fig. 5 (a) A static measurement on the force plate. The ground reaction force (**GRF**) equals the man's weight (**W**). (b) A dynamic measurement on the force plate during normal level walking. The ground reaction force (**GRF**) does not equal the man's weight (**W**).

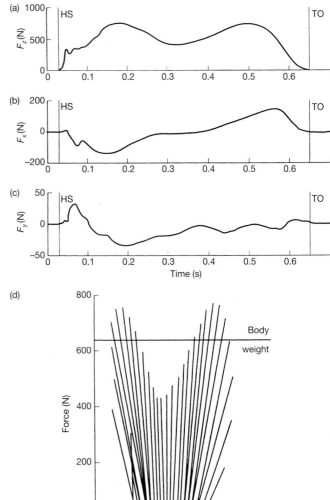

Fig. 6 The ground reaction force during the stance phase of normal gait. (a) The vertical component F_z is positive upward. (b) The fore–aft horizontal component F_x is positive forward. (c) In this case the mediolateral horizontal component F_y is positive laterally. (d) The pattern of ground reaction force vectors as seen in the sagittal plane. HS, heelstrike; TO, toe-off. (Data courtesy of the Oxford Gait Laboratory, Nuffield Orthopaedic Centre NHS Trust, Oxford, UK.)

corner (Fig. 4). Force transducers are mounted on each support in each axis direction (*x, y, z*). Summing the *x, y*, and *z* components of force measured at each corner gives the *x, y*, and *z* components of the ground reaction force. To find the point on the force plate through which the ground reaction force appears to act (the centre of pressure x_p, y_p) and what is called the 'free moment of rotation' about a vertical axis (**M**$_z$), a series of equations must be written and solved.[17] When a person stands perfectly still with both feet on the force plate, the measured ground reaction force will equal the person's body weight (Fig. 5(a)). When a person walks or runs across the force plate, the force measured no longer equals body weight but is an indication of both the mass and the inertia of the body (Fig. 5(b)). Figure 6(a)–(c) shows how the components of the ground reaction force change over time during the stance phase of walking. Figure 6(d) shows a normal pattern of ground reaction force vectors as seen in the sagittal plane;

this plot is known as a Pedotti diagram or a butterfly diagram. In addition to the force plate, instrumentation has been designed to measure the forces applied to the feet during cycling.

Statics versus dynamics

Mechanics deals with bodies either in a state of rest or moving under the action of forces. Statics involves a description of the conditions of force that are both necessary and sufficient to maintain a state of equilibrium. When a body is in equilibrium (either stationary or moving at constant velocity, according to Newton's first law of mechanics), the resultant force and resultant moment acting on it are zero ($\Sigma \mathbf{F} = 0$, $\Sigma \mathbf{M} = 0$).

Moment is the term used to describe the tendency of a force to rotate a body about some axis. The magnitude of a moment **M** is proportional to the magnitude of the force **F** that causes it and to the moment arm d, which is the perpendicular distance from the axis about which rotation occurs to the line of action of the force, or $|\mathbf{M}| = |\mathbf{F}|d$, as shown in Fig. 7(a). The moment produced by two equal and opposite but non-collinear forces (**F** and $-\mathbf{F}$) a distance d apart is known as a couple **C** with magnitude $|\mathbf{F}|d$ (Fig. 7(b)). Notice that the sum of the two forces is zero since they are equal and opposite. There is no tendency for the forces to translate the body, but they do tend to rotate it. Moments and couples are vectors, and their directions are given by the 'right-hand rule' (Fig. 8).

To check whether the sum of the forces acting on a body is zero, the force vectors must be summed either graphically using the 'parallelogram law' (Fig. 3) or algebraically using the force components. In all but the simplest two-dimensional problems, it is more convenient to add the components. This is especially true if a large number of forces is involved and a computer is used to solve any equations. In two dimensions, to check whether the sum of the moments acting on a body is zero, moments about any point must be summed. Clockwise moments must balance counterclockwise moments. In three dimensions, moments about the x-, y-, and z-axes must be considered.

Dynamics is the study of the motion of bodies under the action of force. 'Forward dynamics' is the prediction of motion from known forces, while 'inverse dynamics' is the calculation of forces from known motions. Dynamics involves the tendency of unbalanced forces to translate a body and the tendency of unbalanced moments to rotate a body. From Newton's second law, we know the $\Sigma \mathbf{F} = m\mathbf{a}$, or the acceleration of a particle (or of the centre of mass of a body) is proportional to the resultant force acting on it and is in the direction of

the force. The constant of proportionality is the mass of the particle or body. Note that acceleration, like force, is a vector and has components in the x-, y-, and z-directions. For moments in two dimensions, $\Sigma M_z = I\alpha$ where I is the moment of inertia (or tendency of the body to resist rotation) and α is the angular acceleration. The moment of inertia is usually referred to the centre of mass of the body or segment. An explanation of how it is calculated and how the moment equation changes for three-dimensional motion is beyond the scope of this chapter.[9]

Loads internal to the body

Before finding the forces acting in particular body tissues during activity, it is necessary to quantify the resultant force and moment acting along a limb or at a joint. For static situations, this is relatively easy. A free-body diagram of the body is drawn and an imaginary slice taken through it at the section of interest. This imaginary slice may be through a bone shaft (Fig. 9(a)) or through a joint (Fig. 9(b)). A resultant force **F** and a resultant moment **M** act at this section, and they balance the external loads and segment weights. At a joint these quantities are sometimes called the 'resultant joint force and moment' or the 'intersegmental force and moment'.

The calculated resultant forces and moments at the sections shown in Fig. 9 do not correspond to actual forces and moments, and they cannot be measured with transducers. They are abstract quantities that are often used not as final results but as inputs to a second step—determination of the distribution of these forces and moments among the structures of the body.

In dynamic situations, the calculation of forces and moments within the body is much more difficult since the accelerations of the various body segments must be taken into account. To do this, the body is usually divided up into segments, and the forces, moments, and accelerations of each segment are considered separately. An example of a two-dimensional link-segment model of the lower limb is shown in Fig. 10. The limb is divided into three segments (thigh, shank, foot),

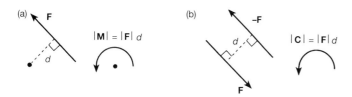

Fig. 7 (a) The Moment **M** of force **F** about a point. The length d is the moment arm of the force **F**. (b) Two equal and opposite but non-collinear forces **F** form the couple **C**.

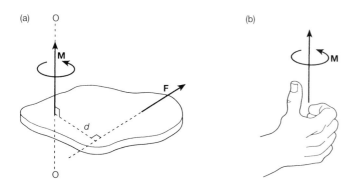

Fig. 8 The 'right-hand rule'. (a and b) The moment **M** of force **F** about O–O is represented as a vector pointing in the direction of the thumb, with the fingers pointing in the direction of the tendency to rotate. (Adapted from reference 8.)

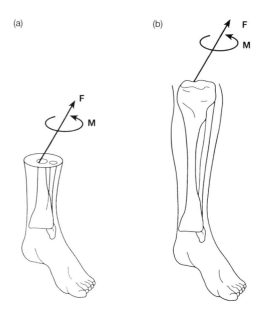

Fig. 9 Resultant force **F** and resultant moment **M** acting at a section (a) through the shank and (b) through the knee. (Adapted from reference 21.)

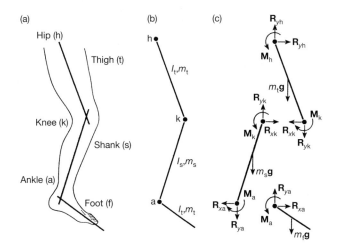

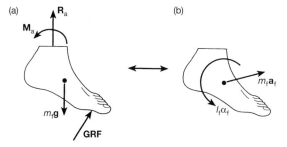

Fig. 11 (a) Free-body diagram and (b) kinetic diagram of the foot during the stance phase of walking.

Fig. 10 (a and b) A sagittal-plane link-segment model of the lower limb. Each link has a mass m_i and a moment of inertia I_i. (c) Free-body diagrams of the three links, each showing the segment weight and the intersegmental forces $\mathbf{F}_i$ and moment $\mathbf{M}_i$. (Adapted from reference 15.)

each with its own mass m_i and moment of inertia I_i (Fig. 10(a)). In this simple model, the links are connected by pins. To draw a free-body of each segment, we disconnect the link-segment model at the joints and draw the resultant force and moment at each joint (Fig. 10(c)). On the foot segment, the resultant joint force $\mathbf{R}_a$ at the ankle has two components, R_{x_a} and R_{y_a}. The resultant joint moment is $\mathbf{M}_a$. On the free-body diagram of the shank segment, $\mathbf{M}_a$ and the components of $\mathbf{R}_a$ are opposite in direction to those drawn on the foot segment. The same is true for the joint reaction force and moment at the knee, as shown on the free-body diagrams of the shank and thigh segments.

In link-segment models of the lower limb, the most distal segment is considered first, followed by the next adjacent segment, moving proximally. Figure 11(a) is a free-body diagram of the foot segment showing all the forces acting on it: the known ground reaction force (GRF), the known segment weight ($m_f\mathbf{g}$), and the unknown joint (ankle) reaction force ($\mathbf{R}_a$) and moment ($\mathbf{M}_a$). Figure 11(b) is a 'kinetic diagram' showing the 'inertial forces' $m_f a_f$ and $I_f \alpha_f$ on the foot. We know from the previous section that, for dynamics in two dimensions $\Sigma\mathbf{F} = m\mathbf{a}$ and $\Sigma M = I\alpha$, so that the diagrams in Figs 11(a) and (b) must be equivalent. When the linear acceleration $\mathbf{a}$ of the centre of mass and the angular acceleration α_f of the foot are known, equations to calculate the unknown joint reaction force components (R_{x_a} and R_{y_a} and the joint reaction moment ($\mathbf{M}_a$) can be written, as will be explained below. Once these are found, the equilibrium of the shank can be considered and, after that, the thigh.

The accelerations needed for a dynamic analysis of a link-segment model can be measured directly using small electronic devices called accelerometers.[22] These are mounted on or strapped to each segment of interest. Three accelerometers mounted at right angles to each other are needed to measure linear accelerations in three dimensions (a_x, a_y, a_z). To quantify the angular accelerations (α_x, α_y, α_z) of a segment, additional accelerometers must be used. The use of accelerometers in biomedical applications is not widespread, possibly because of problems associated with these measurements,[23] such as how to distinguish between the accelerations of the bone and the surrounding soft tissue and how to separate the measured acceleration into its translational, rotational, and gravitational components.

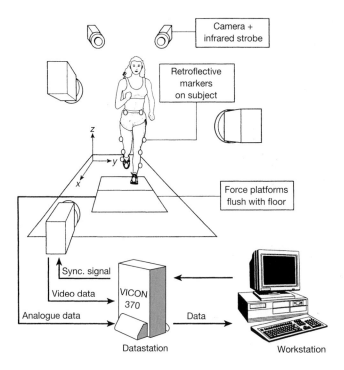

Fig. 12 Schematic diagram of a motion analysis system. (Courtesy of H.S. Gill.)

A second method for finding the accelerations needed for a dynamic analysis of a link-segment model is to measure the sequential positions of each segment and then to differentiate the position data with respect to time, once to obtain segment velocity and twice to obtain segment acceleration. Because measurement errors are magnified in the differentiation process, the position data must first be filtered to remove unwanted noise. Various methods can be used to gather three-dimensional position data. An instrumented spatial linkage,[24, 25] a complex version of the conventional electrogoniometer, can be strapped across a joint to measure the relative positions of the two bones. Magnetic tracking systems[26] are used to measure the position and orientation of a sensor mounted on a segment relative to a magnetic source. Such systems are accurate and easy to use, but it is important to understand the effects that metal in the experimental environment can have on the measurements.

Optoelectronic motion analysis systems (Fig. 12) are also used to collect three-dimensional position data. A minimum of three markers are fixed to each body segment of interest, and the changing positions of the markers are recorded by at least two cameras. Some systems use reflective markers, while others use markers containing light-emitting diodes which flash on and off in sequence. Data are analysed automatically by a computer. A more detailed discussion of motion analysis systems can be found in books on gait analysis.[15, 16, 27]

The problem of indeterminacy

In mechanics, a system is called 'determinate' if the number of equations describing it is the same as the number of unknown quantities (force, position, etc.). When there are more unknown quantities than there are equations, the system is called 'indeterminate' or 'redundant'. In two dimensions, mechanics provides us with three equations: force equilibrium in the x- and y-directions (two equations) and moment equilibrium about an axis perpendicular to the plane of interest (one equation). Therefore with three equations, one can solve for three unknown quantities. In three dimensions, there are six equations: force equilibrium in the x-, y-, and z-directions and moment equilibrium about the x-, y-, and z-axes. Therefore in three dimensions, one can solve for six unknown quantities.

The musculoskeletal system is highly indeterminate. Figure 13 shows as an example a sketch of the knee with its known joint force $\mathbf{F}^k$ and joint moment $\mathbf{M}^k$. Also shown on the drawing are all the unknown forces at the knee: muscle forces $\mathbf{f}^m$, ligament forces $\mathbf{f}^l$ and forces $\mathbf{f}^c$ in the articular cartilage that result from contact between the tibia and the femur. With six equations of equilibrium, it is possible to solve for

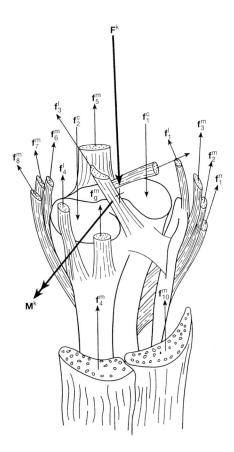

Fig. 13 The indeterminate force system at the knee. Superscripts: k, knee; l, ligament; m, muscle; a, articular cartilage. (Reproduced from reference 28.)

six unknown quantities. The problem is that there are far more than six unknown forces in Fig. 13—the forces cannot be found using the equations of equilibrium alone. In biomechanics, much effort has gone into trying to solve this 'problem of indeterminacy'. Methods involve either increasing the number of equations or decreasing the number of unknowns.

Structures that carry load

In the fields of orthopaedics and traumatology, there is interest in the forces in the bones, muscles, tendons, ligaments, and articular cartilage. These are the tissues that must provide the internal forces and moments discussed above. Muscles produce force and are therefore thought of as 'active' tissues. Bones, tendons, ligaments, and articular cartilage are 'passive' structures, since they take up load only as needed to balance the external, inertial, and muscle forces and moments. Understanding how these tissues produce or carry load can help in calculating the forces within them. For example, knowing that muscles can 'pull' but not 'push', and that ligaments can resist tension but not compression, allows one to reduce the number of unknowns in the indeterminate problem. Theoretical models of the individual tissues can also be formulated. The level of detail required in a model depends, of course, on its final application.

Muscle

As an 'active' tissue, a muscle generates force as a result of neural stimulation. The amount of force that a muscle can produce depends on the lengths and arrangement of its fibres, on its size or physiological cross-sectional area, on its excitability or fibre type, on the contraction velocity and activation level, and on its level of fatigue. Forces produced by the muscles are transmitted by tendons to the skeleton. A muscle that crosses a joint produces a moment about that joint.

It is possible to tell when a muscle is active by detecting with electrodes the electrical signal or electromyogram (EMG) associated with its contraction. In most cases in orthopaedic biomechanics, electrodes placed on the skin (surface electrodes) are used for this measurement. The EMG is then the sum of the electrical signals from all the motor units within the recording area of the electrode. The raw EMG signal varies in amplitude in a seemingly random way above and below a zero level (Fig. 14). In some cases, it is processed (amplified, filtered, etc.) before use. In order to decide whether a given muscle is 'on' or 'off', the processed EMG signal can be compared qualitatively with the raw EMG of the muscle at rest or quantitatively with the processed EMG recorded during a maximum voluntary isometric contraction. This 'on–off' information is used in biomechanics to reduce the number of unknowns in the indeterminate problem.[29] Entire textbooks are devoted to the methods of detecting, processing, and analysing EMGs.[30, 31]

It is tempting to believe that there is a simple relationship between the amplitude of the EMG signal and the force produced by a muscle. For voluntary isometric contractions only, investigators now report either a linear relationship or a more than linear increase of the EMG signal with force.[30] However, the exact relationship depends on the muscle being studied. Complications arise not only because of the complex relationship between the EMG signal and muscle physiology, but also because the EMG signal recorded for any given muscle is affected by the technical details of detection procedure and by physiological events occurring in muscles not being monitored.[30]

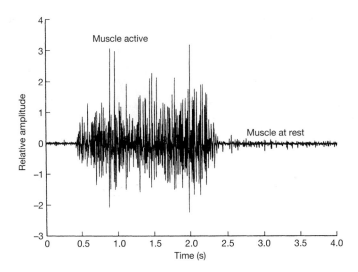

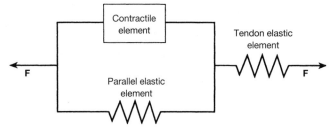

Fig. 16 Hill-type muscle model.

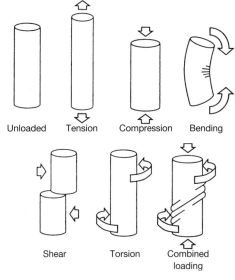

Fig. 14 An EMG signal from the flexor carpi radialis during clenching of the first in a normal subject. Data collected with a surface electrode and sampled at 4 kHz. Periods of rest and activity are evident. (Data courtesy of S. Taffler, Oxford Orthopaedic Engineering Centre.)

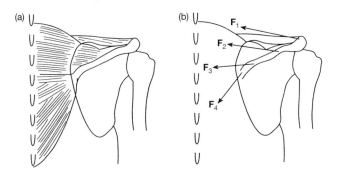

Fig. 17 The types of loads to which bone may be subjected. (Reproduced from reference 3.)

Fig. 15 Representation of muscles with large attachment areas such as the trapezius (a) may need many force vectors (b). (Reproduced from reference 33.)

EMG–force relations for dynamically contracting muscles are rare and controversial.[32]

In many biomechanical models in which a muscle force is unknown, the muscle is represented by a single force vector pointing along the muscle line of action. Many force vectors may be needed for an adequate representation of the mechanical effect of broad pennate muscles with large attachment sites (Fig. 15).[33] In simulations in which muscle forces are prescribed, the simplest and most common model of muscle contraction dynamics is the Hill-type model (Fig. 16). The force produced by the contractile process is attributed to the 'contractile element' and depends on the muscle length, the velocity of contraction, and the muscle activation. Hill's equation[34] is often modified and used to relate these parameters to muscle force.[35] The passive resistance of the muscle to being stretched is represented by a spring, the 'parallel elastic element'. Total muscle force is then the sum of the active and passive elements. Some models include a series elastic element (not shown in Fig. 16) next to the contractile element. The elasticity of the muscle tendon can be included in series with the muscle model (Fig. 16). Storage of energy in the elastic elements is thought to be important in activities such as running and jumping.[36]

Bone

The mechanical functions of the bones of the skeleton are to support and protect the tissues of the body and to function as a lever system on which the muscles can act. As a result of external forces and muscle forces, bones are subjected to all kinds of loading: tension, compression, bending, shear, torsion, and combinations of these (Fig. 17).

For several reasons, bone is difficult to model using the basic techniques of classical mechanics. Even though many bones appear at first to be either simply tubular or plate-like, on closer inspection their detailed geometry is found to be highly complex. Furthermore, most bones have both cortical and trabecular parts, each made up of different proportions and arrangements of organic and inorganic material. As a result, the ability of bone to resist deformation varies throughout its substance.[37]

Since the early 1970s,[38] an advanced computer technique of structural stress analysis called finite-element analysis (FEA) has been used in biomechanics to model bone. In FEA, the geometry of the model is defined first. The model is then divided into a number of sections called 'elements', all of which are connected together at points called 'nodes' (Fig. 18). The solution procedure requires that forces be applied to the model only at the nodes. Distributed forces or pressures

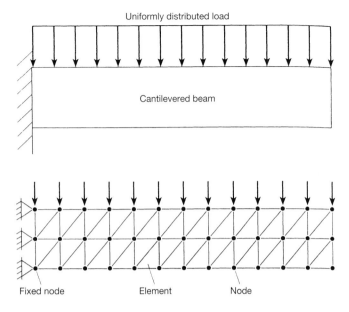

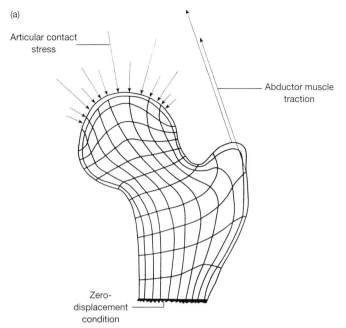

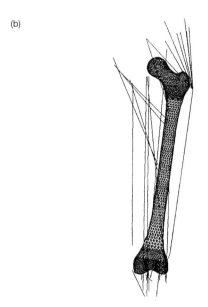

Fig. 18 (a) A uniformly distributed load applied to a cantilevered beam. (b) A simple finite-element model of the beam.

are divided up amongst relevant nodes, usually automatically by the FEA computer program. In order to prevent rigid body motion, a sufficient number of nodes must be fixed or their displacements limited to, say, translation in one direction only. After the material behaviour or stiffness of every element in every direction is defined, the FEA program solves a large number of equations governing force equilibrium at the nodes to find the nodal displacements within the model. From these displacements, strains and stresses can be calculated. The amount of computer time needed to solve an FEA problem depends mainly on the number of nodes and the number of ways in which the nodes can move; it can be quite high for three-dimensional models with complex geometries.

During the first decade of FEA use in orthopaedic biomechanics, work concentrated on the stress analysis of bones, fracture fixation, and artificial joint design and fixation.[39] Most of these highly simplified models were of the lower limb, many involving the proximal femur (Fig. 19(a)) and the femoral component of total hip replacement. During this time, most researchers were still learning the capabilities and limitations of FEA in biomechanics. Since then, increased computer capabilities, more sophisticated FEA computer programs, and a better understanding of FEA overall have led to the development of more realistic models of bone (Fig. 19(b)) and bone–implant interactions.[41] Iterative procedures are now being used to predict the time-dependent mechanical behaviour of bone, to optimize implant design, and to study the relationship between loading and bone shape, bone density, and trabecular architecture. It is also possible to simulate bone growth, maintenance, repair, and remodelling. FEA models of articular cartilage and ligament also now exist. Although FEA is cheap compared with clinical, animal, or laboratory testing methods, the combination of FEA with experimental analyses is many times more powerful than the sum of their individual applications.[41]

Articular cartilage

The articulating surfaces of the bones in a synovial joint are covered with a thin layer of connective tissue known as hyaline articular cartilage

Fig. 19 (a) Two-dimensional finite-element model of a coronal plane section of a proximal femur. (Reproduced from reference 40.) (b) Three-dimensional finite-element model of the femur. Lines of action of the major muscle group forces are shown. (Courtesy of K. Polgar, Oxford Orthopaedic Engineering Centre.)

(a notable exception is the temporomandibular joint in which fibro-cartilage covers the bone ends). The mechanical functions of articular cartilage are to transmit compressive forces across the joint, to distribute the compressive contact force between the bones (by deforming and making the contact area larger), and to allow joint motion with minimal friction and wear.[42]

In some biomechanical models, articular cartilage is considered to be a deformable cushion of linear elastic springs sitting on top of the rigid subchondral bone.[43] It is also possible to allow for the occurrence of tension, compression, and shear (see Fig. 17) within the depths of the cartilage layer. Such models are useful in certain contexts, but they ignore the fact that fluid flow is intrinsically linked to articular cartilage deformation and to its time-dependent responses to loads.[44] Simple single-phase linear viscoelastic models (see below) can be used to take the time-dependency into account but, for a full representation of fluid flow, cartilage must be modelled as at least a biphasic material, with the solid matrix and the interstitial fluid as the two phases.[45, 46] A triphasic theory that combines the biphasic theory with an ion phase, representing the cation and anion of a single salt, has since been developed to study the behaviour of cartilage under chemical and/or mechanical loads.[47] Both analytical and finite-element methods have been used to find solutions to these mathematical models.

Synovial joints have very low coefficients of friction (order of magnitude 10^{-2}) and experience only minimal amounts of wear, even after many decades of use.[48] This is because of the complex lubrication processes involving articular cartilage and synovial fluid. Fluid-film lubrication, in which a thin film of fluid causes surface separation, appears to be the dominant effect. Lubrication occurs by elastohydrodynamic action, in which the bearing surfaces either slide past each other or are squeezed together. The pressure generated in the fluid film supports the load across the joint, but also substantially deforms the articular surfaces and causes fluid to be expelled from the cartilage. Boundary lubrication, in which lubricant is adsorbed on the bearing surfaces, provides additional protection against wear.[48, 49]

Ligaments and tendons

Ligaments and tendons are approximately parallel-fibred collagenous tissues that transmit tensile forces across the joints. A ligament connects one bone to another and functions to guide and limit joint movement. A tendon connects a muscle to a bone across a joint, thereby causing joint motion when the muscle contracts. Tendons also store elastic energy.

In models of the musculoskeletal system, ligaments and tendons are often modelled by a small number of tension-only springs.[50] These can be either linear springs, in which the spring force is directly proportional to the amount of stretch, or non-linear springs, in which the relationship between force and extension is more complicated. It is also possible to model a single ligament as a series of elastic fibres. This gives a better idea of the load distribution across the ligament and of the relationship between ligament structure and function.[51, 52]

Like articular cartilage, ligaments and tendons contain a high proportion of water and so exhibit time- and history-dependent behaviour under load. The quasilinear viscoelastic theory developed by Fung[4] has been used to model these features of the mechanical behaviour of ligaments, tendons, and many other soft tissues. Various extensions to this theory have been proposed, including a finite-element implementation.[53]

Mechanical properties

Almost all work in biomechanics requires some knowledge of the mechanical properties of the tissues of the musculoskeletal system. For instance, when designing a new ligament replacement, it is important to know how much load the natural ligament supports before it breaks and how much deformation it undergoes during loading. Another example is the need to know how bone density relates to bone strength, so that various treatments for osteoporosis can be evaluated

or compared. Finally, many biomechanical models of the musculoskeletal system require mechanical properties, such as tissue stiffness, as input parameters.

Much information about the mechanical properties of tissues comes from tension and compression tests performed using a tensile-testing machine (Fig. 20). The ends of the tissue specimen are held in special clamps, one attached to the rigid base of the testing machine and the other to a moving actuator (in a hydraulically driven machine) or crosshead (in a screw-driven machine). The movement of the actuator/crosshead up or down is usually controlled electronically, and the load applied to the specimen is measured with a load cell attached to the testing machine. Deformation of the specimen can be measured by tracking the movement of the actuator crosshead or by attaching an extensometer or strain gage directly to the specimen. In many cases, however, these methods are not accurate enough, and a noncontact optical method must be used. This typically involves recording on high-speed video the positions of reference marks drawn on the specimen before the start of the test.[54] A computer is usually used to set the test parameters (e.g. the testing speed) and to log the force and displacement data.

The output from any tension or compression test is typically a plot of applied load P versus specimen elongation Δl. Figure 21 shows a plot for a tensile test on a ligament. The 'structural properties' of the entire ligament can be found from such a graph. These include the stiffness (slope of the linear part of the curve), energy absorbed (area under the

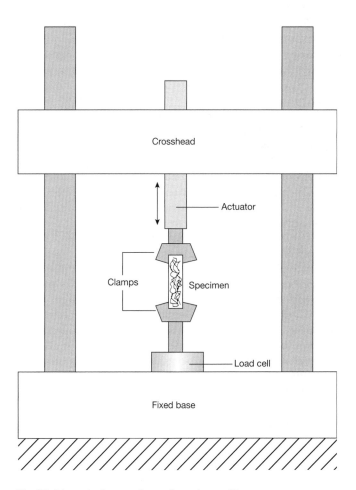

Fig. 20 Schematic diagram of a tensile-testing machine.

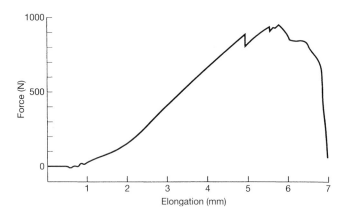

Fig. 21 The force–elongation curve generated from an anterior cruciate ligament tested in tension to failure. (Reproduced from reference 55, based on data from reference 56.)

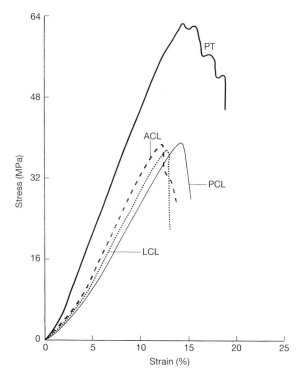

Fig. 22 Typical stress–strain curves for the patellar tendon (PT), anterior cruciate ligament (ACL), posterior cruciate ligament (PCL), and lateral collateral ligament (LCL) fascicle–bone units. Note the much larger elastic modulus and ultimate stress for the PT specimen. (Reproduced from reference 57.)

curve), and ultimate (maximum) load and elongation. These values depend, amongst other things, on the geometry of the tissue, such as its cross-sectional area and length, and on the properties of the tissue substance.

To study the 'mechanical properties' of the ligament tissue alone, it is necessary to calculate and plot a graph of stress versus strain. Stress σ is defined as the load P divided by the cross-sectional area A perpendicular to the load: $\sigma = P/A$. Strain ε is defined as the change in specimen length Δl divided by the original length l: $\varepsilon = \Delta l/l$, Mechanical properties such as the elastic modulus (slope of the linear part of the curve), strain energy density (area under the curve), and ultimate (maximum) stress and strain can be found from a graph of σ versus ε (Fig. 22).

Using the tensile-testing machine shown in Fig. 20 it is possible to obtain the mechanical properties in a single direction. This information would be adequate if the material being tested were isotropic, that is, its mechanical properties were the same in all directions. However, biological tissues are usually anisotropic, which means that they have oriented structural elements (collagen fibres, trabeculae, osteons, etc.) that lead to very different mechanical properties if the tissue is tested in different directions or if different parts of the tissue are tested.[58] As many as 21 independent quantities (elastic constants) could be required for a full description of the behaviour of such materials. Further explanations and details of the structural and mechanical properties of the tissues of the musculoskeletal system are given by Yamada[59] and by Nordin and Frankel.[3]

It is important to recognize that mechanical measurements on tissues are affected by experimental, biological, and external factors.[60] Experimental factors include specimen orientation, strain rate, temperature, and tissue hydration. Biological factors are tissue maturation, age, immobilization, and exercise. Storage by freezing and sterilization are external factors.

Viscoelasticity

In the discussion of the mechanical properties of biological tissues thus far, time has not been mentioned much. Indeed, the mechanical behaviour of engineering materials such as metals and ceramics is usually not time-dependent over the range of operating temperatures. In

contrast, almost all polymers (plastics) and all biological materials exhibit time-dependent or viscoelastic properties.

Viscoelasticity is a mechanical behaviour involving both fluid-like (viscous) and solid-like (elastic) characteristics. The viscoelastic properties of soft tissues, in particular articular cartilage,[49] have received much attention. The main features of viscoelasticity are shown in Fig. 23. Stress relaxation (Fig. 23(a)) is a decrease in stress in a material subjected to prolonged constant strain. Creep (Fig. 23(b)) is an increase in deformation or strain that occurs when a constant load is applied. Hysteresis (Fig. 23(c)) is a characteristic behaviour in which a material property plot follows a closed loop, that is, the loading and unloading curves are not coincident. Because the area under the curve is related to the strain energy, the hysteresis loop indicates that energy is being dissipated, usually as heat. These features of the behaviour of biological materials are rarely taken into account in models of joints and limbs because the duration of the activity being studied is relatively short, the viscoelastic effects are secondary, or inclusion of such effects would make the models too difficult to solve.

Load transmission across joints

A knowledge of the loads transmitted by the anatomic structures at the joints of the body is necessary for, amongst many other things, the design of joint replacements, an understanding of the mechanical factors that may influence the development of osteoarthritis, and the assessment of the effect of tendon transfer operations in the treatment

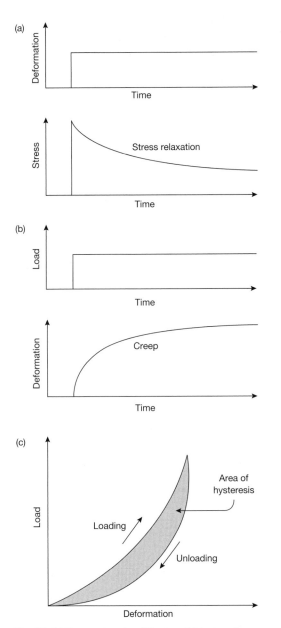

Fig. 23 (a) Stress relaxation; (b) creep; (c) hysteresis.

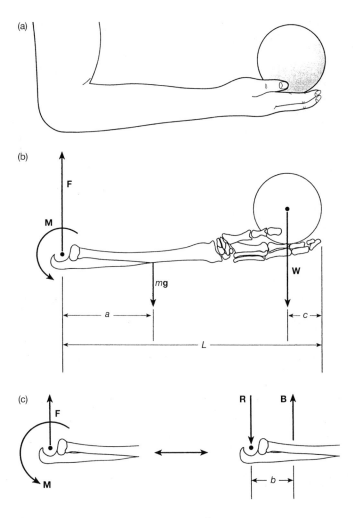

Fig. 24 (a) A heavy ball is held in the hand with the elbow joint flexed to 90° and the forearm parallel to the ground. (b) A free-body diagram of the situation shown in (a). W, Weight of the ball; mg, weight of the forearm and hand; F, intersegmental force at the elbow joint; M, intersegmental moment at the elbow joint. (c) Distribution of F and M amongst the relevant anatomical structures at the elbow joint. B, the biceps muscle force; R, the articular contact force. (Reproduced from reference 61.)

of cerebral palsy. As explained above and illustrated in Fig. 13, the musculoskeletal system is highly indeterminate, and many methods have been used either to increase the number of equations describing the body in question or to decrease the number of unknowns. Rather than describing the details of various joint models and their solution techniques, in this section we use a simple well-known example to illustrate some important points about the loads across joints.

Consider the situation shown in Fig. 24(a) in which a weight is held in the hand with the elbow joint held fixed at 90° flexion and the forearm parallel to the ground. To find the forces transmitted by the anatomical structures at the elbow joint during this activity, it is necessary first to draw a free-body diagram of the forearm (Fig. 24(b)) and to calculate the intersegmental force F and moment M at the elbow. In Fig. 24(b), the weight W of the ball and the weight mg of the forearm and hand both act downwards. In this example, it is obvious

that the force F balances the forces W and mg, and so must act upwards, having a vertical component only. In addition, the moment M must be counterclockwise to balance the moments of W and mg about the centre of the elbow joint. Assuming that the arm belongs to a person of height 170 cm and body mass 60 kg, anthropometric tables[15] can be used to estimate the length and mass of the forearm and hand ($L = 43$ cm, $m = 1.3$ kg) and the distance of their centre of mass from the centre of the elbow joint ($a = 29$ cm). The position of the centre of mass of the ball from the fingertips is estimated to be $c = 9$ cm.

Solving the equations for static force and moment equilibrium in two dimensions gives F = 62.75 N upwards and M = 20.70 Nm counterclockwise. To distribute F and M amongst the anatomical structures of the joint, a model of the elbow joint is needed. Figure 24(c) shows a simple model in which it is assumed that the biceps is the only muscle acting. For the elbow position in Fig. 24(a), it is assumed that the line of pull of the biceps is parallel to the humerus and that its insertion is

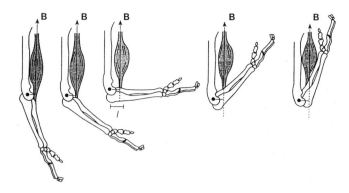

Fig. 25 The biceps (B) at various elbow flexion angles. Note the variations in the moment arm *l* of biceps. (Reproduced from reference **62**.)

$b = 4$ cm from the centre of the elbow joint. It is also assumed that the elbow is a hinge (has a fixed axis of rotation) and that the articular contact force **R** acts vertically at this flexion angle. Using static equilibrium of force and moment in two dimensions (two equations, two unknowns) gives the biceps force **B** = 517 N upwards and the joint reaction force **R** = 454 N downwards.

It is important to note that the magnitudes of both **B** and **R** are larger than the magnitude of the external load **W**. The biceps force **B** is larger because its moment arm *b* is smaller than the moment arm of the external load $(L - c)$. The joint reaction force **R** is larger than **W** because it must balance both **B** and **W**. That the muscle and joint reaction forces are larger than the external loads is true for most joints. Indeed, the joint reaction forces at the hip and knee can be several times body weight. Further details of the elbow problem, together with a summary of joint forces in the upper extremity and the hip joint, are given by An *et al.*[61]

One further important point to note is that the moment arm of a muscle about a joint may change as the joint flexes. This obviously influences the force that it is necessary for a muscle to provide to balance the moment due to an external load. The changing moment arm of the biceps about the centre of the elbow joint is illustrated in Fig. 25.

Conclusions

Much of the progress in the field of biomechanics that has been made over the past half-century has been due to collaborations between scientists, engineers, and clinicians. The scientists and engineers have had to delve into the anatomy and physiology textbooks and the medical literature, while the orthopaedic clinicians have had to return to the mathematics and physics that they studied years before. Both sides have benefited, along with many thousands of patients. This chapter has reviewed and explained some of the fundamental concepts and techniques involved in studying the biomechanics of the musculoskeletal system. It is hoped that clinicians have found this introduction useful and that they will be encouraged to explore the subject further.

References

1. **Williams, P.L., Warwick, R., Dyson, M., and Bannister, L.H.** (1989). *Gray's anatomy*, 37th edn. Churchill Livingstone, London.

2. **Wolff, J.** (1892). *The law of bone remodelling*. Trans. P. Macquet and R. Furlong and reprinted by Springer-Verlag, Berlin, 1986.

3. **Nordin, M. and Frankel, V.H.** (ed.) (1989). *Basic biomechanics of the musculo-skeletal system*, 2nd edn. Lea & Febiger, Philadelphia.

4. **Fung, Y.C.** (1993). *Biomechanics: mechanical properties of living tissues*, 2nd edn. Springer-Verlag, New York.

5. **Nigg, B.M. and Herzog, W.** (ed.) (1994). *Biomechanics of the musculo-skeletal system*. Wiley, Chichester.

6. **Simon, S.R.** (ed.) (1994). *Orthopaedic basic science*. American Academy of Orthopaedic Surgeons, Rosemont, Illinois.

7. **Mow, V.C. and Hayes, W.C.** (1997). *Basic orthopaedic biomechanics*, 2nd edn. Lippincott-Raven, Philadelphia.

8. **Meriam, J.L. and Kraige, L.G.** (1993). *Engineering mechanics*. Vol. 1, *Statics*, 3rd edn. Wiley, New York.

9. **Meriam, J.L. and Kraige, L.G.** (1993). *Engineering mechanics*. Vol. 2, *Dynamics*, 3rd edn. Wiley, New York.

10. **Komi, P.V., Salonen, M., Jarvinen, M., and Kokko, O.** (1987). *In vivo* registration of Achilles tendon forces in man. I. Methodological development. *Int. J. Sports Med.* **8** (Suppl. 1), 3–8.

11. **Beynnon, B., Howe, J.G., Pope, M.H., Johnson, R.J., and Fleming, B.C.** (1992). The measurement of anterior cruciate ligament strain *in vivo*. *Int. Orthopa.* **16**, 1–12.

12. **Cobbold, R.S.C** (1974). *Transducers for biomedical measurements: principles and applications*. Wiley, New York.

13. **Lord, M., Reynolds, D.P., and Hughes, J.R.** (1986). Foot pressure measurement: a review of clinical findings. *J. Biomed. Eng.* **8**, 283–294.

14. **Alexander, I.J., Chao, E.Y.S., and Johnson, K.A.** (1990). The assessment of dynamic foot-to-ground contact forces and plantar pressure distribution: a review of the evolution of current techniques and clinical applications. *Foot Ankle* **11**, 152–167.

15. **Winter, D.A.** (1990). *Biomechanics and motor control of human movement*, 2nd edn. Wiley-Interscience, New York.

16. **Whittle, M.W.** (1996). *Gait analysis: an introduction*, 2nd edn. Butterworth Heinemann, Oxford.

17. **Nigg, B.M.** (1994). Force. In *Biomechanics of the musculo-skeletal system* (ed. B.M. Nigg and W. Herzog), pp. 200–224. Wiley, Chichester.

18. **Hull, M.L. and Davis, R.R.** (1981). Measurement of pedal loading in bicycling. I: Instrumentation. *J. Biomech.* **14**, 843–856.

19. **Newmiller, J., Hull, M.L., and Zajac, F.E.** (1988). A mechanically decoupled two force component bicycle pedal dynamometer. *J. Biomech.* **21**, 375–386.

20. **Ruby, P. and Hull, M.L.** (1993). Response of intersegmental knee loads to foot/pedal platform degrees of freedom in cycling. *J. Biomech.* **26**, 1327–1340.

21. **O'Connor, J.J.** (1991). Load simulation problems in model testing. In *strain measurement in biomechanics* (ed. A.W. Miles and K.E. Tanner), pp. 14–38. Chapman & Hall, London.

22. **Morris, J.** (1973). Accelerometry—a technique for the measurement of human body movements. *J. Biomech.* **6**, 729–736.

23. **Nigg, B.M.** (1994). Acceleration. In *Biomechanics of the musculo-skeletal system* (ed. B.M. Nigg and W. Herzog), pp. 237–253. Wiley, Chichester.

24. **Kinzel, G.L., Hall, A.S., and Hillberry, B.M.** (1972). Measurement of the total motion between two body segments. I: Analytical development. *J. Biomech.* **5**, 93–105.

25. **Kinzel, G.L., Hillberry, B.M., Hall, A.S., van Sickle, D.C., and Harvey, W.M.** (1972). Measurement of the total motion between two body segments. II: Description of application. *J. Biomech.* **5**, 283–293.

26. **An, K.-N., Jacobsen, M.C., Berglund, L.J., and Chao, E.Y.S.** (1988). Application of a magnetic tracking device to kinesiologic studies. *J. Biomech.* **21**, 613–620.

27. **Perry, J.** (1992). *Gait analysis: normal and pathological function*. Slack, Thorofare, NJ.

28. **Crowninshield, R.D. and Brand, R.A.** (1981). The prediction of forces in joint structures: distribution of intersegmental resultants. *Exercise Sport Scie. Rev.* **9**, 159–181.

29. Morrison, J.B. (1968). Bioengineering analysis of force actions transmitted by the knee joint. *Biomed. Eng.* **3**, 164–170.

30. Basmajian, J.V. and De Luca, C.J. (1985). *Muscles alive: their functions revealed by electromyography*, 5th edn. Williams and Wilkins, Baltimore.

31. Loeb, G.E. and Gans, C. (1986). *Electromyography for experimentalists*. University of Chicago Press, Chicago.

32. Herzog, W., Guimaraes, A.C.S., and Zhang, Y.T. (1994). EMG. In *Biomechanics of the musculo-skeletal system* (ed. B.M. Nigg and W. Herzog), pp. 308–336. Wiley, Chichester.

33. van der Helm, F.C.T. and Veenbaas, R. (1991). Modelling the mechanical effect of muscles with large attachment sites: application to the shoulder mechanism. *J. Biomech.* **24**, 1151–1163.

34. Hill, A.V. (1938). The heat of shortening and the dynamic constants of muscle. *Proc. R. Soc. Lond.* **126**, 136–195.

35. Zajac, F.E. (1989). Muscle and tendon: properties, models, scaling, and application to biomechanics and motor control. *Crit. Rev. Bioeng.* **17**, 359–411.

36. Alexander. R.McN. (1988). *Elastic mechanisms in animal movement*. Cambridge University Press, Cambridge.

37. Keaveny, T.M. and Hayes, W.C. (1993). A 20-year perspective on the mechanical properties of trabecular bone. *Trans. ASME: J. Biomech. Eng.* **115**, 534–542.

38. Brekelmans, W.A.M., Poort, H.W., and Slooff, T.J.J.H. (1972). A new method to analyse the mechanical behaviour of skeletal parts. *Acta Orthop. Scand.* **43**, 301–317.

39. Huiskes, R. and Chao, E.Y.S. (1983). A survey of finite element analysis in orthopaedic biomechanics: the first decade. *J. Biomech.* **16**, 385–409.

40. Brown, T.D., Way, M.E., and Ferguson, A.B. (1980). Stress transmission anomalies in femoral heads altered by aseptic necrosis. *J. Biomech.* **13**, 687–699.

41. Huiskes, R. and Hollister, S.J. (1993). From structure to process, from organ to cell: recent developments of FE-analysis in orthopaedic biomechanics. *Trans. ASME: J. Biomech. Eng.* **115**, 520–527.

42. Shrive, N.G. and Frank, C.B. (1994). Articular cartilage. In *Biomechanics of the musculo-skeletal system* (ed. B.M. Nigg and W. Herzog), pp. 79–105. Wiley, Chichester.

43. An, K.-N., Himeno, S., Tsumura, H., *et al.* (1990). Pressure distribution on articular surfaces: application to joint stability and evaluation. *J. Biomech.* **23**, 1013–1020.

44. Mow, V.C., Holmes, M.H., and Lai, W.M. (1984). Fluid transport and mechanical properties of articular cartilage: a review. *J. Biomech.* **17**, 377–394.

45. Torzilli, P.A. and Mow, V.C. (1976) On the fundamental fluid transport mechanisms through normal and pathological articular cartilage during function, I: The formulation. *J. Biomech.* **9**, 541–552.

46. Torzilli, P.A. and Mow, V.C. (1976). On the fundamental fluid transport mechanisms through normal and pathological articular cartilage during function. II: The analysis, solution, and conclusions. *J. Biomech.* **9**, 587–606.

47. Lai, W.M., Hou, J.S., and Mow, V.C. (1991). A triphasic theory for the swelling and deformation behaviors of articular cartilage. *Trans. ASME: J. Biomech. Eng.* **113**, 245–258.

48. Dowson, D. (1990). Bio-tribology of natural and replacement synovial joints. In *Biomechanics of diarthrodial joints*, Vol. 2 (ed. V.C. Mow, A. Ratcliffe, and S.L-Y. Woo), pp. 305–345. Springer-Verlag, New York.

49. Mow, V.C, Proctor, C.S., and Kelly, M.A. (1989). Biomechanics of articular cartilage. In *Basic biomechanics of the musculoskeletal system*, (ed. M. Nordin and V.H. Frankel) 2nd edn , pp. 31–58. Lea & Febiger, Philadelphia.

50. Crowninshield, R.D., Pope, M.H., and Johnson, R.J. (1976). An analytical model of the knee. *J. Biomech.* **9**, 397–405.

51. Zavatsky, A.B. and O'Connor, J.J. (1992). A model of human knee ligaments in the sagittal plane. I: Response to passive flexion. *Proc. Inst. Mech. Eng. Part H: J. Eng. Med.* **206**, 125–134.

52. Zavatsky, A.B. and O'Connor, J.J. (1992) A model of human knee ligaments in the sagittal plane. II: Fibre recruitment under load. *Proc. Inst. Mech. Eng. Part H: J. Eng. Med.* **206**, 135–145.

53. Puso, M.A. and Weiss, J.A. (1998). Finite element implementation of anisotropic quasi-linear viscoelasticity using a discrete spectrum approximation. *J. Biomech. Eng.* **120**, 62–70.

54. Woo, S.L.-Y., Orlando, C.A., Camp, J.F., and Akeson, W.H. (1986). Effect of postmortem storage by freezing on ligament behaviour. *J. Biomech.* **19**, 399–404.

55. Carlstedt, C.A. and Nordin, M. (1989). Biomechanics of ligaments and tendons. In *Basic biomechanics of the musculoskeletal system* (ed. M. Nordin and V.H. Frankel), pp. 59–74. Lea & Febiger, Philadelphia.

56. Noyes, F.R. (1977). Functional properties of knee ligament and alterations induced by immobilization. *Clin. Orthop. Rel. Res.* **123**, 210–242.

57. Butler, D.L., Kay, M.D., and Stouffer, D.C. (1986). Comparison of material properties in fascicle-bone units from human patellar tendon and knee ligaments. *J. Biomech.* **19**, 425–432.

58. Litsky, A.S. and Spector, M. (1994). Biomaterials. In *Orthopaedic basic science* (ed. S.R. Simon), pp. 447–486. American Academy of Orthopaedic Surgeons, Rosemont, Illinois.

59. Yamada, H. (1970). *Strength of biological materials*. Williams and Wilkins, Baltimore.

60. Woo, S.L.-Y., Livesay, G.A., Runco, T.J., and Young, E.P. (1997). Structure and function of ligaments and tendons. In *Basic orthopaedic biomechanics*, 2nd edn (ed. V.C. Mow and W.C. Hayes), pp. 209–252. Lippincott-Raven, Philadelphia.

61. An, K.-N., Chao, E.Y.S., and Kaufman. K.R. (1997). Analysis of muscle and joint loads. In *Basic orthopaedic biomechanics*, (ed. V.C. Mow and W.C Hayes) 2nd edn, pp. 1–36. Lippincott-Raven, Philadelphia.

62. Leveau, B.F. (1992). *William's and Lissner's biomechanics of human motion*, 3rd edn. W.B. Saunders, Philadelphia.

3.2 Locomotion analysis

Richard Brand

Introduction

Doctors have used observation of human movement to interpret disease states for at least as long as recorded history. The skilled clinician often finds qualitative observational analysis critical to establish the presence of disorders, to distinguish between certain classes of conditions, or to ascertain the severity of disease. The notion of using technology to measure quantitatively and record critical clinical information arose in the nineteenth century. However, despite thousands of studies over more than 100 years and despite many technical advances, recorded locomotion analysis beyond the observational has never gained widespread clinical use.

Throughout this chapter the term 'observational analysis' is used to refer to those qualitative assessments that a clinician can routinely perform without technology, while the expression 'locomotion analysis' is used specifically to refer to the various means of quantitatively recording and/or assessing locomotion—obviously, these definitions are quite arbitrary.

Although Borelli's landmark static analysis of human and animal bodies *De Motu Animalium* (published in 1680)[1] implies locomotion (Fig. 1), the first scientific work (i.e. systematic exploration of specific questions) on gait came from the Weber brothers in 1836.[2] (They were not, they stated, particularly interested in locomotion *per se*, but rather decided to explore the issues because they wished to work together, and locomotion was an area where an anatomist and a mathematician could both contribute!) Their tools were limited to clocks (which had recently afforded accuracy in the range of fractions of seconds) and rulers. Not surprisingly, their data concentrated on temporal and distance factors of gait (Fig. 2), although they postulated that normal gait minimizes energy expenditure and argued that the leg acted as a pendulum during swing (a notion still explored today).

The works of subsequent early investigators remained primarily reports of approaches[3–5] or explorations of specific questions,[6] rather than information obtained for an individual patient. Dercum, a neurologist at the University of Pennsylvania, had seen Muybridge's photographs of human motion, including some of patients with various disorders (Figs 3 and 4), and correctly realized that they might provide a more sensitive analysis than the human eye.[7] Collaborating with Muybridge, he commented:[8]

To show how difficult it is to observe a moving limb, even when the movement is slow, it need only be stated that medical writers almost without exception describe this gait [locomotor ataxia] erroneously. Almost all lay stress upon rigidity of the leg and insufficient action of the knee-joint. It needs but a hasty examination of the photographs to show how utterly wrong this view is. Every one of the plates reveals the action of the knee joint, and in fact of all of the joints, to be far in excess of the normal.

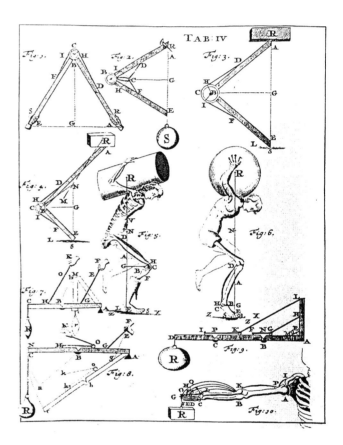

Fig. 1 Borelli used the emerging principles of static analysis to estimate resultant joint as well as muscle forces. While he was not the first to recognize the importance of forces in biological function, his prescient insight provided the first quantitative models of biological organisms. When one recalls that Borelli's work preceded the publication of Newton's *Principia Mathematica*, his approaches appear all the more extraordinary.

This seminal study clearly delineated the potential of locomotion analysis of a single patient for purposes of assessment (i.e. a 'clinical' use), as contrasted with exploring some hypothesis (i.e. a 'scientific' use). This chapter focuses on the former, but it is important to keep in mind that some of the criticisms or problems equally apply to the latter. Furthermore, since many authors provide excellent reviews of observational analysis,[9–11] this chapter will be limited to the use of various recording techniques to provide supplemental information. The fundamental approaches will be reviewed applying those techniques, whilst exploring their capabilities and limitations, providing reasons for the failure of those approaches to achieve widespread clinical use, and criteria required to achieve utility. Current and future

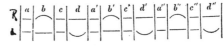

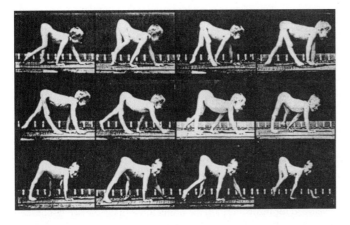

Fig. 2 The Weber brothers made the first quantitative measurements of locomotion parameters, (a) Frontispiece to their seminal work; (b) the relationship of stance and swing phases of gait during level walking, and their overlap. The Weber brothers clearly described the changes in overlap as speed increased.

Fig. 3 Muybridge's photographs of a child with a paralytic disorder walking on all fours because of lower-extremity weakness and (in all likelihood) severe hip flexion contractures.

technology represents an untapped resource to provide critical clinical information.

The modern concepts of locomotion analysis (i.e. kinematics and kinetics) were established by Braune and Fischer in a series of studies begun in the late 1880s and early 1900s.[6] Extending the static analysis of Borelli, and using Newtonian concepts (and their extrapolations), they realized that one could estimate resultant joint forces and moments by treating limb segments as rigid bodies, then ascertaining their displacement histories (i.e. displacements, velocities, and then accelerations and inertial properties (i.e. mass and mass distribution. They accomplished this with a five-part procedure:

1. instrumenting the limb segments with Geisler tubes (Fig. 5(a));
2. recording displacement histories with four camera views (for three-dimensional analysis) with time-lapse photography (Fig. 5(b));
3. ascertaining accelerations by transferring the segment displacements to graph paper and graphically differentiating the curves (Fig. 5(c));
4. estimating segment mass properties using pendulum techniques (Fig. 5(d));
5. computing intersegmental resultant joint forces using equations of motion (Fig. 5(e)).

They realized that the quantities that they computed did not represent the forces on the articular surfaces, but rather resulted from articular, muscle, and ligament forces. They noted that the problem of computing the articular surfaces was redundant (indeterminate) owing to the fact that there were more unknown muscle, ligament, and articular forces than equations of motions. They extensively discussed, but did not solve, the problem (Fig. 5(e)). (Ironically, some contemporary investigators have not recognized the critical distinction between articular forces and intersegmental resultant forces. In a general sense, the two are mathematically linked, but not directly related given that an infinite number of muscle, ligament, and articular force solutions can lead to the same intersegmental result. This error has probably lead to misleading conclusions regarding joint surface responses to forces.) Much of the modern locomotion work described in this chapter builds conceptually on the seminal work of Braune and Fischer.

Locomotion analysis: research versus clinical utility

As implied above, making the distinction between the research and clinical utility of locomotion analysis is critical since such approaches have been very useful to the systematic exploration of well-posed questions, though as yet they have failed to reach widespread clinical utility. The reasons for such divergent applicability arise from distinct requirements of 'clinical' versus 'research' utility.

'Clinical' utility means the study ('testing') of a single patient, and the use of these observations to guide diagnosis, treatment, or prognosis of that patient. Statistical treatment is not generally required, except perhaps to obtain descriptive statistics of multiple trials, or to

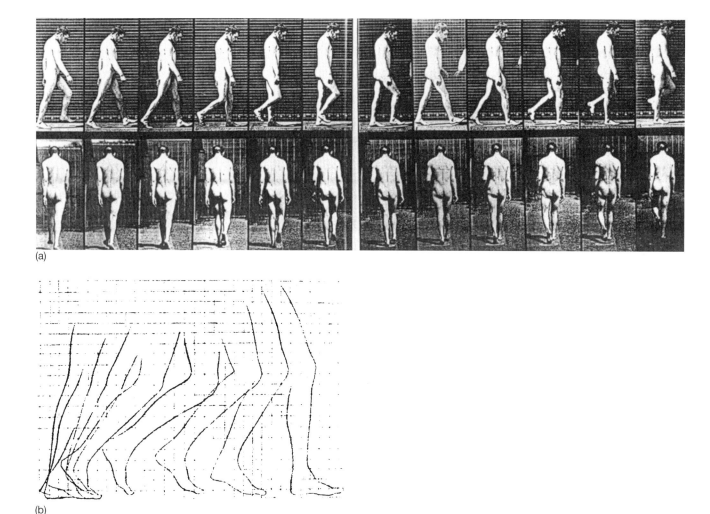

Fig. 4 Dercum's analysis of Muybridge's photographs of a patient with locomotor ataxia. (a) Photograph. (b) Dercum's tracings illustrating knee motion. These recordings disproved the commonly held view of a rigid-knee gait in this disorder.

document that the individual patient's observations fall outside some confidence limits for a 'normal' population.

'Research' or 'scientific' utility means the positing of an explicit hypothesis or question, and the systematic attempts to support or disprove the hypothesis, or unambiguously answer the question. In locomotion analysis, a reasonable number of subjects is required, since all such observations are subject to 'biological' variability and reproducibility of observations must be ensured. (There are times when very specific questions might be answered by single subject studies.) In addition, we generally perform further statistical treatment to make inferences of the (random or nonrandom) observations based upon limited samples.

Although locomotion analysis has always held great promise to aid the clinician, it has never lived up to its promise. Schwartz and his colleagues recognized that 'Measurement is essential for the interpretation of normal and abnormal phenomena of the human body' and that 'Empiricism fostered by trial and error, must continue to govern the therapy of abnormal function until measurement in some form improves the treatment of disabilities affecting the back and lower extremities'.[12–15] They described a series of tools to measure certain gait features, but ultimately admitted that 'All methods heretofore

developed for recording gait, including those that have been published by others and ourselves, have failed to be of practical clinical value'.[14] By 1937, the group had collected various sorts of recordings in over 2500 patients, but still had not documented clinical usefulness.[13]

Much more recently, Cappozo[16] commented on the clinical utility of locomotion analysis following a 3-day conference devoted to the subject: 'From the three-day discussion a state of the art emerged. "A rather disappointing state of the art" was the comment of many observers. It should however be emphasized that the disappointment did not apply to the hardware'. They realized that despite increasing technical sophistication, locomotion analysis had failed to meet its promise.

Means of observation

Concepts of human locomotion analysis arise from the disciplines of kinematics (the branch of mechanics which deals with the motion of bodies) and kinetics (the branch of mechanics which deals with the actions or forces producing motion). Terms specific to the peculiarities of human locomotion (e.g. heel strike) provide a means of communication, although they bear a rather more general connection

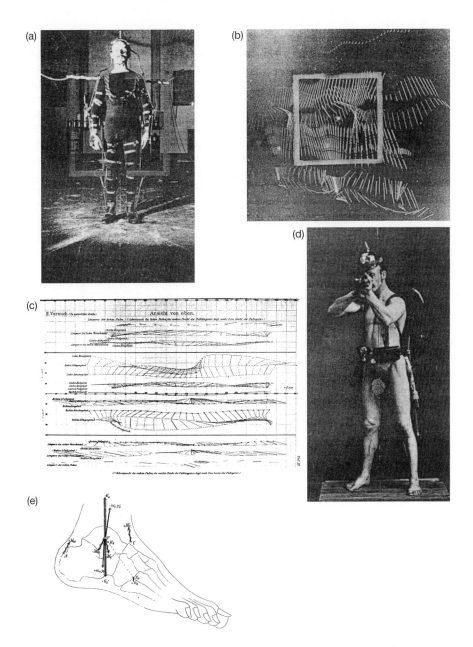

Fig. 5 Critical aspects of the work of Braune and Fischer. (a) Instrumentation of subject's body segments with Geisler tubes. (b) Time-lapse photography from right-oblique camera. (c) Displacement history of body segments as viewed from above. (d) Subject with military gear on a pendulum platform used for ascertaining the overall mass centre of gravity. (e) Illustration of intersegmental resultant force and various muscle forces in one position of the foot during gait.

to well-accepted kinematic concepts. Since the concepts arise from these two disciplines, the means of observation generally include at least some (if not all) elements of motion or force analysis (Table 1). However, the recording of muscle activity (electromyograms) or energy expenditure often provide supplementary (or in some cases critical) information.

Kinematic analysis

Kinematic analysis is the oldest of the approaches, and in its simplest form involves mere observation of movement by the clinician. A skilled clinician can detect many, if not most, of the subtle variations required to make a diagnosis or assessment. For the purposes of this

chapter, 'diagnosis' means making a distinction between various disorders that might explain the array of patient symptoms and signs. Conversely, 'assessment' or 'evaluation' refers to the application of a relative (quantitative or semiquantitative) value to an observation, either in relation to a normal population or the same patient over time. Except in cases where an abnormal movement is so characteristic that it occurs only in a single disorder, locomotion analysis merely allows the clinician to limit the possibilities to one of several disorders. Thus, it does not allow 'diagnosis' in a strict sense. The diagnosis is ordinarily made upon other sorts of observations (e.g. history, neurological examination, laboratory tests, and so on).

The use of recording tools to provide quantitative or semiquantitative measures often increases the resolution of the observation (i.e.

Table 1 Tools of locomotion analysis

Kinematics
Still cameras
Movie cameras
Video recorders
Goniometers
Instrumented walkways
Biplanar roentgen stereophotogrammetry
Videofluoroscopy
Optoelectronic systems
Accelerometers
Foot–floor pressures
Foot–shoe pressures

Kinetics
External forces
Force plates
Instrumented transducers
Internal forces
Instrumented implants
Computation models

Electromyography
Surface electrodes
Intramuscular (fine wire or needle) electrodes

Energetics
Oxygen consumption
Computational models of mechanical energy

certain observations may be made by a tool that cannot be made even by a skilled clinician) or affords the possibility to compare the observation objectively over time (eliminating the need for precise memory). Furthermore, the use of such tools provides a way to ascertain the average response, which might more accurately reflect the disorder than a potentially atypical response.

Many such tools have been developed.[3, 12–15, 17–21] The possibility of capturing movement events increases with the numbers of observations (e.g. frame rate). During the past 20 years, researchers have introduced various techniques, some of which are commercially available. In their simplest form, one merely records patient motion. In their more complicated forms, multiple markers placed upon the body can be tracked by automated or semi-automated (interactive) means in order to quantify limb segment motion histories.

Parameters of kinematic analysis

At the simplest level, temporal and distance features are recorded as a reflection of a recorded displacement history, for example, stride length or cadence in the lower extremity,[22] or object-to-nose time of a finger in the upper extremity. With increasing sophistication, it is possible to record analogue signals reflecting isolated limb segment motions (e.g. joint angles), three-dimensional reconstructions of segment or total body motions, or even the motions of individual bones. In these latter cases, much information is available to the clinician, but one must select those specific features or parameters of greatest interest. Such parameters include three-dimensional joint motion, joint motion (translational or angular) projected on to some plane (e.g. the sagittal or coronal planes), distance between two critical events, time between two events, limb segment velocities, or limb segment accelerations. Clinically useful observations are ordinarily limited to the more obvious and straightforward features.

Limitations of kinematic analysis

Perhaps the most serious limitation of locomotion analysis relates to inherent biological variability. Movements are never quite identical: they change according to the circumstance and mood of the patient, and they may change over time. Such variability relates to the fact that, while the neural system develops limited sorts of strategies for movement, there remains virtually an infinite number of ways to achieve the identical or similar movement. Depending upon the need, one may wish to analyse a single motion, or the means of multiple motions. The infinite number of ways to achieve a given movement (i.e. 'redundancy') relates to mathematical indeterminacy—a state in which there are more unknowns than simultaneous equations and an infinite number of solutions satisfy the equations. About any given joint, there are far more unknown muscle, ligament, capsular, and joint contact forces (or distributions) than equations of motion which those forces must satisfy. Therefore a potentially infinite number of combinations of muscle, ligament, capsular, and joint contact forces may satisfy the precise movement.

A second limitation relates to the first, in that some movements will be altered by a particular environment. Laboratory conditions, which are often strange for a patient, limiting in size or shape, or requiring unaccustomed clothing, may result in more or less subtle alterations in movement for physical or psychological reasons. Furthermore, the application of markers, 'umbilical cords', or recording devices may inhibit normal patterns. Some authors have published sensitivity studies[23, 24] documenting the range of errors created by these and other sources of error. When interpreting published studies, readers should consider the effect of these and additional sources of error or artefact upon the validity of the conclusions.

The measure selected should logically and critically relate to the condition under consideration. For example, measuring knee stance phase flexion–extension in normal level gait will be of little value in a patient with a torn anterior cruciate ligament, since that particular parameter is ordinarily normal (even if another is not) and logically one would not anticipate abnormality.

The measure should clearly distinguish normal and patient populations. For many features, the values for a patient will lie within the considerable normal variability (i.e. confidence intervals) of the measure in a normal population. Furthermore, some parameters (e.g. cadence) vary with age, and many vary with walking velocity.[25, 26] Large databases on the normal population are therefore required that afford appropriate matching.[26, 27] Given the variability of locomotion analysis settings or laboratories, it may be important to ensure that local databases are consistent with published databases or even to ascertain an appropriate database for comparison.

For some techniques (e.g. those involving marker or goniometer placement) intratester variability may be an issue. Kerschot et al.[28] suggested variability of placement of external markers could lead to one standard deviation variability of 2.5° in estimating knee joint flexion extension from interrupted light photography (i.e. potential errors of 5° within two standard deviations). Boone et al.[29] documented substantial variability (e.g. up to 5° or 6°) differences in the measurement of joint angles between different testers, and somewhat less variability with a given tester measuring the same subject at differing times. They suggested that differences of less than 6° in the upper extremity and 5° in the lower extremity in a given subject over time could not be considered a significant change.

Intermarker distance affects the magnitude of potential errors. In general, errors are unlikely to be more than a few degrees if markers upon which the angles are computed are located over long distances (e.g. estimating knee angles from markers near the hip, at the 'knee centre, and at the ankle). However, if markers are located over short distances (e.g. about the foot), the resulting errors might be as much as 10° or 20°. Paradoxically, most sensitivity studies of error have been performed on joints least subject to error.

A reasonable number of trials must be ascertained for each observation. In comparing the reliability of knee joint angles measure by goniometry and interrupted light photography, Kerschot et al.[28] found that one would need to record seven photographic and 20 goniometric gait cycles to achieve one standard deviation of 2°.

More refined techniques generally increase the information available. However, a variety of errors may occur in the various steps required for capturing the additional data, and errors can propagate.[19] For example, relative motion between the soft tissues and bone during movement inevitably limit reliability, since one is generally interested in the movement of the relatively rigid underlying bones, rather than movement of the soft-tissue envelope.[30] Markers closest to the bones with a minimum of underlying soft tissue provide the most reliable (i.e. most repeatable) observations, while those held away from the body segment on sticks and/or with substantial underlying soft tissues are the least reliable. Furthermore, if one is interested in movement of the bones, then one must relate external landmarks to bony landmarks, a potential source of substantial error of some centimetres. One potential way to minimize error from marker movement utilizes redundant markers.[31] To compute full three-dimensional relative motion of two rigid bodies, one must know the displacement histories of a minimum of three landmarks on each rigid body. However, if one uses four, five, six, or more markers on each body segment, it is possible to compute the distance between all pairs of markers. Rigidly attached to rigid body, these would always remain the same, but on a body segment such as the thigh, some may move against the overlying soft tissues. If only one or two move relative to the others, a correction can be made for those that move (or move the greatest), and this reduces the error of computation of the relative motion of the two limb segments.

In contrast to ascertaining times and distances (which may be more or less directly measured), velocities and accelerations are generally computed using smoothed displacement histories.[32] (Accelerations may be directly measured with an accelerometer but, since the accelerations of multiple limb segments are required, this latter method is not generally used for these forms of locomotion analysis.) Many mathematical approaches are available for such processing, and each includes certain assumptions and potential errors. The choice is somewhat arbitrary, but one must know the specific limitations of whatever technique is chosen, and their potential impact on conclusions.

Other errors include (but are not limited to) calibrating the location of markers, errors in identifying markers, and optical distortion in the recording device. Most investigators will systematically identify and explore such potential problems in their own systems, and in most cases these latter do not incur large errors. In assessing the reliability of the observations, these points should always be considered.

Kinetic analysis

Kinetic analysis involves measurement or calculation of the forces causing observed motions. In clinical terms, this means estimating forces external to the body (e.g. foot–floor forces) or internal forces (e.g. joint or muscle forces). The former require various forms of force transducers (Table 1), while the latter typically require computational models, although internal forces have been measured in humans in a very few specific instances.[33, 34]

Parameters of kinetic analysis

In the simplest cases, forces are directly measured using various transducers (e.g. force plates built into the floor, hand grip strength devices). These devices provide analogue or digital records, which can then be analysed in various ways, most often as peak forces. Accelerations may be ascertained from accelerometers attached to limb segments.[35] While the devices themselves are accurate, they may lead to errors when attached to soft tissues rather than rigidly fixed to bone.[36]

In more complex analyses, it is possible to compute various force parameters using linked-segment mathematical models (including certain assumptions regarding system constraints). Perhaps the most common computes the intersegmental resultant forces and moments.[37, 38] The intersegmental forces and moments (sometimes termed simply 'joint forces' or 'joint torques') do not represent forces in any actual joint structures, but rather represent the vector sums of all such forces (muscle, ligament, capsule, joint contact forces) acting about a joint. (Although one should distinguish the intersegmental resultant force from the joint contact force, it is important to realize that the joint contact force is ordinarily reported as a single number (magnitude) or vector, and is therefore itself a 'resultant' since that single force is distributed over the articular surface.)

Models computing the intersegmental resultants require estimates of body segment inertial properties and limb motion (segment accelerations) as well as externally measured forces. Computation of both segment inertial properties and accelerations in turn requires mathematical models, the latter making assumptions about joint constraints (e.g. hinge joint, ball-and-socket joint). Computation of intersegmental joint forces and moments has become a standard procedure in virtually all gait laboratories, partly owing to marketed software capable of computing these quantities. Linked-segment models also allow the computation of mechanical energy.[35, 39–41] However, such analyses have rarely been used for clinical purposes.

Considerably more complex modelling procedures are required to estimate forces in actual anatomical structures.[37, 42] These latter types of model are generally subject to far more assumptions and limitations than those required for estimating the intersegmental resultants, and accordingly are subject to far greater error and question. For virtually all current clinical uses, one need not consider internal forces other than the rather more simply obtained intersegmental resultant forces and moments.

Limitations of kinetic analysis

Ascertainment of external forces can be accomplished with considerable precision using contemporary devices. One need only be aware of the general accuracy of the device (supplied by the manufacturer, or readily ascertained through calibration procedures if custom made). While accelerometers themselves are reasonably accurate, attachment to the soft tissues may introduce error.[36]

Conversely, computation of internal forces (i.e. intersegmental resultant forces and moments) is not so straightforward, although 'turnkey' software packages might lead the unsuspecting user to believe they are. As noted above, the following information or data is required: external forces, limb segment accelerations, and body segment inertial properties. Limb segment accelerations normally arise from processing recorded marker displacement data, but a number of steps are required.

Firstly, one must ascertain the 'joint centre'; not an actual anatomical point, but rather the origin of the required reference frames. Since these are ordinarily anatomically based, the location of specific landmarks must be determined. Obviously, potential errors associated with landmarks (discussed above) apply to these determinations. At the knee, for example, the locations of the medial and lateral epicondyle might be determined, then the midpoint of those two locations selected as the 'joint centre'. However, the ill-defined nature of the epicondyles and overlying soft tissues may create errors of 1 to 2 cm in locating the 'joint centre'. As another example, the 'hip centre' may be ascertained by estimating the location of the anterior superior iliac spine and the symphysis pubis, establishing a co-ordinate system from the plane created by those three points, then the hip centre location estimated as a percentage of the interanterior superior iliac spine distance from the anterior superior iliac spine and that plane. Such approaches are also subject to errors of several centimetres. Data reported by Andriacchi and Strickland[23] suggests variability of between 10 and 20 per cent in some joint moment computations assuming errors in estimating hip centre location of only 1.6 cm. Precise knowledge of all landmarks is obviously required to record displacement histories of limb segments accurately.

Secondly, a model of the limb is needed. Ordinarily a linked-segment model[31] as well as a mathematical technique is used to differentiate the displacement histories to obtain velocities and accelerations.[32] Linked-segment models may make a variety of approximations on joint motions, such as a hinge joint at the knee or a ball-and-socket joint at the hip. Such assumptions affect model results, although typically not in a major way. The mathematical techniques for smoothing displacement data, and then computing velocities and accelerations, can make errors, probably in the range of several to perhaps 10 per cent.

Thirdly, specific inertial properties must be known (e.g. mass centre location, mass distribution). Estimates are ordinarily based upon anthropometric measurements on a given patient, then inputting those measurements into anthropometric models from the literature.[43–46] However, both the initial anthropometric measurements and models are subject to certain assumptions and errors, probably in the range of 10–20 per cent.

All of these uncertainties cause potentially inaccurate computation of the intersegmental joint resultants, and errors may propagate. Unfortunately, such uncertainties are rarely mentioned in current clinically relevant studies or in software documentation. When one interprets the literature on locomotion analysis or the data of a given patient, particularly that related to differences of one kinetic parameter relative to a normal database, one must have an appreciation of the potential for these errors: often the uncertainty of the measure exceeds the difference from patient to normal.

Electromyographic analysis

Electromyography (EMG) provides a valuable tool for ascertaining temporal activation of a muscle during movement. As a clinical tool, one can determine whether or not a muscle is being activated at an expected ('normal') time and duration. In general, the more cyclic and stereotypical the activity, the greater the potential value for a given subject. For less reproducible activities, it is difficult to distinguish normal from abnormal activation patterns. This situation creates a paradox, since many stereotypical activities occur through 'hard-wired' pattern generators in the central nervous system, and are relatively unaffected by many abnormalities (e.g. level gait in a patient with a tear of the anterior cruciate ligament). Those activities that are most likely to result in abnormal EMG patterns are often those that are not stereotypical and that are subject to considerable variability. In these cases, distinguishing a normal from an abnormal EMG may be difficult or impossible.

Parameters of EMG analysis

EMG patterns may be analysed as 'raw' signals, or processed to create 'envelopes' of patterns. All EMG signals are first filtered to exclude motion artefact and eliminate obviously irrelevant signal ('noise'). Typically a 'high-pass filter' eliminates signal below 10–20 Hz (the range of signal from motion artefact) and a 'low-pass filter' eliminates signal above 500–1000 Hz (the level above which there is no substantial energy content). The resulting raw signals per se may be interpreted only qualitatively, typically determining timing of activation during a cycle of some more or less reproducible activity. Onset of activity is ascertained by presuming some threshold of activity. For clinical purposes, such interpretation often suffices.

However, if one must make a quantitative assessment (e.g. Is the signal magnitude greater or lesser after some intervention or is the signal duration different?), then the raw signal may be processed in a variety of ways. Such quantitative assessments are possible only in activities that are reasonably reproducible. Typically this involves rectification (taking the raw signal with its positive and negative voltage signal components and placing all the signal on one side or the other of the zero axis) and then smoothing, filtering, or averaging to create an envelope of activity.[26, 47–49] The resulting envelopes may then be further processed and analysed in a variety of ways.

To compare envelope timing and magnitude directly (and quantitatively), both aspects need to be normalized. Timing is normalized by assuming a constant timing for all activity cycles, then mathematically expanding the shorter ones and contracting the longer ones. Signal magnitude may be normalized in a variety of ways: to the maximum signal observed during the test, to the average of all signals, to the maximum voluntary contraction, or to the magnitude during some standard event (i.e. with a fixed joint moment).[50] Each approach has utility in a given situation, and each has certain associated problems.

Once the individual raw signals are processed and normalized, one may then combine any number of curves (typically a given number of cycles from an individual) into an 'ensemble-averaged' curve.[47, 48] The 'average' curve of a number of individuals may then be used to obtain the average of a sample population ('grand ensemble average'). This latter procedure affords the average curve of a normal population,[26, 27] or the average curve for a patient population when answering a specific research question. Alternatively, one may numerically represent a signal using principal component analysis[51] or cluster analysis.[52] The ensemble-averaging approach is far more common and, in clinical practice, one need only the ensemble average of the given patient, plus that for a large, matched normal population.

With the ensemble averages and their variation, it is possible to determine whether various aspects (parameters) of the ensemble from a given patient differ from those of the normal population. Quantities such as the peak magnitudes, or timing to one or two peaks in a cycle, are commonly used. It is also possible to ascertain merely the percentage of time during a given cycle that a muscle is active. This requires the establishment of a threshold of activity. Sometimes this is merely a fixed per cent (e.g. 5 per cent) of the peak; perhaps a more rational approach is to record system noise over some short time interval (e.g. 10 s) with the subject resting, then process that signal, determine a mean and two or three standard deviations, then presume all signal above those ranges of standard determinations represent 'true' signal, and not noise.[49]

Once specific parameters (e.g. peak magnitude, per cent activation time) are ascertained, differences of a given patient from a normal population may be determined using an appropriate statistical test. When examining populations, rather than individual subjects, it is also possible statistically to determine differences between the pattern of entire envelopes. The Kolmogorov–Smirnov test is one such way to examine pattern differences.[53, 54]

Limitations of EMG analysis

EMG signals merely reflect voltage changes within tissues at the site sampled. Obviously those signals arise from electrical discharge throughout the body (and perhaps 'noise' from the environment, such as lighting). In general, electrical discharge from some distant site (e.g. heart muscle activity) is sufficiently small to create no problem in interpretation. However, discharge from adjacent muscles (cross-talk) is often a substantial problem. Surface electrodes are far more subject to this problem since they generally sample larger volumes of tissue. However, intramuscular electrodes are not entirely free from cross-talk, particularly since the location of the electrode is not always well documented (or documentable): if the intramuscular electrode is very near the interface of two muscles, discharge from both will obviously be sampled. Nonetheless, most investigators consider that intramuscular electrodes are essential for distinguishing the activity of two adjacent muscles, particularly those which may act in concert. Cross-talk may be explored by the clinical observer by having the patient perform activities activating a given muscle of interest though not activating adjacent muscles. For example, the popliteus muscle (which cannot be studied by surface electrodes) is activated by active internal rotation of the tibia on the femur with the subject sitting relaxed with the knee at 90°; the overlying gastrocnemius muscles are not activated in this position.[55] Conversely, when the subject is standing erect and rises on to tiptoes, the gastrocnemius muscles are activated while the popliteus is not. Such tests provide selective activation and ensure a signal is activated when appropriate and silent when appropriate, thus confirming proper electrode placement. One then has some confidence that cross-talk will be minimized when studying other activities.

The specific method of hardware or software filtering or smoothing as well as the number of analysed cycles has a distinct effect on the resulting curves and their statistical analysis. Using a consistent set of data, Gabel and Brand[56] demonstrated that it was possible to obtain statistically significant or statistically insignificant results merely by altering the processing methods. If considerable smoothing is appropriate for the question asked, then perhaps only three cycles of a reproducible activity from a normal subject may suffice.[57] Conversely, smoothing eliminates perhaps biologically important detail from the curves and, if less smoothing is used, up to 20 or more cycles may be necessary.[56]

In determining the percentage of time that a muscle is activated during a given cycle or time of an activity, the per cent activation time will vary depending upon the choice of threshold. That is, a very sensitive threshold will create a greater per cent activation time than a less sensitive threshold. For very repeatable patterns, this will not ordinarily affect the computed activation time substantially but, for non-repeatable patterns, differing conclusions may result depending upon threshold. As a minimum, it is necessary to be sensitive to this issue, and perhaps explore thresholds in a parametric fashion to ascertain sensitivity to the specific question.

As noted above, quantitatively comparing multiple EMG trials of a given individual to some population average requires normalizing. The signal intimately depends upon electrode placement, thickness of overlying soft tissues, amount of perspiration, cleanliness of the electrodes, and so on. Such variables will result in signals of somewhat differing magnitude even when placing the same electrode at the identical site on different days. Thus, normalization is required even to compare signals between test sessions (intrasubject variability). Perhaps the most common method is to compare signal magnitude of some activity to that recorded in multiple trials of a maximum voluntary contraction of the muscle in question. Even this latter quantity will be somewhat variable, and the number of trials needs to be sufficiently large to be representative, but not conducted in such a way as to introduce fatigue. Normalizing to the maximum voluntary contraction allows comparison of magnitude between various activities in a given individual, but it is important to be cautious in interpreting magnitudes between the same (or differing) activities in multiple individuals since the maximum contraction is variable between individuals. That is, one can compare timing parameters of a given patient to a population norm, but perhaps not magnitude parameters. Alternatively, if one normalizes to some activity that is standardized between all subjects (e.g. the activation of the quadriceps muscles resisting a given torque), then some inferences can be made about relative magnitudes.

When applying statistical tests to biological features, one need always ensure coherence of 'statistical' and 'biological' significance: what is statistically significant at some preselected level (e.g. 0.05) may not be biologically or clinically significant and vice versa. Particular care must be taken in interpreting EMG signals with their many layers of processing. The rather sensitive Kolmogorov–Smirnoff test, for example, may show 'statistically significant' (i.e. $p < 0.05$) differences in randomly selected sets of different trials from the same activity of a given subject; such differences can have neither biological nor clinical meaning. However, if care is taken to establish biological or clinical significance at an appropriate level of statistical significance, this is not a problem.

Energy expenditure analysis

For normal subjects, most locomotor functions are metabolically efficient. However, disabled patients often must exert considerable effort. Oxygen consumption allows a reasonably convenient way to assess changes in efficiency over time or occurring as a result of some intervention.[58–63] The measure is a good one in that it takes into account general or systemic factors such as the cardiopulmonary status of the patient. Furthermore, it relates reasonably well to computed mechanical work.[41] However, it is sensitive to such factors as walking speed, and patients must be able to reach a steady state for reasonably accurate measurement. Interestingly, the minimum oxygen consumption for a given individual typically occurs at their self-selected walking speed. As a measure for an individual patient, it is rarely useful, although it has been useful to assess various disabilities and the efficacies of various interventions in large groups of patients.

Processing locomotion data

The various locomotion techniques can quickly generate large amounts of data, even for a single patient. Most of the data is continuous, in the form of a time-varying wave (and cyclic for such activities) pattern. For comparison between trials or subjects, many forms of data must be normalized in the time and magnitude domains. While the former is straightforward, the latter is not (see discussion above on EMG). One must then select from among many specific aspects of the patterns that are believed to reflect the disease state in question, then ascertain how they differ from normal. For example, one might select peak magnitudes, timing of peaks, or areas under curves.

Single or even multiple features rarely correlate in any meaningful way with severity of disease, although there may be crude correlations between severity and a parameter such as walking speed. The reason for this is rather simple: the impact a disease or treatment has upon a patient arises from a complex compilation of many physical, social, and psychological factors. Any single locomotion measure reflects merely 'the tip of the iceberg'.

Recognizing the problem with single locomotion features, several groups have attempted to incorporate more than one. Chao and his colleagues, in a series of papers, introduced a 'performance index' incorporating many features of an analysis of patients with knee disability. A stepwise discriminate analysis selected and weighted seven gait variables out of a potential 43 to create their index.[64] This procedure generally discriminated between normal and abnormal, although not in all cases. The approach seems intuitively promising, but there remain unsolved problems. First, while the index correlated with a Harris Hip Score (an independent functional scale) when all subjects were considered, the performance index of either the normals or patients alone did not correlate with the hip score; furthermore, it failed to discriminate between the least and most affected patients. Second, when they included additional subjects in a study of 243 patients and considered 54 candidate variables, 9, rather than the original 7, were selected by the stepwise analysis, and the weighting factors changed.[65] This means the weighting is sensitive to the specific database. If such features were so sensitive, an impractically large database would be needed to ascertain weighting. Third, the weighting coefficients were different for men and women, again demonstrating sensitivity to subgroups. Finally, when the group developed a third performance index for hip disability,[66] the weighting factors again changed, illustrating a sensitivity to choice of joint. Mittlmeier et al.[67] reported a seemingly more successful effort to establish a performance index of five parameters of dynamic foot contact pressures. In this case, the index did correlate with an independent clinical rating, but sensitivity to the various features was not explored. Thus, while the approach seems promising, sensitivity of the indices to its individual elements and the database require systematic consideration.

Once the clinician establishes a procedure for selecting and processing locomotion events, there remains the task of statistical analysis. Appropriate tests must be made taking into account normalcy of data, and dependence or independence of features. Statistical levels of significance should be established on a rational basis taking into account intra- and intersubject variability, not merely some more or less arbitrary level (e.g. $p = 0.05$). To emphasize a previous point, such statistically significant levels may not be biologically or clinically important and, conversely, statistically insignificant levels may in fact be clinically important.

Requirements for the clinical relevance of locomotion

Given the general failure of locomotion analysis to enter the clinical arena, and all of the cautions noted above, it might be reasonable to ask whether technology can actually achieve clinical utility. The answer is a qualified but definite yes—qualified provided that certain criteria are met.

Doctors order tests for one of five reasons:

1. to distinguish between one of several possible disorders explaining some array of symptoms and signs ('diagnosis');

2. to select the best among several treatment options;

3. to screen asymptomatic patients at high risk for developing some problem for which prophylactic or early treatment is critical to long-term outcome;

4. to predict outcome ('prognosis');

5. to determine the severity of disease or injury ('assessment').

From the standpoint of patient care, there are no other reasons for ordering tests. Legitimate educational or legal reasons may nonetheless affect a decision to order a test. In fact, decisions over whether or not to treat a patient largely arise from the first three reasons. Knowledge of long-term outcome (prognosis) may affect recommendations for the patient's lifestyle and planning, but less often interventions per se. For most medical, administrative (disability ratings), and legal reasons, a clinical assessment is sufficiently precise, and the greater precision of various technical approaches is not required. Disease and injury produce disability as a result of interacting physical and psychological factors, and such factors are more appropriately ascertained by taking a history, observing the overall behaviour of the patient, and conducting an appropriate examination, including observations of patient movement when appropriate.

The 'acid tests' of clinical usefulness of any measure are whether that measure predicts a different outcome than would be predicted without the measure, or whether the measure suggests a different treatment than would be recommended without the measure.

Additional criteria arise from problems recognized with various forms of technology. Schwartz et al.,[14] recognizing some of these problems, suggested the following criteria for 'any method' of recording gait':

• ease

• rapidity

• economy

• a mechanism that would not change the gait

• constancy of recording (unless the gait were changed)

• measures that when changed in the recording reflected real changes in the gait.

Brand and Crowninshield,[68] unaware of Schwartz's suggestions, proposed several similar criteria. The author would add the following:

1. Any technique must be accurate and reproducible.

2. It must not alter the function it intends to measure.

3. The measure must be stable over time (i.e. not vary during a given day or week or time frame within which a disease does not change).

4. The measure must be cost-effective.

5. The measure must be independent of mood, motivation, and pain.

6. The measure should clearly distinguish normal from abnormal.

7. It should not be directly observable by a skilled clinician.

8. It should be reported in a form analogous to an accepted clinical concept.

This list is not all inclusive; others might propose equally important or more important criteria.

Few would argue with some of these criteria, although a brief amplification of some of the others is appropriate. The first four are not likely to be controversial. However, while most investigators demonstrate reproducibility of the measures, few have demonstrated accuracy by an independent 'gold standard'. For some features (e.g. walking speed) this step is unnecessary, but for others (e.g. joint motion) it may be more important owing to greater measurement errors.[28]

There have been few demonstrations of the effect of the measuring system on function, although at least one investigator has documented that intramuscular electrodes do not seriously affect gait. However, most investigators assume the laboratory environment and recording apparatus do not affect any measured parameters.

Features substantially dependent upon the patient's mood or motivation are of limited usefulness because they are not reproducible. Locomotion, to a greater or lesser degree, always depends upon the patient's disposition. Patients with chronically painful conditions may be depressed and will not move as well as they might otherwise.

A clinically useful measure should clearly distinguish normal from abnormal. However, many locomotion features (e.g. walking speed) in large populations are defined by Gaussian or non-Gaussian distributions in which data from normal subjects and diseased or injured patients substantially overlap. When this is the case, then a single measure alone may not help in making clinical decisions. Schneider and Chao[69] reached this conclusion in their study of a variety of parameters of foot–floor reaction force patterns in patients with total knee replacements. Perhaps importantly, they found statistically significant differences with a Fourier analysis of the waveforms. Wong et al.[70] and Woolen et al.[52] suggested that cluster analysis might more clearly distinguish normal from abnormal gait parameters, while Yamamoto et al.[71] reported principal component analysis techniques based upon 10 gait variables that better distinguished normal from abnormal subjects. Thus, it seems the ability to distinguish normal from abnormal may relate to the procedures for processing the data. Yet many studies fail to address this issue adequately.

The seventh criterion (the measure should be non-observable) might be more controversial, although it can be effectively argued. In clinical medicine decisions are rarely based upon single observations, but rather an array of observations. In such a situation, semiquantitative information (i.e. an estimate) of each individual observation usually suffices, assuming that observation can be directly made by the clinician. Adding precision or accuracy (by various technical means) rarely adds value. Conversely, many important functions cannot be readily observed (e.g. a patient's blood sugar, or joint moment, or level of muscle activation), yet be critical in making decisions. In such cases, technology to make the measurements proves most useful.

Finally, it is important to formulate features analogous to clinical concepts. Measures not readily contained within the language of clinical medicine will not be readily accepted.

Each of these criteria alone may not prove critical and for a given measure will not likely be equally important. The point is that the likelihood of usefulness and acceptance will increase as more consideration is given to the various criteria.

At the same time, insuring that a gait measure meets all of these criteria will not insure clinical acceptability for decision-making. Any measure must be adequately validated and clinical usefulness documented. In this context, 'validated' means that the measure correlates well with some more or less independent measure, usually one providing some overall index of function (such as a clinical rating scale). Some years ago my former colleague, Roy Crowninshield, and I went through our files on gait analysis. Among 146 papers, 44 per cent merely described some technique and proposed a potential clinical role, 32 per cent illustrated application with a small number of subjects, 8 per cent proposed a clinical application without illustrative data, and 6 per cent demonstrated an application with a reasonable number of normal subjects or patients. No paper in our files validated the measures!

While clinical rating scales incorporating various features of patient history and examination have been used for decades, few have themselves been validated. (The SF-36 Health Survey represents one such instrument that has been reasonably validated and that has achieved wide use. The SF-36 is perhaps the most widely validated quality-of-life measure.[72] It can be used for virtually any medical condition or intervention.) Brand et at.[73] attempted to validate one gait measure (the centre of pressure path) against an independent functional rating scale. However, our gait measure correlated neither with the scale nor radiographic changes. Furthermore, the measure failed to distinguish patients clearly from normal subjects. We concluded that the centre of pressure path had no utility for the intended purpose.

Clinically confirming the utility of locomotion analysis

As noted above, it is important to remember the 'acid tests' of clinical utility.

1. Does the measure (or group of appropriately combined or analysed features) predict a different outcome than would be predicted without the measure?

2. Does the knowledge of the measure change the clinician's choice of treatment?

A measure that does not meet these tests will never be truly useful nor probably gain wide acceptance.

What strategies, then, can be used to document clinical utility? There are four possible suggestions.

1. Cross-sectional studies of patients in which the clinical evaluation with the measure results in a differently predicted outcome than would be predicted without the measure; such a design might include two clinicians evaluating the same patient.

2. Longitudinal studies that document that the predicted outcome with the new measure is indeed correct.

3. Cross-sectional studies to demonstrate that clinicians recommend differing treatments with and without knowledge of the measure. Again, a multiclinician study evaluating the same patients could be considered.

4.   Prospective randomized longitudinal trials that document that the outcome of treatment (whichever is recommended) is better when the recommendation based upon the new treatment is followed.

In the first and third strategies, one would obviously need two groups of physicians, one with and one without the measure, and both patient and evaluator would need to be blinded with respect to the process of physician decision.

Clinically useful locomotion measures

There are relatively few cases where investigators have addressed clinical utility of locomotion measures in the manner outlined. For illustrative purposes, two such cases are briefly discussed. In both cases, the analysis provided a measure that could not be directly observed by the clinician, and was used to select logically between alternative treatment options, thus meeting the 'acid test'.

It is well known that certain forms of surgery, such as tendon transfers or releases, are not predictable in cerebral palsy. One reason for this is the lack of correlation between presumed muscle strength with voluntary testing and muscle activation during some activities. These patients often do not have sufficient voluntary control to assess muscle strength adequately. In addition, owing to redundancy of muscles, it is difficult to ascertain which muscles are responsible for a given pattern of limb movement. EMGs during gait or upper extremity movements can document which muscles are active at which time and how active they are relative to other muscles, potentially improving our ability to select which patients will benefit from surgery, and which form of surgery is most appropriate. Hoffer and Perry[74] pioneered the use of EMG for this purpose. For example, when the posterior tibial muscle is active throughout gait, lengthening best corrects equinus induced by that muscle. When the muscle is active only during swing, then tendon transfer is the better procedure. A similar approach has been used in ascertaining the best procedure in the upper extremity.[75, 76] However, it is important to be aware that, despite the logic and considerable potential of these approaches, utility has not been documented in large series of patients treated with and without the measure.

High tibial osteotomy is frequently performed when only one compartment of the knee joint has deteriorated because of osteoarthrosis. However, the procedure is not very predictable (particularly compared to total knee replacement) and is not performed as often as it might given greater predictability. Prodromos et al.[77] ascertained that the preoperative adduction moment correlated with outcome: patients with a low adduction moment did significantly better than those with a high adduction moment at an average follow-up of 3.2 years. In a later study with longer follow-up (3.0–8.9 years) of the same patients, all 14 patients in the low adduction group, but only nine of the 14 in the high adduction group, had good or excellent results.[78] This sort of study indeed fulfils some of the criteria outlined in this chapter, and uses some of the validation strategies.

Summary

It is clear that locomotion analysis has not gained widespread clinical use. Using specific criteria to select a potential tool and measure will help to avoid proposing methods that will probably not gain clinical acceptance, but this alone will not guarantee utility. To insure utility (i.e. to select the best among several treatment options and/or to predict outcome), clinical follow-up studies must be pursued to ensure outcomes are actually different with and without the measure or to ensure that doctors select different and more appropriate treatments when they have knowledge of the measure than when they do not. However, when the relevant precautions are taken and the appropriate strategies used, locomotion analysis can provide critical information in the evaluation of a given patient.

Further reading

Allard, P., Stokes, I.A.F., and Blanchi, J.-P. (ed.) (1995). *Three-dimensional analysis of human movement*. Human Kinetics, Champaign, Illinois.

Cappozzo, A., Marchetti, M., and Tosi, V. (1992). *Biolocomotion: a century of research using moving pictures*. Promograph, Rome.

Ducroquet, R., Ducroquet, J., and Ducroquet, P. (1968). *Walking and limping: a study of normal and pathological walking*. Lippincott, Philadelphia.

Groves, R. and Camaione, D.N. (1975). *Concepts in kinesiology*. W.B. Saunders, Philadelphia.

McMahon, T. (1984). *Muscles, reflexes, and locomotion*. Princeton University Press, Princeton.

Nigg, B.M. and Herzog, W. (ed.) (1994). *Biomechanics of the musculo-skeletal system*. Wiley, New York.

Perry, J. (1992). *Gait analysis: normal and pathological function*. Slack, Thorofare, New Jersey.

Rose, J. and Gamble, J.G. (1994). *Human walking*. Williams & Wilkins, Baltimore.

Steindler, A. (1955). *Kinesiology of the human body: under normal and pathological conditions*. Thomas, Springfield, Illinois.

Vaughan, C.L., Murphy, G.N., and du Toit, L.L. (1987). *Biomechanics of human gait: an annotated bibliography*, 2nd edn. Human Kinetics, Champaign, Illinois.

Winter, D.A. (1991). *The biomechanics and motor control of human gait: normal, elderly, and pathological*, 2nd edn. University of Waterloo Press.

References

1.   Borelli, G.A. (1989). *On the movement of animals (De motu animalium*, originally published in 1680), (trans. P. Maquet). Springer-Verlag, Berlin.

2.   Weber, W. and Weber, E. (1836). *Mechanik der Menschlichen Gehwerkzeuge*. Dieterichshen, Buchhandlung, Gottingen.

3.   Carlet, G. (1872). Sur la locomotion humaine. *Ann. Sciences Nat.*, Serie 5.

4.   Marey, E.-J. (1873). De la locomotion terrestre: chez les bipèdes et les quadrupèdes. *J. Anat. Physiol. Normales Pathologiques l'Homme Animaux* **9**, 42–80.

5.   Marey, E.-J. (1895). *Movement*. Heinemann, London.

6.   Braune, W. and Fischer, O. (1895–1901). *Der Gang des Menschen*, Vols I–IV. Teubner. Leipzig.

7.   Dercum, F.X. (1888). A study of some normal and abnormal movements, photographed by Muybridge. In *The Muybridge work at the University of Pennsylvania. The method and the result*, Vol. 9. In *Muybridge's complete human and animal locomotion* (1979). Dover Publications, New York.

8.   Dercum, F.X. (1888). The walk and some of its phases in disease, together with other studies based on the Muybridge investigations. *Trans. Coll. Physicians (Philadelphia)* **10**, 308–338.

9.   Steindler, A. (1955). *Kinesiology of the human body: under normal and pathological conditions*. Thomas, Springfield, Illinois.

10. Ducroquet, R., Ducroquet, J., and Ducroquet, P. (1968). *Walking and limping: a study of normal and pathological walking*. Lippincott, Philadelphia.

11. **Perry, J.** (1992). *Gait analysis: normal and pathological function.* Slack, Thorofare, New Jersey.

12. **Schwartz, R.P. and Heath, A.L.** (1932). The pneumographic method of recording gait. *J. Bone Joint Surg.* **4**, 783–794.

13. **Schwartz, R.P. and Heath, A.L.** (1937). Some factors which influence the balance of the foot in walking: the stance phase of gait. *J. Bone Joint Surg.* **19**, 431–442.

14. **Schwartz, R.P., Heath, A.L., and Wright, J.N.** (1933). Electrobasographic method of gait. *Arch. Surg.* **27**, 926–934.

15. **Schwartz, R.P., Heath, A.L., Misiek, W., and Wright, J.N.** (1934). Kinetics of human gait: the making and interpretation of electrobasographic records of gait. The influence of rate of walking and the height of shoe heel on duration of weight-bearing on the osseous tripod of the respective feet. *J. Bone Joint Surg.* **16**, 343–350.

16. **Cappozzo, A.** (1983). Considerations on clinical gait evaluation. *J. Biomech.* **16**, 302.

17. **Amar, J.** (1916). Trottoir dynamographique C.R. *Hebd. Séances Acad. Sci.* **163**, 130–132.

18. **Amar, J.** (1920). *The human motor.* Routledge. New York.

19. **Allard, P., Blanchi, J.-P., and Aïssaoui, R.** (1995). Bases of three-dimensional reconstruction. In *Three-dimensional analysis of human movement* (ed. P. Allard, I.A.F. Stokes, and J.-P. Blanchi), pp. 19–40. Human Kinetics, Champaign, Illinois.

20. **Cappozzo, A., Marchetti, M., and Tosi, V.** (1992). *Biolocomotion: a century of research using moving pictures.* Promograph, Rome.

21. **Vierordt, K.H.** (1881). *Das Gehen des Menschen in Gesunden und Kranken Zuständen nach selbstregistrirenden Methoden dargestelt.* Laupp, Tubingen.

22. **Gabel, R.H., Johnston, R.C., and Brand, R.A.** (1979). A gait analyzer/trainer instrumentation system. *J. Biomech.* **12**, 543–549.

23. **Andriacchi, T.P. and Strickland, A.B.** (1985). Gait analysis as a tool to assess joint kinetics. In *Biomechanics of normal and pathological human articulating joints* (ed. N. Berme, A.E. Engin, and K.M. Correia da Silva), pp. 83–102. Martinus Nijhoff, Dordrecht.

24. **Bell, A.L., Pedersen, D.R., and Brand, R.A.** (1990). A comparison of the accuracy of several hip joint center location prediction methods. *J. Biomech.* **23**, 617–621.

25. **Crowninshield, R.D., Brand, R.A., and Johnston, R.C.** (1978). The effects of walking velocity and age on hip kinematics and kinetics. *Clin. Orthop. Rel. Res.* **132**, 140–144.

26. **Winter, D.A.** (1991). *The biomechanics and motor control of human gait: normal, elderly, and pathological,* 2nd edn. University of Waterloo Press.

27. **Shiavi, R., Green, N., McFadyen, B., Frazer, M., and Chen, J.** (1987). Normative childhood EMG patterns. *J. Orthop. Res.* **5**, 283–295.

28. **Kerschot, M., Soudan, K., and Van Auderkercke, R.** (1980). Objective recording of human gait, a quantitative evaluation of two techniques: electrogoniometry and interrupted light photography. *Acta Orthop. Belg.* **46**, 509–521.

29. **Boone, D.C., Azen, S.P., Lin, C.-M., Spence, C., Baron, C., and Lee, L.** (1978). Reliability of goniometric measurements. *Phys. Ther.* **58**, 1355–1360.

30. **Lafortune, M.A., Cavanagh, P.R., Sommer, H.J. 3rd, and Kalenak, A.** (1992). Three-dimensional kinematics of the human knee during walking. *J. Biomech.* **25**(4), 347–357.

31. **Kinzel, G.L. and Gutkowski, L.J.** (1983). Joint models, degrees of freedom, and anatomical motion measurement. *J. Biomech. Eng.* **105**, 55–62.

32. **Woltring, H.G.** (1995). Smoothing and differentiation techniques applied to 3-D. In *Three-dimensional analysis of human movement* (ed. P. Allard, I.A.F. Stokes, and J.-P. Blanchi), pp. 79–99. Human Kinetics, Champaign, Illinois.

33. **Kotzar, G.M., Davy, D.T., Goldberg, V.M.,** *et al.* (1991). Telemeterized *in vivo* hip joint force data: a report on two patients after total hip surgery. *J. Orthop. Res.* **9**, 621–633.

34. **Bergmann, G., Graichen, F., and Rohlmann, A.** (1993). Hip joint loading during walking and running measured in two patients. *J. Biomech.* **26**, 969–990.

35. **Cavagna, G.A., Saibene, F.P., and Margaria, R.** (1963). External work in walking. *J. Appl. Physiol.* **18**, 1–9.

36. **Lafortune, M.A., Hennings, W., and Valiant, G.A.** (1995). Tibial shock measured with bone and skin mounted transducers. *J. Biomech.* **28**, 989–993.

37. **Crowninshield, R.D. and Brand, R.A.** (1981). The predictions of forces in joint structures: distribution of intersegmental resultants. In *Exercise and sport science reviews* (ed. D.I. Miller), pp. 159–181. Franklin Institute Press, Seattle.

38. **Andrews, J.G.** (1995). Euler's and Lagrange's equations for linked rigid-body models of three-dimensional human motion. In *Three-dimensional analysis human movement* (ed. P. Allard, I.A.F. Stokes, and J.-P. Blanchi), pp. 145–175. Human Kinetics, Champaign, Illinois.

39. **Elftman, H.** (1939). Forces and energy changes in the leg during walking. *Am. J. Physiol.* **125**, 339–356.

40. **Mansour, J.M., Lesh, M.D., Nowak, M.D., and Simon, S.R.** (1982). A three dimensional multi-segmental analysis of the energetics of normal and pathological human gait. *J. Biomech.* **15**, 51–59.

41. **Burdett, R.G., Skrinar, G.S., and Simon, S.R.** (1983). Comparison of mechanical work and metabolic energy consumption during normal gait. *J. Orthop. Res.* **1**, 63–72.

42. **Zajac, F. and Winters, J.M.** (1990). Modeling musculoskeletal movement systems: joint and body-segment dynamics, musculotendinous actuation, and neuromuscular control. In *Multiple muscle systems: biomechanics and movement organization* (ed. J.M. Winters and S.L.-Y. Woo), pp. 121–148. Springer-Verlag, New York.

43. **Dempster, W.T.** (1955). *Space requirements of the seated operator. WADC Technical Report 55–159.* Wright-Patterson Air Force Base, Dayton, Ohio.

44. **Jensen, R.K.** (1978). Estimation of the biomechanical properties of three body types using a photogrammetric method. *J. Biomech.* **11**, 349–358.

45. **Jensen, R.K. and Fletcher, P.** (1994). Distribution of mass to the segments of elderly males and females. *J. Biomech.* **27**, 89–96.

46. **Hatze, H.** (1979). *A model for the computational determination of parameter values of anthropomorphic segments.* Tegniese Verslag, Pretoria.

47. **Hershler, C. and Milner, M.** (1978). An optimality criterion for processing electromyographic (EMG) signals relating to human locomotion. *IEEE Trans. Biomed. Eng.* **5**, 413–420.

48. **Shiavi, R. and Green, N.** (1983). Ensemble averaging of locomotor electromyographic patterns using interpolation. *Med. Biol. Eng. Comput.* **21**, 573–578.

49. **Jacobson, W.C., Gable, R.H., and Brand, R.A.** (1995). Surface versus fine-wire electrode ensemble-averaged signals during gait. *J. Electromyogr. Kinesiol.* **5**, 37–44.

50. **Yang, J.F. and Winter, D.A.** (1984). Electromyographic amplitude normalization methods: improving their sensitivity as diagnostic tools in gait analysis. *Arch. Phys. Med. Rehabil.* **65**, 517–521.

51. **Wooten, M.E., Kadaba, M.P., and Cochran, G.V.B.** (1990). Dynamic electromyography. I. Numerical representation using principal component analysis. *J. Orthop. Res.* **8**, 247–258.

52. **Wooten, M.E., Kadaba, M.P., and Cochran, G.V.B.** (1990). Dynamic electromyography. II. Normal patterns during gait. *J. Orthop. Res.* **8**, 259–265.

53. **Hoel, P.G.** (1971). *Introduction to mathematical statistics.* Wiley, San Diego.

54. **Limbird, T.J., Shiavi, R., Frazier, M., and Borra, H.** (1988). EMG profiles of knee joint musculature during walking: changes induced by anterior ligament deficiency. *J. Orthop. Res.* **6**, 630–638.

55. **Barnett, C.H. and Richardson, A.T.** (1953). The postural function of the popliteus muscle. *Ann. Phys. Med.* **1**, 177–179.

56. **Gabel, R.H. and Brand, R.A.** (1994). The effects of signal conditioning on the statistical analyses of gait EMG. *Electroencephalogr. Clin. Neurophysiol.* **93**, 188–201.

57. Arsenault, A.G., Winter, D.A., Marteniuk, R.G., and Hayes, K.C. (1986). How many strides are required for the analysis of electromyographic data in gait? *Scand. J. Rehab. Med.* **18**, 133–135.

58. Fischer, S.V. and Gullickson, G. (1978). Energy cost of ambulation in health and disability: a literature review. *Arch. Phys. Med. Rehabil.* **59**, 124–133.

59. Brown, M., Hislop, H.J., Waters, R.L., and Porell, D. (1980). Walking efficiency before and after total hip replacement. *Phys. Ther.* **10**, 1259–1263.

60. McBeath, A.A., Bahrke, M.S., and Balke, B. (1980). Walking efficiency before and after total hip replacement as determined by oxygen consumption. *J. Bone Joint Surg. Am.* **62**, 807–810.

61. DuBow, L.L., Witt, P.L., Kadaba, M.P., Reyes, R., and Cochran, G.V.B. (1983). Oxygen consumption of elderly persons with bilateral below knee amputations: ambulation by wheelchair propulsion. *Arch. Phys. Med. Rehabil.* **64**, 255–259.

62. Nowroozi, F., Salvanelli, M.L., and Gerber, L.H. (1983). Energy expenditure in hip disarticulation and hemipelvectomy amputees. *Arch. Phys. Med. Rehabil.* **64**, 300–307.

63. Pinzur, M.S., Gold, J., Schwartz, D., and Gross, N. (1992). Energy demands for walking in dysvascular amputees as related to the level of amputation. *Orthopedics* **15**, 1033–1037.

64. Chao, E.Y., Laughman, R.K., and Stauffer, R.N. (1980). Biomechanical evaluation of pre- and postoperative total knee replacement patients. *Arch. Orthop. Trauma. Surg.* **97**, 309–317.

65. Laughman, R.K., Stauffer, R.N., Ilstrup, D.M., and Chao, E.Y.S. (1984). Functional evaluation of total knee replacement. *J. Orthop. Res.* **2**, 307–313.

66. Kaufman, K.R., Chao, E.Y.S., Cahalan, T.D., Askew, L.J., and Bleimeyer, R.R. (1987). Development of a functional performance index for quantitative gait analysis. In *Biomedical sciences instrumentation* (ed. J.D. Enderle), pp. 49–55. Instrument Society of America, Research Triangle Park, North Carolina.

67. Mittlmeier, T., Lob, G., Mütschler, W., and Bauer, G. (1989). Assessment of the subtalar joint function after fracture by analysis of the dynamic foot to ground pressure distribution. *Trans. Orthop. Res. Soc.* **14**, 248.

68. Brand, R.A. and Crowninshield, R.D. (1981). Comment on criteria for patient evaluation tools. *J. Biomech.* **14**, 655.

69. Schneider, E. and Chao, E.Y.S. (1983). Fourier analysis of ground reaction forces in normals and patients with knee joint disease. *J. Biomech.* **16**, 591–601.

70. Wong, M.A., Simon, S., and Olsen, R.A. (1983). Statistical analysis of gait patterns of persons with cerebral palsy. *Stat. Med.* **2**, 345–354.

71. Yamamoto, S., Suto, Y., Kawamura, H., Hashizume, T., and Kakurai, S. (1983). Quantitative gait evaluation of hip diseases using principal component analysis. *J. Biomech.* **16**, 717–726.

72. Jaglal, S., Lakham, Z., and Schatzker, J. (2000). Reliability, validity, and responsiveness of the lower extremity measure for patients with a hip fracture. *J. Bone Joint Surg. Am.* **82A**, 955–962.

73. Brand, R.A., Laaveg, S.J., Crowninshield, R.D., and Ponseti, I.V. (1981). The center of pressure path in treated clubfeet. *Clin. Orthop. Rel. Res.* **160**, 43–47.

74. Hoffer, M.M. and Perry, J. (1993). Pathodynamics of gait alterations in cerebral palsy and the significance of kinetic electromyography in evaluating foot and ankle problems. *Foot Ankle*, **4**, 128–134.

75. Hoffer, M.M. (1993). The use of the pathokinesiology laboratory to select muscles for tendon transfers in the cerebral palsy hand. *Clin. Orthop. Rel. Res* **288**, 135–138.

76. Kozin, S.H. and Kennan, M.A.E. (1993). Using dynamic electromyography to guide surgical treatment of the spastic upper extremity in the brain-injured patient. *Clin. Orthop. Rel. Res.* **288**, 109–121.

77. Prodromos, C.C., Andriacchi, T.P., and Galante, J.O. (1985). A relationship between gait and clinical changes following high tibial osteotomy. *J. Bone Joint Surg. Am.* **67**, 1188–1193.

78. Wang, J.-W., Kuo, K.N., Andriacchi, T.P., and Galante, J.O. (1990). The influence of walking mechanics and time on the results of proximal tibial osteotomy. *J. Bone Joint Surg. Am.* **72**, 905–909.

4

General principles

4.1 Classification of soft tissue disorders

Cathy Speed

The challenges

What's in a name? That which we call a rose / By any other name would smell as sweet

(William Shakespeare, Romeo and Juliet (1595), 2.2.43).

Words are, of course, the most powerful drug used by mankind

(Rudyard Kipling, 1865–1936).

Controversy relating to the relevance of taxonomy has complimented literature for centuries and there is clearly varied opinion on the subject in general. Nevertheless, nomenclature in medicine is of paramount importance, as it is by words that we convey our meaning to others, and they to us. Nomenclature is also important in the development of clear case definitions to permit interventional and epidemiological studies of specific complaints.

Box 1 Nomenclature: the insight of Lewis Carroll (1832–1898)

'When I use a word,' Humpty Dumpty said in rather a scornful tone, 'it means just what I choose it to mean—neither more nor less.'

'Then you should say what you mean,' the March Hare went on.

'I do,' Alice hastily replied; 'at least—at least I mean what I say—that's the same thing, you know.'

'Un important, of course, I meant,' the King hastily said, and went on to himself in an undertone, 'important—unimportant—unimportant—important—' as if he were trying which word sounded best.

Although musculoskeletal disorders have been recognized for centuries, the terms 'rheumatology' and 'rheumatologists' were not coined until the 1940s.[1] The terms, of course, arise from the term *rheuma*—a substance that flows—which first appeared in the literature in the first century AD. 'Rheuma' probably derived from *phlegm*, an ancient primary humour believed to originate from the brain and flowing to various parts of the body, causing ailments. From 'rheuma' arose 'rheumatism', introduced into the literature in 1642 by French physician Dr G. Baillou, initially in reference to arthritis. William Heberden used the expression as a 'common name for many aches and pains, which have yet no peculiar appellation, though owing to very different causes'.[2] 'Rheumatism' remains a popular term and, importantly, means different things to different people, including pain associated with movement with no obvious reason, any musculoskeletal complaint, articular complaints, collagen disorders, rheumatic fever, or chorea. *Soft tissue rheumatic disorders* include disorders of tendon, ligament, bursa, joint capsule, fascia, localized lesions of skeletal muscle, and nerve entrapments. Common as these disorders are, they receive scant interest relative to other areas of rheumatology. This perhaps explains why, despite the description by Dixon in 1979 of soft tissue rheumatology as the 'great new frontier land, ill defined and little explained, its features poorly categorized and far from internationally agreed',[3] it has been similarly described in 2001.[4] The slow progress in the development of the field has been partly attributable to difficulties with the description and classification of soft tissue complaints. For example, although the term 'tendinitis' first originated in 1763, and is now known to be frequently incorrect in relation to the underlying pathology, it continues to be used inappropriately. Furthermore, a structured classification system for tendinopathies did not appear until the late twentieth century.[5, 6]

Many complaints have multiple names, and descriptions have moved in and out of fashion. Some complaints are named on the basis of assumed causation, others on historical associations or colloquial terms, and some after the individual who originally described the complaint (Table 1). While some are now well established terms, many give little insight into the site or nature of the condition. In some cases the very existence of the diagnostic entity is questionable. Furthermore, the need for universally accepted diagnostic terminology and criteria has been overlooked.

Table 1 Some examples of limitations in terminology of soft tissue complaints

Limitation	Examples	Preferred terms
Assumed pathology	Tendinitis	Tendinopathy (see below)
	Repetitive strain injury	Non-specific upper limb pain
	Fibrositis	Fibromyalgia
Assumed causation or early associations	Weaver's bottom,	Ischiogluteal bursitis
	Tomato grower's shoulder	Subacromial bursitis
	Golfer's elbow	Lateral epicondylitis
	Tennis elbow	Medial epicondylitis
Named after physician	Gilmore's groin	Sportsman's hernia, athletic pubalgia
Colloquial term	Charley horse/dead leg	Deep intra/inter muscular haematoma of quadriceps

The confusion over the description and classification of soft tissue complaints is an illustration of how poorly understood many of these disorders have been—and in some cases still are. Generally, the understanding of both localized and general soft tissue disorders is in inverse proportion to the number of terms used to describe them. For example, fibromyalgia may initially have been described in the Bible by Job: 'and the days of affliction have taken hold upon me. My bones are pierced in me in the night season; and my sinews take no rest' (*Job* 30: 16–17). In modern times Gower termed it 'fibrositis' (1904) and subsequently it was described by a range of terms (Table 2). Complex regional pain syndromes have a multitude of terms, as will be further discussed in later chapters.

Some of the difficulties with terminology have been confounded by socio-political and legal environments. The prime example is 'repetitive strain injury' RSI, a disorder of epidemic proportions in the 1980s, but, again, the concept was not new. Writer's cramp was described in mail clerks in the British Civil Service in the 1830s, and was attributed by the workforce to the introduction of a new steel nib. Telegraphist's cramp was described in 1908 and was added to the schedule of diseases that were covered by the Workman's Compensation Act of 1906.

The International Classification of Diseases

Diseases of the musculoskeletal system and connective tissue can be found in the manual for the International Classification of Diseases (ICD),[7] first devised over a century ago and regularly updated. Soft tissue disorders are listed in one section and are categorized as 'disorders of muscles' (M60–63), 'disorders of synovium and tendon' (M65–78), and 'other soft tissue disorders' (M70–79). There is an additional section on 'other disorders of the musculoskeletal system and connective tissue' (M95–99). The ICD was devised for epidemiological purposes and for the evaluation of health care, and as a clinical tool it is relatively unhelpful. It can be difficult to find diagnostic entities and there are frequent cross-references and exclusions. It is also non-specific; for example, bursitis, capsulitis, and 'tendinitis' are grouped together as lower limb 'enthesopathies' (M76). Outdated terms such as fibrositis are included (with fibromyalgia listed under 'rheumatism, unspecified' (M79.0)).

A classification system for soft tissue disorders

Local soft tissue disorders

The requirements of a clinically useful disease classification system are that it should be simple, reliable, and clinically relevant. A classification system for soft tissue disorders can be developed based on the site, primary symptoms, clinical findings, and, increasingly, imaging findings (principally ultrasound and magnetic resonance imaging (MRI)).

Since pain is the cardinal symptom of musculoskeletal disease, it has been proposed that soft tissue disorders be classified by the regional site of pain—hence a diagnosis of shoulder pain, back pain, knee pain, etc. Whilst useful for epidemiological surveys, this approach lacks specificity and is not clinically helpful. Just as a cardiologist would not find the diagnosis of chest pain satisfactory, nor should the rheumatologist be content with this approach. 'Every pain has its distinct and pregnant signification if we will but carefully search for it' (John Hilton, *Rest and pain*, 1863).

Nevertheless, the symptom of pain is a useful starting point in a clinical classification system and its site, the specific tissue(s) affected, the degree of pain, and associated symptoms (e.g. instability) represent the initial stages of classification (Fig. 1 & Table 3).

The *duration* of the complaint at presentation is included, where acute can be considered as less than 3 days, subacute 4 days to 6 weeks, and chronic more than 6 weeks.

Next, where possible, the *pathology* and *aetiology* should then be described. Most soft tissue tendon injuries are traumatic in origin. A *macrotraumatic* injury involves a single episode of acute tissue destruction, whereas a *microtraumatic* injury involves either chronic overload or an acute on chronic episode. They may be due to intrinsic and /or extrinsic factors that may result in inflammation, degeneration, tear, or rupture. Most of those factors that predispose to injury have the potential to impair the response to the event(s) and are prime considerations in planning management (Tables 4 and 5).

Rupture of a normal or healthy tendon is rare but occurs in tendons that are already abnormal, for example, due to injury or when there is degeneration within the central tendon substance (which may

Table 2 Some examples of entities with multiple descriptive terms

Example	Other descriptive terms
Non-specific upper limb pain	RSI, work-related upper limb pain, telegraphist's cramp, writer's cramp
Fibromyalgia	Fibrositis, tension myalgia, generalized tendomyopathy, fibromyositis, cervical fibrositis, traumatic fibrositis
Rotator cuff tendinosis	Rotator cuff tendinitis, shoulder pain, impingement syndrome, scapulohumeral periarthritis, peritendinitis calcarea, calcifying or calcified tendonitis
Frozen shoulder	Adhesive capsulitis, Duplay's disease, periarthritis, adhesive bursitis, check rein disorder, etc.

Table 3 Classification of soft tissue pain (adapted from reference 8)

Level	Pain	Performance of task(s)
Mild		
1	None	Does not affect performance
2	With extreme exertion only; not intense; disappears on cessation of activity	Does not affect performance
Moderate		
3	Starts with activity; lasts 1–2 h after cessation of activity	Performance may be affected
4	Starts and progresses with activity; lasts 4–6 h after activity	Performance significantly affected
Severe		
5	Starts immediately upon any activity; major increase in pain on continuing activity; lasts 12–24 h afterwards	Performance may be prevented

Table 4 Aetiological factors in soft tissue injuries

Intrinsic
Age: strength and proprioception decline with age and tissues take
longer to heal
Biomechanical malalignments
Muscle imbalance
Poor technique
Hypermobility
Hypomobility (localized or general)
Poor vascular supply
Disease
Reduced vascularity and impaired innervation
Fatigued muscles (altered movement patterns)

Extrinsic
Equipment
Use Training patterns (volume, content, intensity, timing)
Environment (e.g. extremes of temperature)
Surface
Supervision
Drugs

Others
Immobilization (tissue atrophy, weakness)
Local steroid injection
Nonsteroidal anti-inflammatory drugs (can mask injury)

Table 5 Systemic disorders and drugs associated with tendon disorders

Inflammatory and crystal arthropathies
Any joint pathology that may alter biomechanics
Diabetes mellitus
Oestrogen deficiency (including menopause)
Drugs: glucocorticoids, fluoroquinolone antibiotics, anabolic steroids.
Possibly stress and overtraining: increased circulating glucocorticoids and catecholamines

be subclinical up to the point of rupture). Degenerate tendon rupture can be painless and is often attritional (e.g. long head of biceps or rotator cuff).

Clinical findings are recorded. These, along with knowledge of the pathological features of injury, allow a combined clinical and histological grading of *tendinopathies* (Table 6).

Ligament injuries are graded according to the degree of the sprain, where a 'sprain' represents tissue disruption (Table 7). Complete rupture of a ligament can occur with severe trauma.

Injuries to *muscle* are described as strains and can be graded according to the degree of tissue disruption (Table 8). Injuries can occur to the myotendinous unit or within the muscle belly itself. Muscle injuries often occur in relation to eccentric actions, where the muscle is lengthening while contracting.

Additional clinical features are noted. These address the intrinsic factors that have been described earlier. Information imaging studies and laboratory investigations are also useful.

This information provides the framework of a thorough but simple and logical classification system for local soft tissue disorders (Table 9) that is orientated towards establishing a clinical diagnosis and guiding treatment and further prevention (Fig. 1).

Bursal pathologies are inflammatory in nature ('bursitis'). The term bursa was developed by Monro in 1788 in his atlas that described 40 bursae in the human body. The society of the time, after the second bourgeois revolution, included businessmen and bankers who ensured that lubrication of 'la bourse' (the purse) encouraged a smooth running society. It is now known that there are 78 anatomical bursae on each side of body and these may occasionally communicate with a nearby joint. New ('adventitious' or 'pathological') bursae may develop in response to trauma, infection, or local inflammation. Many bursitides are described according to their common historical associations, for example, 'weaver's bottom' (ischiogluteal bursitis) and 'housemaid's knee' (prepatellar bursitis).

General soft tissue disorders

General soft tissue disorders are frequently characterized by their limited objective clinical signs and a scant knowledge of their aetiology and pathophysiology. Hence classification is rather more simplistic

Table 6 Classification of tendon disorders (adapted from reference 5)

Term	Definition	Histology	Clinical
Paratenonitis[a]	Inflammation of paratenon	Inflammatory cells in paratenon/peritendinous tissue	Swelling, pain, crepitus, local warmth, dysfunction
Paratenonitis + tendinosis	Inflammation of paratenon and intratendinous degeneration	Inflammatory cells in paratenon/peritendinous tissue + fibre disarray, decrease in cellularity, vascular ingrowth, calcification	Swelling, pain, crepitus, local warmth, dysfunction ± nodule
Tendinosis	Intratendinous degeneration due to atrophy (ageing, microtrauma, vascular, etc.)	Fibre disarray, decrease in cellularity, vascular ingrowth, calcification	A nodule and/or point tenderness may be present
Tendinitis	Symptomatic degeneration with vascular disruption and inflammatory response	Acute inflammation Inflammation plus degeneration Calcification and degeneration ± central necrosis and/or interstitial injury	Signs of inflammation or a nodule and/or point tenderness may be present
Tear	Disruption of tendon integrity		Pain, poor response to treatment, weakness, palpable gap

[a] Tenosynovitis is included in this term, as is tenovaginitis, which expresses an additional restriction of the tendon due to scarring or adhesions within the sheath.

Table 7 Ligament injuries

Grade of tear	Description	Clinical findings[a]
I	Microscopic damage to ligament (mid-substance or at bony attachment)	Localized pain and tenderness, pain on stressing ligament, no joint instability
II	Partial tear of ligament (mid-substance or at bony attachment)	Localized pain and tenderness, pain on stressing ligament, mild joint instability with firm end-point
III	Complete tear of ligament (mid-substance or at bony attachment) or bony avulsion	Localized pain and tenderness, bruising, unstable joint, no end-point.

[a] Inflammation may be present.

Table 8 Grading of muscle injuries

Grade of injury	Description	Clinical findings[a]
I	Microscopic damage to muscle or myotendinous unit	Localized pain and tenderness, pain on stretch and stress. Bruising may be evident
II	Partial tear of muscle or myotendinous unit	Localized pain and tenderness, bruising, pain on stretch and stressing. A palpable gap and weakness may be evident
III	Rupture of muscle or myotendinous unit	Localized pain and tenderness, bruising, obvious gap, weakness
IV	Avulsion of tendon attachment to bone	Localized pain and tenderness, bruising, obvious gap, weakness

[a] Inflammation may be present.

than that for local disorders (Fig. 1). In many cases any positive signs must be balanced by corroborative negative signs.

Conclusions

The need for clear, concise, and universally accepted terminology in the description and classification of soft tissue rheumatic diseases is of paramount importance. Confusion in terminology relates to the many perceived complexities of disorders of the soft tissues, and our poor understanding of them.

'What is conceived well, is expressed clearly, / And the words to say it arrive with ease' (Nicolas Boileau, *L'Art poetique*, 1674, 1).

Table 9 Examples of local soft tissue disorders

Site	Tissue	Pathology	Aetiology
Partial tear of the rotator cuff secondary to rotator cuff tendinosis related to instability-associated impingement			
Shoulder	Tendon, rotator cuff	Disruption, inflammation, and degeneration	Impingement, instability
Ankle sprain			
Lateral ankle	Ligaments: anterior talofibular ± calcaneofibular ± posterior talofibular	Disruption, graded I–III, and inflammation	Trauma and, for example, muscle imbalance due to weak peroneals

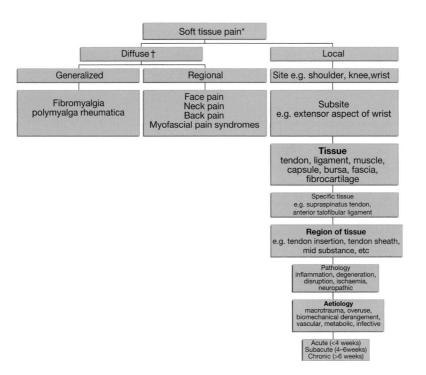

Fig. 1 A classification system for soft tissue disorders.

References

1. **West, S.** (1996). Clasification and Health Impact of the Rheumatic Diseases. In *Rheumatology secrets* (ed. S. West), pp. 1–3. Mosby, St. Louis. Mosby, Philadephia.

2. **William Heberden** (1710–1801). *Commentaries on the history and cure of diseases*, chapter 79. Hafner Publishing Company (1962).

3. **Dixon, A. StJ.** (1979). Soft tissue rheumatism: concepts and classification. *Clinics Rheumat. Dis.* **5**, 739–742.

4. **Hayem, G.** (2001). Tenology: a new frontier. *Joint Bone Spine* **68** (1), 19–25.

5. **Clancy, W. G.** (1990). Tendon trauma and overuse injuries. In *Sports-induced inflammation: clinical and basic science concepts* (ed. W. B. Leadbetter, J. A. Buckwater, and S. L. Gordon) pp. 609–618. American Academy of Orthopaedic Surgeons, Park Ridge, Illinois.

6. **Puddu, G., Ippolitto, E., and Postacchini, P.** (1976). A classification of Achilles Tendon Disease. *Am. J. Sports Med.* **4**, 145–150.

7. **World Health Organization.** (1996). *ICD-10: International classification of diseases and health related problems*, 10th Revision. American Psychiatric Press.

8. **Curwin, S. L.** (1994). The aetiology and treatment of tendinitis. In *Oxford textbook of sports medicine* (ed. M. Harries, C. Williams, W.D. Stanish, and L.J. Micheli), pp. 512–555. Oxford University Press, Oxford.

4.2 The epidemiology of soft tissue rheumatic disorders

Karen Walker-Bone and Cyrus Cooper

Introduction

Soft tissue rheumatic disorders are common—the lifetime prevalence of neck and back pain approach 70 and 80 per cent, respectively. However, the model of traditional rheumatological practice is associated with the management of articular, principally inflammatory, diseases. It is unsurprising, therefore, that a popular misconception has arisen—that the majority of disability from musculoskeletal disorders is caused by inflammatory disease. This chapter will challenge this misconception, describing our current knowledge of the burden of pain and disability in the population arising from soft tissue rheumatic complaints. However, the epidemiology of soft tissue rheumatic disorders is currently poorly characterized for several reasons. Therefore, this review will scrutinize the available epidemiological research, highlight its strengths and weaknesses, and identify those areas in which further research is urgently required.

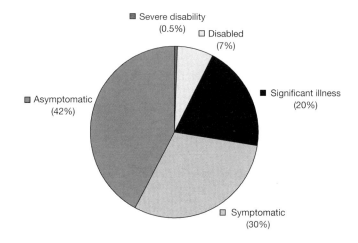

Fig. 1 The impact of musculoskeletal disorders in the general population. (Data adapted from reference 1.)

The impact of soft tissue rheumatic disorders

Figure 1 summarizes the impact of all musculoskeletal disorders in the adult population. While an infrequent cause of mortality, at any one time over half (58 per cent) of the population have musculoskeletal symptoms and, of these, approximately another half (48 per cent) describe themselves as having a significant health problem or disability as a result of these symptoms.[1] However, what is less clear is the proportion of the latter group that have musculoskeletal disability attributable to soft tissue rheumatic disorders. Currently, our best estimate is derived from a combination of population surveys of disability, consultation rates in general practice, consultation rates in secondary care, and time lost from work. However, there is no perfect method of gathering data in any of these settings and it should be borne in mind that there several biases inherent in the available data.

Population surveys of disability

Since the majority of soft tissue rheumatism is self-limiting and non-life threatening, scientific study of these disorders must extend out into the population if reliable estimates of occurrence, impact, and risk factors are to be obtained. Population-based surveys provide estimates of the extent of pain and disability in a given population, but there are difficulties with this type of research. One issue is non-response bias: those individuals who perceive themselves to be disabled are more likely to take part than those who are completely

well, and the prevalence rate obtained may be an overestimate. Another difficulty is that studies that measure self-reported indices of disability yield higher estimates than those that involve disability assessment by independent examiners. One survey in the United Kingdom circumvented these difficulties as far as possible, achieving an above average response rate of 87 per cent and validating the results of the questionnaire survey of self-reported disability by calling a random sample of subjects to take part in an in-depth interview.[2] The derived prevalence estimates suggest that 8 per cent of the adult population, and 30 per cent of individuals aged 75 years or older, have disabling rheumatic diseases. The most commonly reported causes of disability were: arthritis (mainly osteoarthritis), with a prevalence of 47/1000; back or neck disorders, 25/1000; soft tissue disorders, 18/1000; and rheumatoid arthritis, 4/1000. Of those with rheumatoid arthritis, 73 per cent were dependent, making it the most disabling disorder but its relative infrequency in the population meant that its relative ranking as a cause of disablement was low. Similar results have been found in the United States (6.3 per cent of the population aged between 24 and 75 years had joint disease with activity restriction)[3] and Canada, with 7 per cent overall rheumatological disability in the population.[4] Surveys of disability in Western populations suggest that 6–8 per cent of adults are disabled by rheumatic disorders, and that back/neck pain and soft tissue rheumatic are significant contributors to the overall burden of dependence and incapacitating pain.

Consultation rates in primary care

Compared with disorders of any other system, musculoskeletal disorders are the number one reason for consultation within the previous 2 weeks. General practice estimates in the United Kingdom suggest that 15 per cent of the population consult their general practitioner about a musculoskeletal disorder every year.[5] Of these, only 40 per cent are for pain caused by a classifiable arthritis. Of the remaining 60 per cent, half are a result of back pain and the other half are a result of soft tissue rheumatic disorders affecting elsewhere in the musculoskeletal system. Clearly, these data report only on individuals who have sought medical care and there is evidence from population surveys that a significant proportion of those with rheumatic symptoms do not consult about them. In two surveys of shoulder pain, only 40 per cent of subjects aged 70 years or older reported having sought treatment.[6, 7]

Consultation rates in secondary care

Surveys in secondary care rely on the patient having sought medical care, being (more or less) correctly diagnosed, and being referred to the appropriate specialist. The majority of general practitioners will confidently diagnose and treat by injection or physiotherapy most soft tissue rheumatism. Therefore, those referred on for secondary care are likely to represent a severely affected group who have not responded to conventional treatment, or who present diagnostic difficulties. However, there are disparities in the training and exposure of practitioners, so that comparison of rates of referral to secondary care will reflect these differences. Surveys in secondary care are made more complex because there is often a choice of specialist services for referral of these conditions. Patients might be seen in designated clinics run by Accident and Emergency, Rheumatology, or Orthopaedics, or they might be sent to sports injuries clinics, medical osteopaths, or chiropractors. For all these reasons, there are few comprehensive data about consultations in secondary care. A recent survey of rheumatological referrals in Canada found that fibromyalgia, neck and back pain, and local soft tissue rheumatism accounted for 65 per cent of new patient consultations.[8]

Time lost from work

In some countries information on the reason for absence from work for sickness is recorded and can be used to study the profile of diseases in an occupational cohort. Data collected in this way in the United Kingdom between 1988 and 1989 show that low back pain is the single largest among all causes of time lost from work, responsible for about 12.5 per cent of all sick days.[9] Surveys of time lost from work in Sweden since 1961 show that 11–19 per cent of all annual sickness absence days were taken by people with a diagnosis of back pain.[10] After low back pain, neck/shoulder problems are the next most frequent musculoskeletal cause of sickness absenteeism, representing approximately 18 per cent of all sick leave benefit claims for rheumatic disorders in Scandinavia.[11] Clearly, soft tissue rheumatic disorders and, in particular, low back pain account for a considerable proportion of sickness absenteeism.

Classification of soft tissue rheumatic disorders

Sound epidemiological research depends upon reliable case definition and ascertainment. This is notoriously difficult in the field of soft tissue rheumatic disorders. Firstly, these are a heterogeneous group of conditions ranging from precise anatomical or pathological entities such as lateral epicondylitis and carpal tunnel syndrome through to diffuse regional pains classified by putative cause, such as 'repetitive strain injury', 'cumulative trauma disorder', or 'work-related upper limb pain'. For the purposes of research on a large scale in the population or in one or more occupational settings, it is often not practical to undertake rigorous physical examination of all subjects. Consequently, it is often convenient to collect questionnaire-derived data about prevalence of pain, using regional pain sites such as 'shoulder' or 'back'. Of course, people vary widely in their definition of what constitutes shoulder pain or back pain, so that the better surveys are often accompanied by drawings of mannequins to allow the subject to mark the site of their pain, which can then be independently assessed by the investigators. Such surveys have considerably enhanced our epidemiological knowledge of the prevalence and impact of regional pain at some sites. However, these surveys of regional pain do not allow us to examine the relative contributions of specific anatomical or pathological causes or risk factors to the burden of pain at that site.

Classification of upper limb soft tissue rheumatic disorders

Strong case definition ideally involves clear clinical criteria with a patho-anatomical basis. Up until recently, there has only been one condition among all of the soft tissue rheumatic disorders to which this applies—carpal tunnel syndrome, for which there are symptom criteria, clinical provocation tests, electrophysiological investigations, and a known pathology. Unsurprisingly, it is the best-studied soft tissue condition in the epidemiological literature. Other conditions have been reasonably well characterized—lateral epicondylitis, de Quervain's tenosynovitis, and Dupuytren's contracture—but epidemiological research into these conditions has been hampered by a lack of consensus case definitions.

For most of the soft tissue rheumatic disorders, the criteria are based upon the recognition of symptoms and signs and few supporting investigations are available. Consequently, their diagnosis is firmly rooted in the clinical experience and teaching of hospital doctors, based upon severe cases. The limitations of this approach are clear—different doctors may reach different diagnoses. Few investigators have examined the reliability of clinical diagnoses of soft tissue rheumatic disorders, but there have been a small number of studies investigating the between-observer agreement for clinical diagnoses at the shoulder. Currently in the United Kingdom, medical students and trainee rheumatologists are taught the physical examination of the shoulder, based upon the textbook clinical descriptions of Cyriax.[12] However, using such systems, Bamji et al. found that three consultant rheumatologists agreed fully on clinical shoulder diagnoses in 26 patients only 46 per cent of the time.[13] Some improvement was demonstrated when the three consultants agreed on the presence of physical signs together before making their diagnoses, but complete consensus was still only reached 78 per cent of the time. Therefore, not only do clinicians perform their physical examinations differently, but also they clearly place variable diagnostic emphasis on the presence or absence of different physical signs.

However, progress has recently been made towards establishing consensus criteria for the classification of disorders of the upper limb. In 1997, the Health and Safety Executive (HSE) in the United Kingdom convened a core group of experts from the fields of rheumatology, orthopaedic surgery, occupational medicine, epidemiology, physiotherapy, ergonomics, clinical psychology, and general practice. Their expert opinions were collated and reviewed at a consensus conference.[14] A Delphi technique was employed in order to establish consensus diagnostic criteria for eight common specific upper limb disorders and for 'non-specific diffuse forearm pain' (Table 1). In all categories except carpal tunnel syndrome the criteria are wholly clinical, comprising a history component together with one or more physical signs. The agreed definitions cover many important conditions, but do not cover all areas comprehensively. In particular, no criteria were proposed for disorders of the neck that lead to symptoms in the arms or acromioclavicular joint dysfunction, subacromial bursitis, or olecranon bursitis.

These new criteria provide a good starting point for epidemiological investigation of soft tissue rheumatic disorders of the upper limb. However, the criteria offer only a skeletal framework for diagnosis and they fall short of delivering a valid, repeatable, workable protocol that researchers can employ as a tool in population or occupational

Table 1 Diagnostic criteria for upper limb disorders from the Delphi Consensus Workshop, 1997[14]

Disorder	Diagnostic criteria
Rotator cuff tendinitis	History of pain in the deltoid region *and* pain on resisted active movement (abduction, supraspinatus; external rotation, infraspinatus; internal rotation, subscapularis)
Bicipital tendinitis	History of anterior shoulder pain *and* pain on resisted active flexion or supination of forearm
Shoulder capsulitis	History of pain in the deltoid area *and* equal restriction of active and passive glenohumeral movement with capsular pattern (external rotation > abduction > internal rotation)
Lateral epicondylitis	Epicondylar pain *and* epicondylar tenderness *and* pain on resisted extension of the wrist
Medial epicondylitis	Epicondylar pain *and* epicondylar tenderness *and* pain on resisted flexion of the wrist
De Quervain's disease of the wrist	Pain over the radial styloid *and* tender swelling of first extensor compartment *and either* pain reproduced by resisted thumb extension *or* positive Finkelstein's test
Tenosynovitis of wrist	Pain on movement localized to the tendon sheaths in the wrist and reproduction of pain by resisted active movement
Carpal tunnel syndrome	Pain *or* paraesthesiae *or* sensory loss in the median nerve distribution *and one of:* Tinel's test positive, Phalen's test positive, nocturnal exacerbation of symptoms, motor loss with wasting of abductor pollicis brevis, abnormal nerve conduction time
Non-specific diffuse	Pain in the forearm in the absence of a specific diagnosis or pathology (sometimes includes loss of function, weakness, cramp, muscle tenderness, allodynia, slowing of fine movements)

settings.[15] Working from these origins, the first attempt to 'put flesh on the bones' of these new criteria has been made. A systematic examination protocol has been designed that includes inspection and palpation of the neck and upper limbs, measurement of the active and passive range of movement of the neck and shoulders using a hydrogoniometer, clinical provocation tests, and electrophysiological testing (Appendix). It is designed to incorporate all of the information (historical and clinical) required to make each diagnosis using the new HSE criteria. However, it also incorporates other relevant information such as acromioclavicular tenderness and pain in the acromioclavicular joint on adduction of the shoulder, in order to try to be as comprehensive as possible for those specific disorders for which there are currently no HSE criteria.

To date, the new examination protocol has been evaluated for validity and repeatability in a randomly selected group of 88 consecutive referrals at soft tissue rheumatology and orthopaedic clinics.[16] It has been found to be repeatable at the levels of both physical signs and diagnoses and it has been shown to give acceptable diagnostic accuracy compared with rheumatologists' clinical diagnoses. Its reliability in a population setting, where disease is less clear-cut, was also acceptable. The protocol demonstrated good reliability of box physical signs and diagnoses (kappa values 0.2–0.9).[17] It is hoped that this protocol might provide the starting point for a valid, repeatable diagnostic schedule that could be employed in future epidemiological research, representing a significant advance in upper limb musculoskeletal research.

Classification of lower limb soft tissue rheumatic disorders

Lower limb soft tissue rheumatic disorders are also common, but there are currently no agreed systems for classifying these disorders. There are no prospective studies of prognosis and outcome to define useful diagnostic entities. Rheumatology textbooks and expert consensus groups have tended to emphasize the systemic inflammatory conditions that are associated with foot or ankle manifestations, or specific painful conditions of the soft tissues such as plantar fasciitis. Consequently, epidemiological research into lower limb pain remains severely hampered, despite the potential for this being a regional pain syndrome where there could be a huge impact on the prevention and treatment of disability.

Occurrence of soft tissue rheumatic disorders

Incidence

Studying the incidence of soft tissue rheumatic disorders in the general population represents a methodological challenge. Conditions that are minor and self-limiting are unlikely to be identified unless elaborate methods of reporting are used. Furthermore, it can be very difficult to dissociate the 'first-ever' occurrence of conditions that frequently recur. One of the best surrogates for incidence in the general population is obtained from consultations in primary care. In this setting, the most useful frequency measure of incidence is the rate at which 'new episodes' develop, avoiding the difficulty of whether or not this is a 'first-ever' episode.[17] Inevitably, however, these represent an underestimate of the true incidence of the soft tissue rheumatic disorders in the population.

In England and Wales, the National Morbidity Surveys in General Practice provide a unique source of data derived from the continuous surveillance of a defined population.[5] The incidence of all soft tissue rheumatic disorders during 1991–1992 was 262.9 episodes per 1000 person years. Of these, 40.6 per cent were dorsopathies, 29.7 per cent rheumatism (excluding back), and 29.7 per cent sprains and strains. These categories are not based upon any strict diagnostic algorithms so that the criteria employed by the diagnosing physician might differ from subject to subject, but these data currently represent the best estimate of the incidence of soft tissue disorders in the population. Another advantage of this resource is that some comparison can be made across previous surveys from previous decades although there have been alterations to some of the categories for labelling soft tissue rheumatic disorders. One category that has remained unaltered, 'sprains and strains', demonstrated an increase in the number of consultations between the 1981 and 1991 surveys. There are, however, two possible explanations: this may represent a true increase in the incidence of these conditions, or an increased willingness of individuals to consult about these conditions.

Aside from the morbidity surveys in primary care, there have been a small number of surveys of specific soft tissue conditions. An example is the 2-year prospective study conducted by Hamilton of newly presenting humeral epicondylitis in primary care.[19] The incidence rate for first-ever episodes was 4/1000, with a recurrence rate approximating to 50 per cent over 1 year. In an occupational setting, Kurppa et al. evaluated the incidence of tenosynovitis and epicondylitis in a meat-processing factory among workers with strenuous manual jobs and those undertaking non-strenuous work.[20] They found an annual incidence of epicondylitis and tenosynovitis of 1 per cent among those workers doing non-strenuous jobs, but much higher rates of 12.5 per cent were found among meat-cutters, 25 per cent among packers, and 17 per cent among sausage-makers.

Prevalence

Most of the epidemiological research into the occurrence of soft tissue rheumatic disorders has taken place in the form of cross-sectional surveys in the population, primary care, secondary care, or the workplace. Consequently, there is a far richer source of data on the prevalence of these disorders than on the incidence. However, close scrutiny of this literature reveals that prevalence estimates for the same regional pain syndrome frequently vary considerably between studies. There are a number of methodological explanations for this diversity.

Point versus period prevalence

Prevalence estimations rely on identifying the number of subjects within a population who are affected by that disorder, but this can be measured at one point in time (point prevalence), or over a specified time (period prevalence). Study design varies considerably in this type of research and, even when the same parameter is being measured, for example, period prevalence, some studies will use 1 week or 1 month for the period and others much longer times. Recall bias becomes increasingly significant as the specified study period lengthens.

Symptom duration

Case definition must also specify the duration of symptoms required in order for a subject to be classified as a case. Symptoms of longer duration can be expected to differ materially from transient ones and will have a lower prevalence.

Sample size

Larger sample sizes will produce more precise estimates of occurrence rates and are absolutely prerequisite if the occurrence of less common conditions is to be measured.

Surveys of self-reported symptoms versus examination findings

The estimated prevalence of pain and disability is always found to be higher in studies that use self-reported indices, in comparison to those surveys that employ a more objective physical examination. However, the practicalities of large-scale epidemiological research do not always allow for every subject to be individually assessed and this does not make the prevalence estimates any less valid.

Choice of population to survey

Many of the epidemiological studies of soft tissue rheumatic disorders have taken place in occupational settings. Frequently, the prevalence of a particular disorder in one group of workers is compared to that in another group of workers with a different level of exposure, thereby deriving a ratio of risk for the exposed versus the non-exposed subjects. This is an extremely important type of epidemiological research. However, all the subjects in such a survey are *selected*, in the sense that they are working in a certain occupational setting at the time of the survey. Therefore, the prevalence estimates obtained cannot be meaningfully extrapolated to a population sample.

Another difficulty encountered in occupational research is selection bias: the study sample selected for investigation differs systematically from those who were not included. In occupational settings, those individuals who have been worst affected by a disorder caused or exaggerated by that occupation select themselves out of employment and escape observation, resulting in an underestimate of the problem: the 'healthy worker effect'.

Selection bias can also be a feature of population surveys. There will always be a proportion of subjects who do not fill out a questionnaire, or do not take part. Unfortunately, people who perceive themselves as having the conditions under study are more likely to take part than the completely healthy subjects—'non-response bias'. The better population-based epidemiological studies attempt to minimize this bias by reducing the number of non-responders by using several reminders and collecting a small amount of information from the non-responders, to see if they differ in basic demographic details.

Epidemiology of regional pain syndromes

Low back pain

Low back pain is a ubiquitous health problem. It represents the most frequent illness of mankind after the common cold. The majority of back pain (~90 per cent) is simple, or mechanical, in origin and a small proportion is a manifestation of systemic disease. Surveys find different estimates of prevalence, depending on the exact wording of the question. Estimates suggest that 70–85 per cent of the population have back pain at some time in their life,[21] 15–45 per cent have had back pain over the past year, 30–40 per cent in the last month,[22] and 12–30 per cent report some back pain on the day of interview (Table 2).[23]

Table 2 Prevalence surveys of back pain

Study (ref. no.)	Number	Age (years)	Gender	Prevalence (%)		
				Point	Period	Lifetime
Reigo et al.[23]	2000	20–59	M,F	23.0	—	—
Biering-Sorensen[24]	449	30–60	M	12.0	—	62.6
Biering-Sorensen[24]	479	30–60	F	15.2	—	61.4
Frymoyer and Cats-Baril[25]	1221	28–55	M	—	—	69.9
Gyntelberg[26]	—	40–59	M	—	25	—
Hirsch et al.[27]	1193	25–59	F	—	—	48.8
Hult[28]	1193	25–59	M	—	—	60.0
Magora[29]	3316	—	M,F	12.9	—	—
Nagi et al.[30]	1135	18–64	M,F	18.0	—	—
Papageorgiou et al.[31]	1884	>18	M	—	35	59.0
Papageorgiou et al.[31]	2617	>18	F	—	42	59.0
Svensson et al.[32]	716	40–47	M	—	31	61.0
Svensson et al.[32]	1640	38–64	F	—	35	61.0
Valkenburg and Haanen[33]	3091	>20	M	22.2	—	51.4
Valkenburg and Haanen[33]	3493	>20	F	30.2	—	57.8
Walsh et al.[34]	2667	20–59	M,F	—	36	58.3
Urwin et al.[35]	2841	>16	M	—	22	—
Urwin et al.[35]	2911	>16	F	—	24	—

It is unsurprising, therefore, that back pain has massive socio-economic implications. In the United States, it is the most common cause of activity limitation in people under the age of 45 years, the second most frequent reason for visits to a physician, the third most frequent cause of surgical procedures,[20] and the fifth most common reason for admission to hospital. The direct cost of back pain in the United States in 1990 was $24 billion, excluding indirect costs from sickness payments, litigation, and time lost from work. Time lost from work due to back pain is estimated to range from 2 per cent in the past month to 8–20 per cent in the past year and 25–30 per cent at some time in their life.[21] A household survey in the United Kingdom found that 5 million days of work were lost in 1995 due to back pain that the sufferers believed was attributable to work.[36]

Most episodes of back pain are not incapacitating. Over 50 per cent of attacks of back pain settle more or less completely within 4 weeks, but as many as 15–20 per cent of patients continue to complain of symptoms at 1 year.[20] However, the recurrence rate of low back pain is so high that it seems to be part of its natural history. Lifetime recurrences may be as high as 85 per cent.[33] Of people who ever experience an attack of back pain, 70 per cent will suffer three or more recurrences but these tend to occur less frequently with age. Recurrence appears to be more likely in men,[37, 38] if the back pain is associated with sciatic symptoms,[39] if the first episode occurs at a young age (25–44 years),[37, 38] and in certain occupational groups (e.g. nurses[40]). Up to 20 per cent of back pain sufferers (i.e. 5–10 per cent of the population) will continue to have some degree of back symptoms

over long periods of their life. However, the high costs of back pain relate to those who have chronic back pain, estimated to be 3–4 per cent of the population aged 16–44 years and 5–7 per cent of the population aged 45–64 years.[21]

Risk factors for low back pain

As for most other bodily symptoms, women report more back pain than men. The proportion of people reporting back pain increases from early adult life to the late 40s/early 50s and remains relatively constant thereafter. In those who continue to have back pain beyond this age, the symptoms become more frequent and more constant. Obesity and cigarette smoking are independent risk factors for low back pain.[21] Back pain is frequently associated with coexistent disease, depression being the most common co-morbidity. The other known risk factors for low back pain can be divided into occupational and psychological characteristics.

Occupational risk factors for low back pain

There are in excess of 40 articles suggesting a relationship between low back pain and physical workplace factors. There is strong evidence from this vast literature that back pain is associated with heavy physical work, especially lifting.[41] These relationships are exaggerated when a job involves driving or working beyond the employee's physical capabilities or in awkward positions. In particular, driving tractors and other large vehicles that are associated with exposure to whole-body vibration incur additional risk.[42] Physical workload has a dose–response relationship with back pain, with prolonged exposure to the workload (>10 years) increasing the risk further.[43] Workers aged over 45 years who perform heavy duty manual tasks have a 2.5 times greater risk of absence from work due to back pain than workers aged less than 24 years.[37]

The majority of the available epidemiological data on low back pain is from Western countries. Some interesting insight is provided by a recent review of the epidemiology of low back pain in low- and middle-income countries.[44] Wide variation is seen between rates of low back pain, varying twofold or more between low- and high-income countries. However, rates of low back pain are higher in the high-income countries than in the rural low-income countries. For example, rates are 2–4 times higher among Swedish, German, and Belgian populations than among Nigerian, southern Chinese, Indonesian, and Filipino farmers. A trend is observed towards higher rates of back pain among urban workers in poorer countries compared to their compatriots in rural environments. There are obviously methodological variations between the studies in different countries, but these findings seem to suggest that the relationship between back pain and hard physical labour is not entirely clear-cut.

Psychological risk factors for low back pain

Psychological factors are important in low back pain. Anxiety, depression, somatization symptoms, stressful responsibility, job dissatisfaction, mental stress at work, negative body image, weakness in ego functioning, and poor drive satisfaction have all been shown to be associated with the occurrence or persistence of symptoms.[20] Prospective studies have shown that psychological distress predicted the development of new back pain, but the experience of stress, anxiety, and depression is sometimes secondary to back pain. One study

that has attempted to tease out these relationships investigated a group of patients with low back pain on entry into a rehabilitation programme.[45] Of these patients 77 per cent met diagnostic criteria for at least one psychiatric syndrome during their lifetime and, of these, 54 per cent of those with depression, 94 per cent of those admitting substance abuse, and 95 per cent of those with anxiety disorders described these symptoms as predating the onset of their back pain. This suggests that anxiety and substance abuse frequently precede the development of back pain, but that depression may develop before or after chronic back pain. There is a complex interrelationship between psychological and other risk factors and many of the available studies have failed to adequately control for these relationships. However, in their extensive review of the evidence, the National Institute of Occupational Safety and Health (United States) concluded that there is enough evidence to suggest an association between perception of intensified workload, job dissatisfaction, and low job control and back disorders.[41]

Neck pain

Neck pain is a poor relation to low back pain. Although not as common, it is still a frequent human experience that presents similar difficulties in diagnosis and management, but it has received far less attention by way of research and its epidemiology is considerably less well elucidated.

The incidence of acute, self-limiting neck pain and stiffness is not known, but clinical evidence suggests that it is a common problem. Some of the population surveys of the prevalence of neck pain are summarized in Table 3. The point prevalence approximates to 10 per cent (9.5 per cent among men, 13.5 per cent among women). Chronic neck pain is also common—one survey found a prevalence of neck pain

Table 3 Prevalence surveys of neck pain

Study (ref. no.)	Number	Age (years)	Gender	Prevalence (%) Point	Prevalence (%) Period	Prevalence (%) Lifetime
Cunningham and Kelsey[3]	6913	25–74	M,F	10	30	—
Urwin et al.[35]	2841	>16	M	—	14	—
Urwin et al.[35]	2911	>16	F	—	17	—
Takala et al.[46]	1090	40–49	M,F	—	13	—
Takala et al.[46]	1178	50–64	M,F	—	20	—
Jacobsson et al.[47]	445	50–70	M,F	—	6.5	—
Lawrence[48]	1803	15–75	M	9	—	27.8
Lawrence[48]	1572	15–75	F	12	—	33.6
Brattberg et al.[49]	1009	18–84	M,F	—	—	26.0
Makela et al.[50]	8000	>30	M,F	10	41	71
Westerling and Jonsson[51]	2500	18–65	M,F	—	18	—
Van der Donk et al.[52]	5440	20–65	M,F	10	—	—
Cote[53]	2184	20–69	M,F	22.2	—	66.7
Bovim et al.[54]	10000	18–67	M,F	—	34.4	—
Lau et al.[55]	400	>30	M	—	15	—
Lau et al.[55]	400	>30	F	—	17	—

lasting at least 3 months of 71 per cent.[50] The determinants of chronic, mechanical neck pain are incompletely understood. The prevalence increases with age, is higher among women than men of similar ages, and is increased in smokers. One factor of controversial aetiological significance is the presence of radiographic cervical spondylosis (or osteoarthritis), which is highly prevalent beyond the age of 50 years.[48] There are no clinical features that distinguish radiological cervical spondylosis from other causes of chronic neck pain. The only available diagnostic criteria are the radiological features, but these may well only be age-related and the radiological changes correlate only poorly with neck pain.[48, 52] Significantly, one study found that cervical spondylosis is more common among those without neck pain.[56] Poor posture is a commonly hypothesized cause of neck pain, but there is no epidemiological evidence to this effect, perhaps principally because there is no agreed definition of what is constituted by 'poor posture'.

Neck pain leads to significant numbers of physician consultations—16 per cent of a population sample and 18 per cent of an occupational sample reporting recent neck pain had consulted a health care professional about their symptoms.[55, 57] It is not known how frequently neck pain leads to consultations in secondary care, but less than 1 per cent of a population sample with neck pain required operative intervention for their symptoms.[55] Neck pain undoubtedly leads to a significant impact at work—6.5 per cent of working subjects from a population sample with neck pain had required at least 1 day off work (mean days off work 8.8).[55] In Norway, 20 per cent of those reporting neck or shoulder pain occurring at least weekly described themselves as 'seriously hampered or unable to perform ordinary work' as a result of their symptoms.[58] In Sweden, older female workers with physically exhausting occupations, having pain in their neck and/or shoulders, and belonging to the lower social classes were those most likely to have to take time off work due to illness.[51]

Risk factors for neck pain

Neck pain appears to become more common with age and women report this symptom more frequently than men. Trauma, in particular whiplash injury, is an important cause of chronic neck pain. Approximately 0.5–1 per cent of the population have chronic neck pain ascribable to a motor vehicle accident.[59] In Western societies, the incidence of whiplash injuries is about 1/1000 adults in the population per year.[60] Most cases recover but, at 12 months, 20 per cent of patients remain symptomatic and 4 per cent are still suffering severe symptoms. By 2 years, 14 per cent remain symptomatic and a further 4 per cent are severely disabled.

Occupational risk factors for neck pain

Much as for low back pain, occupational factors are implicated in the aetiology of chronic neck pain. Some studies have found an association between the type of occupational work and neck pain: manual workers and office workers are among those who appear to be at highest risk.[61, 62] There appears to be a complex interrelationship among different types of risk factors such as lifting, monotony of work, vibration, and uncomfortable posture, smoking; and psychosocial factors such as work content, social support, and work load.[41] Other studies have implicated self-reported heavy workload and level of education[47] and prolonged extreme flexion of the neck.[63] Importantly, no association has been demonstrated between prolonged sitting at a work station and neck pain.[64]

Psychological risk factors and neck pain

Although studies have attempted to address the influence of psychosocial factors on neck pain, few have controlled adequately for confounding factors. However, several studies have highlighted the importance of locus of control in a job: ability to vary workload, cooperation between employees, perceived workload demands,[65] and little influence on one's own work situation.[66] As with back pain, there is an apparently complex association between mechanical risk factors, trauma, and psychological factors, as suggested by the studies described above. Depression is a frequent co-morbidity.[66]

Shoulder pain

There have been wide variations in the systems of classification used in studying the epidemiology of shoulder disorders. Some studies have used a regional classification: 'neck–arm pain', 'neck–shoulder–upper arm pain', 'cervicobrachial pain'. Such classifications are all likely to be overlapping but not identical in their use. In other studies, the operational definition has been ambiguous. Pope et al. illustrated the difficulties of this type of research: they employed four different definitions of shoulder pain to estimate the occurrence of symptoms derived from answers to a questionnaire about musculoskeletal symptoms.[68] They demonstrated that the 1-month period prevalence of shoulder pain ranged from 31 to 48 per cent in their sample, depending on which of four definitions were employed to the same data. Interestingly, the lowest estimate was obtained by the question that asked directly about shoulder symptoms. This survey illustrates the poor specificity of symptom based definitions of shoulder pain, almost certainly accounting for the wide disparities in prevalence estimates shown in Table 4.

In the general population, around 1 per cent of people experience a new episode of shoulder pain annually, with rates increasing to 2.5 per cent in the fourth and fifth decades of life.[69] The prevalence of shoulder symptoms increases with age, so that around 15–20 per cent of middle and older age groups experience shoulder symptoms in any 1 month. Women report shoulder pain more frequently than men at all ages. In the United Kingdom, some 6.6 per 1000 of the population consult in primary care with a new episode of shoulder pain each year,[5] while the rates of consultation in Dutch general practice are somewhat higher (up to 12–25 per 1000 adults).[72] The apparent wide discrepancy between consultation and prevalence rates is explained partly by the duration of each episode of shoulder pain, and partly by estimates that only 40 per cent of adults consult about each episode of pain.[6]

Risk factors for shoulder pain

Several general medical conditions are associated with shoulder pain, for example, osteoarthritis, stroke, multiple sclerosis, inflammatory arthritis, polymyalgia rheumatica, fibromyalgia syndrome, and diabetes mellitus. However, those studies involving a physical examination component suggest that the majority of shoulder pain is 'non-articular rheumatism' arising from the supporting soft tissues around the joint.[73] Trauma (including contusion, fracture, minor instability, and joint displacement), surgical intervention and intravenous infusion, thoracic kyphosis, reduced mobility of the cervicothoracic spine and adjacent ribs, and impairment of consciousness have all been reported to have a causal relationship with shoulder disorders.[72, 73] Undoubtedly, neck and shoulder pathology overlap

Table 4 Population surveys of shoulder pain

Study (ref. no.)	Number	Age (years)	Gender	Prevalence (%)		
				Point	Period	Lifetime
Cunningham and Kelsey[3]	6913	25–74	M,F	—	6.7	—
Urwin et al.[35]	2841	>16	M	—	14	—
Urwin et al.[35]	2911	>16	F	—	17	—
Takala et al.[46]	1090	40–49	M,F	—	10	—
Takala et al.[46]	1178	50–64	M,F	—	22	—
Jacobsson et al.[47]	445	50–70	M,F	—	6.7	—
Lawrence[48]	3375	15–75	M,F	—	—	16
Makela et al.[50]	8000	>30	M,F	2	—	—
Pope et al.[68]	312	18–75	M,F	20	31–48	—
Allander[69]	15268	40–74	M,F	20	—	—
Chard and Hazleman[70]	318	>70	M	17	—	—
Chard and Hazleman[70]	326	>70	F	25	—	—
Bergenudd et al.[71]	319	53	M	—	13	—
Bergenudd et al.[71]	255	53	F	—	15	—

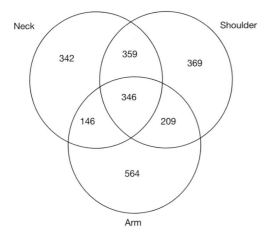

Fig. 2 Prevalence of musculoskeletal complaints of the neck and upper limb in 6913 men from a random population sample in the United Kingdom. (Data from reference 74.)

frequently: almost 40 per cent of adults with shoulder pain reported concomitant neck complaints in a survey in the United States.[74] Figure 2 illustrates this striking overlap in a population survey in the United Kingdom examining the 1-week period prevalence of neck, shoulder, and arm pain—many subjects have pain simultaneously in all three regions.[75]

Psychosocial risk factors for shoulder pain

There is limited evidence from epidemiological studies, but depression, poor coping skills, and catastrophic belief symptoms are implicated in the perpetuation of shoulder pain.[73]

Occupational risk factors for shoulder disorders

Broadly, the occurrence of shoulder disorders depends on the type of work and the population of workers included. The studies in occupational groups are also methodologically heterogeneous: the classification systems are diverse and some involve self-reported symptoms whilst others entail scrupulous physical examination to a predefined algorithm. Consequently, out of 13 reviewed papers examining the occurrence of shoulder disorders in industry, the shipyards, and agriculture, odds ratios vary as widely as 1.9–11.0.[41] Occupational factors that have been implicated are: workplace design, repeated or prolonged elevation of the shoulder, vibration, overuse, high workload, stressful work, monotonous work, poor job satisfaction, lack of autonomy and job control, perceived high demands, isolation and hostility, poor social support, and infrequent breaks. The epidemiological research into shoulder disorders is considerably behind that into back pain, but it is interesting that similar occupational risk factors are being highlighted for both these different regional pain syndromes.

Epidemiology of adhesive capsulitis

Some studies have attempted to differentiate the specific shoulder disorders from each other. Adhesive capsulitis is estimated to affect 2–3 per cent of the general population,[76] and up to 10–20 per cent of the diabetic population.[77] The association with diabetes is not understood, but is more frequently observed in insulin-dependent than non-insulin-dependent diabetics. In diabetic patients, adhesive capsulitis tends to occur at a younger age and is more frequently bilateral.

Epidemiology of shoulder tendinitis

Pathological studies suggest that it is usual, by the fifth decade of life, for the rotator cuff tendons to have developed degenerative changes—characteristically, thinning and fibrillation at the 'critical zone', or hypovascular area of the cuff. Chronic rotator cuff tears are a frequent finding at post mortem. Epidemiological surveys suggest that abnormalities of the rotator cuff tendons are a frequent cause of painful shoulder syndromes,[70, 78] although much of rotator cuff disease may be asymptomatic during life. There have been several studies of shoulder tendinitis among different occupational groups, which have produced widely different estimates of the occurrence of tendinitis in association with types of occupational exposure. However, the case definitions and methodologies employed in these studies vary considerably. Research in this field could be considerably enhanced with the advent of a validated examination protocol that could be employed in different occupational settings.

Elbow pain

There have been few population-based studies into the epidemiology of elbow pain (Table 5). The prevalence of ever having had elbow pain was estimated to be 4 per cent in a population in the United States.[4] However, the 1-year prevalence in a Finnish survey was 7 per cent among 40–50 year olds and 14 per cent among those aged over 50 years.[46] The 1-month prevalence was recently found to be 6 per cent in a population in the United Kingdom.[35]

Epidemiology of lateral epicondylitis

Lateral epicondylitis (tennis elbow) is the most common non-articular disorder of the elbow.[79] Using a case definition of pain lasting for at least 1 month exacerbated by carrying, associated with tenderness over the epicondyle and pain on resisted pronation (similar to the definition in Table 1), a point prevalence of 2.5 per cent was obtained among a population of 31–74 year olds.[69] Using a case definition of reproducible tenderness using direct pressure on the epicondyle, as assessed by an examining physician, a point prevalence of 2 per cent was found among a manufacturing workforce.[80] It is reassuring that the studies with a very precise clinical case definition find lower frequency estimates than the studies of undifferentiated elbow pain.

The only study of the incidence of lateral epicondylitis among tennis players relied on self-reported diagnoses and was retrospective, but found an incidence as high as 9 per cent over the 2-month study period.[81] However, only a small percentage (<5 per cent) of the cases seen in clinical practice have arisen from the sport. The condition appears to peak among 40–60 year olds and is unusual at less than 30 years.[18] Men and women appear to be affected equally. It tends to occur in the dominant arm. The majority of affected individuals are not manual workers or athletes and many cannot describe any precipitating factors.

Lateral epicondylitis is generally considered to be a self-limiting disorder, with improvement occurring over 1 year, with or without treatment.[82] However, there is evidence to the contrary, one study having found that the majority of sufferers from one rheumatology clinic were still symptomatic after 1 year.[83] There is also evidence that this is a relapsing condition. In one study, more than 50 per cent of those individuals followed up over 18 months experienced a recurrence.[18]

Occupational risk factors for elbow pain

There is some evidence to indicate an association between elbow pain and occupation, although whether a particular working activity actually causes lateral epicondylitis or merely aggravates an underlying tendency to the condition is not clear.[41] One cross-sectional survey in the meat-processing industry found that elbow pain occurs more frequently among those with strenuous jobs, such as meat-cutters, sausage-makers, and packers, than among those performing less physically demanding jobs, but that the prevalence of clinically verified epicondylitis was the same for both groups.[81] However, a prospective study in the same industry found a significantly increased risk ratio of incident clinical epicondylitis among sausage-makers and meat-cutters than among office workers.[20]

Epidemiology of carpal tunnel syndrome

Carpal tunnel syndrome results from compression of the median nerve at the wrist, frequently of unknown cause. It is unique among the soft tissue disorders in that the symptoms, signs, and associated electrophysiological abnormalities allow the 'classical case' to be clearly defined. However, in population-based epidemiological research, the case definition becomes much less clear—symptoms without signs, signs with normal tests, and abnormal electrophysiology in asymptomatic individuals. Conceptually, carpal tunnel syndrome represents a continuum of physiology and pathology, not a

Table 5 Prevalence of elbow pain and epicondylitis

Study (ref. no.)	Number	Age (years)	Gender	Prevalence (%) Point	Period	Lifetime
Elbow pain						
Cunningham and Kelsey[4]	6913	25–74	M,F	—	—	4
Urwin et al.[35]	2841	>16	M	—	6	—
Urwin et al.[35]	2911	>16	F	—	6	—
Takala et al.[46]	1090	40–49	M,F	—	7	—
Takala et al.[46]	1178	50–64	M,F	—	14	—
Lateral epicondylitis						
Allander[69]	15268	31–74	M,F	2.5	—	—

dichotomy consisting of those with the disorder and those without. For the purposes of epidemiological research, case definition must be precise at the outset. The more precise the diagnosis, the more selective the picture is likely to be.

Diagnostic criteria for carpal tunnel syndrome

Electrophysiological testing is widely regarded as the 'gold standard' for research into carpal tunnel syndrome. Certainly, these tests have a high level of repeatability and results can be conveniently compared between different centres. However, there is evidence that even the most sensitive tests detect only 90 per cent of 'classical' clinical cases. Unfortunately, clinical provocation tests, including those of Tinel and Phalen, are found to be negative in some individuals with classical symptoms and have been shown to have poor validity against electrophysiology.[84, 85] For example, an occupation-based survey examining the association between symptoms, signs, and electrophysiology found that only 5 per cent of subjects with at least one positive finding met all three criteria.[86] Among the different clinical tests, the use of a hand diagram and Tinel's tests give the highest specificity with respect to electrophysiology.[87, 88]

The majority of validation studies of clinical signs are performed in the secondary care setting, using those who are awaiting carpal tunnel decompression as the 'cases' and asymptomatic subjects as 'controls'. However, one study recently demonstrated that the sensitivity and specificity of the clinical tests vary depending on the comparison group, such that, in those with normal electrophysiology, there are far more likely to be false-positive provocation tests in the presence of hand symptoms than in asymptomatic subjects.[89] This suggests that the clinical tests are rather less likely to be useful discriminators in population-based research than in the more clear-cut hospital-based research. However, one population-based survey of subjects with hand symptoms demonstrated an association between delayed median nerve latencies and self-reported disability,[90] suggesting that, despite the diagnostic difficulties, there is a functionally important entity occurring in these individuals.

Estimates of the incidence of carpal tunnel syndrome in the United States range from 1.25/1000 person years to 3.46/1000 person years.[91, 92] There is a suggestion, from secular trends, that the incidence is increasing although it is not clear if this represents a true change or alterations in the accuracy of diagnosis using electrophysiological techniques.[92] In the United Kingdom, data are available from a large cohort of women who participated in the Oxford Family Planning Association Study.[93] The crude incidence was 1/1000 women-years presenting in secondary care because of symptoms or signs suggestive of carpal tunnel syndrome. In comparison, data from primary care suggest that 2.3/1000 women-years present to primary care with symptoms or signs of carpal tunnel syndrome.[5] The probable explanation for this discrepancy is that less than half of the cases seen in primary care are referred on for hospital management. Furthermore, using a precise case definition of symptoms of pain, tingling, or numbness in the thumb, index, or middle fingers occurring twice a week or more and waking at night, and neurophysiological testing, the point prevalence has been estimated to be 5.8 per cent in women and 0.6 per cent in men.[94] This prevalence exceeds that which would be expected from the incidence rates above, suggesting that a high proportion of individuals with symptoms do not reach medical attention.

Risk factors for carpal tunnel syndrome in the population

Carpal tunnel syndrome is considerably more frequent in women than in men at all ages. Incidence rates in women appear to increase steadily up to a peak at age 45–54 years, followed by a decline thereafter, whilst incidence rates in men appear to increase steadily with age. This female preponderance is unexplained, but hormonal factors may play a part since there is an excess of carpal tunnel syndrome during pregnancy and breastfeeding, after a hysterectomy or oophorectomy, and among women taking the oral contraceptive pill or hormone replacement therapy.[95] Associations are also seen with some other hormonal conditions such as acromegaly, hypothyroidism, and diabetes. Another important risk factor is obesity.[96] Other associations are seen with coexistence of an inflammatory musculoskeletal condition, a family history of carpal tunnel syndrome, and non-participation in sports. Clearly, the associations with endocrine and metabolic disorders and inflammatory arthritis explain only a small proportion of cases and the most important risk factors are female gender and obesity.

Occupational risk factors for carpal tunnel syndrome

The prevalence of carpal tunnel syndrome has been studied more frequently in occupational settings than in the general population. A meta-analysis of these studies has been recently published.[97] Seventeen studies were identified, ranging across several different occupational groups, including aeroplane manufacturing, forestry workers, grocery checkers, and heavy metal workers. There were wide variations between studies for the risk estimates obtained (e.g. ranging from 1.05 in supermarket checkers to 18.75 in forestry workers). The meta-analysis showed that risk estimates were consistently higher in studies of workers in the United States than in European studies, but European studies more consistently relied upon electrophysiological testing. The meta-analysis models showed that force and repetition involved in the occupation were significant risk factors for carpal tunnel syndrome. Other work factors that appear to be important are perception of employer's attention to health and safety, cumulative hours in a job, use of power tools and machinery, exposure to vibration, bending or twisting of an arm or hand, and job control.[41] To date, no associations have been found between use of a keyboard and carpal tunnel syndrome.

Wrist/hand pain

The differential diagnosis of wrist/hand pain is potentially very diverse. Epidemiological surveys estimating period prevalence suggest that 10.5 per cent of the general population have had wrist/hand pain lasting for 1 day or longer in the past month and that 12 per cent have had hand pain lasting for more than a week over the past month.[35] Although such studies do not allow any insight into the type of disorders causing pain, they do suggest that this is a relatively common symptom.

Epidemiology of tenosynovitis/tendinitis of the wrist

To date, there have been no population-based epidemiological surveys of hand/wrist tenosynovitis that have included a physical examination. Data collected from primary care in the United Kingdom suggest that the incidence of tenosynovitis, tendinitis, synovitis, and bursitis combined is 10.9/1000 persons per year.[5] In the US National Health

Interview, 2 per cent of adults reported that a doctor had told them that they had 'tendinitis'.[98] Tenosynovitis is more common in women than men at all ages and the incidence peaks in middle age.

In the spectrum of tenosynovitis, peritendinitis crepitans represents the most clear-cut condition, defined as pain, swelling, and crepitus at the anatomical site where the thumb extensors cross the radial wrist extensors. This disorder may be caused by certain types of occupations and is recognized as a prescribed condition. There have been surveys among several occupational groups. Car factory workers, board manufacturers, sewers, and packers have all been shown to have increased relative risk of developing tenosynovitis when compared with non-manual workers (odds ratios 3.9–8.0).[20, 99, 100] Work combining high force and repetition appears to carry the greatest risk, especially when occupational change necessitates unaccustomed movements, when work is resumed after absence, or when there is direct local trauma.[99]

The number of compensation claims for tenosynovitis is increasing rapidly despite the fact that doctors have been advised against making the diagnosis 'unless they have good evidence that there is inflammation of the synovium around a tendon'.[101] In addition to statutory Department of Social Security claims, workers have also initiated civil cases through the courts for compensation. This area has become further complicated by the unrestricted use of terminology such as 'repetitive strain injury'. Such terms are considered to be best avoided.[102]

Epidemiology of De Quervain's tenosynovitis

Another of the more discrete entities among the spectrum of tenosynovitis is de Quervain's stenosing tenovaginitis (tenosynovitis). This is characterized by thickening and associated synovial inflammation of the fibrous sheath of abductor pollicis longus and extensor pollicis brevis. It is thought to occur most frequently among women aged 30–50 years.[103] There is an association with rheumatoid arthritis, psoriatic arthritis, and other inflammatory arthritides and it may be triggered by direct trauma. It is also described during pregnancy and in the postpartum period.[104] There is limited evidence that this condition may have occupational associations, but the majority of cases are not thought to be related to occupation.[105]

Epidemiology of trigger digit

Trigger finger, or thumb, also known as stenosing digital tenosynovitis, or snapping finger or thumb, is thought to be a repetitive disorder of the hand. The anatomical lesion is a tenosynovitis of the flexor tendon, often associated with a nodule. It has been suggested that this phenomenon occurs more frequently among long distance lorry drivers or those who perform occupational repetitive tasks, but the evidence is inconclusive.[106]

Epidemiology of Dupuytren's contracture

This is a relatively common condition characterized by nodular thickening and contraction of the palmar fascia, drawing one or more fingers into flexion at the metacarpophalangeal (MCP) joints. The classical case, with flexion contractures, is easily recognized. However, early or more minor forms are more difficult to diagnose reliably. Population-based prevalence estimates are shown in Table 6. Clearly, Dupuytren's contracture is more frequent among men than women at all ages and is increasingly common with age. Differences between the

Table 6 Prevalence surveys of Dupuytren's contracture

Study (ref. no.)	Age (years)	Prevalence (%)	
		Male	Female
Hueston[107]	45–59	16.3	13.0
	>60	25.6	20.4
Early[108]	45–54	4.1	0.5
	55–64	10.1	1.4
	65–74	14.1	6.2
	>75	18.1	9.0
Mikkelsen[109]	35–44	1.9	0.2
	45–54	7.5	1.3
	55–64	17.9	2.9
	65–74	30.8	10.1
	75–89	30.5	17.6
Gordon[110]	36–45	6.6	12.6
	46–55	15.4	9.4
	56–65	25.6	23.9
	66–75	26.0	33.0
	76–85	28.7	35.0

population estimates are almost certainly explained by the difficulties in assigning the early or more minor variants to 'case' or 'not case'.

Inheritance, diabetes mellitus, epilepsy, and alcoholism have all been reported as aetiological factors. A pathogenetic role for local repetitive and occupational trauma remains unproven, although one hypothesis is that a single injury or the subsequent immobilization in those who have a predisposition may exacerbate Dupuytren's contracture. Against this, two surveys of merchant mariners and locomotive workers found an incidence among the heavy manual workers similar to that among clerical workers.[106, 111] More recently, exposure to hand-transmitted vibration has been implicated—Dupuytren's contracture occurs more commonly among quarry-drillers and stone-carvers, compared to stone-workers performing manual work but not exposed to vibration.[112]

Epidemiology of hip pain

With the exception of osteoarthritis, there are remarkably few data about the prevalence and causes of hip pain. One survey in the United Kingdom found that 7 per cent of men and 11 per cent of women report pain lasting at least 1 week out of the past month.[35] Prevalence of hip pain increases with age in both sexes, probably reflecting the increasing risk of osteoarthritis.[113] A frequent cause of hip pain is bursitis, which may arise from any of the 18 bursae around the joint. Little is currently known, however, about the epidemiology of hip bursitis.

Epidemiology of knee pain

Knee pain is a common problem. It has been estimated that 10 per cent of adults experience at least 1 month of significant daily knee pain in a year and that 19 per cent of women and 20 per cent of men experienced knee pain over at least 1 week in the past month.[35] The frequency increases with age, from 6 per cent in the third decade of life to 18 per cent in the seventh, with a slight female preponderance. The patient who has mechanical knee pain without effusion or with a non-inflammatory effusion has regional knee pain. Regional knee pain is frequently discordant with radiographic changes even in the older age groups. Anterior knee pain syndrome is a frequent bilateral phenomen described in adolescent girls, rather than boys.

Epidemiology of knee bursitis

There are a number of periarticular knee bursae, including the deep infrapatellar (or retropatellar) bursa, the anserine bursa, and the prepatellar bursa. All are sites associated with acute inflammation, occasionally secondary to infection or gout. However, these sites are also predisposed to inflammation consequent to acute or repetitive trauma—'housemaid's knee' (prepatellar) and 'parson's knee' (infrapatellar). As these eponyms suggest, these are seen most commonly among occupational groups where kneeling is a factor, such as carpet-laying.

Epidemiology of ankle pain

The prevalence of ankle pain in the general population may be as high as 4.1 per cent.[113] There has been very little epidemiological research in this field and there are no consensus systems of classification for ankle disorders. Where studies are performed, foot and ankle pain are frequently 'lumped' together.

Epidemiology of foot pain

A survey in the United Kingdom found that 4.8 per cent of the population have foot problems.[113] Using a broader definition, a rather higher prevalence was found in the United States, where as many as 40 per cent of the population were thought to have 'foot/ankle dysfunction'.[114]

Epidemiology of fibromyalgia syndrome

This syndrome is characterized by chronic generalized musculoskeletal pain. Consensus criteria for this disorder were developed in 1990.[115] However, accurate accounts of the symptoms of this disorder are found in the literature as early as the mid-1800s. Over time, these symptoms have been classified and re-classified as fibrositis, psychogenic rheumatism, myogelosis, and muscle pain syndrome. Consequently, epidemiological research has been difficult, and incomparable between studies. In 1990, the American College of Rheumatology (ACR) defined it as 'bilateral pain, above and below the waist, present for at least 3 months, associated with touch positive tender points positive in a minimum of 11 out of 18 specified locations'. However, these criteria remain controversial since, although they provide a useful means of characterizing and managing individuals in a clinic setting, it is not clear that this is a distinct disease entity. One study in the United Kingdom found that, while tender point counts were higher among those who reported pain and among those with

widespread, as opposed to regional pain, most individuals with chronic, widespread pain had fewer than 11 tender points.[116] It may be that fibromyalgia syndrome represents one end of a continuum of pain and tenderness, so that the strict diagnostic cut-off (i.e. 11 or more tender points indicating fibromyalgia and fewer than 11, not fibromyalgia) might be creating an artificial distinction.[117]

Population-based prevalence estimates from the United States and Sweden found that 2 per cent of the population are affected at any one time.[118, 119] Approximately 1 per cent of those attending primary care, and around 20–30 per cent of those referred to rheumatology clinics in North America, have fibromyalgia.[8] There is a significant female preponderance, such that 80–90 per cent of those diagnosed are female, with a mean age of 30–60 years, and the prevalence increases with age. The identified risk factors include high anxiety and depression levels, low levels of education and family income, and divorce. Associations are seen with sleep disturbance, headaches, irritable bowel syndrome, paraesthesiae, Raynaud's type symptoms, and psychological disorders.

The evidence is increasing that fibromyalgia impacts significantly in Western societies.[120] Most patients report that chronic pain and fatigue adversely affect their quality of life and impair their ability to compete for employment. Such difficulties as poor stamina, reduced physical efficiency, loss of mental sharpness, fear of poor performance, difficulty conforming to usual work hours, and inability to sit or stand for prolonged periods contribute to poor employment records. However, the extent of disability varies from one country to another, probably reflecting different cultural philosophies and socioeconomic factors such as welfare payments. A survey in the United States found that 19.7 per cent of those diagnosed with fibromyalgia had applied for disability payments and 7.3 per cent were in receipt of benefit.[121] Assessment of the extent of disability in chronic pain disorders is notoriously difficult, and rheumatologists generally feel more confident at assessing disability from conditions such as rheumatoid arthritis. However, one study showed that fibromyalgia patients demonstrated functional impairment at work similar to that of those with rheumatoid arthritis.[121] Dysfunction associated with chronic pain conditions correlates poorly with the severity of pain experienced by the sufferer, and this may lead to suspicion that the patient is not genuinely impaired. To date, there is no validated means to assess disability in fibromyalgia, although the Fibromyalgia Impact Questionnaire and the Quality of Life scale are useful. However, the relationship between disability and fibromyalgia is complex—past experiences, education level, motivation, and fatigue are all important components.

Conclusion

Soft tissue rheumatic disorders are common and are, therefore, major contributors to chronic musculoskeletal pain and disability. Despite this, epidemiological research remains sparse and is poorly comparable across studies, due to the lack of a consensus approach to case definition. Good quality research based upon consistent strategies is urgently required in order to better understand the features which predict occurrence and recurrence, leading to the development of prevention strategies and early management techniques in order to reduce this burden in our population.

Appendix: the Southampton examination proforma for surveillance of soft tissue upper limb disorders

MRC
MEDICAL RESEARCH COUNCIL
and

ARC
ARTHRITIS AND RHEUMATISM COUNCIL
FOR RESEARCH

The Southampton
examination proforma for
surveillance of soft tissue
upper limb disorders

EXAMINATION PROFORMA

Interviewer: ☐   Serial No: ☐☐☐☐☐

Date ☐☐ ☐☐ ☐☐
     day month year

Height cms ☐☐☐   Weight kg ☐☐☐.☐

NECK

Range of movement (°)?

		Active Movement
Rotation	right side	☐☐☐
	left side	☐☐☐
Flexion		☐☐☐
Extension		☐☐☐
Lateral flexion	right side	☐☐☐
	left side	☐☐☐

SHOULDERS

Left Side

1 History: Where is the pain located?	Yes	2 Palpation: Where is it maximally tender?	Yes
No pain	☐	No tenderness	☐
Deltoid area	☐		☐
Anterior shoulder	☐		☐
Acromio clavicular joint	☐		☐
Subacromial bursa	☐		☐
Diffuse	☐		☐
Elsewhere?	☐		☐

(describe)_____   (describe)_____

3   Pain on resisted movement?

	Yes
Elbow flexion	☐
Forearm supination	☐
External rotation	☐
Internal rotation	☐
Abduction	☐

Painful arc? No ☐ Yes ☐   **Range of movement (°)?** ☐☐☐ ☐☐☐ ☐☐
☐

(neutral)   (started)   (stopped)

4   Stress test, acromioclavicular joint

Acromioclavicular joint pain on adduction?   No ☐ Yes ☐

5   Range of movement (°)?

	Active Movement	Passive Movement
Abduction	☐☐☐ °	☐☐☐ °
Forward flexion	☐☐☐ °	☐☐☐ °
Extension	☐☐☐ °	☐☐☐ °
External rotation	☐☐☐ °	☐☐☐ °
Internal rotation	☐☐☐ °	☐☐☐ °

SHOULDERS

Right Side

1 History: Where is the pain located?	Yes	2 Palpation: Where is it maximally tender?	Yes
No pain	☐	No tenderness	☐
Deltoid area	☐		☐
Anterior shoulder	☐		☐
Acromio clavicular joint	☐		☐
Subacromial bursa	☐		☐
Diffuse	☐		☐
Elsewhere?	☐		☐

(describe)_____   (describe)_____

3   Pain on resisted movement?

	Yes
Elbow flexion	☐
Forearm supination	☐
External rotation	☐
Internal rotation	☐
Abduction	☐

Painful arc? No ☐ Yes ☐   **Range of movement (°)?** ☐☐☐ ☐☐☐ ☐☐
☐

(neutral)   (started)   (stopped)

4   Stress test, acromioclavicular joint

Acromioclavicular joint pain on adduction?   No ☐ Yes ☐

5   Range of movement (°)?

	Active Movement	Passive Movement
Abduction	☐☐☐ °	☐☐☐ °
Forward flexion	☐☐☐ °	☐☐☐ °
Extension	☐☐☐ °	☐☐☐ °
External rotation	☐☐☐ °	☐☐☐ °
Internal rotation	☐☐☐ °	☐☐☐ °

ELBOWS

Right Side

1 History: Where is the pain located?	2 Palpation: Where is it maximally tender?
Yes	Yes
No pain ☐	No tenderness ☐
Lateral elbow ☐	☐
Medial elbow ☐	☐
Posterior elbow ☐	☐
Other ☐	☐
(describe)_____	(describe)_____

Other observations/procedures:

	No	Yes	Crepitus? Yes
Pain lateral elbow on resisted wrist extension?	☐	☐	☐
Pain medial elbow on resisted wrist flexion?	☐	☐	☐
Swelling over posterior elbow joint?	☐	☐	☐

Left Side

1 History: Where is the pain located?	2 Palpation: Where is it maximally tender?
Yes	Yes
No pain ☐	No tenderness ☐
Lateral elbow ☐	☐
Medial elbow ☐	☐
Posterior elbow ☐	☐
Other ☐	☐
(describe)_____	(describe)_____

Other observations/procedures:

	No	Yes	Crepitus? Yes
Pain lateral elbow on resisted wrist extension?	☐	☐	☐
Pain medial elbow on resisted wrist flexion?	☐	☐	☐
Swelling over posterior elbow joint?	☐	☐	☐

Right side

If the subject has indicated tingling or numbness in the hand(s)/arm(s) in the past 7 days (question 30), indicate where it (they) occured by shading the affected parts on the diagram below.

Diagnosis: classical ☐ probable ☐ possible ☐ unlikely ☐

Left side

If the subject has indicated tingling or numbness in the hand(s)/arm(s) in the past 7 days (question 30), indicate where it (they) occured by shading the affected parts on the diagram below.

Diagnosis: classical ☐ probable ☐ possible ☐ unlikely ☐

FOREARMS AND HANDS: Left side

1. History: location of pain (on movement)?	Palpation: maximum tenderness?	Swelling?
	Yes	Yes	Yes
dorsal forearm	☐	☐	☐
palmar forearm	☐	☐	☐
dorsal wrist	☐	☐	☐
palmar wrist	☐	☐	☐
radial wrist	☐	☐	☐
medial wrist	☐	☐	☐
other	☐	☐	☐
(describe)	(describe)	(describe)

2. Pain on resisted movement?

	No	Yes	Crepitus? Yes
radial wrist	☐	☐	☐
medial wrist	☐	☐	☐
finger extension	☐	☐	☐
finger flexion	☐	☐	☐

3. Hand examination

		No	Yes		No	Yes
Muscle wasting	thenar eminence	☐	☐	hypothenar eminence	☐	☐
Dupuytren's contracture		☐				
Heberden's nodes		☐				

Light touch:

	normal	abnormal			
thumb	☐	☐	Thumb base:	No	Yes
index finger	☐	☐	Pain?	☐	☐
little finger	☐	☐	Tenderness?	☐	☐

	No	Yes
Positive Phalen's test?	☐	☐
Positive Tinel's test?	☐	☐
Weakness of thumb abduction	☐	☐
Pain on resisted left thumb extension?	☐	☐
Positive Finkelstein test?	☐	☐

	No	Yes
thumb opposition	☐	☐

FOREARMS AND HANDS: Right side

1. History: location of pain (on movement)?

	Yes	Palpation: maximum tenderness? Yes	Swelling? Yes
dorsal forearm	☐	☐	☐
palmar forearm	☐	☐	☐
dorsal wrist	☐	☐	☐
palmar wrist	☐	☐	☐
radial wrist	☐	☐	☐
medial wrist	☐	☐	☐
other	☐	☐	☐

(describe)   (describe)   (describe)

2. Pain on resisted movement?

	No	Yes	Crepitus? Yes
radial wrist	☐	☐	☐
medial wrist	☐	☐	☐
finger extension	☐	☐	☐
finger flexion	☐	☐	☐

3. Hand examination

	No	Yes		No	Yes
Muscle wasting thenar eminence	☐	☐	hypothenar eminence	☐	☐
Dupuytren's contracture	☐				
Heberden's nodes	☐				

Light touch:

	normal	abnormal	Thumb base:	No	Yes
thumb	☐	☐	Pain?	☐	☐
index finger	☐	☐	Tenderness?	☐	☐
little finger	☐	☐			

	No	Yes		No	Yes
Positive Phalen's test?	☐	☐			
Positive Tinel's test?	☐	☐			
Weakness of thumb abduction	☐	☐	thumb opposition	☐	☐
Pain on resisted left thumb extension?	☐	☐			
Positive Finkelstein test?	☐	☐			

Fibromyalgia tender spots

(Tick those that are tender)

Electroneurometry

Latency (milliseconds) Sensory	☐	☐	☐
Motor	☐	☐	☐

References

1. Badley, E.M. (1992). The impact of musculoskeletal disorders in the Canadian population. *J. Rheumatol.* **19**, 337–340.

2. Badley, E.M. and Tennant, A. (1993). Impact of disablement due to rheumatic disorders in a British population: estimates of severity and prevalence from the Calderdale Rheumatic Disablement Survey. *Ann. Rheum. Dis.* **52**, 6–13.

3. Cunningham, L.S. and Kelsey, J.L. (1984). Epidemiology of musculoskeletal impairments and their associated disability. *Am. J. Public Health* **74**, 574–579.

4. **Statistics Department, Department of the Secretary of State of Canada** (1986). *Report of the Canadian health and disability survey 1983–1984.* Ministry of Supply and Services, Ottawa.

5. McCormick, A., Fleming, D., and Charlton, J. (1995). *Morbidity statistics from general practice: The 4th National Survey of Morbidity in General Practice*, Series MB5, No. 3. HMSO, London.

6. Chard, M.D., Hazleman, R., Hazleman, B.L., King, R.H., and Reiss, B.B. (1991). Shoulder disorders in the elderly: a community survey. *Arthritis Rheum.* **34**, 766–769.

7. Chakravarty, K.K. and Webley, M. (1990). Disorders of the shoulder: an often unrecognised cause of disability in elderly people. *Br. Med. J.* **300**, 848–849.

8. White, K.P., Speechley, M., Harth, M., and Ostbye, T. (1995). Fibromyalgia in rheumatology practice: a survey of Canadian rheumatologists. *J. Rheumatol.* **22**, 722–726.

9. Frank, A. (1993). Low back pain. *Br. Med. J.* **306**, 901–908.

10. Nachemson, A.L. (1991). Back pain. Causes, diagnosis and treatment. The Swedish Council Technology Assessment in Healthcare, Stockholm.

11. Nygren, A., Berglund, A., and von Koch, M. (1987). Neck-and-shoulder pain, an increasing problem. Strategies for using health insurance to follow trends. *Scand. J. Rehabil. Med.* **32S**, 107–112.

12. Cyriax, J.H. (1982). *Textbook of orthopaedic medicine: diagnosis of soft tissue lesions.* Baillière Tindall, London.

13. Bamji, A.N., Erhardt, C.C., Price, T.R., and Williams, P.L. (1996). The painful shoulder: can consultants agree? *Br. J. Rheumatol.* **35**, 1172–1174.

14. Harrington, J.M., Carter, J.T., Birrell, L., and Gompertz, D. (1998). Surveillance case definitions for work related upper limb pain syndromes. *Occup. Environ. Med.* **55**, 264–271.

15. Palmer, K., Coggon, D., Cooper, C., and Doherty, M. (1998). Work related upper limb disorders: getting down to specifics. *Ann. Rheum. Dis.* **57**, 445–446.

16. Palmer, K., Walker-Bone, K., Linaker, C., Reading, I., Kellingray, S., Coggon, D., and Cooper, C. (2000). The Southampton examination schedule for the diagnosis of musculoskeletal disorders of the upper limbs. *Ann. Rheum. Dis.* **59**, 5–11.

17. Walker-Bone, K., Byng, T., Linaker, C., Reading, I., Coggon, D., Palmer, K., and Cooper, C. (2002). Reliability of the Southampton examination schedule for the diagnosis of upper limb disorders in the general population. *Ann Rheum. Dis.* **61**, 1103–1106.

18. Croft, P. (1993). Soft tissue rheumatism. In *Epidemiology of the rheumatic diseases* (ed. A.J. Silman and M.C. Hochberg), pp. 375–421. Oxford University Press, London.

19. Hamilton, P.G. (1986). The prevalence of humeral epicondylitis: a survey in general practice. *J. R. Coll. Gen. Pract.* **36**, 464–465.

20. Kurppa, K., Viikari-Juntura, E., Kuosma, E., Huuskonen, M., and Kivi, P. (1991). Incidence of tenosynovitis or peritendinitis and epicondylitis in a meat-processing factory. *Scand. J. Work Environ. Health* **17**, 32–37.

21. Andersson, G.B.J. (1999). Epidemiological features of chronic low-back pain. *Lancet* **354**, 581–585.

22. Rosen, M. (Chairman) (1994). *Back pain*, report of a CSAG Committee on back pain, pp. 1–89. HMSO, London.

23. Reigo, T., Timpka, T., and Tropp, T. (1999). The epidemiology of back pain in vocational age groups. *Scand. J. Prim. Health Care* **17**, 17–21.

24. Biering-Sorensen, F. (1989). Low back trouble in a general population of 30-, 50-, and 60-year old men and women. Study design, representativeness and basic results. *Dan. Med. Bull.* **29**, 289–299.

25. Frymoyer, J.W. and Cats-Baril, W.L. (1991). An overview of the incidences and costs of low back pain. *Orthop. Clin. N. Am.* **22**, 263–271.

26. Gyntelburg, F. (1974). One-year incidence of low back pain among male residents of Copenhagen aged 40–59. *Dan. Med. Bull.* **21**, 30–36.

27. Hirsch, C., Jonsson, B., and Lewin, T. (1969). Low back pain symptoms in a Swedish female population. *Clin. Orthop.* **63**, 171–176.

28. Hult, L. (1954). Cervical, dorsal and lumbar spinal syndromes. *Acta Orthop. Scand.* **17** (suppl.), 1–102.

29. Magora, A. (1970). Investigation of the relation between low back pain and occupation. 2. Work history. *Ind. Med. Surg.* **39**, 504–510.

30. Nagi, S.Z., Riley, L.E., and Newby, L.G. Social epidemiology of back pain in a general population. *J. Chronic Dis.* **26**, 769–779.

31. Papageorgiou, A.C., Croft, P.R., Ferry, S., Jayson, M.I.V., and Silman, A.J. (1995). Estimating the prevalence of low back pain in the general population. *Spine* **20**, 1889–1894.

32. Svensson, H.O., Andersson, G.B., Johanssen, S., Wilhelmsson, C., and Vedin, A. (1988). A retrospective study of low back pain in 38- to 64-year old women. Frequency and occurrence and impact on medical services. *Spine* **13**, 548–552.

33. Valkenburg, H.A. and Haanen, H.C. (1982). Low back pain in forty to forty-seven year old men. 1. Frequency of occurrence and impact on medical services. *Scand. J. Rehabil. Med.* **14**, 47–53.

34. Walsh, K., Cruddas, M., and Coggon, D. (1992). Low back pain in eight areas of Britain. *J. Epidemiol. Community Health* **46**, 227–230.

35. Urwin, M., Symmons, D., Allison, T., *et al.* (1998). Estimating the burden of musculoskeletal disorders in the community: the comparative prevalence at different anatomical sites and the relation to social deprivation. *Ann. Rheum. Dis.* **57**, 649–655.

36. Jones, J.R., Hodgson, J.T., Clegg, T.A., *et al.* (1998). *Self-reported work-related illness in 1995. Results from a household survey.* HMSO, London.

37. Rossignol, M., Suissa, S., and Abenhaim, L. (1988). Working disability due to occupational low back pain: three-year follow-up of 2300 compensated workers in Quebec. *J. Occup. Med.* **30**, 502–505.

38. Abenhaim, L., Suissa, S., and Rossignol, M. (1988). Risk of recurrence of occupational low back pain over three-year follow-up. *Br. J. Ind. Med.* **45**, 829–833.

39. Andersson, G.B.J., Svensson, H.O., and Oden, A. (1983). The intensity of work recovery in low back pain. *Spine* **8**, 880–884.

40. Smedley, J., Inskip, H., Cooper, C., and Coggon, D. (1998). Natural history of low back pain. A longitudinal study in nurses. *Spine* **23**, 2422–2426.

41. Bernard, B.P. (ed.) (1997). *Musculoskeletal disorders (MSDs) and workplace factors.* US Department of Health and Human Services, Cincinnati.

42. Bovenzi, M. and Hulshof, C.T.J. (1999). An updated review of epidemiologic studies on the relationship between exposure to whole-body vibration and low back pain. *Int. Arch. Occup. Environ. Health* **72**, 351–365.

43. Krause, N., Ragland, D.R., Greiner, B.A., Fisher, J.M., Holman, B.L., and Selvin, S. (1997). Physical workload and ergonomic factors associated with prevalence of back and neck pain in urban transit operators. *Spine* **22**, 2117–2126.

44. Volinn, E. (1997). The epidemiology of low back pain in the rest of the world. A review of surveys in low- and middle-income countries. *Spine* **22**, 1747–1754.

45. Polatin, P.B., Kinney, R.K., Gatchel, R.J., Lillo, E., and Mayer, T.G. (1993). Psychiatric illness and chronic low back pain. The mind and spine—which goes first? *Spine* **18**, 66–71.

46. Takala, J., Sievers, K., and Klaukka, T. (1982). Rheumatic symptoms in the middle-aged population in south-western Finland. *Scand. J. Rheumatol.* **47** (suppl.), 15–29.

47. Jacobsson, L., Lindgarde, F., Manthorpe, R., and Ohlsson, K. (1992). Effect of education, occupation and some lifestyle factors on common rheumatic complaints in a Swedish group aged 50–70 years. *Ann. Rheum. Dis.* **751**, 835–843.

48. Lawrence, J.S. (1969). Disc degeneration: its frequency and relationship to symptoms. *Ann. Rheum. Dis.* **28**, 121–137.

49. Brattberg, G., Thorslund, M., and Wikamn, A. (1989). The prevalence of pain in the general population. The results of a postal survey in a county of Sweden. *Pain* **37**, 215–222.

50. Makela, M., Heliovaara, M., Sievers, K., Knekt, P., Maatela, J., and Aromaa, A. (1993). Musculoskeletal disorders as determinants of disability in Finns aged 30 years or more. *J. Clin. Epidemiol.* **46**, 549–559.

51. Westerling, D. and Jonsson, B.G. (1980) Pain from the neck–shoulder region and sick leave. *Scand. J. Soc. Med.* **8**, 131–136.

52. Van der Donk, J., Schouten, J.S.A.G., Passchier, J., van Romunde, L.K.J., and Valkenburg, H.A. (1991). The association of neck pain with radiological abnormalities of the cervical spine and personality traits in the general population. *J. Rheumatol.* **18**, 1884–1889.

53. Cote, P. (1998). The Saskatchewan health and back pain survey. *Spine* **23**, 1689–1698.

54. Bovim, G., Schrader, H., and Sand, T. (1994). Neck pain in the general population. *Spine* **12**, 1307–1309.

55. Lau, E.M.C., Sham, A., and Wong, K.C. (1996). The prevalence of and risk factors for neck pain in Hong Kong Chinese. *J. Public Health Med.* **18**, 396–399.

56. Friedenberg, Z.B. and Miller, W.T. (1963). Degenerative disc disease of the cervical spine. A comparative study of asymptomatic and symptomatic subjects. *J. Bone Joint Surg.* **45A**, 1171–1178.

57. Linton, S.J. (1990). Risk factors for neck and back pain in a working population in Sweden. *Work Stress* **4**, 41–49.

58. Hasvold, T. and Johnsen, R. (1993). Headache and neck or shoulder pain—frequent and disabling complaints in the general population. *Scand. J. Prim. Health Care* **11**, 219–224.

59. Bogduk, N. (1999). The neck. *Baillière's Clin. Rheumatol.* **13**, 261–285.

60. Barnsley, L., Lord, S., and Bogduk, N. (1983). The pathophysiology of whiplash. In *Cervical flexion–extension/whiplash injuries* (ed. G.A. Malanga) *Spine [state of the art reviews]* **12**, 209–242.

61. Holt, L. (1971). Frequency of symptoms for different age groups and professions. In *Cervical pain* (ed. C. Hirsch and Y. Zotterman), pp. 17–20. Pergamon Press, New York.

62. Vasseljen, O. and Westgaard, R.H. (1995). A case-control study of trapezius muscle activity in office and manual workers with shoulder and neck pain and asymptomatic controls. *Int. Arch. Occup. Environ. Health* **67**, 11–18.

63. Harms-Ringdahl, K. and Ekholm, J. (1986). Intensity and character of pain and muscular activity levels elicited by maintained extreme flexion position of the lower cervical and upper thoracic spine. *Scand. J. Rehabil. Med.* **18**, 117–126.

64. Kamwendo, K., Linton, S.J., and Moritz, U. (1991). Neck and shoulder disorders in medical secretaries.1.Pain prevalence and risk factors. *Scand. J. Rehabil. Med.* **23**, 127–133.

65. Linton, S.J. and Kamwendo, K. (1989). Risk factors in the psychosocial work environment for neck and shoulder pain in secretaries. *J. Occup. Med.* **31**, 609–613.

66. Eriksen, W., Natvig, B., Knardahl, S., and Bruusgaard, D. (1999). Job characteristics as predictors of neck pain. A 4-year prospective study. *J. Occup. Environ. Med.* **41**, 893–902.

67. Leino, P. and Magni, G. (1993). Depressive and distress symptoms as predictors of low back pain, neck–shoulder pain and other musculoskeletal morbidity: a 10-year follow-up of metal industry employees. *Pain* **53**, 89–94.

68. Pope, D.P., Croft, P., Pritchard, C.M., and Silman, A.J. (1997). Prevalence of shoulder pain in the community: the influence of case definition. *Ann. Rheum. Dis.* **56**, 308–312.

69. Allander, E. (1974). Prevalence, incidence and remission rates of some rheumatic diseases and syndromes. *Scand. J. Rheumatol.* **3**, 145–153.

70. Chard, M.D. and Hazleman, B.L. (1987). Shoulder disorders in the elderly: a hospital study. *Ann. Rheum. Dis.* **46**, 684–687.

71. Bergenudd, H., Lindgarde, F., Nilsson, B., and Petersson, C.J. (1988). Shoulder pain in middle age. *Clin. Orthop.* **231**, 234–238.

72. van der Windt, D., Koes, B.W., Boeke, A.J.P., Deville, W., De Jong, B.A., and Bouter, L.M. (1996). Shoulder disorders in general practice: prognostic indicators of outcome. *Br. J. Gen. Practice* **46**, 519–523.

73. van der Heijden, G.J.M.G. (1999). Shoulder disorders: a state of the art review. *Baillière's Clin. Rheumatol.* **13**, 287–309.

74. Norlander, S., Gustavsson, B.A., Lindell, J., and Nordgren, B. (1997). Reduced mobility in the cervico-thoracic motion segment. A risk factor for musculoskeletal neck–shoulder pain: a two-year prospective follow-up study. *Scand. J. Rheumatol. Med.* **29**, 167–174.

75. Palmer, K., Coggon, D., Kellingray, S., *et al.* (1998). A national survey of occupational exposure to hand-transmitted vibration and associated health effects. In *Proceedings from the PREMUS-ISEOH 1998. The 3rd International Scientific Conference on Prevention of Work-Related Musculoskeletal Disorders*, p. 263.

76. Lundberg, B.J. (1969). The frozen shoulder. *Acta Orthop. Scand.* **119**, 1–59.

77. Bunker, T.D. (1997). Frozen shoulder: unravelling the enigma. *Ann. R. Coll. Surg. England* **79**, 210–213.

78. Vecchio, P., Kavanagh, K., Hazleman, B.L., and King, R.H. (1995). Shoulder pain in a community-based rheumatology clinic. *Br. J. Rheumatol.* **34**, 440–442.

79. Chard, M.D. and Hazleman, B.L. (1989). Tennis elbow—a reappraisal. *Br. J. Rheumatol.* **28**, 186–190.

80. Viikari-Juntura, E., Kurppa, K., Kuosma, E., *et al.* (1991). Prevalence of epicondylitis and elbow pain in the meat-processing industry. *Scand. J. Work Environ. Health* **17**, 38–45.

81. Gruchow, W. and Pelletier, D. (1979). An epidemiologic study of tennis elbow. *Am. J. Sports Med.* **7**, 234–238.

82. Cyriax, J.H. (1982). Diagnosis of soft tissue lesions. II Treatment by manipulation, management and injection. In *Textbook of orthopaedic medicine*, pp. 43–67. Baillière Tindall, London.

83. Binder, A.T. and Chard, M.D. (1983). Lateral humeral epicondylitis—a study of natural history and the effect of conservative therapy. *Br. J. Rheumatol.* **22**, 73–76.

84. De Krom, M.C.T.F., Knipschild, P.G., Kester, A.D.M., and Spaans, F. (1990). Efficacy of provocative tests for diagnosis of carpal tunnel syndrome. *Lancet* **335**, 393–395.

85. Massy-Westropp, N., Grimmer, K., and Bain, G. (2000). A systematic review of the clinical diagnostic tests for carpal tunnel syndrome. *J. Hand Surg. (Am.)* **25**, 120–127.

86. Homan, M.M., Franxblau, A., Werner, R.A., Albers, J.W., Armstrong, T.J., and Bromberg, M.B. (1999). Agreement between symptom surveys, physical examination procedures and electrodiagnostic findings for the carpal tunnel syndrome. *Scand. J. Work Environ. Health* **25**, 115–124.

87. Katz, J.N., Larson, M.G., Sabra, A., Krarup, C., et al. (1990). The carpal tunnel syndrome: diagnostic utility of the history and physical examination findings. *Ann. Intern. Med.* **112**, 321–327.

88. Szabo, R.M., Slater, R.R., Farver, T.B., Stanton, D.B., and Sharman, W.K. (1999). The value of diagnostic testing in carpal tunnel syndrome. *J. Hand Surg. (Am.)* **24**, 704–714.

89. Gerr, F. and Letz, R. (1998). The sensitivity and specificity of tests for carpal tunnel syndrome vary with the comparison groups. *J. Hand Surg. (Br.)* **23**, 151–155.

90. Ferry, S., Pritchard, T., Keenan, J., Croft, P., and Silman, A.J. (1998). Is delayed nerve conduction associated with increased self-reported disability in individuals with hand symptoms? A population-based study. *J. Rheumatol.* **25**, 1616–1619.

91. Stevens, J.C., Sun, S., Beard, C.M., O'Fallon, W.M., and Kurland, L.T. (1988). Carpal tunnel syndrome in Rochester, Minnesota, 1961 to 1980. *Neurology* **38**, 134–138.

92. Nordstrom, D.L., DeStefano, F., Vierkant, R.A., and Layde, P.M. (1998). Incidence of diagnosed carpal tunnel syndrome in a general population. *Epidemiology* **9**, 342–345.

93. Vessey, M.P., Villiard-Mackintosh, L., and Yeates, D. (1990). Epidemiology of carpal tunnel syndrome in women of childbearing age. Findings in a large cohort study. *Int. J. Epidemiol.* **19**, 655–659.

94. De Krom, M.C.T.F., Knipschild, P.G., Kester, A.D.M., Thus, C.T., Boekkooi, P.F., and Spaans, F. (1992). Carpal tunnel syndrome: prevalence in the general population. *J. Clin. Epidemiol.* **45**, 373–376.

95. Solomon, D.H., Katz, J.N., Bohn, R., Mogun, H., and Avorn, J. (1999). Nonoccupational risk factors for carpal tunnel syndrome. *J. Gen. Intern. Med.* **14**, 310–314.

96. Lam, N. and Thurston, A. (1998). Association of obesity, gender, age and occupation with carpal tunnel syndrome. *Aust. NZ J. Surg.* **68**, 190–193.

97. Abbas, M.A.F., Abdelmonem, A.A., Zhang, Z.W., and Kraus, J.F. (1998). Meta-analysis of published studies of work-related carpal tunnel syndrome. *Int. J. Occup. Environ. Health* **4**, 160–167.

98. Kramer, J.S., Yelin, E.H., and Epstein, W.V. (1983). Social and economic impacts of four musculoskeletal conditions. *Arthritis Rheum.* **26**, 901–907.

99. Thompson, A.R., Plewes, L.W., and Shaw, E.G. (1951). Peritendinitis crepitans and simple tenosynovitis: a clinical study of 544 cases in industry. *Br. J. Ind. Med.* **8**, 150–160.

100. Luopajarvi, T., Kuorinka, I., Virolainen, M., and Holmberg, M. (1979). Prevalence of tenosynovitis and other injuries of the upper extremities in repetitive work. *Scand. J. Work Environ. Health* **5** (suppl. 3), 48–55.

101. Barton, N.J. (1989). Repetitive strain disorder. Often misdiagnosed and often not work related. *Br. Med. J.* **299**, 405–406.

102. Diwaker, H.N. and Stothard, J. (1995). What do doctors mean by tenosynovitis and repetitive strain injury? *Occup. Med.* **45**, 97–104.

103. Field, J.H. (1979). De Quervain's disease. *Am. Fam. Physician* **20**, 103–104.

104. Nygaard, I.E., Saltzman, C.L., Whitehose, M.B., and Hankin, F.M. (1989). Hand problems in pregnancy. *Am. Fam. Physician* **39**, 123–126.

105. Barton, N.J., Hooper, G., Noble, J., and Steel, W.M. (1992). Occupational causes of disorders in the upper limb. *Br. Med. J.* **304**, 309–311.

106. Kivi, P. (1984). Rheumatic disorders of the upper limbs associated with repetitive occupation tasks in Finland 1975–9. *Scand. J. Rheumatol.* **13**, 101–107.

107. Hueston, J.T. (1960). The incidence of Dupuytren's contracture. *Med. J. Aust.* **47**, 999–1006.

108. Early, P.F. (1962). Population studies in Dupuytren's contracture. *J. Bone Joint Sur.* **44-B**, 602–613.

109. Mikkelson, O.A. (1972). The prevalence of Dupuytren's disease in Norway. *Acta Chir. Scand.* **138**, 695–700.

110. Gordon, S. (1954). Dupuytren's contracture: the significance of various factors in its aetiology. *Ann. Surg.* **140**, 683–687.

111. Fisk, G. (1985). The relationship of manual labour and specific injury to Dupuytren's disease. In *Dupuytren's disease*, 2nd edn (ed. J.T. Hueston and R.T. Tubiana), pp. 104–105. Churchill Livingstone, Edinburgh.

112. Bovenzi, M., Cerri, S., Merseburger, A., *et al.* (1994). Hand arm vibration syndrome and dose–response relation for vibration induced white finger among quarry drillers and stone carvers. *Occup. Environ. Med.* **51**, 603–611.

113. Badley, E. and Tennant, A. (1992). Changing profile of joint disorders with age: findings from a postal survey of the population of Calderdale, West Yorkshire, United Kingdom. *Ann. Rheum. Dis.* **51**, 366–371.

114. Gould, N., Schneider, W., and Ashikaga, T. (1980). Epidemiological survey of foot problems in the continental United States: 1978–9. *Foot Ankle* **1**, 8–10.

115. Wolfe, F., Smythe, H.A., Yunus, B.Y., *et al.* (1990). The American College of Rheumatology 1990 criteria for the classification of fibromyalgia: a report of the Multicenter Committee. *Arthritis Rheum.* **33**, 160–172.

116. Croft, P., Schollum, J., and Silman, A.J. (1994). Population study of tender point counts and pain as evidence of fibromyalgia. *Br. Med. J.* **309**, 696–699.

117. Croft, P., Burt, J., Schollum, J., *et al.* (1996). More pain, more tender points: is fibromyalgia just one end of a continuous spectrum? *Ann. Rheum. Dis.* **55**, 482–485.

118. White, K., Speechley, M., Harth, M., *et al.* (1996). The London fibromyalgia epidemiology study: the prevalence of fibromyalgia in London, Ontario. *Arthritis Rheum.* **39**, S212.

119. Wolfe, F., Ross, K., Anderson, J., *et al.* (1995). The prevalence and characteristics of fibromyalgia in the general population. *Arthritis Rheum.* **38**, 19–28.

120. Bennett, R.M. (1996). Fibromyalgia and the disability dilemma. A new era in understanding a complex, multidimensional pain syndrome. *Arthritis Rheum.* **39**, 1627–1634.

121. Cathey, M.A., Wolfe, F., and Kleinheksel, S.M. (1988). Functional ability and work status in patients with fibromyalgia. *Arthritis Care Res.* **1**, 85–98.

4.3 History and examination: general principles regarding the diagnosis of soft tissue disorders

Andrew Östör

When in a Search of any Nature the Understanding stands suspended, then Instances of the Fingerpost shew the true and inviolable Way in Which the Question is to be decided. These Instances afford great Light, so that the course of Investigation will sometimes be terminated by them. Sometimes, indeed, these Instances are found amongst that Evidence already set down.

Francis Bacon, *Novum Organum Scientarum.* Section XXXVI,
Aphorism XXI (1620).

Introduction

In all disciplines of medicine the history and examination form the foundation upon which a diagnosis is made. The majority of diagnoses are made after the history alone with physical findings playing a confirmatory role. The level of experience and knowledge base of the clinician has significant bearing on the chance of achieving the correct diagnosis. Further investigations, although helpful, may be time-consuming, expensive, and unnecessary.

The classification of soft tissue disorders, despite great advances in the understanding of their aetiopathogenesis, remains suboptimal and is heavily reliant on the clinical features (see Fig. 1 of Chapter 4.1). The purpose of this chapter is to describe the general principles of history and examination of soft tissue disease. A more detailed approach to the individual conditions will be covered in the relevant chapters. There is a common misconception that cases referred to rheumatologists are complex; however, Rheumatologists' clinics are not filled with unusual cases but with straightforward, misdiagnosed cases that could have been avoided by asking the right questions.[1]

History

The medical history is of paramount importance and its pivotal role cannot be overemphasized. The effectiveness of achieving a diagnosis is greatly improved if patients are allowed time to explain their symptoms in their own words.[2] By interrupting too early, crucial information may be missed, leading to both patient and doctor frustration. Algorithms to aid diagnosis have been developed but it is prudent to be open-minded to the myriad presentations of illness.[1] Occasionally, patients present having already been 'labelled' by another physician and thus the doctors view may be biased from the outset. On the other hand, the patient may present with their own preconceived idea of the diagnosis, this having been formulated by gleaning information from multiple sources notably the burgeoning use of the internet as a reference base. Patients may subsequently have difficulty defining their symptoms adequately and fully. The 'spot'

diagnosis is virtually non-existent in rheumatology. The history at times may be very short, for example, in the case of straightforward de Quervain's tenosynovitis. Alternatively, it may need to be extensive, for example, when systemic disease presents as a soft tissue disease, an example being ankylosing spondylitis presenting as plantar fasciitis.

The history commences with an exploration of the patient's presenting complaint. Pain is the cardinal symptom with varying degrees of stiffness, swelling, weakness, crepitus, clicking, and loss of function. Each of these symptoms will be covered in greater depth further in the chapter, as will pertinent aspects of the past, social, family, sporting, occupational, drug, allergy, and treatment history. Demographic information including the age, sex, and race of a patient has diagnostic significance, for example, in polymyalgia rheumatica, a condition most commonly seen in northern European elderly women.[3] It is during the history that the doctor–patient relationship develops and recognition of both verbal and non-verbal cues is important. The history finishes with an investigation of the patient's attitude to his or her illness and expectations regarding diagnosis and treatment.

Patient symptoms

Pain

Pain is a ubiquitous symptom in soft tissue rheumatism and arises from multiple sources. The physician's understanding of pain, however, encompassing a multitude of complaints, may be quite removed from that of the patient. Some individuals have difficulty in characterizing their symptoms using terms such as ache, soreness, burning, or the more nebulous general discomfort. Equally, patients may describe pain when another sensation is meant such as paraesthesia or stiffness.

Site of pain

Many soft tissue rheumatic conditions are localized and an appropriate starting point is to ask the patient 'Where exactly is the pain?' The patient should then be instructed to point to where the pain originated and to where it is most severe. Localization, however, may be difficult due to multisegmental or overlap innervation of an area or when pain presents in a sclerotomal distribution.[4] Diffuse pain syndromes, in some respects, are easier to identify as pain is felt 'everywhere'.

Severity

Pain severity may be volunteered by the patient but is heavily reliant on psychological factors and can be unhelpful or misleading. Pain scales, however, have been developed and validated such as the Shoulder Pain and Disability Index (SPADI).[5, 6] Excruciating pain (in women equivalent to childbirth without epidural anaesthesia) may occur in crystal disease or after dislocation of a joint due to ligamentous laxity or trauma. Less severe, constant pain is more consistent with a tendinopathy or enthesopathy.

Radiation

Pain radiation may give important diagnostic clues. Pain may radiate in a defined anatomical distribution, for example, radiation into the lateral three and a half digits in carpal tunnel syndrome or a cervical radiculopathy radiating into the shoulder. Pain that spreads in a diffuse, non-anatomical distribution may occur in conditions such as myofascial and complex regional pain syndromes (CRPSs).

Time course

Information about when and what the patient was doing at the time the pain started, what has happened subsequently, and whether the pain is constant or remitting and relapsing allows the clinician to narrow the diagnostic possibilities. Inflammatory pain often develops insidiously over weeks to months whereas pain usually develops immediately following a significant sporting injury. Tendinous injury often has a characteristic pain cycle with pain in a low-grade injury dissipating after a few minutes of activity with a recrudescence at rest. More severe injury leads to constant pain with decreased performance.

Relieving and exacerbating features

Symptoms may fluctuate depending upon posture, movement, activity, rest, and time of the day. Patients usually gain relief by lying on the side counter to that of the pain, for example, in rotator cuff disease or trochanteric bursitis. However, some paradoxically gain relief lying on the symptomatic side. Resting an affected limb usually ameliorates pain in ligamentous and tendinous injuries. The use of analgesics and other medications, including both prescription and non-prescription remedies, is covered further in the chapter.

Stiffness

Generally associated with arthritis, a subjective complaint of prolonged stiffness, the hallmark of inflammatory disease, is not uncommon in soft tissue rheumatism. Pain may be verbalized as stiffness therefore this complaint requires clarification. Stiffness that is worse in the morning and after rest, improving with activity, implies inflammatory disease. This is seen classically in polymyalgia rheumatica where stiffness and pain reach a zenith upon rising in the morning and after prolonged rest. Alternatively, stiffness exacerbated by movement and ameliorated by inactivity suggests degenerative disease such as in rotator cuff pathology and other tendinoses.

Swelling

Akin to stiffness, swelling is a highly significant finding as part of the inflammatory response. However, it may be quite subjective. The complaint of an inability to remove rings, for example, is no substitute for physician-observed swelling and the patient should be encouraged to present if swelling is visible. Despite the lack of objective swelling, it may be considered a real symptom in certain conditions such as fibromyalgia and CRPSs.

Weakness

Patients may describe weakness of an affected area that may be constant or present only when performing particular tasks such as reaching above the head in rotator cuff disease. It is important to

Table 1 Differential diagnosis of weakness

Neurogenic
Individual peripheral nerve lesions
Mononeuritis multiplex
Peripheral neuropathy
Spinal cord disease
Neuromuscular junction, e.g. myasthenia gravis
Myopathic
Congenital (rare)
Hereditary muscular dystrophy, e.g. Duchenne's, myotonic dystrophy
Metabolic
Connective tissue disease, e.g. polymyositis, dermatomyositis
Endocrine disorder, e.g. thyroid disease, Cushing's syndrome
Malignancy associated
Infection, e.g. HIV
Toxic, e.g. alcohol
Drugs
Others: sarcoidosis, osteomalacia, periodic paralysis, inclusion body myopathy
Mechanical
Soft tissue disease—tendinosis, tendonitis, partial or complete tear of tendon

ascertain whether the weakness is due to pain or to structural damage, this being apparent on examination. The differential diagnosis of weakness however is vast (Table 1).

Clicks

When a soft tissue moves over a bony prominence, the production of a click may develop. Clicking may be due to inflammation, instability, a previous tear, or scarring of soft tissues. It may also arise from soft tissues within the joint, as in meniscal damage of the knee, and from changes in bony contour following a fracture. In the absence of other symptoms clicks are of little consequence.

Crepitus

Crepitus, the sound made by the grating of irregular surfaces, is frequently heard but is more common in arthritides. Similar to clicks, crepitus in the absence of other symptoms is of undetermined significance.

Triggering

Triggering is a feature of tendon pathology most commonly due to tendon scarring. It manifests as a feeling of locking, usually of the digits, that may be overcome by effort or by passively moving the joint. The unlocking process may be accompanied by a clicking or snapping sensation.

Discolouration

Colour change is a significant feature of many illnesses including vascular insufficiency and Raynaud's phenomenon as well as in CRPSs. (See Chapters 6.15–6.17.)

Functional impairment

The consequence of many soft tissue diseases is disability and handicap. The World Health Organization has developed an international classification for the terms disease, impairment, disability, and handicap.[7] *Disease* or *disorder* is the medical diagnosis from which the patient suffers, for example, plantar fasciitis. *Impairment* is the manifestation of disease or more simply the symptoms and signs that develop—in the case of plantar fasciitis, pain, stiffness and focal tenderness. *Disability* is the functional limitation imposed by the impairment—in our example difficulty standing and walking. *Handicap* is the impact the disability has on the patient functioning in society, for example, loss of employment and inability to use certain modes of transportation. Handicap also encompasses the effect the disability has on interpersonal relationships. Severe disability, however, may not necessarily cause equally profound handicap. For example, many buildings and trains have access for patients in wheelchairs.

Difficulties may be encountered in areas such as personal hygiene, ambulating, and performance of household chores as well as sexual function. The impact on the patient's work commitments and responsibilities may be dire, for example, when a heavy manual worker is unable to continue their occupation as a consequence of a tendinopathy.

Patients' attitudes, expectations, and responses to illness vary enormously. A trivial matter for the doctor may be a huge burden for the patient and *vice versa*. Occasionally, the patient may have a vested interest in developing illness. It is important to determine whether secondary gain may be attained as a consequence of disease such as for benefit payments or when a child feigns or augments illness to placate feuding parents. This may be particularly prevalent amongst children with complex regional pain syndrome (CRPS).[8]

Due to embarrassment or pride patients may not volunteer information therefore delicate direct questioning is required. It is occasionally necessary to interview family members together with, and then separately from the patient to clarify problems encountered and to highlight any ongoing concerns. An understanding of the effect of disease on marriage is paramount as stresses may develop and insight into the support supplied by a spouse is crucial. Referral to occupational therapy for formal assessment may be required and may uncover significant deficiencies.

Systems review

Certain systemic symptoms, such as fatigue, lethargy, and malaise are common to many rheumatic diseases. Others, such as fever, anorexia, and loss of weight are more sinister and require further questioning. Soft tissue disease may be the presenting feature of an inflammatory disorder such as a spondyloarthropathy (Table 2). Involvement of any specific organ system, whether dermatological, gastrointestinal, ophthalmological, or mucous membrane, warrants more extensive questioning regarding systemic illness.

Family history

Family history of rheumatic disease is important but may not be directly relevant. The focus should be placed on the possibility of hereditary conditions leading to soft tissue disease including HLA-B27 associated spondyloarthropathies, gout, psoriasis, and hypermobility. True hereditary disorders of connective tissue such as Marfan and Ehlers-Danlos syndromes and osteogenesis imperfecta are usually diagnosed in infancy or childhood in the majority of cases. Patients, however, may occasionally display milder phenotypes and present later in life with soft tissue symptoms.[9]

Occupational history

Soft tissue disorders account for a significant amount of time lost from work.[10] This results in a substantial economic burden for the community. In the more mechanized industrial environment heavy manual labour has been replaced by work requiring a higher frequency of movement with repetitive actions of predominantly the upper limb. This type of labour may lead to chronic low-grade trauma resulting in occupational repetitive strain injuries. Ergonomic assessment of the work area may be required to assess contributing factors to soft tissue injury.

Sporting history

Soft tissues are prone to damage in the professional and highly competitive amateur sporting spheres as well as in the occasional sportsperson striving for their personal best. The increased prevalence of soft tissue disease in this population almost certainly resulted in the use of sporting synonyms such as tennis and golfer's elbow for lateral and medial epicondylitis, respectively.[11] A review of the frequency, intensity, and duration of participation in sporting pursuits will aid diagnosis and help to identify precipitating and perpetuating causes. Individuals with mobile joints, whether truly hypermobile or at the upper end of the spectrum of normality, are frequently selected for dance schools and gymnastics and are predisposed to injury.[12]

Medication history

Certain drugs have been implicated in the development of tendon disorders. Enquiry regarding the use of glucocorticoids, fluoroquinolone antibiotics, and anabolic steroids may shed light on an underlying cause for tendon dysfunction.

Past and present treatment

Various treatments are available to ameliorate soft tissue disorders. Enquiry should be made into which medications have been tried, both prescription and over the counter, including doses, efficacy, side-effects, and possible reasons for discontinuation. Poor response to a therapy may have been due to inadequate dosing rather than poor efficacy *per se*. Physical therapies prescribed for soft tissue disease, including exercise, splints, mobility aids, and orthosis, as well as any surgical intervention require documentation. The use of alternative remedies and treatment administered by paramedical health care workers such as chiropractors, osteopaths, myotherapists, and naturopaths is

Table 2 Spondyloarthritides associated with enthesopathies

Ankylosing spondylitis
Psoriatic arthritis
Reactive (Reiter's) arthropathy
Enteropathic arthritis (inflammatory bowel disease associated)
Undifferentiated spondylitis
Juvenile spondyloarthropathy

common,[13] and any intervention may alter the clinical expression of disease and influence patient expectation.

Past medical history

Associated medical conditions that may complicate the disease or the management of soft tissue disorders include peptic ulcer disease, bronchospasm, and medication allergy. Patients may believe they have an allergy to aspirin or aspirin-like compounds but frequently no clear history of an allergic reaction is found with patients rather describing well known side-effects of the medication. This is commonly seen with nonsteroidal anti-inflammatory drug (NSAID) use and complaints of nausea or dyspepsia. Patient education and reassurance that their symptoms are not truly allergic is warranted. In itself asthma is not a contraindication to the use of NSAIDs.

The physical examination

The examination of soft tissue disease stems directly from the information obtained during the history. It not only aids the physician in confirming a diagnosis but also gives information regarding disease activity, functional capacity, asymptomatic pathology, and coexistent disease. In addition, the examination gives meaning to the patient's symptoms by localizing the problem, if possible, to an abnormal anatomical region or structure. A sound knowledge of the anatomy is therefore essential.

An exhaustive examination of the entire musculoskeletal system is unnecessary in most cases as, by its nature, soft tissue disease is usually localized. Any features suggestive of systemic disease or more diffuse pathology, however, warrant more extensive examination. Rarely is the diagnosis reliant predominantly or solely on the examination findings.

A fundamental rule in examination is to adequately expose the affected area. The examination should occur in a warm, well lit, private area with a chaperone occasionally being required. Rheumatologists have been blessed with the opportunity to compare and contrast signs on one side with the contralateral side and this situation should be exploited to the full.

Convention dictates adherence to a specific order of examination, which, in the musculoskeletal system, involves inspection, palpation, movement, measurement (if indicated), functional assessment, special tests, and requesting of appropriate investigations (Table 3).

Table 3 Summary of examination for soft tissue disease

Inspection
Palpation
Movement
Active
Passive
Resisted
Measurement (if indicated)
Functional assessment
Special tests
Investigations

Depending upon the disease process a general and/or neurological examination may be necessary. It should be noted that strictly following the above protocol is not necessary in all situations.

The examination is consciously and subconsciously occurring during the entire patient–doctor interaction. It commences at the very beginning of the review when the patient arises from the waiting room chair and walks into the doctor's office. Vital information may be gleaned by observation at this early stage and whilst taking the history. Facial expressions, for example, can give an insight into the degree to which the patient is experiencing discomfort.

Inspection

General aspects of the examination include body habitus, posture, mobility, and gait. More specific features to observe include asymmetry, muscle wasting (disuse from pain, incapacity, or denervation), swelling (localized or diffuse), and structural abnormality including deformity and malalignment. Other features include discolouration noting particularly any pallor, erythema, mottling, cyanosis, or bruising. Inspection for nodules, suggestive of rheumatoid arthritis, gout, or tendon scarring is required. Note should be made of any nail changes, rashes, excess adipose tissue, and/or features of a peripheral neuropathy or endocrinopathy.

Palpation

Enquiry as to whether the patient has any tender areas should preface palpation. Tenderness is a significant feature and may be localized or diffuse. When localized, a search for the site of maximal tenderness may identify the involved anatomical structure, for example, an inflamed trochanteric bursa. Care should be taken as certain conditions may cause exquisite tenderness such as plantar fasciitis and CRPS.

Temperature change is of paramount importance with a localized increase in warmth being suggestive of inflammation. In this situation infection requires exclusion forthwith.

Deformity may not be apparent on inspection due to overlying muscles and adipose tissue and therefore should be palpated, for example, following subluxation or dislocation or of a joint. Swelling is palpable and may be of soft tissue or bony consistency. Frequently, crepitus may be easier to palpate than to hear. An increase or decrease in moisture of a limb may be indicative of neurovascular compromise, for example, in neuropathy or CRPS. Deeper palpation may detect muscle knots, spasm, guarding, and tenderness. Pulses should be checked.

Movement

Assessment of three specific types of movement is required: active, passive, and resisted movement. Muscle strength can be quantified using MRC guidelines (Table 4).

Active movement testing

This is undertaken by asking the patient to move the body part through its full range of movement without examiner intervention. This type of movement assesses the integrity of muscles, tendons, ligaments, and bones. An appreciation of the quality as well as the quantity of movement may also be assessed. The rhythm, symmetry, and rate of movement can give information regarding flexibility, mobility, and strength.

Table 4 Grades of muscle power (Medical Research Council)

Grade	Definition
0	No movement
1	Visible or palpable flicker of contraction
2	Active movement with gravity eliminated
3	Active movement against gravity
4	Active movement against gravity and resistance but which is weaker than normal
5	Normal power

Passive movement testing

In passive movement testing the patient is asked to relax the involved limb and to refrain from putting in effort whilst the examiner moves the affected limb. It should be noted that some patients find it quite difficult to relax. Passive movement assesses ligaments, joint capsule, fascia, and bursae as well as nerve roots and dura mater, for example, the straight leg raising test for sciatica. Passive movement also gives information regarding the integrity of muscles and tendons. If a complete tear or rupture is present, passive movement will be full unless limited by patient discomfort.

Resisted movement testing

This is the process whereby movement is tested by isometric (i.e. same length) contraction of muscle. Its purpose is to isolate the pathology to a musculotendinous unit. The limb is placed in a neutral or mid-position and the patient is instructed to contract the muscle against resistance until a maximal contraction is achieved. Weakness without pain implies neurological deficit. Weakness with pain implies musculotendinous inflammation or degeneration. Interpretation may be difficult when weakness is due to pain without inherent weakness, for example, in polymyalgia rheumatica.

Goniometry

Formal measurement of the range of movement of a joint with a goniometer, an angle-measuring device, is occasionally employed. However, in practice 'eyeball' estimation is usually sufficient. The clinical relevance of determining the precise angle at which pain is experienced in a condition such as rotator cuff disease, is questionable.

Neurological examination

Depending upon the history and musculoskeletal examination findings, it may be necessary to perform a thorough neurological examination. The standard sequence of neurological examination is adhered to commencing with tone followed by power, coordination, reflexes, and sensation. The sensory component is performed using the modalities of light touch and pinprick.

Special tests

Many soft tissue conditions display features that are detected by special tests. These will be covered in detail in the individual chapters. However, a few examples follow.

Table 5 The nine-point Beighton scoring system for joint hypermobility[a]

Scoring 1 point on each side
Passive dorsiflexion of the fifth metacarpo phalangeal joint to 90°
Apposition of the thumb to the flexor aspect of the forearm
Hyperextension of the elbow beyond 90°
Hyperextension of the knee beyond 90°

Scoring 1 point
Forward trunk flexion placing hands flat on the floor with knees extended

[a] Maximum score 9.

Shoulder instability testing

In young patients presenting with shoulder pain, exclusion of shoulder instability is necessary as a cause for their symptoms that may lead to recurrent dislocation.

Pain provocation tests

These help to localize the pathology to an affected anatomical region, for example, as Finkelstein's test for de Quervain's tenosynovitis or resisted wrist extension for lateral epicondylitis.

Tender and trigger points

Tender and trigger points are phenomena encountered in diffuse pain syndromes. The American College of Rheumatology includes specific anatomical sites for tender points as part of the diagnostic criteria for fibromyalgia.[14] Trigger points, which are not equivalent to tender points, reproduce the diffuse pain experienced by patients with myofascial pain. (See Chapter 6.11.)

Hypermobility testing

Beighton described a nine-point scale for determining joint hypermobility (Table 5).[15] The diagnostic significance is that hypermobile patients may have an underlying connective tissue disorder, such as Ehlers–Danlos syndrome, and are prone to soft tissue injury.

Functional assessment

Despite being left until the end, this is the most important part of the physical examination. Functional capacity, however, is being appraised throughout the interview. Overall function, particularly that of the lower limb, is assessed as the patient gets up from the waiting room chair and walks into the office. Difficulties may be more apparent when an attempt is made to undress or to climb on to the examination couch. Upper limb functional assessment is undertaken by asking the patient to perform specific tasks such as removing glasses or reaching for a wallet. More subtle testing of manual dexterity may be assessed by asking the patient to do up buttons and write. The functional assessment is tailored according to the underlying condition. Referral to an occupational therapist for formal assessment is frequently necessary and enlightening.

Conclusion

Soft tissue disease is common but poorly understood by many health care professionals. Acumen is greatly improved if a careful history and tailored examination is undertaken when assessing soft tissue disease.

Reliance on investigations, in the vast majority of situations, is unnecessary. One of the important features of soft tissue rheumatism is the tendency for resolution and, despite the accelerated pace of life in the twenty-first century, patients should be reassured that their symptoms will improve in time. As physicians we not only have the capacity to ameliorate disease we also have the ability to give meaning to the patients' symptoms, empowering them with an understanding of their malady, undoubtedly improving overall satisfaction.

References

1. Ferrari, R., Cash, J., and Maddison, P. (1996). *Rheumatology guidebook.* BIOS Scientific Publishers Ltd, Oxford.

2. Marvel, M.K., Epstein, R.M., Flowers, K., and Beckman, H.B. (1999). Soliciting the patient's agenda: have we improved? *J. Am. Med. Assoc.* **281** (3), 283–287.

3. Cimmino, M.A. and Zaccaria, A. (2000). Epidemiology of polymyalgia rheumatica. *Clin. Exp. Rheumatol.* **18** (4 suppl. 20), S9–11.

4. Kellgren, J.H. (1938). Observations on referred pain arising from muscle. *Clin. Sci.* **3**, 176–190.

5. Roach, K.E., Budiman-Mak, E., Songsiridej, N., and Lertratanakul, Y. (1991). Development of a shoulder pain and disability index. *Arthritis Care Res.* **4** (4), 143–149.

6. Williams, J.W. Jr, Holleman, D.R. Jr, and Simel, D.L. (1995). Measuring shoulder function with the Shoulder Pain and Disability Index. *J. Rheumatol.* **22** (4), 727–732.

7. World Health Organization (WHO) (1980). *International classification of impairments, disabilities and handicaps.* WHO, Geneva.

8. Coughlan, R.J., Kavanagh, R.T., and Hazleman, B.L. (1995). The clinical features of algodystrophy in childhood. *J. Orthop. Rheumatol.* **8**, 146–150.

9. Grahame, R. (2000). Heritable disorders of connective tissue. *Baillière's Best Pract. Res. Clin. Rheumatol.* **14** (2), 345–361.

10. Adebajo, A.O. and Hazleman, B.L. (1993). Incidence, nature and economic effects of soft tissue injury. In *The soft tissues, trauma and sports injuries* (ed. G.R. McLatchie and C.M.E. Lennox), pp. 3–29. Butterworth-Heinemann, Oxford.

11. Gruchow, H.W. and Pelletier, B.S. (1979). An epidemiologic study of tennis elbow. *Am. J. Sports Med.* **7**, 234–238.

12. Klemp, P., Stevens, J.E., and Isaacs, S. (1984). A hypermobility study in ballet dancers. *J. Rheumatol.* **11** (5), 692–696.

13. Ernst, E. (1998). Usage of complementary therapies in rheumatology: a systematic review. *Clin. Rheumatol.* **17** (4), 301–305.

14. Wolfe, F., Smythe, H.A., and Yunus, M.B., *et al.* (1990). The American College of Rheumatology 1990 criteria for the classification of fibromyalgia. Report of the Multicentre Criteria Committee. *Arthritis Rheum.* **33**, 160–172.

15. Beighton, P., Solomon, L., and Soskolne, C. (1973). Articular mobility in an African population. *Ann. Rheum. Dis.* **32**, 413–418.

4.4 The diagnosis of soft tissue disorders: radiology

Philip Bearcroft

Introduction

A variety of radiological techniques is available for the assessment of soft tissue pathology. Each has certain strengths and advantages that must be seen in the context of the corresponding weaknesses and disadvantages. In the current chapter, each radiological technique will be considered in turn. The technical aspects will be outlined, together with the associated strengths and weaknesses and the specific clinical uses for which the technique is best suited. In the final section, two fundamental principles of imaging will be described. The first is an understanding of the potential harm that a patient might suffer when undergoing a radiological examination and the sources of that harm. The second is an understanding that the result of a radiological test once obtained must be put into a wider context, and a mathematical model will be described to help with this analysis.

Plain radiographs

Technical aspects

A plain radiograph is produced when a film coated in photographic emulsion is exposed to X-rays. X-rays are part of the electromagnetic spectrum of light and possess a short wavelength and therefore high energy. Energy values in the range 60–120 kV are typical for diagnostic radiology. The resulting image, once developed, is a map of X-ray attenuation along the lines radiating from the X-ray point source to the various points on the film, and each point therefore represents a summation of the attenuation of the various structures through which the photons have passed. Different body parts cause varying degrees of X-ray attenuation, varying from high attenuation from bone and calcified structures, through intermediate attenuation from soft tissues, to low attenuation from fat and gas. The resulting contrast on the film produces the image and is determined by the different relative attenuation of the various anatomical structures involved (Fig. 1)

It is an axiom of good radiographic technique that radiographs of extremities should be taken in two orthogonal planes. This is particularly important in cases of trauma when undisplaced fractures might otherwise be missed. For each joint, standard projections have been defined representing a minimum of a frontal and a lateral projection, allowing a standardized technique to be followed.[1] The annotation of the frontal radiograph (e.g. anteroposterior, dorsiplantar, or dorsipalmar) corresponds to the direction of travel that the photons took through the anatomical structure. Therefore, in an anteroposterior view the radiographic film is positioned posterior to the region of interest, and the X-ray tube anterior. Additional or alternative views

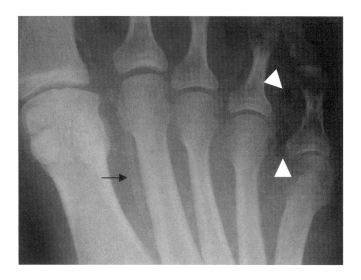

Fig. 1 Soft tissue abscess in a diabetic. Plain film allows differentiation between calcium (vascular calcification, black arrow), soft tissue, and gas (within an abscess, arrowheads).

may be necessary when the anatomical region is complex, or is orientated in a different plane. For example, an axial view of the shoulder is often performed instead of the lateral view as it gives more information about the acromioclavicular joints and acromion. Similarly, an oblique projection is required to evaluate fully the upper sacrum, in the form of an anteroposterior radiograph with 15° to cephalad angulation. A detailed catalogue of imaging projections is beyond the scope of this book, and the interested reader is referred to a suitable book of radiographic positioning.[1]

Variations

Fluoroscopy

In fluoroscopy, the radiographic film is replaced by an image intensifier, which can be likened to a video camera sensitive to the X-ray photons. The resulting image is projected on a TV screen in real time and, as the patient moves, the changes are reflected on the screen. This can be particularly useful in the dynamic assessment of an extremity, but its use in the musculoskeletal system is more usually confined to directing and guiding an interventional procedure, such as an arthrogram (see below).

Digital imaging

More recently, attempts have been made to replace the conventional radiographic film with a reusable suitably sensitized plate that converts the incident X-ray image into a digital image, which can be then be transferred to a computer and viewed on the computer monitor. It should be noted that there are significant advantages to acquiring images with a digital system over and above the convenience of digital storage and archive. For example, a digital plate has a higher latitude to overexposure and underexposure. The images obtained are therefore more consistent, irrespective of the individual radiographic parameters used, and this in turn aids comparison over time when a patient requires serial radiographs. In addition, because the images are digital, they can be manipulated on the computer to enhance fine detail. There are two main ways of achieving the digital image—either indirectly where the exposed plate must itself be processed before the image is composed (*computed radiography*) or directly where the plate is wired to the acquisition computer and the image is read off instantaneously (*direct radiography*). For reporting purposes, the monitors used to display the images are conventionally high quality devices. For review purposes, however, standard computers and monitors are often adequate, and this will form the basis of future hospital-wide developments where radiology departments become 'filmless' and where the images are transmitted via networks to hospital-wide workstations throughout the hospital (picture archive and communication systems (PACS)). To date, over 1000 hospitals worldwide have already made the transition to filmless, or nearly filmless radiology. Of course, the fact that the image is acquired and archived digitally and can be viewed on one or more monitors simultaneously at different sites does not preclude it from also being printed on to film. Many thousands of hospitals have progressed to this lesser level of digital development.

Tomography

In tomography, the tube and film move in opposite directions during a prolonged exposure. The geometry of the movement is such that only a single plane within the imaging volume remains in focus for the whole exposure, and this imaged slice must necessarily be parallel to the film. The technique has largely now been replaced by other tomographic techniques (e.g. computerized tomography (CT) and magnetic resonance imaging (MRI); see below). However, before the advent of these other tomographic techniques, this was a very useful technique in the evaluations of sites of complicated anatomical detail and a variety of devices were invented to maximize the blurring of the structures outside of the slice being imaged.

Strengths

Plain radiography has a historical heritage dating back over 100 years, which is unmatched by any other imaging technique. The raw materials are relatively inexpensive and the radiographic equipment required is universally available worldwide. The resulting image and the underlying bony anatomy are widely recognizable to the referring clinician and the spatial resolution of the image, which is an indication of how small a structure or an abnormality can be determined, is excellent with calcified structures of less than 1 mm readily identifiable.

Weaknesses

Despite the many obvious advantages of plain radiography, the technique suffers one major disadvantage in the context of *soft tissue* imaging, namely, that all structures of soft tissue density have the same attenuation values. Therefore, differences between soft tissue structures will not be shown on plain radiographs in the absence of mineralization or calcification. The majority of soft tissue abnormalities will therefore be invisible on plain radiography alone, and their detection will require the addition of one of the other radiological techniques listed below. The other main disadvantage relates to the ionizing nature of X-ray radiation, an issue that is covered in depth below.

Specific clinical uses

The clinical uses of plain film radiography are particularly diverse. However, because of the clarity with which bony and calcified structures are demonstrated, the main strengths of plain radiography in the musculoskeletal system relate to the detection of osseous abnormalities, particularly fractures and tumours. Although bone abnormalities represent the main focus of plain film radiology, plain films are also vital in the proper evaluation of most soft tissue abnormalities. For example, it is important to visualize the underlying bone when evaluating soft tissue pathology to exclude a primary bony pathology presenting with secondary soft tissue features or, conversely, secondary bone involvement from a soft tissue process. In particular, in the context of soft tissue injury, evaluation of the adjacent bone is mandatory either to exclude bony fracture or tendon–bone avulsion (Fig. 2). The latter is particularly common in the adolescent age group when avulsion at the enthesis at a number of sites causes detachment of the underlying periosteum (Fig. 3). In the earliest stages, these are often successfully treated surgically, but postoperative outcome is impaired if surgery is delayed.[2]

In addition, plain radiography can provide useful diagnostic information in a patient with a soft tissue mass. For example, the mass itself may exhibit areas of calcification such as phleboliths, which are pathognomonic of a haemangioma (Fig. 4), or the typical soft tissue changes of myositis ossificans (Fig. 5). Conversely, there may be

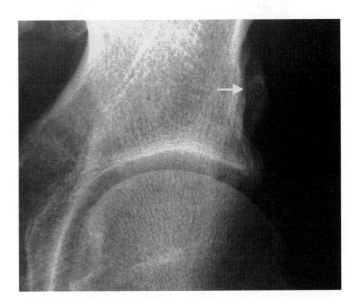

Fig. 2 Chronic avulsive injury of the anterior inferior iliac spine. Repetitive traction at the insertion of rectus femoris has resulted in episodes of partial detachment and repair leading to calcification.

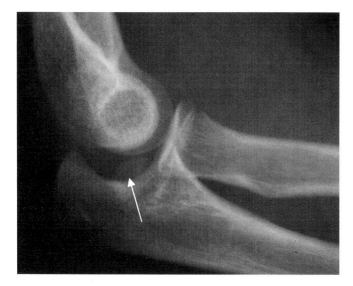

Fig. 3 Avulsed medial epicondyle. A calcified structure is projected over the joint (arrow), representing an avulsed and displaced medial epicondyle following excessive traction on the common flexor origin during a road traffic accident.

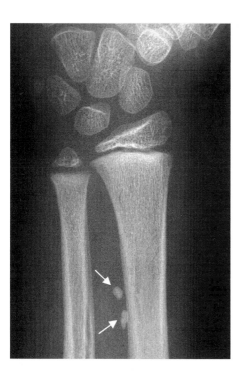

Fig. 4 Haemangioma in the forearm of a child. The presence of two phleboliths within the lesion seen best on a plain film is a pathognomonic feature that indicates that this tumour is a haemangioma.

(a)

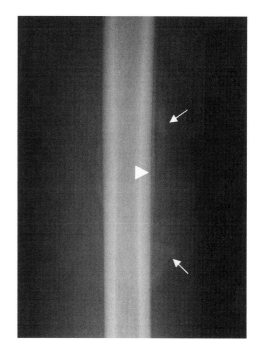

(b)

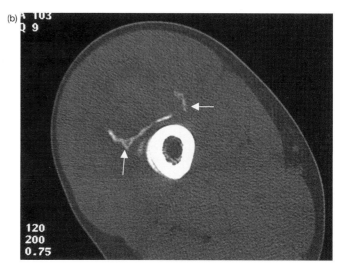

Fig. 5 Myositis ossificans. (a) 2 months after a direct blow to the thigh a calcified structure is seen to arise intimately related to the femur (arrows). The thin line parallelling the cortex of the bone (arrowhead) is a clue that this lesion is arising in the soft tissue adjacent to bone, and not from the bone itself. (b) A CT examination shows the curvilinear nature of the calcification (arrows) that is typical of myositis ossificans.

secondary changes in an adjacent bone that help make the diagnosis (Fig. 6). Furthermore, the relative position of adjacent bones is due to the interposed soft tissues, and abnormality of joint morphology gives indirect information about those interposed soft tissue structures. For example, degenerative joint disease is associated with joint space narrowing, representing cartilage loss.

Summary

Plain radiographs are the 'bread and butter' of a radiology department due to their universal availability and their low cost. They are accurate in diagnosing the majority of bone abnormalities, but are more limited when the pathology arises from soft tissues. They are a useful adjunct to other imaging techniques in the evaluation of soft tissue processes, but it is the remaining imaging modalities considered below that have contributed most to our understanding of soft tissue pathology.

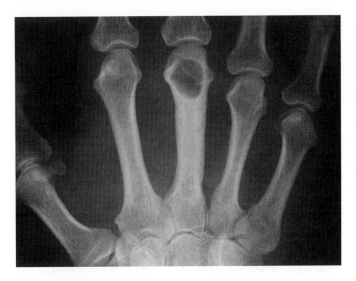

Fig. 6 Implantation dermoid. The patient was a keen gardener and swelling and discomfort after a rose thorn injury to the palm of the hand was ignored for many months.

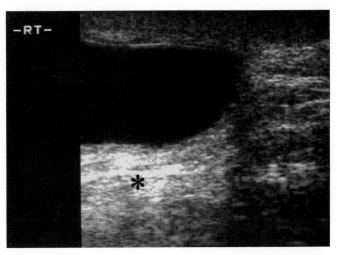

Fig. 7 A cyst in the thigh showing the anechoic fluid and posterior acoustic enhancement.

Ultrasound

Technical aspects

This technique uses high-frequency pulses of sound to generate cross sectional images through the body. The frequency of sound that is used (3–20 MHz) is inaudible to the human ear (range of hearing frequency approximately 10–20,000 Hz) and the sound waves bounce off internal structures. The echoes are received and recorded by the same transducer and converted into an image. Indeed, the transducer can be considered to be the most important part of the ultrasound machine. It converts electrical energy into sound and vice versa, and it is the component that is held in the operator's hand and placed on the patient's skin. A suitable coupling gel is placed between the skin and the transducer to prevent sound waves reflecting from the first interface they meet, namely, the skin surface.

The individual pixels within the image have an intensity that is related to the strength of the echo reflected from the corresponding point in the body, at the relevant distance from the transducer. Reflections will be greatest at interfaces between tissues of differing acoustic impedance and, in general, areas of more detailed anatomical complexity will return a more heterogeneous image, compared to the more uniform image that would correspond to a homogeneous organ or region. The higher the frequency of the sound used, the better the spatial resolution but, conversely, the shallower will be the depth that can be imaged. Frequencies below 7.5 MHz are generally unsuitable for musculoskeletal imaging, and frequencies higher than 20 MHz are likely to lack sufficient penetration depth for anything other than the most superficial structures. In general, a range of transducers are provided with an ultrasound machine and the individual transducer can be selected with a view to the clinical question posed and the depth of the potential abnormality that is suspected. In addition to the frequency of transducer, variation also exists in the design of the transducer shape. For musculoskeletal imaging, a linear array transducer with a flat contact with the skin is preferable.

Unlike in the case of CT, the value of intensity of the pixel in the image is not quantitative. The echogenicity relates to the proportion of incident energy that is reflected. A highly reflective tissue, such as the cortex of bone, returns a great proportion of the incident energy and will be represented as a bright well-defined line. Conversely, little energy is reflected from the homogeneous fluid within a cyst, and the contents of these structures will characteristically be of homogeneous low echogenicity and therefore will appear dark on the resulting image (Fig. 7). In addition, in the latter case energy loss through the cyst will be reduced in relation to the adjacent tissues, and therefore the tissues deep to the cyst will appear brighter (acoustic enhancement) as the remaining energy within the beam is greater (Fig. 7). Because virtually all energy is reflected from bony cortex, ultrasound is not able to visualize structures within bone. It is therefore purely a soft tissue modality.

Variations

Doppler ultrasound

Doppler ultrasound gives information about moving structures. In addition to recording the depth and intensity of echoes returned from the structure being imaged, the transducer also detects any alteration in frequency of the received sound, which would imply that the contents of the corresponding voxels within the sample gate were moving with a vector towards or away from the transducer. For example, blood flow within a vessel can be recorded in graphical format as the Doppler shift as a function of time, and this can be displayed on the screen alongside the image.

Colour Doppler and *power Doppler* techniques are each an extension of the Doppler technique where, rather than a single Doppler gate, every pixel in that part of the image is assessed for a change in the frequency in the reflected sound. A colour map is constructed to represent this directional information where the colour of each pixel corresponds to the size of that frequency change. Furthermore, structures moving towards the probe may be coloured blue and those moving away are red on colour Doppler. Power Doppler has a higher sensitivity for slow flow, but this is at the expense of directional information.

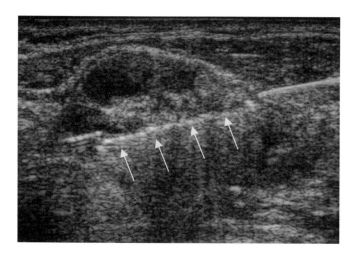

Fig. 8 Soft tissue sarcoma biopsy. Ultrasound is used to guide a biopsy needle (arrows) into the middle of a soft tissue mass allowing a sample sufficient for histological analysis to be obtained percutaneously under local anaesthetic.

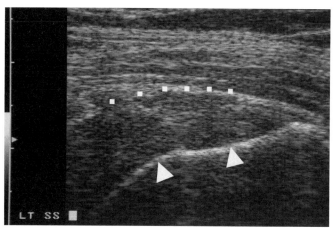

Fig. 9 Normal supraspinatus tendon. The supraspinatus tendon lies between the humeral head cortex (arrowheads) and the subacromial–subdeltoid bursa (dots—collapsed in this normal individual).

Biopsy

Ultrasound can be particularly useful in guiding real-time biopsy of soft tissue masses. With this technique, the position of a needle inserted percutaneously can be tracked as it advances into the lesion of clinical concern and fluid can be aspirated or soft tissue material provided for histology using one of several commercially available core biopsy needles (Fig. 8). In addition to guiding the point of the needle into the lesion, ultrasound is also useful to ensure that vital structures, particularly vessels, can be avoided.

Strengths

Ultrasound enjoys certain unique properties that make it ideally suited to soft tissue imaging. It is non-invasive, does not involve ionizing radiation, is painless to the patient, and has no known side-effects. The machines are universally available, although improvements over the last decade in transducer design mean that some machines are better able to produce the spatial resolution required for adequate musculoskeletal imaging.

Weaknesses

A major weakness of ultrasound is that the accuracy of the results depends upon the operator in a way that is not mirrored with other imaging techniques. The hard copy images are a series of snapshots of what the operator has chosen to demonstrate from the examination. They are difficult to interpret by other people unless a systematic approach to layout has been adopted. Added to this, ultrasound requires a detailed knowledge of anatomy and there is a relatively long and steep learning curve during which the results of the apprentice sonographer may be less than those quoted in the literature. Finally, the technique is not able to visualize bone pathology, and plain film radiographs or other imaging remain necessary to evaluate bony structures.

Specific clinical uses

Shoulder

Sonography has revolutionized the imaging of shoulder pathology, particularly in relation to impingement and rotator cuff disease. The majority of degenerative tears involve the supraspinatus tendon.[3] This tendon is particularly well visualized longitudinally by adopting a sagittal oblique approach with the patient's arm behind the back to bring the tendon forward from underneath the acromion. The normal tendon is represented as a well-defined structure with a convex anterior border with a uniform internal linear anatomical architecture (Fig. 9). With a complete rupture of the supraspinatus tendon with retraction, the deltoid abuts the humeral head with no interposing tendinous structure. A full thickness tear without retraction demonstrates a concave anterior border to the tendon, and the ends of the tendon may be visualized, particularly dynamically as the patient's arm is moved (Fig. 10). Altered signal within the tendon correlates with tendinosis but, as the only finding, is not an indication of a full thickness rotator cuff tear. Partial tears can be visualized as a focal discontinuity in the fibrillar pattern, but the accuracy of ultrasound in this diagnosis is not established. Infraspinatus, subscapularis, the tendon of the long head of biceps, and teres minor muscles can also be evaluated sonographically, although isolated tears in these structures in the absence of supraspinatus damage are not the norm.

Elbow

Although the diagnosis of golfer's elbow and tennis elbow is essentially clinical, ultrasound can be useful in demonstrating the degree of tear, particularly when retraction is present. Ultrasound is also useful in demonstrating intraarticular bodies, although confirming that they are loose can be difficult in the absence of an effusion. In addition, ultrasound can be used to visualize the immature cartilage of the elbow in children, particularly when a cartilaginous fracture or dislocation of the radial head is suspected.

Hand

Soft tissue abnormalities, including the presence of a ganglion, soft tissue material in the carpal tunnel, and tendon pathology, are well

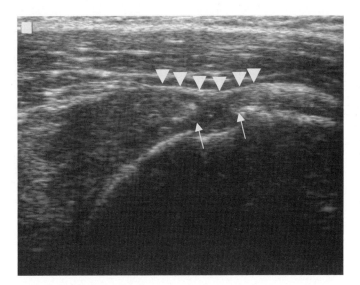

Fig. 10 Supraspinatus tendon tear. The sagittal oblique ultrasound shows the torn ends of the tendon (arrows) and the concave anterior border to the supraspinatus tendon (arrowheads).

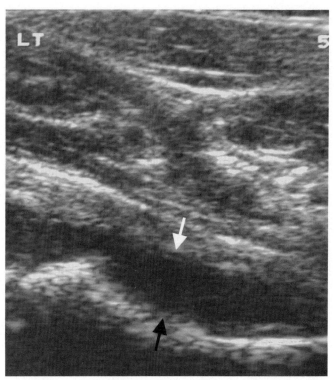

Fig. 12 Hip effusion. The anechoic region between the femoral neck (black arrow) and iliopsoas tendon (white arrow) represents fluid within the joint. This could be aspirated under ultrasound guidance.

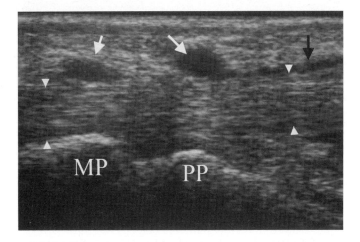

Fig. 11 Tenosynovitis. The flexor digitorum longus tendon of the third digit of the hand (between arrowheads) is normal. Fluid tracking along the tendon sheath (black arrow) and accumulating in small pockets (white arrows) indicates early tenosynovitis.

demonstrated by ultrasound. Ganglia appear as a well defined structure of low echogenicity. Ultrasound is very sensitive in demonstrating pathology within the synovial sheath surrounding tendons, and can pick up tenosynovitis at an early stage (Fig. 11). The technique can also visualize the underlying tendon and quantify the degree of tendonitis. The use of ultrasound in the quantification of erosions, particularly in the context of rheumatoid arthritis, has huge potential future benefit and is the focus of extensive current research.

Hip

Hip pain represents a diagnostic challenge due to the wide variety of potential underlying causes. Ultrasound is useful at all ages. In the neonate, ultrasound is used to detect and quantify developmental dysplasia. In the child ultrasound can detect a hip effusion in the context of reactive synovitis, and ultrasound is used to guide percutaneous hip

aspiration to differentiate synovitis from infection (Fig. 12). In the adult, ultrasound is sensitive at detecting abnormal fluid within the hip, which can be a useful non-specific marker for inflammation, and can also visualize the surrounding musculature to detect avulsion injuries, tendon ruptures, and haematomas. The presence of clicking in association with pain is a common presenting complaint and, in some situations, the structure causing the clicking can be identified, particularly the presence of a snapping iliopsoas band.[4] Fluid within the iliopsoas bursa is another potential mimic of hip pathology, and such bursitis is elegantly demonstrated sonographically.

Knee

Although ultrasound is not a first line investigation in the evaluation of a patient with internal derangement of the knee, soft tissue swelling in relation to the knee, as with other joints, is particularly well demonstrated on ultrasound. The semimembranous–gastrocnemius bursa (Baker's cyst, popliteal cyst) is well demonstrated and, because of the specific configuration where the cyst can be shown to arise between the semimembranosus tendon and the medial head of gastrocnemius (Fig. 13), the diagnosis can be made with certainty. Patellar tendinopathies are also well demonstrated sonographically, although, in general, abnormalities of the patella tendon remain a clinical diagnosis as the tendon is easily palpated.

Foot

Because of the superficial nature of the various tendons that are related to the ankle, ultrasound is ideally suited to their evaluation.

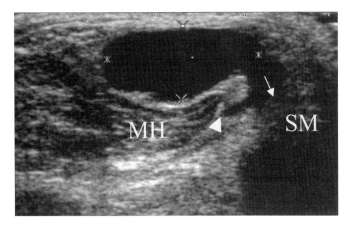

Fig. 13 Baker's cyst. A cystic structure is seen arising (arrowhead) between the medial head of gastrocnemius (MH) and the semimembranosus tendon (SM, arrow). This anatomical arrangement gives the cyst its formal name— the semimembranosus–gastrocnemius bursa.

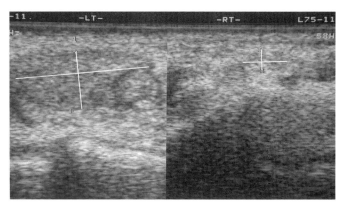

Fig. 15 Peroneal tenosynovitis. Ultrasound shows marked increase in size of the peroneal tendons on the left when compared to the right (white lines indicate cross-sectional area of peroneus longus bilaterally).

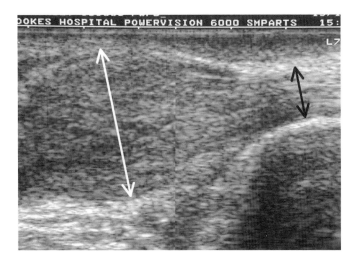

Fig. 14 Gross Achilles tendonitis. 5 cm proximal to the distal insertion of the Achilles tendon, the structure is grossly thickened (white arrowheads) when compared to the normal size expected (black arrowheads). The normal internal parallel fibrillar pattern has been replaced by irregular regions of relative increased and decreased echogenicity indicating severe tendonitis.

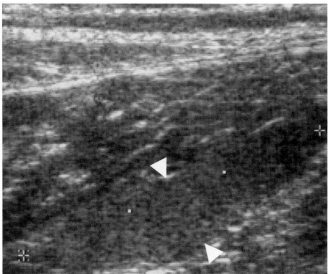

Fig. 16 Calf haematoma. Slow recovery from a calf muscle tear prompted an ultrasound examination, which confirmed the presence of a 3 cm haematoma (between arrowheads) within the medial head of gastrocnemius. This was aspirated under ultrasound guidance allowing more rapid recovery.

The Achilles tendon and the posterior tibial tendons are the most common tendons to be injured and, in addition to diagnosing tendinopathy, ultrasound can be useful in quantifying the degree of damage. This information helps in deciding which patients require surgery and can also help in surgical planning (Figs 14 and 15). Soft tissue abnormalities in relation to the foot and ankle are ideally suited to sonographic evaluation, and a cystic structure is readily differentiated from a solid mass. Specific tumours that are confined to the foot include the presence of a Morton's neuroma, and such lesions can be demonstrated sonographically, although the diagnosis essentially remains a clinical one. Tendons of the foot and toes are occasionally ruptured, and the advent of high-frequency transducers allows even these tiny structures to be followed peripherally to detect disruption, and to identify the anatomical site of the torn ends prior to surgery.

Muscle injuries and tumours

The normal muscle appears as a well-defined arrangement of parallel echogenic structures representing the intermuscular fibrous fascicles and disruption to this arrangement is readily identified. Muscle haematomas, therefore, which may incapacitate otherwise fit individuals, are easily identified and followed up and, if suitable clinically, the collections of fluid can be aspirated under ultrasound guidance (Fig. 16). Soft tissue tumours arising from muscle are uncommon but are important due to the fact that solid muscle lesions are not uncommonly malignant. The accuracy of ultrasound in their detection depends on the nature of the tumour, and an infiltrating lesion with similar sonographic characteristics to the adjacent muscle may be missed on ultrasound. For this reason, although ultrasound is a good initial technique in the evaluation of a soft tissue mass, if the diagnosis is not clear sonographically when the mass is definite clinically, then the

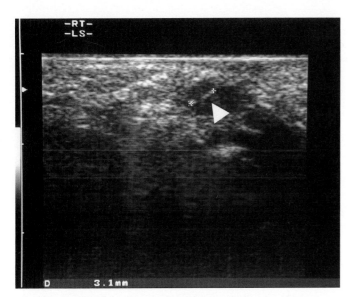

Fig. 17 Foreign body. Ultrasound confirmed the presence of a 3 mm splinter of wood that was successfully surgically excised (arrowhead). The patient presented with a 'synovitis' and was unaware of the initial injury.

patient should be referred for MRI. In many cases, however, a confident diagnosis of a superficial lipoma is made precluding further investigation, as long as the mass is not increasing in size over time.

Foreign bodies

Radio-opaque foreign bodies are readily visualized on plain film radiography. However, a large number of foreign bodes are not radio-opaque and these include wood splinters and thorns. Because these structures have very different acoustic impedance from soft tissues, they are readily identified within the adjacent soft tissue, even when very small (Fig. 17). Lesions down to 1 mm can be seen with an appropriate high-frequency transducer. In addition to demonstrating the presence of a foreign body, its position can be documented. This is particularly important in the case of splinters that enter a tendon sheath, as they are then free to move within the sheath and may be carried to a position some distance away from the entry point. Not uncommonly, a patient with soft tissue inflammation due to a splinter may have no recollection of the injury (Fig. 17).

Summary

Ultrasound is a universally available, cheap, radiation-free form of imaging, ideally suited to soft tissue pathology. The advent of high-frequency transducers over the last decade has revolutionized the application of ultrasound to musculoskeletal imaging and new applications will develop even further over the coming years. In many institutions, ultrasound is the first-line diagnostic technique for the majority of soft tissue injuries. It has no known adverse side-effects.

Magnetic resonance imaging

Technical aspects

Magnetic resonance imaging (MRI) is an imaging modality that does not use ionizing radiation and that can generate cross-sectional images in any arbitrary plane. The images are acquired by placing the patient into a strong homogeneous magnetic field (common systems range in field strength from 0.02 to 1.5 Tesla (T), where 1 T corresponds to approximately 10,000 times the strength of the Earth's magnetic field). In response to the external magnetic field, the body's protons tend to exist in one of two fundamental physical energy states, the difference in energy between those states being related to the strength of the magnetic field. A radiofrequency pulse is applied at exactly the correct frequency to promote some protons from the lower energy state into the higher energy state. Only a tiny proportion of protons are excited in this way, but this is sufficient to generate the image. Subsequently, protons drop from the higher energy state by releasing the extra energy. A *T1-weighted image* is one in which the intensity of each pixel is related to the rate at which protons within the corresponding voxel release this energy to adjacent macromolecules, the so-called *lattice*. Conversely, a *T2-weighted image* is one in which the intensity of each pixel relates to the ability of the protons within the corresponding voxel to release energy to surrounding protons. A *proton density-weighted image* is a corresponding map of the number of protons that are available to absorb energy in this way, and this in turn is related to the quantity of free water. Therefore, the image generated by MRI is a representation of certain fundamental quantum physical characteristics of protons. The interested reader is referred to more detailed texts for an account of how this basic physical property is translated into an image (see Table 1 for a glossary of common MRI terms and descriptions).

The high magnetic field strength associated with conventional magnets, together with the requirement for highly homogeneous field strength across the imaging volume, imposes stringent requirements for the location of MRI systems. Specialized rooms need to be constructed to limit the amount of unwanted external interference from electrical devices elsewhere, and similarly to avoid the magnetic field from the MR system affecting electrical equipment outside the MRI suite. Such building considerations contribute significantly to the cost of installing an MRI system.

Variations

Sequences

Much of the complexity of MRI relates to the profusion of sequences that are available, and further sequences are being developed and improved annually. However, virtually all imaging sequences are based on one of two primary sequences namely the *spin echo* (SE) and *gradient echo* (GE) techniques. In part, the drive to produce further sequences is related to the requirement for reduced imaging times. Traditionally, MRI was a technique where a single series of images took several minutes to be produced, during which time the patient was required to remain still. With increasing speed and sequence development however, this is no longer the case and many images can be obtained in second or subsecond timescales. Nevertheless, most of the sequences used in routine musculoskeletal imaging require acquisition times of several minutes.

In general, T1-weighted sequences are useful for demonstrating and evaluating anatomical structures, but pathological processes are generally not well visualized: an abnormal structure will frequently have a signal on T1-weighted images similar to that of adjacent normal soft tissues and therefore is inconspicuous. On T2-weighted sequences, however, voxels that contain a greater proportion of fluid (usually an indication of pathology such as infection, inflammation,

Table 1 Glossary of terms used in magnetic resonance imaging

Fat saturation. A technique to render the signal from fat dark. On *FSE* T2-weighted images (commonly used in musculoskeletal applications) fat is bright, as is the lesion being evaluated. By selectively darkening the normal adjacent fat, the lesion becomes more conspicuous. An alternative fat saturation technique is *STIR*

FSE (fast spin echo). A technique to increase the speed of a *spin echo* sequence. Can be used with *T1, T2*, or proton-density-weighted images, and with or without *fat saturation*

Gradient. Spatial variation of some physical quantity, such as magnetic field.

Gradient Echo. One of the two fundamental MRI sequences. The term relates to the way that the *protons* are refocused after they have been excited by using a magnetic field *gradient*

PD (proton density or spin density). Density of free water protons in a given volume. It is therefore one of the principal determinants of the strength of the MR signal.

Proton. A positively charged nucleon, that is, a hydrogen nucleus. Although all protons are affected by the magnetic field, it is those hydrogen nuclei that are part of free water molecules that contribute most significantly to the radiological image

Spin. A spin is another name for a *proton*

Spin Echo (SE). One of the two fundamental imaging sequences. In SE imaging, the *protons* are refocused after they have been excited by applying a second radiofrequency pulse

STIR (short T1 inversion recovery). A technique to suppress signal from tissues with a short T1 value. Fat has a particularly short (low) T1 value so STIR is a technique to produce *fat saturation*

T1 (pronounced 'T-one'). Spin–lattice or longitudinal relaxation time measured in milliseconds. A measure of the rate at which excited protons release their energy to surrounding larger macromolecules ('the lattice')

T2 (pronounced 'T-two'). Spin–spin or transverse relaxation time measured in milliseconds. A measure of the rate at which excited protons release their energy to other adjacent protons

tumour etc.) are generally brighter and are therefore conspicuous. A variety of techniques exists to maximize the conspicuity of pathological processes. Central to these is the desire to render the signal from normal structures, such as fat, dark so that an abnormal bright structure on the image will stand out. The majority of MR examinations therefore include some form of *fat saturation*, and the combination of fat saturation with a fast spin echo sequence finds universal acceptance in musculoskeletal imaging. When not available, a useful alternative is the 'short T1 inversion recovery' (STIR) sequence. A further complexity is created, as in many cases there is inconsistency in the terminology used by different competing manufacturers for what is fundamentally the same sequence.

Gadolinium diethylenetriaminepentaacetic acid (Gd-DTPA)

The intravenous injection of Gd-DTPA is used in a way analogous to intravenous (IV) contrast with CT examinations (see below). Gd-DTPA is a paramagnetic agent that increases the rate at which energy can be transferred from protons by acting as a suitable receptacle for that extra energy. The molecule permeates out of the vascular bed at a rate related to the permeability of the structure concerned, and therefore pathological processes, which often are of both increased perfusion and permeability, will frequently enhance more avidly that adjacent normal structures. Combined with T1-weighted sequences therefore, possibly with fat saturation, gadolinium causes an increase in the conspicuousness of a structure that is abnormal. In *MR arthrography*, gadolinium is injected at a lower concentration directly into a joint, and this increases the information available from the examination, albeit at the expense of converting a non-invasive procedure into an invasive one.

Open MR scanning systems

The conventional MR scanning system is comprised of an elongated doughnut-shaped construction that contains the supercooled wire coil that produces the strong magnetic field when an electrical current is passed through it. Such an arrangement was initially the easiest way to achieve sufficiently strong magnetic field strengths. The disadvantage, however, is that the patient has to be passed into the centre of the coil, which resembles a tunnel. Many patients find this uncomfortable, although only a few are overtly claustrophobic, and the geometry means that it is not possible to perform interventional procedures on the patient while they are inside the machine. Developments in coil design have taken several paths over the past 10 years with the development of other geometries including a double-doughnut design that allows the interventionist to access the patient between the doughnuts and a horizontal design where the magnetic field is orientated perpendicular to the floor between two horizontal surfaces with the patient lying in-between.

Niche low-field-strength magnets

These have the potential to revolutionize the availability of MRI. They are self-contained MRI solutions that can literally be wheeled into any medium-sized room, and require no formal installation. Currently, they are only available for the assessment of extremities (wrists, knees, etc.) and they work at a lower field strength (typically 0.02 T). Imaging time is therefore longer, but they are convenient and they open the prospect of installing an MR system near to a casualty department where it can assist in the immediate assessment of trauma victims.

Strengths

The rapid increase in the number of MRI examinations performed for musculoskeletal disorders over the past decade is a testament to the usefulness of the technique in the evaluation of soft tissue abnormalities. This success is due to many factors. MRI is very sensitive in detecting areas of increased free water. Most pathological processes involve either altered morphology of the affected structure or oedema (increased tissue-free water). In addition, the ability to image in any arbitrary imaging plane means that the abnormality can be visualized optimally in relation to adjacent structures. Because of alterations in the signal due to flow, larger vessels are conspicuous without the requirement to inject IV contrast medium. In addition, the combination of a number of series with different imaging parameters allows specific tissue diagnoses to be made The technique appears to be not associated with any biological hazard and, in particular, avoids the use of ionizing radiation (see below).

Disadvantages

The technique relies on expensive hardware and buildings, supported by complicated software and peripherals. The resulting cost has meant that MRI has been slower to be widely implemented than may have been desirable. In addition, the technique involves the patient being passed through a narrow 'tunnel' and, while acquiring the image, the scanning system is noisy. Approximately 1–2 per cent of individuals cannot tolerate the examination due to claustrophobia. Perhaps surprisingly, a significant proportion of patients who have had both MRI and arthrography separately indicate that they preferred the arthrogram, even though it involved an intraarticular injection. Although MRI is acutely sensitive at detecting abnormalities, it is not always associated with specificity. In particular, as most pathological processes involve an increase in the amount of free water, MRI has difficulty in differentiating between them. For example, an ill-defined area of increased signal intensity on T2-weighted sequences, which would indicate increased oedema, may be due to tumour, trauma, infection, or some other injury. For this reason, it is always important to review MR examinations in conjunction with other information, particularly plain film and clinical findings. Table 2 shows the relative MR signal intensity of a variety of tissues, and demonstrates how the combination of T1-, proton density-, and T2-weighted images can be useful to differentiate the constituents of corresponding tissues. Finally, there is a myriad of factors that need to be taken into consideration and to be optimized before the image is produced. These include choice of the appropriate coil, the anatomical plane of imaging, slice thickness, slice spacing, the pulse sequence, two- or three-dimensional acquisition, the specific imaging characteristics, to name but a few. In practice therefore, the combination of options that is eventually chosen will be a compromise and will depend on the clinical context. The specific clinical question must be understood at the time of performing the examination. It is not always possible to return to the images in retrospect and answer a new question that was not considered at the time of imaging.

Specific clinical uses

Hip

Pain arising from the region of the hip may be due to one of a number of causes, including cartilage and labral pathologies of the hip itself, abnormalities arising from adjacent bursae, and avulsion injuries from

Table 2 MR signal characteristics in musculoskeletal imaging

	T1 signal	Proton density signal	T2 signal
Fat	Very high	High	Intermediate
Yellow marrow (fatty)	Very high	High	Intermediate
Red marrow	Intermediate/low	Intermediate/low	Intermediate/low
Muscle	Intermediate	Intermediate	Low
Most tumours	Intermediate/low	Intermediate	Intermediate/high
Tendon/ligament	Very low	Very low	Very low
Cortical bone	Very low	Very low	Very low
Calcium	Low	Low	Low
Fluid (oedema, inflammation, trauma)	Intermediate/low	Intermediate	Intermediate/high
Haemosiderin-containing (e.g. mature haematoma)	Very low in parts	Very low in parts	Very low in parts

the greater trochanter or ischium, or may even be referred from the lumbar spine. For this reason, MR represents a good screening tool for hip pathology. Avascular necrosis is readily diagnosed and staged on MRI, and changes can be seen before plain film abnormalities are apparent. MRI is also useful to follow up postoperatively to confirm that there has been no subsequent progression.

Labral pathology is common and presents with pain, frequently associated with clicking. Plain MR can be useful in evaluating the labrum, but MR arthrography increases the accuracy of the technique. MR is particularly sensitive at detecting fractures, and is capable of detecting a radiologically occult fracture of the neck of the femur immediately after injury, and certainly before a scintigraphic abnormality would be detected.[5] In the future, therefore, MRI may become an appropriate screening tool for the injured elderly patient in whom an occult fracture is suspected, as in this age group in particular scintigraphic abnormalities can remain undetected for 48–72 hours after injury. In addition, stress fractures are well demonstrated on MRI as a linear low-signal structure on all sequences often surrounded by bone marrow oedema when acute (Fig. 18). The distension and oedema associated with bursitis make MR a suitable diagnostic tool for its detection—the iliopsoas bursa and the trochanteric bursa are most commonly affected (Fig. 19).

Knee

It was the early application of MRI to knee pathology, together with the advent of knee arthroscopy, that gave MRI its first widespread appeal. Meniscal and cruciate injuries are demonstrated with high accuracy at all field strengths from 0.2 to 1.5 T.[6] The normal meniscus appears as a 'bow tie' shaped structure in the sagittal plane, comprising anterior and posterior horns, which is of low signal on all sequences. Tears have been variously classified, and appear as an area of high signal on T2*-weighted sequences, which extend to the

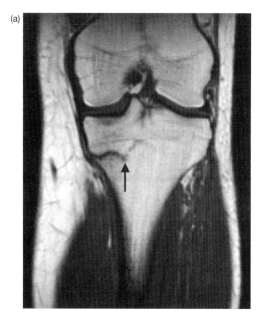

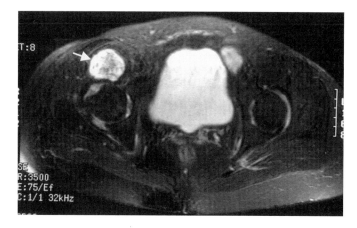

Fig. 19 Iliopsoas bursa. A soft tissue structure is present anterior to the right hip (arrow) that returns increased signal on this T2-weighted-fat saturated image, but appears somewhat heterogeneous.

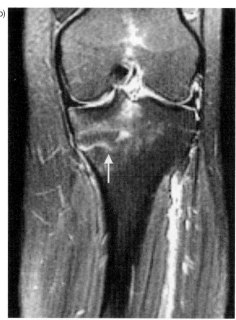

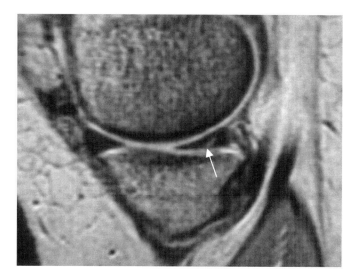

Fig. 20 Meniscal tear. There is an oblique tear through the posterior third of the medial meniscus opening on to the inferior surface (arrow).

Fig. 18 Tibial stress fracture. The fracture line is well demonstrated medially within the tibial plateau in this long distance runner. (a) T1-weighted image and (b) fat-saturated T2-weighted image.

meniscal surface (Fig. 20). The majority of the tears are demonstrated in the sagittal plane, with only a minority being seen only coronally. The cruciate ligaments are intracapsular but extrasynovial and tears are common in the population imaged by MRI (Fig. 21). The accuracy of MRI is in excess of 90 per cent in the demonstration of meniscal and cruciate ligament tears. The collateral ligaments are injured by excess valgus or varus force applied to the knee. Although they are demonstrable on MRI, diagnosis is often clinical but, more importantly, collateral ligament damage is often associated with additional cruciate or meniscal injury. As at other sites, MR is an accurate way to demonstrate fractures that are occult on plain films, including stress fractures in the appropriate circumstance (Fig. 18).

Anterior knee pain requires additional sequences targeting the patella, and chondromalacia patellae is particularly well demonstrated on axial T2-weighted fat-saturated images (Fig. 22). The degree of chondromalacia can be staged relative to whether just the cartilage is involved, or whether the underlying bone is also oedematous.[7] The height of the patella in relation to the tibia is also an important factor in the aetiology of anterior knee pain. The normal craniocaudal position of the patella is such that the length of the patella tendon should be equal to the height of the patella ±20 per cent.[8] A high patella (patella alta) is associated with the development of chondromalacia, whereas a low patella (patella baja) is seen secondary to polio and juvenile chronic arthritis.

Cysts and bursae around the knee are particularly well demonstrated due to the presence of internal fluid. A ganglion cyst is represented as a well-defined, often multiloculated cystic structure, which may have the beaded appearance resulting from the adjacent development of multiple small component cysts, but which does not

(a)

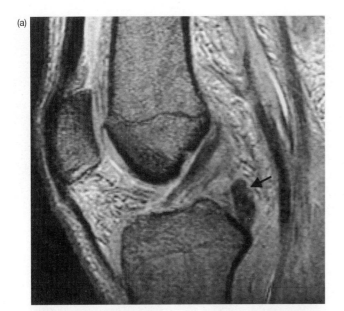

(b)

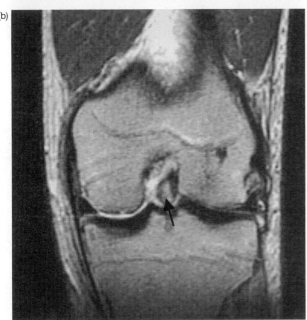

Fig. 21 Chronic posterior cruciate ligament (PCL) tear. (a) Sagittal gradient-enhanced image shows the PCL to be truncated (arrow). (b) The centre returns increased signal on a T2-weighted coronal image (arrow).

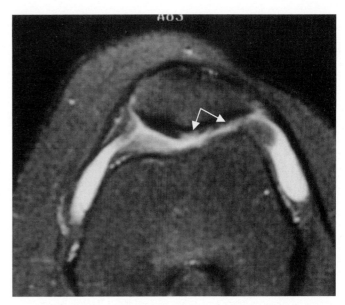

Fig. 22 Chondromalacia patellae. High signal is seen within the cartilage on the posterior aspect of the patella (arrows). The cartilage itself has an irregular contour on the lateral facet when compared to the medial facet. The underlying bone is normal.

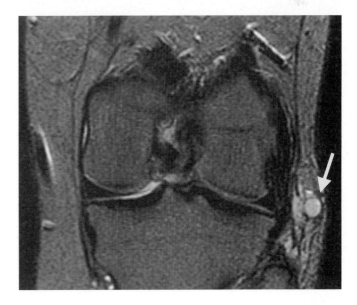

Fig. 23 Ganglion. A well defined structure returning fluid signal is seen lateral to the joint line (arrow). It is not associated with a meniscal tear.

communicate with the joint (Fig. 23). A meniscal cyst develops as a result of fluid being forced through a meniscal tear into the adjacent soft tissues. A necessary prerequisite therefore in the diagnosis of meniscal cyst is the presence of an adjacent meniscal tear (Fig. 24). There are a variety of bursae that exist in relation to the knee, the most common being the semimembranous–gastrocnemius bursa (Fig. 25, Baker's cyst, popliteal cyst), which commonly enlarges, particularly in patients with rheumatoid arthritis and other intraarticular pathology. The patient presents with a soft tissue swelling in the popliteal fossa that may rupture giving an identical presentation to calf deep vein thrombosis. The presence of a semimembranous–gastrocnemius bursa in a child is a separate entity, and usually no associated knee

pathology is presented. Prepatellar bursitis (housemaid's knee) presents with a well-defined fluid-containing structure anterior to the patella, namely, the prepatellar bursa (Fig. 26).

Ankle and foot

The Achilles tendon is the largest and the strongest tendon in the human body. It is formed by the common insertion of the medial and lateral heads of gastrocnemius, soleus, and plantaris. In common with tendon abnormalities elsewhere in the body, the tendon undergoes degeneration with age, and this manifests as tendon swelling in the

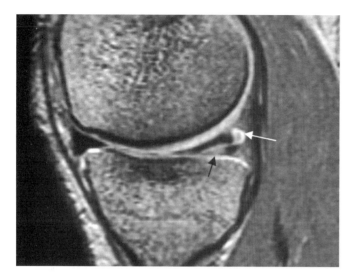

Fig. 24 Meniscal cyst. There is an oblique tear through the middle third of the lateral meniscus (black arrow) with fluid extending through the tear into the meniscal cyst immediately lateral to the meniscus (white arrow).

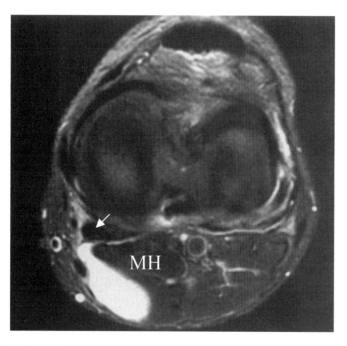

Fig. 25 Baker's cyst. A semimembranosus–gastrocnemius bursa is seen to arise between the semimembranosus tendon (arrow) and the medial head of gastrocnemius (MH). The appearances are analogous to the ultrasound appearances in Fig. 13.

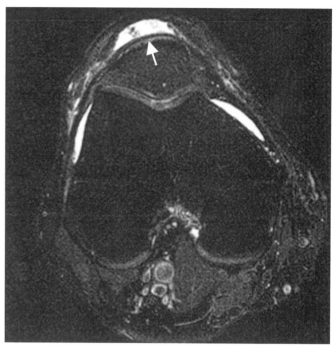

Fig. 26 'Housemaid's knee'. The pre-patellar bursa is enlarged (arrow) on this T2-weighted-fat saturated axial image.

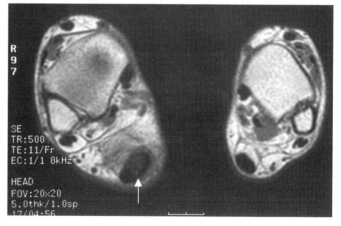

Fig. 27 Achilles tendinosis. The right Achilles tendon is enlarged when compared to the left and returns increased signal internally (arrow). Adjacent fat planes are indistinct.

first instance. Cystic degeneration develops, and this may lead on to fissure and partial tear formation. The weakened tendon is then liable to complete rupture. All of these stages can be demonstrated and differentiated on MRI. In the earlier stages, the normal low signal returned from the tendon is replaced by increased signal on T1- and T2-weighted images and the structure becomes swollen (Fig. 27). The presence of a complete tear is associated with extensive adjacent soft tissue abnormalities, in addition to haematoma formation and tendon

fragmentation (Fig. 28). The posterior tibial, long flexor, and peroneal tendons are also well demonstrated on MRI. Ligament injuries do not themselves necessitate MR examination, but the normal ligament is well demonstrated on MR sequences, and acute injuries, which are associated with oedema, are easily demonstrated. After healing, however, ligament laxity is not an MR diagnosis. Accessory muscles occur at many sites, but the most common such muscle is the accessory soleus muscle where the soleus, instead of joining the gastrocnemius muscles to form the Achilles tendon, inserts separately into the calcaneus. The diagnosis is readily made on axial MRI (Fig. 29).

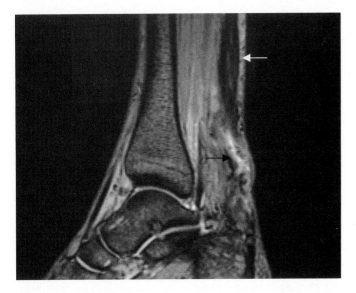

Fig. 28 Complete Achilles tendon rupture. The distal 8 cm of the Achilles tendon is disrupted, with oedema and haemorrhage (black arrow) replacing the normal structure. More superiorly (white arrow) the tendon appears more normal.

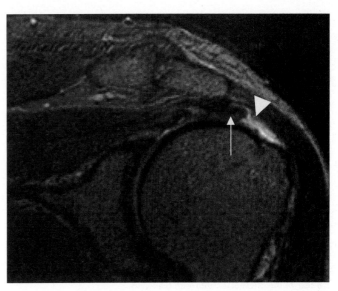

Fig. 30 Full thickness supraspinatus tear. Fat-saturated, coronal oblique, T2-weighted image shows an interruption in the supraspinatus tendon (arrow), with fluid crossing the full width of the tendon (arrowhead).

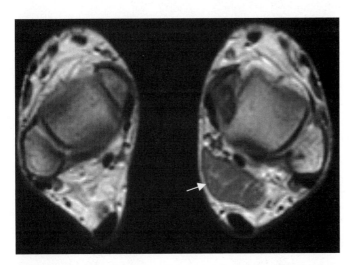

Fig. 29 Accessory soleus muscle. This congenital anomaly presents as a soft tissue mass on the medial aspect of the ankle. The structure returns signal typical for muscle (arrow).

Shoulder

The most common reason for performing MRI of the shoulder is in the context of shoulder impingement, where MRI can accurately differentiate between tendonitis and a full thickness rotator cuff tear. In the former, increased signal within the tendon is demonstrated on both the proton-density- and T2-weighted sequences, but this is ill defined and not intense. In the case of a full thickness tear, however, discrete focal intense high signal is demonstrated on the T2-weighted sequence, and any resulting retraction of the proximal tendon fragment can be well demonstrated and quantified (Fig. 30). The majority of such tears affect the supraspinatus tendon, and secondary signs include fluid within the subacromial–subdeltoid bursa, atrophy of the supraspinatus muscle, cranial migration of the humeral head, and impingement cysts affecting the greater tuberosity of the humerus. In addition to demonstrating tear or tendonitis however, MR can demonstrate the degree of degenerative change affecting the acromioclavicular joint, and the shape of the acromion, both of which are important aetiological factors in the development of a rotator cuff tear.[9]

Calcific tendonitis is essentially a plain film diagnosis, but the area of calcification is well demonstrated on MR as a signal void on all sequences. Glenohumeral joint instability affects a younger age group than affected by impingement and, although bony abnormalities resulting from previous dislocation can be seen on plain MR techniques, the demonstration of the cartilaginous glenoid labrum itself and the important inferior glenohumeral ligament[10] requires MR arthrography.

Elbow

The complicated three-dimensional anatomy of the elbow means that designing imaging protocols for the elbow represent a challenge. Osteochondritis dissecans, commonly occurring in adolescents and young adults, is an important indication for MR of the elbow, where bony fragmentation can be demonstrated and where, more importantly, the integrity of the overlying cartilage can also be assessed. Loose bodies are well demonstrated, particularly in the presence of an effusion. Epicondylitis (tennis elbow, golfer's elbow) can also be detected on MRI, although in general these diagnoses remain clinical, and MR is rarely performed (Fig. 31). Biceps tendon rupture more commonly occurs proximally, resulting in the typical 'popeye' appearance clinically, but tendon injuries at the bicipital tuberosity of the radius are also elegantly demonstrated on MRI.

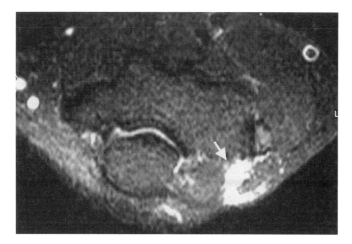

Fig. 31 Lateral epicondylitis. Axial STIR image demonstrates oedema in the insertion of the common extensor origin (arrow) in this patient with a partial tear of the origin associated with tendonitis.

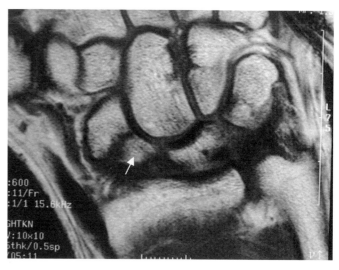

Fig. 33 Scaphoid fracture without avascular necrosis. Coronal T1-weighted image through the wrist shows a fracture through the waist of the scaphoid. The proximal pole of the scaphoid (arrow) returns high signal in keeping with viable fat.

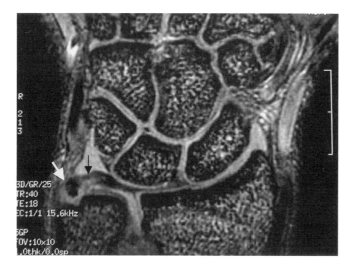

Fig. 32 Intact TFCC and avulsed ulnar styloid. In this patient with symptoms typical of a torn TFCC, the TFCC itself was seen to be intact (black arrow) but the ulna styloid is shown to be detached (white arrow).

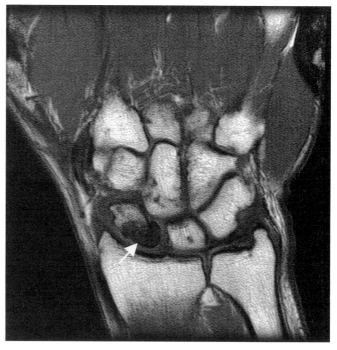

Fig. 34 Scaphoid fracture with avascular proximal pole. The proximal pose is of low signal on this T1-weighted coronal image. This indicates that the marrow therein is non-viable.

Hand and wrist

MR of the wrist has been revolutionized in recent years by the advent of dedicated wrist coils, which are of a small size that can comfortably accommodate only the wrist. The result is increased spatial resolution, which is necessary for assessing the small structures within the wrist. The triangular fibrocartilage complex (TFCC) can be well demonstrated on gradient echo sequences in particular and tears can be detected as an area of high signal across the width of what would otherwise be a low signal structure on all sequences (Fig. 32). Another common indication for MR of the wrist relates to fractures of the scaphoid. MR is sensitive at demonstrating the presence of a fracture, and can do so immediately after injury.[11] More importantly, after a delay of 6 weeks MR can be used to determine the prognosis by

predicting the risk of avascular necrosis of the proximal fragment in cases where non-union has occurred.[12] In situations where the proximal pole is vascular, marrow fat remains alive and the fragment returns high signal on T1-weighted sequences. However, prolonged avascularity results in adipocyte death, and this in turn results in reduced signal on T1-weighted images (Figs 33 and 34).

(a)

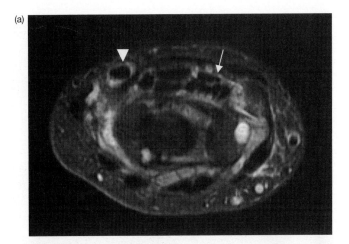

(b)

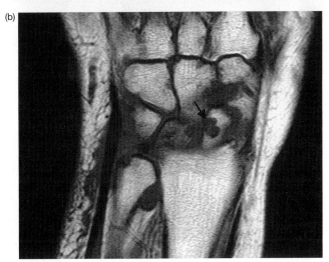

Fig. 35 Rheumatoid arthritis (RA) presenting with carpal tunnel syndrome. (a) Axial fat-saturated T2 image shows diffuse synovitis resulting in increased soft tissue within the carpal tunnel (arrow) together with tenosynovitis (arrowhead). (b) Coronal T1-weighted image confirms the presence of multiple erosions. Subsequent plain film confirmed that some of these erosions could be seen on plain radiograph, but plain films underestimate the extent of erosive change. The diagnosis of RA was confirmed serologically.

Carpal tunnel syndrome remains an electrophysiological diagnosis, although MR can be useful when the diagnosis is established to detect underlying causes, commonly in the form of space-occupying lesions such as ganglia or synovitis within the carpal tunnel (Fig. 35).

Spine

MRI has a pivotal role in the diagnosis of low back pain and demonstrates the soft tissue structures including the intervertebral disc to advantage. The diagnosis of disc prolapse can be made, and the size and extent of the prolapsed disc are well seen, together with the relationship of the protrusion to exiting nerve roots (Fig. 36), information that is not available from plain film radiography. In addition, discitis results in a typical MR appearance where bone marrow oedema is seen within two adjacent vertebral bodies and furthermore, fluid (high signal material on T2) is demonstrated within the intervertebral disc space.

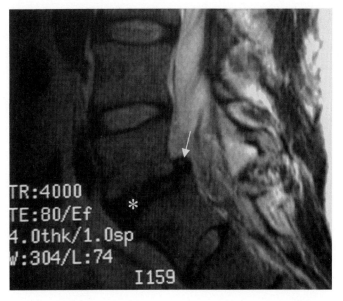

Fig. 36 Prolapsed intervertebral disc. The L5/S1 disc is of reduced signal on this T2-weighted image indicating lack of hydration (*) and there is a disc prolapse posteriorly (arrow) extending into the intervertebral canal at this level. A minor degree of spondylolithesis is associated at the same level, which is degenerative in aetiology.

Soft tissue and bone tumours

Soft tissue and bone tumours represent entirely different entities with different imaging requirements. Nevertheless, MR is uniquely positioned to provide information in both situations that helps to select patients for surgery and provides details necessary for surgical planning. In the case of bone tumours, it is the plain radiograph that is most likely to give the specific diagnosis. MR, however, will give the extent of the lesion, and more accurately demonstrate the degree of adjacent soft tissue involvement (Fig. 37). Nevertheless, it is unwise to review MR images of the bone tumour without having first seen the plain film.

Most soft tissue masses, however, are not demonstrable on plain film radiography unless secondary bone involvement is present, and MR is particularly well suited to their demonstration and evaluation. Certain characteristic features enable an accurate histopathological diagnosis to be made in some situations, such as a lipoma or haemangioma (Fig. 38). In other situations, MR will help to suggest of whether the lesion is aggressive or non-aggressive but in principle remains non-specific from a histological point of view. In these cases the definitive diagnostic technique, once the presence of a solid mass has been confirmed on MR, is biopsy and histology.

Summary

In many situations, MRI has become the cornerstone of imaging for soft tissue abnormalities. Its supreme sensitivity to increased free water makes it able to demonstrate oedema, inflammation, trauma, and degeneration. The pathology can be imaged in the plane that is most suitable, depending on circumstance, and the technique is free of the biohazard associated with ionizing radiation. The equipment is expensive, but the costs are reducing every decade, and this process of cost reduction will continue particularly as applications both inside and outside of musculoskeletal imaging are expanding.

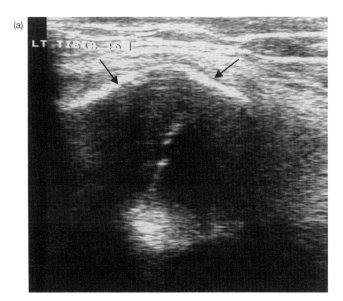

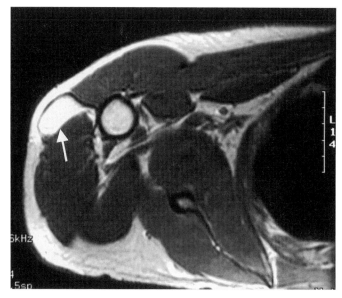

Fig. 38 Lipoma. An abnormal soft tissue mass is arising from the deltoid on the right. It has identical signal characteristics to those of subcutaneous fat, and histologically was proven to be a simple lipoma.

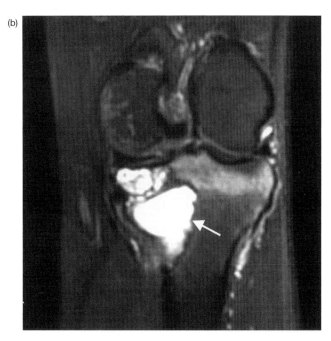

Fig. 37 Giant cell tumour of bone presenting with soft tissue swelling. This patient presented for ultrasound with the presumed diagnosis of pes anserine bursitis. (a) Ultrasound confirmed the presence of an abnormality within the bone and (b) the true extent of the lesion was demonstrated in MRI. The diagnosis of giant cell tumour was made histologically.

Arthrography

Technical aspects

The technique of contrast arthrography was developed at a time when many of the other imaging techniques outlined in this chapter were not available. The technique addressed the fundamental problem with plain radiography, namely, that the latter does not visualize soft tissue structures directly. It achieved this by using the injection of iodinated contrast agents into a joint to distend the joint space. This provides additional information about the soft tissue structures related to the joint either directly by specifically outlining them, or indirectly.[13] Common to all arthrographic contrast agents is the combination of an iodine molecule bound into a larger macromolecule, and it is the bound iodine within the molecule that increases the X-ray attenuation of photons passing through the area injected. The technique is performed with fluoroscopic guidance to ensure that the needle tip lies within the joint to be imaged and, after the contrast injection, plain radiographs are taken using a conventional technique. The details of each injection vary from joint to joint, and the interested reader is referred elsewhere for further details.[13]

The technique is interventional in that it requires the percutaneous insertion of a needle into the joint, and contraindications to arthrography would include the presence of cutaneous or subcutaneous infection overlying the joint, or of a blood dyscrasia that would make haemarthrosis following the injection more likely.

Variations

Double contrast arthrography

This technique is sometimes advocated and involves the injection of a small amount of iodinated contrast material followed by a larger volume of room air. The result is that joint capsule can be lined from inside by contrast material, giving a pseudo three-dimensional effect. In some instances, this enhances the diagnostic information available, particularly in relation to the detection of loose bodies. In addition, either double or single contrast arthrography can be combined with a CT or an MRI examination (CT arthrography or MR arthrography—see below).

Therapeutic arthrography

Arthrography can also be useful as a therapeutic procedure when steroid can be injected into a joint. Although steroid injection is commonly performed using anatomical landmarks and manual palpation, deeper joints such as the hip, sacroiliac, or subtalar joints can be difficult to palpate. When these are the cause of pain, a small amount of contrast can be injected to confirm that the needle tip lies within the joint (Fig. 39), and thereafter a combination of steroid and local anaesthetic can be instilled. The addition of local anaesthetic can be a useful adjunct, as failure of the pain to improve after local anaesthetic injection implies that the pain may not be arising from the suspected joint. For example, hip pain is common and often non-specific with a number of possible causes including lumbar disc pathology. In some circumstances where a total hip replacement is being considered, it may be considered necessary to prove that the pain that the patient is experiencing is truly arising from the hip. In this situation, failure of improvement of the pain temporarily after local anaesthetic has been injected into the hip would imply that the pain may be arising from outside the hip and therefore that a total hip replacement may not be successful in curing the patient's main symptoms.

Strengths

Conventional arthrography is inexpensive, reliable, and universally available. The technique is easily learned and is well tolerated by the patient. Indeed many patients prefer the technique to other imaging techniques such as MRI, although this may be because of the personal contact between clinician and patient.[14] Nevertheless, with the advent of MRI, its use has become more limited to specific indications that are outlined below. Where MRI has become available, the use of arthrography has reduced significantly. For example, knee, wrist, and ankle arthrograms are particularly infrequently performed in institutions with access to MRI.

Weaknesses

In general, the two main weaknesses are, first, that the technique is invasive, requiring direct intraarticular injection and, second, that the information provided is predominantly of an indirect nature—the soft tissues themselves are not directly visualized. In addition, the radiation exposure to the patient consists of the initial fluoroscopy time together with the radiation from the series of plain radiographs that can number up to 10 or so films. Therefore, the technique may result in radiation exposure 5–10 times greater than that attributable to corresponding plain radiography.

Specific clinical uses

Shoulder

The shoulder is a large joint where diagnostic arthrography still plays an important role. The joint is approached anteriorly, and in a single contrast technique 10–15 ml of iodinated contrast is injected into the joint. The concept behind the technique relates to the anatomical fact that the roof of the joint is comprised of the tendons of the rotator cuff, especially supraspinatus and infraspinatus, covered by joint synovial lining. A full thickness rotator cuff tear in one of these tendons associated with capsular damage at that site allows contrast to escape out of the shoulder joint and into the subacromial–subdeltoid bursa (Fig. 40). In a normal individual, there is no communication between these two structures (Fig. 41). The accuracy of shoulder arthrography for the detection of a full thickness tear is excellent.[15] Partial thickness tears, however, are not so readily demonstrated, unless they extend on to the inferior surface of the tendon, a situation that only arises in 20 per cent of partial tears.[16] Therefore, the majority of partial tears remain missed at arthrography. The other main diagnosis that can be made at shoulder arthrography is the presence of capsulitis, where inflammation of the capsule results radiologically in a tight joint of reduced volume. During the procedure, this is manifest as a reduction in the amount of contrast that can be injected into the shoulder before the patient experiences pain. This is followed by early lymphatic filling, a tight joint on visual inspection of the resulting images with obliteration of the axillary recess, and irregularity of the capsular insertion (Fig. 42). Indeed, the distension of the shoulder by iodinated contrast material during the procedure is associated in some with a reduction in the symptoms, and this has led to the suggestion that capsulitis can be

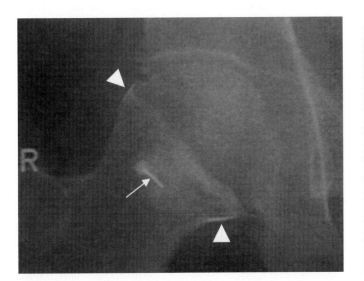

Fig. 39 Fluoroscopic spot film taken during the early stages of a hip arthrogram examination. The needle (arrow) has been inserted and its tip lies within the hip joint. Radiographic contrast has been injected into the joint and outlines the capsule (arrowheads).

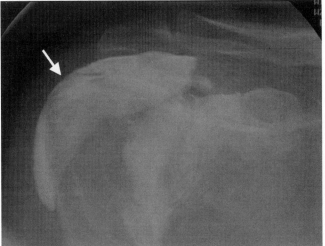

Fig. 40 Full thickness rotator cuff tear. Shoulder arthrogram shows that contrast has escaped from the shoulder joint where it was injected into the subacromial–subdeltoid bursa, the anatomical boundaries of which are well defined (arrow).

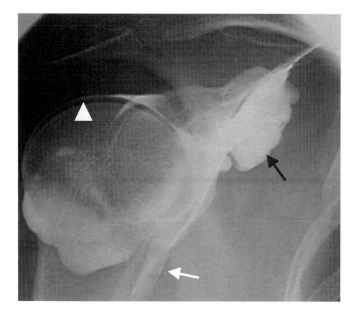

Fig. 41 Normal shoulder arthrogram. Contrast opacifies the joint, and flows into the subcoracoid bursa (black arrow) and the tendon sheath for long head of biceps (white arrow). The articular surface of the humeral head cranially is outlined (arrowhead) and no contrast is seen to escape into the subacromial-subdeltoid bursa.

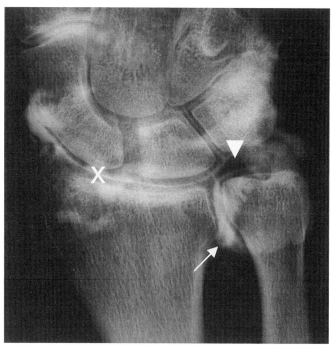

Fig. 43 TFCC tear. In this wrist arthrogram, contrast was injected between the radius and scaphoid (X) and has escaped into the distal radial ulnar joint (arrow) implying that the TFCC is torn. The triangular outline of the TFCC is demonstrated (arrowhead) but the tear itself is not seen.

Elbow and wrist

Plain elbow arthrography is limited in its diagnostic use, but can be useful particularly in conjunction with CT in the evaluation and detection of loose intraarticular bodies (see below). Similarly, in the wrist the diagnosis of TFCC tears can be made reliably by MRI and therefore, where MRI is available, plain arthrography may not be required. When arthrography is performed, perforations through the TFCC can be detected indirectly when contrast injected into the radiocarpal joint is seen to escape into the distal radiocarpal joint (Fig. 43). Additionally, escape of contrast from the radiocarpal articulation into the midcarpal compartment indicates that the either of the scapholunate or lunotriquetral ligaments are disrupted, which is a difficult diagnosis to make at MRI unless the bones are subluxed.

Lower limb

Diagnostic arthrography in the lower limb is not commonly performed if MRI is available, but arthrography can be useful in all joints when loose bodies are suspected, particularly in conjunction with MRI or CT. As indicated, however, fluoroscopic injection of steroid using a modified arthrographic technique is particularly useful in patients with pain arising from the sacroiliac, the hip, and the subtalar joints.

Summary

Arthrography is a technique that involves ionizing radiation and percutaneous joint injection to obtain information, often indirect, about the lining of a joint and periarticular structures. Its role has largely been taken over by other imaging techniques that directly visualize soft tissues but the technique can be combined with CT or MRI to advantage when searching for an intraarticular loose body.

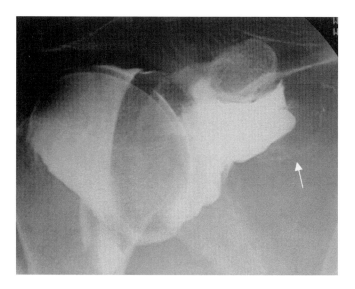

Fig. 42 Capsulitis. Contrast has passed from the joint into the lymphatics (arrow) after only 6 ml of contrast was injected, indicating the presence of severe capsulitis.

treated hydrostatically using this technique.[17] To gain maximal advantage from the injection, however, the patient will be required to exercise to a level that would be beyond most patients' pain thresholds, and therefore manipulation under anaesthetic may be preferred. The injection of steroid after the contrast material, once the diagnosis of capsulitis is established, is theoretically an attractive way to ensure that the inflamed capsular lining receives maximal steroid exposure, but the efficacy of such a technique is not determined.

Computed tomography (CT)

Technical aspects

CT scanning uses ionizing radiation in the form of X-rays to produce multiple parallel cross-sectional images. Unlike in plain radiography where the X-ray tube is stationary and where the resulting image is a projection image, in CT scanning the tube moves during the exposure and produces an axial cross-sectional image. For this reason, it is known as a tomographic technique. CT also differs from conventional radiography in that the resulting image is a digital image that can be stored and manipulated by computer. The CT scanning system measures the attenuation of X-ray photons through the area of interest from a variety of projections, and calculates (reconstructs) a two-dimensional array of numbers, each of which represents the attenuation of an identifiable and specific corresponding volume of the body known as a volume element (*voxel*). This array of numbers can be translated into an image by associating a different grey scale level to each CT number or range of numbers. The resulting picture is made up of numerous picture elements (*pixels*), the darkness of which corresponds to the calculated average amount of radiation absorbed by the corresponding voxel. Of fundamental importance is the concept that the CT density (the value of the number in the CT matrix) is *linearly* proportional to the X-ray attenuation coefficient of the volume elements. Internal calibration of the scanner sets the CT density of water to be defined as 0 Hounsfield units (HU) and that of room air there to be minus 1000 HU. Therefore, although the computed CT values and the visual grey scale associated with them are arbitrary, they remain consistent relatively and are related to the physical attenuation values of the corresponding voxel.

However, the human eye can only distinguish approximately 20 shades of grey although attenuation values can vary from at least −1000 HU to +1000 HU. Typical attenuation values with various body tissues and fluids are listed in Table 3. As most soft tissue and fluid structures range between 0 and 50 HU, therefore, if the entire density scale of 2000 HU were displayed on a single image with 20 shades of grey, then all soft tissue structures would be of a single shade of grey covering 100 HU, and there would be no differentiation between the different soft tissue structures. For that reason, the concept of the 'image window' was developed to facilitate with the viewing of CT images and, at any one time, only a subset of the total values of HUs are represented. Each window has a '*width*' of HUs centred on a '*window level*' representing the centre of the density scale. For extracting maximum information from bony structures therefore, 'bony settings' will be used employing a high window level and a wide window width, whereas, for visualizing soft tissues and for discriminating different soft tissue structures, 'soft tissue settings' would be preferred with a window level of +40 HU and a narrow width of 40 HU (Fig. 44). These alternative methods are

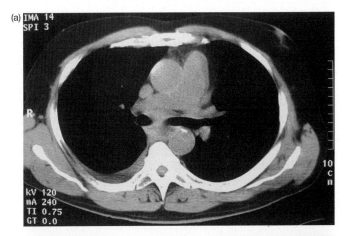

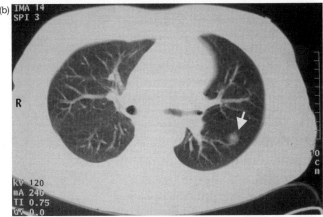

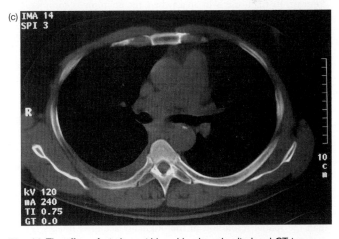

Fig. 44 The effect of window width and level on the displayed CT image. (a) On 'soft tissue settings' differentiation between the various soft tissue structures is optimized, but bony detail is obscured. (b) On 'lung settings' structures within the lung (e.g. vessels and a metastasis—arrow) become clear, which were not seen on soft tissue settings. (c) 'Bone settings' would be required to demonstrate any abnormality within bone. Note that all three images relate to a single radiological acquisition and are different visual representations of the same data.

Table 3 Attenuation values for various body tissues and fluids

Tissue type	Standard value (HU)
Bone (compact)	>250
Bone (spongy)	130 ± 100
Muscle	45 ± 5
Liver	65 ± 5
Fat	−65 ± 10
Lung tissue	−750 ± 150
Blood (venous whole blood)	55 ± 5
Exudate (>30 g protein/l)	>18 ± 2
Transudate (<30 g protein/l)	<18 ± 2

different ways in which the same information can be displayed—a separate patient exposure is not required.

The orientation of the cross sectional image obtained is limited by the geometry of the CT scanning system. At neutral, this represents a transaxial slice and, although the angle can be altered by up to 10–15° by angling the CT scanning system gantry, coronal and sagittal images cannot be obtained directly, unless the patient can be repositioned (an option only available for limited parts of the human body). Alternatively, the axially acquired images may be reconstructed mathematically into alternative planes, as long as no gap existed between the axial slices when they were originally acquired (see below).

Several parameters are selectable by the CT scanning system operator, and some of these have marked effect on the eventual image. The thickness of the slice in particular is of fundamental importance. Typical figures for the slice thickness in soft tissue and bone examinations will vary from 3 to 5 mm and, in general, the thinner the slice the higher the resolution as there is less summation from structures adjacent to the structure of interest. Conversely, the signal-to-noise ratio is lower and more slices will be required to cover a volume of interest, and therefore the radiation dose for the patient will be higher.

CT scanning can be performed in conjunction with the injection of intravenous contrast medium. This iodinated contrast material passes in blood vessels, and permeates into soft tissues in relation to a combination of blood flow and capillary permeability. It causes an increase in the attenuation value of the voxels when imaged, and this information can be used either in relation to detecting differences in regional blood flow and perfusion or by increasing the conspicuousness of small soft tissue lesions that enhance to a different extent to their surroundings.

Variations

CT arthrography

CT arthrography involves the imaging of a joint after the intraarticular injection of iodinated contrast material. This allows soft tissue structures that would otherwise not be seen on CT to be outlined with contrast. Its main use is in areas where the anatomy is complex, and where overlying structures may obscure detail, and it is also often the best way to determine whether a cartilaginous or calcified body within a joint is loose, or whether it is adherent to the capsule or attached to the underlying bone (Fig. 45).

Reconstruction

'Reconstruction' of the axially acquired images into other images takes two forms. *Two-dimensional reconstruction* involves recreating an alternative two-dimensional image in a different plane to the plane of acquisition by taking pixel values from lines in adjacent contiguous axial slices and recreating a further image in the chosen plane (Fig. 46).[18] Spatial resolution in the plane of reconstruction will be limited by the thickness of the axial slices and therefore will be less than the spatial resolution in the originally acquired images. *Three-dimensional reconstruction* involves recreating a surface-shaded virtual image from the original two-dimensional slices. To produce a three-dimensional image of the skeleton the computer picks out only those pixels from contiguous slices that have HU attenuation values that correspond to those of bone. The computer then paints the three-dimensional image by deducing what the image would look like if light were shone on the virtual three-dimensional construction.

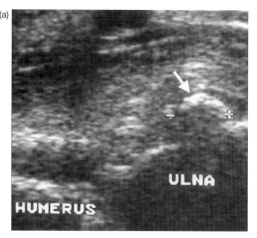

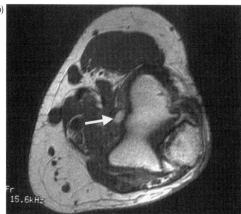

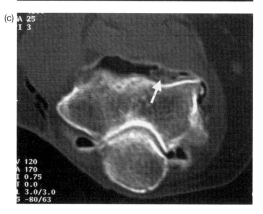

Fig. 45 Intraarticular loose body in the elbow. (a) On ultrasound, a calcified structure is seen anterior to the anterior border of the ulnar (arrow). (b) On MRI the abnormality returns increased signal (arrow). (c). On CT double arthrography, contrast is seen around the abnormality confirming that it is a loose body.

The viewing angle can be altered, as can the angle of 'incident light'. The resulting image can be useful for giving an added insight into the pattern of bony alignment and may help the surgeon in presurgical planning (Fig. 46). However, the reconstruction algorithm will necessarily smooth over discontinuities, and therefore fractures, for example, will be missed on the surface-shaded views, although they will remain readily apparent on the original slices.

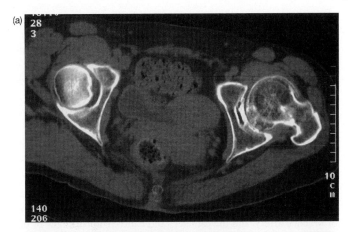

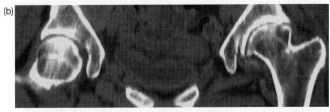

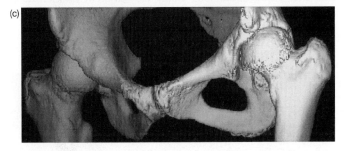

Fig. 46 Developmental dysplasia of the hip. (a) Axial acquired images through the hip demonstrate the degenerative change on the left, together with the anteverted angle of the femoral neck. (b) Reconstructed coronal images show the abnormal morphology of the femoral head, and the degree of joint destruction. (c) Surface-rendered three-dimensional views can be obtained in any projection.

Multiple detector CT scanning systems

The hardware associated with CT scanning systems is improving year by year. The 1990s saw the advent of *spiral CT*, where slip ring technology allowed the tube to continue rotating after 360° and even do so while the table moved. This geometry enabled slices to be obtained more rapidly, with less patient radiation, and allowed reconstruction in sagittal and coronal planes to be more photographically elegant and radiologically useful. The first decade of this century sees further evolution in the form of multiple detectors, which allows multiple slices to be obtained simultaneously from a single rotation of the X-ray tube. This will allow even more rapid imaging, with smoother reconstructions and higher resolution, but will be associated with increased demands on the reconstruction hardware and software, which will in some situations result in an increase in the radiation exposure to the patient.

Strengths

The strength of CT scanning arises from its cross-sectional nature: the problem of overlapping structures that affects plain radiography

acutely is less of a problem with CT. Similarly, unlike plain radiography where the patient may be required to assume an uncomfortable position during the exposure, with CT scanning the patient is required only to lie supine, and remain still during the acquisition of the slices. The CT scanning systems are universally available in developed countries but remain expensive to buy and are not universal in the developing world.

Weaknesses

The fundamental weakness of CT in relation to soft tissue imaging is that soft tissue structures generally all have attenuation values within a narrow range and therefore are not well differentiated from each other, even when the imaging window width is narrow. Similarly, as oedematous fluid and soft tissues have similar values, abnormal oedematous structures may not be conspicuously abnormal on CT. Furthermore, a soft tissue mass or tumour may only be demonstrable on CT by virtue of the fact that either it distorts adjacent fat planes and anatomical structures or it enhances differently from adjacent structures. CT is therefore not the routine method of choice for evaluating soft tissue pathology. The high radiation exposure associated with CT has already been alluded to and is illustrated in Table 4.

The risks associated with the CT imaging are related primarily to the patient's exposure to ionizing radiation. Obtaining images of the extremities is associated with a relatively low patient radiation exposure, conventionally calculated as the 'effective dose equivalent'. However, images acquired of the trunk are associated with a relatively high radiation exposure, particularly when compared with plain radiography (see Table 4). The injection of intravenous contrast may be associated with complications such as minor allergic reactions which can occur in up to 5 per cent of injections with certain ionic contrast agents. More severe allergic reactions resulting in hospital admission and intubation are recognized but uncommon unless there has been a previous documented reaction to contrast material. With ionic contrast agents, up to 1 : 40,000 injections are associated with a sufficiently

Table 4 Typical effective doses from diagnostic medical exposures[a]

Procedure	Typical effective dose (mSv)	Equivalent number of chest radiographs	Approximate equivalent period of natural background radiation[b]
Extremity joint	<0.01	<0.5	<1.5 days
Chest X-ray	0.02	1	3 days
Hip	0.3	15	7 weeks
Pelvis	0.7	35	4 months
Lumbar spine	1.3	65	7 months
Bone scintigram (Tc-99m)	4	200	1.8 years
CT abdomen *or* pelvis	10	500	4.5 years

[a] Source: Reference 20, p. 13.

[b] UK average background radiation, 2.2 mSv per year: regional averages range from 1.5 to 7.5 mSv per year.

severe allergic reaction to result in the patient's death, but this occurrence has become less frequent with the advent of non-ionic contrast agents.[19]

Specific clinical uses

Because the HUs of bone are significantly higher than those of adjacent structures, bony detail and calcification with the structures or calcified abnormalities are particularly well distinguished and differentiated. This confers a major advantage to CT scanning over other imaging techniques in the context of bony *trauma*. Indeed, CT is commonly part of the routine work-up of patients with fractures involving the pelvis or sacrum, and is useful in the evaluation of spinal trauma. CT can also add additional information in cases of trauma to other parts of the body, particularly in those cases where surgical intervention is planned (Fig. 47) or where a stress fracture is suspected.

Inflammatory arthropathies are generally not well visualized with CT, although exceptions exist. In particular, CT can be useful in the evaluation of sacroiliitis although MRI and bone scintigraphy are both sensitive alternative techniques. In addition, CT can be used to guide percutaneous biopsy of either bone or joint in situations such as discitis or sacroiliitis. Such a procedure is not easily performed using plain film fluoroscopy and, similarly, it is not a routine MR technique.

Although CT is not optimal for the routine evaluation of a soft tissue mass, it can be useful in circumstances where calcification within a mass is suspected, or for evaluation the degree of erosion on adjacent bone by the mass. For example, myositis ossificans frequently presents with a soft tissue swelling and the history of previous trauma may be confused or absent. It is the typical development of curvilinear calcification, which will be evident on CT before it is seen on plain radiographs, that allows a definitive diagnosis (Fig. 5). MRI is poor at detecting calcification. In addition, where percutaneous biopsy of a deeply sited soft tissue mass is required, CT often provides the best approach to image guidance.

Summary

CT is a technique that employs ionizing radiation to create a series of radiological slices through the area of interest. The radiation burden to the patient can be significant when the region of interest involves the trunk or torso. Its main use in the musculoskeletal system lies in the evaluation of bony structures, particularly in the context of trauma, or calcification within soft tissue lesions, and to guide intervention. Purely soft tissue abnormalities are often not best evaluated by CT.

Angiography

Technical aspects

Angiography involves the insertion of a thin catheter, up to 1 m long, into the arterial tree. The point of entry is most commonly the femoral or brachial artery, and the catheter can be directed proximally or distally within the arterial tree using real-time fluoroscopic guidance. The injection of contrast material, identical to that used intravenously in other situations such as CT, enables the vascular tree distal to the tip of the catheter to be visualized immediately after injection, followed subsequently by the capillary blush and the venous return of the supplied territory. Abnormal structures, such a tumour or vascular malformation (Fig. 48), have an abnormal capillary architecture and often an increased blood supply and can be well demonstrated angiographically.

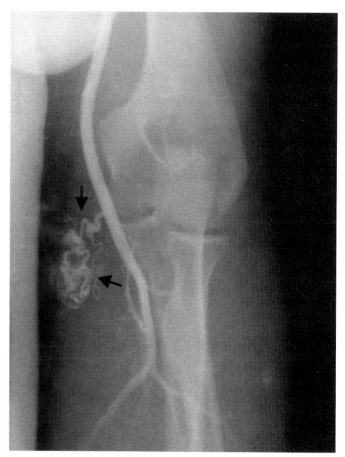

Fig. 48 Arteriovenous malformation. Arteriogram shows contrast filling a soft tissue mass via an abnormal leash of vessels (arrows).

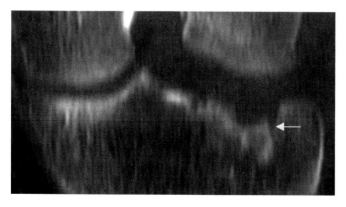

Fig. 47 Central depression fracture of the tibial plateau. Coronal reconstructions from axially acquired CT slices show the extent of the depressed fragment (arrow). This information is useful prior to surgery.

Variations

Intravenous digital subtraction angiography

In this technique the arterial injection is avoided and contrast is injected intravenously, and digital subtraction techniques are used that subtract the image obtained before the contrast was injected from the image obtained afterwards. The difference between the two images is a map of the contrast within the vascular tree at that time.

Super-selective catheterization

Conventional angiography requires the tip of the catheters to be positioned within one of the major arterial branches. With super-selective catheterization, a thinner tube is used and is directed into one of the small subsidiary arteries, which themselves arise from named branch arteries. Super selective catheterization is often the prerequisite to embolization procedures.

Embolization procedures

After a suitable artery has been catheterized, material can be injected with the intention that it is retained within the artery to result in that artery becoming thrombosed. The result is a reduction in the blood supply to the territory supplied by that artery.

Strengths

The use of arteriography is uncommon in the evaluation of soft tissue musculoskeletal pathology, but the main strength relates to the ability to catheterize directly the arteries supplying a tumour or arterial malformation with a view to embolization. In essence, therefore, the strength of arteriography is that it can be used therapeutically. The advent of other imaging techniques has made the use of diagnostic angiography largely obsolete.

Weaknesses

The main weakness relates to the fact that the technique is interventional and only a small territory (namely, that supplied by the artery catheterized) can be imaged at any one time. The complications from arteriography include local bleeding, haematoma, and false aneurysm formation although, with the use of modern techniques and materials, the incidence of complication is low.

Specific clinical uses

The use of arteriography in musculoskeletal soft tissue imaging relates to two specific situations. First, is a situation where a hypervascular soft tissue tumour is being considered for resection. Prior embolization will result in a reduction of the hypervascularity and a consequent reduction in blood loss at the time of surgery. The second indication relates to the management of a lesion that, for reasons of size and position, is considered inoperative, such as a vascular malformation. Reducing the blood flow through the lesion is often associated with a reduction in the patient's symptoms.

Summary

Angiography is a specialized technique that has only certain very specific limited indications. Despite its interventional nature, the modern angiography technique is associated with a low complication rate, and is generally well tolerated by patients. The use of ionizing radiation is unavoidable but, in the extremity in particular, the radiation dose absorbed by the patient remains acceptable.

Other imaging considerations

Radiation dosimetry and risk assessment

The absorption of X-rays by biological tissues happens when an individual X-ray photon interacts either with the atomic nucleus or the electron shell of an atom. The resulting damage at the atomic level may lead to cell death or, alternatively, to altered cell biological characteristics. These would include genetic mutation or the development of a malignant pattern of growth.

It is well documented from experimental studies that irradiation of the gonads of children and adults of reproductive age leads to an increased rate of genetic mutations in both their offspring and also in subsequent generations. The effect is difficult to quantify because of the prevalence of spontaneous mutations that occur with unknown frequency. Nevertheless, it is incumbent upon the technician at the time of exposure to protect the gonads as far as possible from the direct X-ray beam and it is also important that the referring clinician has a suitably high threshold for referring children and patients of child-bearing age for examinations that are known to have a higher absorbent radiation dose (see Table 4). This is particularly the case when the possible benefits from the diagnostic test are low.

Similarly, the fact that malignancy follows ionizing radiation exposure after a long latent period is well known, but the relationship of a given dose of radiation to the resulting risk of subsequent malignancy is not determined. Although it is likely that the effect of radiation is related to radiation dose, it is not clear whether this relationship holds at very low dose rates, or whether there is a threshold below which the risks are reduced. Although a variety of radiation versus risk models have been devised underlining the contentious nature of the subject, it is nevertheless clear that medical diagnostic imaging will result in malignant transformation in a way that is not quantifiable and that is likely to have long latency. One authority puts the risk of malignant change after a patient has had an abdominal CT at 1 in 2000.[20] To an individual who may have more than one anatomical site imaged, possibly on more than one occasion, this becomes a significant risk. Of more importance, however, is the effect of the exposure to a population of patients. For example, an average CT scanning system that images 5000 patients a year must expect every year to produce several malignancies 20–40 years later. Of course, in that time many of the older patients may have died of other causes. However, although in the developed world the total dose absorbed by the population from diagnostic procedures by far exceeds the dose from all other man-made sources of radiation, it still remains lower that the background radiation dose to the population derived from inevitable exposure to naturally occurring radioactive elements that are present in the minerals that make up the Earth's crust.

Ultrasound and MRI do not use ionizing radiation but are also associated with the deposition of energy into the anatomical structure being imaged. This will result in a rise in local temperature. With very high energy ultrasound radiation, this can lead to tissue damage, and indeed this forms the basis of extracorporeal shock wave therapy. Similarly, at high field strength MRI (higher than usually used for routine medical imaging), the increase in temperature is measurable and, in some instances, nerve tingling can also be induced, which can be uncomfortable. Nevertheless, the energies used for diagnostic ultrasound and diagnostic MRI are several orders of magnitude lower than the levels needed to produce any biological effects, so these techniques are generally regarded as being free of risk.

The woman who is known to be pregnant or thinks that she might be so deserves separate consideration. Ultrasound is considered free of risk, and indeed is used worldwide for the evaluation of the fetus in all stages of pregnancy. By comparison to the literally thousands of studies that have been performed to examine the possible hazards of ultrasound during pregnancy, only a few investigations have examined the teratogenic potential of MRI. Although none of these studies have demonstrated an adverse affect on the fetus, controversy and doubt remain. For this reason, the current guidelines of the United States Federal Drugs Administration (FDA) require labelling of MR devices to indicate that the safety of MRI when used to image the fetus and infant has not been established. In Great Britain, the accepted limits of exposure for clinical MRI recommended by the National Radiological Protection Board (NRPB) in 1983, specified that 'it might be prudent to exclude pregnant women during the first three months of pregnancy'. In practice, a risk–benefit assessment must be made and, if an important question can only be answered by MRI, then it may be considered that the benefits outweigh the risks. Techniques that involve ionizing radiation, however, are well known to induce teratogenic effects and, where possible, should be avoided in pregnancy, unless the indication is strong.

MRI is contraindicated for patients who have had certain ferromagnetic materials implanted or foreign bodies, primarily due to possibility of movement or dislodgement of these objects under the influence of the magnetic field. These include certain aneurysm clips or a loose intraoccular body from previous trauma. In addition, electrical currents can be induced in suitable conductors and therefore the presence of a permanent pacemaker device represents an absolute contraindication to MRI. The other potential risk to patients is the acoustic noise produced during an MRI examination. The noise is unavoidable and relates to the activation and deactivation of electrical current in the MR imaging system that induces vibrations of the gradient coils. In practice, disposable earplugs are routinely used and the resulting reduction in perceived noise has the added advantage that the patient is more comfortable during the examination.

Diagnostic accuracy

Fundamental to the interpretation of the results of a diagnostic test is the understanding that every radiological test is imperfect. Quantitative evaluation of diagnostic performance is based on probability statistics and decision theory and the simplest measure of a diagnostic test is its 'accuracy'. This is defined as the number of correct diagnoses made as a proportion of the total sample. A better measure of diagnostic performance is to consider the technique for those with disease (sensitivity) and those who are disease-free (specificity). Sensitivity describes the ratio of patients with diseases that are correctly diagnosed from the referral sample using the established diagnostic criteria. Similarly, specificity is the ratio of patients who are disease-free who are correctly diagnosed from the same sample using the same diagnostic criteria. Sensitivity and specificity can be represented graphically in the form of a receiver/operator characteristic (ROC) curve.[21] The curve represents the way that sensitivity and specificity change as the diagnostic threshold varies. The curves are

calculated by plotting sensitivity against one-minus-specificity for different diagnostic criteria and the area under the ROC curve can be used to compare directly the diagnostic performance of various imaging techniques used for a clinical problem, independent of decision thresholds.[22]

The clinician, however, is not only concerned with the probability that the patient has been correctly diagnosed, but also the probability that the disease can be correctly detected within the sample. The conditional probability that disease exists given a positive or negative result is known as the predictive value.[23] The positive predictive value is defined as the probability that a patient for whom the test is positive for a particular lesion does indeed have that lesion. Conversely, a negative predictive value is the probability that a patient for whom the test is negative is indeed disease-free.

The relevance to the clinician is that few radiological tests have sensitivities, specificities, or predictive values above 95 per cent, and indeed, in many cases, the corresponding values may be between 75 and 95 per cent. It is important therefore to evaluate the radiological test result in relation to the overall clinical context. Statistically, this is quantified by applying *Bayes' theorem*. Although a detailed assessment is outside the scope of this chapter, it is important to note that, when any diagnostic test is positive for a particular condition, the probability that the patient does indeed have that condition is related in equal measure to the sensitivity of the technique and to the *pre-test probability*, which is related to the prevalence of the disease in the population and to the clinician's suspicion that the patient has the particular condition before the diagnostic test was performed. Conversely, the predicative value of a negative test is related to the specificity of the test rather than the sensitivity. Bayes' theorem enables prior assessments about the chances of a diagnosis (pre-test probability) to be combined with the eventual test results to obtain an *a posteriori* assessment about the diagnosis. Indeed, this reflects the procedure of making a clinical judgement where multiple sources of information are combined to develop a final differential diagnosis. Clearly, most clinicians do not go through the mathematics of the process, although Macartney[24] has shown how the formal method closely follows the intuitive approach usually adopted by clinicians. Knill-Jones[25] gives numerous examples of how the diagnoses of a large number of diseases have been formalized and adapted for use with a computer.

To understand the difference between test accuracy and predictive value, consider an example where the prevalence of a certain disease is 1 in 1000, and there is a test that can detect it with a sensitivity of 100 per cent and a specificity of 95 per cent (which would be remarkably good results for a radiological test). An individual has the radiological test and the result is positive for the particular disease. What is the probability that this person has that disease?

The referring clinician might assume the answer would be 0.95 (which is the specificity). This is not the case. Using Bayes' theorem,

The probability that a patient has the disease given a positive test =
(sensitivity × prevalence) divided by
the overall probability of a positive result.

To calculate the probability of a positive result, consider a group of 1000 people in which one person has the disease. The test will certainly detect this one person (sensitivity 100 per cent). However, it will also give a positive result on 5 per cent of the 999 people without the disease (specificity 95 per cent). Thus, the total positives is 1 + (0.05 × 999) which is calculated to be 50.95 and therefore the probability is

50.95/1000 = 0.05095. In this case, therefore, the probability that this patient with a positive test truly has the disease is 2 per cent, which is significantly less than might be imagined intuitively.[26]

The vital message here is that the result of any radiological test, whether positive or negative, must be seen in the light of the patient's clinical circumstances and the pre-test suspicion that the patient has the disease being sought. Specifically, if the pre-test probability is low in the first instance, then care should be exercised when interpreting a positive result and, conversely, when the clinician is confident that a patient has a positive diagnosis, a negative test result should be treated with a degree of caution.

Guidelines

The combination of the ionizing nature of X-rays and the imperfect accuracy sometimes associated with a specific radiological examination has resulted in an interest in the development of guidelines for the use of radiological tests. For example, a clinician is faced by a young individual with 2 weeks of lumbar back pain. Is a lumbar spine series worthwhile? Referring to Table 4, the radiation dose that a patient undergoing a lumbar spine series experiences is equivalent to that of 65 chest radiographs or 7 months of average background radiation in the United Kingdom. In this example, the soft tissue intervertebral disc is the most likely source of the acute pain but the plain radiograph will provide limited information on this structure. Therefore plain radiographs should be used sparingly in the context of back pain and sciatica in the young patient (see reference 20, p. 36). The Royal College of Radiologists (RCR) in the United Kingdom has published a booklet covering guidelines for all routine radiological examinations that aims to clarify the most appropriate use of such examinations.[20] The timeliness of this publication is illustrated by the rapidity with which the guidelines have been taken up internationally.

References

1. Swallow, R.A. and Naylor, E. (ed.) (1996). *Clark's positioning in radiography*, 11th edn. William Heinemann Medical Books, London.
2. Rogers, L.F. (1978). Fractures and dislocations of the elbow. *Semin. Roentgenol.* **13**, 97–101.
3. Kieft, J.J., Bloem, A.L., Razing, P.M., *et al.* (1988). Rotator cuff impingement syndrome: MR imaging. *Radiology* **166**, 211–215.
4. Cardinal, E., Buckwalter, K.A., Capello, W.N., and Duval, N. (1996). US of the snapping iliopsoas tendon. *Radiology* **198**, 521–522.
5. Evans, P.D., Wilson, C., and Lyons, K. (1994). Comparison of MRI with bone scanning for suspected hip fracture in elderly patients. *J. Bone Joint Surg. (Br.)* **76**, 158–162.
6. Cotton, A., Delfaut, E., Demondion, X., *et al.* (2000). MR imaging of the knee at 0.2 and 1.5 T: correlation with surgery. *Am. J. Roentgenol.* **174**, 1093–1097.
7. Ficat, R.P., Phillippe, J., and Hungerford, D.S. (1979). Chondromalacia patellae. A system of classification. *Clin. Orthop.* **144**, 55–68.
8. Insall, J. and Salvati, E. (1971). Patella position in the normal knee joint. *Radiology* **101**, 101–104.
9. Uhthoff, A.K. and Sarkar, K. (1991). Classification and definition of tendinopathies. *Clin. Sports Med.* **10**, 707–713.
10. O'Brien, S.J., Neves, M.C., Arnoczky, S.P., Rozbruck, S.R., Dicarlo, E.F., Warren, R.F., Schwartz, R., and Wickiewicz, T.L. (1990). The anatomy and histology of the inferior glenohumeral ligament complex of the shoulder. *Am. J. Sports Med.* **18**, 449–456.
11. Bretlau, T., Christensen, O.M., Edstrom, P., Thomsen, H.S., and Lausten, G.S. (1999). Diagnosis of scaphoid fracture and dedicated extremity MRI. *Acta Orthop. Scand.* **70**, 504–508.
12. Sakuma, M., Nakamura, R., and Imaeda, T. (1995). Analysis of proximal fragment sclerosis and surgical outcome of scaphoid non-union by magnetic resonance imaging. *J. Hand Surg. Br.* **20**, 201–205.
13. Resnik, D. (1995). Arthrography, tenography and bursography. In *Diagnosis of bone and joint disorders*, 3rd edn (ed. D. Resnick), pp. 277–409. W.B. Saunders Co, Philadelphia.
14. Blanchard, T.K., Bearcroft, P.W.P., Dixon, A.K., *et al.* (1997). Magnetic resonance imaging or arthrography: which do patients prefer? *Br. J. Radiol.* **70**, 786–790.
15. Ahovuo, J., Paavolainen, P., and Slatis, P. (1984). The diagnostic value of arthrography and plain radiography in rotator cuff tears. *Acta Orthop. Scand.* **55**, 220–225.
16. Palmer, W.E., Brown, J.H., and Rosenthal, D.I. (1993). Rotator cuff: evaluation with fat-suppressed MR arthrography. *Radiology* **188**, 683–688.
17. Andrén, L. and Lundberg, B.J. (1965). Treatment of rigid shoulders by joint distension during arthrography. *Acta Orthop. Scand.* **36**, 45–49.
18. Bearcroft, P.W.P. (1998). The use of spiral computed tomography in musculoskeletal radiology of lower limb: the calcaneus as an example. *Eur. J. Radiol.* **28**, 30–38.
19. Dore, C.J., Sidhu, P.S., and Dawson, P. (1995). Corticosteroid prophylaxis in patients at increased risk of adverse reactions to intravascular contrast agents. *Clin. Radiol.* **50**, 198–199.
20. Royal College of Radiologists (RCR) Working Party (1998). *Making the best use of a department of clinical radiology*, 4th edn. RCR, London.
21. Black, W.C. (1990). How to evaluate the radiological literature. *Am. J. Radiol.* **154**, 17–22.
22. Hanley, J. and McNeil, B. (1982). The meaning and use of the area under a receiver operating characteristic (ROC) curve. *Radiology* **143**, 29–36.
23. Rockette, H., Gur, D., and Metz, C. (1992). The use of continuous and discrete confidence judgements in receiver operating characteristic studies of diagnostic imaging techniques. *Invest. Radiol.* **27**, 169–172.
24. Macartney, F.J. (1987). Diagnostic logic. *Br. Med. J.* **295**, 1325–1331.
25. Knill-Jones, R.P. (1987). Diagnostic systems as an aid to decision making. *Br. Med. J.* **295**, 1392–1396.
26. Campbell, M.J. and Machin, D. (1990). *Medical statistics: a common sense approach*, p. 34. John Wylie and Sons Ltd, Chichester.

4.5 The investigation of soft tissue disorders: nuclear medicine

Jane Dutton and Ignac Fogelman

Introduction

The use of nuclear medicine in the investigation of soft tissue rheumatological disorders embraces a wide variety of nuclear medicine methods including specialized techniques such as labelling white cells for imaging, single photon emission computerized tomography (SPECT), and, most recently, positron emission tomography (PET) with ^{18}F-fluorodeoxyglucose. By far the most common scan, however, is the standard planar bone scan with ^{99m}Tc-methylene diphosphonate. This chapter attempts to give an overview of the principles of the methods employed, their indications, and examples of the abnormalities demonstrated or diagnosed by these techniques.

Radionuclide imaging has been available in clinical practice for more than 50 years and, although there have been considerable technical advances giving rise to more aesthetically appealing images and complicated quantitative analysis, the basic principles of the science remain the same.

Basic principles

The essence of nuclear medicine lies in the ability of a gamma camera to detect and accurately locate the site of emission of gamma rays. For our purposes a gamma ray can be considered identical to an X-ray, the main differences occurring at atomic level in the method of production of the radiation. A substance that undergoes radioactive decay by emitting gamma rays can be injected intravenously into the patient and the patient positioned against a gamma camera for image acquisition. The tracer that is administered can be the salt of a radioactive element, for example,^{67}Gallium-citrate or, more frequently, a compound of a radioactive element and a chemical that is known to have a particular biodistribution. An example of the latter is ^{99m}Tc-MDP, the tracer most frequently used for bone scanning. ^{99m}Tc-MDP is an abbreviation for methylenene diphosphonate (a 'bone-seeking' chemical) labelled with 99m-Technetium (radioactive substance with a half-life of 6 h).

The gamma camera is sensitive to radioactivity and can identify the original site of the gamma ray emission within the body. Most modern gamma cameras are able to resolve two points as separate foci when positioned as close as 8 mm. This is comparable with other radiological techniques such as computerized tomography (CT). Thus, an image of the distribution of radioactivity in the body is created as, for instance, injected ^{99m}Tc-MDP will accumulate in bones and joints. Where there is increased metabolic activity in bones, for example, in the normal immature skeleton at growth plates or in the abnormal skeleton at sites of pathology, then this will generally be reflected by increased ^{99m}Tc-MDP uptake at this site (Fig. 1). This will be

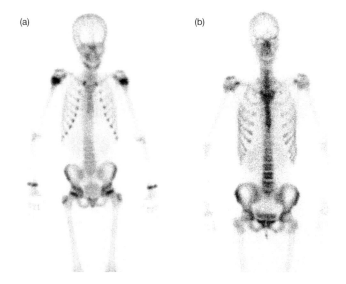

Fig. 1 Normal ^{99m}Tc-MDP bone scan in the (a) immature skeleton and in the (b) mature skeleton. There is increased signal from the growth plates in the growing skeleton.

displayed on the nuclear medicine image as a focal area of increased radioactive signal, or 'hot spot'.

Radionuclide imaging is a sensitive method for detecting pathology but is frequently non-specific in producing a precise diagnosis. Specificity can be improved by combining knowledge of the underlying pathology of the suspected disorder with an understanding of the biodistribution of the radiopharmaceutical. It is always helpful to interact with clinical specialists and to be aware of the results of other imaging studies to ensure the maximum useful information is gained from the nuclear medicine scans.

Technical aspects

Generally, the radiation dose to the patient from nuclear medicine scans is slightly higher than that from radiographs. For example, the dose to a patient from a bone scan using 600 MBq of ^{99m}Tc-MDP (the standard amount of radioactive tracer) is 3 mSv,[1] whereas the dose from a radiograph of the lumbar spine is approximately 2.4 mSv and that from a knee radiograph is approximately 0.01 mSv.[2] It is important, however, to put this in perspective by relating this to natural background irradiation, which gives approximately 2–4 mSv per year.

Hence, the dose from a bone scan or lumbar spine radiographs is equivalent to approximately 1–1.5 years' worth of natural background radioactivity.

The most common radionuclide scan that is likely to be performed for investigation of soft tissue rheumatological disorders is a ^{99m}Tc-MDP bone scan. The tracer is injected intravenously as a small-volume bolus. Information can be acquired from the moment that the patient is injected with tracer—the so-called 'radionuclide angiogram'—which represents the distribution of blood flow in the body. This can be useful when comparing the normal side and the affected limb, and in assessment of more focal vascular abnormalities such as vascular bone tumours. Following this, a single image can be acquired approximately 3–5 min after tracer injection. This image is referred to as the 'blood pool' image and represents the intra- and extravascular distribution of tracer in the imaged body part. The standard bone scan images are acquired at approximately 2–4 h after injection. It takes this duration of time for the soft tissue activity to be cleared producing optimal bone to soft tissue contrast. The precise method by which the tracer is taken up by the bone has still to be elucidated.

When all three sets of images are acquired this is called a three-phase bone scan. Occasionally a fourth phase is performed at 24 h when there is improved ratio of bone to soft tissue uptake of tracer that can make lesions more conspicuous. However, the radioactive count rate from the patient is low at this time (owing to radioactive decay) and the image will be of generally poorer quality. Radioactivity leaves the body by a combination of physical means (radioactive decay) and biological processes. In the case of a ^{99m}Tc-MDP scan, approximately 60–70 per cent of the radioactive tracer is excreted through the urinary tract. Different tracers have different methods of biological excretion just as they have different patterns of radioactive decay. The effective half-life of a tracer, which is the time taken for radioactivity in the body to reduce to half of its initial value, is related to the biological excretion of the tracer as well as the radioactive decay of the tracer.

One of the advantages of using a bone scan to make an assessment of joints is that the entire skeleton can be imaged without any increase in radiation dose to the patient when compared with a scan to look at a few joints only, unlike the acquisition of multiple radiographs. Sometimes, however, when the clinical question is specific to a single limb or joint, a reduced amount of radioactivity can be administered and produce a satisfactory set of images provided that the scan acquisition time is increased accordingly. In other circumstances the amount of radioactivity administered can be increased, for instance, in SPECT imaging. This is a method by which raw image data, acquired with the gamma camera at multiple different angular projections with respect to the patient, is transformed into reconstructed images or tomograms of the body, or body part, in any chosen plane. Usually the orientations of the chosen planes are sagittal, coronal, and axial with respect to standard anatomical positioning. This is very similar to the image representation for X-ray CT, and MRI (magnetic resonance imaging). SPECT images may help to accurately locate abnormalities of tracer uptake that are masked on planar images because of overlying structures.

PET is a newer variant of radionuclide imaging that is not yet readily available in all centres in the United Kingdom but may have more diverse clinical applications other than oncology. Its role in rheumatological disorders has still to be determined. The main difference between PET and standard nuclear medicine techniques is in the type of radioactive photons detected by the camera. As mentioned previously, nuclear medicine gamma cameras detect gamma photons. PET cameras detect positrons, which are essentially high-energy, positively charged electrons that are produced in pairs by radionuclides undergoing a specific form of decay. The positrons in each pair travel in opposite directions (at 180° to each other). The most common PET tracer is ^{18}F-FDG (fluorodeoxyglucose).

Although undoubtedly the most commonly used radioactive tracer in rheumatological disorders is ^{99m}Tc-MDP, there are multiple other valuable tracers. Leucocytes labelled with either ^{99m}technetium or ^{111}indium are used in suspected infection or inflammation.[3–5] ^{67}Gallium-citrate can detect infected or inflammatory foci as well as granulomatous conditions, such as tuberculosis, brucellosis, and sarcoidosis.[6] More recently, ^{201}Thallium chloride and ^{99m}Tc-MIBI (methoxyisobutylisonitrile labelled with Tc-99m) are under evaluation in suspected compartment syndrome in the lower leg.[7] And so the list continues.

Applications

To help demonstrate the applications of radionuclide imaging in soft tissue rheumatology, examples of the pathologies encountered will be given. No apology is made for including examples of non-soft tissue diseases because these may arise in the differential diagnosis of soft tissue pathology. Nuclear medicine techniques, specifically bone scans, may therefore be performed to positively exclude bone or joint pathology rather than to positively diagnose disorders of the soft tissues.

General

Bone scintigraphy is a sensitive but non-specific technique. However, there are many situations when the clinical findings combined with the pattern of bone scan abnormalities will lead to a specific diagnosis. An example of this is the demonstration of increased blood flow, blood pool, and tracer uptake in the scaphoid bone in the context of trauma, representing acute fracture.[8, 9] Negative scintigraphy is equally important since excluding a fracture will shorten the period of immobilization. Studies have shown that bone scanning in the detection of occult scaphoid fracture has a sensitivity of up to 100 per cent and a specificity of 98 per cent with a positive predictive value of 93 per cent and good inter- and intra-observer agreement.[9, 10] MRI has the advantages of detection of soft tissue pathology as well as more precise anatomical definition at the wrist. It avoids the use of ionizing radiation. However, access to MR imaging may be limited and the cost-effectiveness of routine use of MR has to be considered.

Bone scans are not routinely used to demonstrate fractures but can be useful in X-ray negative/equivocal situations such as may be encountered with fractures of the scaphoid, Salter–Harris type growth plate injuries, stress fractures at all sites, and non-displaced fractures (Fig. 2).

Bone scans may also be used to identify complications of fractures including, degenerative arthritis, infection, and avascular necrosis.[11] The latter is demonstrated well with MR scans but can also be diagnosed on bone scintigrams.[12, 13] In the early stages of avascular necrosis, radiographs may be normal but bone scans show reduced signal in the affected bone as a result of ischaemia. As the disease progresses, the osteoblastic response in the surrounding bone is represented as increased vascularity and tracer uptake on the bone scan.[13] In the chronic stages bone scintigraphy is often not indicated as

(a)   (b)

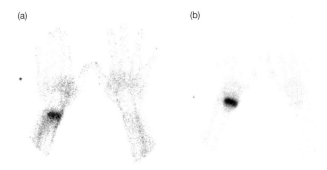

Fig. 2 ^{99m}Tc-MDP bone scan demonstrating (a) increased blood pool and (b) increased bone uptake at the site of an non-displaced fracture of the distal right radius. (The black dot beside the hands marks the right limb.)

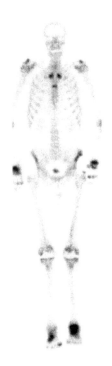

Fig. 3 ^{99m}Tc-MDP bone scan in rheumatoid arthritis. Multiple joints demonstrate increased tracer uptake at the involved joints in a relatively symmetrical pattern. Bilateral knee replacements are present.

radiographs will usually demonstrate destruction with fragmented collapsed bone and sclerosis.

Arthritis is not a routine indication for bone scintigraphy, but it may be performed at the onset of disease to assess the pattern of joint involvement for diagnostic purposes (Fig. 3). Joints that are actively involved will demonstrate increased tracer uptake and, when there is an inflammatory component, increased blood pool is also seen. Several other radionuclide tracers are employed in the evaluation of arthritides, including labelled leucocytes,[4] ^{67}gallium-citrate,[6] and labelled polyclonal human immunoglobulin (HIG).[14] These tracers are taken up at sites of inflammation and some have been shown to be able to identify subclinical disease.[15] This may have implications in assessing response to drug treatment in inflammatory arthritides such as rheumatoid arthritis.

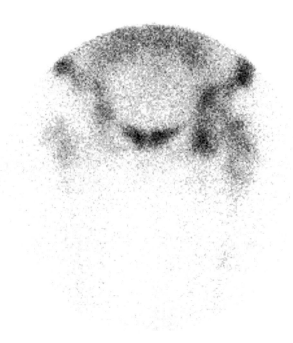

Fig. 4 Anterior view of the pelvis at 24 h after injection of Indium-111 labelled white cells. There is abnormal white cell localization at the site of the infected left hip replacement and in the adjacent soft tissues inferior to the left acetabulum.

A number of tracers may be used in the identification of infection. Often more than one scan is required to improve the specificity of results. Labelled leucocyte scans and ^{67}gallium-citrate scans may be employed with both tracers localizing at sites of infection (Fig. 4), but often a bone scan is performed initially.[16, 17] ^{99m}Tc-MDP demonstrates increased vascularity, blood pool, and bone uptake of tracer in the presence of infection.[18] In septic arthritis, both sides of the joint are affected equally, whereas in osteomyelitis increased tracer uptake is most intense at the affected epiphysis. The situation is more complicated in the clinical situation of suspected infection associated with active synovitis. Radionuclide techniques are of limited value as all of the infection-seeking agents accumulate at sites of active synovitis, so the ability of nuclear medicine to differentiate active synovitis from septic arthritis is poor.

Hand and wrist

^{99m}Tc-MDP bone scans have a somewhat limited role in the diagnosis of soft tissue disorders of the hand and wrist but they can be extremely useful in the exclusion of underlying bone or joint pathology such as fractures, arthritis, avascular necrosis, or tumours. Bone scintigraphy is also a helpful adjunct to clinical acumen in reflex sympathetic dystrophy syndrome (or complex regional pain syndrome-type 1 (CRPS I)) where there is no clearly defined 'gold standard' diagnostic test (see Chapter 6.17).

CRPS I is a complicated syndrome of limb pain, vasomotor disturbances, dystrophic skin changes with swelling, and reduced limb function. It can be difficult to diagnose clinically and different types of diagnostic tools such as thermography and nerve conduction studies amongst others have been employed. Since sympathetically driven vasomotor instability is one of the hallmarks of this disorder, the bone scan should include the blood flow and blood pool phases as well as the standard delayed views (Fig. 5). The specificity and sensitivity of bone scintigraphy results is variable, ranging from 60 to 100 per cent and 85 to 98 per cent, respectively.[19–21] Factors contributing to this variability include differences in patient selection and in criteria used to establish the diagnosis. The most commonly seen bone scan pattern is increased blood flow associated with diffuse increase in tracer uptake in the affected limb and juxta-articular accentuation in tracer uptake at the joints.[19, 20] There is some evidence that the bone scan may be able to indicate the stage of the disease. Work by Demangeat et al., which has been supported by others, describes increased blood flow and pool in the affected limb when imaged within the first 20 weeks of onset of symptoms.[22] After this time the early phases of the bone scan are often unremarkable.

When more focal pathology is suspected in the hand, the lack of anatomical clarity on bone scans can be problematic. Is the abnormal uptake at the joint itself or in the adjacent bone? Which of the carpal bones is demonstrating increased tracer uptake, or is the hot spot in tendon or ligament? These questions can be extremely difficult to answer—hence the emergence of the co-registration scan (Fig. 6). Co-registration can be performed in different ways but in essence

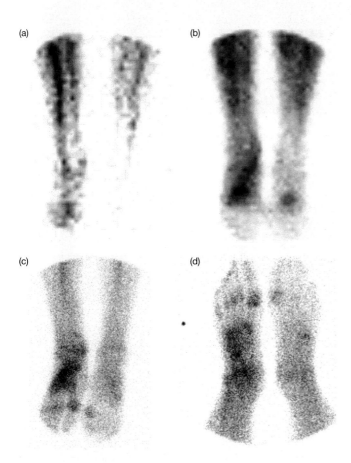

Fig. 5 Selected images from a three-phase ^{99m}Tc-MDP bone scan of the feet. The upper images are (a) summed frames from the dynamic study and (b) blood pool images (right) of the feet, dorsal views. The lower images demonstrate bone uptake of tracer in the feet—(a) dorsal view (b) plantar view. There is increased blood flow, blood pool, and bone uptake of tracer in the symptomatic right foot. This pattern of findings is consistent with the clinical diagnosis of reflex sympathetic dystrophy.

the anatomical precision of a radiograph is superimposed on the functional bone scan image of the hand, demonstrating more clearly the location of the bone scan hot spots.[23]

Shoulders and elbows

Nuclear medicine currently has no role in the confirmation of suspected soft tissue disorders of the shoulder such as rotator cuff pathology. MRI or shoulder arthrography demonstrate rotator cuff tears and any bone spurs that may result in the impingement syndrome.

When shoulder pain is unexplained, bone scintigraphy may be used in the evaluation of suspected infection, avascular necrosis, CRPS I, or overuse injuries. Exercise-induced overuse injuries of the upper limb are seen predominantly in sports such as javelin-throwing, tennis, golf, and weight-lifting (Fig. 7). In weight-lifting, humeral periostitis may be seen at the site of insertion of pectoralis major in the humeral shaft. This is akin to the stress reactions in the tibia described later in this chapter. In asymptomatic individuals, a low intensity focus of ^{99m}Tc-MDP is so frequently seen at the site of insertion of the deltoid muscle in the lateral aspect of the upper humeral shaft that it is considered physiological.

'Golfers' elbow' (medial epicondylitis) and 'tennis elbow' (lateral epicondylitis) can cause well-defined increased blood pool and tracer uptake at the medial and lateral humeral epicondyles, respectively. Stress fractures of the ulnar shaft are mostly seen in body-builders and weight-lifters. Bone scintigraphy is most unlikely to be performed in the evaluation of these injuries, but should be considered where evaluation is difficult or the symptoms are unexplained.

Thoracolumbar spine

Backache is a major cause of morbidity in the United Kingdom accounting for many lost days away from work per year. Frequently, it is self-limiting and current guidelines recommend that specialized imaging such as MR or CT is not performed until a minimum of 6 weeks' duration of symptoms has elapsed in those presenting acutely without neurological signs.[2]

Planar bone scan images of the lumbar spine may be adequate imaging in many cases, for instance in those with known primary malignancy and suspected bony metastatic spread. In adolescents or in those where there is no known underlying pathology, additional SPECT imaging of the lumbar spine can provide valuable extra information (Fig. 8).

SPECT bone scintigraphy has been used to assess disease activity with facet joint arthropathy and with spondylolysis where planar imaging may demonstrate abnormalities but cannot accurately localize the 'hot spot'. In facet joint disease, SPECT bone scanning has been used to identify the site of pain with a view to therapeutic steroid injection.[24] In spondylolysis, increased tracer uptake at the site of the pars interarticularis may indicate healing processes—such patients are managed by rest and the use of a lumbar brace. In the absence of increased tracer uptake, but radiographic proof of spondylolysis, some surgeons would consider surgical intervention to prevent spondylolisthesis.[25]

Bone scanning may be performed in the investigation of discitis. Typically, a 'wafer' pattern of horizontal bands of increased ^{99m}Tc-MDP uptake is seen either side of the affected disc. When infection is suspected in the vertebra itself, bone scans demonstrate markedly abnormal metabolic activity, but white cell scans may give false-negative results with a 'cold' area at the site of infection. The explanation

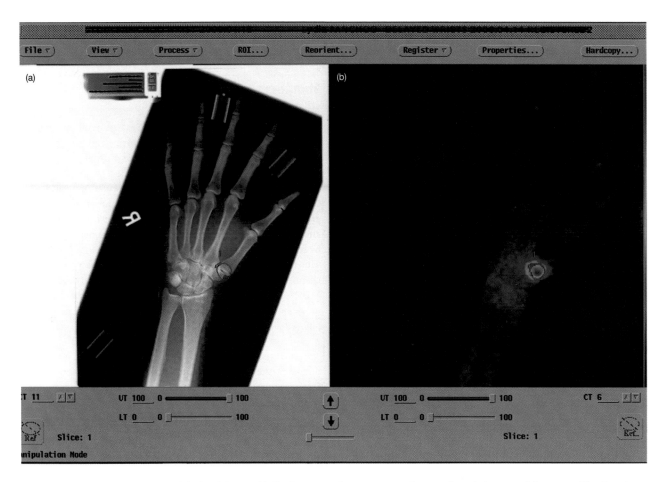

Fig. 6 Example of co-registration image of the hands/wrists. (a) The bone scan shows an intense focus in the radial aspect of the carpus. The three hot spots (blue) external to the patient are radioactive markers used for image alignment. (b) Radiograph of hand. The red outline superimposed from the bone scan image shows that the bone scan activity is localized to the carpometacarpal articulation of the right thumb.

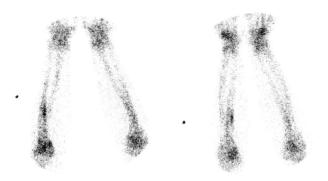

Fig. 7 ^{99m}Tc-MDP scan of the forearms in unilateral ulnar stress fracture. (The black dot external to the patient marks the right limb.) This type of overuse injury is often associated with weight-lifting. This patient's job involved stacking shelves.

for this is not clear, but because of this pitfall some authors advocate the use of ^{67}gallium-citrate in suspected vertebral osteomyelitis.[26]

Pelvis and hips

Bone scintigraphy can be helpful in the evaluation of the acutely painful hip, particularly where radiographs are unremarkable or/and

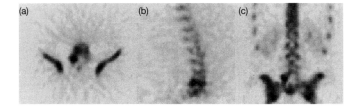

Fig. 8 Selected images of a ^{99m}Tc-MDP bone SPECT scan of the lumbar spine in a young athlete with back pain. (a) Axial, (b) sagittal, and (c) coronal slices at the level of the known spondylolysis demonstrate a focus of increased tracer uptake at the site of the affected pars interarticularis.

ultrasound ± aspiration has not produced a diagnosis (Fig. 9). Infection, avascular necrosis, synovitis, and septic arthritis may produce transient ischaemia resulting in a 'cold' femoral head on bone scan. In the elderly, X-ray-negative/equivocal subcapital fracture of the neck of femur may fail to demonstrate the typical fracture pattern of increased activity on all three phases of the bone scan when performed within a few days of the injury.[27] In a review of bone scans in 2000 patients, Spitz et al. found that fractures of the axial skeleton and shafts of long bones may remain negative on bone scan up to 12 days

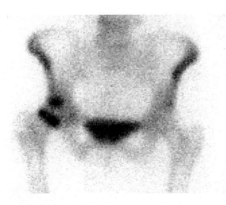

Fig. 9 There is a linear band of abnormal tracer uptake traversing the right femoral neck on this ^{99m}Tc-MDP bone scan in an elderly patient with a painful hip after falling. The pelvis radiograph at the time of injury did not demonstrate the fracture that is clearly visible on the bone scan.

(a)

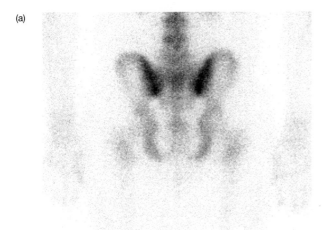

(b)

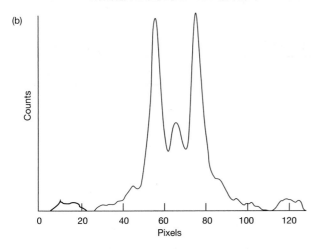

Fig. 10 Bilateral sacroiliitis. (a) The posterior view of the pelvis from the bone scan shows increased tracer uptake at the sacroiliac joints. (b) The graph demonstrates a count profile across the midportion of the sacroiliac joints. The three peaks correspond to the left sacroiliac joint, sacrum, and right sacroiliac joint (from left to right). The ratio of the counts of each sacroiliac peak compared with the sacrum is greater than 2, indicating sacroiliitis.

post-traumatic fracture.[28] Consideration should be given to repeating the bone scan when clinical suspicion of fracture persists but radiographs are consistently negative.

Sacroiliitis can be assessed by bone scintigraphy, often as part of a whole body joint assessment in suspected seronegative arthritis (Fig. 10). The lower synovial portion of the joint is most frequently affected. Visual inspection of the bone scan image may prove satisfactory. However, quantitative analysis can be helpful.

Different methods are used to calculate the sacroiliac joint index, but in principle the intensity of uptake at the joint is compared with that at a non-involved site such as the sacrum.[29, 30] Care has to be taken when examining the scans of adolescents and athletic individuals since physiologically increased uptake may be seen at the sacroiliac joints.[31]

Bone scans can identify exercise-induced pathology in the femur that is not seen on radiographs (Fig. 11). Stress fractures may occur in the shaft or in the femoral neck. When identified, prompt action should be taken to ensure appropriate management with a period of non-weight-bearing to prevent progression to complete fracture. Enthesopathies can also be demonstrated with focal increased tracer uptake at the site of tendon insertion. Trochanteric bursitis produces uptake at the level of the greater trochanter.[32] Adductor strains produce focal uptake in the inferior pubic ramus, presumably occurring by the same method by which plantar fasciitis produces focal calcaneal periostitis at the medial calcaneal tubercle.

Knees

The most common soft tissue disorders of the knee include trauma and derangement of the internal knee stabilizing structures. Whilst

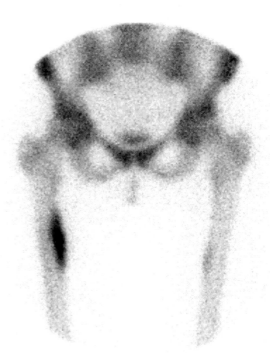

Fig. 11 ^{99m}Tc-MDP bone scan in a female athlete demonstrating increased tracer uptake at the medial aspect of the upper right femoral shaft (and to a lesser extent in the left femoral shaft also) at the site of exercise-induced stress fractures.

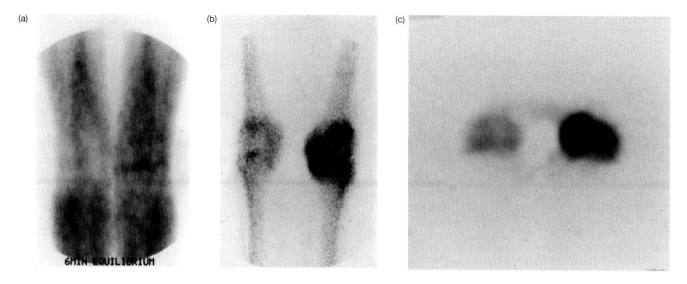

6MIN EQUILIBRIUM

Fig. 12 Selected images from ^{99m}Tc-MDP bone SPECT scan of the knees in a patient with meniscal injury. (a) Early blood pool, (b) delayed anterior view, and (c) an axial slice from the SPECT study demonstrate abnormal activity as in the medial tibial plateau, increased adjacent femoral activity, and increased blood pool as a result of tear of the medial meniscus of the left knee.

arthroscopy allows direct visualization and treatment at the same time, it is invasive, expensive, and may not be indicated or optimal in all circumstances.

With the increasing availability of MRI and its exquisite anatomical definition, the use of bone scanning for imaging internal knee pathology has been superseded in most cases. Nevertheless, the applications of SPECT bone scanning of the knee will be described as this may still be of value where MR is not readily available or contraindicated, or when the result is equivocal.

Ryan *et al.* have described specific patterns of bone scan abnormalities with meniscal tears.[33] They examined a group of 40 patients within 6 months of acute knee injury. With SPECT ^{99m}Tc-MDP imaging, a half-crescent or more of increased activity in the tibial plateau had a sensitivity of 89 per cent. This is similar to the findings of Murray *et al.*[34] Ryan *et al.* also found that the triad of a full crescent of tibial plateau activity, increased blood pool, and tracer uptake in the adjacent femoral condyle gave a specificity of 94 per cent and a positive predictive value of 93 per cent for 'bucket-handle' meniscal tears (Fig. 12).

The same group from Guy's Hospital (London) has also evaluated SPECT imaging with injuries to the anterior cruciate ligament (ACL).[35] Chronic ruptures demonstrate increased activity at the point of insertion of the ACL at the posterior aspect of the lateral femoral condyle, and, less often, at both attachments of the ACL. Scintigraphy can also detect associated injuries to the collateral ligaments and the posterior cruciate ligament as well as the secondary arthritic change in the joint which occurs as a consequence of trauma. These abnormalities, however, are more clearly demonstrated on MR scans, which remain the mainstay of imaging internal knee injuries.

Lower leg

Nuclear medicine has a role in the evaluation of subacute exertional limb pain in the lower leg. The differential diagnosis for this condition includes stress fractures, chronic compartment syndrome, popliteal

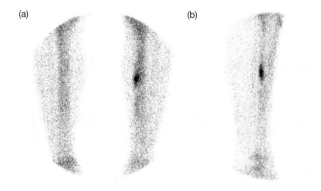

Fig. 13 Tibial stress fracture. ^{99m}Tc-MDP scan ((a) anterior view; (b) medial view) of left leg demonstrating abnormal focus in the posteromedial aspect of the left tibial shaft in the region of the junction of the upper third with the lower two-thirds.

artery entrapment, medial tibial syndrome, muscle tears, and referred pain from other sites such as the lumbar spine.

Bone scans are sensitive in detecting stress fractures.[36] Stress fractures are most frequently seen in runners and may occur in the fibula or, more commonly, in the tibia (Fig. 13). The pathology underlying stress fractures is thought to be multiple microfractures in the cortical bone owing to mechanical stresses and an imbalance between bone resorption and new bone formation in response to continued stress.[37] Typically, a tibial stress fracture is identified on the bone scan as a focus of increased tracer uptake, characteristically located at the posteromedial margin of the shaft of the tibia. Some authors have graded stress fractures according to the bone scan appearances.[38–40] Generally, the smaller, more focal, and less intense abnormalities are considered lower grade, with the high-grade fractures being more intense and extensive abnormalities approaching transcortical thickness of the tibia. The differentiation of stress fracture grade can be

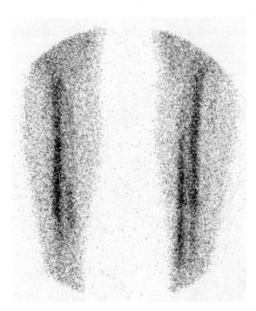

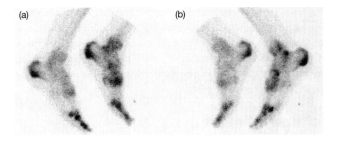

Fig. 15 Bone scan of the feet in a patient with bilateral plantar fasciitis. A black dot marking the right limb is seen in both images. (a) shows left foot medial and right foot lateral projections; (b) shows left foot lateral and right foot medial projections. Note the focal uptake in the calcaneum at the point of insertion of the plantar fascia at the medial calcaneal tubercle.

Fig. 14 Exercise-induced tibial periosteal stress reactions in the tibiae. ^{99m}Tc-MDP scan demonstrating uptake in both tibiae predominantly affecting the anterolateral margin.

important in the management of the patient since duration of rehabilitation appears to correlate with the stress fracture grade. A more extensive (higher-grade) stress fracture of the tibia will generally require a more prolonged rest period than the lesser grades of fracture.[38–40] The location of the abnormality within the tibia also may influence duration of rehabilitation with stress fractures in the anterior cortex of the midtibial shaft being more problematic.

Periosteal stress reactions, which may be diagnosed clinically and demonstrated on nuclear medicine bone scans (Fig. 14), are a less severe form of overuse injury, but can be produced by the same stress factors that result in tibial stress fractures. The bone scan often shows bilateral leg abnormalities with low-grade diffuse tracer uptake tracking along the margin of the tibia, usually as a continuous line giving a 'double stripe' appearance. Periosteal stress reactions and stress fractures may be seen together or may be present individually, but one is not necessarily a precursor of the other.

Bone scans can be helpful in excluding the presence of tibial stress injuries and, under such circumstances, alternative diagnoses are considered. Chronic compartment syndrome in the lower leg is one such consideration. There have been a few preliminary studies using Thallium-201 chloride and ^{99m}Tc-MIBI to assess changes in muscle perfusion on exercise compared with rest with some promising results.[7, 41] Larger and more quantitatively robust studies are required before this method can be considered to compete with the 'gold standard' invasive method of direct measurement of compartment pressure.

Foot and ankle

The feet are exposed to repetitive traumatic insults as a result of weight-bearing and ambulation. Each minor traumatic event is likely to result in altered bone metabolism at the site of injury which may account for the presence of small foci of ^{99m}Tc-MDP uptake in the feet of asymptomatic individuals. At times this can make interpretation difficult.

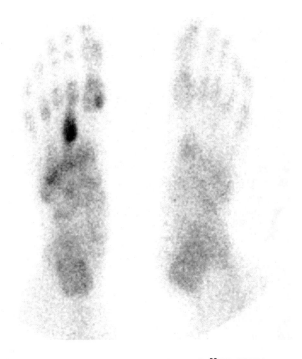

Fig. 16 Metatarsal stress fracture ('march fracture'). ^{99m}Tc-MDP bone scan (plantar view) showing a 'hot spot' in the right foot third metatarsal shaft at the site of the stress fracture.

Nevertheless, bone scintigraphy in the feet is valuable, particularly in suspected plantar fasciitis (Fig. 15), mapping joint involvement in arthritis, and in the investigation of trauma for which radiographs have failed to demonstrate a fracture such as metatarsal stress fractures ('march' fractures; Fig. 16) and fractures of the calcaneum.[42]

When bone scans demonstrate 'hot spots' in the forefoot, anatomical localization is usually straightforward. In the hindfoot, and particularly midfoot, localization can be extremely difficult and is helped by co-registration techniques, similar to those used in the wrist.[43]

Summary

In the diagnosis of soft tissue rheumatological disorders ^{99m}Tc-MDP bone scans are by far the most common nuclear medicine technique employed. The abnormalities demonstrated are frequently not specific for a particular pathology. However, bone scans are highly sensitive and can identify sites of altered bone metabolism before detection by other imaging modalities. In the evaluation of soft tissue disorders, bone scans can help by excluding or confirming underlying bone or joint pathology.

Acknowledgements

We are grateful to Nick Bird for his valuable assistance and expertise in the preparation of the figures.

References

1. Administration of Radioactive Substances Advisory Committee (1998). *Notes for guidance on the clinical administration of radiopharmaceuticals and use of sealed radioactive sources.* Didcot, Oxon: National Radiological Protection Board, Didcot, Oxford shine.

2. Royal College of Radiologists (RCR) Working Party (1995). *Making the best use of a Department of clinical radiology: guidelines for doctors,* 3rd edn. RCR, London.

3. Al-Janabi, M.A., Critchley, M., Maltby, P., *et al.* (1991). Radiolabeled white blood cell imaging in arthritis. Is it a blood pool effect? *Nucl. Med. Commun.* **12**, 1013–1024.

4. Al-Janabi, M.A., Jones, A.K.P., Solanki, K., *et al.* (1988).^{99}Tc^m-labelled leucocyte imaging in active rheumatoid arthritis. *Nucl. Med. Commun.* **9**, 987–991.

5. Schauwecker, D.S. (1989). Osteomyelitis: diagnosis with In-111-labeled leukocytes. *Radiology* **171**, 141–146.

6. McCall, I.W., Sheppard, H., Haddaway, M., *et al.* (1983). Gallium 67 scanning in rheumatoid arthritis. *Br. J. Radiol.* **56**, 241–243.

7. Edwards, P.D., Miles, K.A., Owens, S.J., *et al.* (1999). A new non-invasive test for the detection of compartment syndromes. *Nucl. Med. Commun.* **20**, 215–218.

8. Rolfe, E.B., Garvie, N.W., Khan, M.A., *et al.* (1981). Isotope bone imaging in suspected scaphoid trauma. *Br. J. Radiol.* **54**, 762–767.

9. Tiel-van Buul, M.M.C., van Beek, E.J.R., van Dongen, A., *et al.* (1992). The reliability of the 3-phase bone scan in suspected scaphoid fracture: an inter- and intra-observer variability analysis. *Eur. J. Nucl. Med.* **19**, 848–852.

10. Tiel-van Buul, M.M., van Beek, E.J., Borm, J.J., *et al.* (1992). The value of bone scintigraphy in suspected scaphoid fracture: a statistical analysis. *J. Hand Surg. (Br.)* **18** (3), 403–406.

11. Leslie, I.J. and Dickson, R.A. (1981). The fractured carpal scaphoid: natural history and factors influencing outcome. *J. Bone Joint Surg.* **63B**, 225–230.

12. Reinus, W.R., Conway, W.F., Totty, W.G., *et al.* (1986). Carpal avascular necrosis: MR imaging. *Radiology* **160**, 689–693

13. Duong, R.B., Nishiyama, H., Mantil, J.C., *et al.* (1982). Kienbock's disease: scintigraphic demonstration in correlation with clinical, radiographic and pathological findings. *Clin. Nucl. Med.* **7**, 418–420.

14. Pons, F., Moya, F., Herranz, R., *et al.* (1993). Detection and quantitative analysis of joint activity inflammation with ^{99}Tc^m-polyclonal human immunoglobulin G. *Nucl. Med. Commun.* **14**, 225–231.

15. Soden, M., Rooney, M., Cullen, A., *et al.* (1989). Immunohistological features in the synovium obtained from clinically uninvolved knee joints of patients with rheumatoid arthritis. *Br. J. Rheumatol.* **28**, 287–292.

16. Roddie, M.E., Peters, A.M., Osman, S., *et al.* (1988). Osteomyelitis. *Nucl. Med. Commun.* **9**, 713–717.

17. Schauwecker, D.S. (1989). Osteomyelitis: diagnosis with In-111-labeled leukocytes. *Radiology* **171**, 141–146.

18. Maurer, A.H., Chen, D.C.P., Camargo, E.E., *et al.* (1981). Utility of three-phase skeletal scintigraphy in suspected osteomyelitis. *J. Nucl. Med.* **22**, 941–949.

19. Mackinnon, S.E. and Holder, L.E. (1984). The use of three-phase radio-nuclide bone scanning in the diagnosis of reflex sympathetic dystrophy. *J. Hand Surg.* **9A**, 556–563.

20. Kozin, F., Soin, J.S., Lawrence, M.R., *et al.* (1981). Bone scintigraphy in the reflex sympathetic dystrophy syndrome. *Radiology* **138**, 437–443.

21. Werner, R., Davidorr, G., Jackson, D., *et al.* (1989). Factors affecting the sensitivity and specificity of the three-phase bone scan in the diagnosis of reflex sympathetic dystrophy syndrome in the upper extremity. *J. Hand Surg.* **14A**, 520–523.

22. Demangeat, J-L., Constantinesco, A., Brunot, B., *et al.* (1988). Three-phase bone scanning in reflex sympathetic dystrophy of the hand. *J. Nucl. Med.* **29**, 26–32.

23. Mohamed, A., Ryan, P.J., Lewis, M., *et al.* (1997). Registration bone scan in the evaluation of wrist pain. *J. Hand Surg.* **22B**, 161–166.

24. Dolan, A.L., Ryan, P.J., Arden, N.K., *et al.* (1996). The value of SPECT scans in identifying back pain likely to benefit from facet joint injection. *Br. J. Rheumatol.* **35**, 1269–1273.

25. Dutton, J.A.E., Hughes, S.P.F., and Peters, A.M. (2000). SPECT in the management of patients with back pain and spondylolysis. *Clin. Nucl. Med.* **25**, 93–96.

26. Palestro, C.J. and Torres, M.A. (1997). Radionuclide imaging in orthopedic infections. *Semin. Nucl. Med.* **27**, 334–345.

27. Matin, P. (1979). The appearance of bone scans following fractures, including immediate and long-term studies. *J. Nucl. Med.* **20**, 1227–1231.

28. Spitz, J., Lauer, I., Tittel, K., *et al.* (1993). Scintimetric evaluation of remodelling after bone fractures in man. *J. Nucl. Med.* **9**, 1403–1409.

29. Russell, A.S., Lentle, B.C., and Percy, J.S. (1975). Investigation of sacroiliac disease: comparative evaluation of radiological and radionuclide techniques. *J. Rheumatol.* **2**, 45–51.

30. Davis, M.C., Turner, D.A., Charters, J.R., *et al.* (1984). Quantitative sacroiliac scintigraphy. The effect of method of selection of region of interest. *Clin. Nucl. Med.* **9**, 334–340.

31. Chisin, R., Milgrom, C., Marguiles, J., *et al.* (1984). Unilateral sacroiliac overuse syndrome in military recruits. *Br. J. Med.* **289**, 590–591.

32. Allwright, S.J., Cooper, R.A., and Nash, P. (1988). Trochanteric bursitis: bone scan appearance. *Clin. Nucl. Med.* **13**, 561–564.

33. Ryan, P.J., Taylor, M., and Grevitt, M. (1993). Bone single-photon emission tomography in recent meniscal tears: an assessment of diagnostic criteria. *Eur. J. Nucl. Med.* **20**, 703–707.

34. Murray, I.P.C., Dixon, J., and Kohan, L. (1990). SPECT for acute knee pain. *Clin. Nucl. Med.* **15**, 828–840.

35. Cook, G.J.R., Ryan, P.J., Clarke, S.E.M., *et al.* (1996). SPECT bone scintigraphy of anterior cruciate ligament injury. *J. Nucl. Med.* **37**, 1353–1356.

36. Ammann, W. and Matheson, G.O. (1991). Radionuclide bone imaging in the detection of stress fractures. *Clin. J. Sports Med.* **1**, 115–122.

37. Holder, L.E. (1993). Bone scintigraphy in skeletal trauma. *Radiol. Clin. N. Am.* **31**, 739–781.

38. Zwas, S.T., Elkanovitch, R., and Frank, G. (1987). Interpretation and classification of bone scintigraphic findings in stress fractures. *J. Nucl. Med.* **28**, 452–457.

39. Matin, P. (1983). Bone scintigraphy in the diagnosis and management of traumatic injury. *Semin. Nucl. Med.* **13**, 104–122.

40. Matin, P. (1988). Basic principles of nuclear medicine techniques for detection and evaluation of trauma and sports medicine injuries. *Semin. Nucl. Med.* **18**, 90–112.

41. Takebayashi, S., Takazawa, H., Sasaki, R., *et al.* (1997). Chronic exertional compartment syndrome in lower legs: localization and follow-up with thallium-201 SPECT imaging. *J. Nucl. Med.* **38**, 972–976.

42. O'Duffy, E.K., Clunie, G.P., Gacinovic, S., *et al.* (1998). Foot pain: specific indications for scintigraphy. *Br. J. Rheumatol.* **37**, 442–447.

43. Robinson, A.H., Bird, N., Screaton, N., *et al.* (1998). Coregistration imaging of the foot. A new localisation technique. *J. Bone Joint Surg. Br.* **80**, 777–780.

4.6 Infrared thermal imaging in musculoskeletal conditions

Brian Hazleman

Introduction

Thermal imaging has been used in musculoskeletal conditions for 40 years. It provides sensitive and reproducible means for diagnostic imaging and monitoring treatment. The diagnosis of inflammatory, degenerative, and traumatic conditions is assisted by infrared imaging. Vasospastic conditions affecting the hands can be monitored by thermal imaging using a mild cold stress test and the efficacy of vasoactive drugs proven by this technique.

Modern infrared imaging systems have developed since 1959. Initially the camera systems were slow with limited facilities for display and hard-copy and Polaroid film was used to record the images. The advent of the computer brought about many advances in infrared imaging. These included the facility for measurement of temperature, recording and archiving images and data, and more reliable hard-copy.

Techniques

Modern systems are used to capture a thermal map of skin temperature distribution in a fraction of a second to an accuracy of 0.1 °C.[1] The technique is quantitative, and provides an objective and non-invasive investigation.[2] It is an efficient way to measure the temperature effects of an inflamed joint. After cooling the limb in an ambient temperature of 20 °C, localized areas of heat can be visualized.[3]

Modern thermal imaging systems allow computer image processing facilities for captive storage and image analysis, using a laptop computer or a desk-based microcomputer. In addition, infrared lenses give great flexibility for close up or wide angle views as with a conventional video camera.

Applications

Thermal imaging of the musculoskeletal system provides an objective and sometimes diagnostic tool. It is often possible to identify the site and severity of an inflammatory lesion, with dermal vascular changes that characterize the inflammatory arthritides, and it can also be used in connective tissue disorders such as scleroderma.[4]

Modern scanning equipment can produce a multiple isotherm scan in less than a second. The success of any thermographic investigation depends on intelligent interpretation of the thermogram in terms of heat flow patterns to the skin surface. The integrity of the blood supply to the skin and the thermal properties and metabolism of tissue are the principal factors that determine the surface temperature characteristics. The more removed the skin effect becomes from the pathological process, the more difficult becomes interpretation of the thermographic data. However, once the surface temperature variations have led to a recognition of a lesion, its site, size, and shape can be assessed, and progression or response to treatment can be monitored.

Thermography can only be used as a quantitative measure if rigid control of techniques and of environmental conditions are achieved. Factors that must be controlled include the state of the patient, who should not have had recent physiotherapy or strenuous exercise and must remain in a temperature-controlled room for a period of at least 15 minutes before thermography is performed. The time of day should be constant to avoid the intrinsic diurnal variation, and the position of the patient must be standardized for each area.

Other applications include Paget's disease of bone,[5] stress fractures,[6] neck pain,[7] and low back pain.[8] Thermography has also been used in chronic pain management.[9] Its value has also been demonstrated in soft tissue disorders including enthesopathies,[10] bursitis, tendinitis, and musculo-ligamentous injections.[11]

Stress fractures

Devereaux and colleagues[6] studied 18 patients with shin pain that was clinically considered to be caused by a stress fracture of the tibia or fibula. Patients underwent radiological, thermographic, and scintigraphic studies and a test of ultrasound-induced pain. Of the 15 patients with stress fractures confirmed by scintigraphy, 12 had abnormal thermograms, eight had positive test results for ultrasound-induced pain, and seven had abnormal radiographs. Therefore thermograms were abnormal in 80 per cent of the confirmed stress fractures.

Most stress fractures of the tibia are posteromedial. Previously, because of overlying muscle, thermographic diagnosis has proved difficult. However, with a period of adequate cooling this difficulty can be overcome, allowing the thermogram to detect the increased blood-flow heat associated with the stress fracture.

Tennis elbow

Binder and colleagues[10] during a therapeutic study of 56 tennis-elbow lesions demonstrated a characteristic localized thermographic abnormality in 53 of 56 affected elbows, and only 3 of 60 normal age- and sex-matched controls. Microcomputer analysis of the thermal gradient slope across the abnormal area showed a correlation with clinical state, reflecting recovery and revealing a much small diurnal variation than was seen in the solely temperature-based parameters.

Patellofemoral pain

A study of thermography in patellofemoral pain[12] has shown that the patella is warmer in patients with patellofemoral pain. In thermograms of 30 athletes with normal knees a uniform pattern was noted. Thermography of the normal knee shows on the anterior view that the patella acts as a heat shield; the medial view shows gradual cooling from the thigh and cuff muscle towards the patella. Osteoarthritic knees and rheumatoid knees show a diffuse increase in heat.

The athletes with patellofemoral pain had normal radiographs, including skyline views. On the anterior view the athletes showed an increase of heat medially beside the patella, corresponding to the site of tenderness. The medial view showed an increase in heat arising from the patella and radiating into the vastus medialis muscle.

With physiotherapy exercises and faradic stimulation to the vastus medialis muscle all the patients were asymptomatic at a 3-month follow-up. As symptomatic improvement occurred, the heat abnormalities noted on thermography disappeared.

The pattern described would appear to be diagnostic of patellofemoral arthralgia. Thermography has demonstrated inflammation in the vastus medialis muscle extending to the patellar insertion. In athletes with patellofemoral arthralgia the vastus medialis may be overstretched by overdevelopment of the vastus lateralis. Such a mechanism would explain the pain in athletes who have no evidence of chondromalacia patellae on arthroscopy.

Frozen shoulder and rotator cuff tendinitis

Vecchio and colleagues have evaluated the role of thermography in frozen shoulder and rotator cuff tendinitis.[13] Twenty-eight patients with unilateral frozen shoulder and 86 patients with unilateral rotator cuff lesions had the index shoulder compared with the normal side. Differences in shin temperature distribution were found in 82 per cent of subjects with frozen shoulder, nearly three-quarters of whom had reduced skin temperature. There was no consistent pattern of shoulder skin temperature found in rotator cuff tendinitis patients (49 per cent normal, 28 per cent reduced, 23 per cent increased). Therefore this study suggests that the majority of patients with clinical frozen shoulder have abnormal cool thermographic patterns, but that there is no significant pattern in rotator cuff tendinitis.

Synovitis

The synovitis associated with rheumatoid arthritis and polymyalgia rheumatica has been extensively studied and also evaluated with other techniques, including isotope bone scans.[14, 15] De Silva and colleagues[14] demonstrated that the heat distribution index based on thermal patterns was more reliable and less affected by diurnal variations in joint temperature than the thermographic index, which is based on average skin temperature values. There were significant correlations between clinical assessment, heat distribution index and radioisotopic studies.

Other conditions

Several studies have confirmed that body surface temperature is very symmetrical in normal healthy subjects.[2, 16] This ranges from 0.25 °C mean temperature between contralateral sides to 0.7 °C depending on the site and conditions under which the subject was examined.

Changes to this symmetrical pattern occur in a number of neuromuscular conditions including proximal nerve root compression[17, 18] and nerve entrapment syndromes such as carpal tunnel syndrome.[19, 20] In these conditions there can be significant side to side temperature changes, the affected limb often being colder than the unaffected side. As the condition improves clinically, the objective temperature changes can indicate if the physiological function of the limb is returning to normal, for instance, in Sudeck's atrophy.[21]

In addition, using a provocation test, thermographic changes were demonstrated in keyboard operators with chronic forearm pain.[22] In this condition, which has diverse symptoms, few physical signs, and uncertain pathology, thermography has shown changes supporting the presence of vasomotor changes in repetitive strain injury. After typing, all 10 patients with chronic forearm pain exacerbated by keyboard work had mean temperature readings significantly reduced. Means before typing in this group and 21 asymptomatic controls were similar, although significantly different afterwards. The changes were reproducible and the temperature readings in one patient who became asymptomatic changed significantly at his reassessment. Cooling in symptomatic patients may be secondary to sympathetic overactivity as a result of nocioceptor and mechanoreceptor stimulation leading to a reflex neuropathic state. However, cooling after challenge suggests that it is a result rather than a cause.

The objective assessment of Raynaud's phenomenon by a thermal challenge is of diagnostic value.[23] Treatment with vasoactive drugs such as prostaglandin analogues may also be monitored using a thermal challenge test.[24]

Kyle and colleagues demonstrated that cold stress testing with thermographic assessment differentiated controls from patients with Raynaud's. The normal response to cold stress testing by immersing the hand in cold water is rapid rewarming of the hand, the fingertips being the hottest area of the digits. Sufferers from Raynaud's, in contrast, fail to rewarm, and their fingertips are the coldest area of the digits. Discriminant analysis of the change in temperature of a finger after cold stress, and the mean thermal gradient along the finger during recovery allows accurate measurement to be made. After treatment the patient's discriminant values moved into the normal range.

Investigations of treatment modalities

Treatment modalities have also been evaluated with thermography. Treatments studied include ultrasound, heat treatment, hydrotherapy massage, and exercise.[25] The effects of surgery on skin temperature have also been recorded and skin temperature measurements used for decision-making.[26, 27] These measurements are usually performed in a warmer environment to avoid superficial vascular constriction.

References

1. **Ring, E.F.J. and Dicks, J.M.** (1999). Spatial resolution of new thermal imaging systems. *Thermol. Int.* **9** (1), 7–14.

2. **Salisbury, R.S., Parr, G., De Silva, M., Hazleman, B.L., and Page Thomas, D.P.** (1983). Heat distribution over normal and abnormal joints: thermal pattern and quantification. *Ann. Rheum. Dis.* **42** (5), 494–499.

3. **Devereaux, M.D., Parr, G.R., Thomas, D.P., and Hazleman, B.L.** (1985). Disease activity indexes in rheumatoid arthritis: a prospective comparative study using thermography. *Ann. Rheum. Dis.* **44** (7), 434–437.

4. Howell, K.J., Martini, G., Murray, K.J., Smith, R.E., and Black, C.M. (2000). Infrared thermography for the assessment of localised scleroderma in children. *Thermol. Int.* **10** (4), 204–209.

5. Crisp, A.J., Smith, M.L., Skingle, S.J., Page Thomas, D.P., and Hazleman, B.L. (1989). The localisation of the bone lesions of Paget's disease by radiographs, scintigraphy and thermography: pain may be related to bone blood flow. *Br. J. Rheumatol.* **28** (3), 266–268.

6. Devereaux, M.D., Parr, G.R., Lachmann, S.M., Page Thomas, D.P., and Hazleman, B.L. (1989). The diagnosis of stress fractures in athletes. *J. Am. Med. Assoc.* **252** (4), 531–533.

7. Taylor, A.L., Garroway, M., Carello, R., and Will, K. (1994). Whiplash injuries—an assessment of infrared thermographic change in patients with unilateral upper limb pain. In K. Mabuchi, S. Mizushina, B. Harrison (eds). *Advanced techniques and clinical applications in biomedical thermologies* (ed. K. Mabuchi, S. Mizushina, and B. Harrison), pp. 237–244. Harwood Academic Publishers, Chur/Schweiz.

8. Thomas, D., Cullum, D., Siahamis, G., and Langlois, S. (1990). Infrared thermographic imaging, magnetic resonance imaging, CT scan and myelography in low back pain. *Br. J. Rheumatol.* **29** (4), 268–273.

9. Hooshmand, H., Hashini, M., and Phillips, E.M. (1990). Infrared thermal imaging as a tool in pain management. An 11 year study. Part II: Clinical applications. *Thermol. Int.* **11** (3), 117–129.

10. Binder, A., Parr, G., Page Thomas, D.P., and Hazleman, B.L. (1983). A clinical and thermographic study of lateral epicondylitis. *Br. J. Rheumatol.* **22**, 77–81.

11. Schmitt, M. and Guillot, Y. (1984). Thermography and muscular injuries in sports medicine. In *Recent advances in medical thermology* (ed. E.F. Ring and B. Philips), pp. 439–444.

12. Devereaux, M., Parr, G., Lachmann, S., Page Thomas, D., and Hazleman, B. (1986). Thermographic diagnosis in athletes with patellofemoral arthralgia. *J. Bone Joint Surg.* **68-B**, 42–44.

13. Vecchio, P.C., Adebajo, A.O., Chard, M.D., Page Thomas, D.P., and Hazleman, B.L. (1992). Thermography of frozen shoulder and rotator cuff tendinitis. *Clin. Rheumatol.* **11**, 382–384.

14. De Silva, M., Kyle, V., Hazleman, B.L., Salisbury, R., Page Thomas, P., and Wraight, P. (1986). Assessment of inflammation in the rheumatoid knee joint: correlation between clinical, radioisotopic and thermographic methods. *Ann. Rheum. Dis.* **45** (4), 277–280.

15. Kyle, V., Tudor, J., Wraight, P., Gresham, G., and Hazleman, B. (1990). Rarity of synovitis in polymyalgia rheumatica. *Ann. Rheum. Dis.* **49** (10), 818.

16. Goodman, P.H., Murphy, M.G., Siltanen, G.L., Kelley, M.P., and Ruckesh, L. (1986). Normal temperature symmetry of the back and extremities by computer-assisted infrared imaging. *Thermology* **1**, 195–202.

17. Takahashi, Y., Takahashi, K., and Moriya, H. (1994). Thermal deficit in lumber radiculopathy. Correlations with pain and neurological signs and its value for assessing symptomatic severity. *Spine* **19**, 2443–2450.

18. Kim, Y.S. and Cho, Y-E. (1994). Pre and postoperative thermographic imaging of lumbar disc herniations. In *Advanced techniques and clinical application in biomedical thermologies* (ed. K. Manuchi, S. Mizushina, and B. Harrison), pp. 265–280. Harwood Academic Publishers, Chur/Schweiz.

19. Reilly, P.A., Clarke, A.V., and Ring, E.F. (1989). Thermography in carpal tunnel syndrome. *Br. J. Rheumatol.* **28** (6), 553–554.

20. Tchou, S., Costich, J.F., Burges, R.C., and Wexler, C.E. (1992). Thermographic observations in unilateral carpal tunnel syndrome: report of 61 cases. *J. Hand Surg. Am.* **17**, 631–637.

21. Giodano, N., Battisti, E., Franci, A., Cecconami, L., Magaro, L., Marcucci, P., and Marcolongo, R. (1991). Telethermography in the early diagnosis and clinical-therapeutic monitoring of Sudeck's disease. *Clin. Ther.* **138**, 91–96.

22. Sharma, S.D., Smith, E.M., Hazleman, B.L., and Jenner, J.R. (1997). Thermographic changes in keyboard operators with chronic forearm pain. *Br. Med. J.* **314** (7074), 118–121.

23. Howell, K., Kennedy, L.T., Smith, R.E., and Black, C.M. (1997). Temperature of the toes in Raynaud's phenomenon measured using infrared thermography. *Eur. J. Thermol.* **7** (3), 132–137.

24. Kyle, V., Parr, G., Salisbury, R., Thomas, P., and Hazleman, B. (1985). Prostaglandin E_1, vasospastic disease and thermography. *Ann. Rheum. Dis.* **44** (2), 73–78.

25. Ring, E.F., Barker, J.R., and Harrison, R.A. (1989). Thermal effects of pool therapy on the lower limbs. *Thermology* **3**, 127–131.

26. Wolff, K.D., Telzrow, T., Rudolph, K., Franke, J., and Wartenberg, R. (1995). Isotope perfusion and infrared thermography of arterialised, venous flow-through and pedicled venous flaps. *Br. J. Plastic Surg.* **48**, 61–70.

27. Suominen, S. and Asko-Seljavaara, S. (1996). Thermography of hands after a radial forearm flap has been raised. *Scand. J. Plastic Reconstruct. Surg. Hand Surg.* **30** (4), 307–314.

4.7 The investigation of soft tissue disorders: nerve conduction studies and electromyography

Julian Ray, Brian McNamara, and Simon Boniface

Introduction

In clinical neurophysiology the fundamental principles of neurophysiology are applied to develop clinical methods of objectively testing central nervous system and peripheral nervous system function. The two techniques with most relevance to soft tissue rheumatology are nerve conduction studies (NCS) and electromyography (EMG).[1]

Diagnostic implications in Rheumatology

The management of a number of rheumatological disorders affecting muscle and nerve can be aided by neurophysiological investigation. Clinical examples include:

1. peripheral nerve compression such as carpal tunnel syndrome and ulnar nerve compression at the elbow;
2. nerve root compression and disorders of the brachial or lumbosacral plexus;
3. generalized neuropathies such as polyneuropathies or mononeuritis multiplex;
4. primary muscle diseases such as polymyositis or dermatomyositis.

Electromyography (EMG)

In EMG, the electrical activity emanating from a group of muscle fibres is recorded extracellularly.[2] This can be achieved by placing an electrode on the surface of the skin surface over the muscle or by placing a needle into the belly of the muscle.

EMG equipment consists of needle or surface electrodes, electrical filters, amplifiers, and a display unit. The display unit should allow analysis and storage of the signal that is obtained from the muscle. Most electromyography is performed by placing a needle electrode into the muscle. There are two types of needle electrodes commonly used. Monopolar needles consist of a single stainless steel cannula, which is coated in Teflon except at its tip.[3] Concentric needle electrodes consist of a fine platinum wire electrode, which is insulated and housed in a steel cannula (Fig. 1).[3] The amplifiers, filters, and display unit are usually housed in a single commercially available EMG machine. In modern equipment all patient connections are isolated from the power supply.[3]

Recordings are normally made from each muscle in three positions: at rest; during slight voluntary contraction; and during increasing or full contraction. The clinical neurophysiologist chooses which muscles

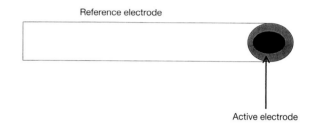

Fig. 1 A schematic diagram of a concentric needle electrode. The outer core of the needle acts as the reference electrode while the inner core acts as an active electrode.

to examine depending on the clinical question that she or he wishes to address.[4]

Nerve conduction studies

In nerve conduction studies the conduction along peripheral nerves is assessed quantitatively. This is achieved by directly recording the activity from the nerve or from a muscle that is supplied by that nerve.[5]

Nerve conduction studies are normally performed using similar apparatus to that required to perform EMG. The activity is recorded using two surface electrodes placed on the skin surface as close as possible to the nerve or muscle that is being examined. The surface electrodes can consist of metal discs or bars attached to the skin surface with conductive paste. Disposable electrodes are also available that use conductive adhesive.[4]

Two stimulating electrodes are placed on the skin close to a nerve. The nerve is electrically stimulated using a short-duration square-wave electrical pulse. For sensory nerves the electrical signal is recorded over the nerve a short distance from the stimulus (Fig. 2). If the direction of conduction along the nerve is in the usual physiological direction of conduction, then the study is *orthodromic*. If it is in the opposite direction, then it is termed *antidromic*. In motor nerve conduction studies the electrical response is recorded over a muscle supplied by that nerve (Fig. 3).[4]

Physiological principles

Electromyography

Activity at rest

Often no spontaneous activity can be recorded from the relaxed muscle. Occasionally, electrical activity generated by the motor

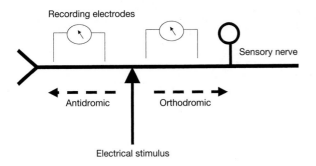

Fig. 2 Schematic diagram of sensory nerve conduction studies. The nerve is stimulated using a square-wave electrical pulse. The compound action potential is recorded using a pair of electrodes placed on the skin surface. If conduction is measured in a distal to proximal direction, the study is said to be orthodromic. If conduction is measured in the opposite direction, it is said to be antidromic.

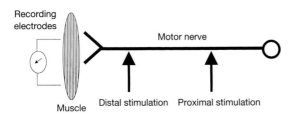

Fig. 3 Schematic diagram showing motor nerve conduction studies. The nerve is stimulated using a square-wave electrical pulse and the compound motor action potential is recorded from a muscle supplied by that nerve. To calculate motor conduction velocity the nerve must be stimulated in two places.

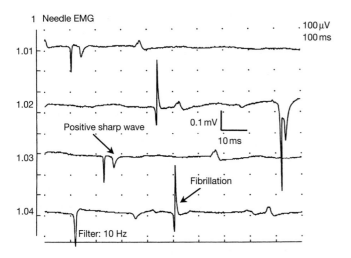

Fig. 4 Fibrillations recorded from the abductor pollicis brevis muscle of a patient with carpal tunnel syndrome. Fibrillations are most commonly a sign of denervation.

Table 1 A selection of the common types of spontaneous activity and some of the associated conditions

Activity	Causes
Myotonia	Myotonic dystrophy
	Myotonia congenita
	Paramyotonia congentia
Complex repetitive discharges	Inflammatory neuropathy
	Denervation
	Thyroid myopathy
	Acid maltase deficiency
Myokymia	Radiation-induced plexopathy
	Radiculopathy
	Entrapment neuropathy
Fibrillations	Denervation
	Inflammatory neuropathy
	Muscular dystrophy
Postitive sharp waves	Denervation
	Inflammatory neuropathy
	Muscular dystrophy

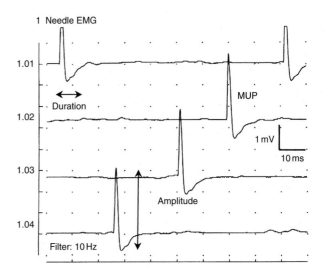

Fig. 5 Normal motor units. MUP, Motor unit action potential.

occur in some primary muscle diseases. *Positive sharp waves* are another feature associated with denervation.[6] Other kinds of abnormal spontaneous activity are summarized in Table 1.

Activity during minimal voluntary contraction

The basic component of the peripheral motor nervous system is the *motor unit*.[7] This consists of a motor neuron, its axon, the neuromuscular junction, and muscle fibres.[7] The extracellular needle EMG recording of a motor unit, the motor unit action potential, is best seen during minimal voluntary contraction.[5] Each motor unit action potential represents the extracellular compound action potential of the muscle fibres in that motor unit, weighted heavily towards the fibres closest to the needle tip.[8]

A normal motor unit action potential (illustrated in Fig. 5), has three phases. The duration and amplitude of each motor unit action

end plates (known as end-plate spikes or end-plate noise) is detected; this is a normal finding.[6] *Fibrillations* are spontaneous depolarization of a single muscle fibre; they have a characteristic appearance (Fig. 4).[6] They are a sign of denervation, although they can also

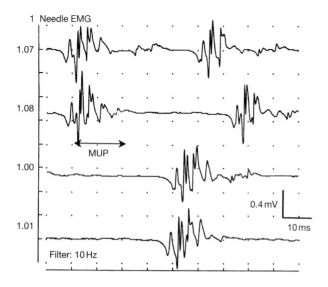

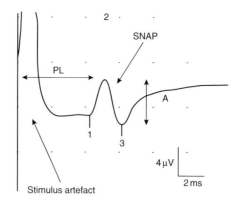

Fig. 7 Sensory nerve action potential (SNAP). This was recorded antidromically from the ulnar nerve of an asymptomatic patient. PL, Peak latency of SNAP; A, amplitude of SNAP. Velocity = distance/PL.

Fig. 6 Neuropathic motor units. These were recorded from the first dorsal interosseous muscle of a patient with ulnar nerve compression at the elbow. They show the characteristic features of increased duration and polyphasia. MUP, Motor unit action potential.

potential varies from muscle to muscle and tables of normal values for the duration and amplitude of motor unit action potentials in each muscle have been compiled. To analyse motor unit action potentials, up to 20 motor unit action potentials are sampled from a particular muscle. The mean duration and amplitude of motor unit action potentials are then compared against the normal values for that muscle. The number of phases in each motor unit action potential is also acquired. The *duration* of each motor unit action potential is determined by the number of fibres in each motor unit and by their dispersion. Most motor unit action potentials are between 5 and 15 ms duration.[8] The *amplitude* of a motor unit is determined by how close the needle tip is to the muscle fibres, the number of fibres in that unit, and the size of the muscle fibres. Most motor unit action potentials have an amplitude of between 100 μV and 2 mV.[8]

The number of *phases* in a motor unit action potential is a measure of synchrony, that is, the extent to which the fibres in a motor unit fire at the same time. In acute denervation, no changes in the amplitude and morphology can be detected.[4] In chronic partial denervation, collateral sprouting occurs from adjacent motor units. Each motor unit contains more muscle fibres and synchrony is lost.[4] The motor unit action potential becomes larger and of longer duration and has an increased number of phases (polyphasia).[4] Neuropathic motor units are shown in Fig. 6. In primary muscle disease, the number of muscle fibres in each motor unit is decreased and synchrony is also lost, so the motor units become smaller, of shorter duration, and polyphasic.[5]

Activity during increasing to maximal strength

In normal subjects if contraction increases, then the firing rate of individual motor units increases, starting at 4–5 Hz and increasing to 30–50 Hz.[9] As strength increases, more motor units begin to fire. During maximal contraction, as more motor units fire at increasing rates, the individual motor action potentials overlap to produce an *interference pattern*, in which no individual motor unit action potentials can be distinguished. In chronic denervation the motor units increase their

firing rate as strength increases. However, since there are fewer motor units available, the individual fast-firing motor units can be distinguished in the interference pattern.[4] In primary muscle disease, since there are fewer muscle fibres in each motor unit, more motor units become recruited earlier and there will be a full low-amplitude recruitment pattern in a weak muscle.[4]

Nerve conduction studies

Sensory nerve conduction studies

The electrical response recorded from the sensory nerve is a compound action potential known as a *sensory nerve action potential* (SNAP; Fig. 7).[5] The time between stimulation of the nerve and recording of the sensory action potential is recorded as the *latency*. The latency may be measured from the first deflection from baseline (onset latency) or the peak (peak latency) of the response. If the distance between the recording and stimulating electrodes, D, is measured, the velocity of sensory nerve conduction is then calculated from the following simple formula

$$\text{Sensory nerve conduction velocity} = D/\text{latency}.$$

The sensory action potential is produced by the summation of all the individual action potentials in the nerve trunk. Its characteristics are determined by the large myelinated fibres only.[5] A reduction in the amplitude of the sensory action potential represents loss of axons in that nerve trunk. A reduction in conduction velocity represents demyelination of the nerve. This can be due to compression of the nerve causing local demyelination or part of a generalized demyelinating neuropathy.[5]

Motor nerve conduction studies

The electrical response is recorded from a muscle supplied by the muscle's relevant nerve and is known as the *compound motor action potential* (CMAP; Fig. 8).[4] The peak or onset latency of the compound action potential is usually recorded. Part of the latency of the compound action potential is due to conduction along muscle fibres and transmission across the neuromuscular junction. Therefore, to calculate the velocity of conduction along the motor nerve, the motor nerve is stimulated at two sites.[4] If the distance between these two sites D, is measured, the velocity of conduction can then be calculated.

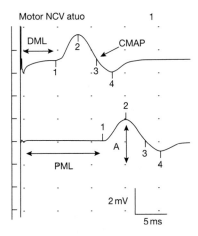

Fig. 8 Compound motor action potential (CMAP). This was recorded by stimulating the median nerve at the wrist and the elbow and recording from abductor pollicis brevis muscle. DML, Distal motor latency; PML, proximal motor latency; A, amplitude of CMAP. Velocity = distance between stimulation sites of DML and PML divided by the difference between the two latencies.

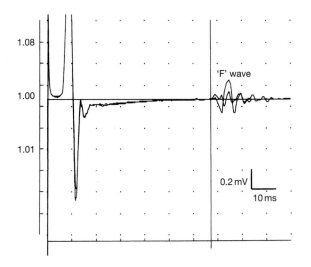

Fig. 9 F-waves. These were recorded by stimulating the posterior tibial nerve at the ankle and recording from the adductor hallicis muscle. The first potential recorded is the compound motor action potential (CMAP). The late-onset F-wave is marked by the linear cursor.

If there is loss of motor axons or damage to anterior horn cells, the amplitude of the response will be reduced.[4] Alternatively, if there is demyelination, the velocity of the response will be reduced.[4] In demyelination there may also be a reduction in amplitude between the proximal and distal stimulation sites (*motor conduction block*). In addition to the orthdromic stimulation of the motor axon resulting in the compound motor action potential, stimulation of a peripheral motor nerve results in antidromic conduction back to the anterior horn cell, which results in a late response known as an *F-wave* (Fig. 9). F-waves are a useful means of assessing conduction in the proximal portion of a motor nerve including its roots. Stimulation of sensory afferents in a mixed nerve sometimes results in a monosynaptic reflex response known as an *H-wave*, which is the electrophysiological equivalent of a tendon reflex.

Clinical indications

Nerve conduction studies

These are helpful in many disorders of the peripheral nervous system. In entrapment neuropathies they help to confirm the involvement of a particular nerve and can be useful in identifying the exact site of entrapment. Nerve conduction studies also help to distinguish disorders of the nerve root from disorders of the brachial or lumbosacral plexus. In generalized neuropathies nerve conduction studies can help to determine whether it is a demyelinating or an axonal neuropathy—this is essential to determining the underlying cause of the neuropathy. Some of the indications for nerve conduction studies and EMG are summarized in Table 2.

Electromyography

EMG is an important part of the assessment of the motor division of the peripheral nervous system and voluntary muscle. It is useful in identifying denervation in diseases of the motor neuron, motor nerve root, or motor axon. It is also an important part of the assessment of primary muscle diseases. Most clinical neurophysiologists perform EMG and nerve conduction studies together as part of a single assessment.

Contraindications

Nerve conduction studies and EMG are relatively safe investigations and there are very few reported instances of serious harm.[10] Some of the potential risks associated with EMG and nerve conduction studies are shown in Table 3. Underlying medical conditions that may predispose to these risks are also shown. Most of these risks are avoidable with a few simple precautions.

Common mistakes made by the referring clinician

Nerve conduction studies and EMG are best considered as extensions of the physical examination. They give information about function in nerve and muscle, but often cannot give a specific pathological diagnosis.[1] For example, electromyography may show signs of denervation in upper and lower limbs: this may be due to a polyradiculopathy or motor neuron disease and the clinician needs to interpret the results in the appropriate clinical context. The best referrals state a clear question.

Table 2 Common indications for nerve conduction studies and EMG

Entrapment neuropathy

Mononeuritis multiplex

Plexopathy

Radiculopathy

Generalized neuropathy

Anterior horn cell disease

Inflammatory myopathy

Muscular dystrophy

Metabolic muscle diseases

Table 3 Hazards of nerve conduction studies and EMG—these are all extremely rare

Risk	Patients at risk	Precautions
Bleeding and sub cutaneous bruising	Prothrombin ratio > 1.5–2.0 Platelets < 300,000/mm³	Do superficial muscles first and examine for bleeding
Transmission of infection	All patients	Use disposable EMG needles Thorough disinfection of electrodes
Electrical hazards	Patients with indwelling catheters Patients connected to multiple electrical devices	Use of equipment that complies with national and international safety guidelines Correct devices Grounding of patient

A referral that states 'arm pain ?cause' is much less likely to produce a meaningful answer than a referral that states 'pain in a C5/C6 distribution, absent biceps jerk, are there signs of radiculopathy or upper trunk plexopathy?'. The latter referral allows the clinical neurophysiologist to concentrate his or her efforts on addressing the most appropriate clinical question.

Additional procedures

Other more specialist procedures that may complement the nerve conduction studies include repetitive nerve stimulation, single-fibre EMG, transcranial magnetic stimulation, and assessment of thermal thresholds.

Repetitive nerve stimulation and single-fibre EMG

In repetitive nerve stimulation, a motor nerve is stimulated at 2–3 Hz for about nine stimuli. The clinical neurophysiologist looks for a reduction in the amplitude of the motor response, which can be a sign of a neuromuscular junction disorder.[11] In single-fibre EMG, pairs of single muscle fibres are examined together. If the neuromuscular junction is functioning normally, then the time between the two fibres firing should be constant, but in neuromuscular junction disorders this time varies considerably (this is described as an increase in 'jitter'), which is a sensitive test for myaesthenia gravis.[12]

Transcranial magnetic stimulation

In transcranial magnetic stimulation (TMS) a magnetic pulse is applied to the scalp surface. This allows non-invasive stimulation of the motor cortex. The conduction time from motor cortex to the spinal cord can be estimated (central motor conduction time). This is useful in distinguishing motor neuron disease from pure lower motor neuron syndromes.[13]

Thermal threshold testing

Conventional nerve conduction studies examine the function of large myelinated fibres only. To diagnose a pure small fibre neuropathy, the ability of the subject to detect heating and cooling is assessed quantitatively. This is known as thermal threshold testing.[14]

Clinical examples

Entrapment neuropathies

The aim of nerve conduction studies in entrapment neuropathies is to confirm the clinical suspicion of neuropathy, to localize the site of nerve compression, and to assess the severity of the neuropathy. The normal procedure is to perform motor and sensory nerve conduction studies on the affected nerve. If possible, the velocity of conduction should be calculated across the site of entrapment and compared with another segment of the same nerve. It is useful to compare the nerve conduction studies with another nerve from the same limb to exclude a generalized neuropathy. As a general rule the first sign is slowing of sensory conduction across the site of entrapment. This is followed by slowing of motor conduction, reduction in the amplitude of the sensory response, reduction of the amplitude of the motor response, and denervation of the affected muscles on needle EMG.[15] Carpal tunnel syndrome and ulnar nerve entrapment at the elbow are the two most common entrapment neuropathies. Other entrapment syndromes and the associated abnormalities on nerve conduction studies and EMG are summarized in Table 4.

Carpal tunnel syndrome

Carpal tunnel syndrome is the most common entrapment neuropathy, occurring in 3 per cent of the general population.[16] The aim of nerve conduction studies is to demonstrate the slowing of median nerve conduction across the carpal tunnel. The following imply median nerve compression in the carpal tunnel: a 10 m/s difference between ulnar and median nerve conduction velocity to the wrist; a reduction in the amplitude of the median nerve sensory action potential; and a reduced motor latency from the wrist to abductor pollicis brevis.[17] Nerve conduction studies from a patient with carpal tunnel syndrome are shown in Fig. 10(a),(b). In severe cases it may also be helpful to perform EMG on abductor pollicis brevis, which may demonstrate signs of denervation. Other procedures that can be performed for carpal tunnel syndrome include recording the motor latency to lumbrical muscles, sensory nerve conduction velocity across the palm to wrist segments, and the detection of bifid sensory wave forms from the fourth finger. If relief of typical symptoms following surgery is taken as a gold standard, then nerve conduction studies for carpal tunnel syndrome have a sensitivity of 85–90 per cent.[18, 19] Although there are significant false-negatives, there are good reasons why all patients should have neurophysiological assessment before surgery. Not all patients present with typical symptoms in a median nerve distribution. There are other causes of sensory symptoms in a median nerve distribution. A thorough neurophysiological assessment can exclude radiculopathy, brachial plexopathy, median nerve entrapment elsewhere in the upper limb, and generalized neuropathies. Neurophysiology is also useful for predicting the prognosis following surgery.[20] Previous nerve conduction studies are an important benchmark for assessing cases where symptoms fail to respond to surgical decompression.

Ulnar nerve entrapment at the elbow

The aim of nerve conduction studies is to confirm the ulnar neuropathy and to localize the site of entrapment. The following are signs of

Table 4 A selection of uncommon nerve entrapment syndromes and the associated electrophysiological signs

Nerve entrapment syndrome	Electrophysiological signs
Common peroneal compression at the fibular head	Slowing of conduction velocity across the fibular head
Entrapment of the posterior tibial nerve in the tarsal tunnel	Reduced mixed nerve responses from medial and lateral plantar nerves
Meralgia paraesthetica	Reduced response from lateral cutaneous nerve of the thigh
Median nerve entrapment by 'ligament of Struthers' at the elbow	Slowing of median nerve conduction from above the elbow to the antecubital fossa
Anterior interosseous nerve entrapment in the forearm	Normal conduction velocity in the nerve trunk from the ante cubital fossa to the wrist. Denervation of flexor digitorum profundus, pronator quadratus, and flexor pollicis longus. Other forearm muscles spared
Median nerve entrapment between the heads of pronator teres muscle	Slowing of median nerve conduction from the ante cubital fossa to the wrist. Denervation of median nerve forearm muscles save pronator teres
Ulnar nerve entrapment in Guyon's canal	Denervation of intrinsic hand muscles. If lesion occurs before bifurcation into superficial and deep branches, will get reduction in ulnar SNAP
Radial nerve compression in the spiral groove	Reduced SNAP from the superficial radial nerve. Denervation of brachioradialis and superficial extensor muscles in the forearm
Posterior interosseus nerve entrapment in the forearm	Normal sensory response from the superficial radial nerve. Denervation of superficial extensors

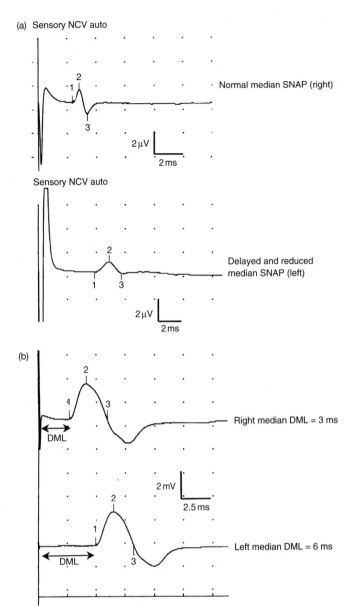

Fig. 10 Carpal tunnel syndrome. (a) Sensory nerve conduction studies. These were recorded by stimulating the median nerve at the index finger and recording at the wrist. The median SNAP is delayed and of reduced amplitude on the symptomatic side. This implies slowing of sensory conduction due to local compression. (b) Distal motor conduction studies. These were recorded by stimulating the median nerve at the wrist and recorded from the abductor pollicis brevis muscle. The distal motor latency (DML) is markedly increased in the affected hand implying slowing of motor conduction across the wrist.

ulnar nerve entrapment at the elbow: an absolute nerve conduction velocity from above the elbow to below the elbow of less than 50 m/s; an above elbow to below elbow segment velocity 10 m/s or more slower than the below elbow to wrist segment; a decrease in compound muscle action potential amplitude from below elbow to above elbow of greater than 20 per cent; mixed nerve action potential of less than 10 µV.[21,22] EMG examination of the first dorsal interosseous muscle and other muscles supplied from the lower trunk of the brachial plexus or C8–T1 nerve roots may help exclude lower trunk plexopathy or cervical radiculopathy.[21] Nerve conduction studies from a patient with ulnar nerve entrapment are illustrated in Fig. 11(a), (b).

Plexopathy and radiculopathy

In nerve root compression there will be signs of chronic partial denervation in the muscles supplied from that nerve root. In suspected radiculopathy at least one muscle innervated by each spinal segment can be examined with needle EMG.[23] Abnormalities can be confirmed if possible by examining another muscle supplied from the same nerve root but from a different peripheral nerve.[23] It may also be helpful to examine paraspinal muscles.[23] At least one sensory and one motor nerve can be examined to exclude an entrapment neuropathy. Nerve root lesions can be distinguished from plexus lesions by sensory nerve conduction studies. For example, in a C5 radiculopathy there will be signs of chronic partial denervation in the biceps brachii muscle but sensory responses from the lateral cutaneous nerve of the arm will be normal, whereas in a lower trunk plexopathy there will be denervation

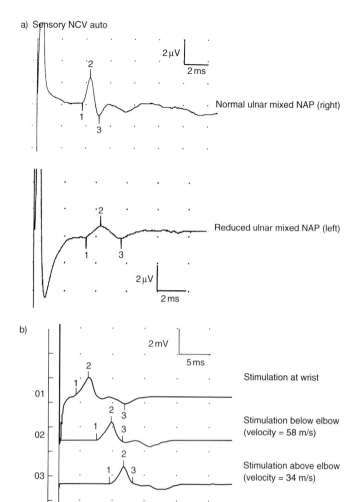

Fig. 11 Ulnar nerve compression at the elbow. (a) Mixed nerve studies. These were recorded by stimulating the ulnar nerve at the wrist and recording over the ulnar nerve above the elbow. There is a significant reduction in the amplitude of the mixed nerve action potential (NAP) on the affected side. (b) Motor study. Recordings were made from the surface of the hypothenar eminence. The ulnar nerve was stimulated at the wrist, below the elbow, and above the elbow. There is significant slowing of motor conduction in the across elbow segment. This implies local demylienation due to compression.

of the biceps and reduced sensory responses because of the position of the dorsal root ganglion.

Generalized neuropathies

In a generalized neuropathy nerve conduction studies will be abnormal in more than one peripheral nerve. One of the most important distinctions is between axonal and demyelinating neuropathies. Some of the causes of demyelinating and axonal polyneuropathies are listed in Table 5. In axonal polyneuropathies there is a symmetrical reduction in motor and sensory amplitudes.[24] Abnormalities of sensory conduction often occur before abnormalities in motor conduction. The reduction in amplitudes is often detected in the lower limbs before the upper limbs. In demyelinating polyneuropathies there is a generalized reduction in conduction velocity.[24] In acquired demyelinating polyneuropathies there may also be motor conduction block and the

Table 5 Common causes of demyelinating and axonal neuropathies

Demyelinating polyneuropathies
Post-infectious inflammatory demyelinating polyneuropathy (Guillian–Barré syndrome)

Chronic inflammatory polyneuropathy

Certain hereditary motor and sensory neuropathies (e.g. HMSN I and HMSN III)

Axonal polyneuropathies
Diabetic polyneuropathy

Uraemic polyneuropathy

Vitamin B_{12} deficiency

Toxic neuropathies
Certain hereditary motor and sensory neuropathies (e.g. HMSN II)

compound motor action potential is often dispersed.[24] In mononeuritis multiplex it is sometimes possible to confirm the involvement of more than one peripheral nerve in the distribution of the patient's signs. However, in a severe mononeuritis multiplex, the neurophysiological signs may be similar to those of a generalized axonal neuropathy.[24]

Primary muscle disease and neuromuscular junction disorders

In most primary muscle diseases the EMG may show the characteristic myopathic features described above.[25] In inflammatory myopathies there may be additional spontaneous activity such as complex repetitive discharges and fibrillations. In Lambert–Eaton myaesthenic syndrome (LEMS) the compound motor action potentials will be small and can be enchanced by tetanic contraction.[26] In myaesthenia gravis the routine EMG examination is usually enchanced by single-fibre EMG or repetitive stimulation.[26]

Summary

The techniques of clinical neurophysiology with most relevance to soft tissue rheumatology are nerve conduction studies and EMG. These are safe investigations that are useful for the investigation of peripheral nerve entrapment syndromes, nerve root compression, disorders of the brachial plexus, generalized neuropathies, and primary muscle disease. More specialized investigations include magnetic stimulation, single-fibre EMG, and thermal threshold testing. To obtain most benefit from neurophysiological tests the referral should be targeted at a clear clinical question. This is often facilitated by discussion of the referral with a clinical neurophysiologist.

References

1. **American Association of Electrodiagnostic Medicine** (1999). The scope of electrodiagnostic medicine. *Muscle Nerve* **8** (suppl.), S5–S12.

2. **Preston, D.C. and Shapiro, B.E.** (1998). Approach to nerve conduction studies and electromyography. In *Electromyography and neuromuscular disorders* (ed. D.C. Preston and B.E. Shapiro), pp. 3–9. Butterworth Heinemann, Boston.

3. **Bischoff, C., Fuglsang-Fredriksen, A., Vendelbo, L., and Sumner, A.** (1999). Standards of instrumentation of EMG. The International

Federation of Clinical Neurophysiology. *Electroencephalogr. Clin. Neurophysiol. Suppl.* **52**, 199–211.

4. Preston, D.C. and Shapiro, B.E. (1998). Fundamentals of electromyography. In *Electromyography and neuromuscular disorders* (ed. D.C. Preston and B.E. Shapiro), pp. 3–9. Butterworth Heinemann, Boston.

5. Preston, D.C. and Shapiro, B.E. (1998). Fundamemtals of nerve conduction studies. In *Electromyography and neuromuscular disorders* (ed. D.C. Preston and B.E. Shapiro), pp. 23–74. Butterworth Heinemann, Boston.

6. Caruso, G., Eisen, A., Stalberg, E., Kimura, J., Mamoli, B., Dengler, R., Santoro, L., and Hopf, H.C. (1999). Clinical EMG and glossary of terms most commonly used by clinical electromyographers. The International Federation of Clinical Neurophysiology. *Electroencephalogr. Clin. Neurophysiol. Suppl.* **52**, 189–198.

7. Myology. (1980). In *Gray's anatomy*, 36th edn (ed. P.L. Williams and R. Warwick), pp. 506–593. Churchill Livingstone, Edinburgh.

8. Stalberg, E., Nandedkar, S.D., Sanders, D.B., and Falck, B. (1996). Quantitative motor unit potential analysis. *J. Clin. Neurophysiol.* **13** (5), 401–422.

9. Sanders, D.B., Stalberg, E.V., and Nandedkar, S.D. (1996). Analysis of the electromyographic interference pattern. *J. Clin. Neurophysiol.* **13** (5), 385–400.

10. American Association of Electrodiagnostic Medicine (1999). Risks in electrodiagnostic medicine. *Muscle Nerve* **8** (suppl.), S5–S12.

11. Preston, D.C. and Shapiro, B.E. (1998). Neuromuscular junction disorders. In *Electromyography and neuromuscular disorders* (ed. D.C. Preston and B.E. Shapiro), pp. 503–524. Butterworth Heinemann, Boston.

12. Stalberg, E. and Trontelj, J.V. (1997). The study of normal and abnormal neuromuscular transmission with single fibre electromyography. *J. Neurosci. Methods* **74** (2), 145–154.

13. Rothwell, J.C., Hallett, M., Berardelli, A., Eisen, A., Rossini, P., and Paulus, W. (1999). Magnetic stimulation: motor evoked potentials. The International Federation of Clinical Neurophysiology. *Electroencephalogr. Clin. Neurophysiol. Suppl.* **52**, 97–103.

14. Jamal, G.A., Hansen, S., Weir, A.I., and Ballantyne, J.P. (1985). An improved automated method for the measurement of thermal thresholds. 1. Normal subjects. *J. Neurol. Neurosurg. Psychiatry* **48** (4), 354–360.

15. Dimitru, D. (1995). Focal peripheral neuropathies. In *Electrodiagnostic medicine* (ed. D. Dimitru), pp. 851–927. Hanley and Belfus, Philadelphia.

16. Atroshi, I., Gummesson, C., Johnsson, R., Ornstein, E., Ranstam, J., and Rosen, I. (1999). Prevalence of carpal tunnel syndrome in a general population. *J. Am. Med. Assoc.* **282**, 153–158.

17. American Association of Electrodiagnostic Medicine (1999). Practice parameter for electrodiagnostic studies in carpal tunnel syndrome. *Muscle Nerve* **8** (suppl.), S141–S143.

18. Concannon, M.J., Gainor, B., Petroski, G.F., and Puckett, C.L. (1997). The predictive value of electrodiagnostic studies in carpal tunnel syndrome. *Plastic Reconstr. Surg.* **100** (6), 1452–1458.

19. Gunnarsson, L.G., Amilon, A., Hellstrand, P., Leissner, P., and Philipson, L. (1997). The diagnosis of carpal tunnel syndrome. Sensitivity and specificity of some clinical and electrophysiological tests. *J. Hand Surg. (Br.)* **22** (1), 34–37.

20. Padua, L., LoMonaco, M., Aulisa, L., Tamburrelli, F., Valente, E.M., Padua, R., Gregori, B., and Tonali, P. (1996). Surgical prognosis in carpal tunnel syndrome: usefulness of a preoperative neurophysiological assessment. *Acta Neurol. Scand.* **94** (5), 343–346.

21. American Association of Electrodiagnostic Medicine (1999). Practice parameter for electrodiagnostic studies in ulnar nerve entrapment at the elbow. *Muscle Nerve* **8** (suppl.), S169–S206.

22. Oh, S.J. (1984). Clinical electromyograpy: nerve conduction studies. University Park Press, Baltimore.

23. Wilbourn, A.J. and Aminoff, M.J. (1998). AAEM minimonograph 32: the electrodiagnostic examination in patients with radiculopathies. American Association of Electrodiagnostic Medicine. *Muscle Nerve* **21** (12), 1612–1631.

24. Kimura, J. (1993). Nerve conduction studies and electromyography. In *Peripheral neuropathy*, 3rd edn (ed. P.J. Dyck and P.K. Thomas), pp. 598–644. W.B. Saunders, Philadelphia.

25. Kimura, J. (1989). Myopathies. In *Electrodiagnosis in diseases of nerve and muscle*, 2nd edn (ed. J. Kimura), pp. 535–557. F.A. Davis, Philadelphia.

26. Kimura, J. (1989). Myaesthenia gravis and other disorders of neuromuscular transmission. In *Electrodiagnosis in diseases of nerve and muscle*, 2nd edn (ed. J. Kimura), pp. 535–557. F.A. Davis, Philadelphia.

4.8 Soft tissue injuries and sport

Cathy Speed

Introduction

Since the health benefits of regular physical activity are well established, it is thus considered to be a physician's responsibility to promote it as part of a patient's health and well-being. This strategy has its challenges, as our society has become more sedentary, having exchanged man's role as a hunter–gatherer for a lifestyle that centres around the laptop, mobile phone, and TV remote control. Children are also less physically conditioned and, within the population as a whole, exercise is often seen as a chore rather than a pleasure.

Although lack of physical activity is still a major public health problem, a sector of society has become 'fitness conscious', and for this group the local gym has been described as the 'cathedral of the modern age'.[1] Organized sport has also come to play a central role in our society, its culture, and in our national identity. This increasing role of sport in Western society and the emphasis that health-care strategies now place on physical activity for health-related benefit highlight the need for the medical profession to possess the expertise needed in dealing with the hazards of physical activity, most commonly musculoskeletal injury.

Sports and exercise medicine

Sports and exercise medicine is a rapidly expanding, multilayered discipline and musculoskeletal medicine is at the core of this due to the frequency and consequences of sport-related musculoskeletal injury. Although the American College of Sports Medicine was not established until 1954, the speciality is not new. Systematic teachings of exercise therapy are found in the Chinese book of Gung Fu (*c.* 1000 BC) and the father of sports medicine was Galen, a Greek doctor who studied in Egypt and then returned to Greece where he was appointed physician to the gladiators in AD 157. This was an ideal place to practise medicine, as there were many injuries, providing plenty of opportunity for Galen to develop his interest in anatomy and his skills as a surgeon. Subsequently, Quintes of Sumer wrote on sport-related injury when he described the treatment of ankle sprain and boxing wounds in the fourth century AD.

Although Pheidippedes inspired Olympic ideals with his run from Marathon to Athens in 490 BC, the importance of the presence of doctors at a marathon was not recognized until the first modern Olympic games in 1896. The first Paralympic games were held in 1948 and the medical care of the disabled athlete has itself become a subspeciality. Olympic competition has been dedicated to the glory of Zeus and the mind, body, and spirit of man—sound principles upon which a sports physician may base his or her practice.

The nature of sports injuries

The specific demands involved in the performance of different sporting activities provide a wonderful insight into the extremes to which the body can be taken in order to achieve a pre-set goal. The musculoskeletal system is a highly integrated system of levers that work as a kinetic chain to overcome inertia. Many sports involve actions that demand a fine balance between the segments of the kinetic chain and an optimal equilibrium between joint mobility and stability. Loss of these unique relationships anywhere along the kinetic chain can result in injury.

Some musculoskeletal injuries are specific to sport, whilst others are also seen in a non-sporting environment, but may differ with respect to their nature of presentation, mechanisms, and management. The spectrum of injuries is wide and, although there are inherent difficulties with injury surveillance, it is clear that injuries are on the increase, with those individuals seeking medical help presenting to casualty, primary care, or to a specialist.

Sports vary in the type and incidence of injuries that are commonly encountered and the reported relative incidences of injury in specific sports vary between studies (Table 1). Most injuries are minor (65 per cent are contusions and/or sprains) and the overall incidence of injury is low (0.8 per cent), with only the minority seeking medical help.[2] The lower limb is most commonly affected. A higher incidence of overuse injuries is seen in older people.

Orava and Puranen performed a large study of top-level athletes aged 20–29 years and recreational athletes aged 30–49 years attending a sports medicine clinic in Finland with overuse injuries.[7] The lower limb was the most common site affected—the knee in 28 per cent, ankle/foot/heel in 21 per cent, and lower leg/shin in 17 per cent. The most common structures involved were: muscles and fascia (27 per cent), tendon insertion (22 per cent); joint surfaces (17 per cent); tendon and tendon sheath (15 per cent); and bursae, bones, and nerves (21 per cent).

Causes of soft tissue injuries in sport

Soft tissue lesions account for more than 80 per cent of injuries and may be related to trauma or, more commonly, to overuse. Intrinsic and extrinsic factors commonly play a role in the development of the injury (Table 2). The physical and psychological characteristics that naturally select an individual to excel at a particular sport are those that may also predispose them to injury. Training and technical errors are the most common precipitants. The principles of training are that

Table 1 Relative incidences of sports injuries (data taken from references 3–6)

Sport	% of participants injured	Incidence/10,000 man hours of play
Soccer	55.8	6.6
English premiership soccer[8]	1.3 injuries per player	
Rugby	53	3.1
Athletics	2.1	1.6
Basketball	1.9	3.5
Ice hockey	12.1	8.6
Mens field hockey	12.1	10.3
Womens field hockey		12.5
Handball	8.1	7.2
Alpine skiing	3.9	3.0
Fitness Training	2.3	1.7
Volleyball	1.2	3.0
Wrestling	0.8	6.3
Gymnastics—apparatus	0.7	1.5
Judo	0.8	2.3
Cricket		2.6
Swimming		0.3
Cycling		1.6
Boxing		1.4
Rowing		1.4
Fencing		4.2
Badminton		1.5
Fitness training	2.3	

Table 2 Factors associated with injury (adapted from reference 8)

Intrinsic	Extrinsic
Age, sex, body habitus	Training
Hypo/hypermobility	Type
Muscle weakness, imbalance	Volume
Adverse biomechanics and malalignments	Intensity
Foot hyper/hypopronation	Frequency
Pes planus/cavus	Technique
Hindfoot varus/valgus	Surface
Tibia vara	Equipment
Genu valgum/varum	Environment
Patella alta/baja	Cold/heat
Femoral neck anteversion	Humidity
Leg length discrepancy	Wind
Medical complaints (e.g. diabetes)	Altitude
	Supervision

many individuals possess such 'adverse' characteristics without any detrimental consequences.

Sports people are often highly motivated individuals, and dedicated to their sport, to the extent that they frequently ignore initial symptoms and continue to train through pain.

The medical approach

The provision of optimal health care to an athlete entails a multidisciplinary approach, with involvement of patient, doctor(s), therapist(s), coach, and others (e.g. parents). Knowledge of the sport or activity is necessary, as many injuries are sports-specific and the mechanism of injury can be unique to that sport. Evaluation commences with a very careful history that will help to identify the structures involved, recent training loads, and the mechanism(s) of the injury. All must be determined for a successful outcome to treatment. A careful training history should be taken and extrinsic causative factors considered. The nature, duration, and progression of symptoms; relieving and exacerbating factors; and previous injuries are all recorded.

The expectations of the patient (e.g. the required level of performance) should also be ascertained. Those of the elite athlete will differ from those of the occasional recreational athlete. Nevertheless, the primary aim of treatment in all cases is to return the patient to full function in their sporting activities.

A thorough examination of the patient includes assessment of the injury and evaluation for intrinsic factors that may be involved. Assessment during the activity that reproduces their symptoms may also be necessary. Equipment such as shoes, rackets or bicycles should also be examined (Figs 2 and 3).

Management of the acute injury usually follows the conventional PRICES regime. The primary aim of initial treatment of both acute and chronic injuries is to control pain so that rehabilitation can take place. Early mobilization is generally encouraged in most injuries. Athletes are well-motivated individuals and this can at times lead to difficulties with compliance, with attempts to progress too quickly. Treatment of the injury proceeds, while ensuring that aerobic capacity is maintained enhances patient compliance and makes a return to sport easier. For example, the patient with a leg injury may be encouraged to use a water vest to allow training in a pool without stressing the injury (Fig. 4).

it is specific to the sport and based upon physiological adaptations as a response to overload, but those adaptations are lost if the training stops. The phenomenon of 'too much, too soon, too often' is all too commonly encountered and musculoskeletal injury is one of the presenting features of the overtraining syndrome. A fine line often exists between excessive overload and that necessary for an optimal adaptive physiological response. Hence, subtle changes in the training pattern, such as the introduction of a new interval session to a runner's weekly programme, may be enough to tip the balance towards injury.

Technical factors may be glaringly obvious, but can be subtle, requiring the use of video analysis and the input of a coach to determine source of the problem (Fig. 1). Equipment errors are also commonly encountered, footwear being the most frequently identified culprit. A pair of running shoes loses half of its cushioning after 300–500 miles, which may be only a few months of a runner's training calendar. Injuries are also seen at the seasonal change when there is a transition from winter training to the track, and both equipment factors (change to spikes) and the change of surface may play contributing roles.

A long list of intrinsic factors have been proposed to predispose to injury, some of which can be corrected. It is important to note that

The running stride. Stance phase 1–3; swing phase 4-11.

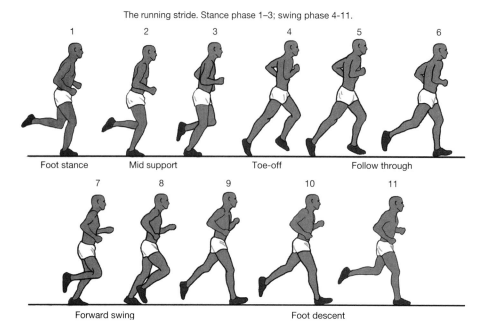

Fig. 1 Subtle abnormalities in running style can lead to injury.

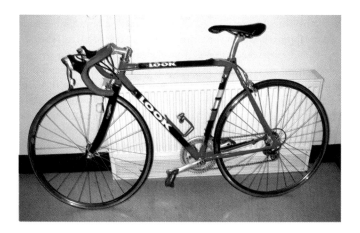

Fig. 2 The setup of a bicycle, including frame size, pedal position, seat height, and angle, and the position of the handlebars and seat are all important in the prevention of injury.

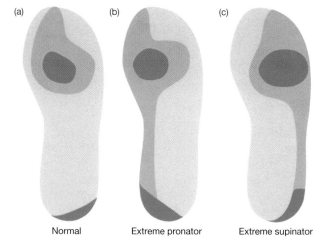

Fig. 3 Equipment should also be examined in the evaluation of a sports injury. For example wear of the sole of a running shoe is indicative of running style.

As is the case with all patients, reassurance, education, explanation, and support are required, but athletes often require additional support, as the psychological sequelae of injury can be significant. Demonstrating an understanding of the psychological impact of injury strengthens the patient–physician relationship. Rehabilitation progresses to sport-specific tasks in a non-competitive environment and then a graded return to sport that is carefully monitored by the medical team and coach. A premature return to competition and/or failure to address the causative factors involved are frequent causes of persisting symptoms.

The physician must also always consider the possibility of a more serious underlying disorder presenting as a sports injury. For example a seronegative arthropathy may present as an Achilles tendinopathy or back pain, arthritis or a septic joint may present with a history of apparent trauma on a sports field, and a chronic 'muscle tear' may disguise a musculoskeletal tumour.

Modification of equipment and associated advice may be necessary. Patients should generally wear a shoe suited to their sport (Table 3). Runners may find it helpful to rotate the shoes they wear during the 'running week'. The use of shock-absorbing insoles may help to improve a cushioning that the shoe provides and orthotics are sometimes of benefit. Patients should be warned to take these with them when they purchase a new pair of shoes and be advised that the most expensive pair of sports shoes is not necessarily the pair that is best suited to their needs!

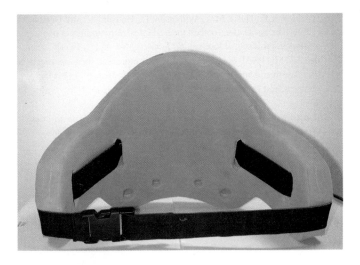

Fig. 4 An aqua vest for water based rehabilitation.

Table 3 Anatomical aspects of the running shoe and errors related to injury

Feature	Common errors
Style	Failure to wear the shoe for the sport
General fit	Too wide, too narrow, Too long, too short
Heel tabs	Too high—Achilles irritation
Toe Box	Too tight, Unsupportive, Worn through
Lacing	None, Too tight / too loose
Sole	Worn through, no grip
Stability	Lacking (can be important in e.g. hyperpronators)
Cushioning	Too little

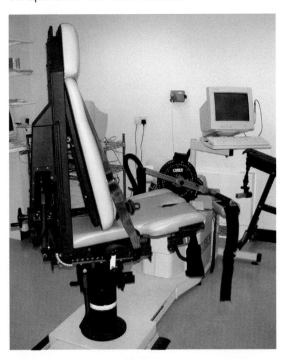

Fig. 5 An isokinetic strength testing system for musculoskeletal evaluation and rehabilitation in particular in relation to sport.

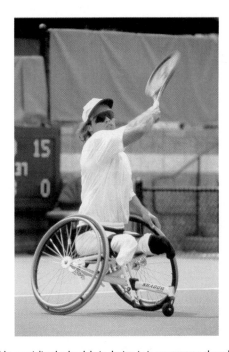

Fig. 6 Highly specialized wheelchair design is important to the wheelchair athlete, but, since the arms become weight-bearing limbs, there is an increased chance of injury.

The disabled athlete

Disabled athletes may have impaired physical, sensory, or cognitive capacity and the majority fit into one or both of the former two groups. Medical management of these athletes is highly specialized, although soft tissue injuries, which represent the most common form of musculoskeletal injury in this group, are often similar in causation to those seen in able-bodied athletes and can be treated using similar approaches. The epidemiology of such injuries is not well defined, but the sports with greatest risk of injury overall to wheelchair athletes include track events, basketball, and road racing. Mechanical inefficiency of locomotion in a wheelchair results in increased demands upon upper limb musculature and greater risk of injury (Fig. 6). Equipment issues, specifically aspects of wheelchair design, may help to reduce this risk (Fig. 7).

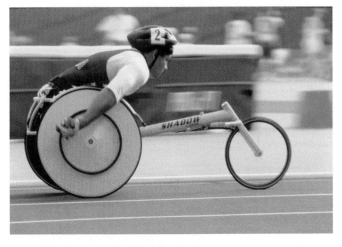

Fig. 7 Disabled individuals participate in sport from grass roots level to international standard. Injuries can arise due to the nature of the chosen sports and the demands imposed upon the musculoskeletal system.

References

1. **Sherry, E.** (1998). Sport and medicine: the human race—a philosophical aside. In *Oxford handbook of sports medicine* (ed. E. Sherry and S.F. Wilson). Oxford University Press, Oxford.

2. **Lawoski, E.R.,** *et al.* (1995). Medical coverage for multi-event sports competition. *Mayo Clin. Proc.* **70**, 549–555.

3. **Weightman, D. and Browne, R.C.** (1974). Injuries in eleven selected sports. *Br. J. Sports Med.* **8**, 183.

4. **Davies, J.E. and Gibson, T.** (1978). Injuries in rugby union football. *Br. Med. J.* **2**, 1759–1761.

5. **Hawkins, R.D., Hulse, M.A., Wilkinson, C., Hodson, A., and Gibson, M.** (2001). The association football medical research programme: an audit of injuries in professional football. *Br. J. Sports Med.* **35** (1), 43–47.

6. **de Loes, M.** (1995). Epidemiology of sports injuries in the Swiss organization 'Youth and Sports', 1987–1989. *Int. J. Sports Med.* **16**, 134–135.

7. **Orava, S. and Puranen, J.** (1979). Athletes' leg pains. *Br. J. Sports Med.* **13**, 92–97.

8. **Renstrom, P.** (1994). An introduction to chronic overuse injuries. In *Oxford textbook of sports* medicine (ed. M. Harries, C. Williams, W.D. Stanish, and L. Michaeli), pp. 531–545.

4.9 Soft tissue disorders in the occupational setting

Philip Helliwell

Introduction

Soft tissue musculoskeletal disorders are common in the community. For example, the point and annual prevalences of low back pain are roughly 20 and 40 per cent, respectively,[1] and the annual prevalences of pain in the shoulder, elbow, and wrist are 40, 12, and 23 per cent, respectively.[2] Even symptoms of such specific conditions as carpal tunnel syndrome are highly prevalent.[3] Since we spend a large part of our waking life at work, it is not surprising that many people attribute these symptoms to their work. The estimated prevalence of self-reported work-related illness, of which back and upper limb pain are by far the most common categories, in Great Britain in 1995 was 2 million people.[4] In the United States, work-related musculoskeletal disorders account for one-third of all occupational injuries reported by employers annually.[5] Low back pain is associated with large personal, social, and economic costs in all industrialized countries.

Many injuries received in the workplace are the result of discrete traumatic events. In these cases there is no doubt as to the cause and effect of the injury but apportioning blame may still be problematical. This chapter is more concerned with symptoms and signs that are not associated with discrete events and are thus more appropriately referred to as cumulative trauma disorders. In these cases there may be doubt about both the existence of the disorder and the causal link to work, as well as the question of blame. Both physical, personal and work-related factors may be important—the former in the occurrence of symptoms, the latter in the presentation. There is continuing argument about the relative importance of these factors.

Showing a causal link between work and soft tissue disorders is fraught with difficulties and studies in this area need to pay particular attention to case definition, exposure estimates, and appropriate controls. Hadler has argued that there is no evidence of a causal link between work and many of the soft tissue disorders.[6] Hadler comments that regional pain is frequent and spontaneous and that work attribution may be misplaced. He also argues that normal, adaptive, physiological responses to physical loads enable us to avoid the proposed pathologies.[7] However, whilst accepting the assertion that good-quality, incontrovertible evidence is lacking, a growing body of cross-sectional and longitudinal studies supports the role of physical, workplace, and psychological factors in the presentation of, and the disability associated with, work-related musculoskeletal disorders.[8]

In this chapter after a brief review of case definitions and putative pathomechanics, a model for understanding and studying these conditions will be presented. The chapter will then consider these disorders in the context of the workplace together with the issues of prevention and compensation.

Case definitions

The US Occupational Safety and Health Administration defines a work-related musculoskeletal disorder as:

- an injury or disorder of the muscles, tendons, ligaments, joints, cartilage, and spinal discs

- diagnosed by a health care professional

- resulting in a positive physical finding or be serious enough to require medical treatment, days off work, or light duties

- directly related to the employee's job

- specifically connected to core activities of the job.

Such explicit criteria do not exist in the United Kingdom outside the courts (see 'Compensation and legal matters'). For the most part rigorous diagnostic and classification criteria are not available.[9] This is largely because of a lack of an accepted 'gold standard' and, in part, because of a lack of agreement about the pathophysiology.[10] Part of the disagreement may result from the use of differing disease models: medical versus biopsychosocial.[11] There is a need for consensus and a uniform approach. A group from the United Kingdom recently published surveillance criteria for a number of upper limb pain syndromes.[12] These criteria were established by consensus by a mixed group of professionals, including rheumatologists, occupational physicians, epidemiologists, ergonomists, and orthopaedic surgeons, actively working in this field. Further work is now needed to examine the reproducibility and utility of these criteria. For example, a recent study of the physical signs contributing to the criteria found interobserver kappa scores of 0.66–1.00.[13] More recently, further consensus criteria have been published detailing criteria for both symptoms alone and symptoms and signs—for each disorder a clinical algorithm is given, although a complete algorithm for 'upper limb pain' would have been more useful for surveillance work.[14] An additional feature of the latter report is the inclusion of evidence for associated work factors.

Some examples of the soft tissue disorders associated with occupation, together with the proposed pathology and associated physical factors, are given in Table 1. This list is not complete but serves mainly for illustration. An interesting but far from exhaustive compilation was attempted by Huskisson and Hart who included such conditions as: 'centenarian hand syndrome' (painful hand associated with much hand shaking), 'miner's elbow' (olecranon bursitis), 'weaver's bottom' (ischial bursitis), and 'policeman's heel' (plantar fasciitis). It is sometimes possible to link these descriptions by pathology, for example, miners and housemaids once had infrapatellar bursitis in common and today tomato trainers and cymbal players may share the affliction of shoulder tendinitis.

Table 1 Some examples of the soft tissue disorders associated with occupation—putative physical, psychosocial, and work factors are listed

Anatomical region (examples)	Pathologies	Physical factors	Psychosocial and work factors
■ Neck (cervicobrachial pain)	■ Osteoarthritis	■ Force	■ Stress
■ Shoulder (cymbal player's shoulder)		■ Repetition	
	■ Tendinitis	■ Posture	■ Low job satisfaction
■ Elbow (tennis elbow)	■ Compression neuropathy	■ Vibration	■ Monotonous work
■ Wrist (carpal tunnel syndrome)	■ Enthesopathy	■ External compression	■ High perceived work rate
	■ Bursitis	■ Friction	■ Time pressures
■ Hand (vibration white finger)	■ Muscle fatigue		■ Low control over the job
■ Low back (regional pain syndrome)	■ Regional pain syndrome		■ Lack of social support by colleagues
■ Hip (farmer's hip)			
■ Knee (housemaid's knee)			
■ Ankle (jogger's ankle)			
■ Foot (policeman's heel)			

Despite issues of case definition the most common disorders seen in the community and in the occupational setting are the so-called non-specific disorders, where no specific pathology can be identified. In the upper limb work attribution is often included in the name with terms such as repetitive strain injury, occupational overuse syndrome, and work-related upper limb disorder. In other anatomical regions the terms are purely descriptive, for example, low back pain and cervicobrachial pain. These conditions are currently described and defined phenomenologically. They may represent one end of a 'pain spectrum'—from regional pain disorders to widespread pain—sometimes defined as fibromyalgia.[15] Efforts have been made to determine the pathophysiology of regional and generalized pain disorders[16, 17] but, in the absence of a unifying concept, these disorders can be managed appropriately by reference to a 'black box' model (see below).

A model for pathogenesis

The features of the biopsychosocial approach have been synthesized in a conceptual model by Armstrong and others for upper limb disorders.[18] This model encompasses external and internal elements and allows for such influences as phenotype and personality on the presentation of pain. Their model is illustrated diagrammatically in Fig. 1. Like any model it not only serves to explain the known facts and observations but also to generate hypotheses suitable for experimental testing. The model provides a useful framework with which to relate certain observations and within which the rationale of treatment can be placed.

Relationship between external factors: dose and response

Physical factors

Most of our knowledge about exposure in occupational arm pain comes from cross-sectional studies. Such studies typically try to answer the questions: 'are certain jobs/actions associated with a higher

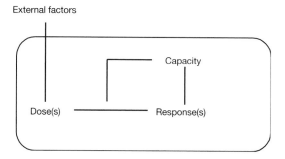

Fig. 1 The proposed model of Armstrong et al.[18] See text for further details.

prevalence of the disorder?' and 'what are the characteristics of these jobs?' However, certain problems accompany cross-sectional studies: it is impossible to imply causality, migration of 'susceptible' workers and persistence of 'robust' workers may confuse the prevalences, and true reference population figures are often unavailable. Nevertheless, a meta-analysis of such studies concluded that soft tissue disorders of the neck and upper limb were strongly associated with jobs involving prolonged abnormal postures, abnormally high forces, or frequent repetition, with pooled odds ratios for pain in the hand and wrist of 9.1 and for carpal tunnel syndrome of 15.5.[14, 19] For low back pain the important physical factors are frequent heavy lifting, prolonged bending and twisting, and whole body vibration.[8, 14, 20]

What are the possible mechanisms by which these physical factors may cause a painful condition? Heavy lifting may damage tissue by imposing loads that exceed the physical capacity of the tissue. A popular concept is that of a 'slipped disc'—an acute intervertebral disc rupture and prolapse in response to a single external event. Whereas there is no doubt that acute severe pain can result from a particular event such as lifting, the evidence that this is frequently due to a disc prolapse is lacking. Indeed, there is better evidence that such an incident is due to a muscle or ligament injury. For example, the pain is often located in these soft tissues, is associated with pain on movement, is not accompanied by any neurological deficit, and gradually improves in 4–6 weeks.

More important, in terms of prolonged exposures, is the phenomenon of creep where a collagenous structure lengthens in response to prolonged loading. The loads responsible for such changes may be much less than the mechanical strength of the tissue or they may be cyclical (e.g. with whole body vibration). The effect is to impart a temporary length change in the tissue (e.g. a ligament) that may in turn alter the biomechanics of the structure to which the tissue contributes. The time course of recovery from these changes may be several hours and an imposed load during this recovery period may subject the other tissues to higher forces than they would otherwise have experienced. Experiments in anaesthetized animals have shown recovery times of 3 h for muscle and 7 h for ligaments after 50 min of cyclic loading.[21]

Whole body vibration may exert other pathophysiological effects according to the acceleration magnitude and the frequency.[22] Single high-amplitude shocks are capable of causing acute damage (e.g. fracture of calcaneum upon jumping from a high wall) but continuous low-amplitude vibration may accelerate creep within tissues, cause muscle fatigue, and may affect blood supply in a mechanism similar to that seen with vibration white finger. Whole body vibration may be of particular importance where the frequency of the vibration coincides with that of the natural frequency of the body (3–8 Hz)—frequencies typically found in vehicle travel. The mechanism by which vibration induces pathological changes remains unclear in the hand–arm vibration syndrome, but studies suggest a clear dose/response relationship.[23]

Finally, pain may be caused by muscle ischaemia. Prolonged submaximal loading can cause a rise in intramuscular pressure and ischaemia. This may occur with sustained muscle contractions of as little as 5 per cent of maximum.[24] In support of this some experimental work has shown a modest rise in muscle enzymes as a result of a submaximal lifting task.[25] In addition, a single study of chronic work-related arm pain found morphological changes in muscles but this study has not been replicated.[26] Our own observations would suggest that abnormal muscle fatiguability may contribute to the pain in work-related non-specific arm pain.[17]

Workplace organization and the individual response

Other external factors may play an important part in the presentation of these disorders, particularly workplace factors such as low job satisfaction and stress. Job satisfaction may be assessed in a number of ways, recording such elements as job control, peer support, staff support, autonomy, work pressure, and physical comfort. Measuring such factors in workers across six government departments in Australia, Hopkins found an association between these factors and arm pain.[27] In a comprehensive review, Bongers *et al.* commented on some of the methodological problems of published studies that have found positive evidence of a relationship between some workplace factors and musculoskeletal symptoms.[28] These workplace factors included monotonous work, high perceived work rate, time pressures, low control over the job, and lack of social support by colleagues. Hypothetically, there are a number of ways in which stress may result in musculoskeletal pain, including increased muscle tension[29] and behavioural changes resulting in misinterpretation of somatic signals.[30] Of course, stress may be a feature outside the workplace and this may influence both the decision to present with pain as well as the resulting disability, including time off work.

Fear may also contribute to symptom presentation. An example of this would be co-workers on a production line discussing injury as a result of the job. The mechanism may be cognitive but the effect may be peripheral. Flor and Turk found specific psychophysical responses in chronic low back pain (increased baseline electromyograph (EMG) activity and increased EMG response to stressors).[31] In relation to upper arm pain, site-specific muscle hyperreactivity in response to non-performance-related stimuli has been found in musicians complaining of performance-related pain.[32]

Coding systems, reporting, and record keeping: surveillance

An internationally agreed taxonomy of soft tissue musculoskeletal syndromes has been published by the World Health Organization (WHO) within the International Classification of Diseases (ICD) and Related Health Problems,[33] but clear definitions of these conditions are not included and some syndromes may be classified under a number of different rubrics. The ICD system and that of the British alternative clinical coding system proposed by Read are seldom used in the occupational setting. The United Kingdom's government household survey codes only by anatomical region.[4] Accepted surveillance criteria may help coding in future studies.[12, 14]

There are, in addition, a number of compensatable disorders prescribed by regulatory authorities (Table 2). These comprise: **A4**, cramp of the hand or forearm due to repetitive movements; **A5–7**, beat conditions, mostly bursitis in miners; **A8**, tenosynovitis; **A11**, vibration white finger; and the recently added **A12**, carpal tunnel syndrome in users of vibrating hand tools. It should be noted that a recent survey revealed considerable professional disagreement about the definitions of these disorders.[34]

Many industries have their own in-house surveillance systems that comprise an essential part of their musculoskeletal disorder prevention and treatment strategy. Such surveillance may vary from passive mechanisms such as routine health checks to unprompted voluntary reporting mechanisms and to regular use of screening questionnaires.[35] In smaller work forces such mechanisms are unlikely to be in place. However, it may be possible to target certain industries that are more likely to produce work-related injuries. These 'high risk' industries involve the physical conditions noted previously and include manufacturing, professional drivers, nurses, visual display unit (VDU) users, foresters and miners.[36]

The United Kingdom's government relies on independent statistics to monitor the burden of work related musculoskeletal disorders.

Table 2 Disorders for which people may apply for Industrial Injuries Compensation Benefit

Category	Disorder
A4	Cramp of the hand or forearm due to repetitive movements
A5–7	Beat conditions, mostly bursitis in miners
A8	Tenosynovitis
A11	Vibration white finger
A12	Carpal tunnel syndrome in users of vibrating hand tools

Essentially there are four methods of surveillance—the first three are likely to be underestimates and the fourth an overestimate. Firstly, there is a legal requirement to report one of the occupational diseases noted in the appropriate schedule. This requirement, introduced in 1996, is known as the Reporting of Injuries, Diseases and Dangerous Occurrences Regulations (RIDDOR). Employers must report cases of occupational disease promptly if they receive a doctor's written diagnosis and the employee's current job involves the corresponding work activity (also defined). The diagnosis, usually made by the employee's personal general practitioner, has to be communicated to the workplace for the system to work properly. Clearly, underreporting will occur with this system particularly since the number of diagnostic categories is limited to the 'prescribable' disorders. In 1998–1999 642 cases were reported in the United Kingdom by this method.[36]

The second source of surveillance criteria is the Industrial Injuries Scheme. This scheme provides statistics on the number of 'prescribed' disorders (noted above). A steady fall in both 'beat' conditions and 'cramp' and 'tenosynovitis' has been recorded since 1992–1993. Approximately 600 cases were recorded under these rubrics in 1997–1998.[36]

Thirdly, occupational physicians working in occupational medicine and a group of interested rheumatologists have for some time been involved in a voluntary reporting scheme for occupational musculoskeletal disorders. The occupational physicians report via the Occupational Physicians Reporting Activity (OPRA) while the rheumatologists report via the Musculoskeletal Occupational Surveillance Scheme (MOSS). Clearly, these figures are incomplete as only a minority of workers have access to an occupational physician and to be reported via MOSS people need to be referred into secondary care. In addition, in the case of MOSS, the figures rely solely on the postconsultation judgement of the rheumatologist. From OPRA the total number of cases reported in 1998 was 5110 of which vibration-associated vascular hand symptoms, other upper limb disorders, and low back pain were the most common categories. The most common occupations were in production engineering (e.g. metal dressing operatives, vehicle assemblers, glass-makers, and press stamping operatives). The industry with the highest estimated incidence was 'insurance and pension funding', presumably associated with keyboard and VDU use. In the same period MOSS rheumatologists reported 2448 cases, with upper limb, neck, low back, and shoulder disorders most frequently reported.

The fourth source of reference is the Labour Force Survey—a large, government-sponsored, household survey in the United Kingdom. Respondents to the main survey are asked about their perception of the occurrence of work-related illness and sent a further questionnaire. In the 1995 survey it was found that musculoskeletal disorders were the most common category of perceived work-related illness with an estimate of 2 million people affected.[4] Many of these conditions were chronic and occurred most commonly in nurses, construction workers, manufacturing processing, and miners. Manual handling, posture, prolonged sitting or driving, and repetitive work were most frequently blamed for the illness.

Primary prevention and screening

Employers, understandably, wish to reduce the incidence of work-related illness and time off work as a result of such disorders. Evidence

from industries that have changed their approach to work-related regional pain[35, 37, 38] suggests that the elements of successful primary prevention include careful attention to work organization, reporting, and ergonomic assessments. The essential features of such a programme are:

- active symptom surveillance
- early assessment and treatment
- education of workers and line managers
- non-adversarial approach
- worker involvement
- ergonomic assessment of jobs—minimization of repetition, force, and prolonged abnormal postures.

Furthermore, legislative recommendations and requirements directly aimed at reducing physical loads are likely to help implementation of these changes.[39, 40] A number of studies have demonstrated the effectiveness of reducing physical exposure by ergonomic and workplace changes.[41] However, the relative importance of the physical, workplace, and psychosocial factors remains controversial.[42]

What individual factors may predispose an individual to develop a work-related musculoskeletal disorder? The model for pathogenesis illustrated in Table 1 incorporates 'internal' factors that can modify the individual response to 'external' events. The simplest way of interpreting this is to consider interindividual differences in anatomical phenotype such as height, weight, and arm reach. Surprisingly, the evidence implicating such factors is weak.[8] For people employed in physical jobs there is evidence that pre-existing capacity (i.e. strength) can influence the development of musculoskeletal pain.[43] As a corollary to this it might be possible therefore to change the worker rather than the job (using a suitable strength-training regime) or to better match the worker based on physical testing. There is some evidence to suggest that pre-employment strength testing with appropriate job matching can reduce the incidence of back pain.[44]

At a more basic level it is tempting to consider differences in collagen structure that might influence an individual's response to, for example, physical loads, manifest as different rates of creep deformation. Bone phenotype may also be important. Some early work suggested that people may differ in their susceptibility to carpal tunnel syndrome—presumably as a result of differing carpal tunnel bony dimensions.[45] Finally, recent evidence suggests that degenerative disc disease may be influenced significantly by heredity.[46]

Individual differences in personality and beliefs are also important both in the development of occupational musculoskeletal disorders[47] and the transition from an acute disorder into a chronic one.[48]

Despite these observations, the evidence for the effectiveness of pre-employment screening is weak.[49] Isometric strength testing was unable to predict low back pain episodes in established workers but the tests were not job-specific.[50] However, it is important to consider other issues here. Firstly, there is the question of discrimination. At present this factor may be influential in preventing the introduction of screening. Secondly, there are issues of disabled employees—in the United Kingdom the Disability Discrimination Act now extends to firms with 15 or more employees and it behoves the employer to make reasonable adjustments to the workplace to accommodate the disabled employee.[51]

Industrial guidelines and requirements

In the United Kingdom a number of government publications are relevant to occupational musculoskeletal disorders. Perhaps of most importance is the Health and Safety at Work Act, 1974. This legislation behoves employers to safeguard the health, safety, and welfare of their employees. Amongst other areas covered by this legislation are the provision and maintenance of safety checks, safe handling of goods, appropriate training, and adequate welfare facilities. The requirements extend to the display of appropriate notices in the workplace and to the appointment of persons competent in health and safety matters. The regulations also cover areas such as workstation design and seating. Much of the relevant material is also available as easy to read booklets published by the Health and Safety Executive (HSE).[52] The HSE has the power to enter a workplace for the purpose of inspection and this is one way in which concerned physicians can exert an effect on an employer they believe not to be complying with the regulations. Nevertheless, it is likely that many small firms are either frankly ignoring the regulations or find them too restrictive to make them economically viable.

Worldwide there is a will to prevent work-related musculoskeletal disorders. In 2000, the US Occupational Safety and Health Administration introduced an ergonomics programme standard for target industries.[5] The programme required employers to check jobs using an ergonomics screening tool with appropriate action triggers. Regrettably, this was rescinded by the Bush administration in 2001, although there remains a commitment to the health and safety of the workforce. In Europe, a campaign called 'Turn your back on work-related musculoskeletal disorders' was chosen as the theme of European Week for Safety and Health at Work for 2000.[53] Of interest, the Manual Handling Regulations introduced in the United Kingdom in 1992 were largely a result of European directives. The situation in Australia, the 'mother' of these disorders following the epidemic in the 1980s, is improving partly as a result of ergonomic changes and partly as a result of changes in compensation procedures but Australia still experiences significant numbers of upper limb injuries/disorders.[54]

Compensation and legal matters

As noted in the previous section, employers have an obligation to keep the workplace safe. Should they not do so and should the worker develop a work-related musculoskeletal disorder then the worker may have the basis for a claim against the employer. However, it is clear that the majority of cases never reach this stage and there is no doubt that in the United Kingdom the process of litigation is prolonged, uncertain, and costly. The situation with certain of the 'prescribed' disorders (noted in the previous section) is different and is a form of 'no-fault' compensation. People who think they have one of these disorders (Table 2) can apply for the Industrial Injuries Benefit. The process requires a government doctor to make the clinical diagnosis and then to make an estimate of the disability—if this exceeds 14 per cent, the person is eligible to claim benefit. A person in receipt of such a benefit is still eligible to work, even in the employment that caused the disorder. If the disability assessment is less than 14 per cent, no benefit is payable, but being in receipt of such an official label may help the person who seeks further compensation in the courts.

A person seeking compensation must first retain a solicitor. A solicitor with an interest in this area will be aware of the legal requirements such as the Health and Safety at Work Act and with the clinical issues such as diagnostic criteria. Medical reports will be necessary and both sides will be anxious to obtain medical evidence that supports their case, although the recent introduction of a single medical expert will obviously change this practice.

When a case comes to court the onus is on the claimant to establish the diagnosis and to prove that this was caused beyond doubt by the workplace. Problems at this stage may occur because of uncertainty concerning the diagnosis of disorders such as low back pain and non-specific upper limb pain.[55] However, a recent judgement has upheld this diagnosis, particularly as a good temporal relationship with an accurately quantified change in work practice was demonstrated.[56] There are two further important elements in the success of a case—proof of negligence in the workplace environment and an appropriate breach of health and safety regulations. Cases may not come to court or ultimately fail for any of the reasons given above, particularly with regard to the diagnosis and the temporal relationship. The court procedure is costly and the projected damages may not be large enough to cover the costs. There is often a considerable delay, partly to allow a more accurate prognosis. For this reason many cases may settle out of court for lesser amounts.

Management—occupational health at the workplace and beyond

The possible pathways of care through which a worker with pain may progress are shown in Fig. 2. In industry the range of occupational health provision varies enormously. Small firms with only a few workers may only have someone who has first aid training. Other, larger firms may have an occupational health department with an occupational health nurse and sometimes a visiting occupational health physician—often a local general practitioner with an interest in occupational medicine. The larger industries will have a staff of physicians, nurses, and ergonomists. However, most of the medical care of occupation-related musculoskeletal disease in the United Kingdom is undertaken by general practitioners who may not have any special interest or training in work-related musculoskeletal disorders. It is for this reason that recent guidelines and algorithms in work-related musculoskeletal disorders have been designed.[57]

For any physician treating these disorders the limitations of focusing treatment purely on the physical aspects of the disorder are apparent from the proposed disease model. Treating the pain while ignoring

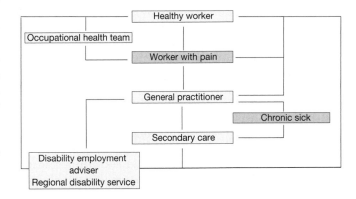

Fig. 2 The pathways of care for a worker with pain.

the associated fear, distress, anxiety, and workplace factors may only temporarily resolve the problem. However, it is in the workplace that this concept must be embraced since professionals working outside generally do not have site access, either because workers are fearful of losing their jobs or because management is worried about professional and legislative interference with the manufacturing process.

Can physicians working in primary and secondary care gain access to and influence the workplace situation? Some firms are willing to allow the physician a site visit but this may do no more than allow the physician to obtain a better understanding of the person's work. If the physician is convinced that the workplace is unsafe or, at least, contravening the regulations of the Health and Safety at Work Act then the physician can contact the local office of the HSE who have the powers to enter and inspect the suspect workplace. If the firm is found to be transgressing, the HSE can impose a fine and insist on reasonable adjustments to the workplace.

In addition, it is possible in the United Kingdom to obtain professional help in these situations by referring the patient (or the patient can refer themselves) to the Disability Employment Adviser (DEA) via the local Job Centre. The DEA works as part of the Employment Service, District Service Team (formerly known as Placement Assessment and Counselling Service (PACT)). This team includes the services of an occupational psychologist. Each region of the Employment Service also has a Regional Disability Service (RDS), which vary across the country in terms of organization and staff. The DEAs will use the RDS when they need more specialist advice, for example, from occupational health physiotherapists, occupational therapists, ergonomists, and technical consultants. A demonstration and assessment area may be available at the RDS. From 2001 an initiative called 'Jobcentre Plus' means some of the functions of the Benefits Agency and the Employment Service will be available together in one building.

The DEA and RDS can carry out work site visits to assess the workplace in relation to the 'disabled' worker. Further, the 'Access to Work' scheme allows the worker to be supported in the workplace. The support may be in the form of fares, aids to employment, and other workplace modifications. Where possible, the costs of these modifications are shared with the employer. The DEA can also negotiate alternative duties and alternative employment—this may be important in getting the disabled worker back to work. Sometimes local training providers may be used where unemployed clients need to update or learn new skills to aid their job search. In addition a 'Job Introduction Scheme' can facilitate the return to work by subsidizing the worker's salary for the first 6 weeks back at work.

The many aspects of the workplace environment may be hard to separate out in a situation where management will often embrace concepts of 'injury prevention' so wholeheartedly that many, probably complementary changes are instituted at once. Changes made at the Ford company plant in the United Kingdom illustrate this point: A package involving education, early reporting, and ergonomic improvements, all in the context of regular meetings of managers, engineers, and doctors, resulted in a striking reduction in reporting of upper limb disorders.[37] However, it is worth noting that, unless such widespread changes are made, ergonomic improvements may not be sufficient in themselves. Pransky et al. illustrate this in reference to two contrasting divisions within the same company, where the division encompassing such elements as effective worker involvement and flexibility had less of a problem with musculoskeletal disorders.[38]

If regional pain symptoms occur and on-site treatment is available, the emphasis should be on early physical treatment and change of work practice. These should be combined with specific ergonomic checks and an assessment of other work elements such as work rate and autonomy. The difficulty arises if the workplace itself has no mechanisms to manage these disorders, as is often the case in a small business. A further problem may reside in the nature of the work—as production demand increases there may be less flexibility in the available job tasks. Additionally, some of the newer occupations such as telephone call centres may have virtually no control over the way in which the job is executed.

Natural history and prognosis—what factors influence chronicity and return to work

There are few studies on the natural history of work-related musculoskeletal disorders. It is possible that the majority of acute cases resolve completely with nothing more than a brief rest and simple analgesics. Some workers may continue working with pain and regard pain as a necessary part of the work. Some will seek medical help or help from the workplace. Psychosocial factors may influence the decision to report pain.

However, some data are available. There is some evidence that active surveillance enables earlier detection of cases and that intervention at this stage has a better outcome.[35, 37] Other figures suggest a poor long-term outcome in terms of continuing symptoms: only 5 of a sample of 181 respondents were symptom-free 3 years after reporting an occupational overuse injury.[58] In terms of employment one-third had changed their jobs. A better outcome was associated with greater social support at home and at work. Possibly, workplace attitudes to regional pain will play a part in influencing the long-term outcome—there are no direct facts but an adversarial attitude to these conditions may have prolonged the outbreak of 'RSI' (repetitive strain injury) seen in Australia in the 1980s.

The persistence of low back pain in primary care can be predicted by psychosocial factors, in particular external locus of control and adverse coping strategies.[48] In an industrial setting Bigos et al. found the only significant predictors of the incidence of back pain over a 2-year period were previous back pain history and perceived adverse working environment.[47] In a further smaller study Symmonds et al. demonstrated that time taken as sick leave can be reduced by the simple introduction of a booklet intended to change beliefs about back pain.[59]

Following a period of sick leave, what factors influence return to work? Undoubtedly the greatest influence is the length of time on sick leave—the longer a worker is off sick with back pain the less likely they will return to work.[60] In a way this factor is self-evident but it illustrates the way in which several factors combine to prevent the long-term sick returning to their job. Recently, a qualitative study of sick-listed workers in Canada found that there were four key features in the process of return to work: someone to understand the problem; learning one's physical limits; the provision of lighter duties; and support from the employer.[61] Further prospective studies in this area are required.

For the minority of cases who progress to chronic pain and significant disability there is evidence that multidisciplinary work rehabilitation programmes improve symptoms, function, and return to work. Such programmes are based on a multifactorial model as outlined previously.

Cognitive behavioural therapy is often a major element of these programmes. The components of cognitive behavioural therapy have been described by Spence[62] and include goal-setting, problem-solving, cognitive restructuring, relaxation, imagery, time management, and assertiveness. The goals include increasing physical activity and social contacts. Cognitive restructuring includes re-education, challenging myths, understanding psychological responses, and reducing maladaptive thoughts.

The evidence for efficacy is strongest in the field of back pain with impressive return-to-work figures.[63] In upper limb disorders, Feuerstein et al.[64] compared 34 subjects with chronic work-related upper extremity disorders referred to their rehabilitation programme with 15 subjects referred but ineligible (for various reasons, including refusal, being referred to other programmes, and high levels of illness behaviour). At 18 months 60 per cent of those completing the original 6-week programme had returned to work, compared to 40 per cent of the 'control' group. Multidisciplinary rehabilitation programmes are expensive and are targeted at a minority of cases, yet it is these few cases that consume so much health care in other ways, so the cost–benefit of such programmes may be favourable.

Research agenda

1. Further data are required on the reliability, sensitivity, and specificity of diagnostic criteria.

2. Longitudinal studies of stable workforces using both inception psychosocial and exposure data in an attempt to identify the most important predictors of the onset and persistence of the disorder.

3. A comparison of the components of rehabilitation—cognitive behaviour therapy, physical training, ergonomic changes, and physical treatments.

4. Given the rapid changes in the nature and pattern of work, in particular higher demands and less flexibility, what can be done to balance output with safety?

5. It could be argued that we now have all the knowledge we need to understand and prevent these disorders. What are the most effective ways of putting this knowledge into practice?

6. Can the diagnosis and management of these conditions across the whole workforce be improved by the introduction of a regionally based occupational health team?

Summary

Regional soft tissue pain is relatively common in the community. However, both specific and non-specific disorders probably occur more often in work involving frequent repetition, high forces, and prolonged abnormal postures. Nevertheless, other factors are involved in the presentation and the continuation of the pain. Notable among these factors are the workplace environment—the attitude to workers and their welfare, the physical conditions, and the design of the job. Most cases seek medical advice from their general practitioner who may not have specific training in this area. The local DST may be able to provide this specialist help. If possible, management should be multidisciplinary, taking a wider look at the problem, although there is some evidence that primary prevention, with active surveillance using sensitive criteria and early intervention, is effective. Rehabilitation programmes for chronic cases need further evaluation.

Acknowledgement

I wish to thank Professor Howard Bird and Ms Gill Gilworth for helpful discussion in the preparation of this chapter.

References

1. Hillman, M., Wright, H., Rajaratnam, G., Tennant, A., and Chamberlain, M.A. (1996). Prevalence of low back pain in the community: implications for service provision in Bradford, UK. J. Epidemiol. Community Health 50: 347–352.

2. Mackay, C., Burton, K., Boocock, M., Tillotson, M., and Dickinson, C. (1998). Musculoskeletal disorders in supermarket cashiers. HSE books, London.

3. Cherniak, M.G. (1996). Epidemiology of occupational disorders of the upper extremity. Occup. Med. 11, 513–530.

4. Jones, J.R., Hodgson, J.T., Clegg, T.A., and Elliott, R.C. (1998). Self-reported work-related illness in 1995. HSE books, London.

5. Occupational Safety and Health Administration (1999). Proposed ergonomics standard. Available from URL: http://www.osha-slc.gov/ergonomics-standard/archive.html (accessed June 2003).

6. Hadler, N.M. (1997). Repetitive upper extremity motions in the workplace are not hazardous. J. Hand Surg. 22A, 19–29.

7. Hadler, N.M. (1993). Occupational musculoskeletal disorders. Raven Press Ltd, New York.

8. Bernard, B.P. (ed.) (1997). Musculoskeletal disorders and workplace factors: a critical review of epidemiological evidences for work-related musculoskeletal disorders of the neck, upper extremity and low back, NIOSH publications 97–141. US Department of Health and Human Services, Washington, DC. Available from: URL: http://www.cdc.gov/ niosh/ergoscil.html (accessed June 2003).

9. Helliwell, P.S. (1996). A review of diagnostic criteria for work-related upper limb disorders. Available from: URL: http://www.hse.gov.uk/hthdir/noframes/musculo/helliwel.htm (accessed June 2003).

10. Helliwell, P.S. (1996). Diagnostic criteria for work related upper limb disorders. Br. J. Rheumatol. 35, 1195–1196.

11. Helliwell, P.S. (1992). Occupational rheumatology: are we using the wrong model? Br. J. Rheumatol. 31, 73–74.

12. Harrington, J.M., Carter, J.T., Birrell, L., and Gompertz, D. (1998). Surveillance case definitions for work related upper limb pain syndromes. Occup. Environ. Med. 55, 264–271.

13. Palmer, K., Walker-Bone, K., Linaker, C., Reading, I., Kellingray, S., Coggon, D., and Cooper, C. (2000). The Southampton examination schedule for the diagnosis of musculoskeletal disorders of the upper limb. Ann. Rheum. Dis. 59, 5–11.

14. Sluiter, J.K., Rest, K.M., and Frings-Dresen, H.W. (2001). Criteria document for evaluating the work-relatedness of upper extremity musculoskeletal disorders. Scand. J. Work Environ. Health 27, Suppl. 1.

15. Wigley, R.D. (1999). Can fibromyalgia be separated from regional pain syndrome of the arm? J. Rheumatol. 26, 515–516.

16. Greening, J. and Lynn, B. (1998). Vibration sense in the upper limb in patients with repetitive strain injury and a group of at risk office workers. Int. Arch. Occup. Environ. Health 71, 29–34.

17. Helliwell, P.S. (1999). The elbow, forearm, wrist and hand. Baillière's Clin. Rheumatol. 13, 311–328.

18. Armstrong, T.J., Buckle, P.A., Fine, L.J., Hagberg, M., Kilbom, A., Kuorinka, I.A.A., Silverstein, B.A., Sjogaard, G., and Viikari-Juntura, E.R.A. (1993). A conceptual model for work related neck and upper limb musculoskeletal disorders. Scand. J. Work Environ. Health 19, 73–84.

19. Stock, S.R. (1991). Workplace ergonomic factors and the development of musculoskeletal disorders of the neck and upper limbs: a meta-analysis. Am. J. Ind. Med. 19, 87–107.

20. Burton, A.K. and Waddell, G. (2000). *Occupational health guidelines for the management of low back pain. Evidence review.* Institute of Occupational Medicine, London.

21. Solmonov, M., Zhou, B.H., Baratta, R.V., Lu, Y., Zhu, M., and Harris, M. (2000). Biexponential recovery model of lumbar viscoelastic laxity and reflexive muscular activity after prolonged cyclic loading. *Clin. Biomech.* **15**, 167–175.

22. Smeathers, J.E. and Helliwell, P.S. (1993). Effect of vibration. In *Mechanics of human joints: physiology, pathophysiology and treatment* (ed. V. Wright and A.E. Radin) pp. 313–339. Marcel Dekker, New York.

23. Bovenzi, M., Franzinelli, A., Mancini, R., Cannava, M.G., Maiorano, M., and Ceccarelli, F. (1995). Dose–response relation for vascular disorders induced by vibration in the fingers of forestry workers. *Occup. Environ. Med.* **52**, 722–730.

24. McGill, S.M., Hughson, R.L., and Parks, K. (2000). Lumbar erector spinae oxygenation during prolonged contractions: implications for prolonged work. *Ergonomics* **43**, 486–493.

25. Hagberg, M., Michaelson, G., and Ortelius, A. (1982). Serum creatine kinase as an indicator of local muscular strain in experimental and occupational work. *Int. Arch. Occup. Environ. Health* **50**, 377–386.

26. Dennett, X. and Fry, H.J.H. (1988). Over-use syndrome: a muscle biopsy study. *Lancet* **1**, 905–908.

27. Hopkins, A. (1990). Stress, the quality of work and repetition strain injury in Australia. *Work Stress.* **4**, 129–138.

28. Bongers, P.M., De Winter, C.R., Kompier, M.A.J., and Hildebrandt, V.H. (1993). Psychosocial factors at work and musculoskeletal disease. *Scand. J. Work Environ. Health* **19**, 297–312.

29. Maeda, K., Hunting, W., and Grandjean, E. (1980). Localised fatigue in accounting machine operators. *J. Occup. Med.* **22**, 810–816.

30. Smith, M.J. and Carayon, P. (1996). Work organisation, stress and cumulative trauma disorders. In *Beyond biomechanics: psychosocial aspects of musculoskeletal disorders in office work* (ed. S.D. Moon and S.L. Sauter), Chapter 2. pp. 23–42. Taylor and Francis, London.

31. Flor, H. and Turk, D.C. (1989). Psychophysiology of chronic pain: do chronic pain patients exhibit symptom specific psychphysiological responses? *Psychol. Bull.* **105**, 215–259.

32. Moulton, B. and Spence, S.H. (1992). Site-specific muscle hyper-reactivity in musicians with occupational upper limb pain. *Behav. Res. Ther.* **30**, 375–386.

33. World Health Organization (WHO) (1992). *International statistical classification of diseases and related health problems*—ICD-10. WHO, Geneva.

34. Diwaker, H.N. and Stothard, J. (1995). What do doctors mean by tenosynovitis and repetitive strain injury? *Occup. Med.* **45**, 97–104.

35. Le Poidevin, J. (1997). Reducing upper limb disorders in the packing line. *IRS Employment Rev.* **256**, 13–15.

36. Health and Safety Executive (1999). *Health and Safety Statistics 1998/9.* HMSO, London.

37. Chatterjee, D.S. (1992). Workplace upper limb disorders: a prospective study with intervention. *Occup. Med.* **42**, 129–136.

38. Pransky, G., Snyder, T.B., and Himmelstein, J. (1996). The organisational response: influence on cumulative trauma disorders in the workplace. In *Beyond biomechanics: psychosocial aspects of musculoskeletal disorders in office work* (ed. S.D. Moon and S.L. Sauter), Chapter 15, pp. 251–262. Taylor and Francis, London.

39. Health and Safety Executive (1990). *Work related upper limb disorders—a guide to prevention.* HMSO, London.

40. Health and Safety Executive (1999). *Getting to grips with manual handling.* HSE Books, London.

41. Grant, C. and Habes, D. (1995). Summary of studies on the effectiveness of ergonomic interventions. *Appl. Occup. Environ. Hyg.* **10**, 523–530.

42. Burton, A.K. (1997). Back injury and work loss—biomechanical and psychosocial influences. *Spine* **22**, 2575–2580.

43. Chaffin, D.B. (1974). Human strength capability and low back pain. *J. Occup. Med.* **16**, 248–254.

44. Chaffin, D.B., Herrin, G.D., and Keyserling, W.M. (1978). Preemployment strength testing: an updated position. *J. Occup. Med.* **20**, 403–408.

45. Murray-Leslie, C.F. and Wright, V. (1976). Carpal tunnel syndrome, humeral epicondylitis, and the cervical spine: a study of clinical and dimensional relations. *Br. Med. J.* **1**, 1439–1442.

46. Sambrook, P.N., MacGregor, A.J., and Spector, T.D. (1999). Genetic influences on cervical and lumbar disc degeneration. *Arthritis Rheum.* **42**, 366–372.

47. Bigos, S.J., Battie, M.C., Spengler, D.M., Fisher, L.D., Fordyce, W.E., Hansson, T.H., Nachemson, A.L., and Wortley, M.D. (1991). A prospective study of work perceptions and psychosocial factors affecting the report of back injury. *Spine* **16**, 1–6.

48. Burton, A.K., Tillotson, K.M., Main, C.J., and Hollis, S. (1995). Psychosocial predictors of outcome in acute and subchronic low back trouble. *Spine* **20**, 722–728.

49. Kuorinka, I. and Forcier, L. (1995). *Work related musculoskeletal disorders (WMSD's): a reference book for prevention.* Taylor and Francis, London.

50. Baltic, M.C., Bigos, S.J., Fisher, L.D., Hansson, T.H., Jones, M.E., and Wortley, M.D. (1989). Isometric lifting strength as a predictor of industrial back pain reports. *Spine* **14**, 851–856.

51. Howard, G. (1997). Legal aspects of musculoskeletal problems in the workplace. *Br. J. Rheumatol.* **36**, 894–903.

52. Health and Safety Executive. Publications available on website. URL: http://www.hse.gov.uk/pubns/hazards.htm (accessed June 2003).

53. European Agency for Safety and Health at Work (2000). *Work related musculoskeletal disorders in Europe*, Factsheet, issue 3. Available from: URL: http://agency.osha.eu.int/publications/factsheets/ (accessed June 2003).

54. Phillips, S. (1999). The continuing problem of occupational overuse syndrome in the office. *Ergonomics Australia* **13**(2), Supplement. Available from: URL: http://www.uq.edu.au/eaol/index9799.html (accessed June 2003).

55. Brahams, D. (1993). Repetitive strain injury. *Lancet* **342**, 1168.

56. Alexander and Others v Midland Bank Plc. Court of Appeal (Civil Division). 22/7/99. Available from Smith Bernal Reporting Ltd., 180, Fleet Street, London EC4A 2HG. URL: http://www.smithbernal.com (accessed June 2003)

57. Graves, R. (2000). *A diagnostic tool for upper limb disorders.* HSE Contract Research Publications, HMSO, London.

58. Kemmelert. K., Orelius-Dallner, M., Kilbom, A., and Gamberale, F. (1993). A three year follow up of 195 reported occupational over-exertion injuries. *Scand. J. Rehabil. Med.* **25**, 16–24.

59. Symmonds, T.L., Burton, A.K., Tillotson, K.M., and Main, C.J. (1995). Absence resulting from low back trouble can be reduced by psychosocial intervention at the work place. *Spine* **20**, 2738–2745.

60. Hunter, S.J., Shana, S., Flint, D., and Tracy, D.M. (1998). Predicting return to work—a long term follow-up study of railroad workers after low back injuries. *Spine* **23**, 2319–2328.

61. Dionne, C.E., Bourbonnais, R., Fremont, P., Rossignol, M., and Stock, S.R. (2000). Predicting 'return to work in good health' among back pain patients in primary care settings: the RAMS prognosis study. Proceedings of Fourth International Forum for Primary Care Research on Low Back Pain, Eilat, Israel, March 2000.

62. Spence, S.H. (1989). Cognitive behaviour therapy in the management of chronic occuptional pain of the upper extremity. *Behav. Res. Ther.* **27**, 435–446.

63. Mayer, T.G., Gatchel, R.J., Kishino, N., Keeley, J., Capra, P., Mayer, H., Barnett, J., and Mooney, V. (1985). Objective assessment of spine function following industrial injury—a prospective study with comparison group and one-year follow-up. *Spine* **10**, 482–493.

64. Feuerstein, M., Callan-Harris, S., Hickey, P., Dyer, D., Armbruster, W., and Carosella, A.-M. (1993). Multidisciplinary rehabilitation of chronic work related upper extremity disorders. *J. Occup. Med.* **35**, 396–403.

4.10 Soft tissue disorders in chronic disability

Stephen Kirker

Introduction

Following the success of disease-modifying drugs and joint replacement surgery for rheumatic diseases, most severe chronic disability is now due to neurological disorders, in particular, stroke and multiple sclerosis. Spinal cord and traumatic brain injuries, cerebral palsy, muscular dystrophies, motor neuron disease, poliomyelitis, and chronic peripheral neuropathies are less common causes. Soft tissue pain in these conditions is associated with muscle weakness, poor support of joints, altered muscle tone, and abnormal posture.

Soft tissue disorders in disability associated with specific medical complaints

Shoulder pain after hemiplegia

Incidence/prevalence

Shoulder pain is one of the most common complications of hemiplegia. It may occur in 85 per cent of cases with spasticity and 18 per cent of those with flaccidity[1] and is more common on the left side.[2] Shoulder pain on movement, subluxation, and malalignment is a strong predictor of poor recovery and longer hospital stay.[3]

Aetiology

The cause of shoulder pain after hemiplegia is not clearly established, but is likely to be multifactorial. In the flaccid limb it may result from subluxation and stretching of the capsule, although a review of hemiplegic patients with subluxation indicated that pain was related to range of movement but not degree of subluxation.[2] In the spastic limb it may result directly from spasm especially in internal rotator and adductor muscles: the humerus may also be pulled up and impinge on the rotator cuff. Thermography usually shows 1–5 °C cooling around the hemiplegic shoulder but this is not related to function or pain,[4] so this finding is insufficient to justify a diagnosis of reflex sympathetic dystrophy. Neurophysiological studies have detected abnormalities of the axillary, musculocutaneous, radial, median, and particularly the suprascapular nerve around subluxed shoulders, but it is not clear whether this represents the cause or the effect of the subluxation.[5, 6] Therapy involving large-range passive movements using an overhead pulley was associated with a higher incidence of shoulder pain than movements limited by the therapist.[7]

Management

The very wide range of approaches to treatment and prevention of shoulder pain after hemiplegia (175 different approaches are described in a recent review of current practice in reference 8) is an indication of the limited effectiveness of many and the paucity of evidence on which to base one's management. The options have recently been reviewed.[9] Avoidance of additional injury to the shoulder from carers pulling the patient up by the hemiplegic arm[10] and good support of the arm on a pillow or wide armrest at the correct height are important and, when there is subluxation, additional support may be simply provided by strapping over the shoulder.[11] In practice, the adhesive bandages tend to stretch, so they may need to be replaced more often than is comfortable. Elastic supports that grip the upper arm tightly are difficult to get on and off and can increase hand oedema, which may outweigh their limited effectiveness.

The Wilmer carrying orthosis (available from Ambroise UK Ltd, 1st Floor, Samson House, Bow St, Langport, Somerset TA10 9PR. www.ambroise-uk.com), which pushes the humeral head up from below rather than pulling it up by skin traction, avoids compression of the upper arm and also supports the forearm and hand (Fig. 1), but prevents elbow extension. Functional electrical stimulation may be useful in the short term,[12] but its effects may not persist after it is withdrawn. A small study found that repeated intraarticular steroid injections eased pain.[13] Spasticity in specific muscles around the

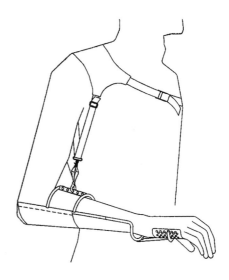

Fig. 1 Wilmer elbow orthosis.

shoulder can be treated with botulinum toxin injections or alcohol nerve blocks, but these come with the potential hazard of iatrogenic subluxation.

Spasticity

Pain associated with spasticity in upper motor neuron lesions of all types is often eased by reducing the overactivity of the relevant muscles. However, this spasticity may not be controlled with oral muscle relaxants, which may cause sedation in large doses. Injections of botulinum toxin into the painful muscles may relieve the pain within 24 hours,[14] and this benefit may last until the paralysing effect wears off after 8–16 weeks.[15] The injections may need to be repeated but, if the spastic muscles are stretched daily and, when tolerated, held in the stretched position for over 6 hours a day by a resting splint, the spasticity and pain may be controlled for longer periods with less frequent injections. This is most practical with soleus, gastrocnemius, tibialis posterior, biceps, brachialis, and the long wrist and finger flexor muscles.

Painful dystonias, such as torticollis and writers cramp, also respond well to botulinum toxin, but it has had a much less convincing effect in pain due to tension headache, fibromyalgia, and myofascial syndromes.[16]

Pain in poliomyelitis

The majority of patients have pain in their joints and muscles more than 30 years after poliomyelitis, with increasing weakness in previously affected muscles in 82 per cent and previously unaffected muscles in 58 per cent.[17] Limbs affected by polio in childhood usually don't grow to the same length as those on the other side. When this affects the lower limb, the pelvic obliquity and abnormal gait due to the muscle weakness may cause premature degenerative changes in the back and pain. Some of this may be prevented or eased by correcting leg length discrepancies with a shoe raise, but the greater symmetry when standing must be balanced against the increased difficulty of swinging through a longer leg.

Pain in the thigh or hip may develop due to overuse of proximal muscles substituting for weak distal muscles in the calf.[18] An ankle foot orthosis that prevents dorsiflexion can reduce the tendency for the knee to flex when standing and may increase confidence and reduce falls. The UTX Swing (available from Ambroise UK Ltd, 1st Floor, Samson House, Bow St, Langport, Somerset TA10 9PR. www. ambroise-uk.com) is a knee–ankle–foot orthosis that locks the knee in extension at heel strike, through the stance phase of gait, and when standing, but allows the knee to bend normally during swing phase. This maintains a more normal looking and energy-efficient gait than walking with a locked knee.

Patients are often only just managing to stand and walk by the time they seek any medical attention or bracing, and any minor alteration (due to even minor trauma, change in orthosis, footwear, or surgical intervention)[19] may make them immobile. Support of weak joints with appropriate orthoses is very useful and may prevent injury and progressive deformity and prolong independent mobility.[20] Progressive deformities, for example, genu recurvatum, may be more easily prevented if bracing is started early, but at this stage, the brace may not enhance the patient's function so there may be little motivation to wear it. If it is heavy, uncomfortable, or cosmetically unacceptable it won't be worn. New materials such as carbon fibre may be moulded to the shape of the patients limb and are much thinner and lighter than older leather and metal callipers.[21] Gait analysis to check the angle of the joints and direction of the ground reaction forces at different phases of gait will facilitate correct alignment of the orthosis, which is particularly important when trying to enhance the function of a very weak limb.

Many people with a history of polio can improve muscle strength and cardiovascular conditioning with an exercise programme.[22, 23] Muscles with stable, mild to moderate weakness can be exercised with care. They should probably not be significantly fatigued, so exercising three times per week for periods of 10–20 minutes with frequent rests is preferable to more sustained exercise. Progressive resistance exercises with gradually increasing weights may be used to maintain and possibly gain strength.

Elective functional surgery, for example, to stabilize knees,[24] is most appropriately done by surgeons with some experience and, as polio has become less common in developed countries, these are few and far between. Medical, surgical, orthotic, and physiotherapy experience tends to be concentrated in supraregional (http://www.ott.zynet.co.uk/polio/lincolnshire/directory/clinics.html#clinics_UK) and national centres (e.g. Lane-Fox Unit, St Thomas' Hospital, Lambeth Palace Road, London SE1 7EH. http://www.hospital.org.uk/ lane_fox_ respiratory_unit/welcome.html), and their advice may be helpful to clinicians elsewhere who are dealing with particular difficulties or contemplating surgery.

Heterotopic calcification

Heterotopic ossification (HO) is the formation of mature lamellar bone in soft tissues, where bone is not normally found. It occurs most commonly after acquired brain or spinal cord injuries and acetabular fractures and, to a lesser extent, after elective hip and shoulder surgery and occasionally after burns. The reported incidence after traumatic brain injuries varies from 11 to 76 per cent, and is more likely with more severe injury, increasing age, and (in spinal cord injuries at least) the presence of spasticity and pressure sores.[25]

It develops as a result of trauma induced by passive movements carried out on joints where contractures have started to develop.[26, 27] Pluripotential stem cells differentiate into osteoid-producing cells and the resultant osteoid is then calcified.

The clinical features are localized swelling, redness, and heat and the differential diagnosis includes deep venous thrombosis, pressure sore, infection, tumour, and reflex sympathetic dystrophy. It may also present as a pyrexia of unknown origin. It is associated with a hypercoaguable state, which persists despite warfarin therapy until markers of HO activity subside to normal.[28]

Alkaline phosphatase, erythrocyte sedimentation rate (ESR), and urinary prostaglandin E2 are elevated early in the condition. More specific and localizing changes are seen on ultrasound,[29] and three-phase isotope bone scanning before calcification is visible on plain X-rays approximately 31 days after injury. Ultrasonography has the advantage of avoiding radiation, being relatively specific and excluding coincidental thrombosis.

Treatment is primarily preventative. Attempts have been made to inhibit stem cell differentiation with radiation within 5 days of injury, with rather ambiguous results.[30] Indomethacin for 6 weeks[31] or ketorolac for 5 days[32] after injury have been used to inhibit osteoid generation with similarly ambiguous results, less expense, and greater morbidity.

Diphosphonates inhibit calcification of osteoid. Intravenous and then oral etidronate rapidly reduces swelling and oedema after positive isotope scans and only 3 per cent of spinal injury patients subsequently develop HO.[33]

Treatment options for established HO are limited. Surgical excision has traditionally been postponed until the new bone is fully mature and markers of disease activity have returned to normal, for example, after 18 months, because of rapid recurrence following earlier surgery. However excision 3–10 months after injury may be more successful with prophylactic radiation and indomethacin.[34, 35] Patients with cognitive or severe neurological deficits are much less likely to retain the range of movement achieved soon after surgery.

Diltiazem has been reported to assist resorption of calcinosis in connective tissue disease,[36, 37] but there have been no reports of its effectiveness in HO.

Soft tissue disorders: aids and appliances

Soft tissue disorders in individuals with chronic disability may be helped by—or arise due to—aids and appliances.

Amputation

Soft tissue complaints following amputation can be divided into those related to the underlying disease or injury that led to the amputation and the associated altered mobility and those problems related to wearing a prosthesis. This description will concentrate on lower limb amputations, but the principles also apply to upper limb amputations.

Complaints related to amputation and altered mobility

Self-propelling a wheelchair, transferring in and out of it, pulling up to stand on one leg, and hopping, or later walking, with crutches often lead to upper limb pain, as described in earlier sections. Any pre-existing joint or soft tissue complaints will be aggravated by these manoeuvres and, to a lesser extent, by pulling on the prosthesis and tightening any suspension straps. If the amputation was for a complication of diabetes, the remaining foot is likely to suffer from a similar degree of small vessel disease and neuropathy and 20–45 per cent of unilateral amputees become bilateral amputees, usually within 1 year.[38, 39] Ulceration may be delayed or prevented by regular footcare and provision of a pressure-relieving (e.g. total contact) insole and appropriate footware.[40]

Pain in the stump may be due to the same processes as may occur in an intact leg, and should be treated similarly. Such processes include inflammatory and degenerative arthritis; deep venous thrombosis; bacterial infection in soft tissues, bone, joints, and around prosthetic joints or bypass grafts; ischaemia; sciatica; and pressure sores.

Most people feel the limb is still present after an amputation (phantom sensation) but reassurance is sufficient treatment and potentially sedative drugs are not necessary. After an amputation, many patients initially, but a fewer later, have unpleasant feelings such as pins and needles, cramp, vice-like compression, contortion, burning, or their prior ischaemia. This phantom pain responds poorly to opiate and other analgesics, but better to Gabapentin, Carbamazepine,

and Amitryptaline.[41] Patients complain less about it with time and when artificial limb wearing allows a return to a more normal lifestyle. This reflects a reduction in severity or frequency and improved acceptance of the pain and of doctors' limited ability to influence it.

In the absence of complications such as falls, infections, and haematomas, an elective amputation stump is usually non-tender after 2–3 weeks. Localized tenderness after this may be due to the general disorders mentioned above, but may also be due to increased sensitivity over the cut ends of large nerves, particularly the sciaticnerve after a transfemoral amputation or the posterior tibial or lateral peroneal nerves after a transtibial amputation. All patients develop neuromas when the nerves are cut, but only a small proportion develop pain and tenderness. These may grow to 3 cm in diameter and become palpable, but are most clearly demonstrated by magnetic resonance imaging (MRI), which may also distinguish them from thrombosed veins and lymph nodes.[42] Adjustment of the prosthesis should be tried first and gabapentin may help, but surgical excision is often more effective. They may recur.

Complaints related to prosthesis

Soft tissue problems due to wearing and walking with a prosthesis may be divided into local stump problems due to direct pressure or contact with the socket, problems with the suspension belts or sleeves proximal to the stump, and distant musculoskeletal pains due to altered biomechanics of gait. Patients quickly identify problems caused by a prosthesis if it settles when they wear another one. These should be addressed by their prosthetist.

Stump–socket interface problems cause well localized discomfort aggravated by weight-bearing and relieved by taking the prosthesis off. Poor socket fit or poor suspension causing pistoning during gait leads to local friction with skin reddening, blistering, and eventual ulceration. Prolonged friction may lead to adventitious bursae developing over bony prominences, for instance, at the fibula head, end of the tibia, or tibial tubercle in transtibial stumps or lateral femoral condyle in knee disarticulation stumps.[43] If the prosthesis can be corrected, or the patient dissuaded from the particular activity that promoted the bursae's formation, these may resolve spontaneously or with an injection of steroid, but they may become chronic or infected, justifying surgical excision after treatment of the acute infection. The underlying bone may be smoothed at the same time to prevent recurrence.

In most transtibial prostheses, the majority of the patient's weight is taken through a bar that presses against the patellar tendon, and none of their weight should be taken through the end of the stump. However, if the skin at the end of a transtibial stump is completely unsupported by the socket, intradermal oedema develops. This may progress over hours or days through reddening, soft tissue swelling, blistering, and ulceration: this characteristically occurs in a circle and is called terminal congestion. It may be prevented by putting some soft foam in the end of the socket, which applies sufficient pressure to the end of the stump to counteract the hydrostatic pressure in the capillaries.

Lower limb prostheses are designed to facilitate walking, and the necessary weight-bearing shelf at the top of a transfemoral prosthesis is often uncomfortable to sit on, particularly on a hard chair. Many patients take them off for long journeys or when relaxing in the evening at home. Similarly, the elastic waist belt or more rigid metal and leather pelvic band may uncomfortably compress the abdomen or press on the lower ribs, particularly in women with osteoporotic collapse of the lumbar vertebrae. These patients are the least likely to be strong or agile enough to manage alternative methods of suspension and those who cannot walk independently may find limb-wearing more trouble than it is worth. They should discuss this with their prosthetist, who may be able to improve their comfort.

Musculoskeletal pains in the knee, hip, contralateral leg, and back may develop many years after successful walking with a prosthesis. These may be aggravated by an asymmetrical gait, leg length discrepancy, malalignment causing knee hyperextension or lateral flexion, and loss of the normal shock- and torque-absorbing properties of the foot, ankle, and knee. Many of these factors can be addressed by prosthetic adjustments or the use of sophisticated components that more completely compensate for the amputated limb, and patients should see their prosthetist before embarking on any course of treatment.

Pain associated with orthoses and switch use

The International Standards Organization defines an orthosis as an externally applied device used to modify the structural or functional characteristics of the neuromusculoskeletal system. Orthoses support existing function, whereas prostheses, such as an artificial leg, replace the missing or damaged part.

Orthoses should not be painful and, if they are uncomfortable, their fit, alignment, and design should be reviewed by an orthotist to ensure that the most appropriate materials and techniques have been used. Adequate correction and stabilization may not be achievable without correction of underlying fixed contractures, bony deformities, and spasticity. Discomfort associated with using orthoses may be reduced if the limb or trunk position can be maintained with lower corrective forces—this situation particularly arises in cerebral palsy, head injury, and incomplete spinal cord injuries, where the orthosis is working against spastic muscles. Botulinum toxin or intrathecal baclofen may weaken these overactive muscles and allow the desired posture to be maintained with less pressure.[44]

Patients with a limited repertoire of movements may develop pain from overuse or straining to reach a poorly positioned switch. Patients with quadriplegia due to spinal cord injury or cerebral palsy who use switches mounted on a headrest to control their wheelchair, computer, or environmental control unit may develop neck pain, and those with continuous movements due to generalized dystonia or athetosis may even develop cervical spondylotic myelopathy. Where possible, the underlying movement disorder should be addressed pharmacologically but the type and position of the switches should also be reviewed by the rehabilitation engineer or occupational therapist. This equipment can be controlled by movements of the tongue, chin, eyes, lips, or voice, and changing to one or more different types of switch may relieve or prevent discomfort.

Crutches, walking sticks, and compression neuropathies

Chronic use of a walking stick, crutch, or wheelchair is associated with median nerve compression at the wrist.[45] In a population of post-polio patients, 49 per cent complained of wrist pain and 22 per cent had carpal tunnel syndrome. The relative risk of getting carpal tunnel syndrome with use of both wheelchair and walking aid was five. In a group of chronic stroke patients, Tinel's sign was observed in 58 per cent of hands contralateral to a disused hemiparetic hand and in 31 per cent of hands contralateral to a functioning hemiparetic hand.[46]

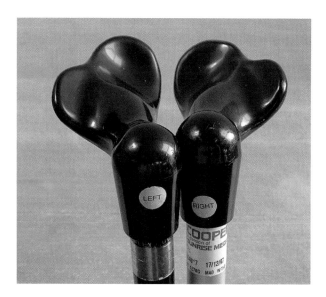

Fig. 2 Fischer handles.

More proximal compression neuropathies are well known complications of axillary crutch use. This typically involves the posterior cord of children, causing wrist drop, when it usually resolves in 3 months.[47] Suprascapular neuropathy has been attributed to improper use and inadequate instruction.[48] Elbow crutches can compress the ulnar nerve,[49] which may also be affected by prolonged bed rest with repeated elbow propping.

While walking stick use may cause neuropathies, it does not appear to cause osteoarthritis.[50] The most effective way of relieving wrist pressure and pain associated with a walking aid is to take the body weight through the forearms on gutters, which may be attached to crutches or walking frame. Walking sticks or crutches with wide contoured handles (Fig. 2) increase the weight-bearing area and so reduce local pressure on some areas of the palm.[51] This is of particular benefit to patients with wasting of the small hand muscles and frail, bony hands who may also find these easier to grip. Peak forces on upper limb joints when walking with an aid may be reduced by a shock absorber. This advanced feature is incorporated in some hiking poles with a walking stick type handle (e.g. Leki Wanderfreund Antishock: Ardblair Sports Importers Ltd, Yard Road, Blairgowrie, Scotland PH10 6NW. www.leki.com; available from camping shops). Similar spring-loaded devices can be used to replace the distal section of conventional crutches, and thicker rubber ferrules, which claim to have a similar effect, can be put on ordinary walking sticks.

Wheelchair use and pressure relief

Discomfort associated with prolonged wheelchair use may reflect the underlying medical condition, but may be aggravated by the type, size, or shape of wheelchair. The great majority of wheelchairs are designed for mobility rather than for comfortable prolonged sitting. Hence, they may be folded and dismantled to be lifted into a car, and have a fixed seat and back rest angle to keep their weight as low as possible. These features may compromise comfort, particularly for patients who are unable to move around within the chair or independently move to another chair. For people who will be spending long periods resting in their chair, but for whom independent mobility, compact size, and light weight are less important, upholstered, tilting, reclining wheelchairs with head-rests and elevating leg-rests are available (e.g. Cirrus from Gerald Simonds Healthcare, 9 March Place, Gatehouse Way, Aylesbury, Bucks HP19 3UG. Tel: 01296 436557 or Rea Comfort from Scandinavian Mobility UK Ltd, Unit C Tyson Courtyard, Weldon South Industrial estate, Corby, Northants NN18 8AZ. Tel: 01536 267660). These generally have to be purchased privately, but in the United Kingdom National Health Service (NHS) wheelchair clinics can often supply simpler reclining wheelchairs with additional padding and elevating leg rests when necessary.

Most dimensions of a wheelchair can be chosen or adjusted to optimize comfort, posture, stability, or manoeuvrability, and the final size will be a compromise among all of these factors. For instance, lengthening the wheel base to increase stability makes it harder to self-propel and get over kerbs, and shortening it makes the chair more likely to tip over backwards. Discomfort in a chair may be due to incorrect footrest heights, sagging seat or back canvas, a back rest that is too low, or a seat that is too deep. Most of these problems can be easily addressed by the NHS wheelchair clinic or private supplier. Patients who have difficulty self-propelling, due to weakness, pain in their back or arms, or shortness of breath, may benefit from an electric wheelchair. A limited range of indoor and larger indoor–outdoor electric chairs is available on free long-term loan from NHS wheelchair clinics, and a much wider choice may be purchased from the many independent suppliers.

All un-upholstered wheelchairs should be supplied with a seat cushion. The simplest is 2 inch foam in a waterproof cover, which provides some comfort rather than having any formal pressure-relieving properties. Patients at risk of pressure sores should be supplied with (often much more expensive) pressure-relieving cushions, for example, RoHo, which uses the dry flotation system (Raymar, Unit 1, Fairview Industrial Estate, Reading Road, Henley on Thames RG9 1HE. Tel: 01491 578446), or Jay 2, which uses gel in bags on a contoured base (Gerald Simonds Healthcare, 9 March Place, Gatehouse Way, Aylesbury, Bucks HP19 3UG. Tel: 01296 436557).[52] Foam cushions get flattened with use and may need to be replaced each year. Dry flotation cushions are often overinflated, which reduces their pressure-relieving effect and makes them feel unstable to sit on. The patient should sit *in* these cushions, with only a finger breadth between their skin and the seat base, rather than *on top of* them. Gel pads need to be massaged each day and occasionally leak, but are less likely to be incorrectly used.

Patients with spinal cord injuries are taught to relieve the pressure on the ischial tuberosities and sacrum when sitting to prevent pressure sores developing. Most do this by lifting themselves by pressing down with their hands on the armrests or tyres of their wheelchairs. This may lead to median nerve compression over time, and sacral pressure may also be relieved, without this risk, by leaning as far forward as possible.

Soft tissue disorders in chronic disability: carers

Soft tissue pains in carers of people with disabilities are common: health and safety regulations now forbid much manual handling and lifting of patients by professional carers, but these are rarely applied by informal and family helpers. Some pain in the back and other areas may be prevented by using optimal transfer techniques, for example, a sliding board or mechanical hoists. Car seats are available that rotate to facilitate entry, or slide out on to a special base to form a wheelchair. It is easier to lift a folded wheelchair on to a wheelchair rack mounted on the back of the car than to put it in the boot, but many people are reluctant to display this obvious sign of disability.

Manual wheelchairs can sometimes be adjusted to make them more comfortable and easier for carers to manage, by optimizing the push handle height, fitting a stepping bar, rear-mounted hand brakes, and choosing castor sizes that are appropriate for the usual surface. Attendant-controlled electric-powered wheelchairs for outdoor use, or motors that can be clipped on to manual chairs, are manufactured, but rarely available from NHS wheelchair services.

Occupational therapists in hospitals, health centres, social services, Disabled Living Centres (Disabled Living Foundation, 380–384 Harrow Rd, London W9 2HU http://www.dlf.org.uk/advice/centre/dlccmap.htm) or specialist referral centres (The Mary Marlborough Centre, Nuffield Orthopaedic Centre, Headington, Oxford. OX3 7LD Tel: 01865 227600. www.noc.org.uk/SerARef/MMC/Mary Marlborough.htm) can advise on specific adaptations and equipment.

References

1. Van Ouwenaller, C., Laplace, P.M., and Chantraine, A. (1986). Painful shoulder in hemiplegia. *Arch. Phys. Med. Rehabil.* **67** (1), 23–26.
2. Ikai, T., Tei, K., Yoshida, K., Miyano, S., and Yonemoto, K. (1998). Evaluation and treatment of shoulder subluxation in hemiplegia: relationship between subluxation and pain. *Am. J. Phys. Med. Rehabil.* **77** (7), 421–426.
3. Roy, C.W., Sands, M.R., Hill, L.D., Harrison, A., and Marshall, S. (1995). The effect of shoulder pain on outcome of acute hemiplegia. *Clin. Rehabil.* **91** (1), 21–27.
4. Thurston, N.M., Kent, B., Jewell, M.J., and Blood, H. (1986). Thermographic evaluation of the painful shoulder in the hemiplegic patient. *Phys. Ther.* **66** (9), 1376–1381.
5. Chino, N. (1981). Electrophysiological investigation on shoulder subluxation in hemiplegics. *Scand. J. Rehabil. Med.* **13** (1), 17–21.
6. Cheng, P.-T., Lee, C.-E., Liaw, M.-Y., Wong, M.-K., and Hsueh, T.-C. (1995). Risk factors of hemiplegic shoulder pain in stroke patients. *J. Musculoskeletal Pain* **3** (3), 59–73.
7. Kumar, R., Metter, E.J., Mehta, A.J., and Chew, T. (1990). Shoulder pain in hemiplegia. The role of exercise. *Am. J. Phys Med. Rehabil.* **69** (4), 204–208.
8. Pomeroy, V.M., Niven, D.S., Barrow, S., Farragher, E.B., and Tallis, R.C. (2001). Unpacking the black box for nursing and therapy practice for post-stroke shoulder pain: a precursor to evaluation. *Clin. Rehabil.* **15**, 67–83.
9. Royal College of Physicians (RCP) (2000). *National clinical guidelines for stroke.* RCP, London. www.rcplondon.ac.uk/ceeu_stroke_home.htm
10. Wanklyn, P., Foster, A., and Young, J. (1996). Hemiplegic shoulder pain (HSP): natural history and investigation of associated features. *Disabil. Rehabil.* **18** (10), 497–501.
11. Ancliffe, J. (1992). Strapping the shoulder in patients following a cerebrovascular accident (CVA): a pilot study. *Aust. J. Physiother.* **38**, 37–41.
12. Chantraine, A., Baribeault, A., Uebelhart, D., and Gremion, G. (1999). Shoulder pain and dysfunction in hemiplegia: effects of functional electrical stimulation. *Arch. Phys. Med. Rehabil.* **3**, 328–331.
13. Dekker, J.H.M., Wagenaar, R.C., Lankhorst, G.J., and de Jong, B.A. (1997). The painful hemiplegic shoulder: effects of intra-articular triamcinolone acetonide. *Am. J. Phys. Med. Rehabil.* **76**, 43–48.

14. Barwood, S., Baillieu, C., Boyd, R., Brereton, K., Low, J., Nattrass, G., and Graham, H.K. (2000). Analgesic effects of botulinum toxin A: a randomized, and placebo-controlled clinical trial. *Dev. Med. Child Neurol.* **42** (2), 116–121.

15. Hyman, N., Barnes, M., Bhakta, B., Cozens, A., Bakheit, M., Kreczy-Kleedorfer, B., Poewe, W., Wissel, J., Bain, P., Glickman, S., Sayer, A., Richardson, A., and Dott, C. (2000). Botulinum toxin (Dysport®) treatment of hip adductor spasticity in multiple sclerosis: a prospective, randomised, double blind, placebo controlled, and dose ranging study. *J. Neurol. Neurosurg. Psychiatry* **68** (6), 707–712.

16. Porta, M. (2000). A comparative trial of botulinum toxin type A and methylprednisolone for the treatment of myofascial pain syndrome and pain from chronic muscle spasm. *Pain* **85** (1–2), 101–105.

17. Wekre, L.L., Stanghelle, J.K., Lobben, B., and Øyhaugen, S. (1998). The Norwegian Polio Study 1994: a nation-wide survey of problems in long-standing poliomyelitis. *Spinal Cord.* **36** (4), 280–284.

18. Perry, J., Fontaine, J.D., and Mulroy, S. (1995). Findings in post-poliomyelitis syndrome: weakness of muscles of the calf as a source of late pain and fatigue of muscles of the thigh after poliomyelitis. *J. Bone Joint Surg.* **77A**, 1148–1153.

19. Moran, M.C. (1996). Functional loss after total knee arthroplasty for poliomyelitis. *Clin. Orthop.* (**323**), 243–246.

20. Waring, W.P., Maynard, F., Grady, W., *et al.* (1989). Influence of appropriate lower extremity orthotic management on ambulation, pain, and fatigue in a postpolio population. *Arch. Phys. Med. Rehabil.* **70**, 371–375.

21. Heim, M., Yaacobi, E., and Azaria, M. (1997). A pilot study to determine the efficiency of lightweight carbon fibre orthoses in the management of patients suffering from post-poliomyelitis syndrome. *Clin. Rehabil.* **11**, 302–305.

22. Gawne, A.C. (1995). Strategies for exercise prescription in post-polio patients. In *Post polio syndrome* (ed. L.S. Halstead and G. Grimby), pp. 141–164. Hanley and Belfus, Philadelphia.

23. Fillyaw, M.S., Badger, G.J., Goodwin, G.D., Bradley, W.G., Fries, T.J., and Shukla, A. (1991). The effects of Long-Term non fatiguing resistance exercises in subjects with post-polio syndrome. *Orthopedics* **14**, 1253–1256.

24. Men, H.X., Bian, C.H., Yang, C.D., Zhang, Z.L., Wu, C.C., and Pang, B.Y. (1991). Surgical treatment of the flail knee after poliomyelitis. *J. Bone Joint Surg. Br.* **73** (2), 195–199.

25. Lal, S., Hamilton, B.B., Heinemann, A., and Betts (1989). Risk factors for heterotopic ossification in spinal cord injury. *Arch. Phys. Med. Rehabil.* **70**, 387–390.

26. Daud, O., Sett, P., Burr, R.G., and Silver, J.R. (1993). The relationship of heterotopic ossification to passive movements in paraplegic patients. *Disabil. Rehabil.* (**3**), 114–118.

27. Michelsson, J.E. and Rauschning, W. (1983). Pathogenesis of experimental heterotopic bone formation following temporary forcible exercising of immobilized limbs. *Clin. Orthop.* **176**, 265–272.

28. Perkash, A., Sullivan, G., Toth, L., Bradleigh, L.H., Linder, S.H., and Perkash, I. (1993). Persistent hypercoagulation associated with heterotopic ossification in patients with spinal cord injury long after injury has occurred. *Paraplegia* **31** (10), 653–659.

29. Thomas, E.A., Cassar-Pullicino, V.N., and McCall, I.W. (1991). The role of ultrasound in the early diagnosis and management of heterotopic bone formation. *Clin. Radiol.* **43** (3), 190–196.

30. Moore, K.D., Goss, K., and Anglen, J.O. (1998). Indomethacin versus radiation therapy for prophylaxis against heterotopic ossification in acetabular fractures: a randomised, and prospective study. *J. Bone Joint Surg. Br.* **80** (2), 259–263.

31. Matta, J.M. and Siebenrock, K.A. (1997). Does indomethacin reduce heterotopic bone formation after operations for acetabular fractures? A prospective randomised study. *J. Bone Joint Surg. Br.* **79** (6), 959–963.

32. Pritchett, J.W. (1995). Ketorolac prophylaxis against heterotopic ossification after hip replacement. *Clin. Orthop.* **314**, 162–165.

33. Banovac, K. and Gonzalez, F. (1997). Evaluation and management of heterotopic ossification in patients with spinal cord injury. *Spinal Cord* **35** (3), 158–162.

34. Freebourn, T.M., Barber, D.B., and Able, A.C. (1999). The treatment of immature heterotopic ossification in spinal cord injury with combination surgery, and radiation therapy and NSAID. *Spinal Cord* **37** (1), 50–53.

35. McAuliffe, J.A. and Wolfson, A.H. (1997). Early excision of heterotopic ossification about the elbow followed by radiation therapy. *J. Bone Joint Surg. Am.* **79** (5), 749–755.

36. Oliveri, M.B., Palermo, R., Mautalen, C., and Hubscher, O. (1996). Regression of calcinosis during diltiazem treatment in juvenile dermatomyositis. *J. Rheumatol.* **23** (12), 2152–2155.

37. Palmieri, G.M., Sebes, J.I., Aelion, J.A., Moinuddin, M., Ray, M.W., Wood, G.C., and Leventhal, M.R. (1995). Treatment of calcinosis with diltiazem. *Arthritis Rheum.* **38** (11), 1646–1654.

38. Little, J.M., Petritsi-Jones, J., Zylstra, P., Williams, R., and Kerr, C. (1973). A survey of amputations for degenerative vascular disease. *Med. J. Aust.* **1**, 329–334.

39. Greant, P. and van den Brande, P. (1990). Amputation in elderly and high risk vascular patients. *Ann. Vasc. Surg.* **4** (3), 288–290.

40. Patout, C.A., Birke, J.A., Horswell, R., Williams, D., and Cerise, F.P. (2000). Effectiveness of a comprehensive diabetes lower-extremity amputation prevention programme in a predominantly low-income African-American population. *Diabetes Care* **23** (9), 1339–1342.

41. Danshaw, C.B. (2000). An anesthetic approach to amputation and pain syndromes. *Phys. Med .Rehabil. Clin., N. Am.* **71** (3), 553–557.

42. Boutin, R.D., Pathria, M.N., and Resnick, D. (1988). Disorders in the stumps of amputee patients: MR imaging. *Am. J. Roentgenol.* **171** (2), 497–501.

43. Ahmed, A., Bayol, M.G., and Ha, S.B. (1994). Adventitious bursae in below knee amputees. Case reports and a review of the literature. *Am. J. Phys. Med. Rehabil.* **73** (2), 124–129.

44. Pierson, S.H., Katz, D.I., and Tarsy, D. (1996). Botulinum toxin A in the treatment of spasticity: functional implications and patient selection. *Arch. Phys. Med. Rehabil.* **77** (7), 717–721.

45. Werner, R., Waring, W., and Davidoff, G. (1989). Risk factors for median mononeuropathy of the wrist in post-poliomyelitis patients. *Arch. Phys. Med. Rehabil* **70** (6), 464–467.

46. Sato, Y., Kaji, M., Tsuru, T., and Oizumi, K. (1999). Carpal tunnel syndrome involving unaffected limbs of stroke patients. *Stroke* **30** (2), 414–418.

47. Raikin, S. and Froimson, M.L. (1997). Bilateral brachial plexus compressive neuropathy (crutch palsy). *J. Orthop. Trauma* **11** (2), 136–138.

48. Shabas, D. and Scheiber, M. (1986). Suprascapular neuropathy related to the use of crutches. *Am. J. Phys. Med.* **65** (6), 298–300.

49. Malkan, D.H. (1992). Bilateral ulnar neuropraxia: a complication of elbow crutches. *Injury* **23**, 426.

50. Wright, V. and Hopkins, R. (1993). Osteoarthritis in weight-bearing wrists? *Br. J. Rheumatol.* **32**, 243–244.

51. Sala, D.A., Leva, L.M., Kummer, F.J., and Grant, A.D. (1998). Crutch handle design: effect on palmar loads during ambulation. *Arch. Phys. Med. Rehabil.* **79** (11), 1473–1476.

52. Medical Devices Agency (1997). *Wheelchair cushions, static and dynamic*, Evaluation no. PS4. HMSO, Norwich.

4.11 Special groups

Cathy Speed

Introduction

Every patient is, of course, unique. Nevertheless, it is helpful to discuss the features of specific groups that are important in the consideration of soft tissue disorders. These include the old, the young, dancers, musicians, and individuals with inflammatory arthritides or enthesopathies.

Older people

With the ever-increasing age of our population, special consideration of soft tissue complaints in older people is warranted. Older people are physiologically, structurally, and psychosocially different from younger adults in their predisposition and response to injury. Along with a greater predisposition to general medical problems and a range of cardiovascular, respiratory, renal, metabolic, and neuropsychiatric changes, a number of musculoskeletal changes occur. Many of these are at least in part related to a decline in activity levels and therefore perhaps the greatest threat to the older person is a sedentary lifestyle.

Ageing is associated with a decline in strength, related to a decline in muscle mass, a decrease in size and number of muscle fibres (especially type II fibres, as opposed to the type I fibre atrophy of disuse), suboptimal contractility properties of muscle, slowing in nerve conduction, and alterations at the neuromuscular junction (Fig. 1).

A general reduction in the tensile load applied to tendons due to reduced muscle mass and strength does, at least in theory, have deleterious effects upon tendons and, indeed, changes in ligament and tendon are noted with ageing. There is reduced collagen turnover and increased stabilization of cross-links and therefore an increase in the stiffness of soft tissues. Collagen fibre thickness is diminished and water and glycosoaminoglycan (GAG) content declines. The result is a greater potential for injuries, including tendinosis and rupture of tendons and ligaments (Fig. 2). Bony resorption at tendon insertions also increases the susceptibility to avulsion injuries.

A number of additional factors contribute to this susceptibility to musculoskeletal injury. These include slowing in reaction time, postural malalignments, altered balance and proprioception, degenerative and inflammatory joint problems, declines in hearing and/or vision associated with an unsteady gait, and cognitive decline.

It appears that many of the changes in the soft tissue components of the musculoskeletal system are partly related to disuse, and are potentially reversible—at least to some extent—with exercise. Significant increases in muscle strength and function have been demonstrated even in the very old.

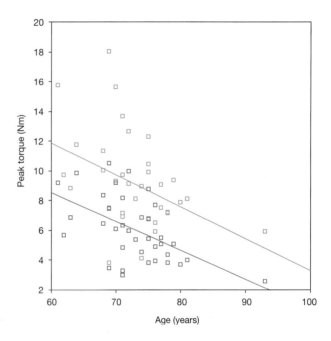

Fig. 1 Muscle strength with increasing age. Scatterplot and regression lines of concentric knee peak torque (Nm) (open squares) and eccentric knee peak torque (Nm) (filled squares) against age (years). (Cambridge, UK.)

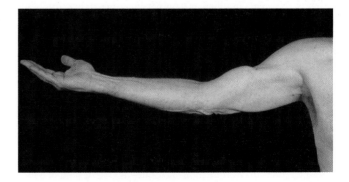

Fig. 2 Older people are more prone to degenerative soft tissue lesions. Rupture of the long head of biceps.

Once a soft tissue injury has been sustained, recovery time is prolonged. There is a dampening of all three (the inflammatory, proliferative, and remodelling) phases of the body's normal response to injury. Soft tissue complaints in older people can have devastating consequences and may be the determining factor in an individual's degree of dependence. Such complaints therefore warrant prompt and thorough attention. It is important for the physician to beware of ageism, and to give careful consideration to any injury, avoiding simply attributing musculoskeletal symptoms to 'wear and tear'.

Careful consideration must also be given in planning therapy in older people. Adequate pain relief may be vital in maintaining function but the use of medications such as nonsteroidal anti-inflammatory drugs (NSAIDs) is associated with a higher incidence of side-effects. The increased incidence in coexisting medical complaints makes interaction with other medications more likely. Tendon rupture after local corticosteroid injection may be more likely due to the presence of degenerative changes, and healing times are prolonged.

Rehabilitation programmes must take account of factors that may lead to a reduced capacity to adapt and respond to a treatment programme, including cognitive decline, altered proprioception, expectations, and motivational and psychosocial issues. Such factors can lead to difficulties with compliance, with the patient either expecting 'too much, too soon', or not persevering with the treatment plan.

Regardless of age, the most effective strategy of managing injuries is prevention. The importance of emphasizing health-related physical activity is widely recognized. Patient education on warm-up/down, stretching, posture, aerobic activities (preferably weight-bearing) involving large muscle groups and a strengthening programme should all be reinforced (Table 1).

Children and adolescents

Soft tissue musculoskeletal complaints in children are usually related to activity (Fig. 3). Different injury patterns occur at different ages, probably reflecting relative strengths of adjacent structures at the particular skeletal age.

The immature musculoskeletal system differs significantly from that of the mature individual (Fig. 4 & Table 2). Open growth plates are vulnerable to different types of injury, the nature of which varies with age, growth rate, and in the presence of a disease process. The characteristics of periosteum and articular cartilage are also different from those of adults.

Additional factors can also play significant roles. Flexibility is usually greater in the child, and there is a greater incidence of hypermobility, which is associated with a higher risk of injury and a longer healing time. On the other hand, growth spurts can lead to muscle–tendon imbalances across joints leading to local injury or to non-specific pain (previously termed 'growing pains'). Growth spurts also result in reduced flexibility, with lengthening of the musculotendinous unit lagging behind elongation of bone, with resulting stresses applied in particular to the musculotendinous attachments.

Biomechanical problems are also common in young people and can increase the stresses upon these tissues and commonly contribute to shin and/or anterior knee pain. Growth spurts and weight gain can cause alterations in co-ordination and centre of gravity, both of which make the child more susceptible to injury.

Lack of supervision or inadequate matching in contact sports, when matching is performed by age rather than height, weight, development,

Table 1 Recommendations for strength training for older people.[1]

Use major muscle groups, 8–10 exercises

Gradual warm-up and stretching of 10 minutes

Lift at moderate speeds, through full range of motion

Avoid Valsalva manoeuvre while lifting

Recommended weight is one that can be lifted 10–15 times, which is the number of repetitions per set that should be performed

Up to 2–3 sets per session

Less than 60 minutes per session

2–3 days per week, allow 2 days recovery time

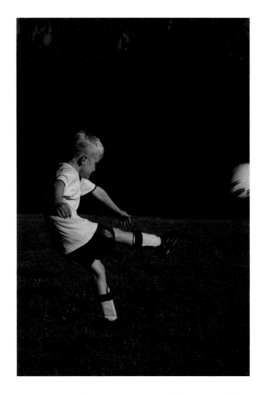

Fig. 3 Although they have a vulnerable musculoskeletal system, children should be encouraged in their enthusiasm for sport.

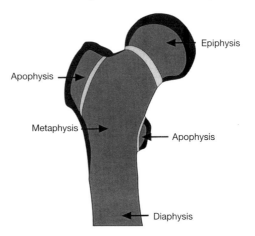

Fig. 4 Growing bone has growth plates which are weaker than the surrounding bone and are vulnerable to injury. Epiphysis: at end of long bone. Apophysis: attachment of musculotendinous unit.

and maturity, are further contributing factors to injury. Psychological factors, motivation, and parental/peer pressure may be positive or negative influences (Fig. 5).

Injuries in children and adolescents can affect the growth plate (physis), since the growing cartilaginous physis resists less force than the bone surrounding it. Specific areas of the physis can be affected, in particular, the epiphysis and the apophysis.

Injuries can be acute or related to overuse (Table 3). Where acute injuries occur in the prepubescent child, ligamentous injuries are more likely, as the bone is usually stronger than soft tissues. At the time of the adolescent growth spurt, however, physeal injuries may occur, as the ligaments may be stronger during this period. At all ages, the possibility of a fracture must be considered. Notably, x-rays can be inconclusive in this group.

Overuse injuries in relation to repetitive microtrauma are increasingly recognized, often in relation to heavy training in sports. Injuries include tendinitis, bursitis, and physeal and osteochondral injuries. Apophyseal injuries (apophysitides) include small avulsions at the

Table 2 The immature musculoskeletal system and injury

Feature	Relevance
Open growth plates	Susceptible to injury with potential serious consequences
Growth spurts	Muscle–tendon imbalances Stress on musculotendinous units as growth lags behind that of bone Reduced flexibility Altered co-ordination
Thicker, highly vascular, periosteum	Stabilizes bone (intact or fractured) Heals quickly
Long bones more porous and more plastic	May bend rather than fracture
Thicker articular cartilage	Prone (reasons unknown) to chondral/osteochondral injuries

Table 3 Examples of injuries in response to specific mechanisms in children versus adults

Force	Child	Adult
Acute injuries		
Traction: ankle inversion injury	Fibula physeal fracture	Ankle sprain
Shear/bending: medial knee/thigh injury	Medial collateral ligament	Femoral fracture
Compression: from fall on to outstretched hand.	Salter fracture of distal radius	Scaphoid fracture
Chronic injuries		
Traction: patellar ligament/tendon	Osgood–Schlatter/ Sinding–Larsen– Johansson disease	Patellar tendinopathy
Compression (and possibly shear)	Growth arrest of distal radius in young gymnasts	Osteoarthritis

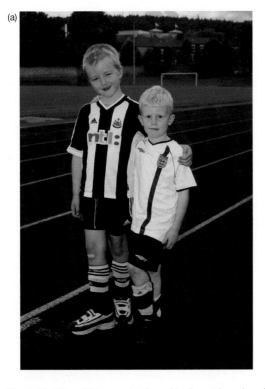
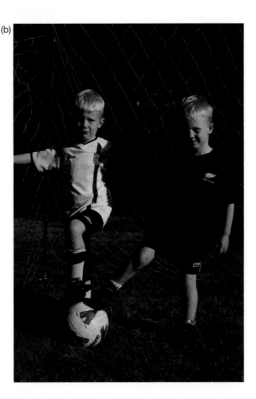

Fig. 5 Matching children on height and body weight rather than age is important in the prevention of injury. The two boys in (a) are the same age, whereas those in (b) differ by 18 months.

Table 4 Common sites of traction apophysitis (adapted from references 2)

Eponym	Site	Clinical features	Management
Thrower's elbow disease	Elbow, medial epicondyle	Medial epicondyle is last elbow growth plate to close. Associated with overuse and poor technique in throwing or racket sports	Reduce repetitive use; Modify technique
Osgood–Schlatters disease	Tibial tubercle/patellar tendon	Boys especially 13–14 years; girls 10–11 years	Reduce activity initially. Quadriceps strengthening and progressive stretching
Sindig–Larsen–Johansson disease	Infrapatellar pole (patellar tendon	Tender inferior patellar pole and radiographic evidence of small bony avulsion	If acute may require cast immobilization
Sever's disease	Os calcis (achilles insertion)	Relative increase in tightness of gastrocnemius/soleus and weakness of dorsiflexors	Supervised flexibility, training dorsiflexion strengthening; Orthotics may help
Accessory navicular syndrome	Navicular (posterior tibial tendon insertion)	Painful apophysitis, often associated with pes planus and secondary pain due to irritation of soft tissues by prominent navicular	Modify footwear; orthotics

weaker bone–cartilage junction due to repetitive traction stresses, with subsequent repetitive rehealing (Table 4). These include Osgood–Schlatter's disease at the knee, Sever's disease at the heel, and iliac crest apophysitis disease at the pelvis.

Management of soft tissue complaints in children and adolescents

Although the principles of management are the same, the treatment of soft tissue complaints in children differs from that in adults in several respects. The use of NSAIDs is generally discouraged, although they may be necessary in severe cases or where rehabilitation is being inhibited. The use of local corticosteroid injections is strongly discouraged. The use of modalities such as ultrasound should be avoided near open growth plates, but the use of electromuscular stimulation is allowed.

Rehabilitation, as with adults, forms the core of the management regime, but must be modified to suit the child. Children have a short attention span, and sessions should be kept short. It is important to ensure that they understand and comply with the rehabilitation process. Feelings of invulnerability (or, in some, vulnerability) and peer pressure may affect compliance. Hence, the programme must be supervised, concise, motivating, fun, goal-orientated (with incentives if necessary), simple, and effective.

Flexibility and strengthening should form part of the programme and it must be remembered that muscles may be relatively short compared to long bones.

Those children with hypermobility need much counselling, reassurance, and supervised rehabilitation. If strength training is considered, the child must adhere to light weights, and move through a limited range of motion.

Those children going through growth spurts also need much explanation and reassurance that, for example, the sudden changes in coordination that have occurred are temporary.

Strength training in childhood

Strength training in childhood is becoming increasingly popular as part of general conditioning and sport-specific training and can form an important part of a rehabilitation programme. It is safe, providing guidelines are followed (Tables 5 and 6).

There is no evidence that strength training during childhood places the individual at greater risk of musculoskeletal injury than participation in other sports and activities, nor that pre-pubertal children are at any greater risk of strength-training-related injury than are older children or adults. There is also no evidence of subclinical injury. Provided that stretching exercises are included, there are no detrimental effects upon flexibility.

Dancers

Dance is both an art form and a sport and dancers are both artists and athletes. Recognition of this apparent dichotomy has led to improvements in the management and prevention of injuries in dancers. Many of the issues that are important in the medical management of dancers are those that are important to other athletes, but there are additional important features with which the treating medical team should be familiar.

Dance, of course, can take many forms, including classical ballet, contemporary dance, and jazz dance, which tends to be fast paced, ballistic, and dynamic in nature. Classical ballet is the foundation of much professional dance training and follows a 400-year tradition that brings inherent reluctance for change in the demand for inclusion of many movements and regimes that are extremely demanding on even the most suited physique. Hence, more injuries are seen in classical ballet than in other forms of dance. Dance training begins at an early age, when the immature skeleton is particularly vulnerable to injury. Selection of physique is rigorous: a slim, small physique; generally good flexibility with a large range of motion at the hip joint; a long and flexible spine; high-arched feet and long Achilles tendons. A slight degree of knee hyperextension is considered to be aesthetically desirable. Those with extreme generalized hypermobility are discouraged from pursuing a career in dance.

Much of ballet training is performed at the barre, a wooden wall-mounted bar, 3.5 feet from the floor, held on to by the dancer to maintain balance. The dancer commences the class here, with flexibility exercises that increase in speed and complexity. Exercise in the five

Table 5 Guidelines for strength training in childhood[3]

A strength training programme should:

Be supervised

Part of an overall conditioning programme

Involve balanced, progressive resistance exercises

Include an appropriate warm-up and cool down

Involve, if appropriate, sport-specific exercises appropriate to the level of physical and psychological maturity of the individual

Pay close attention to proper technique: avoid the Valsalva manoeuvre, hyperventilation, and back hyperextension

Emphasize dynamic concentric contractions as opposed to eccentric overload exercises

Emphasize high repetitions at low resistance

Each exercise should be taken through the full range of motion for maximum muscle development and maintenance of flexibility

Competition weight-lifting, power-lifting, and body-building should be avoided

Maximal lifts should not be performed until skeletal maturity is reached

---

Table 6 Strength training in childhood: a sample programme[3]

1–3 sets of 6–10 exercises per session
2–3 sessions per week with at least 1 rest day between
20–60 minutes per session

Progressive resistance

- Start at no resistance/weight until proper technique achieved
- Then initiate resistance at 6-repetition level
- Advance to 15 repetitions
- Weight gradually increased in 1–3 pound increments until child can just do 6 repetitions
- Advance again to 15 repetitions before increasing weights

---

basic positions are performed to strengthen the foot muscles, the turn-out muscles, and the torso (Fig. 6). Symmetrical, centred movements, essential for proper execution of more difficult jumps, balance movements, and turns, are emphasized.

The turn-out position ideally requires external hip rotation of 180° and it is important to ensure that there is no inadvertent flexion or abduction at the hip. Stretching of the internal rotators helps. Errors in turn-out are common sources of injury. Such errors include attempts to increase the turn-out through increasing the lumbar lordosis and 'rolling in', involving forced eversion and pronation of the foot (Fig. 7). The results are a spectrum of injuries, including flexor hallucis longus tendinitis, anterior and medial knee pain, and spinal pain.

Once a dancer has the strength and technique to perform consistently away from the barre and is adequately developed (usually aged 11–12 years), dancing *en pointe* (on toes) is commenced (Fig. 8).

Most soft tissue dance injuries are related to overuse and are due to errors in technique and training. For example, the constant repetition of a particular piece of choreography, with which the dancer is usually unfamiliar, can lead to fatigue and then injury. Examples of common dance-related injuries include chronic tendinopathies (Achilles, flexor hallucis longus (FHL), sartorius), snapping hip, jumper's knee, trochanteric bursitis, piriformis syndrome, metatarsalgia, and Morton's neuroma.[4] Anterior knee pain is common and is usually related to vastus medialis obliquus insufficiency, external rotation of the lower leg to compensate for inadequate external rotation of the hips, and to sliding across floor in jazz and modern dance. Bony injuries can also occur and must be considered in the differential diagnosis of any injury. These include stress fractures and ankle impingement.

The aim of treatment is to return the dancer to full performance. Management of dance injuries involves attention to the injury itself and correction of the underlying cause(s). The physician and therapists must understand the nature of the dance programme and movements, the psychological impact of injury, and the external pressures (financial, teachers, and peers) that may affect compliance with rehabilitation. Other medical problems need to be investigated, including malnutrition, low body mass, and menstrual irregularities, which may add to the risk of injury and delay healing. The emphasis

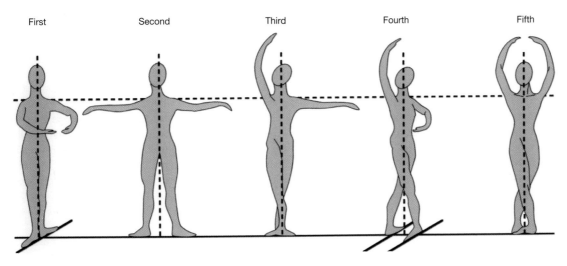

Fig. 6 The basic five positions of classical dance. The plie then involves external rotation of the lower extremities, extreme plantar flexion of the toes and simple knee flexion, with the weight on the metatarsal heads.

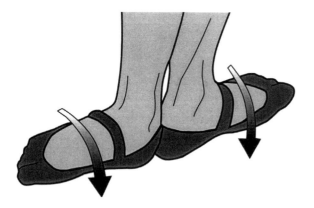

Fig. 7 'Rolling in' is a common error in technique that results in a number of lower limb injuries.

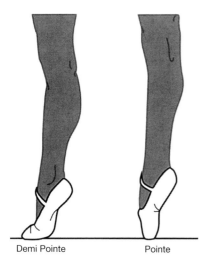

Demi Pointe   Pointe

Fig. 8 Demipoint involves extreme plantar flexion of the toes, with the knees flexed to 90°, and the weight on the metatarsal heads. Pointe involves standing on the tips of the toes.

must be on education and prevention and planning a year-round conditioning and flexibility programme.

Musicians

Musicians and in particular professional musicians, form a special group of individuals, who are highly motivated, dedicated, and goal-orientated. They suffer from a range of soft tissue disorders, some of which are found in the general population and some of which are not. A minor ailment may result in an inability to perform at high level and therefore musicians are commonly more sensitive to a developing condition than others.[5]

Musicians frequently begin to play their chosen instrument(s) at an early age and this may influence the development of posture and the musculoskeletal system, such that the individual is anatomically 'shaped' to their instrument. Mild postural spinal deformities are common and include thoracic kyphosis and prominence of the

scapula in 45 per cent and scoliosis (thoracic, lumbar, or thoracolumbar) in 11 per cent, with the greatest incidence being seen in harpists. Violinists are noted to have a higher left shoulder than right, a longer right upper extremity, and reduced internal rotation of the shoulder. The latter is also reduced in bassists (15 per cent). Cellists have a longer left hand than right, violists a longer left middle finger, and harpists a narrower first web space in both hands.[6] Muscle imbalances are inevitable, due to the physical demands placed upon very specific muscle groups. Hypermobility, localized or generalized, is also common in musicians and may be beneficial with respect to playing but detrimental if symptoms occur due to associated joint subluxation or tendinopathy. Acquired ligamentous laxity, due to long-term ligamentous and capsular stretching, may also occur.

The onset of musculoskeletal symptoms may be associated with the length of time that musicians have been playing—those starting at an earlier age presenting later, possibly due to early adaptive changes in the musculoskeletal system. As is the case with athletes, the better trained the musician is, the less likely is injury to occur. Good technique and efficient use of involved muscles while maintaining optimum posture are all important. Fluctuation of playing schedules, excessive playing, and, in particular, a sudden increase in unfamiliar and/or technically demanding repertoire may also contribute to injury.

Musculoskeletal complaints in musicians are common, with up to 78 per cent being affected at some stage in their career, with women and string and keyboard players more commonly affected. Different instruments and playing positions make different demands on joints and may contribute to the variance in the incidence of musculoskeletal symptoms among musicians. Spinal complaints are the most common, and tendinopathies and bursitis are the most frequently noted disorders in the upper limb (36 per cent).[5–8] 'Overuse syndrome', a form of work-related upper limb pain, is common and attributed to the stresses of repetitive complex movement patterns while supporting the instrument, often in awkward positions. Women are more commonly affected than men and the site of symptoms varies according to the instrument involved. String players report symptoms in their flexors and extensors and in the muscles used to put the fingering hand into the ulnar-deviated position and to spread the fingers. Keyboard players report symptoms in the wrist and finger extensors and the lumbricals (in particular, the ring and little fingers) of both hands, and in the interossei of the right hand (Figs 9 & 10). Oboists, clarinettists, and players of the English horn all may report symptoms in the first web space due to static loading in supporting the instrument.[8]

Management involves relative rest from exacerbating activities (playing) and attention to technique, workload, and postural, ergonomic, and musculoskeletal faults. Rehabilitation is progressive but slow, and playing is reintroduced with short sessions of easy familiar pieces. Relaxation techniques and a long-term conditioning programme should also be emphasized. Ergonomic changes may be simple, such as using a neck strap to support a guitar, or orthotic devices to modify the hand position and grip of the instrument. Postural training, including Pilates or the Alexander technique, is of vital importance. Encouragement and support are also vital and will aid compliance, which may be limited by the need for musicians to earn their living.

Entrapment neuropathies are common complaints in musicians, partly because symptoms are noted early. Errors in technique can lead to neural stretching due to traction, friction from repetitive motion, and/or compression from hypertrophied forearm musculature. Since

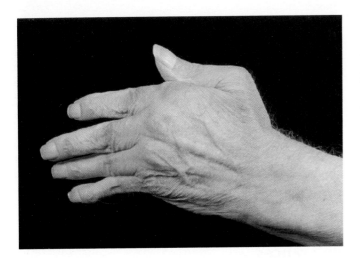

Fig. 9 The rheumatoid hand, with small muscle wasting and MCPJ subluxation and ulnar drift. Inflammation, lengthening, and suboptimal mechanics of extensor and flexor tendons contribute to the deformities.

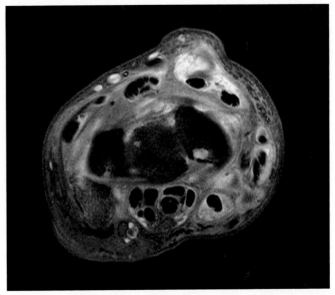

Fig. 10 T2 FSW Fat sat Axial MRI of a rheumatoid wrist, showing extensor tenosynovitis.

symptoms may only be noted when playing, electrodiagnostic confirmation can be difficult. Treatment involves the strategies used in non-musicians, in addition to assessment for technical and ergonomic faults.

Focal motor dystonias consist of abnormal muscle spasms and/or posturing of isolated muscle groups, triggered by voluntary movements. This may only be apparent during playing unless the complaint is severe. Up to a quarter of individuals may have an underlying disorder (metabolic, genetic), but the remainder are idiopathic and the pathogenesis is unknown, although considered to be central in origin. The condition is slowly progressive and potentially devastating for the professional musician as there is no effective cure, although providing some sensory or proprioceptive input may help.

Inflammatory arthritis and enthesopathies

Soft tissue lesions (in particular tendinopathies and bursitides) in individuals with inflammatory arthritides are common and can occur at any stage of the disease, due to primary inflammation (tenosynovitis, bursitis), attrition secondary to local inflammation or sharp bony prominences, deranged biomechanics, or drugs (local or systemic corticosteroids). Infiltration of tendons by rheumatoid nodules has also been described.[9] Soft tissue lesions are also frequently overlooked by both patient and physician due to (a) the focus of attention being placed on articular manifestations of the disease, (b) difficulties in examination of musculotendinous units due to the presence of advanced deformities, and (c) occasionally due to neurological involvement. Nevertheless, the consequences of such lesions can be significant when combined with the other sequelae of the disease.

Tendinopathies are commonly seen in ensheathed tendons: the extensor tendons of the wrist are frequently affected early but may present only after rupture has occurred. Extensor pollicis longus at Lister's tubercle and extensor digiti minimi usually are the earliest to rupture, although rupture of the latter may pass unnoticed because extensor digitorum communis (EDC) extends all four fingers simultaneously. Valeri *et al.*[10]

studied tendon involvement at the wrist in rheumatoid arthritis (RA) and noted low grades of peritendinous effusion to be more common in the volar compartment, whereas moderate and high degrees of tendon sheath fluid collection and/or pannus and signs of tendinitis were more frequent in the dorsal and ulnar tendon sheaths.

Posterior tibial tendon disease symptoms including lengthening, tenosynovitis, tears, and rupture, contribute to flat foot deformity in the disease (Fig. 11).[11] Other tendons not invested within a tendon sheath are also commonly affected. Imaging studies in patients with RA have demonstrated structural alterations in the rotator cuff, tenosynovitis of the long head of the biceps, and subacromial bursitis.[12, 13] Stiskal *et al.* suggested that rheumatoid Achilles tendinopathy can be distinguished from degenerative tendinopathy in patients with chronic pain of the heel using magnetic resonance imaging (MRI).[12] Inflammation of the retrocalcaneal bursa and the absence of enlargement of the tendon combined with the presence of intratendinous signal alterations are characteristic findings of rheumatoid Achilles tendinopathy.

Education on joint protection and effective control of rheumatoid disease is the priority in the prevention of soft tissue complications. Splinting in severe tenosynovitis and the use of specialized footwear and orthoses are helpful in this context. Local corticosteroid injections also play a role in the treatment of tenosynovitis and bursitis, although repeated injections increase the risk of tendon rupture. Where rupture has occurred, prompt repair and/or tendon transfer is usually indicated to prevent function limitation. Additional surgery may be necessary to remove bony prominences contributing to tendon attrition. Reconstruction is not possible in some cases due to the advanced disease within the tendon substance. In some cases surgery is not necessary—for example, mallet finger. Flexor tendon ruptures within the finger have a poor prognosis, although fortunately they are less common than extensor ruptures.

Entrapment neuropathies, in particular carpal and tarsal tunnel syndromes, are frequent manifestations of RA and occur due to compression by local synovitis or due to biomechanical changes as a

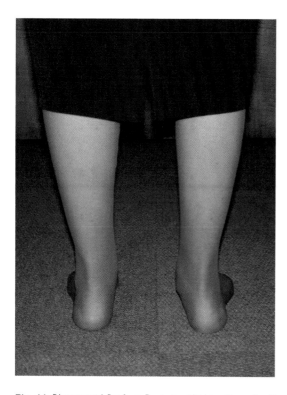

Fig. 11 Rheumatoid flat foot. Posterior tibial tendinopathy disease is one of many soft tissue manifestations of rheumatoid disease.

Table 7 Disorders in which enthesopathies are a feature

Seronegative spondyloarthropathies

Diffuse idiopathic skeletal hyperostosis

SAPHO (synovitis, acne, pustulosis, hyperostosis, osteitis)

Calcium pyrophosphate dihydrate and hydroxyapaptite deposition diseases

Acromegaly and other endocrinopathies

Chronic retinoid toxicity

Fluorosis (chronic fluoride intoxication)

consequence of the disease. Other disorders can mimic entrapment neuropathy, including a mononeuritis multiplex, nerve root compression, and brachial plexopathy. Treatment includes management of the inflammatory process and correction of biomechanical abnormalities as appropriate. Surgical decompression may be necessary.

Ligamentous involvement in RA is also common. This is most commonly a feature of the synovitic process eroding ligament, bone, and cartilage, and contributes to instabilities of areas such as the cervical spine, knee, and carpus. Attenuation of ligaments due to

biomechanical aberrations and direct injury as a result of reduced proprioception also can occur.

An *enthesopathy* is a disorder of a tendon, ligament, or capsule on to bone and may be traumatic, inflammatory, metabolic, or degenerative in nature. Enthesopathies occur at distinct sites: at synovial joints; at cartilaginous articulations; at extraarticular sites, including syndesmoses. They are a feature of a number of disorders (Table 7). The pathology of enthesopathies has been reviewed earlier.

Patients with enthesopathies may report few or no symptoms or may be severely affected. Those patients with seronegative spondyloarthropathies commonly develop severe and often unremitting inflammatory 'enthesitis'. Treatment includes anti-inflammatory approaches, physiotherapy, and, where appropriate, second-line drugs.

References

1. **Snell, E.D. and Dimeff, R.J.** (1996). The geriatric athlete. In *ACSM essentials of sports medicine* (ed. R.E. Sallis and F. Massimino), pp. 99–109. Mosby, St Louis.

2. **Perry, D.J.** (1998). Sports medicine: the clinical spectrum of injury. In *Rheumatology*, 2nd edn (ed. J.H. Klippel and P.A. Dieppe), pp. 4–17. Mosby, London.

3. **Harris S.S.** (1996). Strength training for children and adolescents. In *ACSM essentials of sports medicine* (ed. R.E. Sallis and F. Massimino), pp. 504–508. Mosby, St Louis.

4. **Shon, L.C. and Weinfeld, S.B.** (1996). Lower extremity musculoskeletal problems in dancers. *Curr. Opin. Rheumatol.* **8**, 130–142.

5. **Lockwood, A.H.** (1989). Medical problems of musicians [review]. *N. Engl. J. Med.* **320** (4), 221–227.

6. **Bejjani, F.J., Gross, M.S., and Brown, P.** (1984). Occupational hand disorders in musicians. *J. Hand Surg. Am.* **9**, 225.

7. **Bejjani, F.J., Stuchin, S., and Brown, P.** (1984). Occupational disorders of string players, pianists, harpists and guitarists. *J. Bone Joint Surg Orthop. Trans.* **8**, 133.

8. **Bejjani, F.J., Kaye, G.M., and Benham, M.** (1996). Musculoskeletal and neuromuscular conditions of instrumental musicians. *Arch. Phys. Med. Rehabil.* **77**, 406–413.

9. **Kotob, H. and Kamel, M.** (1999). Identification and prevalence of rheumatoid nodules in the finger tendons using high frequency ultrasonography. *J. Rheumatol.* **6**, 1264–1268.

10. **Valeri, G., Ferrara, C., Ercolani, P., De Nigris, E., and Giovagnoni, A.** (2001). Tendon involvement in rheumatoid arthritis of the wrist: MRI findings. *Skeletal Radiol.* **30** (3), 138–143.

11. **Coari, G., Paoletti, F., and Iagnocco, A.** (1999). Shoulder involvement in rheumatic diseases. Sonographic findings. *J. Rheumatol.* **26**, 668–673.

12. **Bare, A.A. and Haddad, S.L.** (2001). Tenosynovitis of the posterior tibial tendon. *Foot Ankle Clin.* **6**, 37–66.

13. **Stiskal, M., Szolar, D.H., Stenzel, I., Steiner, E., Mesaric, P., Czembirek, H., and Preidler, K.W.** (1997). Magnetic resonance imaging of Achilles tendon in patients with rheumatoid arthritis. *Invest. Radiol.* **32** (10), 602–608.

5

Principles of management

5.1 The management of pain in soft tissue disorders: pharmacological agents

Mark Abrahams and Rajesh Munglani

Introduction

The perception of pain is a physiological protective mechanism designed to act as a warning that tissue damage, has occurred, to encourage prevention of further damage and to allow the healing process to be completed. The persistent pain associated with soft tissue disorders, however, may serve no useful biological purpose. Frequently, the patient will experience pain when there is no evidence of injured tissue. Alternatively, significant irreversible tissue damage may be present but unresponsive to normal tissue healing processes. Pain sensation in these situations is, therefore, redundant. Unlike acute pain, which can serve as an indicator of disease severity or progression, the intensity of persistent pain often bears no relationship to the underlying disease process.

Pharmacological treatment of soft tissue pain in the recent past followed guidelines set out in the World Health Organization's (WHO) analgesic ladder (Fig. 1).[1] The progression of analgesia described by the WHO is of limited usefulness in the treatment of chronic pain disorders, however, due to the reduced effectiveness of simple and opioid analgesics in neuropathic pain. Co-analgesic agents such as the antidepressants and anticonvulsants were originally used as adjuncts to standard analgesic regimens, but have gradually gained more prominence, and are now regarded as the mainstay of pharmacological treatment for chronic pain. As we understand more about the physiological processes producing persistent pain in soft tissue disorders, we are able to treat painful conditions with greater confidence of success.

This chapter is aimed at summarizing the pharmacological therapies currently available for the treatment of pain associated with soft tissue disorders, and will focus on the methodology underlying the use of different drug classes, as well as presenting important or novel therapeutic agents. It should be noted that much of the evidence for the efficacy of treatment in chronic pain comes from studies of neuropathic pain disorders, and not specifically soft tissue disorders. Nevertheless, it is fair to assume that different neuropathic conditions have similar underlying pathology and, in general, drug efficacy is interchangeable.

Nonsteroidal anti-inflammatory drugs and paracetamol

Since the synthesis of salicylic acid in 1874 by Kolbe as an antipyretic agent, a vast number of aspirin-like drugs have been synthesized and exploited for their antipyretic, anti-inflammatory, and analgesic properties. These drugs have had a long-established role in the treatment of acute pain, but their benefit in chronic pain is less certain, with efficacy only proven in chronic inflammatory musculoskeletal pain, although their use in cancer pain is widely recognized.[2]

Nonsteroidal anti-inflammatory drugs (NSAIDs) impair the synthesis of prostaglandins by inhibiting the cyclo-oxygenase enzyme (Fig. 2). Prostaglandins have an important role in the generation of pain and, in particular, the establishment of hyperalgesia, both at the peripheral nociceptor and at the level of the spinal cord. After tissue injury, the local synthesis of prostaglandins is increased, and extracellular concentrations of prostaglandins and a number of other inflammatory mediators (including bradykinin, histamine, serotonin, adenosine, catecholamines, cytokines, and potassium, and hydrogen ions) increase around the site of the peripheral nociceptor. The effect of these substances is to lower the threshold potential of the peripheral nociceptor, thus increasing its response to a given stimulus or causing it to respond to a lower, previously subthreshold, stimulus. In addition,

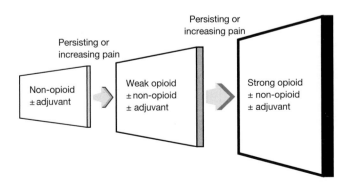

Fig. 1 The WHO analgesic ladder. (Adapted from reference 1.)

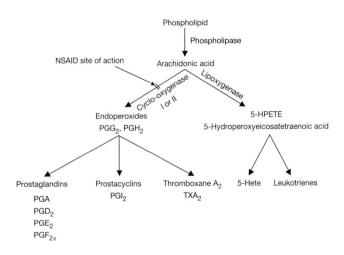

Fig. 2 Prostaglandin synthesis. Nonsteroidal anti-inflammatory drugs impair prostaglandin synthesis by inhibiting the cyclo-oxygenase enzyme.

prostaglandins act to increase the sensitivity of 'silent' polymodal nociceptors.[3] These receptors are present in tissues throughout the body, but have high threshold potentials and are normally quiescent. The release of prostaglandins following tissue trauma causes these receptors to become sensitive to a variety of different stimuli, resulting in a net increase in the frequency of impulses reaching the dorsal horn.[4] Prostaglandins have also been shown to facilitate nerve growth factor-mediated expression of tetrodotoxin-insensitive (TTXi or TTXr) sodium channels.[5, 6] Increased expression of these channels may contribute to the peripheral nociceptor sensitization seen in chronic pain states.

Prostaglandins (PG) also have an important role in the development of central sensitization. PGE_2 activates EP_2 receptors at the dorsal horn, enhancing neurotransmitter release from the primary afferent fibres, while $PGF_{2\alpha}$ activates EP_3 receptors, causing increased postsynaptic responsiveness.[7–9]

The discovery in 1991 of the existence of a second isoform of the cyclo-oxygenase enzyme has increased our understanding of the side-effect profiles of the different NSAIDs and led to the development of cyclo-oxygenase-2-specific inhibitors (COX-2 inhibitors). The COX-1 enzyme is present in most tissues and is responsible for the normal homeostatic functions of prostaglandins. These include prostacyclin-induced protection of the gastric mucosa, the maintenance of normal blood flow in the kidney, and the preservation of normal platelet function. Inhibition of COX-1 function, therefore, is responsible for the major side-effects of NSAID therapy. Though present constitutively in the kidney, brain, and lungs and the dominating isoform in the spinal cord,[10] the COX-2 enzyme is expressed in most tissues at fairly low concentrations. The production of cytokines in inflammation, however, induces synthesis of the enzyme, and levels in tissue are greatly increased leading to augmented prostaglandin production.[11] Prostaglandin synthesis at the dorsal horn is mediated by constitutive COX-2, and it is clear that many NSAIDs act centrally to inhibit this isoenzyme, even when administered systemically.[12]

COX-2 appears to be co-localized with neuronal nitric oxide synthase (nNOS) at the level of the dorsal horn, and some of the aspirin-like drugs may interfere with this system.[13] Synergism with central opioid receptors may also play a role in the analgesic effects of NSAIDs. The central actions of diclofenac and ketorolac are suppressed by opioid receptor antagonists,[14] suggesting that structural differences in NSAIDs may be responsible for alternative modes of action. These opioid receptor interactions may also explain the incidence of psychotropic side-effects in some patients treated with NSAIDs.

The side-effect profiles of different NSAIDs depend largely upon their distribution in the body, and upon their selectivity for the COX-1 or COX-2 enzyme isoforms (Fig. 3). Highly protein-bound acidic drugs like the NSAIDs are distributed preferentially to tissues with a lower pH, such as inflamed tissue, the wall of the upper gastrointestinal tract, and the renal collecting ducts, while neutral drugs like paracetamol and phenazone distribute quickly throughout the body and can permeate the blood–brain barrier easily.[15] Aspirin and indomethacin have greater selectivity for the COX-1 enzyme, and are thus associated with an increased risk of gastrointestinal tract damage. By contrast, drugs more potent against COX-2 than COX-1, such as etodolac and meloxicam, are less damaging to the gastric mucosa. COX-2-specific inhibitors, such as celecoxib and rofecoxib and the newer drugs valdecoxib and parecoxib, have significantly better gastrointestinal side-effect profiles.[16–18] Note, however, that renal side-effects are not

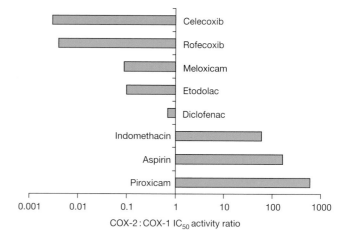

Fig. 3 Comparison of NSAID selectivity for COX-1 and COX-2. The COX-2 : COX-1 IC_{50} (log concentration that inhibits 50 per cent) activity ratio indicates the relative selectivity of NSAIDs for the COX-1 and COX-2 enzymes. Drugs with high ratios, such as piroxicam, are more selective for the COX-1 enzyme and have a greater incidence of gastrointestinal bleeding and perforation with long-term therapy.

significantly reduced with the COX-2 inhibitors due to the constitutive presence of the cyclo-oxygenase-2 enzyme in the kidney.

NSAIDs and paracetamol: principles of drug therapy in soft tissue disorders

NSAIDs and paracetamol are among the most widely-prescribed drugs in soft tissue disorders, yet there is sparse evidence of their efficacy in chronic pain states. Studies consistently show little or no benefit in the treatment of neuropathic pain and the authors would suggest that drugs with such adverse side-effect profiles should be avoided. However, there is evidence that NSAIDs are effective in diminishing hyperalgesia in soft tissue disorders with an inflammatory component[19] and controlled use of nonsteroidal drugs in these circumstances would seem appropriate. In addition, it should be recognized that many predominantly non-inflammatory conditions undergo phases of inflammatory change. Osteoarthritis, for example, though regarded as a non-inflammatory condition, is characterized by episodes of inflammatory change in soft tissues where focal synovial hyperplasia occurs along with mononuclear cell infiltrates. NSAIDs are an important part of the treatment of pain during such acute exacerbations of the disease. A small number of patients with soft tissue disorders do seem to gain a sustained analgesic effect from nonsteroidal drug usage. Whether their disease process has a significant inflammatory component or whether they have idiosyncratic reactions to some of the NSAIDs is uncertain and, unfortunately, such patients are very difficult to predict.[20] A carefully controlled trial of NSAID therapy may be justified in patients with uncontrolled pain, but the physician should be prepared to discontinue therapy if no benefit is gained. Equally, there are many patients on long-term NSAID therapy who may be able to discontinue their medication without any deterioration in symptoms. NSAIDs and paracetamol are still perceived as first-line treatments for the pain associated with cancer syndromes as part of a multimodal approach to analgesia. Their efficacy in these circumstances, however, has not been examined adequately in clinical trials.

Nonsteroidal anti-inflammatory drugs

There are a large number of NSAIDs available for use in soft tissue disorders, and the prescription of one drug rather than another is often dependent upon individual physician preference, frequently guided by anecdotal evidence or personal perception of improved efficacy or side-effect profile. The choice of drug, administration route, and dose should be targeted at gaining maximum efficacy with minimum side-effects.

NSAIDs differ in their pharmacokinetic properties, and this should be taken into account when choosing a nonsteroidal agent for long-term use in soft tissue pain. The oxicams (e.g. piroxicam, tenoxicam) are metabolized slowly and have a high degree of enteropathic circulation. Consequently, they have long elimination half-lives (but also higher incidences of gastrointestinal and renal side-effects). Their main indication is for persistent pain associated with chronic illnesses. However, successful treatment with NSAIDs requires careful titration of the drug dose to obtain optimal analgesia, and NSAIDs with shorter half-lives are more suited to dosage adjustment.

Analgesic efficacy

Although reviews in the medical literature frequently compare the potency of different NSAIDs, in practice such differences are unimportant. That one drug is found to be more effective than another simply implies that a more optimal analgesic dose of the drug was given. There is no consistent evidence, either in acute or in chronic pain, that a particular drug provides superior analgesia.[21–23] Thus, the dose of a NSAID should be titrated until adequate analgesia is obtained. As common side-effects are also dose-dependent, dosage is often limited before analgesic concentrations are reached. The most important factor determining choice of agent must, therefore, be variations in the side-effect profiles of different drugs.

Side-effects of NSAIDs

As explained previously, the dose-dependent side-effects common to NSAIDs are due to the inhibition of normal prostaglandin protective mechanisms (Table 1). The most important adverse effect, damage to the gastroduodenal tract, is predominantly caused by inhibition of the COX-1 isoenzyme, and the risk of gastrointestinal damage depends largely upon the relative selectivity of different drugs for the COX-1 compared to the COX-2 enzyme (Fig. 3). Thus, drugs like naproxen, etodolac, and diclofenac have better gastrointestinal side-effect profiles than piroxicam or indomethacin. The risk of gastric ulceration can be as high as 47 per cent for some drugs,[24] and physicians should consider prophylactic use of misoprostol or H2 antagonist drugs to protect against gastric and duodenal ulcers, respectively. Alternatively, prodrugs such as benzoxaprofen bypass the stomach and have a reduced incidence of gastric damage.

COX-2-selective inhibitors such as celecoxib and rofecoxib have been shown to have analgesic efficacy with greatly reduced gastrointestinal side-effects (see below). Research has shown that different enantiomer forms of some NSAIDs have different effects. The S enantiomer of the drug, flurbiprofen, is responsible for anti-inflammatory and analgesic actions and is ulcerogenic, while the R form blocks nociception and has very little effect on gastrointestinal mucosa. The development of more specific drugs may lead to better side-effect profiles.

Routes of administration of NSAIDs

Systematic reviews show no advantage of parenteral administration of NSAIDs over the enteral route[23, 25] and drugs should be given orally

Table 1 Adverse effects of nonsteroidal anti-inflammatory drugs

Gastrointestinal toxicity
Nausea and vomiting
Dyspepsia
Diarrhoea
Gastric irritation, superficial gastric erosions
Peptic ulceration (usually antral and prepyloric)
Gastrointestinal bleeding

Renal toxicity
Reduced renal blood flow
Reduced glomerular filtration rate
Medullary ischaemia
Tubular necrosis
Acute renal failure

Haematological toxicity
Impaired platelet aggregation
Prolonged bleeding time

Respiratory adverse reactions
Bronchospasm
Exacerbation of asthma

Other adverse effects
Drowsiness, confusion
Rashes, hypersensitivity reactions
Tinnitus, dizziness, deafness
Convulsions
Hyperpyrexia

when possible. The topical route of administration is an exception, however, and systemic reviews have shown that they are effective as analgesics for musculoskeletal pain with a lower incidence of gastrointestinal side-effects.[25, 26]

Paracetamol (acetaminophen)

The major advantage of paracetamol over the NSAIDs is its relative lack of side-effects, and this justifies its use as a first-line analgesic drug. It can be used as the sole analgesic agent, or synergistically with nonsteroidal drugs and has effective analgesic and antipyretic properties, though very weak anti-inflammatory action. Paracetamol acts centrally as a COX-3 inhibitor but has very little action on peripheral COX. It has also been shown to produce central nociception by interfering with the neuronal nitric oxide system.[13] Its major drawback is the liver toxicity seen in acute overdose due to the accumulation in the liver of benzoquinones.

There are many compound preparations available containing paracetamol and *weak* opioids. Meta-analysis shows little difference between the analgesic effects of these preparations and of paracetamol alone in acute pain, except for the preparations containing 60 mg codeine.[25] However, opioids like codeine have little efficacy in the chronic pain associated with soft tissue disorders and are associated with a high incidence of constipation, and such preparations should be avoided.

Cyclo-oxygenase 2 inhibitors

The drugs celecoxib and rofecoxib and the newer preparations valdecoxib and parecoxib are selective for the cyclo-oxygenase 2 isoform of the enzyme. These drugs have been shown to be effective analgesics,[27–30] but have greatly reduced gastrointestinal side-effects.[16, 18, 31]. As the COX-2 isoenzyme appears to be responsible for prostaglandin-induced central sensitization, it is hoped that selective drugs may be more effective in chronic pain. However, it is not yet certain that the current drugs adequately penetrate into the spinal cord.

Opioids

Although opioid drugs are accepted as the mainstay drug therapy for the management of cancer pain, their role in the treatment of non-cancer pain, particularly the neuropathic pain associated with many soft tissue disorders, is still to be established. The reasons for the apparent reluctance of physicians to prescribe opioids for non-cancer pain (and for the suspicions of many patients who are offered the drugs) can be due to experience of genuine problems associated with long-term opioid use in patients, and widespread perceptions of opioids as dangerous and addictive drugs. In addition, these drugs are believed by many physicians to be ineffective for the treatment of neuropathic pain.

The view that opioids are ineffective in relieving neuropathic pain stems from a combination of anecdotal reports and misplaced evidence from badly designed studies.[32] A series of randomized controlled studies in the last decade examining use of intravenous and oral opioids for the treatment of chronic neuropathic pain of different pathologies confirmed that opioids do have analgesic efficacy in neuropathic pain, in particular, inflammatory pain.[33–39] Many studies show that neuropathic pain conditions require higher than normal doses of opioid to obtain analgesia. This could be explained by chronic stimulation of endogenous opioid systems in patients with longstanding pain leading to changes in opioid receptor regulation, and by the activation of endogenous anti-opioid systems in these patients utilizing N-methyl-D-aspartate (NMDA)-, cholecystokinin-, and orphanin FQ/nociceptin-based mechanisms.

A distinction should be made between 'efficacy' and 'usefulness'. Although opioids have proven efficacy in chronic pain, the benefits of therapy must be weighed against the considerable incidence of side-effects and the risk, in those patients (and physicians) who perceive opioid therapy as definitive or 'end-stage' treatment, of neglecting other pain-coping strategies. Opioid therapy should be seen as an adjunct to other pharmacological and non-pharmacological treatment.

Tolerance, dependence, and addiction

When discussing the use of opioids for chronic pain disorders, many physicians quote fear of tolerance, dependence, and addiction as a major factor influencing their decision to prescribe.

Tolerance indicates the need to increase the dose of a drug with time to achieve the same effect, and is due to a number of physiological mechanisms. The NMDA–nitric oxide cascade appears to play an important part, and the combination of opioids with NMDA receptor antagonists has been shown to significantly inhibit the development of tolerance.[40–42] In practice, tolerance is not usually a problem unless side-effects prevent further escalation of the drug dose. In addition, studies in cancer pain show that, with long-term use of opioids, the rate of rise in drug dose decreases with time and most patients' dose requirements stabilize.[43]

Dependence is related to tolerance and implies changes in opioid receptor regulation and expression with prolonged drug use. Again, it is not usually a problem in clinical practice, unless the drugs are discontinued abruptly, triggering withdrawal reactions. Reactions can be avoided by reducing the drug dose gradually at the end of treatment by about 50 per cent every 2 days. Patients on long-term opioid therapy should not be given mixed agonist/antagonist drugs, as they can precipitate withdrawal.

Addiction is a behavioural problem characterized by drug-seeking activity in the individual in order to experience its psychic effects. Although it can happen, patients treated with opioids for chronic pain conditions very rarely become addicted to the drugs.[44] It is difficult to predict which patients are at risk of addiction, but it is prudent to check for a history of drug dependence and to select patients carefully before commencing long-term opioid therapy.

Side-effects of opioid therapy

Agonist activity at opioid receptors mediates a number of dose-related side-effects that can become problematic with long-term therapy. The most frequently occurring adverse reactions are respiratory depression and constipation (Table 2).

Respiratory depression is mediated predominantly through opioid μ_2 receptors, and is frequently encountered when inappropriate doses of opioids are administered for acute pain. In the chronic pain setting, however, respiratory depression is rarely seen, especially outwith certain at-risk patient groups. This can be explained in part by the practice of slow titration of the opioid dose and the preference for the oral route of administration in chronic pain patients. Sedation occurs at doses significantly lower than that causing respiratory depression. Opioid-induced respiratory depression is due to inhibition of respiratory drive, producing a reduced ventilatory response to carbon dioxide. Opioids should be used with care in patients with pulmonary disease, especially in patients who tend to retain carbon dioxide, in the elderly, and in those patients with liver or renal impairment. Particular care must be taken when titrating doses of drugs with long terminal half-lives such as methadone, and when administering opioids via the intrathecal route, particularly in the opioid-naïve patient.

Table 2 Adverse effects of opioid analgesics

Respiratory effects
Respiratory depression

Gastrointestinal effects
Constipation
Nausea and vomiting
Delayed gastric emptying

Central nervous system effects
Sedation
Drowsiness
Euphoria, dysphoria
Addiction
Tolerance and dependence
Tremor
Mioisis

Cardiovascular effects
Bradycardia
Hypotension

Gastrointestinal side-effects of opioids include constipation, nausea, and vomiting. Constipation results from brain and myenteric plexus μ_2-receptor-mediated inhibition of gastrointestinal transit. Nausea and vomiting are caused by stimulation of the chemoreceptor trigger zone.

Other side-effects include bradycardia, miosis, and reductions in basal metabolic rate and temperature. Opioids have also been shown to suppress cytokine function as well as inhibiting stress-induced release of corticotrophin from the pituitary gland.

Mechanism of action of opioids

Opioids produce their effects via action at specific G protein-coupled receptors in the brain, spinal cord, and peripheral nervous system. There are three major classes of opioid receptor: δ-opioid (OP_1, DOR), κ-opioid (OP_2, KOR), and μ-opioid (OP_3, MOR), which correspond to their endogenous ligands, enkephalin, dynorphin, and β-endorphin, respectively. Although studies suggest the existence of subtypes of all three major opioid receptor groups, the evidence is controversial and, as yet, of little practical value. The discovery of two new receptors (or receptor subtypes) may be important. The widespread opioid receptor-like type 1 (ORL_1) is related to κ-receptors and has an endogenous ligand, orphanin FQ.[45] Agonists at this receptor produce analgesia at the spinal level. Studies in knockout mice also suggest that the morphine metabolite, morphine-6-glucuronide, acts upon a distinctive receptor, M6G, in the central nervous system producing potent analgesia.

Stimulation of opioid receptors generally causes hyperpolarization of the nerve membrane, via G-protein-coupled inhibition of adenyl cyclase, by the inhibition of voltage-gated calcium channels and the activation of inwardly rectifying potassium channels. The result is a physiological antagonism of the transmission of pain. Synthesis, expression, and activation of peripheral opioid receptors in damaged tissue are stimulated by the action of inflammatory mediators, perhaps explaining the improved efficacy of opioids in chronic pain disorders with an inflammatory component.[46–48]

Opioids: principles of drug therapy in soft tissue disorders

Though recognized as an important part of the treatment of cancer pain, the use of opioids in chronic non-malignant pain is still to be firmly established, despite evidence of its efficacy in some patient groups.[33, 49] There is a growing consensus, however, that opioid therapy can be a valid adjunct to other analgesic strategies in the treatment of chronic pain, and should not be confined to patients as a last resort when other therapies have failed. As some painful conditions respond better than others to opioids, a trial of drug therapy is useful to determine efficacy. Trials of intravenous patient-controlled opioid analgesia are a preferred technique but are dependent upon available resources.[49] Gourlay and Cherry describe guidelines on the use of strong opioids in chronic non-malignant pain that take the form of a contractual agreement between physician and patient emphasizing goal-orientated therapy.[50] They stress that the opioids are to be given initially for a limited period of time, and that extension of treatment is subject to the patient attaining proscribed targets, such as increased mobilization or a return to work. Treatment is also discontinued if the patient displays drug-seeking or non-productive behavioural changes.

Route of administration of opioids

While the parenteral route of administration of opioids is useful in acute pain, in chronic pain disorders, conventional enteral administration is generally sufficient and may be more convenient for the patient. Drug dosages should reflect bioavailability, and the physician must be prepared to alter dosages if converting from one route to another. Important exceptions to the preference for enteral administration of opioids are the administration of intrathecal and epidural opioids, and the application of transdermal fentanyl patches (see below).

The high numbers of opioid receptors present at the dorsal horn of the spinal cord mean that, when compared to systemically administered drug, opioid drugs delivered epidurally or intrathecally can produce equivalent analgesia, but with substantial reductions in dose.[51] The main indication for the use of continuous epidural or spinal opioids in chronic pain is the patient who gains considerable analgesic benefit from opioid therapy, but in whom treatment is limited by the intolerable adverse effects of high-dose systemic opioids.[52, 53] Indwelling epidural and spinal catheter techniques can be associated with significant morbidity, particularly the risk of infection, and the administration of epidural or intrathecal opioids can also produce serious adverse reactions, including nausea and vomiting, pruritis, and urinary retention. Respiratory depression can be a life-threatening complication, especially with intrathecal delivery of opioids and with opioid-naïve patients. Treatment should be established in a fully monitored clinical setting, and drug dose carefully titrated for analgesic effect. In practice, adverse effects tend to diminish with prolonged therapy, and the development of tolerance means that drugs have to be given in increasing doses.

Highly lipid-soluble drugs like fentanyl are less effective when given by the epidural or intrathecal route as they are rapidly absorbed systemically, and less-soluble drugs like morphine are preferable if a more prolonged action is desired. As a rough guide, intrathecal doses of 1–2 per cent, and epidural doses of 10–20 per cent of the former total daily parenteral (intravenous or subcutaneous) opioid can be given.

Individual opioid agents

The classification of drugs as *weak* opioids or *strong* opioids is arbitrary and not of great practical value in the treatment of chronic pain. In general, less potent opioid drugs like codeine and dextropropoxyphene have little place in the management of patients with chronic pain disorders, as the higher doses required for analgesic efficacy in chronic pain are associated with intolerable side-effects, particularly constipation, nausea, and vomiting. At lower doses, drugs often have little effect, and can frequently be discontinued without an increase in pain. The exception to this rule is tramadol, which may have non-opioid mechanisms of action, making it more suitable for use in neuropathic pain.

Tramadol

The analgesic action of tramadol results from a weak agonist action at μ-opioid receptors combined with an inhibition of noradrenaline (norepinephrine) and serotonin reuptake. These two mechanisms act synergistically to produce pain relief,[54, 55] and are responsible for its analgesic efficacy in neuropathic pain.[37, 56] Common adverse reactions include nausea and dizziness and can be minimized by titrating the dose upwards over several days.[57] Tramadol also benefits from a low record of abuse and, because of its mode of action, can be safely combined with NSAID therapy.[58] It can rarely cause seizures, and should be used with caution in susceptible patients.

Morphine

Morphine is still the strong opioid of choice globally and is the standard by which other opioids are compared. Standard preparations of morphine need to be given at 4-hourly intervals, but the development of slow-release formulations has allowed dosing intervals of 6–12 h. These slow-release preparations take about 2.5 h to reach peak plasma concentrations of morphine. Morphine is metabolized in the liver to its main metabolites, morphine-3-glucuronide and morphine-6-glucuronide (M6G). M6G contributes to the analgesic action of morphine, particularly when blood levels increase with chronic dosing, and can cause nausea, vomiting, and respiratory depression. Accumulation of M6G in renal failure can lead to excessive sedation and prolonged drug action.

Modified-release preparations are generally started at a dose of 20–30 mg twice daily, and can be adjusted at 48-hour intervals until analgesic efficacy occurs.

Methadone

Methadone combines μ agonist activity with NMDA channel blocking properties and inhibition of serotonin reuptake. This combined action makes it a particularly useful drug for use in neuropathic pain.[53] High protein binding and slow liver metabolism give it an extremely long half-life, allowing less frequent dosing, but giving an increased risk of drug accumulation. Analgesia lasts 6–12 h, but can be much longer with chronic administration. It should be started at a dose equivalent to one-tenth of the previous total daily morphine dose, and titrated slowly upwards until adequate analgesia is obtained. Patients who obtain poor analgesia from large doses of morphine often require very low doses of methadone with few adverse effects to achieve the same pain relief.[53]

Transdermal fentanyl

Transdermal fentanyl patches have been used in cancer pain for some time, and can be a convenient way of providing opioid-based analgesia for patients with non-malignant chronic pain. Fentanyl is a potent μ-receptor agonist with high lipid solubility. Transdermal fentanyl is less constipating than morphine. Once the patch is applied, it takes 3–24 h to reach effective plasma concentrations of fentanyl, and steady-state concentrations are reached after 36–48 h.[59] The initial dose of fentanyl can be calculated using a morphine:fentanyl ratio of 100:150:1. Studies suggest that the patch should be changed every 2 days. Once the patch is removed, the elimination half-life of fentanyl is about 24 h.[60]

Co-analgesic agents

Antidepressants

When Paoli et al.[61] first started using antidepressants in patients with chronic pain in 1960, the drugs were intended to treat the reactive depression associated with the pain, rather than the pain itself. It was noted, however, that the patients were reporting a significant improvement in their pain after commencing the antidepressant medication. There is no doubt that a minority of patients with chronic pain are clinically depressed, and that the analgesic response to antidepressants tends to be more pronounced when the onset of the depressive illness precedes or coincides with the onset of pain. It was suggested that the pain experienced by these patients was a somatic expression of their

depressive illness. However, it was subsequently realized that antidepressant drugs have analgesic action in persistent pain states that is separate from their antidepressant action and independent of the affective state of the patient.[62, 63] The onset of the analgesic effect occurs at a much earlier stage than the antidepressant effect (3–7 days rather than 3 weeks) and, indeed, may occur without significant antidepressant response (perhaps suggesting that the therapeutic range for analgesic action is lower than that for antidepressant action). Similarly, antidepressant drugs have been shown to create powerful analgesic effects in patients with no evidence of clinical depression.

Antidepressants work by altering the activity of monoamine neurotransmitters in the brain by blocking the presynaptic reuptake of serotonin and noradrenaline. The acute effect is to increase synaptic levels of monoamines. Chronic administration modulates neurotransmitter action by altered regulation of monoamine receptors or by an action on co-modulators, including substance P, thyrotrophin-releasing hormone (TRH)-like peptides, and gamma aminobutyric acid (GABA). The side-effects of antidepressants, particularly the older tricyclic antidepressants (TCAs), are mostly related to interaction with other receptor groups in the central nervous system. Thus, antagonist activity at anticholinergic muscarinic receptors, H_1 and H_2 receptors, and α_1 and α_2 receptors leads to anticholinergic, antihistaminergic, and antiadrenergic side-effects (Table 3). The TCAs have also been shown to display calcium channel blocking effects and inhibition of prostaglandin synthetase,[64, 65] and may induce endogenous opioid peptide release producing effects at the δ-opioid receptor.[66]

Different classes of antidepressant agents have been used in chronic pain conditions with varying degrees of success. Analgesic efficacy has been noted for tricyclic and heterocyclic antidepressants, selective serotonin reuptake inhibitors, serotonin–adrenaline reuptake inhibitors, and monoamine oxidase inhibitors. Most clinical trials have studied the effects of the older TCAs in chronic pain, and these are still considered to be first-choice agents.

In persistent pain states, the dorsal horn neurons are sensitized, increasing the probability that sensory input into the spinal cord will lead to the activation of neurons carrying pain sensation to the cortex. This sensitization is caused by anatomical and physiological changes in the nerve pathways, which include altered receptor expression, and

Table 3 Adverse effects of tricyclic antidepressant drugs

Anticholinergic effects
Dry mouth
Constipation
Palpitations, cardiac tachyarrhythmias
Urinary retention
Precipitation of glaucoma
Blurred vision

α-receptor blockade
Orthostatic hypotension

Central nervous system adverse effects
Sedation
Tremor
Convulsions
Confusional states

Other adverse effects
Weight gain
Rashes/hypersensitivity reactions

result in an imbalance in the excitatory and inhibitory control of the dorsal horn neurons. As a number of different types of receptor are affected by these changes, it is perhaps not surprising that older, less-specific antidepressants such as amitriptyline are more effective in the treatment of chronic pain than newer, more selective drugs such as the selective serotonin reuptake inhibitors, fluoxetine or paroxetine. A study by Max et al., however, which used an active placebo with anticholinergic and sedative action designed to mimic the side-effects of amitriptyline, still showed a significant improvement in pain with amitriptyline but not with the placebo.[62] This may suggest that altered regulation of synaptic monoamine levels, and the subsequent effect on descending inhibitory pathways do contribute to the analgesic action of these drugs.

Although the monoamine oxidase inhibitors have proven efficacy in the treatment of chronic pain, they must be used with great care because of their pharmacological interactions with other drugs, their side-effects, and the necessity of dietary restrictions. Successful and safe treatment requires familiarity with drug effects and interactions, and careful patient selection and education. We would suggest that use of these drugs remains restricted to prescription by psychiatric physicians.

Tricyclic antidepressants: principles of drug therapy in soft tissue disorders

There are well over 100 published trials examining the use of TCAs in chronic pain. Around 50 of these trials are controlled studies, the vast majority of which show a significant analgesic effect when compared to placebo. Most clinical trials report a reduction of pain from moderate or severe to mild in about two-thirds of patients given drug treatment with TCAs. It is rare to obtain complete pain relief. There is very little evidence that a particular TCA has superior analgesic efficacy, and the choice of TCA should be tailored to the specific needs of a particular patient. Thus, patients with poor sleep patterns may benefit from an antidepressant agent with more pronounced sedative effects. Intolerance to particular adverse effects, for example, dry mouth, may warrant a change to a TCA with a better side-effect profile, for example, desipramine or maprotiline.

In general, the adverse effects of the TCAs are mild and tend to diminish with continued use. Tolerance to the daytime sedation frequently encountered when the drug is first taken can occur within days, and the patient should be encouraged to persevere with treatment. Tolerance to antimuscarinic side-effects, including dry mouth and constipation, can take several weeks to develop. Orthostatic hypotension due to α-adrenergic blockade can be troublesome, especially in the elderly, and drugs like imipramine with potent α-antagonist activity should be avoided (Table 4). Nortriptyline has a better

cardiovascular side-effect profile and is recommended in at-risk patients. Surgical support stockings can help to an extent and, in severe cases, the use of mineralocorticoid agents may be considered. Cardiac effects of the TCAs are due to anticholinergic and quinidine-like properties and are generally only seen in overdose situations, but the drugs should be used with caution in elderly patients and patients with cardiac risk factors. In trial patients, delerium and drowsiness are the most common reasons for discontinuation of treatment.

The relative frequency of adverse effects, albeit mild and transient ones, can lead to problems with patient compliance, particularly when the patient does not perceive immediate analgesic benefit after taking the drug. Patients should be warned of the more common side-effects but reassured that they will diminish with time. Education of the patient is essential. They should be informed that the analgesic effects of the antidepressant medication may take days or weeks to develop, and that the drug must be taken on a regular basis to have effect. It is not uncommon for patients to report taking the medication intermittently as a supplement to simple analgesics 'when the pain is bad'. Crucial to ensuring patient compliance is the need to emphasize that the drugs are being given to the patient for their analgesic effects and not for their antidepressant properties.

Abrupt withdrawal of the antidepressant drugs should be avoided as it can cause a variety of unpleasant symptoms, thought to be related to rebound cholinergic activity. These include vivid dreams, restlessness, and gastrointestinal hyperactivity. These symptoms can be minimized if the drug dose is reduced gradually over a period of 5–10 days.

Amitriptyline

Evidence for the efficacy of amitriptyline in the treatment of chronic pain has been supported by trials in disorders as diverse as osteoarthritis, rheumatoid arthritis, fibromyalgia, diabetic neuropathy, chronic facial pain, and postherpetic neuralgia. It blocks the reuptake of noradrenaline to a greater extent than serotonin, and is a potent antagonist at muscarinic and α_1-adrenergic receptors, giving rise to the most frequently occurring side-effects of dry mouth and sedation. It should be avoided in patients with narrow-angle glaucoma. Other common adverse effects include constipation, urinary retention, and weight gain.

Studies generally show median analgesic doses of 50–75 mg, but there is wide variation in the patient population, and patients may require much smaller or larger doses to gain analgesic efficacy. As with other TCAs, the severity of side-effects can be reduced by gradually increasing the dose given. A starting dose of 25 mg (10 mg in the elderly) is usually given at night to minimize daytime sedation, and can be increased by 10–25 mg every 7–10 days until analgesia occurs, or dose escalation is limited by unacceptable side-effects. Again, the patient can be reassured that adverse effects do tend to diminish with time. The co-prescription of stool softeners and methylcellulose mouth spray may help reduce symptoms.

Nortriptyline

This is primarily a noradrenaline reuptake blocker and is the active metabolism of amitriptyline. It has mild sedative and antihistaminergic activity, but is associated with less cardiovascular and antimuscarinic effects, making it a useful drug for use in elderly patients.

Imipramine

This well-studied drug inhibits noradrenaline reuptake to a greater extent than serotonin and is thought to be less sedating than amitriptyline, with a lower incidence of orthostatic hypotension.

Table 4 Comparison of adverse reactions of tricyclic antidepressant drugs

Drug	Sedative effects	Anticholinergic potency	Orthostatic hypotension
Amitriptyline	High	High	High
Trimipramine	High	Moderate	Moderate
Doxepin	High	Moderate	Moderate
Trazodone	High	Low	Moderate
Imipramine	Moderate	High	Moderate
Nortriptyline	Moderate	Moderate	Low
Clomipramine	Moderate	Moderate	Moderate
Desipramine	Low	Low	Low

Desipramine and maprotiline

These are relatively pure noradrenaline reuptake blockers, and are associated with better side-effect profiles than the older, mixed drugs. Desipramine has little antimuscarinic and antihistaminergic activity, and is less sedating than amitriptyline. Maprotiline is a tetracyclic agent with little antimuscarinic activity, fewer cardiac side-effects, but moderate sedative action. The analgesic efficacy of both desipramine and maprotiline has been demonstrated in controlled trials. The drugs are probably less effective than amitriptyline. However, a study comparing amitriptyline with maprotiline for the treatment of postherpetic neuralgia showed a small number of patients who responded to maprotiline but not to amitriptyline, suggesting that for some patients, noradrenaline-based inhibitory pathways predominate.[67]

Selective serotonin reuptake inhibitors

Although selective serotonin reuptake inhibitor drugs have been studied in a variety of chronic pain conditions, results have generally been disappointing, and many trials did not support the clinical use of the drugs.

Anticonvulsants

There are many similarities between pathological processes causing the neuropathic pain associated with many soft tissue disorders and those causing seizure activity in neurons in epilepsy. Both conditions are characterized by hyperexcitable neurons that display spontaneous or paroxysmal action potential activity, and by the activation of NMDA receptors centrally, leading to oversensitivity of the normal nerve pathways. The activation of NMDA receptors causes wind-up in neuropathic pain and kindling in epilepsy.

Recognition of the similarities between epileptiform activity and the spontaneous neuronal activity witnessed in some pain syndromes led to the successful use in 1962 of carbamazepine for the pain associated with trigeminal neuralgia.[68] Since then, the anticonvulsant agents have been extensively used in a wide variety of neuropathic pain syndromes, particularly those associated with 'lancinating' or 'shooting' pain. Animal studies have shown that peripheral nerve fibres in persistent pain syndromes have altered expression of certain ion channels, particularly novel sodium channels,[69] and *N*-type calcium channels.[70, 71] This would suggest that anticonvulsant agents that block sodium or calcium channels might have analgesic efficacy in a much broader range of neuropathic pain syndromes, and in inflammatory pain states.[72, 73]

Carbamazepine

Carbamazepine is well-established as the first-line treatment for trigeminal neuralgia, but it also has efficacy in the treatment of neuropathic pain caused by a number of other pathologies. Carbamazepine's ability to block sodium channels (like other anticonvulsant agents) is frequency-dependent. This means that it preferentially blocks spontaneously active fibres conducting abnormal pain sensation, while sparing normal nerve conduction.

Older studies showing efficacy in disorders such as trigeminal neuralgia and painful diabetic neuropathy suffered from poor study methodology, but results have been confirmed by newer and better-designed trials.[74–78] Carbamazepine has also been found to be effective in carpal tunnel syndrome, suggesting possible efficacy in other nerve entrapment neuropathies.[79]

Carbamazepine can be given in tablet or chewable tablet form at a start dose of 200 mg twice daily, gradually increasing to a therapeutic dose of 800–1200 mg daily in divided doses, although studies have suggested doses up to 2400 mg daily. Blood levels of 4–10 µg/ml are thought to be within the therapeutic range. The major adverse effects are somnolence, dizziness, and gait disturbance, but the drug has also been known to cause haematological problems such as thrombocytopenia and pancytopenia. For this reason, baseline haematological studies should be performed and repeated regularly at the start of treatment and intermittently once treatment has been established.

Phenytoin

The analgesic effect of phenytoin is thought to be due to suppression of sodium channels and inhibition of presynaptic glutamate release. Randomized studies have been conducted on patients with painful diabetic neuropathy and cancer pain, but have given conflicting results.[80, 81] The usual adult starting dose is 100 mg two to three times daily and is associated with adverse effects that include hirsutism, ataxia, diplopia, and confusion. Gingival hyperplasia can occur with long-term use.

Valproic Acid

Valproate works by prolonging repolarization of voltage-gated sodium channels and by increasing GABA levels in the brain. It has been shown to relieve pain in 50–80 per cent of patients with trigeminal neuralgia, but data from good clinical trials are sparse. It may have a useful role in treatment of migraines and head and neck pains. The usual starting dose is 15 mg/kg/day, and this can be increased weekly by 5–10 mg/kg/day to a maximal dose of 60 mg/kg. Side-effects of nausea, vomiting, anorexia, and diarrhoea tend to lessen with time. Other adverse effects include sedation, ataxia, rashes, transient alopecia, weight gain, and liver damage. Liver function tests should be monitored during treatment.

Benzodiazepines

The GABA-A agonists, lorazepam, clonazepam, and nitrazepam have all been used in neuropathic pain, but failed to demonstrate analgesic properties in clinical trials.

Lamotrigine

This newer anticonvulsant agent works, again, by blocking voltage-dependent sodium channels and inhibiting glutamate release at the dorsal horn. Studies have shown analgesic efficacy in the treatment of neuropathic pain refractory to therapy with carbamazepine and phenytoin, in trigeminal neuralgia, HIV-associated painful sensory neuropathy, and painful diabetic neuropathy.[82, 83] Studies have used daily doses of 50–400 mg, and it is believed that the higher doses may be more beneficial. Adverse effects of dizziness, somnolence, constipation, nausea, and diplopia were tolerated better when the dosage was escalated slowly.

Gabapentin

Gabapentin was developed as a structural GABA analogue, but has no direct action on GABA receptors or metabolism. It is thought to have a central site of action and may work by binding to the $\alpha_2\delta$ subunit of voltage-dependent calcium channels, blocking calcium influx into the neuronal cell.[84] The development of gabapentin as an analgesic agent has been a major advance in the treatment of neuropathic pain. Large-scale studies have shown gabapentin to be effective in the treatment of neuropathic pain associated with diabetic neuropathy and postherpetic neuralgia,[85, 86] and a further randomized control trial has shown similar efficacy to amitriptyline in diabetic neuropathy peripheral pain.[87] Studies also showed that patients treated with gabapentin had improvements in some measures of quality of life, including sleep and mood.

The dose of gabapentin can be escalated over a period of 2 weeks from 900 to 3600 mg daily, administered in three divided doses. Most studies show analgesic efficacy with daily doses greater than 1800 mg. Analgesia seems to be maintained for the duration of treatment.

The major advantage of gabapentin over other co-analgesic agents used in the treatment of neuropathic pain is the relative lack of adverse effects associated with drug treatment. The main side-effects, dizziness and somnolence, tend to diminish with time, and the drug is associated with few drug interactions. This gives a strong argument for its use as a first-line treatment in neuropathic pain, particularly in the elderly patient, and may justify its expense when compared to other co-analgesic agents. Another GABA analogue drug, pregabalin, may have similar actions and is likely to be more efficacious.

Local anaesthetic agents

The use of local anaesthetic peripheral and regional nerve blocking techniques is a recognized treatment modality in the chronic pain associated with soft tissue disorders, and will be covered in Chapter 5.5. The rationale behind the use of nerve blockade in chronic pain is to disrupt the peripheral nervous input that may be partly responsible for the maintenance of central sensitization at the dorsal horn. Recently, the lidocaine patch has been used in postherpetic neuralgia to block peripheral sensitization, and may have a place in the treatment of other chronic pain disorders. In addition, the ability of low-concentration, systemically administered local anaesthetic agents to block sodium channels can be used to target the increased expression of sodium (and other) ion channels found in chronic pain conditions. This is similar to the rationale behind the use of anticonvulsant agents. In clinical practice, this is most commonly achieved by the use of lidocaine infusions, and the administration of oral sodium channel blockers such as mexiletine.

Local anaesthetic agents work by binding and inhibiting voltage-gated sodium channels. Sodium channels alternate between three different conformational states—resting, open, and inactivated. As local anaesthetics bind open and inactivated channels more readily than resting channels, they have greater affinity for frequently activated channels that spend less time in a resting state. This frequency-dependency is responsible for the anti-arrhythmic action of local anaesthetic agents and for their ability to target nociceptor fibres in chronic pain conditions. Local anaesthetics also inhibit, to a lesser extent, potassium and calcium channels, nicotinic acetylcholine receptors, and β-adrenoceptors.

Local anaesthetics consist of an aromatic ring connected via an ester or amide link to a hydrocarbon chain containing a tertiary amino group. The aromatic ring confers a degree of lipid solubility to the molecule, while the amino group can exist as a neutral free-base form or can gain a proton, becoming positively charged. At higher tissue pH, larger proportions of the free-base form occur, making the local anaesthetic agent more soluble. More lipophilic agents such as bupivacaine,

ropivacaine, and etidocaine bind to receptor sites on sodium channels more readily, increasing their potency. Lipid solubility also correlates with increased protein binding and duration of action. Local anaesthetics are stereospecific with the $R(+)$ stereoisomers showing greater potency than the $S(-)$ stereoisomers. These differences are more pronounced in cardiac conduction tissue, when local anaesthetic agents are more likely to bind to the inactivated sodium channels, than in nerve tissue, where they have greater affinity for sodium channels in the open state. Thus, new anaesthetic agents such as ropivacaine and levobupivacaine are formulated as the $S(-)$ isomer to reduce cardiac toxicity without significantly decreasing their ability to block peripheral nerve conduction.

Smaller nerve fibres are more susceptible to blockade by local anaesthetic, and anaesthetic agents are more likely to block small Aδ and, to a lesser extent, C fibres carrying pain sensation than large motor fibres. Thus, there is an inherent degree of differential blockade. This preferential blockade of sensory fibres is more pronounced at low anaesthetic concentrations and with agents such as bupivacaine and ropivacaine.

Increasing systemic concentrations of local anaesthetic lead to central nervous system (CNS) and cardiovascular system toxicity. As blood concentrations rise, initial disruption of inhibitory fibres in the CNS causes unopposed excitation, leading to symptoms such as circumoral and peripheral paraesthesia, tinnitus, visual abnormalities, muscular twitching, and, eventually, seizures. Higher blood concentrations cause progressive blockade of excitatory fibres in the CNS, causing respiratory depression and coma, and cardiovascular system toxicity, causing conduction defects and cardiac arrest. With more potent agents like bupivacaine, CNS and cardiovascular toxicity occur at lower blood concentrations. In addition, with racemic bupivacaine, the difference between a blood concentration that causes seizures and that causing cardiac arrest is greatly diminished.

Topical lidocaine

A topical lidocaine patch preparation, Lidoderm, has recently been approved by the United States Food and Drug Administration (FDA) for the treatment of postherpetic neuralgia. The patch consists of an adhesive dressing infused with a preparation containing 5 per cent lidocaine (700 mg per patch), and has shown reasonable efficacy in clinical trials with minimal systemic absorption of the local anaesthetic agent.[88–91] It is thought to work by local action on peripheral nociceptors, blocking transmission of impulses to the dorsal horn and, consequently, decreasing peripheral maintenance of central sensitization. Its ease of use and lack of side-effects may encourage use in postherpetic neuralgia as well as other neuropathic pain disorders.

Lidocaine infusion

Intravenous infusions of lidocaine have been used in the treatment of chronic pain for over 10 years and were first noted to be effective in the treatment of painful diabetic neuropathy.[92] Since then, they have been studied in many neuropathic pain disorders, including fibromyalgia, facial pain, and cancer pain. Results show that intravenous lidocaine is an effective analgesic, particularly in pain associated with nerve injury.[25] In a clinical trial studying its use in fibromyalgia, lidocaine was found to give significantly better pain relief than placebo, but the effect tended to be short-lived, with analgesia lasting up to 1 week after the infusion.[93] Studies using lidocaine infusions for cancer pain showed no significant effect.

Lidocaine infusion is clearly an impractical method of long-term treatment for neuropathic pain, and it tends to be used to identify a subpopulation of patients with neuropathic pain who respond to local anaesthetic agents. Susceptible patients can be commenced on a trial of oral local anaesthetic therapy with drugs such as mexiletine.

There are significant dangers associated with the intravenous infusion of local anaesthetics, and trials must be performed in a clinical setting with fasted patients, immediate access to resuscitation drugs and equipment, full monitoring, and a clinician with skills in resuscitation that should include intubation and ventilation and a familiarity with the particular problems associated with local anaesthesia toxicity. Studies show efficacy with an intravenous dose of 5 mg/kg given over at least 30 minutes.[25] The patient must be continuously monitored for signs and symptoms of toxicity. Electrocardiogram (ECG) monitoring throughout is mandatory. Minor adverse effects are common and include circumoral paraesthesia, drowsiness, and nausea. The infusion rate may be reduced. Worsening symptoms or the presence of motor effects such as weakness, dysarthria, or tremor necessitate discontinuation of the infusion. Similarly, evidence of ECG changes, fitting, or significant drop in blood pressure warrant immediate withdrawal from treatment.

Mexiletine

Patients who respond to lidocaine infusion may be started on a trial of its oral analogue, mexiletine. Again, mexiletine showed most benefit in patients with nerve injury pain, but analgesia also occurred in pain due to diabetic neuropathy.[94, 95] A trial studying mexiletine therapy in spinal cord injury dysaesthetic pain showed no benefit.[96]

Studies showed greatest efficacy in higher doses of 675–750 mg/day, but these doses were also associated with more side-effects, including nausea, constipation, and tremor.

Atypical analgesic drugs

Adrenoceptor agonists

α_2-Adrenoceptor agonist drugs were originally introduced as antihypertensive agents, but their sedative and antinociceptive effects were soon recognized. The α_2-adrenoceptors are present throughout the nervous system, but are especially abundant in primary sensory afferent terminals, the superficial laminae of the spinal cord, and brainstem nuclei, including the locus ceruleus. Presynaptic activation of α_2-adrenoceptors inhibits noradrenaline release from the nerve terminal, producing sympatholytic effects, but may also enhance the release of acetylcholine, producing cholinergic side-effects such as dry mouth and blurred vision. Activation of central postsynaptic α_2-adrenoceptors increases potassium conductance, causing hyperpolarization and reduced excitability of the nerve cell. The α_{2A} receptor subtype is thought to be responsible for the analgesic action of adrenoceptor agonists such as clonidine,[97] but action at other receptors including serotonin, acetylcholine, and imidazoline may be important. α_{2B} receptors mediate hypertension and vasoconstriction and antagonism of these receptors is responsible for the major side-effects of the agonist drugs.

Clonidine

Clonidine has agonist activity at α_2 and imidazoline receptors and is an effective analgesic when given intravenously or via the epidural or intrathecal routes. Oral preparations also exist, and are well-absorbed, with 75–95 per cent bioavailability. Clonidine's greater potency when given centrally means that analgesic efficacy can be obtained with smaller doses, reducing the incidence of side-effects. Clonidine has been shown to augment the analgesic potency of epidural local anaesthetic agents and opioids, and has proven efficacy in chronic pain disorders including cancer pain.[98, 99]

Epidural and intravenous doses of clonidine are similar, with typical adult doses of 150–500 μg. This compares to an intrathecal dose of 50 μg. The intravenous drug should be given as a slow infusion to minimize the risk of sudden hypotension.

The major side-effects are sedation and hypotension. The latter is caused primarily by central sympatholysis, and may be compounded by concomitant bradycardia. Chronic administration leads to a risk of rebound hypertension if withdrawn suddenly.

NMDA receptor antagonists

The development and maintenance of central sensitization in chronic pain disorders is dependent upon the function of dorsal horn NMDA receptors. These receptors govern the opening of a postsynaptic ion channel permeable to calcium (II) and other ions. Ion channel activation is subject to partial depolarization of the postsynaptic membrane, caused by prior excitation of other postsynaptic receptors. Continued release of glutamate from the peripheral nerve terminal due to high-frequency nociceptor stimulation, results in the opening of the NMDA receptor channel, causing a massive influx of calcium into the dorsal horn neuron. This depolarizes the postsynaptic membrane, generates a prolonged reduction in the threshold potential, and activates several intracellular secondary messenger systems, leading to augmented protein synthesis, altered expression of receptor proteins, and the production of local regulating factors including NOS and nerve growth factor.

These changes lead to sensitization of the dorsal horn neurons, altered receptor expression, structural changes to nerve pathways, and activation of high-threshold wide dynamic range neurons in the dorsal horn, and are ultimately responsible for the phenomena of spontaneous ongoing pain, allodynia, hyperalgesia, and wind-up seen in chronic pain conditions.

NMDA receptor antagonists have been proven to prevent the development of the above changes in acute pain models, but also have a place in treatment of established chronic pain syndromes, and have proven efficacy in peripheral and central neuropathic pain, muscular pain, ischaemic pain, and cancer pain. The major factor limiting their widespread use is the occurrence of dose-limiting side-effects, including sedation, nausea, dissociative reactions, dizziness, and visual distortions.

Ketamine

Ketamine has been used as an anaesthetic agent for over 30 years and it was recognized from very early on that subanaesthetic doses produced analgesia. Ketamine is a non-competitive NMDA antagonist that acts at the phencyclidine (PCP)-binding site in the NMDA receptor.[100] There is a close correlation between analgesic efficacy and serum concentrations of ketamine but, in general, doses of less than one-fifth the anaesthetic dose (serum concentrations less than 1 μmol/L) are sufficient to give some pain relief. The drug can be given using various routes of administration but trials most frequently report the use of intravenous boluses of 0.1–0.45 mg/kg, followed in some studies by infusions of around 5–7 μg/kg/min. One double-blind study in a patient with glossopharyngeal neuralgia reports statistically significant pain relief following 10 2-day treatments with oral ketamine at a dose of 60 mg six times daily.[101] Controlled studies show good analgesic efficacy in peripheral and central neuropathic pain, fibromyalgia, and chronic ischaemic pain. Some case studies report analgesic effects lasting several weeks following treatment with ketamine.

Psychotomimetic adverse effects include unpleasant dreams, hallucinations, visual and auditory disturbances, cognitive impairment, and disturbed proprioception and limit the value of ketamine as an analgesic agent. However, promising results have been obtained using a combination of low-dose ketamine and opioid. Ketamine appears to have a synergistic action with opioids and interferes with mechanisms giving rise to tolerance. The use of low-dose ketamine–opioid combinations in patients with cancer pain has given good analgesia, with dramatic decreases in the daily dose of opioid.[40–42]

Other NMDA-receptor antagonists

The NMDA-antagonists dextromethorphan and amantadine have shown effectiveness in patients with central and peripheral neuropathic pain syndromes, diabetic neuropathy, postherpetic neuralgia, and cancer pain, and are thought to have better side-effect profiles compared to ketamine. Amantadine, in particular, has shown analgesic efficacy with minimal adverse effects. In one study in patients with cancer pain, the most severe side-effect reported after successful treatment with infusions of amantadine (200 mg over 3 h) was dry mouth.

Recent evidence shows that the opioid agent, methadone, has NMDA-antagonist properties, explaining effectiveness in the treatment of chronic pain.[53]

Capsaicinoids

The nociceptive effects of capsaicin have been known about for more than 50 years, but it is only in recent years that the idea (and eventual cloning) of a specific vanilloid receptor has been accepted. The effect of vanilloid receptor activation is to produce a non-selective increase in cation permeability at a specific channel in the peripheral nociceptor membrane. Depolarization of the membrane leads to increased sensitivity of the peripheral nociceptor, and augments release of neurokinins at the nerve terminal. The immediate pain precedes a transient period of antinociception caused by desensitization of the neuron. Further degeneration of neuronal axons and nerve terminals can lead to long-term impairment of nociception, and is the basis for the use of capsaicin in chronic pain conditions.

Capsaicinoids are thought to be more useful for the burning pain associated with noxious C-fibre signalling, and have been used clinically in conditions as diverse as postmastectomy pain syndrome, postherpetic neuralgia, peripheral neuropathy, arthritis, and bony fractures. Clinical trials using topically applied capsaicin cream show good results for pain due to diabetic neuropathy, postherpetic neuralgia, and pain after nerve injury.[102–106] Previous studies used capsaicin concentrations of less than 1 per cent. However, recent studies using much higher concentrations (7.5–10 per cent) of capsaicin under regional anaesthetic are very promising, with pain relief reported to last for several months following a single treatment.[107]

Cannabinoids

The endogenous cannabinoid system is thought to have a physiological role in the tonic regulation of pain thresholds. There is good evidence that cannabinoid receptor agonists induce selective inhibition of nociceptive processing through the activation of CB_1 receptors in the spinal cord and thalamus,[108, 109] and may have a synergistic action with opioids, perhaps by inducing the release of κ opioids.[110–112]

However, despite the initial promise that cannabinoids may contribute greatly to our ability to treat pain, initial studies in humans have been disappointing, with cannabinoids showing similar efficacy to codeine, but with more problematic CNS side-effects.[113] Most of the studies performed so far have been in acute pain conditions, and judgement in chronic pain should be reserved until more studies are available.

Other drug classes

GABA-B receptor agonists

The skeletal muscle relaxant, baclofen, is an agonist at GABA-B receptors and has been shown to give significant pain relief in trigeminal neuralgia.[114, 115] It is also used frequently in patients with chronic pain associated with muscular spasm, for example, lower back pain. Dosing is usually started at 5 mg 2–3 times daily and gradually increased until effective. Some patients require more than 100 mg daily. Adverse effects include sedation, drowsiness, and hypotonia.

Corticosteroids

Corticosteroids have been used in the treatment of chronic pain conditions, both systemically and as an adjunct to local anaesthetic nerve blocking techniques. The mechanism of action is unknown, but may involve anti-inflammatory actions or direct alteration in nerve function. An important mode of action in soft tissue disorders may relate to a reduction in oedema around damaged nerves. The use of systemic corticosteroids is associated with major adverse effects and should probably be confined to cancer patients.

Sympathetic blockers and calcitonin

Patients with soft tissue disorders often have pain that is closely related to sympathetic nervous system activation. Such sympathetically mediated pain has been shown to respond to sympathetic blockers such as guanethidine and to treatment with calcitonin.[116, 117] Such treatment, however, is not supported by clinical trials in large groups of patients though reports of individual dramatic responses are common.

Conclusion

Pharmacological treatment is an important part of the multimodal approach to the management of chronic pain associated with soft tissue disorders. Our knowledge of the physiological processes that cause pain has improved our understanding of the mechanisms of action of available drugs, and enabled us to utilize the different drugs in the most effective ways. The expansion of pain physiology has also exposed a vast array of new therapeutic targets for future drug development.[118] Drugs acting at many of these targets are already in advanced stages of development. We can be confident that pharmacological agents will become even more important at providing successful treatment of pain associated with soft tissue disorders in the future.

References

1. World Health Organization (WHO) (1996). *Cancer pain relief*, 2nd edn. WHO, Geneva.

2. Takeda, F. (1991). WHO cancer pain relief programme. *Pain Res. Clin. Management* **4**, 467–474.

3. Neugebauer, V., Geisslinger, G., *et al.* (1995). Antinociceptive effects of R(−)- and S(+)-flurbiprofen on rat spinal dorsal horn neurons rendered hyperexcitable by an acute knee joint inflammation. *J. Pharmacol. Exp. Ther.* **275**, 618–628.

4. Weissman, G. (1993). Prostaglandins as modulators rather than mediators of inflammation. *J. Lipid Med.* **6**, 275–286.

5. England, S., Bevan, S., and Docherty, R.J. (1996). PGE2 modulates the tetrodotoxin-resistant sodium current in neonatal rat dorsal root ganglion neurones via the cyclic AMP-protein kinase A cascade. *J. Physiol. (London)* **495**, 429–440.

6. Akopian, A.N., Sivilotti, L., and Wood, J.N. (1996). A tetrodotoxin-resistant sodium channel expressed by sensory neurones. *Nature* **379**, 257–262.

7. Malmberg, A.B., Rafferty, M.F., and Yaksh, T.L. (1994). Antinociceptive effect of spinally delivered prostaglandin E receptor antagonists in the formalin test on the rat. *Neurosci. Lett.* **173** (1–2), 193–196.

8. Minami, T., Uda, R., Horiguchi, S., Ito, S., Hyodo, M., and Hayaishi, O. (1994). Allodynia evoked by intrathecal administration of prostaglandin E2 to conscious mice. *Pain* **57** (2), 217–223.

9. Nicol, G.D., Klingberg, D., and Vasco, M.R. (1992). Prostaglandin E2 increases calcium conductance and stimulates release of substance P in avian sensory neurons. *J. Neurosci.* **12**, 1917–1927.

10. Beiche, F., Scheuerer, S., Brune, K., Geisslinger, G., and Goppelt-Struebe, M. (1996). Up-regulation of cyclooxygenase-2 mRNA in the rat spinal cord following peripheral inflammation. *FEBS Lett.* **390**, 165–169.

11. Feng, L., Sun, W., Xia, Y., *et al.* (1993). Cloning two isoforms of rat cyclooxygenase: differential regulation of their expression. *Arch. Biochem. Biophys.* **307**, 361–368.

12. Geisslinger, G. and Yaksh, T.L. (2000). Spinal actions of cyclooxygenase inhibitors. In *Proceedings of the 9th World Congress on Pain*, Vol. 16 (ed. M. Devor, M.C. Rowbotham, and Z. Weisenfeld-Hallin), pp. 771–785. IASP Press, Seattle.

13. Bjorkman, R., Hallman, K.M., Hedner, J., Hedner, T., and Henning, M. (1994). Acetaminophen blocks, spinal hyperalgesia induced by NMDA and substance, P. *Pain* **57**, 259–264.

14. Uphouse, L.A., Welch, S.P., Ward, C.R., Ellis, E.F., and Embrey, J.P. (1993). Antinociceptive activity of intrathecal ketorolac is blocked by the kappa-opioid receptor antagonist, nor-binaltorphimine. *Eur. J. Pharmacol.* **242**, 53–58.

15. Brune, K., Rainsford, K.D., and Schweitzer, A. (1980). Biodistribution of mild analgesics. *Br. J. Clin. Pharmacol.* **10** (suppl 2), 279–284.

16. Schnitzer, T.J., Truitt, K., Fleischmann, R., Dalgin, P., Block, J., Zeng, Q., Bolognese, J., Seidenberg, B., and Ehrich, E.W. (1999). The safety profile, tolerability, and effective dose range of rofecoxib in the treatment of rheumatoid arthritis. *Clin. Therapeut.* **21** (10), 1688–1702.

17. Langman, M.J., Jensen, D.M., Watson, D.J., Harper, S.E., Zhao, P.L., Quan, H., Bolognese, J., and Simon, T.J. (1999). Adverse upper gastrointestinal effects of rofecoxib compared with NSAIDs. *J. Am. Med. Assoc.* **282** (20), 1929–1933.

18. Silverstein, F.E., Faich, G., Goldstein, J.L., Simon, L.S., Pincus, T., Whelton, A., Makuch, R., Eisen, G., Agrawal, N.M., Stenson, W.F., *et al.* (2000). Gastrointestinal toxicity with Celecoxib vs nonsteroidal antiinflammatory drugs for osteoarthritis and rheumatoid arthritis: the CLASS study: a randomised controlled trial. *J. Am. Med. Assoc.* **284** (10), 1247–1255.

19. Justins, D. (1996). Basic principle of chronic pain management. In *pain—an updated review* (ed. J.N. Campbell), pp. 255–267. IASP Press Seattle.

20. Bradley, J.D., Brandt, K.D., Katz, B.P., *et al.* (1992). Treatment of knee osteoarthritis: relationship of clinical features of joint inflammation to the response to a nonsteroidal antiinflammatory drug or pure analgesic. *J. Rheumatol.* **19**, 1950–1954.

21. Riedermann, P.J., Bersinic, S., Cuddy, L.J., Torrance, G.W., and Tugwell, P.X. (1993). A study to determine the efficacy and safety of tenoxicam versus piroxicam, diclofenac and indomethacin in patients with osteoarthritis: a meta-analysis. *J. Rheumatol.* **20**, 2095–2103.

22. Eisenberg, E., Berkey, C., Carr, D.B., Mosteller, F., and Chalmers, T.C. (1994). Efficacy and safety of nonsteroidal antiinflammatory drugs for cancer pain: a meta-analysis. *J. Clin. Oncol.* **12**, 2756–2765.

23. Tramer, M.R., Williams, J.E., Carroll, D., *et al.* (1995). Comparing analgesic efficacy of non-steroidal anti-inflammatory drugs given by different routes in acute and chronic pain. A qualitative systematic review. *Acta Anaesthesiol. Scand.* **42**, 71–79.

24. Stalnikowicz, R. and Rachmilewitz, D. (1993). NSAID-induced gastroduodenal damage: is prevention needed? *J. Clin. Gastroenterol.* **17**, 238–243.

25. McQuay, H.J. and Moore, R.A. (1998). *An evidence-based resource for pain relief*. Oxford Medical Publications, Oxford.

26. Moore, R.A., Tramer, M.R., Carroll, D., Wiffen, P.J., and McQuay, H.J. (1998). Quantitative systematic review of topically applied non-steroidal anti-inflammatory drugs. *Br. Med. J.* **316**, 333–338.

27. Lane, N.E. (1997). Pain management in osteoarthritis: the role of COX-2 inhibitors. *J. Rheumatol.* **24** (suppl. 49), 20–24.

28. Malmstrom, K., Daniels, D.O., Kotey, P., Seidenberg, B., and Desjardins, P.J. (1999). Comparison of Rofecoxib and Celecoxib, two cyclooxygenase-2 inhibitors, in postoperative dental pain: a randomized, placebo- and active-comparator-controlled clinical trial. *Clin. Therapeut.* **21** (10), 1653–1663.

29. Fricke, J., Morrison, B.W., Fite, S., Sandler, M., Yuan, W., Howard, C., and Seidenberg, B. (1999). MK-966 versus naproxen sodium 550 mg in post-surgical dental pain. *Clin. Pharmacol. Therapeut.* **65** (2), 118.

30. Brown, J., Morrison, B.W., Christensen, S., Dunkley, V., Turpin, M., Sandler, M., Yuan, W., Lesneski, L., and Seidenberg, B. (1999). VIOXX 50 mg versus ibuprofen 400 mg in post-surgical dental pain. *J. Clin. Pharmacol.* **39** (9), 974.

31. Watson, D.J., Harper, S.E., Zhao, P.L., Quan, H., Bolognese, J., and Simon, T.J. (2000). Gastrointestinal tolerability of the selective cyclooxygenase-2 (COX-2) inhibitor rofecoxib compared with nonselective COX-1 and COX-2 inhibitors in osteoarthritis. *Arch. Intern. Med.* **160** (19), 2998–3003.

32. Arnér, S. and Meyerson, B.A. (1988). Lack of analgesia effect of opioids on neuropathic and idiopathic forms of pain. *Pain* **33**, 11–23.

33. Rowbotham, M., Reisner-Keller, L., and Fields, H. (1991). Both intravenous lidocaine and morphine reduce the pain of post-herpetic neuralgia. *Neurology* **41**, 1024–1028.

34. Kupers, R.C., Konings, H., Adriaensen, H., and Gybels, J.M. (1991). Morphine differentially affects the sensory and affective pain ratings in neurogenic and idiopathic forms of pain. *Pain* **47**, 5–12.

35. Dellemijn, P.L. and Vanneste, J.A. (1997). Randomized double-blind active-placebo-controlled crossover trial of intravenous fentanyl in neuropathic pain. *Lancet* **349**, 753–758.

36. Changes in pain, mood, and sensation from i.v. fentanyl in patients with PHN. October. 1997; 16th Annual Scientific Meeting.

37. Harati, Y., Gooch, C., Swenson, M., Edelman, S., Greene, D., *et al.* (1998). Double-blind randomized trial of tramadol for the treatment of the pain of diabetic neuropathy. *Neurology* **50**, 1842–1846.

38. Krames, E. (1996). Intraspinal opioid therapy for chronic nonmalignant pain: current practice and clinical guidelines. *J. Pain Symptom Manage.* **11**, 333–352.

39. Watson, C.P. and Babul, N. (1998). Efficacy of oxycodone in neuropathic pain: a randomized trial in postherpetic neuralgia. *Neurology* **50**, 1837–1841.

40. Yang, C.Y., Wong, C.S., Chang, J.Y., and Ho, S.T. (1996). Intrathecal ketamine reduces morphine requirements in patients with terminal cancer pain. *Can. J. Anaesth.* **43**, 379–383.

41. Wong, C.S., Lu, C.C., Cherng, C.H., and Ho, S.T. (1997). Pre-emptive analgesia with ketamine, morphine and epidural lidocaine prior to total knee replacement. *Can. J. Anaesth.* **44**, 31–37.

42. Chia, Y.Y., Liu, K., Liu, Y.C., Chang, H.C., and Wong, C.S. (1998). Adding ketamine in a multimodal patient-controlled epidural regimen reduces post-operative pain and analgesic consumption. *Anesth. Analg.* **86**, 1245–1249.

43. Brescia, F., Portenoy, R., Ryan, M., Krasnoff, L., and Gray, G. (1992). Pain, opioid use, and survival in hospitalized patients with advanced cancer. *J. Clin. Oncol.* **10**, 149–155.

44. Porter, J. and Jick, J. (1980). Addiction is rare in patients treated with narcotics. *N. Engl. J. Medi.* **302**, 123.

45. Meunier, J.C. (1997). Nociceptin/orphanin FQ and the opioid receptor-like ORL 1 receptor. *Eur. J. Pharmacol.* **340**, 1–15.

46. Stein, C. (1995). The control of pain in peripheral tissue by opioids. *N. Engl. J. Med.* **332**, 1685–1690.

47. Schafer, M., Carter, L., and Stein, C. (1994). Interleukin-1β and corticotrophin releasing factor inhibit pain by releasing opioids from immune cells in inflamed tissues. *Proc. Nat Acad. Sci., USA* **91**, 4219–4223.

48. Hassan, A.H.S., Ableitner, A., Stein, C., and Herz, A. (1993). Inflammation of the rat paw enhances axonal transport of opioid receptors in the sciatic nerve and increases their density in the inflamed tissue. *Neuroscience* **55**, 185–195.

49. Jadad, A., Carroll, D., Glynn, C., Moore, R., and McQuay, H.J. (1992). Morphine sensitivity of chronic pain: a double-blind randomized crossover study using patient-controlled analgesia. *Lancet* **1**, 1367–1371.

50. Gourlay, G.K. and Cherry, D. (1991). Response to controversy corner: 'can opioids be successfully used to treat severe pain in non-malignant conditions?'. *Clin. J. Pain* **7**, 347–349.

51. Cousins, M.J. and Mather, L. (1984). Intrathecal and epidural administration of opioids. *Anesthesiology* **1**, 276–310.

52. Hogan, Q., Haddox, J., Abram, S., Weissman, D., Taylor, M., and Janjan, N. (1991). Epidural opiates and local anaesthetics for the management of cancer pain. *Pain* **46**, 271–279.

53. Morley, J. and Makin, M. (1998). The use of methadone in cancer pain poorly responsive to other opioids. *Pain Rev.* **5**, 51–58.

54. Raffa, R.B., Friderichs, E., Reimann, W., *et al.* (1992). Opioid and nonopioid components independently contribute to the mechanism of action of tramadol, an 'atypical' opioid analgesic. *J. Pharmacol. Exp. Ther.* **260**, 275–285.

55. Desmeules, J.A., Piguet, V., Collart, T., and Dayer, P. (1996). Contribution of monoaminergic modulation to the analgesic tramadol. *Br. J. Clin. Pharmacol.* **41**, 7–12.

56. Sindrup, S.H., Andersen, G., Madsen, C., Smith, T., Brøsen, K., and Jensen, T.S. (1999). Tramadol relieves pain and allodynia in polyneuropathy: a randomized, double-blind, controlled trial. *Pain* **83**, 85–90.

57. Ruoff, G.E. (1999). Slowing the initial titration rate of tramadol improves tolerability. *Pharmacotherapy* **19**, 88–93.

58. Desmeules, J.A. (2000). The tramadol option. *Euro. J. Pain* **4** (suppl. A), 15–21.

59. Gourlay, G.K., Kowalski, S.L., Plummer, J.L., Cherry, D.A., Gaukroger, P., and Cousins, M.J. (1989). The transdermal administration of fentanyl in the treatment of post-operative pain: pharmacokinetic and pharmacodynamic effects. *Pain* **37**, 193–202.

60. Portenoy, R.K., Southam, M.A., Gupta, S.K., *et al.* (1993). Transdermal fentanyl for cancer pain. *Anaesthiology* **78**, 36–43.

61. Paoli, F., Darcourt, G., and Cossa, P. (1960). Note préliminaire sur l'action de l'imipramine dans les états douloureux. *Rev. Neurol.* **102**, 503–504.

62. Max, M.B., *et al.* (1987). Amitriptyline relieves diabetic neuropathy pain in patients with normal or depressed mood. *Neurology* **37**, 589–596.

63. Sharav, Y., *et al.* (1987). The analgesic effect of amitriptyline on chronic facial pain. *Pain* **31**, 199–209.

64. Peroutko, S.J., Banghart, S.B., and Allen, G.S. (1984). Relative potency and selectivity of calcium antagonists used in the treatment of migraine. *Headache* **24**, 55–58.

65. Krupp, P. and Wesp, M. (1975). Inhibition of prostaglandin synthetase by psychotropic drugs. *Experientia* **31**, 330–331.

66. Gray, A., Spencer, P., and Sewell, R. (1998). The involvement of the opioidergic system in the antinociceptive mechanism of action of antidepressant compounds. *Br. J. Pharmacol.* **124**, 669–674.

67. Watson, C.P., Chipman, M., Reed, K., *et al.* (1992). Amitriptyline versus maprotiline in postherpetic neuralgia: a randomized double-blind crossover trial. *Pain* **48**, 298–336.

68. Blom, S. (1962). Trigeminal neuralgia: its treatment with a new anticonvulsant drug. *Lancet* **1**, 839–840.

69. Waxman, S. (1999). The molecular pathophysiology of pain: abnormal expression of sodium channel genes and its contribution to hyperexcitability of primary sensory neurones. *Pain* **6**, S133–S140.

70. Matthews, E. and Dickenson, A.H. (1999). Plasticity in the effects of the N-type calcium channel blocker, ω-conotoxin GVIA on dorsal horn neuronal activity in normal and neuropathic rats. In *Abstracts—9th World Congress on Pain*. IASP Press, Seattle.

71. Cizkova, D., Marsala, M., Stauderman, K., *et al.* (1998). Calcium channel α1B subunit in spinal cord/DRG of normal and nerve-injured rats. In *Abstracts—9th World Congress on Pain*. IASP Press, Seattle.

72. Chapman, V. and Dickenson, A.H. (1997). Inflammation reveals inhibition of noxious responses of rat spinal neurones by carbamazepine. *Neuroreport* **8**, 1399–1404.

73. Stanfa, L.C., Singh, L., William, R.G., and Dickenson, A.H. (1997). Gabapentin, ineffective in normal rats, markedly reduces C-fibre evoked responses after inflammation. *Neuroreport* **8**, 587–590.

74. Wilton, T. (1974). Tegretol in the treatment of diabetic neuropathy. *S. Afr. Med. J.* **27**, 869–872.

75. Vilming, S.T., Lyberg, T., and Lataste, X. (1986). Tizanidine in the management of trigeminal neuralgia. *Cephalalgia* **6**, 181–182.

76. Lindstrom, P. and Lindblom, U. (1987). The analgesic effect of tocainide in trigeminal neuralgia. *Pain* **28**, 45–50.

77. Lechin, F., van der Dijs, B., Lechin, M.E., *et al.* (1989). Pimozide therapy for trigeminal neuralgia. *Arch. Neurol.* **46**, 960–963.

78. Gomez-Perez, F.J., Choza, R., Ríos, J.M., *et al.* (1996). Nortriptyline–fluphenazine vs. carbamazepine in the symptomatic treatment of diabetic neuropathy. *Arch. Med. Res.* **27**, 525–529.

79. Facchetti, D., Chiroli, S., Bascelli, C., *et al.* (1999). Gabapentin (GBP) versus carbamazepine in conservative treatment of carpal tunnel syndrome [abstract]. *Neurology* **52** (suppl. 2), 203.

80. Yajnik, S., Singh, G.P., Singh, G., and Kumar, M. (1992). Phenytoin as a coanalgesic in cancer pain. *J. Pain Symptom Manage*, **7**, 209–213.

81. Webb, J. and Kamali, F. (1998). Analgesic effects of lamotrigine and phenytoin on cold-induced pain: a crossover placebo-controlled study in healthy volunteers. *Pain* **76**, 357–363.

82. Luria, Y., Brecker, C., Daoud, D., *et al.* (1999). Lamotrigine in the treatment of painful diabetic neuropathy: a randomized, placebo-controlled study. In *Proceedings of the 9th World Congress on Pain* (ed. M. Devor, M.C. Rowbotham, and Z. Weisenfeld-Hallin). IASP Press, Seattle.

83. Eisenberg, E., Alon, N., Avraham, I., Daud, D., and Yarnitski, D. (1998). Lamotrigine in the treatment of diabetic neuropathy. *Eur. J. Neurol.* **5**, 167–173.

84. Gee, N.S., Brown, J.P., Dissanayake, V.U.K., *et al.* (1996). The novel anticonvulsant drug gabapentin (Neurontin) binds to the alpha-2-delta subunit of a calcium channel. *J. Biol. Chem.* **271**, (10), 5768–5776.

85. Backjona, M., Beydoun, A., Edwards, K.R., Schwartz, S.L., Fonseca, V., Hes, M., LaMoreaux, L., and Garofalo, E. (1998). Gabapentin for the symptomatic treatment of painful neuropathy in patients with diabetes mellitus: a randomized controlled trial. *J. Am. Med. Assoc.* **280** (21), 1831–1836.

86. Rowbotham, M., Harden, N., Stacey, B., Bernstein, P., and Magnus-Miller, L. (1998). Gabapentin for the treatment of postherpetic neuralgia: a randomised controlled trial. *J. Am. Med. Assoc.* **280** (21), 1837–1842.

87. Morello, C.M., Leckband, S.G., Stoner, C.P., Moorhouse, D.F., and Sahagian, G.A. (2000). Randomised double-blind study comparing the efficacy of gabapentin with amitriptyline on diabetic peripheral neuropathy pain. *Arch. Intern. Med.* **159** (16), 1931–1937.

88. Argoff, C.E. (2000). New analgesics for neuropathic pain: the lidocaine patch. *Clin. J. Pain* **16**, S62–S66.

89. Rowbotham, M.C., Davies, P.S., and Fields, H. (1995). Topical lidocaine gel relieves postherpetic neuralgia. *Ann. Neurol.* **37**, 246–253.

90. Rowbotham, M.C., Davies, P.S., Verkempinck, C., and Galer, B.S. (1996). Lidocaine patch: double-blind controlled study of a new treatment method for post-herpetic neuralgia. *Pain* **65**, 39–44.

91. Galer, B.S., Rowbotham, M.C., Perander, J., and Friedman, E. (1999). Topical lidocaine patch relieves postherpetic neuralgia more efficiently than a vehicle topical patch: results of an enriched enrollment study. *Pain* **80**, 533–538.

92. Kastrup, J., Peterson, P., Dejgard, A., Angelo, H., and Hilsted, J. (1987). Intravenous lidocaine infusion- a new treatment of chronic painful diabetic neuropathy? *Pain* **28**, 69–75.

93. Sörenson, J., Bengtsson, A., Bäckman, E., Henriksson, K.G., and Bengtsson, M. (1995). Pain analysis in patients with fibromyalgia. *Scand. J. Rheumatol.* **24**, 360–365.

94. Dejgard, A., Peterson, P., and Kastrup, J. (1988). Mexiletine for treatment of chronic painful diabetic neuropathy. *Lancet* **2**, 9–11.

95. Oskarsson, P., Lins, P.E., and Ljunggren, J.G. (1997). Mexiletine Study Group. Efficacy and safety of mexiletine in the treatment of painful diabetic neuropathy. *Diabetes Care* **20**, 1594–1597.

96. Chiou-Tan, F.Y., Tuel, S.M., Johnson, J.C., Priebe, M.M., Hirsh, D.D., and Strayer, J.R. (1996). Effect of mexiletine on spinal cord injury dysthesthetic pain. *Am. J. Phys. Med. Rehabil.* **75**, 84–87.

97. Stone, L.S., Broberger, C., Vulchanova, L., *et al.* (1998). Differential distribution of α2A and α2C adrenergic receptor immunoreactivity in the rat spinal cord. *J. Neurosci.* **18**, 5928–5937.

98. Eisenach, J.C., Rauck, R.L., Buzzanell, C., and Lysak, S.Z. (1989). Epidural clonidine analgesia for intractable cancer pain: phase 1. *Anesthesiology* **71**, 647–652.

99. Eisenach, J.C., DuPen, S., Dubois, M., Miguel, R., and Allin, D. (1995). Epidural Clonidine Study Group. Epidural clonidine analgesia for intractable cancer pain. *Pain* **61**, 391–399.

100. Anis, N.A., Berry, S.C., Burton, N.R., and Lodge, D. (1983). The dissociative anaesthetics, ketamine and phencyclidine, selectively reduce excitation of central mammalian neurones by N-methyl-D-aspartate. *Br. J. Pharmacol.* **79**, 565–575.

101. Eide, P.K. and Stubhaug, A. (1997). Relief of glossopharyngeal neuralgia by ketamine-induced N-methyl-D-aspartate receptor blockade. *Neurosurgery* **41**, 505–508.

102. Bernstein, J.E., Korman, N.J., Bickers, D.R., Dahl, M.V., and Millikan, L.E. (1989). Topical capsaicin treatment of chronic postherpetic neuralgia. *J. Am. Acad. Dermatol.* **21**, 265–270.

103. Watson, C.P. and Evans, R.J. (1992). The post-mastectomy pain syndrome and topical capsaicin: a randomised trial. *Pain* **51**, 375–379.

104. Capsaicin Study Group (1991). Treatment of painful diabetic neuropathy with topical capsaicin. A multicentre, double-blind, vehicle-controlled study. *Arch. Intern. Med.* **151**, 2225–2229.

105. Nolano, M., Simone, D.A., Wendelschafer-Crabb, G., Johnson, T., Hazen, E., and Kennedy, W.R. (1999). Topical capsaicin in humans: parallel loss of epidermal nerve fibers and pain sensation. *Pain* **81**, (1–2), 135–145.

106. McCleane, G. (2000). Topical application of doxepin hydrochloride, capsaicin and a combination of both produces analgesia in chronic human neuropathic pain: a randomized, double-blind, placebo-controlled study. *Br. J. Clin. Pharmacol.* **49** (6), 574–579.

107. Robbins, W.R., Staats, P.S., Levine, J., *et al.* (1998). Treatment of intractable pain with topical large-dose capsaicin: preliminary report. *Anesth. Analg.* **86**, 579–583.

108. Tsou, K., Lowitz, K.A., Hohmann, A.G., Martin, W.J., Hathaway, C.B., Bereiter, D.A., and Walker, J.M. (1996). Suppression of noxious stimulus-evoked expression of fos protein-like immunoreactivity in rat spinal cord by a selective cannabinoid agonist. *Neuroscience* **70**, 791–798.

109. Martin, W.J., Hohmann, A.G., and Walker, J.M. (1996). Suppression of noxious stimulus-evoked activity in the ventral posterolateral nucleus of the thalamus by a cannabinoid agonist: correlation between electrophysiological and antinociceptive effects. *J. Neurosci.* **16**, 6601–6611.

110. Smith, P.B., Compton, D.R., Welch, S.P., Razdan, R.K., Mechoulam, R., and Martin, B.R. (1994). The pharmacological activity of anandamide, a putative endogenous cannabinoid, in mice. *J. Pharmacol. Exp. Ther.* **270**, 219–227.

111. Welch, S.P., Thomas, C., and Patrick, G.S. (1995). Modulation of cannabinoid-induced antinociception after intracerebroventricular *versus* intrathecal administration to mice: possible mechanisms for interaction with morphine. *J. Pharmacol. Exp. Ther.* **272**, 310–321.

112. Welch, S.P. and Eads, M. (1999). Synergistic interactions of endogenous opioids and cannabinoid systems. *Brain Res.* **848** (1–2), 183–190.

113. Campbell, F.A., Tramer, M.R., Carroll, D., Reynolds, D.J.M., Moore, R.A., and McQuay, H.J. (2001). Are cannabinoids an effective and safe treatment option in the management of pain? A qualitative systematic review. *Br. Med. J.* **323**, 13–16.

114. Fromm, G.H. and Terrence, C.F. (1987). Comparison of L-baclofen and racemic baclofen in trigeminal neuralgia. *Neurology* **37**, 1725–1728.

115. Fromm, G.H., Terrence, C.F., and Chattha, A.S. (1984). Baclofen in the treatment of trigeminal neuralgia: double-blind study and long term follow up. *Ann. Neurol.* **15**, 240–244.

116. Gobelet, C., Waldburger, M., and Meier, J.L. (1992). The effect of adding calcitonin to physical treatment of reflex sympathetic dystrophy. *Pain* **48**, 171–175.

117. Jaeger, H. and Maier, C. (1992). Calcitonin in phantom limb pain: a double blind study. *Pain* **48**, 21–27.

118. Abrahams, M.J. and Munglani, R. (2000). Emerging therapeutic strategies for chronic pain. *Emerging Drugs* **5**, 385–413.

5.2 Therapeutic modalities

Cathy Speed

Introduction

Therapeutic modalities may be defined as thermal, mechanical, electrical, or electromagnetic energies used for the treatment of medical complaints. A range of such modalities is used in the treatment of soft tissue complaints, including thermal agents, ultrasound, and electrical agents (Table 1). In this chapter, the basis for the use of specific modalities and the existing evidence relating to their clinical effects are outlined.

Thermal agents

Cryotherapy

Cryotherapy involves the application of cold in the temperature range 32–65 °F to have therapeutic effects upon tissue to a depth of 5 cm (Table 2). Cryotherapy may be delivered in the form of ice packs, ice immersion, ice bags, or ice massage, with the aim of limiting the effects of the acute injury upon a tissue (Table 3). Standard treatments last for 15–20 minutes. During this time, cell metabolism is reduced by almost 20 per cent, considered to be beneficial by reducing the hypoxic

damage by the inflammatory process. Inflammation is nevertheless an important component of the healing process and excessive use of cold is inappropriate. Treatment is usually applied every 2 h, although controlled continuous treatment can be delivered via cold therapy units. Cryotherapy is continued during the acute phase of the injury, which may vary in duration between individuals.

Cryotherapy is generally safe, but frostbite with excessive or inappropriate use has been reported. The risk is increased by the use of reusable cold packs that contain antifreeze and are stored below freezing and by failure to place a moist towel between the ice pack and skin.

Heat

Many of the effects of heat upon tissue are the opposite to those of cold. Heat therapy can be superficial, where the skin temperature is raised to 104–113°F and tissue of depths less than 2 cm are heated, or deep, penetrating to 5 cm. Heat is avoided in acute injuries on the basis that it will promote the inflammatory response and increase cell metabolism. With the initial application of heat, the skin temperature rises rapidly for the first 10–15 minutes, until vasodilatation balances the heat being delivered and the patient may (falsely) believe that the modality has cooled. With continued application of a heat at a stable temperature, rebound vasoconstriction may occur as a protective mechanism.

Superficial heat treatment in the form of packs, an infrared lamp, or paraffin bath is usually applied for 15–20 minutes and can be repeated several times daily. Deep heat treatment can be delivered using shortwave diathermy or some of the other devices described below.

Table 1 Therapeutic modalities in soft tissue injuries

Thermal agents—cold
Packs, immersion, bags, controlled therapy units

Thermal agents—heat
Superficial
    Heat packs/lamps
    Paraffin baths
    Immersion

Deep
    Shortwave diathermy
    Ultrasound
    Laser

Ultrasound
Ultrasound
Phonophoresis
Extracorporeal Shock Wave Therapy (ESWT)

Electrical agents
Neuromuscular Electrical Stimulation (NMFS)
Transcutaneous Electrical Stimulation (TENS)
Interferential
Iontophoresis

Others
Laser

Table 2 Local effects of thermal agents

Cold	Heat
Vasoconstriction	Vasodilatation
Reduced cellular metabolic rate	Increased cellular metabolic rate

Reduction in inflammation
    Reduced inflammatory mediators
    Reduced prostaglandin synthesis
    Reduced capillary permeability
	Increase in inflammation
	    Increased inflammatory mediators
	    Increased capillary permeability

Decreased pain
    Reduced sensitivity of
      afferent neurones
    Reduced sensitivity of
      muscle spindles
	Decreased pain
	    Stimulates free nerve endings,
	      blocking pain pathways

Decreased muscle spasm	Decreased muscle spasm

Table 3 Indications/contraindications for the use of thermal agents in soft tissue injuries

Cold	Heat
Indications	
Acute injury	Subacute/chronic injuries
Acute/chronic pain	Subacute/chronic pain
After initial rehabilitation sessions	Subacute/chronic muscle spasm
Muscle spasm	Soft tissue stiffness, joint contractures
	Resolution of haematomas
Contraindications	
Open wounds	Acute injuries
Circulatory insufficiency	Open wounds
Sensory deficit	Circulatory insufficiency
Raynaud's phenomenon	Sensory deficit
	Neoplasms

Short-wave diathermy

Short-wave diathermy delivers high frequency electromagnetic energy that is absorbed by tissues, resulting in a heating effect. Treatment is delivered in either continuous or pulsed forms, with the former causing greater heating effect. Fat and muscle, having a high water content, are selectively heated at depths of up to 5 cm.

Short-wave diathermy is used in deep-seated injuries, including bursitis, muscle injuries, and some tendinopathies. Contraindications include local ischaemia, circulatory disturbance, sensory deficit, pregnancy, bleeding disorders, malignancy, and sensitive areas.

Ultrasound

With the exception of thermal agents, ultrasound is the most commonly used modality in the management of soft tissue complaints.[1]

Characteristics of therapeutic ultrasound

Ultrasound is a form of acoustic energy, consisting of inaudible high-frequency mechanical vibrations that may produce thermal or non-thermal effects upon the tissue. Ultrasound waves are created when a generator produces electrical energy that is converted to acoustic energy through mechanical deformation of a piezoelectric crystal located within the transducer. Ultrasound causes molecular collision in a medium, which allows its transmission by propagation of the wave through vibration of molecules, and a progressive loss of the intensity of the energy due to absorption and/or dispersion occurs with passage through the tissue (*attenuation*).

Therapeutic ultrasound has a frequency range of 0.75–3 MHz, with most ultrasound units set at a frequency of 1 or 3 MHz. Ultrasound at a frequency of 1 MHz is absorbed primarily by tissues at 3–5 cm depth. The lower the frequency of the waves, the greater the depth of penetration and the lower the absorption. Ultrasound at a frequency of 1 MHz is thus recommended for deeper injuries, particularly in those patients with considerable subcutaneous fat, whereas a frequency of 3 MHz is suggested for more superficial lesions at depths of 1–2 cm.

The greater the density of the medium (tissue), the faster is the velocity of the ultrasound wave travelling through it. Low absorption (and therefore high penetration) of ultrasound waves is seen in tissues that are high in water content (e.g. fat), whereas absorption is higher

in those tissues rich in protein (e.g. skeletal muscle). Tissues are characterized by their *acoustic impedance*, the product of their density and the speed at which ultrasound will travel through them. When travelling through more than one tissue, some of the ultrasound will be transmitted to the next tissue and some will scatter at the boundaries that separate them: the larger the difference in acoustic impedance, the greater the scattering. The percentage of energy reflected at the soft tissue/fat interface is 1 per cent as compared to 40 per cent at the soft tissue/bone interface.[2] When ultrasound energy reflected at tissue interfaces meets further waves being transmitted, a standing wave (hot spot) may be created, which has potential adverse effects upon tissue. This can be minimized by ensuring that the apparatus delivers a uniform wave, using pulsed waves (see below), and moving the transducer during treatment.

Since almost all energy is reflected away at the soft tissue/air interface, coupling media, in the form of water, oils, and most commonly gels, prevent reflection of the waves by excluding air from between the transducer and patient. Different media have different impedances. The criteria for any coupling medium are that its acoustic impedance should be similar to the impedance of the transducer, that it absorbs little of the ultrasound passing through it, that it remains free of air bubbles, and that it allows easy movement of the transducer over the skin surface.

The larger the diameter of the effective radiating area of the face of the transducer, the more focused the beam of ultrasound produced. Within this beam, energy is not evenly distributed, the greatest non-uniformity occurring close to the transducer surface (near zone). The variability of the beam intensity is termed the beam non-uniformity ratio (BNR)—this should optimally be 1:1 but, failing this, should be less than 8.

Therapeutic ultrasound can be pulsed or continuous. The former has on/off cycles and the amount of energy being delivered can be varied by adjusting the duration of either part of the cycle. Continuous ultrasound has a greater heating effect but either form at low intensity will produce non-thermal effects.

Ultrasound 'dosage' can also be varied by alteration of its amplitude and intensity. Various definitions of ultrasound intensity exist and machines differ with respect to the definition chosen for their intensity setting (Tables 4 and 5).

Modified forms of ultrasound

Modified forms of ultrasound include *phonophoresis* and *extracorporeal shock wave therapy* (ESWT). Phonophoresis involves the use of ultrasound energy and its effects upon cell permeability for the transdermal delivery of low molecular weight drugs. ESWT involves high-energy, focused ultrasound energy delivered using a modified lithotripter and is described further below.

The physiological effects of ultrasound

Ultrasound may induce thermal and non-thermal physical effects in tissues (Table 6). When it is applied for thermal effects, non-thermal effects will also occur but, through alteration of the dose parameters, non-thermal effects can be achieved in the absence of thermal effects. Reported thermal effects of ultrasound upon tissue include increased blood flow, reduction in muscle spasm, increased extensibility of collagen fibres, and a pro-inflammatory response. It is estimated that thermal effects occur with elevation of tissue temperature to 40–45 °C for at least 5 minutes.[3] Excessive thermal effects, seen in particular with higher ultrasound intensities, may damage the tissue. The use of

Table 4 Definitions used in ultrasound therapy [1]

Term	Definition
Power	Total amount of energy in an ultrasound beam (watts)
Acoustic impedance of a tissue	The product of the density of the tissue and the speed that ultrasound will travel through it
Attenuation	Progressive loss of energy during passage through tissue
Beam Nonuniformity Ratio (BNR)	The variability of the beam intensity: the ratio of the maximal intensity of the transducer to the average intensity across the transducer face
Coupling medium	Substance that prevents the reflection of ultrasound at the soft tissue/air interface
Duty cycle	The percentage of time ultrasound that is delivered over one on/off cycle
Standing wave (hot spot)	Created when reflected ultrasound meets further waves being transmitted, with potential adverse effects on tissue
Intensity (common examples):	
Spatial averaged intensity (SA_I)	Intensity averaged over the area of the transducer. Calculated by dividing the power output by the effective radiating area of the transducer head
Spatial peak intensity (SP_I)	The maximum intensity over time
Temporal peak intensity (or pulsed averaged intensity)	The peak intensity during the on period of pulsed ultrasound
Temporal-averaged intensity (TA_I)	The average power during the on/off periods of pulsed therapy
Spatial-averaged temporal peak intensity (SATP)	The maximum intensity occurring during a single pulse

Table 5 Some variables that may affect the dosage of ultrasound delivered to target tissue

Frequency

Walength

Intensity

Amplitude

Effective radiating area of transducer head

BNR

Continuous/pulsed therapy

Coupling medium

Tissue composition

Movement of transducer

Table 6 Proposed effects of therapeutic ultrasound

Thermal effects
Increase in tissue extensibility
Increase in blood flow
Modulation of pain
Mild inflammatory response
Reduction in joint stiffness
Reduction of muscle spasm

Non-thermal effects
Cavitation
Acoustic microstreaming
Cavitation and acoustic microstreaming in combination may result in stimulation of fibroblast activity, increase in protein synthesis, increased blood flow, tissue regeneration, bone healing

ultrasound in subacute or chronic conditions aims to relieve pain and spasm, and to increase tissue extensibility in the 10 minutes after heating, before the tissue cools. This may be of use in combination with stretching exercises to achieve optimal tissue length. Lengthening with thermal doses of ultrasound has been demonstrated in the ligament of normal knees[4] and in scar tissue.[5]

It has been suggested that the non-thermal effects of ultrasound are more important in the treatment of soft tissue lesions than are thermal effects.[6] These non-thermal properties of ultrasound include *cavitation* and *acoustic microstreaming*. Cavitation is the formation of gas-filled bubbles that expand and compress due to ultrasonically induced pressure changes in tissue fluids.[7] As a result there is increased flow in the surrounding fluid. Stable (regular) cavitation is considered to be beneficial to injured tissue, whereas unstable (transient) cavitation is considered to cause tissue damage.[7]

Acoustic microstreaming, the unidirectional movement of fluids along cell membranes, occurs due to the mechanical pressure changes within the ultrasound field. Microstreaming may alter cell membrane structure, function, and permeability,[8] which has been suggested to stimulate tissue repair.[6] Effects of cavitation and microstreaming that have been demonstrated *in vitro* include stimulation of fibroblast repair and collagen synthesis, tissue regeneration, and bone healing.[9, 10] Adverse effects of ultrasound have also been reported.

Most of our knowledge of the effects of ultrasound on living tissue is gained through *in vitro* studies or in animal models and many have focused in particular upon skin wounds and ulcers. It has been suggested that ultrasound interacts with one or more components of inflammation, and earlier resolution of inflammation,[11] accelerated fibrinolysis,[12] stimulation of macrophage-derived fibroblast mitogenic factors,[13] heightened fibroblast recruitment,[14] accelerated angiogenesis,[15] increased matrix synthesis, more dense collagen fibrils,[16] and increased tissue tensile strength,[9] have all been demonstrated *in vitro*. Such findings provide a rationale for the use of ultrasound to promote and accelerate tissue healing and repair. However, as has been detailed in earlier chapters, the pathophysiology of many soft tissue lesions (in particular, tendinopathies) and the mechanisms of healing of such lesions are poorly understood in comparison to those of the skin. The effects of ultrasound upon these processes are not yet known.

Research on the use of ultrasound specifically in tendon healing is minimal and relates only to animals. Using a range of regimes, variable increases in the tensile strength and the energy absorption, increased mobility, and improved alignment of collagen fibrils reduced inflammatory infiltrate and scar tissue of tenotomized rabbit and cockerel tendons[17] but not in others.[18–20] These findings not only demonstrate the variety of therapeutic regimes (and definitions of treatment intensities), but also the conflicting evidence that exists on the issue of the use of therapeutic ultrasound in tendon lesions, even in animal studies. Caution must be exercised in extrapolating these results to human tendon lesions, as differences exist between species in the types of collagen in tendon.

The evidence for clinical effect

Gam and Johanssen reviewed 293 papers published between 1953 and 1993 to evaluate the evidence of effect of ultrasound in the treatment of musculoskeletal pain.[21] Twenty-two trials of a variety of soft tissue disorders comparing ultrasound treatment with sham-ultrasound treated, non-ultrasound treatment, and untreated groups were found. The studies were generally found to be methodologically lacking. Data from 13 studies were presented in a way that made pooling possible; no evidence was found for pain relief with ultrasound treatment. Further papers have been published on the subject of ultrasound treatment upon soft tissue lesions, but few have added any support for the use of ultrasound.[22, 23]

There has been some suggestion that ultrasound may be of particular use in the early stages after injury, whereas many studies have evaluated more chronic lesions (or are unspecified in duration). This has been addressed in part by the use of delayed onset muscle soreness (DOMS) as a clinical model of acute inflammation. A reduction in pain and tenderness and increased muscle strength with pulsed ultrasound in DOMS in the quadriceps has been reported[24] but other studies have refuted this.[25, 26]

It is apparent that, although ultrasound is used extensively in soft tissue injuries and there are rational theories for its use, sound evidence for its effectiveness in such conditions is lacking. While *in vitro* studies have demonstrated many of the effects described earlier to occur, these have failed to translate into *in vivo* success. The absence of evidence for benefit for ultrasound in soft tissue lesions may be due to a true lack of effect, but poor study design or technical factors may play a role (Table 7). Inadequate calibration of machines has also been noted.[27]

Extracorporeal shock wave therapy (ESWT)

Extracorporeal shock waves are focused, single-pressure pulses of microsecond duration delivered using either an electromagnetic or electrohydraulic generator. They represent one of the most effective approaches to the treatment of renal calculi. More recently, ESWT has

Table 7 Possible reasons for the apparent lack of effect of therapeutic ultrasound in soft tissue lesions

Study design
Insufficient blinding
Dissimilar groups at baseline, inadequate sample sizes
Varied outcome measures, withdrawal from treatment
Loss to follow-up
Inadequate duration of follow-up
Wide spectrum of pathologies within study group

Dosage of ultrasound
Varied between studies
Varied between treatments
Inappropriate dose

Inadequate calibration of machinery
Inappropriate dose

Inappropriate/inadequate coupling medium
Inadequate delivery of ultrasound to injured site

True lack of effect

been used in the treatment of a number of musculoskeletal conditions, including insertional disorders such as calcifying tendonitis, plantar fasciitis, and lateral epicondylitis, at doses of 10–20 per cent of those used in lithotripsy of renal calculi.[28–30] The rationale for such an approach is the stimulation of soft tissue healing, reduction of calcification, inhibition of pain receptors, or denervation to achieve pain relief, although the true effects have not been established. Hardware, doses, and treatment protocols vary and there is a need for studies of different regimes in specific musculoskeletal conditions. There is evidence of benefit of ESWT in calcifying tendinitis of the rotator cuff. Loew *et al.* reported relief of pain in a significant number of patients with calcifiying tendinitis after one or two high-energy (EFD 0.3 mJ/mm^2) ESWT treatments administered under local anaesthetic infiltration. No improvements were noted in low dose and control (no treatment) groups 3 months after treatment.[31] Improvement in constant score was also significant with high-dose treatment and improvements correlated with reduction in calcification. There is also some evidence for benefit in chronic plantar fasciitis with treatment under local anaesthetic with shockwaves delivered using a electrohydraulic generator.[32] Evidence of benefit in other soft tissue disorders, including lateral epicondylitis and non-calcifying rotator cuff tendinosis, is lacking.[33, 34]

Electrical agents

Electrical agents have been used in the management of painful conditions since circa 2500 BC. Stone carvings from this time have been found in Egyptian tombs, depicting the application of local fish to painful areas of the body. Such fish contained organs that produced an electric charge (e.g. *Malapterurus electricus*). However, it was not until the mid-eighteenth century that electrical stimulation was delivered using manmade devices.[35] The field received little attention until the publication of the gate theory in 1965,[36] after which further interest in the use of electrical agents for pain control began to develop.

Several indications have been proposed for the use of electrical agents in the treatment of soft tissue injuries (Table 8). Electrical

Table 8 Therapeutic uses of electrical currents in soft tissue injuries

Pain control

Reduction of muscle spasm

Limitation of disuse atrophy

Re-education of muscle contraction

Promote local blood flow

Reduction of oedema

Promotion of tissue healing

stimulation may be used for analgesic effects and to stimulate muscle contractions, to limit disuse atrophy during the initial phase post-injury, to reduce oedema, to promote local muscle blood flow, and to maintain range of motion. Soft tissue healing may be enhanced but, although evidence exists for benefit in superficial wounds, benefits in soft tissue musculoskeletal injuries are unproven.

A number of different forms of electrical stimulation are in common use in the management of soft tissue complaints. The dose of the electrical current being delivered varies according to the characteristics of the electrical generator, the frequency and amplitude of the current, the tissues through which it is passing, and whether the current is pulsed or continuous. Where the current is pulsed, dose is influenced by the pulse attributes (pulse frequency, period, duration, etc. as described in relation to ultrasound). The size, position, number, and orientation of the electrodes, the space between them, and the degree of contact with the skin also influence the 'dose' of current being applied. Muscle is most effectively stimulated by application of the electrodes to motor points. Larger electrodes produce stronger but less selective contractions. The optimal interelectrode distance varies according to the site stimulated.

Neuromuscular electrical stimulation (NMES)

NMES aims to stimulate and re-educate muscle, to limit atrophy, to maintain range of motion, and to reduce muscle spasm and involves high-amplitude, longer-pulse duration. It is particularly useful in the early phases after injury/operation and is superior to no exercise at all in terms of improved local blood flow and reduced oedema. In the less acute patient it is not a substitute for active rehabilitation. Daily treatments can be given but the response of the patient should be closely monitored. Contraindications include avulsions and musculotendinous lesions if it is considered that any increase in muscle tension may be detrimental.

Transcutaneous electrical nerve stimulation (TENS)

In addition to neuromuscular stimulation, electrical stimulation may result in a reduction in pain in a format of lower-intensity, high-pulse frequencies. TENS is a process that uses an electrical current, applied through surface electrodes applied to the skin, to alter the perception of pain. The mechanism of pain reduction depends upon the characteristics of the current and includes action on central mechanisms (release of endogenous opiates) and stimulation of the gate control mechanism. A variety of approaches to electrode placement has been described but direct placement over or around the painful site is common practice.

High-frequency (conventional) TENS involves pulses at high frequency and short duration and selectively stimulates A-δ fibres,

closing the pain pathway gate to painful stimuli but opening it to sensory information. Onset of pain relief occurs within the initial 10 minutes of treatment and may persist for minutes to hours afterwards.

Low-frequency TENS, involving higher intensity but lower-frequency shorter-duration pulses, results in pain relief probably as a result of release of β-endorphins from the pituitary. Relief of pain may take longer to occur than with high-frequency TENS, but may be longer lasting. However, no overall difference in the degree of pain relief between the two types has been demonstrated. Since some degree of motor stimulation occurs, low-frequency TENS is best avoided in the acute phase of a musculotendinous injury.

A third and final form of TENS involves stimulation at high-intensity, high-pulse frequency and long duration (*brief-intense TENS*). Analgesia appears to be achieved through action at brainstem level, ultimately resulting in inhibition of release of substance P. Pain relief is generally of short duration.

The use of TENS units for pain control has several advantages. They are safe, non-addictive, easy to use, patient-operated, and portable. Side-effects are possible—they may cause skin irritation and, of course, may not be effective. They should not be used in a patient with a pacemaker or an arrhythmia and must be used with caution in those with epilepsy. The patient should not operate a machine or drive during use. Although there is a theoretical risk of thermal burns, the risk is negligible.

When a TENS unit is given to a patient for pain control, specific instructions should be given with respect to application of electrodes, treatment time, intensity, pulse frequency, potential adverse reactions, and care of the machine.

Initial treatment should be less than 30 minutes and the response (including adverse reactions) should then be evaluated. Provided the patient has tolerated the therapy, treatments can subsequently last up to an hour at a time, with a minimum of 30 minutes break at a time. The intensity is one that produces strong tingling or buzzing under the electrodes, without discomfort. Recommendations for electrode positioning include: placement over or close to the painful area, over motor points, over a peripheral nerve supplying the cutaneous area over the site of pain, or over the paraspinal region, or over peripheral nerves that supply the dermatome or myotome of the site of pain. Ultimately, the choice of the type of electrode placement depends upon the condition involved and patient preference and, at times, a degree of trial and error.[37] Unilateral or bilateral placement may be selected, and a minimum interelectrode distance of the diameter of the electrode is recommended.[38] Some units require the use of gel for skin contact and tape to secure the electrodes. A diary of pain levels and machine use is often helpful in evaluating the response.

Interferential stimulation

Interferential therapy involves the generation of two alternating sine waves, one at constant high frequency and the other at variable frequency. This results in easy penetration of tissues, whereupon the interference between the two waves results in (proposed) biological effects upon tissues. These effects are suggested to include analgesia, neuromuscular stimulation, and reduction of oedema although, as is the case with so many modalities, evidence is lacking.

Iontophoresis

Iontophoresis involves the use of low-voltage electrical current to deliver medication into the skin or subcutaneous structures. Such medications include anaesthetics, analgesics, and nonsteroidal anti-inflammatory drugs (NSAIDs). The transdermal route has obvious advantages over the systemic route, but there is no evidence for benefit from this approach.

Laser therapy

The use of laser (*light amplification by stimulated emission of radiation*) to cut and destroy tissue is well established. The same electromagnetic radiation, at much lower intensities, can elicit non-destructive physiological responses in tissues in the absence of significant heating ('cold laser' therapy). This phenomenon forms the basis for the use of 'laser therapy' in the management of a variety of soft tissue complaints.

An assortment of devices exists, including helium–neon, infrared diodes, argon, and krypton lasers, with the former two types of apparatus being the most commonly used. Treatment times are short (e.g. 30 seconds), with an output power in the range 1–75 mW, and treatment can be delivered as either pulsed or continuous, using a static or dynamic technique.

The proposed effects of laser therapy are analgesia and tissue healing, with the latter resembling the non-thermal effects proposed for therapeutic ultrasound. Laser energy commonly penetrates tissues at a depth of a few millimetres, although it is possible to stimulate tissues at a depth of up to 15 mm below the skin. Beneficial effects upon tissue healing are proposed to occur through stimulation of cellular and chemical aspects of the healing process, particularly in the early phases. Pain reduction may also take place through reduction of muscle spasm or altering nerve conduction velocity.[39] Nevertheless, the clinical utility of laser therapy remains unestablished.

Summary

A vast number of therapeutic modalities for the treatment of soft tissue complaints are in widespread use. Whilst there are numerous physiological rationales proposed for their use, further clinical research is needed to define their role(s) more clearly in the management of these conditions.

References

1. **Speed, C.A.** (2001). Therapeutic ultrasound in soft tissue lesions. *Rheumatology* **40** (12), 1331–1336.
2. **McDiarmid, T. and Burns, P.N.** (1987). Clinical applications of therapeutic ultrasound. *Physiotherapy* **73**, 155.
3. **Prentice, W.E.** (1994). *Therapeutic modalities in sports medicine*, 3rd edn. Mosby, St Louis.
4. **Ellis, D.G.** (1969). Cross-sectional area measurement for tendon specimens: a comparison of several methods. *J. Biomech.* **2**, 175–186.
5. **Noyes, F.R., Torvik, P.J., Hyde, W.B., and DeLucas, J.L.** (1974). Biomechanics of ligament failure II. An analysis of immobilisation exercise and reconditioning effects in primates. *J. Bone Joint Surg. (Am.)* **56**, 1406–1418.
6. **Dyson, M. and Suckling, J.** (1978). Stimulation of tissue repair by ultrasound: a survey of the mechanisms involved. *Physiotherapy* **64** (4), 105–108.
7. **Wells, P.N.T.** (1977). *Biomedical ultrasonics.* Academic Press, London.
8. **Dyson, M.** (1987). Mechanisms involved in therapeutic ultrasound. *Physiotherapy* **73** (3), 116–120.
9. **Dyson, M. and Luke, D.A.** (1986). Induction of mast cell degranulation in skin by ultrasound. *IEEE Trans. Ultrasonics, Ferroelectrics, Frequency control* **UFFC-33**, 194.
10. **Pilla, A.A., Figueiredo, M., Nasser, P., et al.** (1990). Non-invasive low intensity pulsed ultrasound: a potent accelerator of bone repair. *Proceedings of the 36th Annual Meeting, Orthopaedics Research Society, New Orleans 1990.*
11. **Young, S.R. and Dyson, M.** (1990). Effect of therapeutic ultrasound on the healing of full-thickness excised skin lesions. *Ultrasonics* **28** (3), 175–180.
12. **Harpaz, D., Chen, X., Francis, C.W., et al.** (1993). Ultrasound enhancement of thrombolysis and reperfusion *in vitro. J. Am. Coll. Cardiol.* **2**, 1507–1511.
13. **Young, S.R. and Dyson, M.** (1990). Macrophage responsiveness to therapeutic ultrasound. *Ultrasound Med. Biol.* **16** (8), 809–816.
14. **Young, S. and Dyson, M.** (1990). The effects of therapeutic ultrasound on the healing of full thickness excised skin lesions. *Ultrasonics* **28**, 175–180.
15. **Young, S.R. and Dyson, M.** (1990). The effect of therapeutic ultrasound on angiogenesis. *Ultrasound Med. Biol.* **16** (3), 261–269.
16. **Friedar, S.A.** (1988). A pilot study: The therapeutic effect of ultrasound following partial rupture of achilles tendons in male rats. *J. Orthop. Sports Phys. Ther.* **10**, 39.
17. **Enwemeka, C.S.** (1989). The effects of therapeutic ultrasound on tendon healing. A biomechanical study. *Am. J. Phys. Med. Rehabil.* **68**, 283–287.
18. **Gan, B.S., Huys, S., Sherebrin, M.H., and Scilley, C.G.** (1995). The effects of ultrasound treatment on flexor tendon healing in the chicken limb. *J. Hand Surg. (Br.)* **20** (6), 809–814.
19. **Turner, S.M., Powell, E.S., and Ng, and C.S.** (1989). The effect of ultrasound on the healing of repaired cockerel tendon: is collagen cross-linkage a factor? *J. Hand Surg. (Br.)* **14** (4), 428–433.
20. **Roberts, M., Rutherford, J.H., and Harris, D.** (1982). The effect of ultrasound on flexor tendon repairs in the rabbit. *Hand* **14**, 17–20.
21. **Gam, A.N. and Johannsen, F.** (1995). Ultrasound therapy in musculoskeletal disorders: a meta-analysis. *Pain* **63**, 85–91.
22. **Green, S., Buchbinder, R., Glazier, R., and Forbes, A.** (1998). Systematic review of randomised controlled trials of interventions for painful shoulder: selection criteria, outcome assessment and efficacy. *Br. Med. J.* **316**, 354–360.
23. **Van der Heijden, G.J.M.G., van der Windt, D.A.W.M., and de Winter, A.F.** (1997). Physiotherapy for patients with shoulder disorders: a systematic review of randomised controlled clinical trials. *Br. Med. J.* **315**, 25–30.
24. **Hasson, S., Mundorf, R., Barnes, W., Williams, J., and Fujii, M.** (1990). Effect of pulsed ultrasound versus placebo on muscle soreness perception and muscular performance. *Scand. J. Rehabil. Med.* **22** (4), 199–205.
25. **Craig, J.A., Bradley, J., Walsh, D.M., Baxter, G.D., and Allen, J.M.** (1999). Delayed onset muscle soreness: lack of effect of therapeutic ultrasound in humans. *Arch. Phys. Med. Rehabil.* **80** (3), 318–323.
26. **Ciccone, C., Leggin, B., and Callamaro, J.** (1991). Effects of ultrasound and trolamine salicylate on delayed-onset muscle soreness. *Phys. Ther.* **71**, 666.
27. **Pye, S.D. and Milford, C.** (1994). The performance of ultrasound physiotherapy machines in Lothian Region, Scotland, 1992. *Ultrasound Med. Biol.* **20** (4), 347–359.
28. **Thiel, M.** (2001). Application of shock waves in medicine. *Clin. Orthop. Rel. Res.* **387**, 18–21.
29. **Delius, M.** (1994). Medical applications and bioeffects of extracorporeal shock waves. *Shock Waves* **4**, 55–72.
30. **Ogden, J.A., Alvarez, R., Levitt, R., and Marlow. M.** (2001). Shock wave therapy (orthotripsy) in musculoskeletal disorders. *Clin. Orthop. Rel. Res.* **387**, 22–40.
31. **Loew, M., Daecke, W., Kusnierczak, D., Ranmauzaden, M., and Ewerbeck, V.** (1999). Shockwave therapy is effective for chronic calcifying tendinitis of the shoulder. *J. Bone Joint Surg.(Br.)* **81-B**, 863–867.

32. Ogden, J.A., Alvarez, R., Levitt, R., Cross, G.L., and Marlow, M. (2001). Shock wave therapy for chronic proximal plantar fasciitis. *Clin. Orthop. Rel. Res.* **387**, 47–59.

33. Speed, C.A., Richards, C., Nichols, D., Burnet, S., Wies, J.T., Humphreys, H., and Hazleman, B.L. (2002). Extracorporeal shock-wave therapy for tendonitis of the rotator cuff: A double-blind, randomised, controlled trial. *J. Bone Joint Surg. (Br.)* **84**, 509–512.

34. Speed, C.A., Nichols, D., Richards, C., Humphreys, H., Wies, J.T., Burnet, S., and Hazleman, B.L. (2002). Extracorporeal shock wave therapy for lateral epicondylitis. A double blind randomised controlled trial. *J. Orthop. Res.* **20**, 895–898.

35. Wesley, J. (1759). *The desideratum: or electricity made plain and useful by a lover of mankind and of common sense.* Baillière, Tindall and Cox, London.

36. Melzack, R. and Wall, P.D. (1965). Pain mechanisms: a new theory. *Science* **150**, 971–979.

37. Walsh, D.M. (1997). The clinical application of TENS. In *TENS: clinical applications and related theory* (ed. D.M. Walsh), pp. 103–124, Churchill Livingstone, London.

38. Mannheimer, J.S. and Lampe, G.N. (1984). *Clinical transcutaneous nerve stimulation.* F.A. Davis, Michigan.

39. Basford, J.R. (1993). Laser therapy: scientific basis and clinical role. *Orthopedics* **16** (5), 541–547.

5.3 Local injections for soft tissue lesions
Cathy Speed

Introduction

Injections of corticosteroids into articular and extraarticular structures began soon after their introduction for the treatment of rheumatoid arthritis in the 1950s. They rapidly became one of the most commonly utilized treatment approaches in the management of soft tissue disorders, in particular, chronic tendon lesions, and have remained so ever since. Corticosteroid injections have little or no role to play in most acute injuries nor in the management of ligament or muscle injuries and offer no advantage over dry needling in myofascial pain. Hence their use in chronic tendinopathies and in cases of bursitis will form the focus of this chapter.

The rationale for corticosteroid injections in tendon lesions

Corticosteroid injections are generally considered to be useful on the basis that they will have an anti-inflammatory effect. While this may be relevant to some lesions (e.g. a chronic bursitis), this is not always the case. Tendinopathies are an extremely varied group of lesions and the structure and pathologies of such lesions have been described in detail in earlier chapters. In many cases (in particular, tendinosis), evidence for inflammation is lacking and, although most histopathological studies to date have included end-stage lesions, it is not clear whether the degenerative features noted are preceded by an inflammatory phase.[1] Other mechanisms of tendon pain in the absence of inflammation may include irritation of mechanoreceptors by vibration, traction, or by shear forces and triggering of nociceptive receptors by neurotransmitters such as substance P and by biochemical irritants such as chondroitin sulfate.[2–4] The effects of corticosteroid upon these processes are undetermined.

Clinical evidence

The consensus of rheumatological opinion is that corticosteroid injections can be helpful in the management of specific soft tissue lesions. Nevertheless, although the literature is abundant with publications relating to the use of corticosteroid injections in the management of chronic soft tissue lesions, there is scant good evidence of beneficial effect in many cases.[5, 6] This may be associated with the methodological limitations of some studies and further research in this area is still desperately required.

There is evidence to support treatment with local corticosteroid injections in trigger finger,[7, 8] a condition where chronic inflammation has been demonstrated.[2] In a double-blind randomized placebo-controlled trial, Murphy et al. compared local injection of betamethasone plus lignocaine in 14 subjects with lignocaine alone in 10 control subjects.[7] At 3 weeks follow-up, 10 subjects in the treatment group were asymptomatic versus 2 in the control group. In another double-blind placebo-controlled trial of local injection of methylprednisolone acetate plus lignocaine with lignocaine alone in 41 subjects with trigger finger, Lambert et al. found a significant improvement (physician rated) in 60 per cent of the treatment group versus 16 per cent in the control group at 1 month follow-up.[8]

There is also evidence for short-term benefit of subacromial corticosteroid injections in rotator cuff tendinosis with respect to range of motion, but not pain. Effectiveness in the longer term is unknown and there are currently insufficient data of adequate quality upon which to base a recommendation for practice. There is evidence that local corticosteroid injection provides early pain relief in patients with lateral epicondylitis, but the long-term outcome is similar to that with non-steroidal anti-inflammatory drugs (NSAIDs) and simple analgesics.[9] The sole prospective double-blind randomized controlled trial addressing the effectiveness of corticosteroid injections in Achilles paratenonitis showed no benefit (with respect to pain, tenderness, and return to normal activity) of peritendinous methylprednisolone (40 mg) and marcaine over marcaine injections alone in 28 subjects.[10]

Accuracy of injection may be important. Even in the hands of musculoskeletal specialists, only a minority of injections for shoulder pain are performed accurately (29 per cent of subacromial and 42 per cent of intraarticular injections) and outcome appears to significantly correlate with accuracy of injection.[11] Zingas et al. demonstrated similar results in subjects with de Quervain's tenosynovitis.[12] For this reason, the use of ultrasound guided injection is becoming popular.[13]

Adverse effects of corticosteroid injection

The overall incidence of side-effects after local corticosteroid injection for tendon lesions is unknown. Similarly, the relevance of the steroid used, the tissue involved, the extent of the injury, the phase of healing at the time of injection and post-injection events—particularly loading of the tissue—remains undetermined. Studies on animal models have demonstrated adverse effects of intratendinous corticosteroid on the biomechanical properties of tendons.[14, 15] Such effects include inhibition of the formation of adhesions, granulation, and connective tissue, reduced tendon mass, and decreased biomechanical integrity with decreased load to failure.[14, 15] The biomechanical effects of peritendinous corticosteroid upon human tendons, as used in clinical practice, are unestablished. Complete tendon rupture with loading after steroid injection is recognized, although the literature is limited to case reports and rigorous studies have not been performed.

Sepsis is reported in 1 in 17–50,000 intraarticular/soft tissue injections.[16] Other commonly reported side-effects include tissue atrophy, facial flushing, post-injection flare, and hypersensitivity reactions.[17] Resuscitation facilities should be available, in the event of a rare severe reaction.

Recommendations for use of local corticosteroid injections in tendinopathies

There are no universally accepted recommendations for the use of local corticosteroid injections. There is no consensus of opinion with respect to environment (operating theatre, treatment room, clinic), the wearing of gloves, shaving of skin, the use of local anaesthetic, the safe number of injections at one site, nor the appropriate interval between injections.[16] Some suggestions by the author for the use of corticosteroid injections for chronic tendinopathies, in the face of a relative vacuum of evidence, are given in Tables 1 and 2.

Agents differ with respect to their potency and solubility, the latter inversely correlating with the duration of action (Table 3).[17] There are few data on the absorption of corticosteroids from peritendinous injections, but methylprednisolone acetate remains in plasma for a mean of 16 days after periarticular injection.[18] Short- or moderate-acting, more soluble preparations (e.g. hydrocortisone, methylprednisolone)

Table 1 Indications and contraindications to corticosteroid injection in soft tissue lesions[a]

Indications
Reserve for chronic injuries, after a failure of intensive use of other approaches for *at least* 2 months
Use when rehabilitation is inhibited by symptoms

Contraindications
If pain relief and anti-inflammatory effects can be achieved by other methods
Local or systemic infection
Coagulopathy
Tendon tear (?)

[a] Local corticosteroid injections are often unnecessary and should be avoided in the younger patient.

Table 2 Suggestions for the use of local steroid injections in tendinopathies

- Informed consent should be obtained from the patient, who must be willing to follow post-injection guidelines (Table 3)
- The practitioner should have full knowledge of the local anatomy
- Prepare carefully and thoroughly, and ensure landmarks have been identified.
- Select the finest needle that will reach the lesion
- Decide beforehand whether you aim to infiltrate around that affected area or just inject a bolus at one defined spot. Bolus injections include intra-articular, bursal, and subacromial injections
- The practitioner's hands and the patients skin should be cleansed and a no-touch technique used
- Use short/medium acting corticosteroid preparations in most cases, with local anaesthetic
- Inject efficiently: pass the needle gently but swiftly through necessary tissue planes to the affected area.
- When the needle is guided to a bony landmark, *touch* rather than *hit* bone, to avoid periostitis
- Injection should be peritendinous; avoid injection into tendon substance
- Injections should *not* be painful and should *not* require much pressure
- The minimum interval between injections should be 6 weeks
- Use a maximum of three injections at one site
- Soluble preparations may be useful in those patients who have had hypersensitivity/local reaction to previous injection
- Details of the injection should be carefully recorded
- Do *not* repeat if two injections do not provide at least 4 weeks relief

Table 3 A comparison of injectable corticosteroids

Preparation	Potency[+]	Concentration (mg/ml)	Solubility (% wt/vol)	Onset of action	Dose
Hydrocortisone acetate (Hydrocortistab)	1	25	0.002	Variable	5–25 mg
Prednisolone acetate (Deltastab)	4	25	0.001	Variable	5–25 mg
Methyprednisolone acetate (Depomedrone)	5	20, 40, 80	0.001	1–5 days	20–80 mg
Tramcinalone acetonide (Adcortyl, Kenalog)	5	10, 40	0.004	Variable	5–40 mg
Betamethasone sodium phosphate/acetate	25	6	NA	2–24 hours	0.25–2 mg
Dexamethasone phosphate	25	4	0.01	2–24 hours	N/A
*Triamcinalone hexacetonide	5	20	0.0002	Variable	*N/A

*Insolubility makes it unsuitable for use in soft tissue injections.
[+]Hydrocortisone equivalents (per mg).
NA not available.

are recommended for soft tissue injections on the basis of likelihood of fewer side-effects. Agents with low solubility should not be used for this purpose.

Local anaesthetic mixed with the corticosteroid is usually used in soft tissue injections, based on the rationale of patient comfort and increasing the volume of the injection for wider dispersion. However, common as this practice is, some manufacturers advise against mixing agents because of the theoretical risk of clumping and precipitation of steroid crystals. There is no evidence that injection of local anaesthetic in advance of the corticosteroid is beneficial, nor of a difference in outcome between the addition of long-acting versus short-acting anaesthetic.

Local steroid injections in the vicinity of the Achilles or patellar tendon and in the circumstances of a tear are frequently discouraged due to the concerns with respect to rupture of heavily loaded tendons and/or impairment of tissue repair where disruption is already present.

Corticosteroid injections in other disorders

Bursitis

Most uncomplicated episodes of bursitis will settle with relative rest, removal of the causative factor(s), protection (such as elbow pads), and NSAIDs if necessary. Occasionally, aspiration of the bursa may be required and in itself may provide symptomatic relief. Intrabursal injection of corticosteroid may settle inflammation, but should be used only in resistant cases and where the clinician is confident that infection is not present. Crystal-associated bursitides are particularly painful and the threshold for the use of corticosteroids is therefore reduced. Side-effects of steroid injections include cutaneous atrophy and introduction of sepsis. Surgical intervention is rarely necessary.

Neuromas

Local corticosteroid and anaesthetic injections (hydrocortisone 10–25 mg + 1 ml 1% lignocaine) are also useful in the medical management of neuromas, in particular, interdigital neuromas of the feet. Surgery is considered if the patient fails to respond to an initial corticosteroid injection.

Myofascial disorders

Local corticosteroid injections have no role in the management of fibromyalgia. They have been recommended in the treatment of trigger points in myofascial pain syndromes, but the author does not consider them to offer any advantage over dry needling, which is discussed in Chapters 5.4 and 6.12.

Local anaesthetic injections

Local anaesthetic injections can be extremely useful for diagnostic purposes.[19] Even in this area of diagnostic imaging, detection of pathology does not necessarily implicate it as the source of the symptoms. Infiltration around the area of interest and immediate reassessment of the patient can therefore be invaluable. For example, Neer's test involves a subacromial injection of local anaesthetic as a diagnostic tool to differentiate rotator cuff impingement from other causes of shoulder pain, with improvement in pain and active and passive range of movement seen with impingement, but not other disorders, after injection.

Suprascapular nerve block

Suprascapular nerve blocks are arguably the most useful nerve block to the rheumatologist and are used in the patient with severe shoulder pain. The suprascapular nerve is a mixed nerve formed by fibres from the C5 and C6 (and in some individuals C4) nerve roots. It passes postero-inferiorly from the brachial plexus, under the coracoclavicular ligament, and through the suprascapular notch. It provides sensory innervation to the shoulder joint and motor supply to the spinati. The injectate can consist of corticosteroid and anaesthetic or just anaesthetic. The procedure is described further below.

Summary

Local corticosteroid injections currently play a major role in the management of many chronic soft tissue lesions, in particular, tendinopathies and their popularity is likely to continue. Further evidence for benefits with their use and greater insights into their effects upon tissue are needed.

Guidance for specific injections

Table 4 gives some post-injection guidelines and Table 5 gives needle gauges commonly used in the United Kingdom.

Table 4 Post-injection guidelines

- Warn the patient of early post-injection local anaesthesia, to avoid initial overuse
- Advise a minimum post-injection rest of 2 weeks and avoid heavy loading for 6 weeks
- The patient should inform the doctor if there is any suggestion of infection or other significant adverse event

Table 5 Needle sizes and colours in common use in the United Kingdom

Gauge	Colour	Thickness (mm)	Length (cm)
19G	White	1.1	4
21G	Green	0.8	4
23G	Blue	0.6	3
25G	Orange	0.5	2
Spinal needle 22G[a]	Black	0.8	4 or 7.5

[a] A range of spinal needles are available in different gauges.

Shoulder region
Glenohumeral joint

- *Corticosteroid.* 40 mg methylprednisolone + 2–3 ml lignocaine (1 per cent)
- *Needle.* 21G.

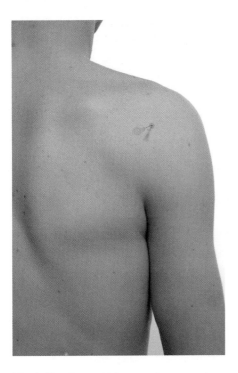

Fig. 1 Glenohumeral joint posterior approach.

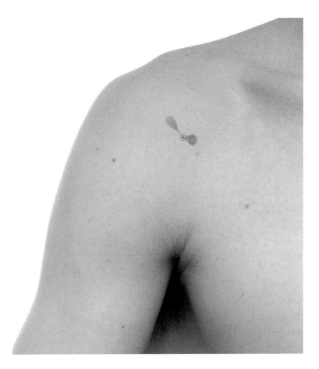

Fig. 2 Glenohumeral joint anterior approach.

Posterior approach (Fig. 1)

This is considered to be easier and safer than the anterior approach. The patient is sitting with the arm resting on the arm of the chair. The physician palpates the coracoid process with the index finger of the free hand with the thumb resting on the posterior edge of the acromion. The needle is inserted 1 cm below and 1 cm medial to the posterior edge of the acromion, aiming towards the coracoid process, aiming to touch bone at the articular space.

Anterior approach (Fig. 2)

The patient is sitting with the arm resting on the arm rest of the chair and the forearm in the sagittal plane. The coracoid process is identified and the needle is inserted 1 cm distal and 1 cm lateral to it. Capsular resistance is felt prior to entering the joint.

Subacromial space (Fig. 3)

* *Corticosteroid.* 40 mg methylprednisolone and 1–2 ml 1 per cent lignocaine

* *Needle.* 22–23G.

Approach

Identify the lateral edge of the acromion. A posterolateral approach is easiest. The needle is directed anteromedially under the acromion.

Bicipital tendon sheath

* *Corticosteroid.* 20 mg methylprednisolone

* *Needle.* 23–25G.

Approach

Identify the bicipital tendon, marking the skin. The needle is directed superiorly along the sheath and injection performed under no resistance.

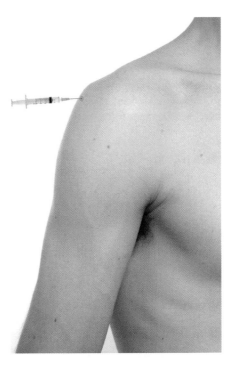

Fig. 3 Subacromial space.

Acromioclavicular joint (Fig. 4)

* *Corticosteroid.* 20 mg methylprednisolone

* Needle. 25G.

Approach

The joint is in the sagittal plane, and is runs obliquely medially. A small gap may be palpated at the anterior margin of the joint.

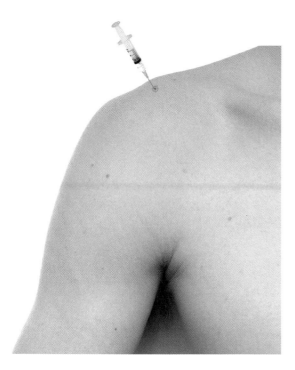

Fig. 4 Acromioclavicular joint.

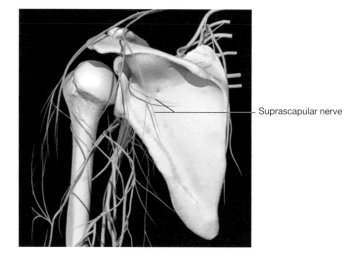

Fig. 5 Suprascapular nerve.

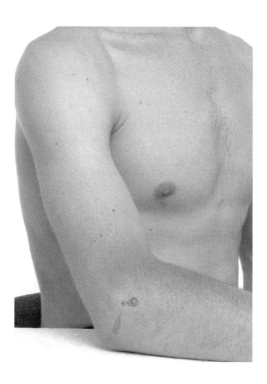

Fig. 6 Lateral epicondylitis.

An anterosuperior approach is easiest. The patient sits with the arm hanging at the side. The needle angle is approximately 30° from the vertical plane. If entry to the joint is difficult, apply traction to the arm. Aspirate prior to injection. The joint will typically only accept 0.5 ml fluid.

Suprascapular nerve block (Fig. 5)

• *Anaesthetic/steroid.* 3 ml lignocaine (1 per cent) or 40 mg methylprednisolone (1 ml) + lignocaine 1 per cent (2 ml)

• *Needle.* 22G spinal needle, 7.5 cm length.

Approach

The patient is seated with the arm hanging loosely by their side. Identify landmarks: the spine of the scapula and the acromion. Mark the site where a vertical line that bisects the spine of the scapula. Mark another point 2–3 cm above and lateral to this point. The patient then places the ipsilateral hand on the opposite shoulder, to reduce the chance of pneumothorax. The skin is prepared. The needle is inserted forward and downward until it makes contact with the body of the scapula (at a depth of approximately 2 cm). 'Walk' the needle supero-medially along the scapula, until it walks off the scapula and into the suprascapular notch. If the notch cannot be identified, then walk the needle superolaterally. *Note* that the suprascapular artery and vein also run through the notch and the lung is also in close proximity. Therefore once in the notch, aspirate prior to injection. Monitor the patient afterwards to observe for any adverse signs. Warn the patient that, since the nerve has been blocked and sensation therefore lost, he or she might not be aware of further damaging the shoulder and of burns through heat modalities and must therefore take special care.

Elbow region

Lateral epicondylitis (Fig. 6)

• *Corticosteroid.* 25 mg hydrocortisone + 2 ml 1 per cent lignocaine

• *Needle.* 23–25G.

Approach

The patient sits with the forearm supported and the elbow in 90° flexion. Identify the site of maximal tenderness. The needle is inserted vertically and directed towards this site until it touches bone. Slightly

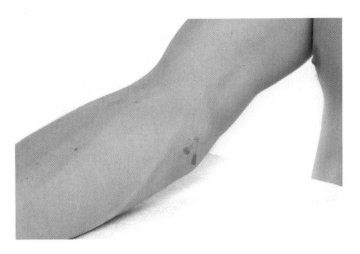

Fig. 7 Medial edpicondylitis.

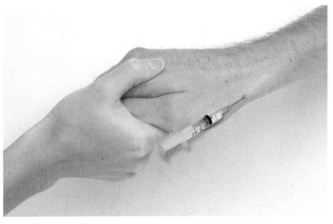

Fig. 8 DeQuervains tenosynovitis.

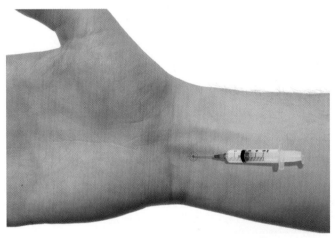

Fig. 9 Carpal tunnel.

withdraw the needle and then infiltrate in a fan shape deeply around the tenoperiosteal junction and surrounding tissues. Avoid superficial injection.

Medial epicondylitis (Fig. 7)

- *Corticosteroid.* 25 mg hydrocortisone + 2ml 1 per cent lignocaine

- *Needle.* 23G.

Approach

The patient sits or lies with the adducted arm resting on a cushion and the elbow extended. The needle is inserted perpendicular to the medial epicondyle until bone is encountered, then withdrawn slightly and the area of the tenoperiosteal junction is infiltrated.

Olecranon bursa

- *Corticosteroid.* 12.5–25 mg hydrocortisone

- *Needle.* 23G.

Approach

Lateral through normal skin, aiming at centre of bursa.

Wrist area

DeQuervain's tenosynovitis (Fig. 8)

- *Corticosteroid.* 25 mg hydrocortisone (or 10 mg methylprednisolone) + 1 ml lignocaine (1 per cent)

- *Needle.* 23–25G.

Approach

This is an intrasheath injection. The patient sits with the hand held in mid-supination and the thumb relaxed in slight flexion. The gaps between abductor pollicis longus and extensor pollicis brevis can be identified. The needle is aimed at the radial styloid and the sheath is felt to distend with the injection.

Carpal tunnel (Fig. 9)

- *Corticosteroid.* 20 mg methylprednisolone

- *Needle.* 23G.

Approach

The patient sits with the forearm supported in the supinated position. The tendons of flexor pollicis longus and flexor digitarum profundus are identified. The needle is inserted at an angle of 45°, just medial to the palmaris longus tendon, at the level of the distal palmar crease, to a depth of 1 cm to lie under the midpoint of the retinaculum. The patient is asked to flex the fingers to ensure the needle is not in a tendon (there should be no needle movement). Also ensure there is no paraesthesia in the median nerve distribution (reposition the needle if this occurs). The steroid should flow without resistance on injection.

Fingers

Flexor tendon sheath (trigger finger, flexor tenosynovitis) (Fig. 10)

- *Corticosteroid.* 25 mg hydrocortisone (or 10 mg methylprednisolone) + 0.5–1 ml 1 per cent lignocaine

- *Needle.* 25G.

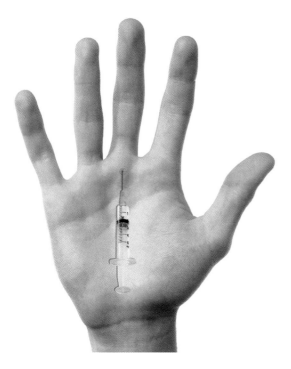

Fig. 10 Flexor tendon sheath (trigger finger, flexor tenosynovitis).

Approach

The needle is inserted, as appropriate, just proximal to the palmar crease of index finger, just distal to the palmar crease of middle, ring, or little fingers, or just distal to the palmar crease of the thumb. Direct the needle proximally at 45° and ask the patient to flex the finger: minimal movement of the needle should be felt. Reattach the syringe and inject into the sheath.

Hip region

Trochanteric bursitis (Fig. 11)

- *Corticosteroid.* 40 mg methylprednisolone + 2–3 ml lignocaine (1 per cent)

- *Needle.* 1.5–2 inch 22G (use a spinal needle if necessary).

Approach

The patient lies on the opposite side with the hip slightly flexed. Identify the greater trochanter by palpating along the femur. It is in a line approximately 10 cm distal to the iliac tubercle, which is the highest point on the iliac crest. Also identify the site of maximal tenderness, usually at the posterior aspect of the greater trochanter. Direct the needle vertically to the site of maximum tenderness, making contact with the periosteum of the greater trochanter. Withdraw the needle very slightly away from the periosteum and infiltrate the surrounding area with the steroid and lignocaine.

Psoas bursa

The author usually performs this under ultrasound control.

- *Corticosteroid.* Depomedrone 20 mg + 1 ml lignocaine (1 per cent)

- *Needle.* Spinal, 21G, 7.5 cm.

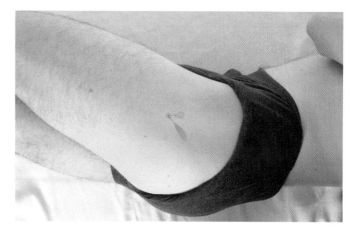

Fig. 11 Trochanteric bursitis.

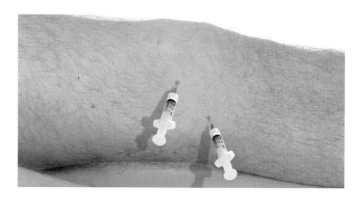

Fig. 12 Knee and anserine bursitis.

Approach

The patient lies supine. A point three fingerbreadths distally and three finger breadths lateral to the femoral pulse at the level of the inguinal ligament is identified. This should be in line with the anterior superior iliac spine. The needle is inserted at an angle of 45° cephalad and 45° medially, under the femoral vessels to touch the femoral neck. It is withdrawn slightly, aspiration is attempted, and then the injection is performed.

Hip adductor tendons

- *Corticosteroid.* 25 mg hydrocortisone (or 20 mg methylprednisolone) and 1–2 ml lignocaine (1 per cent)

- *Needle.* 23G.

Approach

The patient lies supine with the leg supported in slight abduction and external rotation. The tendon and its insertion are identified. The needle is directed towards the insertion until it touches bone. It is withdrawn slightly and the area infiltrated.

Knee region

Anserine bursitis (Fig. 12)

- *Corticosteroid.* 25 mg hydrocortisone and lignocaine (1 per cent)

- *Needle.* 23G.

Approach

The patient sits with the knee supported in extension. Identify the common tendon of sartorius, gracilis, and semitendinosis medially just below the joint line. The tender bursa is deep to this. The needle is directed vertically to touch the periosteum, then withdrawn very slightly back, and the injection is performed.

Iliotibial band bursitis

* *Cortocosteroid.* 25 mg hydrocortisone

* *Needle.* 23G.

Approach

The patient sits with the knee supported in extension. The bursa is identified deep to the iliotibial band above the lateral femoral condyle. The needle is directed into the bursa to touch periosteum, withdrawn slightly, and the injection is performed.

Foot

Plantar fascia (Fig. 13)

* *Corticosteroid.* 25 mg hydrocortisone (or 20 mg methylprednisolone) + 1–2 ml lignocaine (1 per cent)

* *Needle.* 22G.

Approach

Use a medial approach, directing the needle towards the medial calcaneal tuberosity. The injection is performed near to the bony surface at the fascial origin.

Morton's neuroma

* *Corticosteroid.* 25 mg hydrocortisone + 1 ml lignocaine (1 per cent)

* *Needle.* 23–25G.

Approach

Identify the site of maximal tenderness. Direct the needle in a plantar direction through the resistance of the intermetatarsal ligament.

Rare injections

The following injections are indicated only rarely.

Retrocalcaneal bursa

This injection should be used only in very resistant retrocalcaneal bursitis in the patient with a spondyloarthropathy, in the absence of tendinosis on ultrasound. Injection is performed under ultrasound guidance by an experienced practitioner. The bursa frequently communicates with the peritendinous tissue.

* *Corticosteroid.* 25 mg hydrocortisone + 1 ml lignocaine (1 per cent)

* *Needle.* 22G.

Approach

A lateral approach into the bursa is taken with the foot in slight plantar flexion.

The sheath of the tendon of tibialis posterior (Fig. 14)

This injection is indicated only in very resistant tenosynovitis, usually in those with an inflammatory arthritis. When performed, ultrasound-guided injection by an experienced physician is strongly recommended. The artery and nerve are in close proximity and there is the additional risk of tendon rupture as this is a loaded tendon. Fluid should be evident within the sheath prior to injection.

* *Corticosteroid.* 20–40 mg methylprednisolone

* *Needle.* 22G.

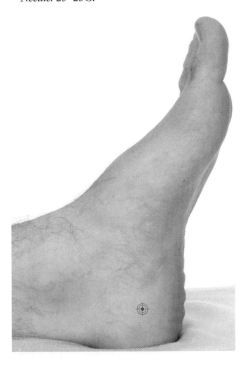

Fig. 13 Plantar fascia.

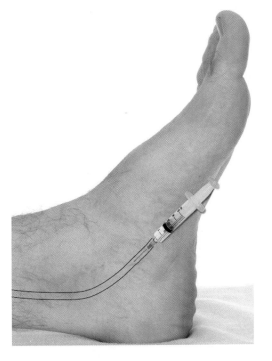

Fig. 14 The sheath of the tendon of tibialis posterior.

Approach

The patient lies supine, with the affected leg resting on the contralateral knee. The needle is inserted three fingerbreadths above the medial malleolus. Aspirate first to ensure the posterior tibial artery has not been punctured. The injectate should be felt distending the sheath.

Infrapatellar bursitis

This injection is used only in very resistant cases and in the absence of patellar tendinosis on ultrasound. Peritendinous leakage is a hazard, as the tendon is heavily loaded. A week of rest after injection is mandatory.

- *Corticosteroid.* 25 mg hydrocortisone and 1 ml lignocaine (1 per cent)

- *Needle.* 23G.

Approach

The patient sits with the knee supported in slight flexion. It is inserted from the medial side horizontally, behind the tendon and into the centre of the bursa.

Hamstrings insertion and ischiogluteal bursitis

These are best injected under ultrasound control.

References

1. Speed, C.A. (2001). Fortnightly review: corticosteroid injections in tendon lesions. *Br. Med. J.* **323** (7309), 382–386.

2. Jósza, J. and Kannus, P. (1997). Overuse injuries of tendons. In *Human Tendons* (ed. J. Jósza and P. Kannus), pp. 164–253. Human Kinetics, New York.

3. Gotoh, M., Hamada, K., Yamakawa, H., *et al.* (1998). Increased substance P in subacromial bursa and shoulder pain in rotator cuff disease. *J. Orthop. Res.* **16**, 618–621.

4. Benazzo, F., Stennardo, G., and Valli, M. (1996). Achilles and patellar tendinopathies in athletes: pathogenesis and surgical treatment. *Bull. Hosp. Joint Dis.* **54**, 236–240.

5. Green, S., Buchbinder, R., Glazier, R., and Forbes, A. (2000). Interventions for shoulder pain. *Cochrane-Database-Syst-Rev.* **2000** (2): CD001156.

6. Speed, C.A. and Hazleman, B.L. (2000). Shoulder pain. *Clinical evidence*, Issue 4. BMJ Press, London.

7. Murphy, D., Failla, J.M., and Koniuch, M.P. (1995). Steroid versus placebo injection for trigger finger. *J. Hand. Surg.* **20A**, 628–631.

8. Lambert, M.A., Morton, R.J., and Sloan, J.P. (1992). Controlled study of the use of local steroid injection in the treatment of trigger finger and thumb. *J. Hand Surg.* **17B**, 69–70.

9. Hay, E.M., Paterson, S.M., Lewis, M., Hosie, G., and Croft, P. (1999). Pragmatic randomised controlled trial of local corticosteroid injection and naproxen for treatment of lateral epicondylitis of elbow in primary care. *Br. Med. J.* **319**, 964–968.

10. DaCruz, D.J., Geeson, M., Allen, M.J., and Phair, I. (1988). Achilles paratendonitis: an evaluation of steroid injection. *Br. J. Sports Med.* **22**, 64–65.

11. Eustace, J.A., Brophy, D.P., Gibney, R.P., Bresnihan, B., and FitzGerald, O. (1997). Comparison of the accuracy of steroid placement with clinical outcome in patients with shoulder symptoms. *Ann. Rheum. Dis.* **56** (1), 59–63.

12. Zhingis, C., Failla, J.M., and Van Holsbeeck, M. (1998). Injection accuracy and clinical relief of de Quervain's tendinitis. *J. Hand Surg.* **23A**, 89–96.

13. Balint, P. and Sturrock, R.D. (1997). Musculoskeletal ultrasound imaging: a new diagnostic tool for the rheumatologist? *Br. J. Rheumatol.* **36** (11), 1141–1142.

14. Kapetanos, G. (1982). The effect of the local corticosteroids on the healing and biomechanical properties of the partially injured tendon. *Clin. Orthop.* **163**, 170–179.

15. Ketchum, L.D. (1971). Effects of triamcinalone on tendon healing and function. *Plast. Reconstr. Surg.* **47**, 471.

16. Haslock, I., Macfarlane, D., and Speed, C. (1995). Intra-articular and soft tissue injections: a survey of current practice. *Br. J. Rheumatol.* **34**, 449–452.

17. Consumers' Association (1995). Articular and periarticular corticosteroid injections. *Drugs Ther. Bull.* **33** (9), 67–70.

18. Mattila, J. (1983). Prolonged action and sustained serum levels of methylprednisolone acetate. *Clin. Trials J.* **20**, 18–23.

19. Kannus, P., Jarvinen, M., and Niittymaki, S. (1990). Long- or short-acting anesthetic with corticosteroid in local injections of overuse injuries? A prospective, randomised, double-blind study. *Int. J. Sports Med.* **11**, 397–400.

5.4 Acupuncture and trigger point needling

Mike Cummings

Introduction

Historical perspective

Fossil evidence of trepanning indicates that man has used physical therapies in the treatment of disease since Neolithic times (circa 10,000 to 3500 BC). Whilst the Chinese are reputed to have evidence of the use of acupuncture from bone etchings dating back to 1600 BC, the recent discovery of Ötzi, the Tyrolean iceman, dates the use of a therapeutic needling technique in Europe to 3200 BC.[1] It is clear that acupuncture-like therapies have developed independently in different civilizations around the world, and this is probably due to late evolutionary features in the mammalian nervous system, combined with intelligence, and the consequent use of tools, in humans.

Children learn at a very early age to rub energetically directly over the site of an acute pain to reduce the noxious sensation. In the case of a more chronic discomfort from aching, 'knotted' muscle, we tend to massage the local tissues more deeply and vigorously even though doing so may temporarily exacerbate the discomfort. This is likely to be conditioned behaviour resulting from the analgesic effect of somatic sensory stimulation. With the development of stone tools it is easy to hypothesize a progression of therapeutic techniques that resulted ultimately in piercing the skin and muscle at a site of chronic pain. It may be that successful treatment of myofascial pain by piercing the body at the site of tenderness not only encouraged the practice, but also led to the recognition of areas of the body that were most likely to harbour these tender points. In some parts of the world people developed superficial techniques of scratching or cauterizing the skin, whereas in the Far and Middle East the technique of acupuncture developed. (Fig. 1(a),(b) shows contemporary acupuncture needles used by the author.)

Traditional theories

The development of acupuncture points probably resulted from clinical observation that certain places in the body were more likely to harbour tender points than others and that treating these points by pressure or piercing could relieve pain and various other non-painful symptoms. Early physicians would also have noted that careful examination of the body surface revealed tender points in healthy subjects. Consistent patterns of pain referral from myofascial trigger points and the relief resulting from needling these and other muscle points would have led them to make links between some of the points. Radiation patterns of painful medical conditions such as sciatica, other radiculopathies, and possibly the consistent rashes of herpes zoster would have added to the impression that the established points were connected. These hypotheses do not explain the location of all acupuncture points, nor the paths of all the meridians, but there is clearly

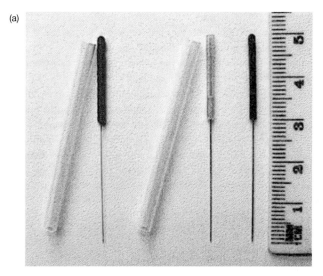

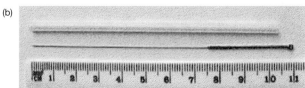

Fig. 1 Contemporary stainless steel acupuncture needles used by the author. (a) Three standard length (30 mm) needles suitable for most purposes. From left to right the needle diameter increases; 0.16 mm (left), 0.25 mm (centre), 0.3 mm (right). The finer needles require guide tubes for insertion through the skin. (b) A 75 mm needle, the length required for needling deep points in the gluteal region.

considerable overlap between myofascial trigger points and acupuncture points,[2] and between the pain referral patterns of the former and meridians (see fig. 1, Chapter 6.12).

Acupuncture was probably used pragmatically by the Chinese and others for centuries before it became systematized within a documented form of medicine some 2000 years ago.[3] The theories that developed were influenced by rational observations imposed upon a limited clinical knowledge base and within the philosophical framework of Taoism. The tendency towards syncretism resulted in the adoption and inclusion of many different theories, and over the centuries this has resulted in the development of a complex system of medicine. Whilst it can be initially unpalatable to the sceptical western scientist, closer inspection reveals that traditional Chinese medicine is built on a series of logical assumptions and, although some of these are clearly wrong, many may still represent valid clinical observations.

Western medical acupuncture

Western acupuncture is a term with a variety of potential meanings. The most literal interpretation invokes thoughts of geographical boundaries, but the term was probably introduced to distinguish a developing system of needle therapy from its traditional philosophical roots, which happened to be in the East.

Filshie and Cummings interpret 'Western medical acupuncture' as the scientific application of acupuncture as a therapy following orthodox clinical diagnosis.[4] It is important to note that the scientific evaluation of acupuncture is not restricted to the West,[5] and that therefore adherence to a geographical definition is inappropriate. Probably a more accurate description of 'Western medical acupuncture' is as a modern scientific approach to therapy involving dry needling of tissues that has developed from the introduction and evaluation of traditional Chinese acupuncture in the West.

The modern scientific method was established by Galileo in the seventeenth century when he introduced systematic verification through planned experiments to the existing ancient methods of reasoning and deduction. This system was adopted by the scientific community throughout the globe and, with only the addition of statistical analysis, it remains established practice today. The ethical practice of medicine requires the practitioner to understand and use scientific method.

Research

Methodological difficulties in acupuncture studies

The principal methodological difficulties in acupuncture studies are concerned with controls and blinding.[6] For a placebo control to be credible the subjects receiving it must believe that they have had an active treatment, identical to, or at least equivalent in potency to, the active intervention. Ideally, for any needling therapy, the control should involve an inactive form of needling, but it seems clear that a needle placed anywhere in the body is likely to have some neurophysiological effect,[7] perhaps simply as a result of the noxious stimulus.[8] A recent innovation in needle design may have overcome this problem by simulating needle penetration in a credible and reproducible way.[9, 10] A convincing control procedure should result in blinding of the subject, but it is impossible to blind an experienced therapist who is performing both real and sham needling techniques. A common way of reducing bias in this situation is to use a blind assessor.

Evidence for needling in myofascial pain

A recent systematic review of 23 randomized controlled trials conclusively shows that, when treating myofascial pain with trigger point injection, the nature of the injected substance makes no difference to the outcome, and that there is no therapeutic benefit in wet over dry needling.[11] These conclusions are supported by all the high quality trials in the review.[12–20]

The review did not find any rigorous evidence that needling therapies have a specific effect in myofascial pain. However, only two of the trials that met the inclusion criteria were designed in a way to provide such evidence.[17, 21] Chu reported results from only 52 per cent of the trial participants, and the study was of poor quality.[21] McMillan et al.[17] used potentially active interventions as controls, which by

design stimulated the same cutaneous receptive field as the test intervention. From a neurophysiological view, all three groups in this trial were needled or injected in about the same place, and they all improved significantly. The authors of the review conclude:

The hypothesis that needling therapies have specific efficacy in the treatment of myofascial pain is not supported by the research to date, but this review suggests that any effect derived from these therapies is likely to be derived from the needle, rather than from either, an injection of liquid in general, or any substance in particular. All groups in the review in whom trigger points were directly needled showed marked improvement in their symptoms; therefore further research is urgently needed to establish the specific effect of trigger point needling, with emphasis on the use of an adequate control for the needle.

Evidence for needling in other soft tissue disorders

There have been few randomized controlled trials of needling therapies in other soft tissue disorders, excluding local steroid injections, which are dealt with in Chapter 5.3. Molsberger and Hille demonstrated a significant analgesic effect ($p < 0.01$) compared with placebo immediately after a single, non-segmental acupuncture needle stimulus in 48 patients with chronic 'tennis elbow pain'.[22] However, whilst this trial revealed a specific analgesic effect from needling, it does not imply that the intervention would be efficient in treating chronic lateral epicondylitis. By contrast, the recent study by Kleinhenz et al., using a novel placebo needle, demonstrated a useful treatment effect from acupuncture needling in 52 sportsmen with rotator cuff tendonitis.[10] It is unclear whether the specific effect of acupuncture needling is limited to analgesia, or whether there is enhanced tissue healing, as has been demonstrated in animal studies.[23, 24] Irrespective of this, needling should not be used as the only intervention in conditions that require physical rehabilitation in addition to symptom control.

A recent systematic review concluded that real acupuncture was better than sham acupuncture in the treatment of fibromyalgia.[25] However, as the authors admit, only one high-quality randomized controlled trial was found. Deluze et al. found that electroacupuncture was significantly better than a minimal superficial electroacupuncture treatment in relieving the symptoms of fibromyalgia.[26] It was a methodologically sound trial, but it has not been repeated, and electroacupuncture is not currently a popular choice of therapy in fibromyalgia.

Mechanisms

Neurophysiology of needling

The therapeutic effects of needling are mediated through stimulation of the peripheral nervous system, and so can be abolished by local anaesthetic.[27, 28] In particular, stimulation of Aδ or type III afferent nerve fibres has been implicated as the key component in producing analgesia.[29] The therapeutic effects of needling can be divided into four categories based on the area influenced: local; segmental; heterosegmental; and general.

Local effects

Release of trophic and vasoactive neuropeptides including neuropeptide Y (NPY), calcitonin gene-related peptide (CGRP), and vasoactive intestinal peptide (VIP) has been demonstrated.[30, 31] It is likely that the release of CGRP and VIP from peripheral nerves stimulated by needling results in enhanced circulation and wound healing in rats,[23, 24] and equivalent sensory stimulation has proved effective in human patients.[32]

Segmental effects

Through stimulation of high-threshold ergoreceptors in muscle, needling can have a profound influence on sensory modulation within the dorsal horn at the relevant segmental level. C fibre pain transmission is inhibited via enkephalinergic interneurons in lamina II, the substantia gelatinosa (Fig. 2). Bowsher reviewed the basic science literature that supports this mechanism,[33] and White appraised both experimental and clinical evidence.[34] Segmental stimulation appears to have a more powerful effect than an equivalent stimulus from a distant segment, in modulating pain,[35, 36] local autonomic activity,[37] and itch.[38] Aδ or type III afferent nerve fibres can be stimulated by superficial needling as well as by needling deeper tissues, but it seems that segmental stimuli from the latter (usually muscle) have a more powerful effect.[36, 38, 39]

Heterosegmental effects

Whilst segmental stimulation appears to be the more powerful effect, needling anywhere in the body can influence afferent processing throughout the spinal cord. The needle stimulus travels from the segment of origin to the ventral posterior lateral nucleus of the thalamus, and projects from there to the sensory cortex. Collaterals in the midbrain synapse in the periaqueductal grey (PAG), from where inhibitory fibres descend, via the nucleus raphe magnus, to influence afferent processing in the dorsal horn at every level of the spinal cord. Serotonin is the prominent neurotransmitter in the caudal stages of this descending pathway, and the fibres synapse with the enkephalinergic interneurons in lamina II (Fig. 3). A second descending system from the PAG travels via the nucleus raphe gigantocellularis: its fibres are noradrenergic, and their influence is mediated directly on lamina II cells, rather than via enkephalinergic interneurons. Diffuse noxious inhibitory controls (DNIC) is the term introduced by Le Bars et al. to define a third analgesic system, which is induced by a noxious stimulus anywhere in the body.[8] Heterosegmental needling exerts influence through all three mechanisms to different degrees,[33, 34] and possibly through others, as yet undefined.

General effects

These are more difficult to define, and there is clearly some overlap with heterosegmental effects. The latter term is used here to denote effects mediated at every segment of the spinal cord, as opposed to effects mediated by humeral means or by influence on higher centres in the central nervous system (CNS) controlling general responses. Acupuncture needling has proven efficacy in the treatment of nausea and vomiting.[40] There is some evidence that it results in increased release of corticosteroids,[41] and early indications suggest that it may stimulate oxytocin, resulting in analgesia, sedation, and relaxation.[42] There is a substantial body of work that indicates the importance of β-endorphin and other endogenous opioids in acupuncture analgesia,[43] and, subsequently, correlations have been identified between the endorphin-releasing effect of acupuncture and that of prolonged exercise.[44] Further correlations in terms of neuropeptide

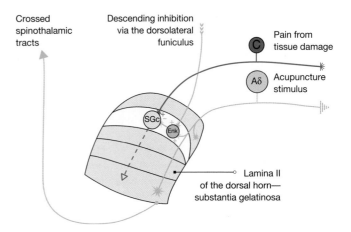

Fig. 2 Segmental analgesia mediated via an enkephalinergic interneuron in the substantia gelatinosa.

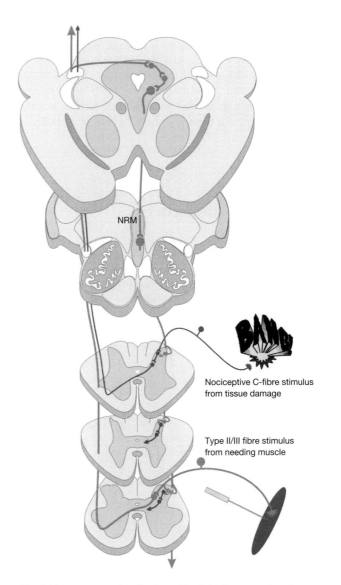

Fig. 3 Heterosegmental analgesia mediated via the serotoninergic descending inhibitory system. PAG, Periaqueductal grey; NRM, nucleus raphe magnus.

release have been noted,[45] and recently it has been suggested that chronic activation of opioid systems by exercise, or potentially by acupuncture, may mediate enhanced immunity, with decreased upper respiratory infections and protection against some forms of cancer.[46]

Needling of trigger points

The mechanism of action of direct needling in the deactivation of trigger points is undetermined. Despite the fact that a causal relationship has not been established between direct needling of trigger points and improvement in symptoms, a discussion of the potential mechanisms involved may still be useful in developing future research questions. Simons et al. comment on the results of two trials that compare direct dry and direct wet needling of trigger points[47, 48] and concludes that the critical therapeutic factor in both techniques is mechanical disruption by the needle.[49] The common factor is certainly needle insertion into the trigger point. However, Hong has demonstrated the importance of stimulating a local twitch response in achieving an immediate effect[47] and with Simons cites evidence that the local twitch response is mediated by a segmental spinal reflex.[50] Fine et al. performed a rigorous experimental study, in which trigger points were subject to direct wet needling, and clearly demonstrated that an opioid mechanism was involved in trigger point pain relief.[51] In light of this evidence it seems more likely that the needle works through sensory stimulation than through mechanical disruption, and this would be consistent with the mechanism of action of acupuncture analgesia.[33, 34, 43]

Technique

Western medical acupuncture

Safety aspects

Acupuncture involves the insertion of, usually stainless steel, needles into the body. Whilst it is often perceived by the general public as 'natural' and 'safe', along with many complementary therapies, it is neither natural nor completely safe. As with any needling therapy the serious risks are associated with the transmission of blood-borne infection and direct trauma. Rampes and Peuker categorize adverse events associated with acupuncture as follows:[52]

1. delayed or missed diagnosis;

2. deterioration of disorder under treatment;

3. pain;

4. vegetative reactions;

5. bacterial and viral infections;

6. trauma of tissues and organs;

7. miscellaneous.

If acupuncture is performed as a therapy by an orthodox medical practitioner within his or her sphere of competence, the first two categories will be avoided.

Persistent pain attributed to acupuncture treatment is rare, but temporary exacerbation of the presenting complaint for a day or so is common.

Vegetative reactions include syncope and sedation. Syncope can be largely avoided by treating patients lying on an examination couch.

However, very occasionally a profound sinus bradycardia will result in loss of consciousness of a patient who is lying down. In all such anecdotal case reports heard by the author, the patient has recovered spontaneously within a few minutes. Sedation is relatively common, and occurs in perhaps 20 per cent of patients after their first two treatments. In perhaps 5 per cent of patients there is always some degree of sedation associated with acupuncture treatment. Sedation is rarely seen as an adverse event by patients, and is only of concern in terms of driving home or operating machinery after treatment.

Infections associated with acupuncture treatment are uncommon but nearly always serious when they occur. Two cases of fatal staphylococcal septicaemia have been reported in debilitated patients following the use of indwelling needles.[53] In two other reports the patients survived,[54, 55] but only after serious illness, and in one case the patient survived disseminated intravascular coagulation.[55] A streptococcal toxic shock-like syndrome has been attributed to acupuncture in two reports—one had a fatal outcome[56] and the other required amputation for the associated superficial fasciitis.[57] Bacterial endocarditis has been reported on three occasions following the use of indwelling needles in patients with valvular heart disease.[58–60] Other infections complicating acupuncture include perichondritis from the use of press needles in the ear, numerous cases of hepatitis from contaminated needles, a few speculative cases of the acquired immune deficiency syndrome, and isolated reports of spinal, meningeal, and joint infections.[52]

Traumatic complications of acupuncture needling are avoidable, and on occasion they have been fatal. Six cases of direct injury to the heart or pericardium have been reported, two of which resulted in death from cardiac tamponade. Over 90 incidents of pneumothorax have been recorded in scientific publications, of which two were fatal. Trauma to abdominal viscera, peripheral nerves, the CNS, and blood vessels have been described. Peuker et al. review the traumatic complications of acupuncture, and conclude that therapists need to know human anatomy.[61]

Point selection

The two main themes in western medical acupuncture are dry needling of trigger points and segmental acupuncture. The latter is defined as the technique of needling an area of the soma innervated by the same spinal segment as the disordered structure under treatment. As the conditions covered in this text are almost wholly related to somatic pathology, which is often localized, point selection is relatively straightforward. Based on neurophysiological and clinical evidence,[33–39] the main principle in point selection is to stimulate the soma as close as is practical to the seat of the pathology, or at least within the same segment. Local trigger points, tender points, or acupuncture points are chosen (Fig. 4), and often these will overlap so that the key point to stimulate is a trigger point (which is tender by definition) at the site of an acupuncture point (Fig. 5). If the key element of the somatic pathology is a myofascial trigger point, this is arguably the only point that it is necessary to treat. In most other cases the analgesia afforded by local needling can be enhanced by using one or more points at a distance from the pathology, in addition to the relevant local points (Lundeberg, personal communication 1999). Distant points are chosen because they stimulate the appropriate segment, or because they are conveniently located and known to generate strong needling sensation (heterosegmental acupuncture). In individual cases point selection may be modified by the need to avoid local conditions:

- skin infection
- ulceration
- moles and tumours
- varicosities

or by the need to avoid regional conditions:

- hydrostatic oedema
- lymphoedema
- anaesthetic areas

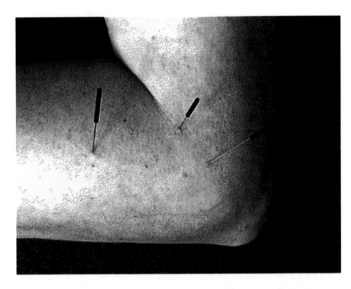

Fig. 4 Typical local needling for the elbow. The needles are in a trigger point in the middle finger extensor (left), the acupuncture point LI11 (middle), and a tender point in the common extensor attachment (right).

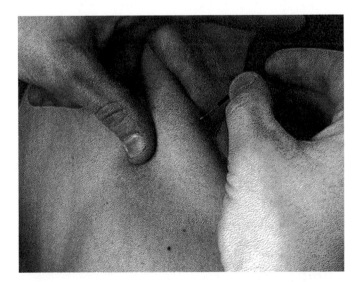

Fig. 5 Needling of a trigger point in the upper free border of trapezius at the site of the acupuncture point GB21. Note that the needle is directed at a tangent to the rib cage, and a fold of soft tissue is pinched up between the thumb and middle finger of the left hand to control the needle tip position—both manoeuvres reduce the risk of trauma to the pleura.

- hyperaesthetic areas
- ischaemia.

As a general rule, therapeutic needling should be performed in healthy tissue.

Needle technique

Sterile, single-use, disposable needles should always be used. In most cases acupuncture needling involves stimulation of muscle tissue. Needling of muscle produces a characteristic sensation, often described as a dull, diffuse ache, pressure, swelling, or numbness, which can be referred some distance from the point of stimulation. Needling of most other tissues of the soma, such as skin, ligament, tendon, periosteum, and fascial layers, produces relatively localized and often sharp sensations. If the aim is to stimulate a point in muscle, a rapid insertion through the skin and superficial layers minimizes discomfort for the patient. Practitioners who are learning the technique find that the use of an introducer facilitates a rapid, often painless insertion. If an introducer is not used, the practitioner will stretch the skin over the point during insertion. Once through the skin, the needle should be rapidly advanced to the desired position or muscle layer, and is then stimulated by rotation back and forth combined with a varying degree of 'lift and thrust' (slight withdrawal and reinsertion) until the desired sensation is achieved. If constant stimulation of the needle is required, an electrical stimulator can be used. For the latter technique, usually a minimum of two needles are inserted and a specially designed electroacupuncture device is used to deliver the electrical stimulus.

Dry needling of trigger points involves a very similar procedure, although the practitioner will often lift and thrust the needle to a greater degree and with a fanning technique, aiming to hit the trigger point precisely. When the needle directly impinges on the trigger point, a local twitch is often seen or felt in the associated band of muscle, and the symptoms derived from that point are reproduced (Fig.6).

In clinical practice a wide variety of needling techniques has been described. These range from superficial needling to periosteal needling, with a variety of intermediate depths in muscle. Superficial needling of acupuncture points is common in Japanese forms of acupuncture, and Baldry describes a superficial needling technique exclusively over trigger points.[62, 63] Periosteal needling was first described by Mann, although he, like most western practitioners who came after him, uses a variety of techniques.[64, 65] As suggested above, muscle is the most common site of stimulation. Depth and strength of needling in this tissue ranges from brief, superficial stimulation of the muscle surface to deep, repetitive intramuscular stimulation. The latter is not uncommon in Chinese acupuncture, but is also promoted by some practitioners in the West, in particular by Gunn, who targets motor points and paraspinal muscles.[66, 67]

Clinical aspects

There is a range of different responses to acupuncture treatment, from no effect in 5 or 10 per cent of the population at one end, to profound analgesia and improved well-being, in a similar proportion, at the other end. Empirical observation suggests that about 70 per cent of the population have a useful response. Patient selection will clearly influence success, and a healthy patient with a short-lived myofascial pain syndrome is much more likely to have a beneficial outcome than a debilitated patient with a chronic, ill-defined, and complex problem.

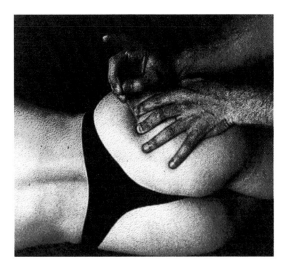

Fig. 6 Needling a trigger point in gluteus medius. The taut band of muscle is fixed between the index and middle fingers of the left hand, and a long needle is tapped through the skin with the aid of an introducer. The needle will then be inserted to the necessary depth and fanned from side to side with a variable degree of 'lift and thrust' until a twitch is felt or the pain referral is produced.

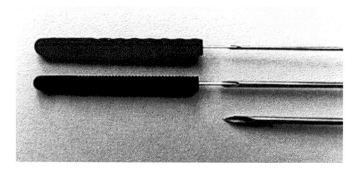

Fig. 7 Acupuncture needles are much finer than the hypodermic needles used for trigger point injections. The hypodermic needles shown are 27G (top right), 22G (centre right), and for comparison a 21G (bottom right) needle used for standard venesection. The acupuncture needles are 0.16 mm (top left) and 0.3 mm (centre left) in diameter, and easily fit within the shaft of the hypodermic needles, as illustrated.

It is difficult to define a 'dose' for acupuncture treatment, because on many occasions a judicious single needle insertion may have the same effect as 10 or more needles left in place for 20 min, and similar-strength, sequential treatments often have increasing potency in the early stages of a course of treatment. Experimental work does appear to support a type of dose–response relationship for sensory stimulation (Lundeberg, personal communication 1997), but it is unlikely to be linear. There is probably a stepwise increase in potency down the following list:

1. superficial, heterosegmental needling with minimal sensation;

2. superficial, segmental needling with minimal sensation;

3. deep, heterosegmental needling with strong sensation;

4. deep, segmental needling with strong sensation;

5. deep, segmental needling with electrical stimulation sufficient to cause muscle contraction.

Whilst acupuncture is likely to do more than simply offer pain relief, the standard pattern of effect from treatment is most easily appreciated in terms of analgesia. There may be little or no effect after the first session, as the practitioner will usually start with gentle treatment. This is to avoid aggravating the complaint in those most sensitive to needling. The initial response is seen within the first 72 hours after treatment, and its onset is often not perceived until the day after needling. Repeat treatments are performed either bi-weekly or weekly, and the interval can be lengthened with the response. Typically, there is a progressive increase in the quality and duration of the effect following repeated sessions and, in chronic pain states, symptom control can be maintained for some patients with relatively infrequent treatments, perhaps every 4–6 weeks.

Trigger point injection

Despite the evidence that injection of trigger points confers no therapeutic advantage over dry needling,[11] the former is still practised widely.[49] Hong suggests that the only reason for using an injection of local anaesthetic rather than dry needling is to reduce post-needling soreness.[47] However, his comparison was made using a hypodermic needle, which is likely to cause more damage with its cutting edge than a solid acupuncture needle (Fig. 7).

The technique of trigger point injection is very similar to that of acupuncture dry needling of trigger points described above. The differences are that the hypodermic needle is often inserted at a shallow angle, rather than perpendicular to the skin, and that small quantities of local anaesthetic are injected each time a local twitch occurs or there is patient recognition of their referred pain. Hong describes injecting 0.02–0.05 ml of 5 per cent lidocaine on each of 20–60 insertions into the trigger point zone using a 1.25-in. 27G needle.[47] On each withdrawal the needle is retained in the subcutaneous tissue to avoid the discomfort of repeated insertion through the skin. He uses a 'fast-in fast-out' technique, which is a modification of the injection technique for trigger points originally described by Travell and Simons.[49]

Prognosis

As there is such limited evidence from controlled trials of the specific efficacy of needling techniques, simple audit and experience of practitioners must be called upon as a guide. Prognosis in myofascial pain syndromes is discussed briefly in Chapter 6.12, but it should be noted here that they appear to respond very well to direct needling of the relevant trigger points, with a successful outcome reported in 90 per cent or more of cases.[68] Musculoskeletal pain in general is helped by acupuncture in 70 per cent of cases but, in some of the more difficult enthesopathies, response rates may be only 40–60 per cent, and in many such cases adequate advice and rehabilitation is as important as the symptomatic treatment mediated through the needle.

Summary

Needling therapies have been applied to the treatment of soft tissue disorders for thousands of years, and the techniques used today probably do not differ dramatically from those applied to Ötzi in 3200 BC. Empirical evidence suggests that direct needling of trigger points is probably the most valuable needling technique, but definitive research to establish the specific action of the needle is still sought. All doctors who treat musculoskeletal dysfunction would find the technique of needling trigger points useful, but adequate knowledge of anatomy and infection control procedures is essential.

References

1. Dorfer, L., Moser, M., Bahr, F., Spindler, K., Egarter-Vigl, E., Giullen, S., et al. (1999). A medical report from the stone age? *Lancet* **354** (9183), 1023–1025.

2. Melzack, R., Stillwell, D.M., and Fox, E.J. (1977). Trigger points and acupuncture points for pain: correlations and implications. *Pain* **3** (1), 3–23.

3. Veith, I. (1972). *The Yellow Emperor's classic of internal medicine*. University of California Press, Berkeley.

4. Filshie, J. and Cummings, T.M. (1999). Western medical acupuncture. In *Acupuncture—a scientific appraisal* (ed. E. Ernst and A.R. White), pp. 31–59. Butterworth Heinemann, Oxford.

5. Han, J.S. and Terenius, L. (1982). Neurochemical basis of acupuncture analgesia. *Annu. Rev. Pharmacol. Toxicol.* **22**, 193–220.

6. Lewith, G.T. and Vincent, C.A. (1998). The clinical evaluation of acupuncture. In *Medical acupuncture, a Western scientific approach* (ed. J. Filshie and A.R. White), pp. 205–224. Churchill Livingstone, Edinburgh.

7. Lewith, G.T. and Machin, D. (1983). On the evaluation of the clinical effects of acupuncture. *Pain* **16** (2), 111–127.

8. Le Bars, D., Dickenson, A.H., and Besson, J.M. (1979). Diffuse noxious inhibitory controls (DNIC). I—Effects on dorsal horn convergent neurones in the rat; II—Lack of effect on non-convergent neurones, supraspinal involvement and theoretical implications. *Pain* **6** (3), 305–327.

9. Streitberger, K. and Kleinhenz, J. (1998). Introducing a placebo needle into acupuncture research. *Lancet* **352** (9125), 364–365.

10. Kleinhenz, J., Streitberger, K., Windeler, J., Gussbacher, A., Mavridis, G., and Martin, E. (1999). Randomised clinical trial comparing the effects of acupuncture and a newly designed placebo needle in rotator cuff tendinitis. *Pain* **83** (2), 235–241.

11. Cummings, T.M. and White, A.R. (2001). Needling therapies in the management of myofascial pain: a systematic review. *Arch. Phys. Med. Rehabil.* **82** (7), 986–992.

12. Mendelson, G., Selwood, T.S., Kranz, H., Loh, T.S., Kidson, M.A., and Scott, D.S. (1983). Acupuncture treatment of chronic back pain. A double-blind placebo- controlled trial. *Am. J. Med.* **74** (1), 49–55.

13. Kuang, X., Su, Y., and Guo, H. (1996). [Study on combined acupunctural and general anesthesia in pneumonectomy]. *Chung Kuo Chung Hsi I Chieh Ho Tsa Chih* **16** (2), 84–86.

14. Lao, L. (1996). Acupuncture techniques and devices. *J. Altern. Complement. Med.* **2** (1), 23–25.

15. Vilholm, O.J., Moller, K., and Jorgensen, K. (1998). Effect of traditional Chinese acupuncture on severe tinnitus: a double-blind, placebo-controlled, clinical investigation with open therapeutic control. *Br. J. Audiol.* **32** (3), 197–204.

16. Cooper, R.A., Henderson, T., and Dietrich, C.L. (1998). Roles of non-physician clinicians as autonomous providers of patient care [see comments]. *J. Am. Med. Assoc.* **280** (9), 795–802.

17. McMillan, A.S., Nolan, A., and Kelly, P.J. (1997). The efficacy of dry needling and procaine in the treatment of myofascial pain in the jaw muscles. *J. Orofacial Pain* **11** (4), 307–314.

18. Tfelt-Hansen, P., Lous, I., and Olesen, J. (1981). Prevalence and significance of muscle tenderness during common migraine attacks. *Headache* **21** (2), 49–54.

19. Tschopp, K.P. and Gysin, C. (1996). Local injection therapy in 107 patients with myofascial pain syndrome of the head and neck. *ORL J. Otorhinolaryngol. Rel. Spec.* **58** (6), 306–310.

20. Wheeler, A.H., Goolkasian, P., and Gretz, S.S. (1998). A randomized, double-blind, prospective pilot study of botulinum toxin injection for refractory, unilateral, cervicothoracic, paraspinal, myofascial pain syndrome. *Spine* **23** (15), 1662–1666.

21. Chu, J. (1997). Does EMG (dry needling) reduce myofascial pain symptoms due to cervical nerve root irritation? *Electromyogr. Clin. Neurophysiol.* **37** (5), 259–272.

22. Molsberger, A. and Hille, E. (1994). The analgesic effect of acupuncture in chronic tennis elbow pain. *Br. J. Rheumatol.* **33** (12), 1162–1165.

23. Jansen, G., Lundeberg, T., Kjartansson, J., and Samuelson, U.E. (1989). Acupuncture and sensory neuropeptides increase cutaneous blood flow in rats. *Neurosci. Lett.* **97** (3), 305–309.

24. Jansen, G., Lundeberg, T., Samuelson, U.E., and Thomas, M. (1989). Increased survival of ischaemic musculocutaneous flaps in rats after acupuncture. *Acta Physiol. Scand.* **135** (4), 555–558.

25. Berman, B.M., Ezzo, J., Hadhazy, V., and Swyers, J.P. (1999). Is acupuncture effective in the treatment of fibromyalgia? *J. Fam. Pract.* **48** (3), 213–218.

26. Deluze, C., Bosia, L., Zirbs, A., Chantraine, A., and Vischer, T.L. (1992). Electroacupuncture in fibromyalgia: results of a controlled trial. *Br. Med. J.* **305** (6864), 1249–1252.

27. Chiang, C.Y., Chang, C.T., Chu, H.L., and Yang, L.F. (1973). Peripheral afferent pathway for acupuncture analgesia. *Sci. Sin.* **16**, 210–217.

28. Dundee, J.W. and Ghaly, G. (1991). Local anesthesia blocks the antiemetic action of P6 acupuncture. *Clin. Pharmacol. Ther.* **50** (1), 78–80.

29. Chung, J.M., Fang, Z.R., Hori, Y., Lee, K.H., and Willis, W.D. (1984). Prolonged inhibition of primate spinothalamic tract cells by peripheral nerve stimulation. *Pain* **19** (3), 259–275.

30. Dawidson, I., Angmar-Mansson, B., Blom, M., Theodorsson, E., and Lundeberg, T. (1998). The influence of sensory stimulation (acupuncture) on the release of neuropeptides in the saliva of healthy subjects. *Life Sci.* **63** (8), 659–674.

31. Dawidson, I., Angmar-Mansson, B., Blom, M., Theodorsson, E., and Lundeberg, T. (1998). Sensory stimulation (acupuncture) increases the release of vasoactive intestinal polypeptide in the saliva of xerostomia sufferers. *Neuropeptides* **32** (6), 543–548.

32. Lundeberg, T., Kjartansson, J., and Samuelsson, U. (1998). Effect of electrical nerve stimulation on healing of ischaemic skin flaps. *Lancet* **2** (8613), 712–714.

33. Bowsher, D. (1998). Mechanisms of acupuncture. In *Medical acupuncture, a Western scientific approach* (ed. J. Filshie and A.R. White), pp. 69–82. Churchill Livingstone, Edinburgh.

34. White, A.R. (1999). Neurophysiology of acupuncture analgesia. In *Acupuncture—a scientific appraisal* (ed. E. Ernst and A.R. White), pp. 60–92. Butterworth Heinemann, Oxford.

35. Chapman, C.R., Chen, A.C., and Bonica, J.J. (1977). Effects of intrasegmental electrical acupuncture on dental pain: evaluation by threshold estimation and sensory decision theory. *Pain* **3** (3), 213–227.

36. Lundeberg, T., Eriksson, S., Lundeberg, S., and Thomas, M. (1981). Acupuncture and sensory thresholds. *Am. J. Chin. Med.* **17** (3–4), 99–110.

37. Sato, A., Sato, Y., Suzuki, A., and Uchida, S. (1993). Neural mechanisms of the reflex inhibition and excitation of gastric motility elicited by acupuncture-like stimulation in anesthetized rats. *Neurosci. Res.* **18** (1), 53–62.

38. Lundeberg, T., Bondesson, L., and Thomas, M. (1987). Effect of acupuncture on experimentally induced itch. *Br. J. Dermatol.* **117** (6), 771–777.

39. Ceccherelli, F., Gagliardi, G., Visentin, R., and Giron, G. (1998). Effects of deep vs. superficial stimulation of acupuncture on capsaicin-induced edema. A blind controlled study in rats. *Acupuncture Electrother. Res.* **23** (2), 125–134.

40. Vickers, A.J. (1996). Can acupuncture have specific effects on health? A systematic review of acupuncture antiemesis trials. *J. R. Soc. Med.* **89** (6), 303–311.

41. Roth, L.U., Maret-Maric, A., Adler, R.H., and Neuenschwander, B.E. (1997). Acupuncture points have subjective (needing sensation) and objective (serum cortisol increase) specificity. *Acupuncture Med.* **15** (1), 2–5.

42. Uvnas-Moberg, K., Bruzelius, G., Alster, P., and Lundeberg, T. (1993). The antinociceptive effect of non-noxious sensory stimulation is mediated partly through oxytocinergic mechanisms. *Acta Physiol. Scand.* **149** (2), 199–204.

43. Pomeranz, B. (1997). Acupuncture analgesia—neurophysiological mechanisms. International Congress: Sensory Stimulation in Pain and Diseases, Karolinska Institutet, Nobel Forum, Stockholm, Sweden.

44. Thoren, P., Floras, J.S., Hoffmann, P., and Seals, D.R. (1990). Endorphins and exercise: physiological mechanisms and clinical implications. *Med. Sci. Sports Exer.* **22** (4), 417–428.

45. Bucinskaite, V., Theodorsson, E., Crumpton, K., Stenfors, C., Ekblom, A., and Lundeberg, T. (1996). Effects of repeated sensory stimulation (electro-acupuncture) and physical exercise (running) on open-field behaviour and concentrations of neuropeptides in the hippocampus in WKY and SHR rats. *Eur. J. Neurosci.* **8** (2), 382–387.

46. Jonsdottir, I.H. (1999). Physical exercise, acupuncture and immune function. *Acupuncture Med.* **17** (1), 50–53.

47. Hong, C.Z. (1994). Lidocaine injection versus dry needling to myofascial trigger point. The importance of the local twitch response. *Am. J. Phys. Med. Rehabil.* **73** (4), 256–263.

48. Skootsky, S.A., Jaeger, B., and Oye, R.K. (1989). Prevalence of myofascial pain in general internal medicine practice. *West. J. Med.* **151** (2), 157–160.

49. Simons, D.G., Travell, J.G., and Simons, P.T. (1991). *Travell and Simons' myofascial pain and dysfunction. The trigger point manual.* Vol. 1. *Upper half of body*, 2nd edn. Williams and Wilkins, Baltimore.

50. Hong, C.Z. and Simons, D.G. (1998). Pathophysiologic and electrophysiologic mechanisms of myofascial trigger points. *Arch. Phys. Med. Rehabil.* **79** (7), 863–872.

51. Fine, P.G., Milano, R., and Hare, B.D. (1988). The effects of myofascial trigger point injections are naloxone reversible. *Pain* **32** (1), 15–20.

52. Rampes, H. and Peuker, E. (1999). Adverse effects of acupuncture. In *Acupuncture—a scientific appraisal* (ed. E. Ernst and A.R. White), pp. 128–152. Butterworth Heinemann, Oxford.

53. Pierik, M.G. (1982). Fatal Staphylococcal septicemia following acupuncture: report of two cases. Occurrence of Staphylococcal septicemia following acupuncture emphasizes need for thorough medical evaluation before such procedures. *R. I. Med. J.* **65** (6), 251–253.

54. Doutsu, Y., Tao, Y., Sasayama, K., Inoue, Y., Yamashita, K., Shigeno, H. *et al.* (1986). [A case of Staphylococcus aureus septicemia after acupuncture therapy]. *Kansenshogaku Zasshi* **60** (8), 911–916.

55. Izatt, E. and Fairman, M. (1977). Staphylococcal septicaemia with disseminated intravascular coagulation associated with acupuncture. *Postgrad. Med. J.* **53** (619), 285–286.

56. Onizuka, T., Oishi, K., Ikeda, T., Watanabe, K., Senba, M., Suga, K., *et al.* (1998). [A fatal case of streptococcal toxic shock-like syndrome probably caused by acupuncture]. *Kansenshogaku Zasshi* **72** (7), 776–780.

57. Harada, K., Suzuki, T., Suzuki, A., Obana, M., Matsuoka, Y., Irimajiri, S., *et al.* (1997). [Toxic shock-like syndrome after acupuncturation]. *Kansenshogaku Zasshi* **71** (10), 1066–1070.

58. Jefferys, D.B., Smith, S., Brennand-Roper, D.A., and Curry, P.V. (1983). Acupuncture needles as a cause of bacterial endocarditis. *Br. Med. J. (Clin. Res. Ed.)* **287** (6388), 326–327.

59. Lee, R.J. and McIlwain, J.C. (1985). Subacute bacterial endocarditis following ear acupuncture. *Int. J. Cardiol.* **7** (1), 62–63.

60. Scheel, O., Sundsfjord, A., and Lunde, P. (1991). [Bacterial endocarditis after treatment by a natural healer]. *Tidsskr. Nor. Laegeforen* **111** (22), 2741–2742.

61. Peuker, E.T., White, A.R., Ernst, E., Pera, F., and Filler, T.J. (1999). Traumatic complications of acupuncture, therapists need to know human anatomy. *Arch. Fam. Med.* **8**, 553–558.

62. Baldry, P.E. (1996). *Acupuncture, trigger points and musculo-skeletal pain* 2nd edn. Churchill Livingstone, Edinburgh.

63. Baldry, P.E. (1998). Trigger point acupuncture. In *Medical acupuncture, a Western scientific approach* (ed. J. Filshie and A.R. White), pp. 33–60. Churchill Livingstone, Edinburgh.

64. Mann, F. (1998). A new system of acupuncture. In *Medical acupuncture, a Western scientific approach* (ed. J. Filshie and A.R. White), pp. 61–66. Churchill Livingstone, Edinburgh.

65. Mann, F. (2000). *Reinventing acupuncture: a new concept of ancient medicine*, 2nd edn. Butterworth Heinemann, Oxford.

66. Gunn, C.C. (1989). *Treating myofascial pain, intramuscular stimulation (IMS) for myofascial pain syndromes of neuropathic origin.* University of Washington, Seattle.

67. Gunn, C.C. (1998). Acupuncture and the peripheral nervous system. In *Medical acupuncture, a Western scientific approach* (ed J. Filshie and A.R. White), pp. 137–150. Churchill Livingstone, Edinburgh.

68. Cummings, T.M. (1996). A computerised audit of acupuncture in two populations: civilian and forces. *Acupuncture Med.* **14** (1), 37–39.

5.5 Neural blockade

Carol Chong and Rajesh Munglani

Introduction

Neural blockade is very commonly performed for the diagnosis and treatment of chronically painful conditions. In this chapter the rationale for the use of neural blockade and why it may fail will be explained. In addition, mention is made of the commonly performed blocks and the evidence for their continued use.

How neural blockade may work

It was once thought that blocking a nerve would simply block afferent noxious input, hence decreasing pain levels. In fact, the situation is actually more complex due to the complex neurobiological changes that occur when acute pain becomes chronic.

The neuroplasticity of the central nervous system in response to pain is better understood and it is now known that certain receptors in the periphery such as adenosine triphosphate (ATP), neurokinin-1, neuropeptide Y, and 5 hydroxytryptamine are associated with nociceptors. Tissue or peripheral nerve injury that causes the release of substances such as histamine and bradykinins results in activation of a complex cascade of events within the peripheral nerve and spinal cord. There is release of substance P, glutamate, and calcitonin gene-related peptide (CGRP), which leads to activation of N-methyl-D-aspartate (NMDA) receptors.

Secondary messengers such as prostaglandins, calcium, and c-*fos* are activated and there is a decrease in gamma aminobutyric acid (GABA). GABA is an inhibitory neurotransmitter, which is also found in laminae 2 of the spinal cord. A reduction in GABA levels makes the spinal cord more excitable. There is a proliferation of sodium channels on the injured nerves, which increases its excitability. This causes an increase in cholecystokinin levels in the spinal cord and therefore makes the cord more receptive to input. New nerve contacts such as A beta fibres are formed between the deep to more superficial laminae 1 and 2. Therefore, mechanical stimuli such as light touch can be interpreted as pain (allodynia).

Concurrently, there is evidence of sympathetic nerve 'baskets' forming in the dorsal root ganglia as well as activation of adrenoreceptors peripherally and centrally. This may be the basis for sympathetically maintained pain. For an in-depth review of these mechanisms, the reader is referred to references 1–4.

Diagnostic and therapeutic blockade

Neural blockade for chronic pain procedures can be diagnostic or therapeutic. The success of such nerve blocks depends on the level of neurobiological change that has occurred (Table 1).[15]

A diagnostic block is performed with local anaesthetic and allows us to predict the response to a more permanent procedure. An example of this is lumbar facet joint injections for back pain. Local anaesthetic can be used to block the medial branch of the posterior primary ramus that supplies the joint. If this is successful, we could proceed to radiofrequency denervation of the joint.

Therapeutic blockade can be performed in more than one way.

1. The addition of corticosteroids to the local anaesthetic may prolong the block in certain ways. It is known that phospholipase-A2 leaks out of intervertebral discs when they herniated or rupture and causes nerve root irritation. The use of steroids in epidurals for sciatica is said to have an antiphospholipase-A2 effect and may bring about early resolution of symptoms. In some studies the use of epidural or dorsal root ganglion blocks reduces the requirement for subsequent surgery in proven lumbar disc prolapse.[6]

2. More permanent blockade can be achieved with neurolytic techniques and these include the use of agents such as phenol or alcohol, radiofrequency denervation, pulsed radiofrequency, and cryotherapy. This will be discussed in more detail below.

Neural blockade procedures in chronic pain aim to decrease nociceptive input into the dorsal horn. It is thought that, if a nerve is quiescent for some time, peripheral sensitization can be reversed.[7]

Why do nerve blocks fail?

There are several reason why neural blockade may fail. First, it may be a failure of technique. The placement of the needle may be inaccurate or incorrect solutions may be used. Second, patient selection is very important. There will certainly be anatomical variation amongst patients. It is also evident that there are certain patients in whom interventional therapy will not be successful. Such patients may have other components to their pain that need to be addressed such as psychological issues, external stressors, or different agendas. Hogan has suggested the use of placebo-controlled intervention to enable better selection of patients,[8] although this in itself may be problematic and not practical. The placebo effect seen in patients who have had chronic pain procedures is quoted as as high as 60 per cent (this is twice the 'normal' placebo response).[3] Predicting which patients will have a placebo effect is not possible.[9] The placebo 'success' of a diagnostic block may account for why some definitive neurolytic procedures sometimes fail to work. Furthermore, it is known from studies of acupuncture that the insertion of a needle itself is an active event (see Chapter 5.4).

When a nerve is injured, impulses flow towards the spinal cord (orthodromic) and towards the tissues that it innervates (antidromic). Blocking a nerve proximal to the lesion may not reduce pain because antidromic peripheral sensitization is not block (Fig. 1).

Alternatively, nerve block distal to the dorsal root ganglion that has 'nociceptive activity' may not succeed because of orthodromic impulses.

Table 1 Neurobiological changes occurring in chronic and cancer pain and implications for neural blockade (Adapted from reference 5)

Neurobiological change	Clinical result	Implications regarding neural blockade
Tissue damage causing release of inflammatory mediators	Peripheral sensitization; altered sensitivity of high threshold nociceptors results in primary hyperalgesia (thermal and mechanical)	May lead to central sensitization
Continued nociceptive C fibre input; cumulative depolarization; increased membrane excitability within spinal cord	Central sensitization: recruitment of low threshold Aβ sensory fibres to nociceptive dorsal horn neurons; secondary hyperalgesia	1. Potential benefit of preemptive analgesia; 2. Failure of peripheral nerve block to reduce pain
Nerve lesion; ongoing C fibre input from site of injury and or dorsal root ganglion	Neuropathic pain	Block proximal to lesion may not reduce pain; false conclusion that this nerve is not source of pain
Nerve lesion; decreased inhibition	Deafferentation pain	1. Risk that neurolytic block itself may produce pain; 2. Receptive field expansion
Nerve lesion, Aβ neuron's central terminals sprout to superficial laminae of dorsal horn	Touch-evoked allodynia	Diagnosis with differential nerve-fibre block
Nerve lesion-sprouting of sympathetic fibres around dorsal root ganglion cells	Sympathetic fibres activity; A fibre activity	Therapeutic role for sympathetic blocks

Achieving neural blockade

Neural blockade is achieved using local anaesthetic solutions that reversibly block sodium channels and hence nociceptive impulses. This is commonly performed for diagnostic purposes. It is not understood why the duration of analgesia obtained can sometimes exceed the duration of action of the local anaesthetic. Abram[7] has suggested that intensed and prolonged blockade of sodium channels may cease or reduce ectopic nerve activity. He also suggested that cessation of nociceptive input into the dorsal horn temporarily by local anaesthetics may lead to a reversal of dorsal horn changes seen in chronic pain. The duration of prolonged local anaesthetic action rarely exceeds 3–4 weeks and repeated blocks with local anaesthetic alone are not recommended in non-malignant pain.[10, 11] The use of corticosteroids with local anaesthetics for neural blockade is thought to work by reducing local inflammation from nerve or tissue injury as well as inhibiting membrane conductance and hence spontaneous neuronal discharge particularly, at neuromas.[3]

More permanent neural blockade can be achieved with cryotherapy. This technique utilizes compressed nitrous oxide or carbon dioxide administered via a probe that delivers it at a low temperature of approximately $-50\,°C$. This technique produces varying degrees of nerve injury and regeneration is likely to recur.[12]

Neurolytic agents such as phenol or alcohol are also used to achieve permanent neural blockade. Although neuritis results from either agent,

it is said to occur less commonly with phenol.[3, 9] Large volumes of phenol are toxic systemically and therefore, for blockade of larger plexuses such as the coeliac plexus, alcohol is used.[3] In practice, neurolytic agents such as phenol and alcohol are seldom used for non-malignant pain. There is an increasing role for radiofrequency ablation in this area (see below). Surgical ablation of nerves rarely works as this can lead to the formation of neuromas with ectopic activity or deafferentation pain. When some afferent input is removed, the cells that responded to this stimulus can become hypersensitive to any other afferent stimuli and, further, their original area of reception may expand in size.[5]

Types of blockade

Neural blockade can be achieved in a great many ways. Here, we have divided them into neuraxial blockade (blockade occurring in the intrathecal or epidural space) and other types. These are listed below. This is schematically represented in Fig. 2.

1. Neuraxial blocks

   (a) epidurals approached via the caudal, lumbar, or transforaminal route;

   (b) intrathecal, single shot techniques or via implantable catheters or pumps.

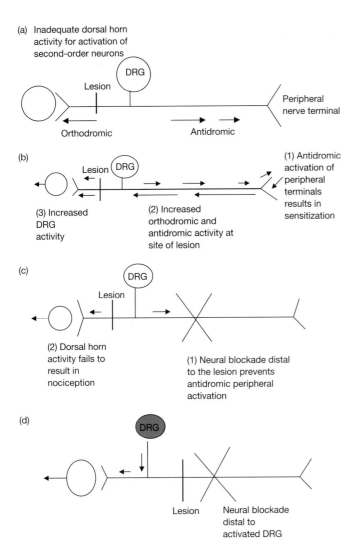

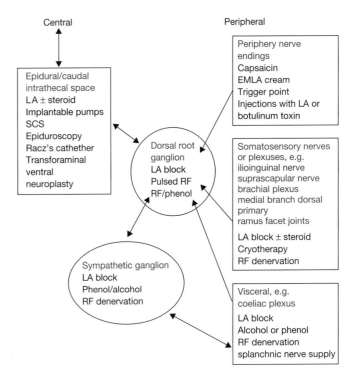

Fig. 1 (a) Proximal nerve root lesion results in orthodromic and antidromic activity. (b) Antidromic activity causes increased orthodromic activity and central sensitizaion. (c) Distal block breaks the vicious circle and pain relief ensues. (d) In situations where dorsal root ganglion (DRG) activity is activated a block distal to DRG may not block pain impulses. (Parts (a)–(c) are adapted from reference 5.)

Fig. 2 Possible sites for neural blockade. LA, Local anaesthetic; RF, radiofrequency; SCS, spinal cord stimulator; EMLA, eutetic mixture of local anaesthetic.

2.   Other

(a) somatosensory peripheral nerve blocks, for example, supra-scapular nerve or ilioinguinal nerve blocks;

(b) facet joint injections at cervical, lumbar, or thoracic level;

(c) sacroiliac joint injection;

(d) facet or sacroiliac joint denervation;

(e) sympathetic blocks, for example, stellate or lumbar;

(f) sympathetic denervation;

(g) dorsal root ganglion blockade.

Neuraxial blockade

The epidural and intrathecal space lends itself to blockade quite easily. The spinal cord ends at L2 in adults and, therefore, intrathecal block-ade is achieved below this level.

Although commonly done for anaesthesia, 'spinals' can be used for chronic problems as implantable systems have become available to allow the continuous delivery of a drug into the intrathecal space. Examples of this include baclofen for spasticity in multiple sclerosis or an opioid delivery in chronic pain syndromes. Intrathecal baclofen has also been used with success in patients with complex regional pain syndrome (reflex sympathetic dystrophy).[13] Intrathecal alcohol and phenol are used in selective pains associated with malignancy and lim-ited duration of life and can be simple and elegant ways of reducing severe symptoms.

Epidurals can be done at any level and are most commonly done in the caudal or lumbar space for sciatica. The caudal space is entered at the sacral hiatus and does not require a loss of resistance technique. However, the placement of a needle in the caudal space is occasionally difficult in adults and the use of radiological help is sometimes necessary. There is also need for a rather large volume of local anaesthetic solution and steroid to enable deposition at the relevant nerve roots.

Current evidence shows that epidural steroids are of benefit in recent onset radicular leg pain but this benefit is not sustained.[14] There is no evidence that epidural steroids are effective in the management of back pain without nerve root irritation.[15] Abram[16] has highlighted the variations in practice of this procedure and that it is of benefit in those mainly with radicular involvement, disc herniation, and a positive sci-atic stretch test. Prolonged symptomology, previous back surgery, and spinal stenosis were associated with lower rates of success.

It is also possible to perform selective nerve root injection for sci-atica. This is achieved using fluoroscopy and via a transforaminal approach. The proponents of this practice suggest that a more con-centrated dose of steroid is deposited at the correct level and that less local anaesthetic is used. Ries and colleagues[6] performed a randomized controlled trial on 50 patients with radicular pain and radiological evidence of nerve root compression. They were randomized into two groups: those whose nerve roots were injected with bupivacaine and steroid and these injected with bupivacaine alone. Ries *et al.* found that a statistically significant proportion of patients who had had nerve root injections with steroid did not progress to surgery.

In another randomized controlled trial of 60 patients with fibrosis following back surgery, patients were randomized to those receiving: local anaesthetic and hyaluronidase; local anaesthetic, hyaluronidase, and steroid; and local anaesthetic and steroid alone. These injections produced analgesia at 1 month but their effects at 6 months were less pronounced. There was no statistical difference between the three groups at 3 months.[17]

Neuraxial blockade carries with it certain risks, which are listed here.

1. Local anaesthetic toxicity. Inadvertent intravascular injection or a large volume of local anaesthetic given intrathecally. This would lead to convulsions and cardiac arrhythmias, possibly cardiac arrest.

2. Hypotension from blocking the sympathetic system.

3. Nerve root injury.

4. Bleeding or spinal haematoma, particularly in those who are anti-coagulated.

5. Post-dural-puncture headache.

6. Infection leading to meningitis.

7. Neurotoxicity. Intrathecal steroids may cause arachdoinitis.[18]

With all the above in mind, it is imperative that these procedures be performed by experienced staff with full resuscitation facilities available.

In recent years the technique of epiduroscopy via the sacral canal has evolved using fibreoptic devices to allow visualization of the epidural space and localization of scar tissue. A catheter is then passed through the scope to the scar tissue and neurolysis is achieved usually using a mixture of local anaesthetic, hyaluronidase, saline, and corticosteroid.[19] At 1 year, those undergoing epiduroscopy were much better than those who had not (unpublished observations), but the long-term results were not known. However, much scar tissue in the epidural space is said to occur ventrally and it is felt that Racz's technique[19] does not always achieve ventral catheter placement. Hammer and Rainwater have described a technique of transforaminal ventral epidural neuroplasty.[20]

There are other methods to neural blockade centrally. These are achieved either via implantable catheters in the intrathecal space as mentioned above or via spinal cord stimulators. These are electrodes placed in the epidural space that can be programmed to stimulate the dorsal columns. In accordance with Melzack and Wall's gate-controlled theory of pain,[21] stimulation of the larger Aα and Aβ fibres inhibits nociceptive signals arriving via Aδ and C fibres. There is also suggestion that nociceptive inhibition may be mediated by an increase in GABA and other neurochemical changes.[22]

Myerson and Linderoth[23] have recently reviewed this topic and state that the best evidence for spinal cord stimulator use is in neuropathic pain or complex regional pain syndromes. The evidence for its use in back pain is unconvincing.[4] The use of such implantable, programmable systems carries quite significant cost implications.

Peripheral somatosensory nerve blocks

It is possible to block the specific somatosensory nerves in the periphery and this is usually achieved with local anaesthetic and steroid. Examples of this are suprascapular nerve blocks for shoulder problems and ilioinguinal nerve blocks for chronic post-hernia repair pain. We are not aware of any randomized controlled trials that have compared such injections with a placebo.

The median nerve is commonly blocked in carpal tunnel syndrome and some authors have reported success rates of 77 per cent.[24] Injection of the median nerve with local anaesthetic and steroid is more successful then injection with local anaesthetic alone.[4] However, good analgesia with median nerve blocks does not predict accurately the response to subsequent neuroablative techniques.[8]

In the acute situation, local anaesthetic blocks of the brachial plexus or femoral nerves are commonly undertaken for postoperative analgesia using local anaesthetic alone. However, catheter techniques to the somatic plexuses have also been described to enable prolonged analgesia in malignant or non-malignant chronic pain. The placement of such catheters may be complicated by infection or dislodgement.

Trigger points

Trigger point injections with local anaesthetic plus or minus steroid is commonly done for myofascial pain. A series of trigger point injections may be useful in this condition as the destruction of mature myocytes by local anaesthetic encourages subsequent growth of new ones.[25] However this technique does not seem to be useful in patients with fibromyalgia.[26]

In recent years, the use of botulinum toxin has been reported for trigger point injections in myofascial pain syndrome. In a randomized, double-blind study of 33 patients, Wheeler *et al.*[27] compared two strengths of botulinum toxin type A with placebo. There was no stastically significant benefit but a high number of patients were asymptomatic after a second injection of botulinum toxin, 100 units. More recently, Porta[28] has shown better results for botulinum toxin when compared with local anaesthetic and methylprednisolone. There was no placebo group in this study.

Spinal nerve blocks

Facet joint injections

It is thought that 15–40 per cent of patients with low back pain may suffer from facet joint arthropathy.[29,30] Half of patients who complain of neck pain after whiplash may actually be suffering from cervical facet joint pain. There are no specific clinical or radiological tests that can predict facet joint pain. However, it is common that these patients complain of pain with extension and twisting and may be tender over the affected facet joints. The sciatic stretch test is usually negative.

It is possible to perform facet joint injections by blocking the medial branch of the posterior primary ramus or to inject the joint itself. Both techniques require the use of an image intensifier to locate the target points precisely. Although facet joint injections with local anaesthetic and steroid are commonly performed in chronic pain practice, Cousins and Walker argue that there is a lack of effective sustained outcome for this procedure.[14] In fact, many authors would argue that diagnostic medial branch blockades are easier to perform and less likely to rupture the joint. This is usually done with view to radiofrequency destruction of the nerve at a later date (discussed below). However, there are many centres in the United Kingdom that do not have access to radiofrequency equipment. The success of patients who have had lumbar and cervical facet joint injections varies enormously and is quoted as between 16 and 86 per cent.[8] Such variation implies differences in patient selection, technique, and medication. Radiofrequency of the nerve supply to the lumbar and cervical facet joints seems to obtain at least 50 per cent pain relief in 45 per cent of patients.[31]

Facet joint injections are relatively safe procedures when done with radiographical assistance. As with all injections in the back, there is a risk of intrathecal or vascular injection, nerve injury, and bleeding, but these are rare.

Radiofrequency lesioning

Radiofrequency denervation involves passing a current down a probe at the correct site to create a thermal lesion in the surrounding tissue. This technique has been practised for the last 20 years. There are generators nowadays that allow stimulation of the point at frequencies to test sensory and motor components of a nerve. This increases the safety of this procedure. Generators also allow us to control the temperature and duration of the lesion. The probes used are insulated and pass down needles no larger than ones that were used for diagnostic blockade with local anaesthetic. Until recently, it was felt that the temperature achieved was very important to the lesion. However, during radiofrequency, the tissues around the tip of the electrode are exposed to a concentrated electromagnetic field and it is thought that this field may contribute to the clinical effects of radiofrequency quite independently from heat.[32]

Therefore the technique of pulsed radiofrequency has been developed to deliver this electromagnetic field to the tissues without heating them above 42 °C (the temperature above which cell death results).

Both radiofrequency and pulsed radiofrequency have many applications in chronic pain and these are considered below. Most of these procedures should be preceded by a diagnostic block with local anaesthetic. In an ideal world this would include a diagnostic block with placebo but, for ethical, practical, and logistical reasons, this is difficult to achieve. These techniques are usually performed as outpatient procedures with the patient awake or lightly sedated. This is because verbal contact should be maintained to help localization of the nerve when stimulated prior to lesioning.

Lumbar, cervical, or thoracic facet denervation

There are now several studies that show good results with lumbar or cervical facet denervation.[33–35] Van Kleef et al. have demonstrated that radiofrequency denervation of lumbar facet joints can alleviate pain and improve function. However, the numbers in this prospective randomized study were small.[36] Cho and colleagues[37] studied 324 patients and found that 96 per cent reported no back pain after a year. However, thoracic facet denervation is less promising.[38]

Dorsal root ganglion blockade

The dorsal root carries nociceptive Aδ and C fibres from the periphery. There is also evidence of sympathetic nerve baskets growing in

dorsal root ganglion.[39,40] Nakamura et al.[41] have shown that the afferent pain pathways from the lower intervertebral discs may travel via sympathetic fibres at L2 nerve root level. Therefore pulsed radiofrequency of the dorsal root ganglia at L2 has been used for chronic lower back pain.[42]

Sympathetic ganglia or nerve denervation: stellate ganglion, sphenopalatine, lumbar or thoracic sympathetic lesions, and splanchnic nerve lesions

Blocking sympathetic nerves or ganglia may be useful in patients with an element of sympathetically maintained pain. This is seen in a variety of conditions including complex regional pain syndrome, phantom limb pain, and neuropathic pain. Sympathetically mediated pain is diagnosed if the patient responds to a test with either intravenous phentolamine or local anaesthetic blocks. The use of local anaesthetic blocks in diagnosing sympathetic pain is an area of controversy as local anaesthetic may inadvertently spread on to somatosensory nerves resulting in false-positives.[43] There have been several good reviews on this topic recently (references 44–47; also see also Chapter 6.16). It is important to note that very few randomized controlled trials have been done to evaluate the usefulness of these blocks.

Sphenopalatine ganglion block

This is located posterior to the middle turbinate and these cells communicate with the trigeminal and facial nerves as well as carotid plexus. Radiofrequency of this ganglion has also been described and may be useful for the treatment of atypical facial pain.

Stellate ganglion block

This ganglion receives sympathetic fibres from T1–2 (head and neck) and T8–9 (upper limb). The stellate ganglion often fuses with the first thoracic ganglion and lies over C7 to T1. There are two common techniques to block the stellate ganglion. The first uses Chaussignac's tubercle (transverse process of C6) and the second is a more medial approach to the anterolateral border of C7.

This block is achieved with 5–10 ml of local anaesthetic. A rise in temperature of the upper limb was thought to indicate successful sympatholysis. The success rate even in the hands of experienced operators is 75 per cent.[48] Neurolytic blockade runs the risk of permanent side-effects such as Horner's syndrome. Therefore, radiofrequency lesioning of the stellate ganglion has been described and a retrospective analysis has shown its efficacy is similar to that of other ways of blocking the stellate ganglion.[49]

Thoracic sympathetic block

The thoracic sympathetic chain lies near the somatic nerves as they arise from the intravertebral foramen. There is a 4 per cent incidence of pneumothorax even in experienced hands.[50] Although this block historically has few indications, one of the authors (R.M.) has found that discogenic cervical pain does respond to T2 sympathetic blockade or radiofrequency.

Coeliac plexus block

The coeliac plexus lies anterolateral to the aorta and receives fibres from T5 to T12 which pass through splanchnic nerves. It innervates all abdominal viscera except for part of the transverse colon, descending colon, rectum, and pelvic viscera. Blockade can be achieved using local anaesthetic with or without steroid and also neurolytic agents such as phenol or alcohol. Neurolytic coeliac blocks work for 6–12 months before the nerves regenerate.

Prithvi Raj et al.[50] recently described successful splanchnic nerve radiofrequency lesioning as an alternative to coeliac plexus blockade for abdominal pain.

Lumbar sympathetic block

Preganglionic sympathetic neurons arise form the anterolateral dorsal horn from T10 to L2–3 and pass through the white rami and sympathetic trunk to the sympathetic and sacral ganglia. These then usually join the L1–5 and S1–3 spinal nerves by way of the grey rami or form a diffuse plexus around the iliac arteries. Preganglionic fibres for the visceral structures synapse commonly in T10–12 and L1 ganglia and then join the aortic and hypogastric plexus to supply the kidney, ureter, bladder, distal transverse colon, rectum, prostate, testicle, cervix, and uterus.

Patients often respond to a diagnostic local block but only 30 per cent respond to the subsequent neurolytic blockade, with duration of action of 6–12 months. This block is usually made at L3 level to avoid permanent damage to the genitofemoral nerve. Successful radiofrequency of the lumbar sympathetic chain has also been described.[49]

Intravenous regional anaesthesia

It is possible to achieve neural blockade using an intravenous regional anaesthesia technique. This is commonly also used for sympathetically maintained pain. Guanethidine is a commonly used drug and acts by depleteing nerve endings of noradrenaline stores and prevents reuptake. Other drugs that have been used include bretylium, ketorolac, phentolamine, reserpine, and ketanserin. This technique's advantages are that it is easy to perform and can be done in an anticoagulated patient. Possible complications include hypotension and neuropraxia from the cuff. Results of these studies are controversial and, recently, randomized, controlled trials by Jadad et al.[51] and Kaplan et al.[52] have failed to show any benefit.

Summary

In this brief chapter, the variety of neural blockade procedures that are practised in chronic pain management have been briefley reviewed. The evidence for use of steroid injections (apart from epidural steroids for radicular pain) appears inconclusive at present. Older neuroablative techniques utilizing phenol or alcohol are fraught with permanent adverse effects such as inadvertent spread to other sites or toxicity, though there is probably place for intrathecal or epidural phenol/alcohol in selected pains of malignant origin. There is growing evidence for the use of radiofrequency denervation techniques in carefully selected patients.

References

1. Besson, J.M. (1999). Pain: the neurobiology of pain. Lancet 353 (19164), 1610–1615.
2. Munglani, R., Hunt, S.P., and Jones, J.G. (1997). The spinal cord and chronic pain. In Anaesthesia review, Vol. 12 (ed. L. Kaufman and R. Ginsburg), pp. 53–76.
3. Munglani, R. (1998). Recent advances in chronic pain with special reference to back pain. In Anaesthesia review, Vol. 14 (ed. L. Kaufman and R. Ginsburg), pp. 153–174. Churchill Livingstone, New York.
4. Siddall, P.J., Hudspith, M.J., and Munglani, R. (2000). Sensory systems and pain. In Foundations of anaesthesia (ed. H. Hemmings and P. Hopkins), pp. 213–232. Mosby, St. Louis.
5. Lamacraft, G. and Cousins, M. (1997). Neural blockade in chronic and cancer pain. Int. Anesthesiol. Clin. 35, 131–153.
6. Ries, K.D., et al. (2000). The effect of nerve-root injections on the need for operative treatment of lumbar radicular pain. J. Bone Joint Surg. 82 (11), 1589–1593.
7. Abram, S.E. (2000). Neural blockade for neuropathic pain. Clin. J. Pain 16, 56–61.
8. Hogan, Q.H. and Abram, S.E. (1997). Neural blockade for diagnosis and prognosis. Anesthesiology 86 (1), 216–241.
9. Liberman, R. (1964). An experimental study of the placebo response under three different situations of pain. J. Psychiatr. Res. 2, 233–246.
10. Johansson, A. and Sjolund, B. (1996). Nerve blocks with local anesthetics and corticosteroids in chronic pain: a clinical follow-up study. J. Pain Symptom Manage. 11, 181–187.
11. Donner, B., et al. (1998). Long-term effects of nerve blocks in chronic pain. Curr. Opin. Anaesthesiol. 11 (5), 523–532.
12. Patt, R.B. and Cousins, M.J. (1998). Techniques for neurolytic neural blockade. In Neural blockade in clinical anaesthesia and management of pain, 3rd edn. (ed. M.J. Cousins and P.O. Bridenbaugh), pp. 1007–1061. Lippincott-Raven Publishers, Philadelphia.
13. Van Hilten, B.J., et al. (2000). Intrathecal baclofen for the treatment of dystonia in patients with reflex sympathetic dystrophy. N. Engl. J. Med. 343 (9), 625–630.
14. Cousins, M.J. and Walker, S. (2001). Chronic pain: management strategies that work. Anesth. Analg. 92 (suppl. 3), 15–25.
15. Koes, B.W., et al. (1995). Efficacy of epidural steroid injections for low back pain and sciatica: a systematic review of randomised clinical trials. Pain 63, 279–288.
16. Abram, S.E. (1999). Treatment of lumbosacral radiculopathy with epidural steroids. Anesthesiology 91, 1937–1941.
17. Devulder, J. (1999). Nerve root sleeve injections in patients with failed back surgery syndrome: a comparison of three solutions. Clin. J. Pain 15 (2), 132–135.
18. Nelson, D.A. (1993). Intraspinal therapy using methylprednolone acetate. Twenty-three years of clinical controversy. Spine 18, 278–286.
19. Racz, G.B. and Holubec, J.T. (1998). Lysis of adhesions in the epidural space. In Techniques of neurolysis (ed. G.B. Racz), pp. 57–62. Kluwer Academic Publishers, Boston.
20. Hammer, M. and Rainwater, S. (1996). Lysis of anterior epidural adhesions using a transforaminal approach for failed back surgery. Int. Spinal Injection Soc. Sci. Newsl.
21. Melzack, P. and Wall, P.D. (1965). Pain mechanisms: a new theory. Science 150, 971–978.
22. Stiller, C.N., et al. (1996). Release of gamma-amino butyric acid in the dorsal horn and suppression of tactile allodynia by spinal cord stimulation in mononeuropathic rats. Neurosurgery 39, 367–375.
23. Myerson, B. and Linderoth, B. (1999). Electric stimulation of the central nervous system. Pain 1999—an updated review (ed. M. Max), pp. 269–280. IASP Press, Seattle.
24. Dammers, J.W. (1991). [Carpal tunnel syndrome.] Ned. Tijdschr Geneeskd. 135 (5), 193–194.
25. Hogan, Q., et al. (1994). Local anesthetic myotoxicity: a case and review. Anesthesiology 80, 942–947.
26. Kraus, H. and Fischer, A.A. (1991). Diagnosis and treatment of myofascial pain. Mt Sinai J. Med. 58, 235–239.
27. Wheeler, A.H., et al. (1998). A randomised, double-blind, prospective pilot study of botulinum toxin injection for refractory, unilateral,

cervicothoracic, paraspinal, myofascial pain syndrome. *Spine* **23** (15), 1662–1666.

28. **Porta, M.** (2000). A comparative trial of botulinum toxin type A and methylprednisolone for the treatment of myofascial pain syndrome and pain from chronic muscle spasm. *Pain* **8** (1–2), 101–105.

29. **Schwarzer, A.C.,** *et al.* (1994). Clinical features of patients with pain stemming from the lumbar zygapophysial joints. Is the lumbar facet syndrome a clinical entity? *Spine* **19**, 1132–1137.

30. **Aeschback, A. and Mekhail, N.A.** (2000). Common nerve blocks in chronic pain management. *Anesthesiol. Clin. N. Am.* **18** (2), 429–457.

31. **North, R.B.,** *et al.* (1994). Radiofrequency lumbar facet denervation: analysis of prognostic factors. *Pain* **57**, 77–83.

32. **Sluijter, M.,** *et al.* (1998). The effects of pulsed radiofrequency fields applied to the dorsal root ganglion—a preliminary report. *Pain Clin.* **2** (2), 109–117.

33. **Lord, S.,** *et al.* (1996). Percutaneous radiofrequency neurotomy for chronic cervical zygapophyseal joint pain. *N. Engl. J. Med.* **335**, 1721–1726.

34. **Tzaan, W.C. and Tasker, R.R.** (2000). Percutaneous radiofrequency facet rhizotomy—experience with 118 procedures and reappraisal of its value. *Can. J. Neurol. Sci.* **27**, 125–130.

35. **Dreyfuss, P.,** *et al.* (2000). Efficacy and validity of radiofrequency neurotomy for chronic lumbar zygapophysial joint pain. *Spine* **25**, 1270–1277.

36. **van Kleef, M.,** *et al.* (1999). Randomized trial of radiofrequency lumbar facet denervation for chronic low back pain. *Spine* **24** (18), 1937–1942.

37. **Cho, J.,** *et al.* (1997). Percutaneous radiofrequency lumbar facet rhizotomy in mechanical low back pain syndrome. *Stereotact. Funct. Neurosurg.* **68**, 212–217.

38. **Stolker, R.J.,** *et al.* (1993). Percutaneous facet denervation in chronic thoracic spinal pain. *Acta Neurochir.* **122**, 82.

39. **Chung, K.,** *et al.* (1997). Sprouting sympathetic fibers form synaptic varicosities in the dorsal root ganglion of the rat with neuropathic injury. *Brain Res,* **75**, 275–280.

40. **McLachlan, E.M., Janig, W., Devor, M., and Michaelis, M.** (1993). Peripheral nerve injury triggers noradrenergic sprouting within dorsal root ganglia. *Nature* **363**, 543–545.

41. **Nakamura, S.I.,** *et al.* (1996). The afferent pathways of discogenic low-back pain. Evaluation of L2 spinal nerve root infiltration. *J. Bone Joint Surg. Br.* **78** (4), 606–612.

42. **Sluijter, M.E.** (2000). The role of radiofrequency in failed back surgery patients. *Curr. Rev. Pain* **4** (1), 29–53.

43. **Hogan, Q.H.** (1997). Neural blockade for diagnosis and prognosis. *Anesthesiology* **86**, 216–241.

44. **Harden, R.N.** (2001). Complex regional pain syndrome. *Br. J. Anaesth.* **87**, 99–106.

45. **Stanton Hicks, M.,** *et al.* (1998). Complex regional pain syndrome: guidelines for therapy. Consensus report. *Clin. J. Pain* **14**, 155–166.

46. **Baron, R., Fields, H.L., Jänig, W., Kitt, C., and Levine, J.D.** (2002). National Institutes of Health Workshop: Reflex sympathetic dystrophy/complex regional pain syndromes – state of the science.

47. **Drummond, P.D.** (2001). Mechanism of complex regional pain syndrome: no longer excessive sympathetic outflow? *Lancet* **359**, 168–170.

48. **Stanton-Hicks, M.,** *et al.* (1996). Use of regional anaesthesia in the diagnosis of reflex sympathetic dystrophy and sympathetically maintained pain. In *Reflex sympathetic dystrophy: a reappraisal* (ed. W. Jänig and M. Stanton-Hicks), pp. 217–237. IASP Press, Seattle.

49. **Forouszanfar, T.,** *et al.* (2000). Radiofrequency lesions of the Stellate ganglion in chronic pain syndromes: a retrospective analysis of clinical efficacy in 86 patients. *Clin. J. Pain* **16** (2), 164–168.

50. **Prithvi Raj, P.,** *et al.* (1999). The development of a technique for radiofrequency lesioning of splanchnic nerves. *Curr. Rev. Pain* **3**, 377–387.

51. **Jadad, A.R., Carroll, D., Glynn, C.J., and McQuay, H.J.** (1995). Intravenous sympathetic blockade for pain relief in reflex sympathetic dystrophy: a review and a randomized double blind crossover study. *J. Pain Symptom Manage.* **10**, 13–20.

52. **Kaplan, R., Claudio, M., Kepes E., and Gu, X.F.** (1996). Intravenous guanethidine in patients with reflex sympathetic dystrophy. *Acta Anaesthesiol. Scand.* **40**, 1216–1222.

5.6 The management of soft tissue disorders: the role of the physiotherapist

Glenn Hunter

Introduction

Physiotherapy can be defined as a health care profession with an emphasis on the analysis of movement, based on the structure and function of the body, and the use of physical approaches to the promotion of health, and the prevention, treatment, and management of disease and disability.[1] This definition places the emphasis on physical treatments, such as manipulation, massage, and exercise, that have been valued as 'healing' arts for centuries[2] and have been the mainstay of the physiotherapy profession since its formation as a professional organization in 1894.[3]

In the early years the development of the physiotherapy profession was predominantly influenced by the medical profession and, consequently, many of the treatments have developed on the basis of the medical model of disease. In this model treatments tend to be directed towards the pathology rather than to the nature of the individual hosting the disease.[2] More recently, the physiotherapist's clinical reasoning has broadened to incorporate psychological and social aspects of dysfunction. Consequently, the biopsychosocial model of dysfunction rather than the pure medical model more closely represents the physiotherapist's approach to the management of soft tissue dysfunction. Using this model the physiotherapist aims to assess the patient's response to pain and dysfunction, and treatment is integrated with the individual's beliefs and behaviour.[4]

Physiotherapists play an extensive and essential role in many health care teams: intensive care, burns, paediatrics, neurology, mental health, orthopaedics, rheumatology, and community and sports medicine form a non-exhaustive list. Because of the diverse nature of the expertise of the physiotherapist it is important when discussing physiotherapy, particularly in the light of research evidence, to define what aspect of physiotherapy is being evaluated. This chapter will focus on the role of the physiotherapist in the management of soft tissue dysfunction.

Soft tissue dysfunction is defined by the author as the inability of a soft tissue or tissues to function optimally in a desired environment or situation. In the medical model of soft tissue dysfunction, the dysfunction may be seen to relate to a specific identifiable pathology, for example, a valgus force applied to the flexed knee may result in a sprain of the medial ligament and treatment would be directed to this site. The assumption would be that, once the pathological reaction in the medial ligament has resolved, 'normal function' would return. The physiotherapist is aware, however, that a local site soft tissue dysfunction can have more global influences and these may prolong the dysfunction even when the pathology has resolved. For example, the soft tissue dysfunction may be due to local effects, such as a healing or degenerative process, or changes in tissue mechanics such as increased stiffness. Changes may, however, also be occurring at a neurophysiological level, for example, the persistent transmission of nociceptive information in the spinal cord following soft tissue injury may produce central sensitivity, whereby the

alteration in the sensitivity of the relay cells in the spinal cord produces hypersensitivity in the region of the lesion. Changes may also occur at the higher centres in terms of mood, motivation, and the cognitive experience of dysfunction. These local and global effects influence the clinical reasoning of the physiotherapist.

The basis of the physiotherapeutic management of soft tissue dysfunction is the principle of adaptation. Adaptation can be defined as 'an inherited or acquired modification in organisms that makes them better suited to survive . . . in a particular environment'.[5] In relation to this chapter it is assumed that asymptomatic soft tissues and associated neurophysiological and higher centre influences have adapted to their functional environment. When the tissues fail to adapt to the environment, dysfunction may occur. Here the aims of the physiotherapist are to establish why failure to adapt has occurred, to identify the system(s) responsible for the dysfunction, and to provide a stimulus that will promote adaptation so the patient can return to 'normal' function in their desired environment.

The stimuli for adaptation can be very diverse, but typically include aspects of manual therapy, exercise therapy, electrotherapy, and psychosocial interaction. In certain cases, despite appropriate stimuli, the patient may be unable to adapt to physiotherapeutic management. This may be due to a structural dysfunction that prohibits the restoration of 'normal' movement or due to a disease that results in a progressive decline in function. Here the aim is to provide a stimulus to maintain or retard a gradual decline in function rather than to restore 'normal' function. In some cases the patient may not be able to adapt to their environment and, in this case, the physiotherapist alongside the occupational therapist aims to modify the environment to suit the patient's needs.

As well as the treatment of dysfunction, physiotherapists also play an important role in the prevention of soft tissue dysfunction in terms of identifying those at risk and promoting behaviours that may decrease the risk of injury such as adequate warm-up prior to activity, stretching to prepare for activity, or modifying the environment to make it safer.

This chapter will expand on the above and begin by addressing the assessment process typically used by the physiotherapist in the management of soft tissue dysfunction. Management strategies in relation to manual therapy, modalities, and exercise therapy will be addressed with the emphasis being placed on the rationale behind the clinical reasoning process used by the physiotherapist.

The assessment of soft tissue dysfunction

General principles

During human movement the soft tissues of the body, are subjected to mechanical loads that manifest as tensile, compressive, and shear forces.[6] Soft tissue dysfunction manifests when either the applied forces are greater than the mechanical properties of the tissue, or the mechanical properties of the tissue have decreased in relation to normal loading parameters,[7] or a combination of excessive loading and decreased mechanical properties occurs.

All three of these scenarios may result from macro- or microtrauma. Macrotrauma occurs when there is a gross mismatch between the load and the tissue's mechanical properties resulting in the immediate onset of tissue dysfunction and symptoms. Microtrauma occurs when there is a lesser mismatch between the force and the tissue's mechanical properties, but repetitive stimuli with inadequate rest periods result in the gradual onset of dysfunction.

Following dysfunction, the ability of the tissue to tolerate force decreases, resulting in decreased movement and hence decreased load being applied to the tissue. The antalgic removal of the load from soft tissue appears to be detrimental in terms of the tissue's biomechanical properties.[8–12] Load removal is beneficial in the short term as a means of controlling the inflammation and pain response. It should be noted, however, that prolonged episodes of decreased tissue loading have profound negative effects on tissue function as well and cardiovascular, psychological, and emotional changes (Table 1).

The major emphasis of physiotherapeutic management is to promote adaptation in order to restore the patient's ability to withstand the specific demands of functional loading and to restore the kinetic environment in which the tissue has to function. In order to achieve this aim the physiotherapist bases the treatment approach on a detailed assessment process.[13]

Assessment process

The physiotherapist generally spends 30–60 minutes on the initial assessment of the patient, as the assessment process forms a critical part of patient management.

The assessment proceeds through a subjective and objective format to try and identify why the patient is failing to adapt to his or her desired environment. The subjective component is the verbal component of the assessment where the patient provides an account of his or her complaint in relation to a series of structured questions. In the objective component of the assessment, clinical tests are applied to the patient to attempt to measure the effect of the dysfunction on movement and to formulate a hypothesis that fits with the subjective information with regard to the nature of the patient's complaint. The main aspects of the assessment process are presented below; a more extensive review of this area can be obtained from reference 13.

Table 1 Negative effects of decreased loading on tissue mechanics

Tissue	Effect
Joint capsule	Periarticular fibrosis leading to decreased range of motion and potential irreversible changes
Ligaments	Decreased collagen thickness and tensile properties
Bone	Decreased bone mineral density
Muscle	Decreased muscle mass, muscle strength, and increased in connective tissue content

Subjective examination

The subjective examination commences with an invitation to the patient to give a brief summary of his or her current problems in terms of what it is the patient experiences and where it is experienced. The therapist attempts to determine the kind of disorder and the associated experience for the patient, for example, pain, stiffness, giving way, instability, weakness, loss of sensation, loss of function. These experiences are translated into anatomical, pathological, and biomechanical models that are used to aid the diagnostic process.

During the questioning, the patient's movements and static positions are observed, as they may relate to positions that relieve the tension of the affected tissue and thus aid the diagnostic process. For example, a patient suffering from neural dysfunction in the upper limb may sit with the shoulder girdle elevated and the neck side flexed towards the painful side to relieve the tension on the problematic nerve root.

The patient's symptoms are explored on the basis of the area involved, nature, behaviour, and irritability.

Area

The patient identifies the area of the symptoms and states whether they are deep or superficial. The locations of the patient's symptoms are drawn on to a body chart and, if there is more than one symptomatic area, relationships between these areas are explored. For example, a patient presenting with low back pain and leg pain would be asked if the leg and back pain occur at the same time, if they are independent, or if one precedes the other. The patient ranks the symptomatic areas in terms of severity using a Likert scale, where a vertical line is drawn on a horizontal scale that ranges from no pain to the worst pain that can be imagined. This score serves as a marker that can be used to assess the value of a treatment protocol. Asymptomatic areas are also typically marked with a tick on the body chart so that changes in the initial pattern can be clearly identified and that the therapist can be sure at a later date that the patient at that time was asymptomatic in these areas of the body chart.

The physiotherapist analyses the area of the patient's symptoms with regard to the tissues that are under the symptomatic area, and what structures in other areas could refer pain to this area. These tissues will be tested in the objective examination. Careful attention is paid to areas of paraesthesia or anaesthesia and these are accurately marked on the body chart and monitored during the following treatment sessions.

Behaviour

The patient characterizes the symptoms and their behaviour in terms of being constant, constant but variable, or intermittent. Symptoms that have mechanical behaviour are typically intermittent and are aggravated by activity and eased by rest. In this case the physiotherapist asks the patient to demonstrate the aggravating movement(s) and analyses the movement in terms of what effect it has on a particular tissue. For example, a patient with an injury to the anterior talofibular ligament of the ankle joint may indicate that plantar flexion and inversion of the ankle joint aggravates their symptoms. Pain-relieving postures are also explored as these may be used as treatment positions if the symptoms are particularly irritable. The frequency and duration of the intermittent symptoms are established to give a 24-hour pattern that can be used to measure the effect of a treatment protocol.

Table 2 Factors that by their nature may influence the objective examination

Personality characteristics, e.g. stoics versus complainers
Pain thresholds
Attitudes towards treatment
Ethnicity and social grouping
Familial or genetic components to the disorder
Healing rate
Stability of the symptoms
Inflammatory or degenerative pathology

Table 3 Intrinsic factors in the aetiology of soft tissue dysfunction

Somatotype
Age and gender
Personality
Previous dysfunction
Genetic predisposition to injury
Posture and body mechanics, e.g. hyper- or hypomobility, bone mineral density, leg length difference, foot pronation and supination, muscle imbalance, decreased muscle control

Attention is paid to the current pattern of the symptoms, that is, are they static, improving, or worsening?

Particular consideration is paid to pain at rest that is worse at night. Though this may be due to the acute inflammation occurring in the early stages of soft tissue injury, it may also indicate more sinister pathology such as a tumour. This pattern of presentation warrants referral for further investigations.

Nature

This refers to circumstances that by their nature may limit or influence the objective examination or treatment protocol. Examples of these are presented in Table 2.

Irritability

It is important to establish the irritability of the symptoms with regard to the amount of activity required to produce them, the degree of pain that ensues, and the time it takes for the symptoms to decrease. This information guides the therapist as to how much treatment may be applied without exacerbating the patient's symptoms. It is also a useful guide to measure the effect of a treatment protocol.

History of the present condition

The aetiology and consequences of the present condition are explored in relation to what happened, when it happened, what the patient experienced, and what the patient did about it. Any treatments that the patient has received are rated in terms of the patient's perception of their effectiveness.

Careful attention is paid to the mechanics of injury, which are explored from a biomechanical perspective. Information relating to the magnitude, direction, frequency, and duration of force application helps to guide the physiotherapist in forming a hypothesis regarding the site and aetiology of tissue dysfunction.

Due to the multifactorial nature of the forces that are applied to body tissues, it is difficult to be precise regarding the exact cause of dysfunction and it is important to note that the majority of proposed causal relationships should be interpreted as being conjectural.[14] Allowing for this limitation, aetiological factors are explored in relation to intrinsic, extrinsic, and task-related factors in order that these factors can be addressed to decrease the risk of re-injury. The extrinsic factors are typically explored in the subjective component of the examination, whereas intrinsic and task-related factors are explored during the objective phase of the examination. Watson provides an excellent review of this area.[15]

Intrinsic factors

These relate to attributes inherent in the person that predispose them to dysfunction. Examples are presented in Table 3.

Though many plausible aetiological theories link intrinsic factors to soft tissue dysfunction (e.g. it is plausible to assume that a large leg length difference may be associated with low back pain), the majority of the hypotheses lack causal support in the scientific literature. Extensive work is required in this area before more confidence is gained in using these hypotheses as part of the clinical reasoning process. An important component of assessing the credibility of intrinsic factors relates to establishing the validity and repeatability of these intrinsic measurements and care should be taken over utilizing information from tests that have poor repeatability and validity.[16, 17] Atkinson and Nevill[18] provide an excellent review of issues relating to repeatability and George et al.[19] provide an excellent review of issues relating to validity.

An example of the association that may be made by the physiotherapist between intrinsic factors and tissue dysfunction involves the assessment of gait and, in particular, the action of the foot during the gait cycle. Using Achilles tendinopathy as an example, the physiotherapist makes static and dynamic assessments of foot function. In particular, the physiotherapist may note that the foot excessively pronates in terms of the range, speed, and rate of motion. This movement involves a reduction in the height of the longitudinal arch of the foot and associated eversion of the subtalar joint. The physiotherapist may reason that the altered subtalar motion alters the loading parameters in the Achilles tendon and may relate to decreased flexibility of the calf complex. With the assumption that a 'tight' calf complex may be associated with increased pronation, stretching exercises may be prescribed to increase the range of dorsiflexion at the ankle joint and hence decrease the pronation and the possible stress in the Achilles tendon.

Extrinsic factors

These are factors external to the patient and examples are presented in Table 4. In contrast to intrinsic factors where the physiotherapist often applies physical measures to correct these factors, with extrinsic factors the physiotherapist provides advice rather than treatment. For example, in relation to a sports person, the advice may relate to the type of training surface, or equipment such as choice of running shoe or racquet, or the use of protective equipment.

Task-related factors

These factors relate to the performance of an activity and examples are presented in Table 5. The assessment incorporates aspects such as an analysis of task performance, intensity, and duration, and the rest periods involved.

Table 4 Extrinsic factors in the aetiology of soft tissue dysfunction

Direct external force applied to the body

Environmental factors—weather, temperature, humidity, wind, type of surface, altitude

Equipment

Psychological influences

Social influences

Table 5 Task-related factors in the aetiology of soft tissue dysfunction

Technique

Preparation

Duration of the task

Intensity of the task

Frequency of the task

Table 6 Key points regarding joint protection—advice given to rheumatology patients

Pain management advice: respect acute pain exacerbation by resting

Maintain activity during remissions

Develop a realistic balance between activity levels and rest

Avoid activities and position that may lead to deformity, e.g. ulnar deviation or sustained knee flexion

During the performance of activities consider the following:
When carrying loads distribute the load over the largest joint rather than the hands, e.g. use the forearm or palms to carry the object rather than the fingers

Avoid heavy loads

Avoid sustained or repetitive activities: varying positions or movements avoids fatigue and tissue overload

Evaluate a task consider how it is possible to make the task simpler and how you can make it more efficient

Summary

The incorporation of intrinsic, extrinsic, and task-related factors forms the basis of ergonomics, and it is becoming commonplace for the physiotherapist to perform ergonomic assessments in industry and sport with the aim of reducing the incidence of soft tissue injury. An example of this approach is the management of soft tissue dysfunction in rheumatoid arthritis, where the physiotherapist gives advice regarding joint protection. Here the aim is to prevent any deterioration of soft tissue function. Advice is given about reducing joint stress and therefore inflammation and pain, and task-related advice is given about energy conservation and improving functional endurance (Table 6). In this context the physiotherapist typically performs an assessment of the patient with an occupational therapist so that the management programme incorporates and relates to activities of daily living. Splinting may also be used to decrease the joint stresses during periods of exacerbation.

The majority of advice given to patients requires a behavioural change and, if approaches are to be successful, the long-term compliance of the patient has to be obtained. Though education may lead to an attitudinal change in patients,[20] the physiotherapist typically uses cognitive behavioural strategies such as verbal and written information, demonstrations, goal setting, and small group work as this has been suggested to be the most effective way of ensuring compliance.[21]

Social and family history

Social, family, and work-related issues are explored. These may have relevance in terms of the contribution of familial traits to disease and the influence of social and financial pressures on timescales for return to work. This aspect, along with psychological issues, forms an important component of the biopsychosocial model of assessment that is discussed later in the chapter.

Past medical history

The past medical history is used to assess the patient's suitability for physiotherapeutic management. Issues in relation to previous treatments for this condition, the patient's general health, fractures, surgical procedures, and contraindications to treatment are explored.

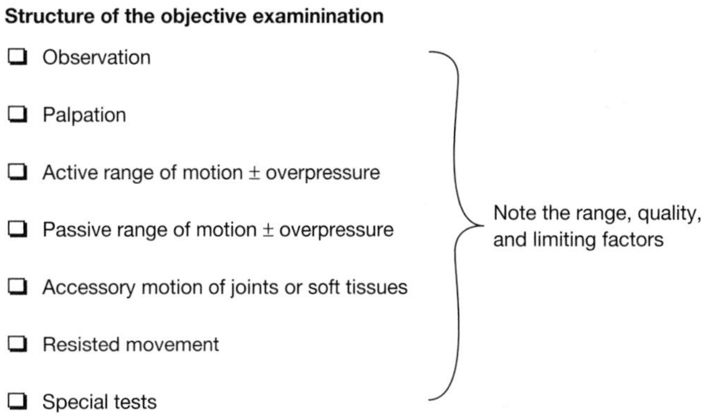

Structure of the objective examinination

❑ Observation

❑ Palpation

❑ Active range of motion ± overpressure

❑ Passive range of motion ± overpressure

❑ Accessory motion of joints or soft tissues

❑ Resisted movement

❑ Special tests

Note the range, quality, and limiting factors

Fig. 1 Components of the objective examination.

Drug history

A full drug history is taken to establish the suitability for particular treatments. The dosage can also be used as a guide to the severity of the patient's symptoms and as an index of the effectiveness of a treatment protocol as the patient may, for example, report a decrease in the use of analgesics as the symptoms decrease with treatment.

Objective examination

Assumptions are made on the basis of information from the subjective assessment as to the possible site of the dysfunction. Observation, palpation, and movement tests are used to identify the site of tissue dysfunction (Fig. 1). The movement tests apply stresses to tissues to assess the response to loading, and typically involve physiological joint movements (movement that occur at joint that are under voluntary control), or accessory joint movements (movements occurring at joint and soft tissues that are not under voluntary control). In particular the range, quality and the limiting factors to the movement are noted.

An example of this process in relation to the assessment of dysfunction in the rectus femoris muscle would be to initially apply the

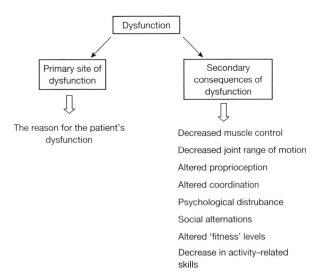

Fig. 2 The primary and secondary consequences of dysfunction.

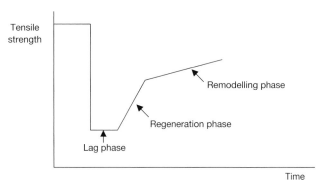

Fig. 3 The stages of the healing properties in relation to the development of tensile strength.

Table 7 Factors influencing the healing process

Local factors	Systemic factors
Type of injury	Age
Location of injury	Disease
Blood supply	Nutritional status
Infection	Hormones
Movement	Medication
Previous tissue trauma	Temperature
	Oxygen levels

physiological joint movements of knee flexion, hip extension, and a posterior pelvic tilt to apply a tensile force to the rectus femoris. The range, quality, and limiting factors to the movement are noted. Accessory movement (movement of the tissue on palpation) of the rectus femoris is then assessed and, again, the range, quality, and limiting factors to the movement are noted. The physiological joint movements and accessory soft tissue movements are then combined, with the range, quality, and limiting factors being noted. Finally, isometric, concentric, and eccentric muscle contraction in combination with accessory soft tissue motion is evaluated.

During the objective examination the physiotherapist uses a series of special tests that help to elicit precautions and contraindications to physiotherapeutic management, for example, vertebral artery tests are conducted prior to cervical mobilization and skin sensation is tested prior to the use of electrotherapeutic modalities.

At the end of the assessment process the physiotherapist has an understanding of the aetiology of the injury and the area, nature, behaviour, and the presentation of the patient's symptoms. This information is used in the clinical reasoning process to form a hypothesis regarding the primary site responsible for the dysfunction. The physiotherapist also identifies the secondary consequences that are associated with the primary site of dysfunction (Fig. 2).

The treatment strategy for the management of soft tissue dysfunction is to address the primary site and secondary factors concurrently, ensuring that the selected approaches do not aggravate the primary site of dysfunction.

The management of soft tissue dysfunction

In the management of soft tissue dysfunction due to soft tissue trauma, a therapeutic stimulus is usually applied to favourably influence the healing process. Critical to this approach is an understanding of the stages of the healing process and the clinical implications of each stage.

The primary site of dysfunction and the healing process

In the early stages in the management of soft tissue dysfunction there is a tension between mobilization and immobilization. In general, the favoured approach is early mobilization on the basis that prolonged immobilization may produce atrophy of cartilage, bone, muscles, tendons, and ligaments,[22, 23] whereas the benefits of early mobilization have been demonstrated in relation to the knee,[24] muscle,[11] tendon,[25] and ligament.[26]

During the healing process the restoration of mechanical tissue properties passes through three phases, termed the lag phase, the proliferation or regeneration phase, and the remodelling phase (Fig. 3). These phases are not clearly delineated in terms of their timescale and the length of each phase is influenced by many factors (Table 7). The physiotherapist uses assumptions drawn from an understanding of these stages in the clinical reasoning process. These assumptions are illustrated below.

Lag phase

This phase typically lasts approximately 4–6 days.[27] During this time the inflammatory reaction prepares the wound for the regeneration phase[27] and involves a combination of vascular, cellular, homeostatic, and immune processes, with humeral and neural mediators serving as control mechanisms for this phase. The vascular events involve vasoconstriction followed by vasodilatation along with increased vasopermeability (regulated by chemical mediators such as bradykinnins, serotonin, histamine, and prostaglandins), platelet adherence, and the activation of a clotting cascade involving fibrin and fibroconnectin.[27] The consequence of these reactions is the production of the classical inflammatory signs of pain, redness, heat, swelling, and loss of function. Inflammation is rather spuriously looked upon as undesirable. However, without it the tissue would not heal and the defence system of the body would be inert.

The healing process typically begins 24 h post-injury with the arrival of the macrophage,[27] and from this time until the regeneration phase begins the wound is vulnerable with regard to further loading as a weak fibrin 'scaffolding' holds the wound edges together.[28] Excessive loading can easily disrupt this fragile tissue bond and further exacerbate the inflammatory reaction.

The lag phase and clinical reasoning

Because of the inflammatory reaction and the weak tensile properties of the wound, the therapeutic intention during this period is to control the inflammatory reaction using rest, ice, compression, elevation, and movement protection as prolonged inflammation may lead to excessive scar tissue formation. Electrotherapy modalities such as laser, ultrasound, transcutaneous electrical nerve stimulation (TENS), and pulsed short-wave may by used during the lag phase because of their proposed effects on the cellular membrane and macrophage activity.

The amount of loading is also controlled as this stage relates to a chemical model of dysfunction, where chemical mediators predominate and, therefore, early aggressive movement can exacerbate the reaction, resulting in excessive scar tissue formation. Taping may be used during this time period to exert compression and to protect the dysfunctional tissues from excessive load.

Regeneration phase

This phase commences approximately 5 days post-injury and lasts for approximately 10–12 weeks depending on the degree of the original trauma.[27] During this time period collagen synthesis predominates and, consequently, it is the period of the greatest increase in the tensile strength of the wound.[27]

Fibroblasts facilitate the formation of collagen and the amount, direction, and type of collagen combined with collagen cross-linkages influence the mechanical properties of the tissue.[29] In the early stages of collagen synthesis, type III collagen predominates, resulting in a weak tissue that is vulnerable to excessive loading. By approximately day 12, type III collagen begins to be replaced with type I collagen, which is a more mature and stronger form of collagen.[30]

Because of the tendency during this period for the formation of randomly orientated collagen fibres, which restore structure but hinder function,[31] careful loading of the tissue during this phase may promote more functional characteristics of the collagen synthesis,[32] facilitating optimal collagen alignment,[33] and reducing the time period for the following remodelling phase.[34]

The regeneration phase and clinical reasoning

The therapeutic intention during this phase is to gradually introduce some load into the tissue to promote the functional formation of scar tissue. Loading appears to be important in influencing collagen and ground substance interaction. For example, glycosaminoglycans, such as hyaluronic acid, appear to facilitate matrix composition and influence the scar tissue architecture.[35] However, it is important to delay loading as early loading may lead to enhanced type III collagen

production and a weaker tissue than that produced by mobilization at the optimal time period.[11]

During this phase the physiotherapist carefully applies progressive force to the tissue being guided by the pain response of the patient. This movement may be applied manually or using exercise, with functional motion being the main influence on the choice of the exercise. Great care is taken during this stage because, although the injured area has the greatest amount of collagen, its tensile strength is only approximately 15 per cent of that of normal tissue.[36]

Electrothermal modalities such as ultrasound and laser may be used in this phase because of their proposed action on collagen synthesis.

Remodelling phase

This phase commences when collagen synthesis matches collagen lysis. The tensile strength of the wound increases but at a slower rate than during the regeneration phase. The number of fibroblasts, macrophages, myofibroblasts, and capillaries decreases and the water content of the tissue declines. In combination, the tensile strength of the wound increases due to the formation of intra- and extramolecular cross-linkages that stabilize over time.[34] These links strengthen the wound but also lead to adhesions that, combined with the gradual decrease in the water content of the scar, result in a stiffer scar with decreased compliance.[29] The tendency for the wound to contract may last for 6–12 months.[34]

The remodelling phase and clinical reasoning

The therapeutic intention during this phase is to load the wound to promote functional healing of the scar tissue and to help promote a compliant rather than stiff scar. A stiff scar results in increased tension in the area on motion which may relate to the pain experienced by the patient. Heating the tissue via thermal modalities or exercise is used to decrease tissue stiffness prior to mobilization.

Two theories attempt to explain the orientation of collagen fibres in scar tissue. The first is the induction theory, which suggests that the scar attempts to mimic the characteristics of the tissue it is healing.[37] The second is the tension theory, which suggests that the internal and external stresses placed on the injured area during the remodelling phase determine the final tissue structure.[38] This theory is supported by the work of Arem and Madden[39] who indicate that the two most important variables responsible for the successful tissue remodelling are: (1) the phase of the repair process in which the mechanical forces were introduced and (2) the nature of the applied forces.

The rationale for loading in the regeneration and remodelling phases is the tension theory of collagen synthesis.

As well as the influence of loading on the wound, the pattern of collagen synthesis is also strongly influenced by the oxygen levels in the area with collagen synthesis being oxygen-dependent, and collagen lysis not.[40] This forms part of the basis for the use of pressure garments in the treatment of burns with the rationale that low oxygen levels influence the process of collagen synthesis towards lysis, which results in a softer and less bulky scar.

Degenerative pathology

Evidence is accumulating to suggest that many supposed inflammatory lesions, for example, Achilles 'tendonitis', may, in certain cases, be degenerative rather than inflammatory.[41] It has been suggested that these degenerative changes may be evident in one-third of tendons in the healthy urban population over the age of 35.[42] These changes manifest as non-inflammatory intratendinous collagen degeneration resulting in fibre disorientation, a relative absence of tenocytes, scattered vascular ingrowth, and increased interfibrillar glycosoaminoglycans.[43] The collagen fibres become thin and frayed and lose their parallel orientation[44, 45] and, in combination, the tenocytes isolated from these areas produce increased quantities of type III collagen, which has a reduced load-bearing capacity compared to that of type I collagen and, consequently, the tissue is likely to fail earlier with mechanical loading.[46]

Degenerative pathology and clinical reasoning

The therapeutic intention during this time period is to apply a load to the affected area to promote adaptation in the area of dysfunction. This adaptation may relate to the movement initiating an inflammatory reaction, which may be absent in the tissue, or by some other mechanism yet to be identified. The load may be applied manually, but eccentric exercise shows promise as a mechanism for the management of tendinopathy (see later).

Treatment approaches

Many treatment approaches may be applied by the physiotherapist in the management of soft tissue dysfunction. They may be broadly classified as electrothermal modalities, manual therapy, and exercise therapy. Some are directed at the primary site of tissue dysfunction, typically electrothermal modalities, and others such as manual therapy and exercise therapy are directed at addressing both the primary and secondary consequences of injury.

Electrothermal modalities

The physiotherapist may choose to promote tissue adaptation by the use of electrothermal agents. These agents may be used in isolation, but are often used as an adjunct to other treatments. The physiotherapist has a large range of modalities to choose from and only a limited number are considered here. For a more extensive review the reader is referred to reference 47.

Transcutaneous electrical nerve stimulation (TENS)

TENS is the term used for the application of electrical stimulation for pain control and its use is indicated in the acute stages of soft tissue injury (the lag phase) to control the pain associated with the inflammatory reaction or for the management of chronic pain (Fig. 4). TENS is thought to provide pain control on the basis of gate control and opium-mediated control.

The gate control theory postulates that painful stimuli are transmitted to the spinal cord via small-diameter, slow-conducting nociceptive nerve fibres with little or no myelin, that is, Aδ and C fibres. This relay is thought to be inhibited by the activity of large-diameter, fast-conducting highly myelinated proprioceptive sensory nerve fibres (Aβ fibres).[48] The electrical current is thought to stimulate the Aβ fibres and therefore activate the substantia gelatinosa to inhibit the transmission of nociceptive impulses by T cells. There is also some evidence to indicate that TENS can modulate the transmission of impulses carried by small-diameter slow-conducting nociceptive fibres.[49] The opiate-mediated control theory postulates that TENS controls pain by the release of endogenous opiates.[50]

Clinically, the physiotherapist manipulates the current, waveform, pulse duration, amplitude, frequency, on and off times, ramp, total

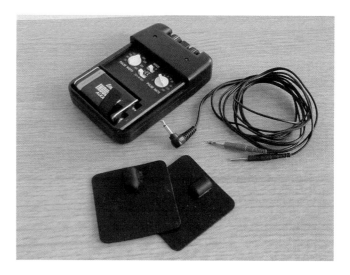

Fig. 4 Transcutaneous electrical nerve stimulator (TENS) unit.

treatment times, and electrode placement until the appropriate combination is found for the patient. Electrode configuration is important and this is determined by a process of trial and error. Locations around the painful site, over the exit of an involved nerve root from the vertebral column, along the course of a nerve, and trigger or acupuncture points are tried. Occasionally, the opposite side of the body may be used, for example, with phantom limb pain.

Usually, sensory level stimulation is used whereby the intensity of the electrical current is increased to the point of mild discomfort and sustained at this point for a period of time. During this time period the intensity may need to be increased due to accommodation of the neural tissue to the stimulus. The decrease in the nociceptive response is quick. However, the effect tends to last for less than 1 hour after the stimulation ceases.[51]

The precautions with regards to the use of TENS involve electrode placement in the area of the carotid sinus, use in a patient with a demand-type pacemaker, undiagnosed pain, patients known to have a hyposensitive area, and during pregnancy other than in labour and delivery.

Pulsed short-wave diathermy

This modality involves the application of pulsed short-wave (10–100 MHz frequency and 3–30 m wavelength) electromagnetic energy to the tissue (Fig. 5). The typical short-wave band is 27.12 MHz.

When the short wave is applied at low average intensity with short pulse duration and a low duty cycle, any transient heating is dissipated. Because of the relatively athermal nature of this modality, the physiotherapist may use this modality in the early stages of the healing process.

The exact mechanism of action is speculative though current theories relate to modification of the ion binding and cellular function by the incident electromagnetic fields and the resulting electric currents.[52] The contraindications and precautions relate to tumours, metallic implants, foreign bodies, acute haemorrhage, cardiac pacemakers, and altered sensation.

Ultrasound

Therapeutic ultrasound (Fig. 6) is generated by applying a high-frequency alternating electrical current to a crystal located in the

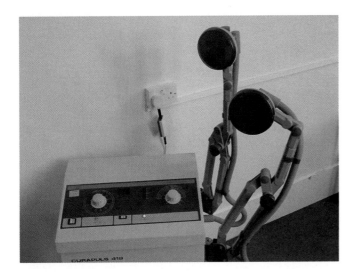

Fig. 5 Pulsed short-wave unit.

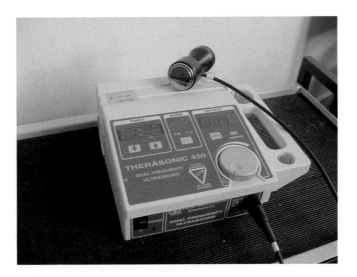

Fig. 6 Ultrasound unit.

ultrasound transducer. The crystal has piezoelectric properties, which cause it to respond to the current by expanding and contracting and generating an ultrasound wave.

The ultrasound wave generated for therapeutic use has a frequency of 0.7–3.3 MHz in order to maximize energy absorption at a depth of 2–5 cm of soft tissue.[47] The ultrasound wave may be used in a continuous or pulsed mode and is applied to the patient via the use of a contact medium such as water or gel.

The therapeutic effects of ultrasound may be divided into thermal and non-thermal effects.

Thermal effects Thermal effects are influenced by the type of tissue and the frequency, duration, and intensity of the ultrasound. The increase in tissue temperature is claimed to accelerate the metabolic rate, reduce pain and muscle spasm, alter nerve conduction velocity, increase circulation, and increase soft tissue extensibility.

The thermal effects are used for pain relief and also prior to soft tissue mobilization. Here the effect is greater for tissues possessing a high collagen content as this type of tissue has a high absorption coefficient

and therefore absorbs more of the ultrasound wave. For example, the soft tissue temperature (in muscle) has been shown to increase by 0.2 °C per minute with ultrasound delivered at 1 W/cm^2 at 1 MHz.[53] On this basis the heating effect is mainly used on muscle, ligaments, and tendons as an adjunct to soft tissue mobilization. In this way the increase in tissue temperature affects tissue extensibility resulting in an increase in the tissue length for the same force of stretch plus a reduced risk of tissue damage.[54]

Non-thermal effects Here the ultrasound wave is pulsed and the therapeutic effects are thought to be due to mechanical events such as cavitation, microstreaming, and acoustic streaming rather than thermal effects. In particular, pulsed ultrasound has been shown to increase intracelluar calcium,[55] increase cell membrane permeability,[56] increase mast cell degranulation,[57] increase macrophage activity,[58] and increase protein synthesis by fibroblasts.[59] As these effects are important chemical components of tissue healing, the assumption is that ultrasound positively influences these processes. The pulsed mode may be used for pain control whereby stimulation of the cutaneous thermal receptors and/or increased tissue temperature or changes in nerve conduction may decrease the pain.

Ultrasound may also be used in combination with topical drug preparations, the preparation being added to the contact medium— this is called phonophoresis. The proposed mechanism of action was thought to relate to a driving force generated by the ultrasound, which propelled the drug though the skin. However, ultrasound exerts only a few grams of force, and it is now thought that any effects relate to increasing the permeability of the stratum corneum.[60]

The proposed benefits of this approach over the oral route include increased drug concentration at the delivery site, avoidance of gastric irritation, and avoidance of first-pass metabolism at the liver. Drugs delivered in this manner become systemic and hence contraindications for systemic drugs also apply to this mode of delivery. It is important that a drug is not delivered by phonophoresis if the patient is receiving the drug of the same type by another route. Byl provides a good review of the principles of phonophoresis.[61]

Contraindications and precautions relate to growing epiphysis, the pregnant uterus, testicular tissues, pacemakers, altered sensation, metallic implants, and fracture sites.

Cryotherapy

Cold therapy can be applied by a variety of means, for example, ice packs, gel packs, ice massage, cold compression units, vapo-coolant sprays, and typically is applied for 20–30 minutes ideally every 3–4 waking hours in the inflammatory phase.

In each case it is typically used in the acute stages of soft tissue injury with the aim being to control inflammation, pain, and oedema. In the more chronic stages post-injury, it may be used for its pain and muscle spasm/spasticity-relieving effects, which may facilitate the restoration of normal movement.

The proposed mechanism of action of ice relates to haemodynamic, neuromuscular, and metabolic processes.

Haemodynamic effects Ice is thought to decrease the intravascular pressure by reducing blood flow into the area via vasoconstriction and increased blood viscosity. It also increases capillary permeability by reducing the release of vasoactive substances such as histamine. These effects are thought to be useful in the inflammatory phase to regulate the amount of oedema formation. Though ice is often applied on the basis of haemodynamic effects, cold-induced vasodilatation is not a consistent response to prolonged cold application.[62]

In order to reduce oedema, ice is typically used in combination with compression, as compression increases the hydrostatic gradients from the tissue to the circulation, thus helping to force fluid into the vessels by increasing the interstitial hydrostatic pressure. The compression may be used during cold application or after the application of ice using foam pads or chiropody felt.

Neuromuscular effects Nerve conduction velocity decreases in proportion to the degree and duration of the temperature change.[63] This affects both sensory and motor nerves but has the greatest effect on myelinated and small fibre nerves and least effect on conduction by unmyelinated and large fibres.[64] Hence the Aδ fibres, which are small-diameter myelinated pain-transmitting fibres, demonstrate the greatest decrease in conduction velocity in response to cooling.

Metabolic effects Cold decreases the rate of all metabolic reactions and therefore is used in the acute stages post-injury to acute inflammatory reaction. On this basis ice may be more effective if it is used on the principle of preventing secondary hypoxia rather than the vasodilatation/constriction model commonly applied in physiotherapy.[65]

Ice may also be useful in the management of joint disease associated with rheumatoid arthritis where cartilage-degrading enzymes such as collagenase, elastase, hyaluronidase, and protease have been shown to be inhibited by decreases in joint temperature of 30 °C or lower.[66]

Laser

A laser (Fig. 7) generates a beam of electromagnetic radiation with wave lengths ranging from 100 nm to 1 mm. Laser light differs from ordinary light in that the waves are of the same frequency (monochromatic), are all in phase with each other (coherent), and exhibit minimal divergence (directional).

Lasers tend to be of two types, helium–neon (He–Ne) lasers, which emit visible red light with a wavelength of 633 nm, and gallium-arsenide (GaAs) lasers, which emit infrared radiation with a wavelength of 830 nm.

The frequency of the laser light, as well as the type of tissue being irradiated, determines the depth to which the light penetrates.[67]

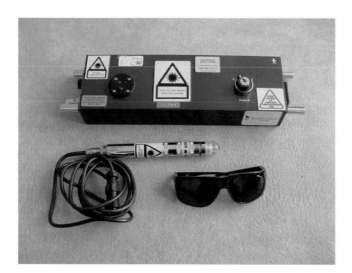

Fig. 7 Laser unit.

However, the depth of penetration of all lasers is limited to a few millimetres. Deeper physiological effects are thought to occur as the photon energy is thought to promote chemical reactions that mediate processes at a distance from the site of application.

The intensity of the laser influences its clinical effects. High-intensity lasers are called 'hot' lasers and they heat and destroy tissue and are typically used to cauterize and make incisions during surgery. Cold lasers are used in rehabilitation and generally output laser light with less than 500 mW power, at around 50 mW/cm^2 power density and with an energy density of less than 35 J/cm^2. Evidence suggests that these levels of electromagnetic energy may be biostimulative and facilitate healing.[68]

The therapeutic effect of cold lasers is thought to relate to alteration of biochemical, physiological, and/or proliferative activities by affecting intercellular communication with short-term activation of the electron transport chain, increased adenosine triphosphate (ATP) synthesis, and a reduction in cellular pH being popular theories of mechanism of action.[69] These biochemical and cellular changes are believed to cause the increases in macrophage and lymphocyte activity that have been observed with laser application.[70] Clinically, the therapist would use lower energy density ranges in the acute phase and higher doses for more chronic conditions.

Studies into the effectiveness of low-level laser yield controversial results but a recent meta-analysis suggested that low-level laser was more effective than placebo for the treatment of musculoskeletal disorders.[71] Contraindications and precautions relate to no application directly to the eye, pregnancy, photosensitive patients, and active infection.

Manual therapy

Once the area of dysfunction has been identified by subjective and objective testing, mobilization techniques may be used to either favourably influence the healing process or restore soft tissue mobility. These techniques are applied in the regeneration and remodelling phase to influence the development of the mechanical properties of the tissue to a level that is compatible with the potential imposed demands, for pain relief, and to restore soft tissue mobility.

Many schools of manual therapy exist, some based on joint principles and others on soft tissue principles, but all involve the application of force to the body tissues to try and restore function. The majority of the literature relating to manual therapy appears to concentrate on its use in relation to the management of low back pain, where the current evidence indicates it has value, particularly in the first 6 weeks after the onset of low back pain.[72] There are, however, many clinical presentations of low back pain, and the physiotherapist conducts a detailed assessment to decide if manual therapy is appropriate for the particular patient's presentation. In applying manual techniques the physiotherapist considers the magnitude, direction, type, rate, frequency, and duration of the force and does this on the basis of the information gleaned from the subjective and objective examination and on the response of the patient. The magnitude of the force varies from gentle small oscillatory movements called 'mobilizations' used to address irritable and painful lesions on the basis of the pain gate theory, to rapid high-velocity short-duration techniques referred to as 'manipulation'.

Recently, the use of manual therapy in relation to the management of low back pain has been challenged by the biopsychosocial model of dysfunction.[73, 74] In this model the use of manual therapy may be seen to reinforce the patient's negative response to dysfunction as it is a passive technique in that the patient does not play an active role in the treatment. The patient may welcome the attention and the attitude of giving the physiotherapist the problem to 'sort out'. On this basis, the physiotherapist is careful to ensure that manual therapy is not applied in circumstances where it would reinforce negative responses to dysfunction.

A branch of manual therapy relates to the direct management of soft tissue dysfunction where soft tissue mobilization techniques are applied to soft tissues to facilitate a return to function. The application of soft tissue mobilization techniques is based on knowledge of tissue mechanics and the key principles and clinical relevance are summarized below.

Biomechanical properties of soft tissue

The mechanical properties of tissues are usually investigated by assessing their response to compressive, shear, and tensile loading. Data about tensile testing feature highly in the clinical reasoning process and relate to tests involving the progressive application of tensile load to a tissue and measuring the resultant change in tissue length (Fig. 8).

The main features gleaned from load deformation analysis used in the clinical reasoning process are these

1. The slope of the linear portion of the curve is called the *elastic modulus*. This represents the stiffness of the tissue.[75] The stiffer the tissue the steeper the slope and consequently a decreased range for a given force results. The physiotherapist would apply techniques to decrease the tissue stiffness such as heat followed by sustained mobilization techniques.

2. The area under the curve represents the energy that is delivered to the tissue during the deformation. This energy is termed *strain energy* and may be useful in improving the efficiency of movements as part of the stretch shorten cycle (where eccentric to concentric muscle activity occurs).[76, 77] If the strain energy exceeds the mechanical properties of the tissue then either micro- or macrotrauma may occur and tissue damage results.[78] Following injury the tissue architecture is less able to with stand the stress of tensile loading. Mobilization techniques facilitate the ability of the tissue to withstand the applied energy,[79] and the therapist gradually increases the amount of mechanical energy applied to the patient's tissues as the symptoms resolve and function improves.

3. The stiffness of the tissue and the energy stored is influenced by the tissue's *viscoelastic properties*.[80] Viscoelasticity is a property of soft tissues whereby the strain induced in the tissue is dependent on the loading rate of the applied stress (Fig. 9). In general, the faster the

rate of loading the stiffer the tissue becomes. This increase in stiffness involves the viscous component of the soft tissue and is thought to be due to interaction between collagen fibre and ground substance.[81] The ability of the tissue stiffness to increase with increased rates of loading is a valuable attribute in tendons.[82] The clinical relevance lies in the need to increase the rate of loading as a component of the rehabilitation programme to allow the tissue to withstand the larger forces that occur with faster rates of loading.

4. The *load deformation curve* can be divided into two regions—the elastic and plastic regions. Loading the tissue within the elastic region results in non-permanent changes in tissue length. Loading the tissue within the plastic region results in permanent deformation of the tissue, which is therapeutically desirable when a decrease in tissue motion relates to the patient's symptoms. Heat is usually applied followed by a controlled stretch for a sustained of time to cause plastic deformation, as is used in some splinting techniques.

5. *Hysteresis* is a phenomenon associated with energy loss exhibited by viscoelastic materials when they are subjected to loading and unloading cycles.[83] An elastic material would demonstrate identical load deformation curves in the loading and unloading phases. However, with viscoelastic materials the curves of the two phases are not identical (Fig. 10). The area between the unloading and

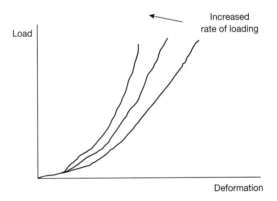

Fig. 9 The effect of changing the rate of loading on the response of the tissue. Viscoelastic response—increased stiffness with increased rates of loading.

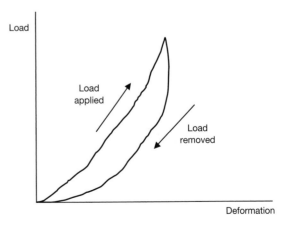

Fig. 10 The energy lost exhibited by viscoelastic materials when subjected to loading and unloading cycles—hysteresis.

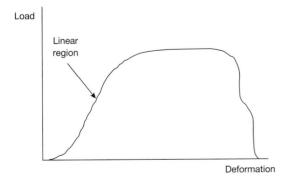

Fig. 8 Load deformation curve.

loading curves represents the energy that is lost due to mechanical damage to the tissue and from internal friction.[75] The energy absorbed by the tissue represents the stimulus that produces the therapeutic effect.

6. *Creep* is characterized by a continued deformation at a fixed load.[84] When the load is applied the material will deflect until an equilibrium point is reached (Fig. 11). The clinical application of a constant low load over a prolonged period takes advantage of the creep response and is useful for increasing soft tissue mobility.[85] For example, serial splinting utilizes this principle to increase range of motion.

7. *Stress relaxation* results in a decrease in the amount of force required over time to hold a tissue at their required length (Fig. 12). The decrease in tissue tension over time may contribute to a decreased pain response in the patient and an increased range of motion.

In summary, the manual therapy is applied to alter the response of the tissue to loading. The alteration of the tissue's mechanical properties typically results in a decrease in the patient's symptoms. The link between altered tissue biomechanics and pain is a complex one. However, a summary of the rationale is presented in Fig. 13.

Manual therapy and neural dynamics—adverse neural dynamics
Recently, the manual techniques used by the physiotherapist have incorporated an approach that acknowledges the role of altered neural

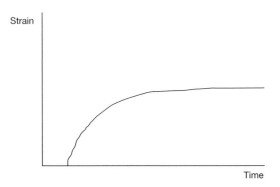

Fig. 11 Creep effects resulting from deformation occurring during the application of a fixed load.

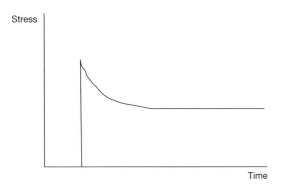

Fig. 12 Stress relaxation resulting from a decrease in stress during constant deformation.

motion and physiology in the production of soft tissue dysfunction. This concept is known as adverse neural dynamics.

During human motion the nervous system moves against adjacent tissue and is subjected to compressive and tensile forces. An alteration in the ability of the neural system to tolerate these forces has been suggested as a contributing factor in musculoskeletal dysfunction.[86] The concept of altered neural motion being associated with dysfunction is not new and manifests in everyday orthopaedic practice with the straight leg raise test,[87] passive neck flexion test,[88] and prone knee bend test.[89] The altered mechanical stresses in the nervous system are intimately linked to neurological and physiological events and the assessment of neural dynamics forms a key part of the physiotherapist's consideration in musculoskeletal assessment.

In this approach the physiotherapist examines the compliance and 'function' of the nervous system with regard to motion by applying a sequence of passive testing procedures each subjecting a particular aspect of the neural system to sliding, elongation tension, and pressure alterations. The quality of motion and response of the patient to the testing procedure are noted and related to the patient's symptoms.

An example of the application of the use of neurodynamic approaches to the management of soft tissue dysfunction is the use of upper limb test 2 in the assessment and management of lateral epicondylitis of the elbow. Here the patient lies supine and the physiotherapist performs a series of movement tests involving the cervical spine, shoulder girdle, shoulder joint, elbow, forearm, wrist, and fingers to try to reproduce the patient's symptoms. The assumption is that, with the elbow extensors under tension in the position of elbow extension, forearm pronation, wrist flexion, and ulnar deviation and finger flexion, the additional side flexion of the cervical spine away from the affected side, and shoulder girdle depression on the affected side increase the mechanical influence on the radial nerve and may thus replicate the patient's symptoms. If the symptoms are reproduced in this position, and then cervical side flexion towards the affected side and shoulder girdle elevation on the affected side decrease the symptoms, the physiotherapist may assume that there is a neural component to the patient's symptoms, as the symptoms are provoked by cervical and shoulder girdle movement rather than by elbow or wrist motion. In this case the physiotherapist may incorporate cervical

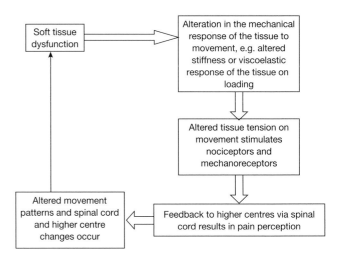

Fig. 13 The rationale for soft tissue mobilization—altered tissue mechanics and pain hypothesis.

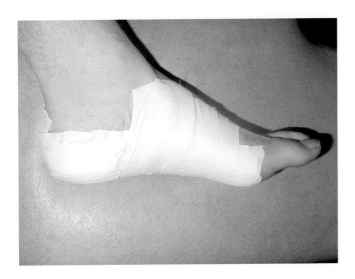

Fig. 14 The use of tape to decrease the loading in the plantar fascia.

spine and shoulder girdle movements in the management of lateral epicondylitis to promote adaptation in the radial nerve components with regard to sliding, elongation tension, and pressure alterations. Butler[90] provides an extensive review of this area.

Taping and bracing
Taping is a manual skill that may be used to facilitate the rehabilitation programme. It is used to hold dressings in place, apply compression during the acute phase of injury, guide and restrict motion to protect injured structures from further trauma, and to offer sensory input to provide proprioceptive input (Fig. 14).

Taping is often used in clinical practice to facilitate the rehabilitation process by reducing pain and thus reflex inhibition. In this case the patient may experience pain on motion that is producing reflex inhibition of a muscle group that is required to produce or control the movement. For example, the quadriceps may be reflexly inhibited in a patient with anterior knee pain. Here the physiotherapist may apply tape to the patella to attempt to reduce tension of load on the symptomatic area, which may reduce the pain and hence allow the patient to recruit the quadriceps during functional activity. This is reviewed in reference 91.

Exercise therapy
Exercise therapy is an essential part of the management of soft tissue dysfunction. In contrast to manual therapy and electrothermal modalities where the patient is usually passive, exercise therapy actively involves the patients in the rehabilitation process, as they become responsible for their dysfunction, being less reliant on the therapist.

A variety of exercise protocols are used to address the secondary consequences on dysfunction, such as altered muscular control, proprioception, and coordination. In each case the exercise regime begins with simple movements, progressing to more complex and eventually functional motion as the pathology allows. Examples are presented below.

Muscular control
This is addressed by the use of resistance exercise with the goals being to restore muscular strength, power, endurance, and muscle control to levels that are compatible with 'normal' function.

Decreased muscular control commonly occurs due to reflex inhibition[92] in relation to joint effusion and pain. It is important to eliminate the cause of the reflex inhibition, as failure to do this will retard muscular development. Following this the active muscle is subjected to progressive resistance from an outside force.

Many exercise protocols exist but common features relate to the following three components; the type of exercise, the type of muscular contraction, and the type of resistance.

Type of exercise
A typical progression is from endurance exercise involving low loads with lots of repetitions to strength exercise involving increased loads with less repetitions, to power exercise involving increased speed.

Type of muscular contraction
Isometric exercise, which involves muscular contraction without joint movement, is used in the initial stages of rehabilitation, as there is less chance of increasing joint irritability. Strength developments, however, appear to be joint-angle-specific. Progression is to dynamic exercise, where joint movement is involved. Concentric exercise progresses to eccentric exercise.

Eccentric exercises (exercises that involve the active lengthening) of the muscle tendon unit have become popular for the management of tendon dysfunction. The basis for this is that active lengthening of the muscle tendon unit results in higher tensile forces and eventually increased tensile properties of the tendon.[93] This increase in tensile properties allows the tissue to withstand more strain energy during the stretch shorten cycle.[94]

Eccentric exercise may also address fatigue-related dysfunction, which is important as fatigue reduces the ability of the muscle tendon unit to attenuate strain energy. Eccentric exercise may also prepare the tendon for rapid unloading, which has been associated with injury as sudden force release is hypothesized to break interfibrillar links, as the shearing forces within the tendon are large.[94]

The clinical use of eccentric protocols was pioneered in the literature by Stannish et al.[93] who reported on a prospective study on 200 patients suffering from chronic Achilles tendonitis with a mean duration time from onset of 18 months. The study indicated that the regime used had a favourable effect in 87 per cent of the subjects but it should be noted that the study had no randomization or control group and used a multiple intervention programme involving the use of static stretching pre- and post-exercise and ice.

Niesen-Vertommen et al.[95] used 17 subjects and, though there was no statistical difference in the outcome, the data suggest that eccentric exercise was more influential on decreasing the pain scale scores than the concentric protocols.

More recently, Alfredson et al.[96] conducted a prospective study into the effect of heavy-load eccentric calf muscle training in 15 patients with Achilles tendonitis. In contrast to other studies this one used purely eccentric exercise with patients raising up on the good side and lowering down on the bad side.

The patients were selected from a group waiting for Achilles tendon surgery and they were subjected to an eccentric programme. The group was compared to 15 patients also on the list who progressed to surgery. The study found that all of the eccentric group at 12 weeks were back to their pre-injury levels with full running activity and the effects in terms of pain reduction and prevention of strength deficits were better than in those who went on to surgery. The eccentric group also achieved better results in half the time of the surgical group (12 weeks versus 24 weeks, respectively).

To summarize, there is evidence of a pre-experimental nature to suggest that eccentric exercise may be beneficial in the management of Achilles tendonitis. Better research designs using a true experimental design are required to give more causal inference to the data currently presented and the exact mechanism of action requires further study.

Type of resistance

A variety of methods are used to apply resistance such as manual techniques and mechanical devices, for example, free weights, pulley systems, isokinetic machines, elastic tubing, springs, and sand bags. Hydrotherapy is particularly useful in the early non-weight-bearing stages of rehabilitation.

As well as developing muscular strength, power, and endurance, particular emphasis is placed on developing muscle control. This relates to an aspect of physiotherapy known as muscle imbalance and is based on the concept that certain muscles have a primary role as stabilizers during movement, others primarily move the joint, and others serve a combined role. Alteration of this pattern due to pain or reflex inhibition results in an imbalance in the normal motor control pattern and hence dysfunction. Physiotherapists apply very specific stability protocols with the aim being to restore optimal motor control. For example, O'Sullivan et al.[97] demonstrated a statistically significant effect in the utilization of exercises to target the anterolateral abdominal muscles and the multifidus, over general spinal exercises, in patients with chronic low back pain due to spondlylolysis and spondylolithesis.

Proprioception and coordination

Here exercises are used to 'stress' the proprioceptive system. Simple balance exercises are progressed on the basis of decreasing the base of support and increasing the displacement of the bodies' centre of gravity until the patients is challenged by the dynamic and complex motor patterns of 'normal' function.

Functional exercises

The SAID principle states that an important principle in rehabilitation is one of specific adaptation to imposed demands.[98] This implies that the body tissues only adapt to specific imposed demands. On this basis the ultimate aim of the exercise programme is to use exercises that are functional in nature as these mimic the typical demands placed on the tissue by the patient. On this basis the physiotherapist will gradually increase the functional demands on a patient by utilizing progressive exercises that mimic the functional activity to which the patient is to return.

Biopsychosocial model of tissue dysfunction

In contrast to the pathology-based approaches mentioned above, particular emphasis has recently been given to the biopsychosocial model of patient care. This model was first introduced in 1977[99] and incorporates aspects of physical dysfunction, beliefs, coping strategies, distress, illness behaviour, social interaction, and influences as part of the patient assessment. The model adds to the perspective of the more traditionally used biomedical model, where treatment is based on the premise that disease is a manifestation of underlying pathology and

management is directed at the pathology to produce a cure.[100] This model views pain as equating to disability and fails to acknowledge the complex human responses to pain and disability (Table 8).[4]

During the assessment process the physiotherapist seeks to identify 'red flags', which indicate pathology more appropriately addressed by the medical model, and 'yellow flags', which indicate psychosocial factors that may be risk factors for the development of chronic dysfunction (Fig. 15).

In relation to chronic soft tissue pain and disability the literature implies that psychosocial factors may be more important than physical factors in predicting the outcome.[73, 74] The influence of negative psychosocial influences on dysfunction typically manifests as fear avoidance behaviour, where movement is avoided due to the misplaced anticipation of pain.[101, 102] The consequences of this are illustrated in Fig. 16. The physiotherapist typically applies the more physical aspects of treatment in the early stages of dysfunction[103] and takes a more hands-off approach in the more chronic stages of the dysfunction.[104]

Table 8 The medical model of treatment

Action	Outcome
Identification of illness patterns and resultant behaviour	Symptoms
Objective examination to identify pathology	Diagnosis
Treatment is directed to the underlying pathology	Treatment
Assumption is that illness patterns and behaviour will resolve	Cure

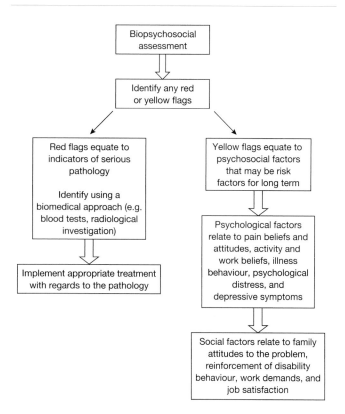

Fig. 15 Summary of the biopsychosocial model of assessment—red and yellow flag identification.

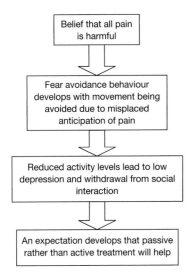

Fig. 16 The effect of negative psychosocial influences on dysfunction—fear avoidance behaviour.

General exercise programmes are used where positive behaviours relating to physical activity (e.g. adherence to exercise quotas) are praised with positive feedback and attention, whereas learned pain behaviour is ignored and treated with the withdrawal of any positive feedback.[105] By applying this strategy it is thought that correct pain beliefs, behaviours, and coping strategies are instilled in the patient.

It should be noted that much of the current evidence regarding the biopsychosocial model relates to chronic low back pain and that identification of yellow flags does not indicate what treatment should be given to a patient—it only highlights the potential barriers to treatment. More evidence is required to indicate whether addressing psychosocial factors is more effective than passive treatments

Conclusion

This chapter has focused on some of the models of reasoning used by the physiotherapist in the management of soft tissue dysfunction. In the light of evidence-based approaches, much research is underway to support, refute, and modify these models. While this research continues, the physiotherapist will continue to play an essential role in the management of soft tissue dysfunction. Through the process of a thorough assessment and the application of appropriate stimuli using electrothermal, manual therapy, exercise, and psychosocial interaction, the physiotherapist aims to promote adaptation in the patient or patient's tissues to restore the patient's ability to function in his or her desired environment. Of particular relevance to soft tissue management is the accumulating evidence supporting the need for early mobilization and tissue loading. With a sound training in these principles the physiotherapist provides a secure guide through this process.

References

1. **Chartered Society of Physiotherapy (CSP)** (2000). *Standards of physiotherapy practice.* CSP, London.
2. **Pratt, J.W. and Mason, A.** (1981). *The caring touch.* Heyden, London.
3. **Roberts, P.** (1994). Theoretical models of physiotherapy. *Physiotherapy* **80** (5), 361–366.
4. **Waddell, G.** (1987). A new clinical model for the treatment of low back pain [review]. *Spine*, **12** (7), 632–644.
5. **Collins** (1999). *Collins English Dictionary—millenium edition.* Harper Collins.
6. **Nordin, M. and Frankel, V.** (1989). Basic biomechanics of the musculoskeletal system, 2nd edn, pp. 9–16. Lea and Febiger, London.
7. **Leadbetter, W.B.** (1992). Cell–matrix response in tendon injury. *Clin. Sports Med.* **11**, 533–578.
8. **Forrester, J.C., Zenefeldt, B.H., Hayes, T.L., and Hunt, T.K.** (1970). Wolf's law in relation to the healing skin wound. *J. Trauma* **10** (9), 770–779.
9. **Burroughs, P. and Dahners, L.E.** (1990). The effect of enforced exercise on the healing of ligament injuries, *Am. J. Sports Med.* **18**, 376–378.
10. **Dahners, L.E. and Padgett, I.** (1990). The effect of joint motion on collagen organization in healing ligaments. *Trans. Orthop. Res Soc.* **15**, 511.
11. **Javinen, M.J. and Lehto, M.U.K.** (1993). The effects of early mobilization and immobilization on the healing process following muscle injuries. *Sports Med.* **15** (2), 78–89.
12. **Muneta, T., Lewis, J., and Stewart, N.** (1993). Effects of controlled load on graft healing: auto vs allograft. *Trans. Orthop. Res. Soc.* **18**, 4.
13. **Maitland, G.** (1991). *Peripheral manipulation*, pp. 13–46. Butterworth-Heinemann, London.
14. **Meeuwisse, W.H.** (1994). Assessing causation in sports injury: a multifactorial model, *Clin. J. Sports Med.* **4**, 166–170.
15. **Watson, A.W.S.** (1997). Sports injuries: incidence, causes, prevention. *Phys. Ther. Rev.* **2**, 135–151.
16. **McPoil, T.G. and Cornwall, M.W.** (1994). The relationship between static lower extremity measurements and rearfoot motion during walking. *J. Orthop. Sports Phys. Ther.* **24** (5), 309–314.
17. **Buckley, E.R. and Hunt, D.C.** (1997). Reliability of clinical measurement of sub-talar joint movement. *Foot Ankle Int.* **18** (4), 229–232.
18. **Atkinson, G. and Nevill, A.M.** (1998). Statistical methods for assessing measurement error (reliability) in variables relevant to sports medicine. *Sports Med.* **26** (4), 217–238.
19. **George, K., Batterham, N., and Sullivan, I.** (2000). The concept and assessment of validity in clinical research. *Phys. Ther. Sport.* **1**, 19–26.
20. **Hammond, A.** (1994). Joint protection behavior in patients with rheumatoid arthritis following an education program: a pilot study. *Arthritis Care Res.* **7**, 5–9.
21. **Hammond, A.** (1996). Rheumatoid arthritis. In *Occupational therapy and physical dysfunction: principles, skills and practice*, 4th edn (ed. A. Turner, M. Foster, and S. Johnson), pp. 747–765. Churchill Livingstone, London.
22. **Józsa, L., Reffy, A., Jarvinnen, M., et al.** (1998). Cortical and trabecular osteopenia after immobilization: a quantitative histological study of the rat knee. *Int. Orthop.* **12** (2), 169–172.
23. **Kannus, P., Józsa, L., Renstrom, P., et al.** (1992). The effects of training, immobilization and remobilization on musculoskeletal tissue 1: training and immobilization. *Scand. J. Med. Sci. Sports* **2** (3), 100–118.
24. **Woo, S.L.-Y. and Hilderbrand, K.A.** (1997). Healing of ligament injures: from basic science to clinical practice. *Baillière's Clin. Orthop.* **2** (1), 63–79.
25. **Mortenson, N.H., Skov, O., and Jenson, P.E.** (1999). Early motion of the ankle after operative treatment of a rupture of the Achilles tendon: a prospective, randomized clinical and radiographic study. *J. Bone Joint Surg. (Am.)* **81** (7), 983–990.
26. **Kannus, P. and Renstrom, P.** (1991). Treatment for acute tears of the lateral ligaments of the ankle, operation, cast or early controlled mobilization? *J. Bone Joint Surg. (Am.)* **73** (2), 305–312.
27. **Barlow, Y. and Willoughby, J.** (1992). Pathophysiology of soft tissue repair. *Br. Med. Bull.* **48** (3), 698–711.
28. **Wahl, S.M., Wong, H., and McCartney-Francis, N.** (1989). Role of growth factors in inflammation and repair. *J. Cell Biochem.* **40**, 193–199.
29. **Evans, P.** (1980). The healing process at a cellular level: a review. *Physiotherapy* **66** (8), 256–259.

30. Martinez-Hernandez, A. and Amenta, P.S. (1990). Basic concepts in wound healing. In *Sport induced inflammation* (ed. W.B. Leadbetter, J.A. Buckwalter, and S.L. Gordon), pp. 55–101. American Academy of Orthopaedic Surgeons, Park Ridge, Illinois.

31. Gomez, M.A., Woo, S.L-Y., Amiel, D., and Harwood, F. (1991). The effects of increased tension on healing medial collateral ligaments. *Am. J. Sports Med.* **19**, 347–354.

32. Arem, A.J. and Madden, J.W. (1976). Effects of stress on healing wounds: 1. Intermittent noncyclical tension. *J. Surg. Res.* **20**, 93–102.

33. Loitz, B.J., Zernicke, R.F., Vailas, A.C., Kody, M.H., and Meals, R.A. (1989). Effects of short term immobilization versus continuous passive motion on the biomechanical and biochemical properties of the rabbit tendon. *Clin. Orthop. Rel. Res.* **244** (7), 265–271.

34. Currier, D.P. and Nelson, R.M. (1992). *Dynamics of human biologic tissues.* F.A. Davis, Philadelphia.

35. Hardy, M. (1989). The biology of scar formation. *Phys. Ther.* **69**, 1014–1024.

36. Levenson, S. (1962). Practical applications of experimental studies in the care of primary closed wounds. *Am. J. Surg.* **104**, 273–282.

37. Madden, J. (1976). Wound healing: the biological basis of hand surgery. *Clin. Plast. Surg.* **3**, 3–11.

38. Alvarez, O.M. (1986). Wound healing. In *Dermatology in general medicine*, 3rd edn (ed. T. Fitzpatrick), pp. 321–336. McGraw-Hill, New York.

39. Arem, A.J. and Madden, J.W. (1976). Effects of stress on healing wounds: 1. Intermittent noncyclical tension, *J. Surg. Res.* **20**, 93–102.

40. Currier, D.P. and Nelson, R.M. (1992). *Dynamics of human biologic tissues.* F.A. Davis, Philadelphia.

41. Kannus, P. (1997). Tendon pathology: basic science and clinical applications. *Sports Exerc. Injury* **3** (2), 62–75.

42. Kannus, P. and Józsa, L. (1991). Histopathological changes preceding spontaneous rupture of a tendon. A controlled study of 891 patients. *J. Bone Joint Surg. (Am.)* **73**, 1507–1525.

43. Józsa, L. and Kannus, P. (1997). *Human tendons*, p. 576. Human Kinetics, Champaign, Illinois.

44. Movin, T., Gad, A., Reinholt, F.P., and Rolf, C. (1977). Tendon pathology in long standing achillodynia. Biopsy findings in 40 patients. *Acta Orthop. Scand.* **68** (2), 170–175.

45. Astrom, M. and Rausing, A. (1995). Chronic Achilles tendinopathy. A survey of surgical and histopathological findings. *Clin. Orthop.* **316**, 151–164.

46. Chan, B., Chan, K.M., Maffulli, N., Webb, S., and Lee, K.K.H. (1997). Effect of basic fibroblastic growth factor. An *in vitro* study of tendon healing. *Clin. Orthop.* **342**, 239–247.

47. Cameron, M.H. (1999). Physical agents in rehabilitation: from research to practice, pp. 273–302. W.B. Saunders Co, Philadelphia.

48. Melzack, R. and Wall, P.D. (1965). Pain mechanisms: a new theory. *Science* **150**, 971–979.

49. Hollman, J.E. and Morgan, B.J. (1997). Effect of transcutaneous electrical nerve stimulation on the pressor response to static handgrip exercise. *Phys. Ther.* **77**, 28–36.

50. Chung, J.M., Fang, Z.R., Cargill, C.L., *et al.* (1983). Prolonged naxolone-reversible inhibition of the flexion reflex in the cat. *Pain* **15**, 35–53.

51. Almay, B.G.L., Johansson, F., vonKnorring, L., *et al.* (1985). Long term high frequency transcutaneous electrical nerve stimulation (hi-TENS) in chronic pain. Clinical response and effects on CSF-endorphins, monoamine metabolites, substance P like immunoreactivity (SPLI) and pain measures. *J. Psychosomatic Res.* **29**, 247–257.

52. Markov, M.S. (1995). Electric current electromagnetic field effects on soft tissue: implications for wound healing. *Wounds* **7** (3), 94–110.

53. Draper, D.O., Castel, J.C., and Castel, D. (1995). Rate of temperature increase in human muscle during 1 MHz and 3 MHz continuous ultrasound. *J. Orthop. Sports Phy. Ther.* **22** (4), 142–150.

54. Lehmann, J.F., Masock, A.J., Warren, C.G., *et al.* (1970). Effects of therapeutic temperatures on tendon extensibility. *Arch. Phys. Med.* **51**, 481.

55. Mortimer, A.J. and Dyson, M. (1988). The effect of therapeutic ultrasound on calcium uptake in fibroblasts. *Ultrasound Med. Biol.* **14** (6), 499–506.

56. Dinno, M.A., Crum, L.A., and Wu, J. (1989). The effect of therapeutic ultrasound on electrophysical parameters of frogs skin. *Ultrasound Med. Biol.* **15** (5), 461–470.

57. Fyfe, M.C. and Chahl, L.A. (1982). Mast cell degranulation. A possible mechanism for the action of therapeutic ultrasound. *Ultrasound Med. Biol.* **8** (suppl. 1), 62.

58. Young, S.R. and Dyson, M. (1990). Macrophage responsiveness to therapeutic ultrasound. *Ultrasound Med. Biol.* **16** (8), 809–816.

59. Harvey, W., Dyson, M., Pond, J.B., *et al.* (1975). The stimulation of protein synthesis in human fibroblasts by therapeutic ultrasound. *Rheumatol. Rehabil.* **14**, 237.

60. Bommannan, D., Okyuyama, H., Stauffer, P., *et al.* (1992). Sonophoresis, I: The use of high frequency ultrasound to enhance trans dermal drug delivery. *Pharmacol. Res.* **9**, 559–564.

61. Byl, N.N. (1995). The use of ultrasound as an enhancer for transcutaneous drug delivery: phonophoresis. *Phys. Ther.* **75** (6), 535–553.

62. Weston, M., Taber, C., Cassagranda, L., *et al.* (1994). Changes in local blood volume during cold gel application to traumatized ankles. *J. Orthop. Sports Phys. Ther.* **19** (4), 197–199.

63. Lee, S.M., Warren, M.P., and Mason, S.M. (1978). Effects of ice on nerve conduction velocity. *Physiotherapy* **64**, 2–6.

64. Douglas, W.W. and Malcom, J.L. (1955). The effect of localized cooling on cat nerves. *J. Physiol.* **130**, 53–54.

65. Knight, K. (1995). *Cryotherapy in sports medicine*, pp. 85–98. Human Kinetics, Champagne, Illinois.

66. Harris, E.D. and McCroskery, P.A. (1974). The influence of temperature and fibril stability on degradation of cartilage collagen by rheumatoid synovial collagenase. *N. Engl. J. Med.* **290**, 1–6.

67. King, P.R. (1989). Low level laser therapy—a review. *Lasers, Med. Sci.* **4**, 141–150.

68. Basford, J.R. (1989). Low energy laser therapy: controversies and new research findings. *Lasers, Surg. Med.* **9**, 1–5.

69. Karu, T.I. (1989). Molecular mechanisms for the therapeutic effects of low intensity laser radiation. *Lasers, Life Sci.* **2**, 53–74.

70. Young, S., Bolton, P., Dyson, M., *et al.* (1989). Macrophage responsiveness to light therapy. *Lasers, Surg. Med.* **9**, 497–505.

71. Beckerman, H., Bde Bie, R.A., Bouter, L.M., *et al.* (1992). The efficacy of laser therapy for musculo-skeletal and skin disorders: a criteria based meta analysis and randomized clinical trials. *Phys. Ther.* **72** (7), 483–491.

72. Goldby, L.J. (1997). Low back pain: the evidence for physiotherapy. *Phys. Ther. Rev.* **2**, 7–11.

73. Hope, P. and Forshaw, M.J. (1999). Assessment of psychological distress is important in patients presenting with low back pain. *Physiotherapy* **85** (10), 563–570.

74. Burton, A.K., Tillotson, K.M., Main, C.J., and Hollis, S. (1995). Psychosocial predictor of outcome in acute and sub-chronic low back trouble. *Spine* **20** (6), 722–728.

75. Burstein, A.H. and Wright, T.M. (1994). *Fundamentals of orthopedic biomechanics*, pp. 97–129. Williams and Wilkins, Baltimore.

76. Blanpied, P.B., Levins, J.A., and Murphy, E. (1995). The effects of different stretch velocities on average force of the shortening phase in the stretch shorten cycle. *J. Orthop. Sports Phys. Ther.* **21** (6), 345–353.

77. Fukashiro, S., Komi, P.V., Järvinen, M., and Miyashita, M. (1995). *In vivo* Achilles tendon loading during jumping in humans. *Eur. J. Appl. Physiol. Occup. Physiol.* **71**, 453–458.

78. Wilson, A.M. and Goodship, A.E. (1994). Exercise induced hyperthermia as a possible mechanism for tendon degeneration. *J. Biomech.* **27**, 899–905.

79. Woo, S.L.-Y., Gomez, M.A., Sites, T.J., and Newton, P.O. (1987). The biomechanical and morphological changes in the medial collateral ligament of the rabbit after immobilization and remobilization. *J. Bone Joint Surg.* **69A** (8), 1200–1211.

80. Threlkeld, A.J. (1992). The effects of manual therapy on connective tissue. *Phy. Ther.* **72** (12). 893–902.

81. Binkley, J. (1989). Overview of ligament and tendon structure and mechanics: implications for clinical practice. *Physiother. Canada* **41** (1), 24–30.

82. Oakes, B. (1994). Tendon ligament basic science. In *Oxford textbook of sports medicine* (ed. M. Harries, C. Williams, W.D. Stanish, and L.J. Micheli), pp. 493–511. Oxford University Press, New York.

83. Soderberg, G.L. (1997). *Kinesiology: application to pathological motion*, 2nd edn, p. 107. Williams and Wilkins, Baltimore.

84. Taylor, D.C., Dalton, J.D., Seaber, A.V., and Garrett, W.E. (1990). Viscoelastic properties of muscle tendon units: the biomechanical effects of stretching. *Am. J. Sports Med.* **18** (3), 300–309.

85. Carlstedt, C.A. and Nordin, M. (1989). Biomechanics of tendons and ligaments. In *Basic biomechanics of the musculo-skeletal system*, 2nd edn (ed. M. Nordin and V.H. Frankel), pp. 65–67. Lea and Febiger, Philadelphia.

86. Butler, D.S. and Gifford, L. (1989). The concept of adverse mechanical tension in the nervous system. Part one: Testing for 'dural tension'. *Physiotherapy* **75** (11), 622–628.

87. Breig, A. and Troup, J. (1979). Biomechanical considerations in the straight leg raising test. *Spine* **4** (3), 242–570.

88. Adams, C. and Logue, V. (1971). Studies in cervical spondylotic myelopathy. 1. Movement of the cervical roots, dura and cord, and their relation to the course of the extrathecal roots. *Brain* **94**, 557–568.

89. O'Connel, J. (1946). The clinical signs of meningeal irritation. *Brain* **69**, 9–21.

90. Butler, D. (1991). *Mobilization of the nervous system*. Churchill Livingstone, Edinburgh.

91. McDonald, R. (1994). *Taping techniques: principles and practice.* Butterworth Heineman, Oxford.

92. Stokes, M. and Young, A. (1984). The contribution of reflex inhibition to arthrogenous muscle weakness. *Clin. Sci.* **67**, 7.

93. Stanish, D.W., Rubinovich, R.M., and Curwin, S. (1986). Eccentric exercise in chronic tendinitis. *Clinical Orthop. Rel. Res.* **208**, 65–68.

94. Curwin, S.L. (1998). The etiology and treatment of tendinitis. In *Oxford textbook of sports medicine* (ed. M. Harries, C. Williams, W.D. Stanish, and L.J. Micheli), pp. 610–624. Oxford University Press, Oxford.

95. Niesen-Vertommen, S.L., Taunton, J.E., Clement, D.B., and Mosher, R.E. (l992). The effect of eccentric versus concentric exercise in the management of Achilles tendonitis. *Clin. J. Sports Med.* **2** (2), 109–113.

96. Alfredson, H., Pietila, T., Jonsson, P., and Lorentzon, R. (1998). Heavy load eccentric calf muscle training for the treatment of Achilles tendonosis. *Am. J. Sports Med.* **26** (3), 360–366.

97. O'Sullivan, P.B., Twomey, L., and Allison, G. (1995). Evaluation of specific stabilising exercise in the treatment of chronic low back pain with radiological diagnosis of spondylolysis or spondylolithesis. *Proceedings of the Manipulative Physiotherapy Association of Australia, Perth, Australia.*

98. Kegerreis, S. (1983). The construction and implementation of functional progression as a component of athletic rehabilitation. *J. Orthop. Sports Phys. Ther.* **5**, 14–19.

99. Engel, G. (1977). The need for a new medical model: a challenge for biomedicine, *Science* **196**, 129–136.

100. Bolton, J.E. (1997). Future directions for outcomes research in back pain. *Eur. J. Chiropract.* **45**, 57–64.

101. Main, C.J. and Watson, P.J. (1995). Screening for patients at risk of developing chronic incapacity. *J. Occup. Rehabil.* **5** (4), 207–217.

102. Klenerman, L., Slade, P.D., Stanley, I.M., Pennie, B., Reilly, J.P., Atchinson, L.E., Troup, J.F.D., and Rose, M.J. (1995). The prediction of chronicity in patients with an acute attack of low back pain in a general practice setting. *Spine* **20** (4), 478–484.

103. Twomey, L. and Taylor, J. (1955). Spine update: exercise and spinal manipulation in the treatment of low back pain. *Spine* **20** (5), 615–619.

104. Harding, V.C. de C. and Williams, A. (1995). Extending physiotherapy skills using a psychological approach: cognitive–behavioral management of chronic pain. *Physiotherapy* **81** (11), 681–687.

105. Klaber Moffet, J.A. and Richardson, P.H. (1995). The influence of psychological variables on the development and perception of musculoskeletal pain. *Physiother. Theory Pract.* **11**, 3–11.

5.7 The role of the occupational therapist and ergonomy

Alison Hammond and Rachel Batteson

Introduction

Of all soft tissue complaints, occupational therapists treat soft tissue disorders of the upper limb most frequently, and in particular those considered to be work-related upper limb disorders (WRULDS). This is therefore the main focus of this chapter. There is considerable debate about the aetiology of upper limb pain and whether this is related to frequent repetitive movements of the upper limb (which can occur occupationally as well as in other daily activities) or, at the other extreme, is a localized form of a fibromyalgia-type syndrome of multiple aetiology. A recent population-based study of working individuals with forearm pain identified a multifactorial aetiology for forearm pain (Table 1).[1]

Different upper limb disorders can variously be attributed to physiological, mechanical, psychosocial, and/or environmental factors. Rehabilitation should therefore be within a biopsychosocial model—assessing the individual's problems holistically and addressing all these potentially contributory factors.

Definitions

As will be discussed, occupational therapy focuses on *rehabilitation* of the individual with a disability or illness back, within his or her normal environment(s), to maximum independence in activities of daily living, leisure, and work.

The occupational therapist assesses the physical, psychological, and social functions of the individual, identifies areas of dysfunction, and involves the individual in a structured programme of activity to overcome disability. The activities selected will relate to the consumer's personal, social, cultural, and economic needs and will reflect the environmental factors that govern his/her life.[2]

There is a growing interface between the two professions of occupational therapy and ergonomy, with common ground in 'health care ergonomics',[3] to maximize preventative and rehabilitative strategies to reduce both the occurrence and severity of soft tissue disorders. Increasingly, occupational therapists specializing in hand therapy have undertaken postgraduate training in ergonomics and are able to combine the approaches of the two professions in assessment and treatment.

Ergonomy

Ergonomics (*ergon* = work, *nomos* = law: also called *human factors engineering*) is the study of work performance. 'Human factors (ergonomics) is a body of knowledge about human abilities, human limitations and other human characteristics that are relevant to design. Human factors engineering (ergonomics implementation) is the application of human factors information to the design of tools, systems, tasks, jobs and environments for safe, comfortable and effective human use'.[4] It is concerned with human interactions with environments, which can include psychological and social factors affecting work performance within organizations, as well as physical factors (such as vibration, climate (indoor and outdoor), lighting, noise, and the effects of contaminants), and organizational factors (such as shift work, workloads, management styles, accidents, safety, motivation, and alienation). Good ergonomic design optimizes the relationship between the person and his/her environment and so works preventatively (Table 2). Ergonomists are increasingly becoming involved in the modification and design of equipment, buildings, vehicles, and systems for people with disabilities and the elderly in order to enhance quality of life and potential for independent living.[5]

Approaches used in occupational therapy and ergonomy

Occupational therapy approaches

Treatment is implemented using appropriate frames of reference, the *biomechanical* and *rehabilitative* being the most commonly used in the treatment of soft tissue disorders. The biomechanical frame of reference is applied to improve active and passive range of movement, strength, stability, and endurance through the use of graded physical activity. The rehabilitative frame of reference is applied both during the treatment stage to facilitate independence and, when the individual is making no further gains in physical ability, to maximize independence through adapted activity, assistive equipment, or physical assistance. A cognitive behavioural approach may also be used to assist

Table 1 Factors implicated in occupational forearm pain

Mechanical factors: repetitive movements of the arms and wrists; lifting and carrying weights

Work-related psychosocial factors: poor levels of satisfaction with support from supervisors and colleagues primarily, as well as rarely being able to make one's own decisions

Presence of other painful areas: e.g. shoulder pain, back pain, or widespread pain

Illness behaviour

Table 2 Ergonomic concerns

Design of work stations, seating, person–machine interfaces (displays and controls), tools, and products to fit the normal anthropometric dimensions for the population under consideration, as well as for the range of normal visual, auditory, cognitive, and other physical abilities

Design of instructional manuals, signs, and warning systems

Evaluation of the work postures, muscle activity, and speed of work required in specific work tasks to assess whether they are within normal human work capacity

Evaluation of the working environment and organization to identify stress factors

Design of tasks, equipment, and systems to meet Health and Safety legislation

Identification of actual and potential hazards in the workplace and conduction of risk or safety assessments

people to cope with pain and to alter behaviour patterns (both physical and psychosocial) that may be precipitating and exacerbating the conditions.

Occupational therapists involved in the treatment of soft tissue disorders will apply these principles during assessment and treatment. Occupational therapy intervention is centred on the individual's roles, occupations, and activities to enable the individual to become a confident performer in his/her daily life.[6] Interventions are focused on maximizing abilities in work, recreational pursuits, self-care and domestic activities, and psychosocial status. They also focus on modifying tasks and the person's environment in relation to his/her abilities and enabling the person to interact successfully in his/her sociocultural environment.

The patient forms a partnership with the therapist and intervention is jointly directed.[6] Occupational therapists may apply a variety of client-centred models of occupational therapy (OT) in their assessment and treatment. The primary aim is to help the person gain his/her highest functional level, that is, to maximize his/her occupational performance, to his/her satisfaction. Strategies can include education, modification of occupation(s) and environment(s), exploration of alternative tasks/life roles, provision of aids and equipment, and management/supervision of others completing difficult occupations. Treatment programmes are graded and dependent on the individual, the nature of the disorder, the treatment being carried out by other professions, the priorities identified by the individual, and the facilities within the department. Interventions include everyday activities (simulation of activities of daily living, work, and leisure appropriate to the individual), purposeful activity, and creative activities and non-purposeful, preparatory activities to maximize ability.

Ergonomic approaches

A number of approaches are applied in ergonomics, based upon biomechanical principles. There are two broad approaches:

Injury prevention approaches focus on ensuring the worker, task, and environment are matched in order to prevent or limit the development of soft tissue and other injuries. For example, one of these is the occupational biomechanics approach that aims to improve workers' occupational performance whilst achieving the organization's goals.[7] This includes personnel selection criteria and training, hand tool design guidelines, workplace and machine control layout guidelines, seating design guidelines, and materials handling limits. Another is the ergonomic tool kit approach[8] that focuses on workplace-based ergonomics of workstation design and modification, altering work

processes and considers organizational factors as well as workers' stress levels, comfort, and safety.[9]

Vocational rehabilitation approaches treat people who have already developed injuries and disabilities. These reflect the merging of ergonomics and rehabilitation. For example, the functional approach[10] encompasses both preventative and rehabilitative approaches. This includes work analysis, functional capacity evaluation, injury prevention education, pre-work screening, ergonomic adaptations, modified work and return-to-work programmes, and injury management and prevention.

Assessment

Occupational therapy assessment

Therapists assess the person's physical, functional, cognitive, psychological, and social abilities, within the context of his/her physical and sociocultural environment and the requirements of his/her roles and occupations (i.e. everyday activities). The assessment procedure used by occupational therapists working with musculoskeletal disorders is the same regardless of the location of the disorder, although specific tests may vary according to its nature and location. The assessment procedure described below focuses on the upper extremity.

Sources

The majority of individuals with soft tissue disorders referred to an occupational therapist will be treated as out-patients, and are referred from orthopaedic, rheumatology, or hand clinics or by general practitioners (GPs).

Gathering information

Prior to the initial assessment, the occupational therapist should supplement the information provided in the referral from both medical notes and multidisciplinary team members on the person's medical history and previous and concurrent treatment.

Initial assessment

This allows the therapist to establish a rapport with the person. This is essential as the quality of the therapeutic relationship can impact on the success of the intervention strategy, which may extend over many weeks. The initial assessment provides an opportunity to gain insight into the individual's perspective of their disorder, how it presents, and its effect on physical, psychological and social aspects of their lifestyle.

Both affected and unaffected upper limbs are assessed to allow comparison of what normal function and appearance are for the individual.

The history of onset and the nature of the condition are discussed. A description of the nature of the pain including the distribution, severity, type, aggravating factors, and strategies that provide relief should be discussed. Visual analogue pain scales may be used before and after treatment and provide subjective information on the amount of pain experienced. The McGill pain scale (short form)[11] incorporates 15 descriptors of the sensory and affective dimensions of pain. A visual analogue scale and present pain intensity provide a measure of the intensity of the pain experienced. The scale takes 2–5 minutes to complete.

Physical examination commences with observation. The patient is observed in relation to how he/she is responding to the presence of the condition and his/her posture. The condition and colour of the skin may indicate if the limb has been used normally. For example, a person with a manual occupation may have calluses over the metacarpal heads, which may be less pronounced on the affected limb suggesting an interference with activities at work. The condition of the nails, hair, and pulps of the fingers, the location and extent of deformity and muscle wasting, and whether the circulation is intact or compromised are all evaluated.

Palpation and handling of the patient should be gentle and slow. A verbal commentary on the assessments and movements conducted should precede any examination. The temperature of the skin, which may indicate infection or poor circulation, sweat pattern, and condition of any scars are also noted during examination.

Range of movement is then evaluated. Active and passive ranges of movement of the upper limb are assessed using a goniometer following standardized methods, with proximal joints supported as necessary, and preferably performed by the same therapist at each assessment to maximize reliability. Sensory examination should record responses as intact and accurate, impaired, or absent.[12] This includes assessment of light touch, pressure, pain, temperature, two-point discrimination, proprioception, and stereognosis (i.e. the ability to identify objects from touch alone). Findings can be recorded on outline drawings of the upper limb.

Light touch and pressure can be tested using cotton wool and the fingertip or using Semmes–Weinstein monofilaments. The original Semmes–Weinstein kit includes 20 monofilaments, and there is also a 'mini kit', which has a five-filament hand set. The reliability of the test has been established and it is considered to yield sensitive and accurate results. The monofilaments provide a method of determining normal versus abnormal sensibility at the sensitivity threshold.[13, 14]

Manual muscle testing is assessed using the Oxford Grading Scale to test muscle power.[12] Various forms of grip strength are assessed in the patient with an upper limb disorder, including power grip, tip, tripod, and lateral pinch. The Jamar dynamometer and B + L hydraulic pinch gauge have high calibration and accuracy and are the instruments of choice.[15–17] The American Society of Hand Therapists (ASHT) has developed a standardized arm position for use with the Jamar dynamometer that should be used to ensure consistency of results.[17] Each grip should be repeated three times with 15 seconds intertrial rest to avoid fatigue. The mean for each grip is then calculated.

The location, extent, classification (primary or secondary), and duration of oedema need to be established.[18] A visual record of any oedema can be recorded on a simple line drawing of the upper limb. A tape measure or volumeter using water displacement can be used to measure oedema in the hand. The involved and uninvolved hand should be assessed. The dominant hand will displace 15–20 ml more than the non-dominant hand.

Functional assessment is then performed. The impact of the disorder on the individual's ability to carry out activities of daily living should be evaluated, including personal and domestic activities, work, and leisure. The affected areas will be dependent on the individual, his/her roles, responsibilities, and occupations. Environmental factors may also influence the individual's performance. Assessment may be specific targeting the area of dysfunction, for example, a work assessment. Alternatively, standardized assessments may be used, as described in Table 3.

McPhee[24] reviewed hand function tests concluding that 82 per cent used time as the critical measure. However, this was not considered to be an accurate indication of hand function. Relatively few tests examine the method of task completion or simulate heavier activities reflective of a work environment. He recommended that no single test be used exclusively for all conditions but that each test must be evaluated to ensure that the most appropriate test for that diagnostic group and person is used.

Psychosocial assessment should be conducted, as the psychological impact of any disorder is not always proportional to the extent of the injury. Psychological effects can determine the success of a treatment programme, especially if motivation, confidence, and self-esteem are affected. Cultural and religious background may also affect the individual's reaction to the disorder. Methods of assessment include informal psychological assessment during the initial assessment, for instance, noting the person's reaction to their injury, assessing motivation, confidence, and self-esteem through therapist–patient interaction. Standardized assessments measuring anxiety may also be used when necessary, such as the hospital anxiety and depression scale (HAD).[25] This is a 14-item scale with seven items relating to anxiety and depression, respectively. It is a self-report scale and uses a four-point Likert scale with responses ranging from 'none' to 'unbearable'.

Work assessment (or functional capacity evaluation) is commonly conducted with people returning to work. This should include a worksite job analysis (see 'Ergonomic assessment') to identify the job requirements the person is being rehabilitated back to, e.g. the need for manual dexterity, balance, or repetitive reaching. Without a jobsite evaluation to investigate the cause or factors contributing to the condition, therapy may just be treating the symptoms not the cause. The work assessment can also include a wide range of activities conducted in the occupational therapy department to simulate the person's normal task demands. For example, the patient's ability to: handle objects, reach, push, pull, lift, carry, perform twisting movements, feel objects, and crawl and climb and the patient's manual dexterity and eye–hand–foot co-ordination are tested.[26] Activities may be simulated using a variety of methods.

1. Tasks available in the department, for example, printing, woodwork, the Baltimore therapeutic equipment (BTE). The BTE machine has a range of interchangeable handles and tools attached to a lever arm allowing a variety of hand and arm actions to be exercised using increasing ranges of movement, levels of resistance, and speed. The integral computer enables a varying programme of activity to be set and analysis of progress.

2. VALPAR Corporation work samples (VCWS). This includes a series of activities. For example, VCWS 1 tests the person's abilities

Table 3 Standardized Assessments suitable for use with WRULDS

Assessment	Type	Description	Time to complete (min)
Disabilities of Arm, Shoulder and Hand Questionnaire (DASH)[19]	Self-report	30 compulsory items: including functional, physical, social, and psychological items. Additional optional section for sports and performing arts. Five-point Likert scale each item. Gives a total score	10
Neck and Upper Limb Index (NULI)[20]	Self-report	20 items: physical task ability, effect of disorder on work, psychosocial impact, sleep, and negative effects of condition. Seven-point Likert scale each item. Gives a total score and four subscales—physical, psychosocial, work, and sleep status	10
Sollerman Hand Function Test (SFHT)[21]	Observation of performance	20 simulated activities of daily living (e.g. opening door, fasten zip, pour water). Scoring is a combination of time taken to perform each task and quality of grip used (rated on a 0–4 scale)	30
Sequential Occupational Dexterity Assessment (SODA)[22]	Observation of performance	12 simulated activities of daily living (e.g. writing, pick up envelope, use a telephone). Six are unilateral and 6 bilateral. Scoring is based on quality of grip function (rated on a 0–4 scale), plus person's perceived difficulty and pain level during performance	30
Jebsen Hand Function test (JHFT)[23]	Observation of performance	Seven grip activities (e.g. pick up small objects, writing, stacking checkers). Each subtest performed separately with left and right hands. Score is the time taken to perform test	10

to work with small tools (screwdrivers, pliers) during six timed exercises—five assembly and one disassembly. This allows the therapist to evaluate: motor co-ordination, manual dexterity, tolerance of frustration, and performance in repetitive tasks. VCWS 9 evaluates the person's ability to work at four different heights: overhead; shoulder; waist; and crouching. It involves transferring items and screwing these into place at these heights. This allows observation of ability to reach, handle, co-ordinate, and of dexterity and moving between different heights.

This information will be used to formulate a treatment plan and act as a baseline against which repeat assessments are compared until discharge. Where it is suspected or known that the disorder is caused or exacerbated by work activities, the OT assessment should be supplemented by more detailed ergonomic assessment.

Ergonomic assessment

Ergonomists and occupational therapists interested in work rehabilitation are skilled in applying ergonomic principles for both injury prevention and the modification of work for the injured worker. A worksite job analysis is essential to identify what may be potential stresses promoting upper limb disorders. Data is obtained through observation, interviews with workers and managers, organizational documentation, and consideration of Health and Safety at Work legislation.

Factors to be considered in an ergonomic assessment

Numerous factors are considered in any assessment. These include force, frequency, and duration of specific tasks, postures, stress, and personal factors.

Table 4 Personal factors affecting risk of musculoskeletal disorders

Previous injury or illness affecting tissues

Poor levels of physical fitness

Increasing age

Anthropometric characteristics of the individual (e.g. height, weight, and reach in relationship to the work environment, seating, and equipment).

Training provided—which can help increase strength and endurance for the task

Personality and psychosocial factors: those with a higher external locus of control and depression have been found to experience musculoskeletal discomfort more frequently

Leisure pursuits: causative factors can arise from hobbies involving repetitive actions, e.g. running, knitting, playing musical instruments

Other factors: e.g. smoking has been associated with musculoskeletal discomfort, which may be because it correlates with other associated factors such as poor physical fitness

The force required to be applied during a heavy or difficult task can result in physical strain as the required force may be either beyond what a muscle can apply or because limb or equipment positioning means the muscle cannot exert its strength effectively. Inadequate tool or equipment design can also result in excessive force being applied, particularly if the working posture necessary does not allow easy application of force. If the muscle's maximum tolerance is exceeded at one event or with repeated exposure, damage to tissues can occur.

Frequency and duration of task performance also affect ability. Performing certain actions repeatedly or for long durations can result in muscle fatigue. This is relieved by rest, but if this is insufficient and actions are continuously repeated, then pathological changes can occur. Pain may then recur more frequently and so require longer rest periods for recovery.

Certain postures can occlude blood flow, increase pressure on nerves and other tissues, stress joints, or require high muscle force to be maintained. Workers with neck and shoulder pain have been found to perform shoulder abduction and forward neck flexion more frequently and for longer.[27] Postures potentially causing discomfort include: extreme postures at the end of range of the joint; postures allowing gravity to act about a joint and so further increasing load on muscles and tissues (e.g. working in elevation); and non-extreme postures that affect normal musculoskeletal geometry and thus increase stress on tendons (e.g. working in ulnar or radial deviation of the wrist, which reduces the efficiency of wrist muscles). Examples of potentially harmful postures include: overreaching; loading in an uneven manner; wrist extension/flexion; reaching behind or above shoulder level or behind the torso; and performing static work above the level of the heart. The layout of the workplace may also cause postural constraints. Marras and Schoenmarklin[28] identified risk factors for carpal tunnel syndrome based on frequency of wrist flexion/extension, angular velocity, and acceleration.

Stress can generate muscle tension that can add to the physical demands already placed on muscles from jobs. For example, tasks requiring greater cognitive or visual demands can increase neck and shoulder muscle activity.[29] There is a higher incidence of musculoskeletal pain amongst those with lower job satisfaction and higher work and life stress. Stress factors related to workload can cause pain as well as damage to interpersonal relationships and social structures within the work environment. A climate of distrust, fear of being inadequate, and unwanted overtime can all increase stress and thus muscle tension.

A variety of personal factors can also increase the risk of musculoskeletal disorders, as described in Table 4. These factors are all considered during the formal assessment of the following.

Job purpose and task analysis

This includes identification of the requirements of a job. For example, the purpose of a check-out operator's job is to ensure the speedy sale of products. It includes welcoming customers, moving items across a conveyor belt, scanning bar codes, weighing goods, working on a till, packing items, ensuring correct payment (including credit card authorization and signature checking), and providing correct change and receipts. All of this is carried out whilst maintaining a friendly approach to the customer, and working at speed to reduce customer waiting time and queues. In task analysis, each task in the job must be analysed to identify work positions and potentially stressful movements. Details of task analysis methods are provided later.

Job organization and structure

This includes identifying hours per shift, the shifts worked, breaks, rest periods, job rotation, piece work, job-rate quotas (e.g. output per hour), production incentives, work pace and frequency of work cycles (i.e. the number of times per hour a job task is performed), and work schedule. Excess speed of work and long shifts with inadequate rest breaks can cause and exacerbate injuries.

Tools and equipment

Tools and equipment should suit the anthropometric dimensions and strength of the individual. This includes assessing the weight and size of tools and considering the use of power tools to reduce the force needed, along with evaluating the even balance of tools in the hand. The friction and slip resistance of grasping surfaces, size, shape and thickness of handles, their surface materials and compressibility, the hand–tool position, and resultant posture of tools in the hand should all be assessed, as appropriate designs can reduce force and torque requirements necessary to operate these. Safety glove use and fit should be considered, as poorly fitting or cumbersome gloves can increase risk of injury. The ability to use both hands to operate equipment will reduce force requirements. The edges and corners of tools and equipment and the provision of padding should be considered to prevent injuries from catching these.

Manual materials handling

This includes lifting of loads—their force, size, weight, and stability, location of loads in relation to the worker, the amount of twisting, bending, and overhead reaching required, location of handles, lifting frequency, and mechanical aid availability. Manual handling regulations should be followed to reduce injury risk.

Workstation design

This includes evaluating the location, height, and adjustability of tables, work surfaces, and shelving which should be within the person's 'reach envelope' (i.e. the space within which the upper limb can be comfortably extended and used). The freedom of the worker's movements, and the positioning of controls, tools, and equipment within the work area should be such that the visual and physical reach (forward flexion and elevation of the upper limb) and postures required during work are within the person's capacity. Workstation design should reduce or eliminate bending and twisting at the wrist, reaching above the shoulder, static muscle loading, full extension of the arms, and raised elbows. Barriers or obstacles in the work area should be absent.

Working position

For seated work the chair should be adjustable in height to suit the person, the depth and width of the seat pan should fit his/her dimensions, and arm and foot rests be provided. The chair should be manoeuvrable and comfortable with lumbar support with an adjustable back rake angle. The workstation should be evaluated in relation to the chair.

For standing work, the type of standing surface should be assessed. The use of cushioned shoes and anti-fatigue mats should be considered to reduce pressure, and workstation design in relation to the standing position should be assessed. Rails and sit–stand chairs with footrests can help reduce pressure when standing. The inclusion of stretch breaks and analysis of work postures to avoid overreaching in the work station design are needed.

Physical demands

The physical demands of a job must be analysed. The following should be recorded: work postures; frequency and repetitiveness of movements; frequency of bending of specific joints; the maximum reach required; the forcefulness and suddenness of movements; frequency of finger pinching; sustained muscle contraction; and the need to maintain specific postures for long periods.

Environmental factors

Poor lighting and illumination, vibration, excess temperature and humidity, high noise levels, and poor air quality and circulation can all influence stress levels and discomfort during work, which increase muscle tension.

Controls and displays

The ease of use, reach, size, shape, and colour of controls and display boards must be considered. Placement of guards to prevent accidental use and feedback mechanisms available to indicate if these are activated should be recorded, as should the viewing distance and angle to see controls and quality of lighting levels.

Psychosocial environment

This also influences stress levels. Thus, job complexity; monotony and repetition, peer and social support, worker autonomy, accuracy requirements, excessive task speed or load, sensory deprivation, or isolation should all be evaluated.

Further details and specific checklists are available.[9, 30]

Task analysis

There are several methods of task analysis, including hierarchical, verbal, and a variety of others.

Hierarchical task analysis

In this form of analysis, the main objective(s) of the worker (or system) is identified. Observation of the worker(s) (or system) is conducted to identify and describe the tasks involved to achieve this objective. The subtasks required for each are also identified, providing a detailed plan of each task in terms of work conditions, skills and equipment required, actions required, complexity, timing, and order, and the tasks' relationships to each other. Decomposition analysis can also be used to identify categories within tasks, such as cues for initiating actions, controls used, decisions made, actions taken dependent on differing decisions, feedback given, and common errors made, with repeat or correcting actions necessary.[31] A flow diagram is produced linking each task to gain an overview of the job being analysed. Work cycles are timed to identify the speed with which each task must be done, the frequency of tasks within a given time period or work day, and the frequency and duration of rest periods (scheduled and non-scheduled). Each task and subtask can then be analysed in terms of force, repetition, duration, speed, and posture required to identify any potentially causative or exacerbatory factors.

Examples of structured methods of analysing work positions, posture and movement are, first, the Ovaco Working Posture Analysis System (OWAS) developed by the Finnish Institute of Occupational Health. This classifies postures into four categories based on the positions of back, arms, and legs. Second, there is the Rapid Upper Limb Assessment,[32] where postures are classified into categories using a checklist and weighted in terms of forces used and frequency of posture adoption. These are both best applied by videorecording workers performing the activity and later analysing the types of postures and percentage of time spent in each (e.g. bent/twisted posture, fixed posture, extreme reach of limbs, static muscle work above heart level, repetitive force applied with extremities, extreme range of motion of wrists, etc.).

Verbal protocol analysis

This explores the mental processes required during tasks and is more difficult to assess. It requires the worker to 'think out loud' and explain the cognitive tasks and decisions made with each subtask of the activity.[33] This can help explain why certain postures and repetitions are performed.

Other methods of task analysis

A variety of rating scales can be used alongside task analysis to obtain workers' opinions on: pain experienced during tasks, for example, Borg's perceived pain scale;[34] body mapping to identify location of pain; perceived exertion, for example, Borg's perceived exertion scale;[35] and occupational stress indicators, for example, the Demand/Control Questionnaire,[36] which evaluates job psychological demands and personal authority over decisions to give a psychosocial stress index.

Recommendations for referral to an occupational therapist or ergonomist

Occupational therapists focus on the individual and maximizing his/her physical, functional, psychological, and social abilities in order to assist people in managing their everyday activities successfully (activities of daily living (ADL), work, and leisure). The appropriate problems for referral to an OT or ergonomist specializing in vocational rehabilitation of injured workers are described in Table 5.

Referral for ergonomic assessment and intervention is appropriate when the soft tissue disorder is suspected as either being caused or exacerbated by the person's work and it is considered that modification of the work environment or work practices will enable the worker to function more effectively without recurrence of the condition.

Treatment approaches used by occupational therapists in soft tissue disorders

Occupational therapists use a range of treatment approaches for soft tissue disorders. The approach used is dependent on the nature and extent of the disorder, medical management including any protocols for treatment, and intervention being carried out by other professions. An outline of the common approaches used is provided below.

Table 5 Indications for referral to an OT/ergonomist

Problem area
Physical changes
Deformity
Decreased range of movement
Sensory changes
Decreased muscle strength
Oedema
Psychological changes
Pain
Loss of confidence/self-esteem
Anxiety/depression as a result of the disorder
Functional changes
Loss of ability to perform:
Self-care activities
Domestic activities
Work activities
Leisure activities
Life roles

Use of splints

Occupational therapists provide a range of splints. These may be either prefabricated or custom-made for the individual. The majority of splints provided for soft tissue disorders are static, that is, without any moving parts. The purpose of splinting is highlighted in Table 6.

Custom-made static splints are usually made from low-temperature thermoplastics, for example, Easi-form, Aquaplast, and Orthoplast. The material is heated and then moulded to the individual, and secured using straps (e.g. using Velcro). The individual is given instructions as to when the splint should be worn, how to remove and replace it, and how to check the skin for any pressure areas. The splint is usually checked at each out-patient appointment to ensure it fits correctly. Precise alterations can be made to thermoplastic splints using spot heat if necessary.

Prefabricated splints are usually made from soft materials, for example, neoprene. They are commercially manufactured in standard sizes and in a wide variety of designs. Minor adjustments can be made if necessary to maximize comfort. Again, instructions on use, removal, reapplication, and likely complications should be discussed with the individual. These splints should also be reviewed at out-patient appointments for comfort and fit. See Table 7 for a summary of splints used.

Table 6 Static splinting (see references 12, 37, and 38)

The purpose of static splinting is to:
Immobilize or limit joint activity
Provide protection
Position and maintain correct joint alignment
Maintain improvement gained through passive stretching or activity
Provide stability to joint(s), therefore facilitating function
Arrest developing contractures

Table 7 Summary of examples of splints used for soft tissue disorders

Splint	Classification	Disorder
Wrist immobilization splint	Static	WRULD Carpal tunnel syndrome Reflex sympathetic dystrophy Wrist extensor tendinitis
Hand immobilization splint	Static	WRULD Tenosynovitis
Thumb immobilization splint	Static	Soft tissue inflammation De Quervain's disease Gamekeeper's thumb
Hand-based splints	Static	Trigger finger
Counterforce bracing	Static	Lateral epicondylitis
Drop-out splint	Static	Ulnar nerve entrapment
Semi-flexible support	Static	Tenosynovitis Tendonitis Carpal tunnel syndrome Gamekeeper's thumb

Management of oedema

An inactive hand left in a dependent position is likely to become oedematous.[18] If oedema persists for more than 2 or 3 weeks, scarring may become extensive as all tissues, vessels, nerves, joints, and intrinsic muscles are exposed to reduced nutrition and elasticity.[39] It is therefore essential that oedema is treated effectively and efficiently in the early stages. Occupational therapists utilize a number of strategies such as patient education, elevation, compression, massage, exercise, and splinting.

Patient education is provided to increase the individual's awareness of the effects of persistent oedema. The importance of movement and compliance with a 'home programme' of activity and exercise is discussed. Elevation can be achieved by encouraging the individual to position the hand above shoulder height when possible, for example, at night in bed. External compression therapy is one of the most common strategies for treating oedema.[40] The compressive force exerted pushes the fluid proximally into the venous and lymphatic system.[39] Methods of compression include Coban wrapping, ace bandaging, string wrapping, lycra gloves, and custom-made garments.[39] Exercise increases the blood flow and therefore reduces oedema by facilitating venous return.[41] The activity-based 'exercise' chosen will use creative and therapeutic activities and be appropriate and meaningful to the individual. This may address more than one aim of treatment. Retrograde centripetal massage increases venous and lymphatic drainage.[39] The pressure exerted should be released at the end of each stroke to maximize effectiveness.[42] Brennan and Weitz[43] consider that, if this is coupled with compression, effectiveness is increased. Splinting may be used if a 'rest/activity' regime is necessary. Periods of activity are alternated with rest periods during which a static splint would be used to 'rest' the hand.

Activity-based approaches

Occupational therapists use a variety of techniques to achieve the overall aim of treatment, which is to restore the individual to their previous level of independence. These techniques include everyday activities and purposeful and non-purposeful activity.

Everyday activities

These include those activities that are part of the individual's normal lifestyle and are incorporated into the occupational therapy treatment programme. These can include self-care and domestic tasks and work and leisure activities. They should be familiar, meaningful, and purposeful to the individual and completed in the appropriate environment with attention to context. Examples are domestic tasks performed in the individual's home environment, and work hardening carried out at work. These may also be performed in a simulated setting, such as an occupational therapy department, although it is preferable when possible to do this in the environment and context familiar to the person.

Purposeful and non-purposeful activity

These include the use of creative activities (e.g. woodwork, pottery, computing, exercises for leisure, printing, gardening, decorating, repair work, office work). The purposeful activities selected for use are those that support the person's life roles and increase his/her ability to perform everyday activities, for example, simulation of aspects of work in the occupational therapy department. This method of treatment is used extensively as it does not require the occupational therapist to treat the individual in his/her own enviromnent, thus reducing costs and increasing the range of available activities.

Non-purposeful activities include the use of preparatory techniques that may be used by occupational therapists as a 'warm-up' to the treatment programme. Techniques included are use of therapeutic putty, massage, active and passive range of movement exercises, progressive resistive exercises, and 'remedial games' (e.g. adapted solitaire, which has larger pieces, and/or a Velcro base attaching to the game board, which increases the resistance requied to move pieces). These techniques are often used as a precursor to purposeful and everyday activities as the person is building up his/her dexterity and muscle strength.

A carefully formulated programme of activity is developed to increase duration, repetition, and resistance in the range of activities used, based on detailed activity analysis of the selected activities and the person's own interests. Strength, endurance, and range of movement are built up and/or alternative methods of task performance identified when necessary.

Joint protection/ergonomic modifications

Repetitive action may contribute to soft tissue disorders such as tenosynovitis, carpal tunnel syndrome, tennis elbow (lateral epicondylitis), De Quervain's disease, and some injuries to the shoulder.[44] In a case control study of 580 people with upper limb soft tissue disorders, thumb conditions were significantly associated with higher rates of pinching, wrist flexion, and maintaining a fixed bent thumb position at work. Other movements and postures associated with upper limb conditions were higher rates of repetitive palmar gripping, repeated elbow flexion accompanied by the use of force, and repeated shoulder rotation with an elevated arm.[44] Such movements can equally occur during household, do-it-yourself, and leisure activities, as well as at work, and thus non-occupational factors can also cause and contribute to these conditions.

During upper limb and work assessments, the therapist can identify if there are specific movements involved in work, leisure, and activities of daily living exacerbating pain and contributing to sustaining the condition. Joint protection is an approach, applying ergonomic principles, originally developed for arthritic conditions,[45, 46] which can be applied to soft tissue disorders.[47, 48] Strategies are described in Table 8.

The aim is to reduce pain and improve other symptoms, such as fatigue, to maintain or improve function, and to improve or limit progression. By providing the person with practical strategies to manage their condition, it should also assist in improving psychological aspects, such as self-efficacy and perceived control. The strategies described in Table 8 can be illustrated by protection measures commonly recommended for soft tissue injuries. For example, protection measures for the hand and wrist include the following.[45–49]

Biomechanics and weight distribution

The patient should use stronger, larger muscles and joints to perform activities, distribute weight of items over the palms (preferably of both hands) rather than using lateral or pulp pinch grips if possible, and use the palms and forearms rather than fingers to carry heavy items. Objects should be grasped with the whole hand and fingers.

Table 8 Joint protection/ergonomic modification strategies

Respect for pain, i.e. using this as a warning sign to either modify or cease activity as appropriate

Modifying movement patterns and postures that are precipitating and/or exacerbating symptoms (see below)

Use of assistive devices or labour-saving gadgets to reduce muscular effort and stress on tissues

Work simplification: modifying activities to alter task structure (e.g. task components, repetition and force) and/or the environment, e.g. the location of the activity/objects in relation to the person

Energy conservation: balancing work and rest and light with heavy activities; taking regular short rest breaks during activity (e.g. 2 minutes in every 10–20 depending on the activity); 'microbreaks' and ensuring a good sleep regime

Maintaining strength and range of movement through regular aerobic exercise and prescribed exercises appropriate to the condition

Avoiding strain

For example, by avoiding heavy lifting and strong grips by pushing, sliding, using trolleys or wheeled equipment, padding items, and using a relaxed grip where possible instead. This avoids sustained or repetitive postures and intrinsic-plus grasp (e.g. as in holding a book or writing) and keeping the fingers flexed. For example, a steering wheel can be padded with a texturized wheel cover to both enlarge grip, enable a more relaxed grip, and reduce slippage between the wheel and the hands. The person should avoid staying in one position for too long, for example, by bending and straightening the wrists and fingers often during use. They should rest the hand in an open not a clenched position.

Tools and aids

These include kitchen assistive devices, power tools, office aids, and expanded and textured handles to avoid repetitive hand clenching or strong gripping actions. These can help reduce the use of the fingers in pinching, hitting, moving, and pulling actions.

Similarly, protection measures for the neck and shoulders can include the following.

Biomechanics and weight distribution

The person should avoiding jutting of the head, particularly when at visual display units (VDUs), when watching television, or doing close work. The body and work activities should be positioned so as to keep the neck straight. Using high back chairs with adequate head and shoulder support and avoiding stressful neck positions (e.g. using one pillow, sleeping on the side or back; using cervical rolls to support the neck whilst sleeping) all help. Overreaching should also be avoided by positioning objects nearer to hand and using stepstools for higher items.

Use of tools and aids

Using speaker phones or headsets for telephone calls reduces neck strain, as does ensuring VDUs, desks, and chairs are correctly positioned and at correct height to maintain correct alignment.[50]

A variety of texts provide further advice on, for example, VDU assessment and modification.[50]

Patient education and rehabilitation programmes

Making the lifestyle and ergonomic changes recommended by occupational and physiotherapists is not easy. People are being advised to use strategies such as joint protection, energy conservation, work simplification and activity modification, and exercise (upper limb specific and aerobic), as well as other lifestyle changes (such as eating a healthier diet and stopping smoking, which can also help). The health belief model[51, 52] suggests that people are unlikely to make major changes in their health behaviours unless they perceive sufficient 'perceived threat' from the condition, that is, symptoms are sufficiently interfering in their current lifestyle to limit or prevent meaningful and necessary activities and will continue to do so in future. Even with sufficient threat, there may be a range of barriers limiting change. Psychological factors, such as insufficient self-efficacy, use of negative coping strategies, and poor perceived control of the condition, all limit adherence. Other factors playing a role include lack of social support from others, educational limitations, and other practical issues such as the time to practise and develop sufficient skills, the ability to develop new daily routines to accommodate behaviours, conflicting demands on time, and the pace of activity at work, leisure, or home.

Education is most commonly provided individually using a combination of verbal instructions and written support information with discussion, demonstration, and practice.[53] Patient education by the OT is focused upon patient insight and motivation into the need and mechanisms for change, initiating these alterations and integrating them into daily life. This may require a range of other cognitive and psychological strategies to manage stress, time, and assertiveness training to communicate effectively with others in their environment. It will include information on the aetiology, clinical features, and presentation of the disorder as well as known factors causing or exacerbating the condition and the theoretical basis behind the recommended treatment strategies.

Educational interventions have been demonstrated to alter the frequency of 'risk' movements in the industrial setting, at least over the short term.[54] Poor compliance with educational programmes in such settings is associated with difficulty with integrating changes such as postural alterations into the work setting, although this is less of a problem in those with ergonomic equipment and adapted work stations. Job demands may also prevent implementation of changes.

There is considerable evidence that work-related soft tissue injuries are not wholly or solely due to physical factors. Work-based and personal stress may be both causative and exacerbatory. Education programmes should therefore also include strategies to identify causes of stress and how to manage stress through using cognitive approaches. Whilst much education and training is individually based, group education programmes have the potential to maximize providing this range of approaches cost-effectively and to facilitate improving self-efficacy through modelling. Peer reinforcement also encourages greater adherence with goal-setting and homework programmes, and there is evidence from arthritis education research that, the longer the group programme, the more effective it will be in facilitating behavioural change and improving outcome.

Few studies have been conducted of educational and rehabilitation programmes in soft tissue disorders. Barthel et al.[55] conducted a retrospective case review with 24 people with 'upper extremity repetitive use syndrome'. They received 1–33 OT sessions (treatment was usually two to three times per week) consisting of ergonomic training (joint protection, energy conservation, and work simplification), stretching, soft tissue mobilizations, graded therapeutic exercise, work simulation with graded work hardening, use of heat and ice, and home exercise programmes. A few with substantial tenderness were provided with resting splints, although these were mainly avoided. A job site evaluation with ergonomic modifications was conducted. Psychological pain management was provided to seven patients and drug therapy as necessary. Six patients were rated by a physician and an OT as having resolved symptoms, 13 as having moderate improvement, and five had minimal or no improvement. Thus 19 of the 24 participants had some improvement.

Feuerstein et al.[56] evaluated a 4–6-week daily therapy programme in a non-randomized controlled trial. This included: warm-up and daily physical conditioning exercises aimed at improving aerobic capacity, muscle strength, and flexibility, particularly in the upper limb (1.5 hours); work hardening simulating the individual's job demands (1 hour); pain and stress management; and an ergonomic analysis. In comparison to a control group receiving usual care, those attending the programme had significantly higher return to work rates 18 months later. However, the design used a control group not eligible for the programme (due to attending other programmes, lack of insurance cover, refusal to participate, or high levels of illness behaviour) and follow-up points varied between 3 and 35 months in both groups.

Cognitive behavioural therapy (CBT) intervention, including goal-setting, cognitive restructuring, relaxation, and assertiveness training has also been evaluated in soft tissue, upper limb disorders. A 2-year follow-up of a randomized controlled trial of individual CBT, group CBT, and wait list control groups identified no differences in return to work rates, although there was significantly improved ability to cope with pain in both CBT groups.[57, 58]

Provision of orthoses

A variety of splints can be provided, some examples of which are given below.

Ulnar nerve entrapment at the elbow

A 'drop-out' splint has been developed for the treatment of ulnar nerve entrapment at the elbow. 'Drop-out' means that the splint allows movement into extension but restricts flexion. Its purpose is to immobilize the elbow in moderate extension, whilst preventing flexion greater than 45°. Prolonged or repetitive elbow flexion aggravates the source of compression, and therefore splinting in extension reduces the nerve irritation.[59]

The splint was designed because patient acceptance of the long arm splint also used in this condition has been poor, especially if the patient is required to wear it during daily activities. The drop-out splint allows some elbow extension and forearm rotation, and wrist movement is not restricted.[59] This splint has been evaluated with 51 patients over 2 years: 24 per cent experienced complete resolution of symptoms; 33 per cent were still wearing the splint; 24 per cent required surgical intervention; and 19 per cent were lost to follow up. The results identified that patient compliance improved by 50 per cent and need for surgery reduced by 50 per cent.[59]

In addition to provision of a drop-out splint, patients would also participate in a structured programme of intervention including activities to maintain range of movement, strength, and endurance, activity modification, and activities of daily living that might include tasks carried out at home, work, or during leisure pursuits.

Semi-flexible support splints

This splint was designed to limit extremes of motion and provide support to soft tissues. It was originally designed for soft tissue disorders such as tenosynovitis and tendinitis but has been used with carpal tunnel syndrome and is therefore a useful adjunct to occupational therapy intervention for any soft tissue disorders.[60] The splint ensures that 'safe wrist motion' is maintained and allows 5° of flexion, 30° of extension, 10° of radial deviation, and 15° of ulnar deviation. These ranges of motion have been determined as 'functional wrist motion' in a study to measure the range of movement necessary to perform activities of daily living.[61]

The splint was evaluated with 73 patients, 41 of whom completed a self-report questionnaire. Of these, 92 per cent considered the support useful during work and non-work activities, and especially useful when writing and driving. It therefore provides additional support for an injured worker who is able to return to work before full resolution of symptoms has occurred.[60] Additional therapy intervention will include: activity to maintain and improve range of movement, strength, and endurance; activities of daily living including home, work, and leisure; activity modification; and patient education.

Summary

The limited research on occupational therapy programmes suggests that, for those with upper limb disorders (which may be work-related), a combined approach of patient education; exercise; work assessment and work hardening; joint protection; energy conservation and work simplification training; ergonomic adaptations at home and work; splinting; and cognitive-behavioural therapy improves coping with pain, return to work rates, and ability to continue in work. However, there has been little research into the effectiveness of such programmes and good quality randomized controlled trials are required.

References

1. **MacFarlane, G.J.**, et al. (2000). Role of mechanical and psychosocial factors in the onset of forearm pain: prospective population based study. Br. Med. J. **321**, 1–5.

2. **College of Occupational Therapists (COT)** (1994). *Core skills and a conceptual foundation for practice: a position statement.* COT, London.

3. **Berg Rice, V.J.** (1998). *Ergonomics and therapy: an introduction.* In *Ergonomics for therapists*, 2nd edn. (ed. K. Jacobs), pp. 3–19. Butterworth Heinemann, Boston.

4. **Chapanis, A.** (1991). To communicate the human factors message, you have to know what the message is and how to communicate it. *Hum. Factors Soc. Bull.* **34**, 1–4.

5. **Nickerson, R.S.** (1992). *Looking ahead: human factors challenges in a changing world.* Erlbaum, Hillsdale, New Jersey.

6. **Hagedorn, R.** (1997). *Foundations for practice in occupational therapy.* Churchill Livingstone, Edinburgh.

7. **Chaffin, D.B. and Anderson, G.B.** (1991). *Occupational biomechanics,* 2nd edn. John Wiley and Sons, New York.

8. **Burke, M.** (1998). *Ergonomics tool kit: practical applications.* Aspen Publications, Gaithersburg, Maryland.

9. **Jacobs, K.** (1999). *Ergonomics for therapists,* 2nd edn. Butterworth Heinemann, Boston.

10. **Isernhagen, S.J.** (ed.) (1995). *The comprehensive guide to work injury management.* Aspen Publications, Gaithersburg, Maryland.

11. **Melzack, R.** (1987). The short form McGill Pain Questionnaire. *Pain.* **30**, 191–198.

12. **Boscheinen-Morrin, J., Davey, V., and Conolly, W.B.** (1992). *The hand: fundamentals of therapy,* 2nd edn. Butterworth Heinemann, Oxford.

13. **Bell-Krotoski, J.** (1999). Research in clinical testing of sensibility: a personal journey. *B. J. Hand Ther.* **4** (1), 13–22.

14. **Bell-Krotoski, J. and Tomancick, E.** (1987). The repeatability of the Semmes–Weinstein monofilaments. *J. Hand Surg.* **12A**, 155–161.

15. **Mathiowetz, V., Weber, K., Volland, G., and Kashman, N.** (1984). Reliability and validity of grip and pinch strength evaluations. *J. Hand Surg.* **9A**, 222–226.

16. **Bohannon, R.W.** (1986). Test–retest reliability of hand held dynamometry. *Phys. Ther.* **66**, 206–209.

17. **Solgaard, S., Kristiansen, B., and Jensen, J.S.** (1984). Evaluation of instruments for measuring grip strength. *Acta Orthop. Scand.* **55**, 569–572.

18. **Palmanda, M., Shah, S., and O'Hare, K.** (1999). Hand oedema: pathophysiology and treatment *Br. J. Hand Ther.* **4** (1), 26–32.

19. **Hudak, P.L., Amadio, P.C., and Bombardier, C.** (1996). Development of an upper extremity outcome measure: the DASH (disabilities of the arm, shoulder and hand). *Am. J. Ind. Med.* **29**, 602–608.

20. **Stock, S.R., Streiner, D., Reardon, R., Darzins, S., Dilworth, P., Tugwell, P., and Loisel, P.** (1995). The impact of neck and upper limb musculoskeletal disorders on the lives of affected workers: development of a new functional status index. *Qual. Life Res.* **4** (5), 491.

21. **Sollerman, C. and Ejeskar, A.** (1995). Sollerman hand function test. A standardised method and its use in tetraplegic patients. *Scand. J. Plast. Reconstr. Hand Surg.* **29**, 168–175.

22. **van Lankveld, W., van't Pad Bosch, P., Bakker, J., Terwindt, S., Franssen, M., and van Riel, P.** (1996). Sequential occupational dexterity assessment (SODA). A new test to measure hand disability. *J. Hand Ther.* **9** (1), 27–32.

23. **Jebsen, R.H., Taylor, N., Tieschmann, R.B., Trotter, M.J., and Howard, L.A.** (1969). An objective and standardised test of hand function. *Arch. Phys. Med. Rehabil.* **50**, 311–320.

24. **McPhee, S.D.** (1987). Functional hand evaluations: a review. *Am. J. Occup. Ther.* **41** (3), 158–163.

25. **Zigmond, A.S. and Snaith, R.P.** (1983). The hospital and anxiety depression scale. *Acta Psychiatrica Scand.* **67**, 361–370.

26. **Schultz-Johnson, K.** (1995). Upper extremity functional capacity evaluation. In *Rehabilitation of the hand: surgery and therapy,* 4th edn. (ed. J.M. Hunter), pp. 1739–1775. C.V. Mosby Co, St Louis.

27. **Sakakibara, H., Miyao, M., Kondo, T., Yamada, S., Nakagawa, T., and Kobayashi, F.** (1987). Relation between overhead work and complaints of pear and apple orchard workers. *Ergonomics* **30**, 805–815.

28. **Marras, W.S. and Schoenmarklin, R.W.** (1993). Wrist motions in industry. *Ergonomics* **36**, 241–251.

29. **Westgard, R. and Bjorklund, R.** (1987). The generation of muscle tension additional to body posture. *Ergonomics* **30**, 911–923.

30. **Ranney, D.** (1997). *Chronic musculoskeletal injuries in the workplace.* W.B. Saunders, Philadelphia.

31. **Kirwan, B. and Ainsworth, L.K.** (1992). *A guide to task analysis.* Taylor and Francis, London.

32. **McAtamney, L. and Corlett, E.N.** (1993). A survey method for the investigation of work related upper limb disorders. *Appl. Ergonom.* **24**, 91–99.

33. **Militello, L.G. and Hutton, R.J.** (1998). Applied cognitive task analysis (ACTA): a practitioner's toolkit for understanding cognitive task demands. *Ergonomics* **41** (11), 1618–1641.

34. **Borg, G.** (1982). Psychological basis of perceived exertion. *Med. Sci. Sports Exerc.* **4**, 377–381.

35. **Borg, G.** (1985). *An introduction to Borg's RPE-scale.* Cornell University Press, Ithaca, New York.

36. **Karasek, R.A.** (1979). Job demands, job decision latitude and mental strain. Implications for job re-design. *Adm. Sci. Q.* **24**, 285–307.

37. **Canon, N.M.** (1985). *Manual of hand splinting.* Churchill Livingstone, Edinburgh.

38. **Barr, N.R. and Swann, D.** (1988). *The hand: principles and techniques of splint-making.* 2nd edn. Butterworth, London.

39. **Hunter, J.M.** (ed.) (1995). *Rehabilitation of the hand: surgery and therapy,* 4th edn. C.V. Mosby Co, St Louis.

40. **Newman, G.** (1988). Which patients with arm oedema are helped by intermittent external pneumatic compression therapy? *J. R. Soc. Med.* **81**, 377–379.

41. **McMeeken, J.** (1994). Tissue temperature and blood flow: a research based overview of electrophysical modalities. *Aust. J. Physiother.* **40**, 49–57.

42. **Downer, A.H.** (1988). *Physical therapy procedures,* 4th edn. Thomas, Springfield, Illinois.

43. **Brennan, M.J. and Weitz, J.** (1992). Lymphoedema 30 years after radical mastectomy. *Am. J. Phys. Med. Rehabil.* **71**, 12–14.

44. **English, C.J., et al.** (1995). Relations between upper limb soft tissue disorders and repetitive movements at work. *Am. J. Ind. Med.* **27**, 75–90.

45. **Cordery, J. and Rocchi, M.** (1998). Joint protection and fatigue management. In *Rheumatologic rehabilitation,* Vol. 1. *Assessment and management* (ed. J. Melvin and G. Jensen), pp. 279–322. American Occupational Therapy Association, Bethesda, Maryland.

46. **Melvin, J.** (1989). *Rheumatic disease: occupational therapy and rehabilitation,* 2nd edn. F.A. Davis Co, Philadelphia.

47. **Sheon, R.P.** (1985). A joint protection guide for nonarticular rheumatic disorders. *Postgrad. Med.* **77** (5), 329–335.

48. **Sheon, R.P.** (1997). Repetitive strain injury: 2. Diagnostic and treatment tips on six common problems. *Postgrad. Med.* **102** (4), 72–88.

49. **Sheon, R.P., Moskowitz, R.W., and Goldberg, V.M.** (1996). *Soft tissue rheumatic pain: recognition, management and prevention,* 3rd edn. Williams and Wilkins, Baltimore.

50. **Keller, K., Corbett, J., and Nichols, D.** (1998). Repetitive strain injury in computer keyboard users: pathomechanics and treatment principles in individual and group intervention. *J. Hand Ther.* **11** (1), 9–26.

51. **Rosenstock, I.M.** (1988). Adoption and maintenance of lifestyle modifications. *Am. J. Prev. Med.* **4** (6), 349–352.

52. **Innes, E.** (1997). Education and training programs for the prevention of work injuries: do they work? *Work* **9**, 221–232.

53. **Lawler, L.L., et al.** (1996). Educational techniques used in occupational therapy treatment of cumulative trauma disorders of the elbow, wrist, and hand. *Am. J. Occup. Ther.* **51** (2), 113–118.

54. **Dortch, H.L. and Trombley, C.A.** (1990). The effects of education on hand use with industrial workers in repetitive jobs. *Am. J. Occup. Ther.* **44** (9), 777–782.

55. **Barthel, R.H., et al.** (1998). Presentation and response of patients with upper extremity repetitive use syndrome to a multidisciplinary rehabilitation program: a retrospective view of 24 cases. *J. Hand Ther.* **11**, 191–199.

56. **Feuerstein, M., et al.** (1993). Multidisciplinary rehabilitation of chronic work-related upper extremity disorders. *J. Occup. Med.* **35** (4), 396–403.

57. **Spence, S.H.** (1991). Cognitive behavioural therapy in the treatment of chronic, occupational pain of the upper limbs: a 2 year follow-up. *Behav. Res. Ther.* **29** (5), 503–509.

58. Spence, S.H. (1998). Cognitive–behaviour therapy in the management of upper extremity cumulative trauma disorder. *J. Occup. Rehabil.* **8** (1), 27–45.

59. Harper, B.D. (1990). The drop out splint: an alternative to the conservative management of ulnar nerve entrapment at the elbow. *J. Hand Ther.* **3** (4), 199–201.

60. Henshaw, J.L., Walker Satren, J., and Wrightsman, J.A. (1989). The semi-flexible support: an alternative for the hand injured worker. *J. Hand Ther.* **2** (1), 35–40.

61. Palmer, A.K., Werner, F.W., Murphy, D., and Glisson, R. (1985). Functional wrist motion: a biomechanical study. *J. Hand Surg.* **10A** (1), 39–46.

5.8 The management of soft tissue disorders: the role of the podiatrist

Trevor Prior

Introduction

Whilst the role of the podiatrist in the management of skin lesions has been established for many years, this role in the management of soft tissue and skeletal abnormalities has only recently been appreciated. This chapter attempts to outline the role of the podiatrist and the treatment methods/modalities available. It is not intended to describe the conditions that are covered elsewhere in this book but the management of these conditions will be outlined.

Podiatry is the more universal term for chiropody and, whilst both terms arise from the Greek language, chiropody relates to hand (*cheir*) and foot (*pous*). More accurately podiatry relates to foot and healing (*iatreia*). Dorland's illustrated medical dictionary defines podiatry as 'The specialised field that deals with the study and care of the foot, including its anatomy, pathology, medical and surgical treatment, etc. Formerly called Chiropody.'

Podiatry training includes general training in the management of conditions of the foot and leg, medical and surgical implications and complications, pathology, physiology, anatomy, and biomechanics/gait analysis.

Patient assessment

Whilst the podiatrist generally concentrates on conditions of the lower limbs, a more general assessment is required to enable an accurate diagnosis and treatment plan. This should include a detailed history of the presenting problem, previous medical/surgical conditions, current medication, allergies, and family and personal social history. A functional enquiry and modified systems review completes this detailed assessment. Although all of this information is not essential for the treatment of routine skin and nail problems, it is necessary for more complex cases. In addition to the information obtained from this inquiry, specific factors relating to the foot are also assessed (see below).

Structure and function

Information relating to the site and extent of skin and nail abnormalities and assessment of structural alignment (podiatric biomechanical evaluation) is recorded. Although gross findings (e.g. arch height, heel position) will provide an indication of the biomechanical function of the foot, more specific analysis can be undertaken to determine more detailed function.

Podiatric biomechanics is a specific entity and was founded on the work by Root *et al.*[1, 2] in the 1960s. This has been the commonly quoted concept of foot function in many texts and papers, although there has been no significant scientific evidence to validate their observations.

Indeed, it is fair to say that foot function is still relatively poorly understood and many myths still exist. However, the management of pathology with orthoses designed around the podiatric concepts has become established and the underlying principles are therefore worth noting.

Podiatric biomechanics—traditional theory

Root *et al.*[1, 2] base their concepts on an ideal neutral position for the foot and thus the ideal position during walking. Their observations concluded that pronation and supination motion within the subtalar joint occurred in a one-third to two-third ratio, respectively. The neutral position of the subtalar joint was deemed to occur when it was neither pronated nor supinated (Fig. 1). Whilst they traditionally described this position as being assessed by measuring the range of motion (and thus calculating the 1 : 2 ratio), many practitioners utilize palpation of the head of the talus to help determine this position. The latter technique assumes that talonavicular joint congruency occurs when the subtalar joint is in neutral. However, neither technique has been validated. Bailey *et al.*[3] studied this relationship utilizing tomograms to assess the range of motion. Whilst the average relationship demonstrated a one-third to two-third ratio, intersubject variability was demonstrated.

Once the subtalar joint has been placed into its neutral position, placing a dorsal force on the lateral aspect of the forefoot locks the midtarsal joint. This then allows the practitioner to assess the relationship of the posterior aspect of the heel to the lower one-third of the leg and the forefoot to the rearfoot. The heel should be parallel to the leg and the forefoot parallel to the rearfoot as a position of inversion or eversion would result in abnormal function to allow ground contact. Thus, when standing, the perfect foot in neutral would have the heel parallel to the lower third of leg and at a right angle to the ground with the forefoot parallel to the rearfoot (Fig. 2).

According to Root *et al.*,[2] the stance phase of the gait cycle can be divided into heel strike, foot flat, midstance, heel lift, and toe off. Pronation of the foot occurs following heel strike so that the foot is mobile and able to adapt to varying terrain. By contrast, at toe off, the foot is supinated to provide a rigid lever for propulsion. Furthermore, as the foot is passing from a pronated to supinated position, it must pass through neutral. This should occur at midstance or the point at which the two medial malleoli are level. Thus, any positional or soft tissue abnormality that prevented this alignment would predispose to abnormal function and injury. Excessive pronation (eversion, abduction, and dorsiflexion), particularly into late stance, would predispose to instability and thus soft tissue overload (Fig. 3). This can be further aggravated by posterior muscle inflexibility, particularly of the calf muscle complex. Normal function requires adequate calf muscle flexibility to allow ankle joint dorsiflexion. Ten degrees of ankle dorsiflexion past vertical (90°) is deemed to indicate normal motion with the

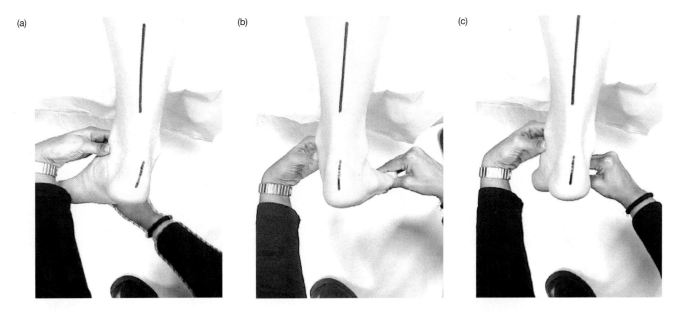

Fig. 1. (a) Maximum supination with lateral talar head prominence. (b) Maximum pronation with medial talar head prominence. (c) Subtalar neutral with neither medial nor lateral prominence.

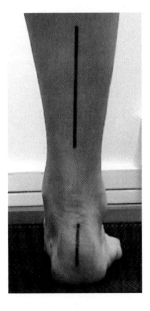

Fig. 2. With the subtalar joint in neutral and the midtarsal joint maximally pronated, the bisection of the leg and heel are parallel and perpendicular to the weightbearing surface. The forefoot and rearfoot are parallel.

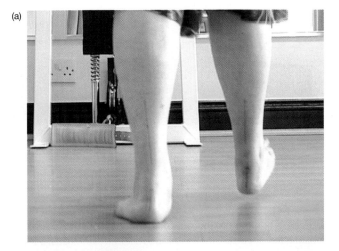

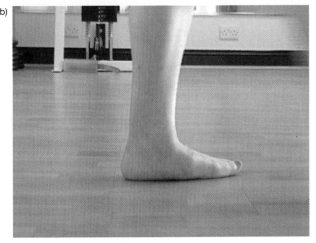

Fig. 3. Excessive mid to late stance pronation with rearfoot eversion (a) lowering of the medial longitudinal arch and jamming of the first ray (b).

knee extended. Limited motion will cause a pronatory force on the foot (as dorsiflexion is a component of this motion), predisposing to injury (Fig. 4).

However, the degree of pronation occurring during walking has been challenged. There is sufficient evidence to indicate that, whilst the heel is in contact with the ground, the heel remains everted.[4, 5] Thus, a pronated position is normal on a flat surface and further studies are required to determine the extent at which pronation becomes clinically significant.

(a)

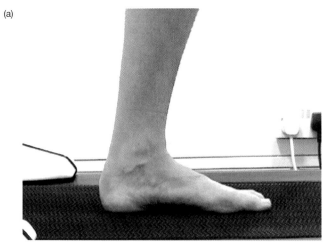

(b)

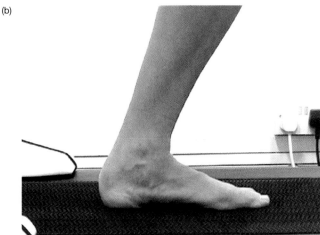

Fig. 4. (a) Adequate calf flexibility allows 10° of ankle joint dorsiflexion. (b) Inadequate flexibility or excessive dorsiflexion will cause pronation of the foot.

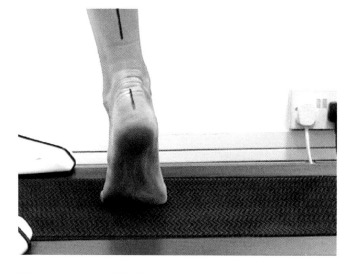

Fig. 5. Dorsiflexion of the foot over the toes at the MTPJs tightens the plantar fascia, plantarflexes the first metatarsal and inverts the foot.

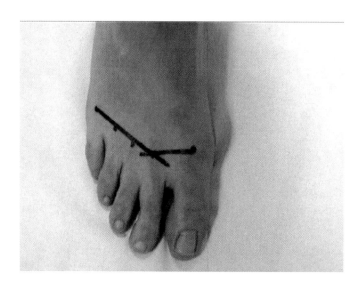

Fig. 6. The oblique (low gear) axis through metatarsals 2–5 and the transverse (high gear) axis through metatarsals 1–2.

Root *et al.*[2] suggest that orthoses be prescribed when an abnormal relationship exists to try and control the position of the foot. Whilst pronation has not been directly linked to specific pathologies, a number of papers note that orthoses are indicated for limiting this motion as part of the treatment programme for a range of conditions.

These concepts, despite the challenges, have formed the traditional basis for podiatric biomechanics. However, there are other concepts utilized, an understanding of which enables further detailed assessment of foot function with some indication to the underlying abnormalities.

Anatomical function

In the 1950s an anatomist, Hicks,[6, 7] demonstrated how joints rotated around axes of motion. He also discussed the complex anatomy of the plantar fascia, describing how it arose from the plantar aspect of the calcaneus and inserted via the plantar fat pad and flexor apparatus into the proximal phalanges of the toes. He observed that dorsiflexion of the toes resulted in plantar flexion of the metatarsals due to the tension placed in the plantar fascia. He termed this the 'tie bar system'. As more motion is available in the first metatarsal compared to the lesser metatarsals, there is greater plantar

flexion of the first metatarsal—hence a rise in the medial longitudinal arch. This in turn will cause an external rotation of the leg via the subtalar joint. During gait, this will happen following heel lift as the foot dorsiflexes over the toes (Fig. 5). He concluded that this occurred in the absence of muscle function as it occurred in paralytic feet.

Another anatomist, Bojsen-Muller,[8] considered this mechanism further. He describes the axes of the metatarsophalangeal joints (MTPJs) at the forefoot. He described two axes, the oblique (low gear) and transverse (high gear), and observed the effect on foot function when subjects toed off through either axis (Fig. 6).

Toe off through the low gear axis required the first toe to plantar flex to stabilize the foot, prevented first MTPJ dorsiflexion, and resulted in no tension observed in the plantar fascia or peroneus longus tendon. By contrast, toe off through the high gear axis resulted in first MJPJ dorsiflexion, plantar flexion of the first metatarsal with tension in the plantar fascia and peroneus longus tendon (which helps to stabilize the plantarflexed first ray against the ground). As the peroneus longus tendon pivots around the cuboid, tension will cause a small rotation of the cuboid allowing the bony process on the plantar medial aspect of the cuboid to become opposed to a notch in the calcaneus. Bosjen-Muller described this as closed packing of the calcaneocuboid joint. It would therefore follow that adequate first ray plantar flexion is necessary to allow normal peroneus longus function and assist with rearfoot stability.

Although there are no normal data relating to the optimum angle of the low and high gear axis, it follows that these angles and MTPJ function have the ability to affect foot function and rearfoot position during walking and running. Furthermore, an internal or external leg position will alter the angle of the foot in relation to the line of progression, in turn affecting the relative position of the low and high gear axes.

Subtalar axis variation

Kirby[9, 10] described a further method of assessing foot function in relation to the subtalar joint axis. He observed that palpation of the foot beneath the first metatarsal head generally resulted in inversion or supination of the foot whilst pressure beneath the fifth MTPJ generally resulted in eversion or pronation of the foot. Thus, by working across the foot, one can find a point at which the foot neither pronates nor supinates. Kirby[9, 10] surmises that this point lies on the subtalar joint axis (Fig. 7). By repeating the process at three different levels along the course of the foot, the subtalar joint axis can be plotted in the transverse plane. Kirby[9, 10] describes foot function in terms of equilibrium of forces across the subtalar joint axis rather than relating to one given position of the joint (i.e. subtalar joint neutral). Any force, muscle/tendon activity, and ligamentous support medial to the axis will result in a supination moment, whilst force lateral to the axis will result in a pronation moment. On weight bearing, all of these factors will reach a point of equilibrium when standing still.

In order to change the position of the foot one must increase the supination or pronation moment accordingly. This concept is useful in understanding how orthoses can relieve discomfort without changing foot position.

If one considers a patient with pain in the sinus tarsi and a maximally pronated foot, this pronation will cause compression within the sinus tarsi. If a further pronatory force is applied to the sinus tarsi, say 10 N, no movement will occur but further compression and discomfort will occur. An orthotic that applies a 10 N supinatory moment to the rearfoot will not alter the position of the foot but will reduce the compressive force by 10 N. This may be sufficient to relieve discomfort.

Kirby[9, 10] has noted that, whilst there is a normal position for the subtalar joint axis in the transverse plane, the axis can become medially or laterally deviated. When this occurs, the pronatory or supinatory moments become greater, respectively. This will affect the rotational equilibrium across the joint and result in abnormal function. Kirby[11] describes a technique for producing orthoses that greatly increases the supinatory moment at the rearfoot to address feet that have a medially deviated subtalar joint axis. Whilst this concept is based around basic physics, there is little scientific validation.

Sagittal plane theory (functional hallux limitus)

By contrast, Dananberg[12–14] described abnormalities within the sagittal plane. Expanding on the work by Perry[15], Dananberg[12–14] noted that there is far greater motion in the sagittal plane than in the transverse and frontal planes combined. In order for normal sagittal plane motion to occur there must be adequate first MTPJ and ankle joint motion.

Perry[15] describes how the body pivots over a stable foot. She describes the heel, ankle, and forefoot rocker phases that occur during the stance phase of gait. The heel rocker phase represents heel contact to foot flat, with the ankle rocker representing the midstance phase as the tibia advances over the stationary foot. Finally, the metatarsal

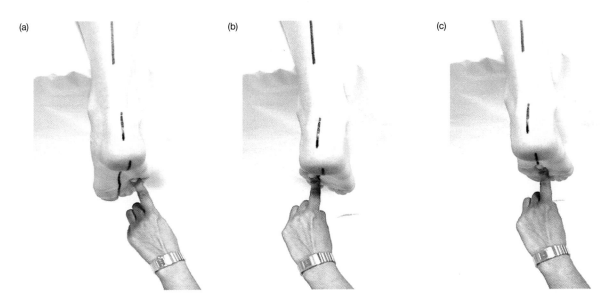

(a)   (b)   (c)

Fig. 7. Force applied to the foot will cause: (a) supination if medial to the axis, (b) pronation if lateral to the axis, (c) neither pronation nor supination when on the axis.

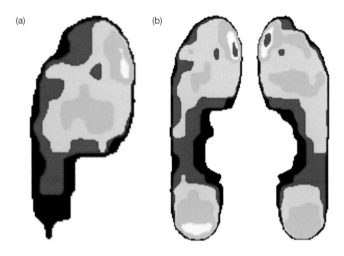

Fig. 8. Force pressure analysis demonstrating reduced load beneath the first MTPJ with increased load beneath the central metatarsals and Hallux, consistent with a functional Hallux Limitus. Midstep (a), both feet (b).

rocker represents dorsiflexion of the MTPJs from heel lift to toe off. As the foot moves from the ankle rocker to the forefoot rocker phase the heel lifts from the ground. Whilst the ankle is initially slightly dorsiflexed, it must plantar flex following contralateral heel strike to allow the weight-bearing leg to proceed into swing. Ankle joint plantar flexion can only occur if there is adequate dorsiflexion at the first MTPJ. Dananberg[12–14] has observed, via video and force platform analysis, that first MTPJ dorsiflexion can be reduced for a short period of time during walking (Fig. 3 and 8). As there is normal first MTPJ dorsiflexion available on non-weight-bearing examination, he terms this condition functional hallux limitus.

He likens the effect of this limited motion to an individual walking into a brick wall. Whilst body weight is driving forward the blockage in the first MTPJ dorsiflexion counteracts forward progression. The only way the body can continue to progress forward over the foot is for the knee to flex early. This in turn prevents hip extension in latter stance.

As the hip flexors are the primary initiators of gait, reduced hip extension prevents them gaining mechanical advantage in order to accelerate the leg into swing. As a result, the whole gait cycle is interrupted predisposing to instability of the foot, leg, and lower back. Treatment for this problem is geared towards facilitating sagittal plane motion, specifically first MTPJ dorsiflexion and ankle joint plantar flexion. Danaberg[12–14] reports that in-shoe pressure analysis is often required to accurately design orthoses to achieve this function.

Once again, there is little direct scientific evidence of the underlying principle. However, Dananberg and Guiliano[16] have performed a controlled study to assess the benefit of orthoses designed in this fashion for patients with chronic lower back pain. This study demonstrated a significant improvement in symptoms for patients receiving orthoses.

Ankle push off power

Ankle push off power, described by Kirtley,[17] is the method by which the lower limb is advanced into swing. By using kinematic and kinetic data it can be demonstrated that ankle joint plantar flexion just prior to swing occurs at a high velocity over a short period of time, thus

producing a high level of power. As this coincides with a concentric contraction of the calf muscle complex, this represents an active push off into the swing phase. However, the power generated at this stage is not transferred to the upper leg or trunk and thus is concentrated at accelerating the lower leg (shank) into swing. For this to occur, there must be adequate ankle joint plantar flexion and thus MTPJ dorsiflexion. Kirtley[17] indicates that anything that limits this function (e.g. limited motion, painful conditions/lesions beneath the MTPJs) will reduce ankle push off power. As the amount of power generated is directly related to walking speed (increased power = increased velocity), walking speed can be used to gauge efficiency. This would appear to support the concepts proposed by Dananberg[12–14].

Podiatric biomechanics—a functional concept based on the underlying principles

Although the underlying concepts described above have not been scientifically validated, combining the principles outlined enables the practitioner to consider the three dimensional aspect of foot function and thus begin the process of prescribing treatment.

If one utilizes the principles described, a potential model of function can be described. At heel contact the subtalar joint pronates due to ground reaction force. This enables the foot to become mobile and thus adapt to varying terrains and contribute to shock absorbency. The ability to adapt is less important in today's society as the majority of people walk on hard flat surfaces. However, this causes a repetitive type of function thousands of times daily that has the potential to cause pathology if excessive function occurs.

This motion is controlled by eccentric contraction of tibialis posterior and is accompanied by internal rotation of the leg and knee flexion. These motions are, in turn, controlled by eccentric contraction of the muscles of the leg and thigh. The body then pivots forward over the weight-bearing foot, thus requiring adequate ankle joint dorsiflexion, which is accompanied by knee extension. Ground reaction forces are sufficient at this stage to maintain the foot in a pronated position.

As the swing leg advances past the weight-bearing foot, the force beneath the heel begins to reduce which allows the process of re-supination to begin. A number of factors can combine to allow this process, which include the continued external rotation of the weight-bearing leg due to swing limb advancement, an initial dorsiflexion at the lesser MTPJs (low gear\axis), elastic recoil within tibialis posterior, and calf muscle contraction.

If sufficient re-supination occurs, actual heel lift (i.e. when the heel is no longer contacting the ground) will be accompanied by a transfer to the first-second MTPJ axis (high gear). Dorsiflexion of the first MTPJ will initiate the windlass mechanism (tightening of the plantar fascia) and thus plantar flexion of the first metatarsal, which, in turn, will be stabilized against the ground by peroneus longus. This will facilitate supination of the foot and the peroneus longus will cause closed packing of the calcaneocuboid joint, thus stabilizing the foot.

If sufficient motion occurs at the MTPJs this will allow the knee and hip to be extended in latter stance. Thus, swing is initiated by ankle push off power accelerating the shank and the hip flexors accelerating the thigh.

Optimum foot function should allow the individual to walk/run between two points with the minimum of energy expenditure. The above sequence of events would enable sufficient control/support as the foot accepts weight, appropriate positioning as the body pivots forward over the foot, and the initiation of swing. As the swing limb passes the weight-bearing foot, gravity/momentum then pulls the body forward—hence an efficient gait.

Foot and leg interaction

Evidence derived from studies utilizing video analysis provides a further insight to the relationship between foot and leg function. It has been demonstrated that there is a high correlation between rearfoot motion and tibial rotation.[18] However, whilst analysis of leg rotation with shoes with varying angular wedges does alter tibial function, this does not alter knee kinematics,[19] with the hip allowing the greatest degree of frontal plane motion.[20] Thus, it would appear that motion of the foot does alter tibial position with this rotation being resolved at the level of the hip. Of course, this is likely to affect the timing of knee function and reiterates the need for considering foot and leg function together rather than as separate entities.

Video analysis

Video analysis has become very popular in the analysis of foot and ankle mechanics, but studies that have attempted to relate static measures to dynamic function have been unable to demonstrate any conclusive link. This leads some authors to conclude that static measures are of little use.

Slow-motion video analysis enables a more accurate assessment of function given the speed at which the events of the gait cycle occur. From a practical perspective, a single camera for specific views (e.g. frontal or sagittal plane) enables this clinical assessment. In order to scientifically evaluate angles during gait, a synchronized two-camera system is a minimal requirement. Furthermore, when significant rotations occur (e.g. the tibia and calcaneus following heel lift), at least a three-camera system is required. These views can then be digitized and the resulting angles calculated. The complexity of the process and relative cost of equipment render the latter two techniques impractical for clinical purposes and they tend to be reserved for research.

Whichever system is used, the camera(s) needs to be positioned in an appropriate position to allow recording. This should generally be at a perpendicular to the plane being assessed (e.g. frontal, sagittal, or transverse) to minimize parallax error with the camera set to record the desired anatomical structures. When more than one camera is utilized, these will be positioned at set angles to ensure repeatability and accurate assessment. In many clinical environments, the motion will be recorded on a treadmill although this can be on a natural surface if a sufficiently large area is available. In certain situations, it may be preferable to record the subject in his/her working/performing environment (e.g. running the bend on a track). Adequate lighting is essential when analysing slow-motion/frame advance as this will often appear darker.

It is possible to perform split-screen analysis whereby different camera views are seen on one screen. Thus, video analysis is useful to gain a perspective of function both barefoot and shod and walking and running. Whilst it is difficult to assess rearfoot function with orthoses within the shoe (due to the heel counter), a sagittal assessment can be of use.

Video analysis can also be of use to assess the benefit of varying footwear. This is of particular benefit when assessing running shoes. The angle of the shoe to leg can indicate if sufficient support is provided (Fig. 9).

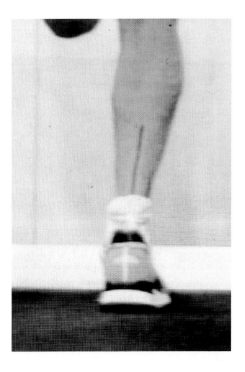

Fig. 9. The rearfoot angle between the leg and running shoe. This demonstrates a shoe with good control.

Computerized force analysis

Advances in sensor technology have resulted in the development of various systems that allow the forces beneath the foot to be analysed during walking and running. These can be in the format of a pressure platform, whereby the patient walks over a fixed plate, or an in-shoe system (insoles containing force sensors are placed within the shoe). Generally, the sensor resolution is greater for the platform system and it allows assessment of function without the influence of footwear. Whilst tests can be performed with shoes, this is more accurately achieved by using an in-shoe system. Furthermore, the in-shoe system allows more accurate assessment of the effect on function of orthoses within the shoe.

These systems allow analysis of the basic distribution of force beneath the foot, the dynamic loading pattern, and the rate at which the force progresses through the step. The systems calculate a centre of pressure line, which essentially represents the balance point of the force under the foot at each scan. Whilst some practitioners utilize this to help assess motion, this line can vary considerably between each step and its use has been questioned. The force/time curve is calculated by totaling the force beneath the foot at each scan. By analysing the shape and symmetry of the curve for each foot an indication of function and symmetry can be appreciated (Fig. 10).

These systems can be of use in evaluating basic function, the effect of surgery, and the effect of footwear and orthoses. However, some limitations still exist. The majority only record vertical forces thus missing the shear component. The sampling frequency (i.e. the number of frames recorded per second) determines the activity analysed with a minimum of 100 MHz required for running for scientific studies. These problems aside, this technology is an extremely useful

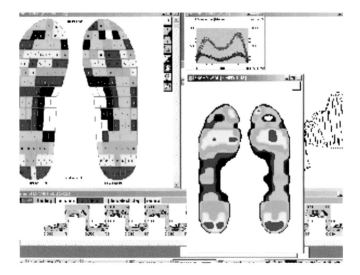

Fig. 10. A representation of the data available from an inshoe pressure analysis using the Pedar system (Novel GMBH, Germany).

adjunct for clinical assessment with slower sampling rates still providing sufficient data for clinical evaluation.

Assessment: conclusion

In summary, many of the principles undermining the assessment of foot function still require scientific validation. The use of more advanced assessment techniques helps to provide more objective assessment, although the interpretation of the events is still subjective in nature. Since orthoses can provide benefit in a range of conditions, further studies are required to improve our understanding of basic function and thus enable the prescription of orthoses that more accurately restore normal function.

The podiatrists' approaches to soft tissue disorders

Once the underlying structure and function have been assessed, attention must be paid to addressing any perceived imbalances. Podiatrists utilize a range of techniques, some of which overlap with those of other professionals. However, these factors need consideration if the treatment is to prove successful and a multidisciplinary approach is the general rule.

The manual techniques utilized by podiatrists are focused upon here.

Manipulation

Gentle manipulation of the foot and ankle can be extremely useful in providing a rapid return to more normal function, thereby facilitating the benefit of other modalities. Limitation of motion can be a particular problem with chronic conditions due to pain-induced inhibition. The primary sites for mobilization are the first MTPJ and metatarsal, the talonavicular joint, cuboid, and ankle joint/fibular. The latter is extremely important for normal function. The talus is wider anteriorly compared to posteriorly. Therefore, in order for the ankle joint to dorsiflex adequately, the fibula must externally rotate to allow this

motion. A failure of this motion can limit dorsiflexion with its resultant effect on function. Mobilization of the ankle joint and fibula can facilitate improved function.

Flexibility and strengthening

Flexibility exercises are a fundamental component of podiatric treatment. If the underlying soft tissue structures are too inflexible to allow normal function, this must be addressed prior to the issue of orthoses, or the orthoses modified to allow for the inflexibility. Attention is directed to all the appropriate muscle groups, although hamstring and calf muscle inflexibility are of particular importance. Inflexibility of these groups can increase the pronatory force on the foot, predisposing to injury. General stretching techniques are covered elsewhere but the author has found the use of a stretching board of particular use for improving calf muscle flexibility.

Strengthening exercises are often recommended, particularly for foot inversion, eversion, dorsiflexion, and plantar flexion. If weakness (endurance, strength, and power) is present, this should be restored to ensure normal intrinsic function. These can be provided by simple weight-bearing exercises, although these are often more effective when used with resistive bandages.

Support

If abnormal function has been observed, this can be addressed by controlling the position of the foot. In cases of acute injury or significant pain, immobilization may be necessary to adequately rest the area. This can be achieved by the application of a foot or below-knee cast or the use of a removable walking boot. The latter are particularly useful as they provide excellent support, can have orthoses incorporated within the boot, enable local treatment and controlled exercises, and are socially more acceptable.

In the majority of cases, simple strapping to support the affected structure or control basic foot position can be of particular benefit to assess the effect on function and the benefit to the patient. In some instances, strapping alone can be sufficient, although conversion to orthoses may prove necessary. In certain situations, strapping may be the only effective means of providing support during activity (e.g. ballerinas, gymnasts, etc.).

Dorland's illustrated medical dictionary defines orthoses as 'an orthopaedic appliance or apparatus used to support, align, prevent, or correct deformities or to improve the function of moveable parts of the body'. Thus, orthoses utilized by podiatrists are many and varied. Simple support can be achieved by combining various soft clinical padding materials (e.g. felt, swanfoan, etc.) to either re-distribute pressure from painful areas or control the position of the foot and digits. The use of synthetic padding materials and coverings enables a more durable yet soft device with similar function, to be provided. The use of mouldable silicone materials that harden by addition of a catalyst is of particular benefit for digital abnormalities.

In general, control of foot function for biomechanical abnormalities is achieved by the use of wedges and blocks of varying angles and thickness in an attempt to restore foot function. These devices include simple insole bases with pre-formed wedges adhered, pre-formed orthoses that provide standard control (Fig. 11(a)) and custom-made devices moulded to an impression of the foot. Whilst the traditional moulded devices are made to a plaster cast of the foot,

(a)

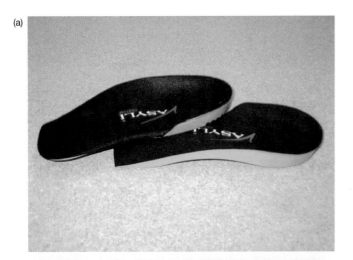

(b)

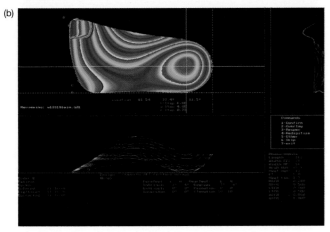

Fig. 11. (a) Pre-made orthoses.** (b) Computer representation of a cadcam orthotic.

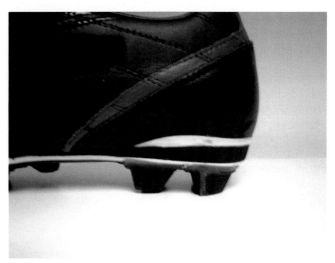

Fig. 12. A football boot with a built-in heel raise.

newer technology has resulted in the ability to scan the cast or foot enabling the production of computer generated moulds and orthoses (Fig. 11(b)).

Once again, the thickness and density of material can vary considerably. In general terms, a soft device must be thicker to achieve the same result as that made from a harder device. In theory, the harder device is deemed to provide more control although this has not been proven. In practice the density and thickness of material used is determined by the desired effect of the orthosis, the type of footwear and activity, and patient preference.

Footwear is an essential component of the podiatric management plan. Patients participating in sport often forget the importance of their footwear in daily activity. Whilst the level of activity is clearly higher during most weight-bearing sports, the low-grade, repetitive nature of everyday walking should not be underestimated. If these forces, repeated thousands of times per day, are not sufficient to cause injury, they may be sufficient to prevent the injury from resolving. The optimum shoe should have adequate depth, length, and width around the toes. As this would cause the foot to slip around in the shoe, an appropriate fastening (lace or adjustable strap) is necessary.

Similarly, the appropriate shoe should be worn for sport. Unfortunately, many recreational sports people often perform in inappropriate footwear. Whilst cross-trainers may be okay for light activity and general gym work, they are often inadequate for running. It is worth visiting a shop that specializes in the footwear for the given sport to ensure that appropriate advice is obtained. Many podiatrists are able to recommend shops in the local area.

However, even with the most appropriate shoe, orthoses and shoe modifications may prove necessary. Patients with a significant limb length discrepancy will require shoe adaptations if it is to be controlled accurately. Some shoe types may predispose to injury by the nature of the design. A good example is the football boot that is traditionally flat-soled. This will increase the stress to the calf muscle/Achilles tendon complex and may aggravate injury. Many of these can be adapted to have a heel built into the shoe (Fig. 12).

Given the lack of access to prescription-only medications, podiatrist's use of these modalities is relatively limited. However, the administration of a local anaesthetic as a local infiltration or ankle block can be of benefit to aid diagnosis or break the pain cycle. Furthermore, many podiatrists administer injectable corticosteroids that are obtained either by a local standing order or via a prescription from the patient's general practitioner. Generally, these are used after other treatment modalities, exercises, and orthoses have been implemented. If conservative measures fail, then surgical intervention may be indicated.

Guidelines for referral

Many soft tissue abnormalities of the leg, pelvis, and spine may benefit from a biomechanical/gait analysis to determine any contributing factors. This may be in the form of predisposing to the injury or delaying resolution. Clearly, knowledge of the injury mechanism and nature of the injury would help determine the appropriateness of the referral. Advice on footwear, appropriate exercises, and orthoses would form part of the overall treatment plan.

Conclusion

This chapter has outlined the role of the podiatrist, the underlying principles of treatment, and treatment options. It is clear that further research is required to improve the understanding of normal foot function. Only then, will the effect of orthoses be more thoroughly understood and applied.

However, it is clear that modification of foot and leg function is one of the components of injury management. The inclusion of a podiatrist within the health care team enables a comprehensive approach to patient management.

References

1. **Root, M.L., Orien, W.P., and Weed, J.H.** (1997). Clinical biomechanics: Normal and abnormal function of the foot, Vol 1. Clinical Biomechanics Corp.

2. **Root, M.L., Orien, W.P., and Weed, J.H.** (1997). Clinical biomechanics: Normal and abnormal function of the foot, Vol 2. Clinical Biomechanics Corp.

3. **Bailey, D.S., Perillo, J.T., and Forman, M.** (1984). Subtalar joint neutral, a study using tomography. *J. Am. Podiatr. Med. Assoc.* **4**(2), 59–64.

4. **McPoil, T. and Cornwall, M.W.** (1994). Relationship between subtalar joint neutral position and pattern of rearfoot motion during walking. *Foot Ankle* **15**(3), 141–145.

5. **Pierrynowski, M.R. and Smith, S.B.** (1996). Rearfoot inversion/eversion during gait relative to the subtalar joint neutral position. *Foot Ankle* **17**(7), 406–412.

6. **Hicks, J.H.** (1953). The mechanics of the foot; I. The joints. *J. Anat.* **87**, 345–357.

7. **Hicks, J.H.** (1954). The mechanics of the foot; II. The plantar aponeurosis and the arch. *J. Anat.* **88**, 25–31.

8. **Bojsen-Moller, F.** (1979). Calcaneocuboid joint and stability of the longitudinal arch of the rearfoot at high and low gear push off. *J. Anat.* **1**, 165–176.

9. **Kirby, K.A.** (1987). Methods for determination of positional variations in the subtalar joint axis. *J. Am. Podiatr. Med. Assoc.* **77**(5), 228–234.

10. **Kirby, K.A.** (1989). Rotational equilibrium across the subtalar joint axis. *J. Am. Podiatr. Med. Assoc.* **79**(1), 1–14.

11. **Kirby, K.A.** (1992). The medial heel skive technique, improving pronation control in foot orthoses. *J. Am. Podiatr. Med. Assoc.* **82**(4), 177–188.

12. **Dananberg, H.J.** (1986). Functional hallux limitus and its relationship to gait efficiency. **76**(11), 648–652.

13. **Dananberg, H.J.** (1993). Gait style as an etiology to chronic postural pain; Part I. Functional hallux limitus. *J. Am. Podiatr. Med. Assoc.* **83**(8), 433–441.

14. **Dananberg, H.J.** (1993). Gait style as an etiology to chronic postural pain; Part II. Postural compensatory process. *J. Am. Podiatr. Med. Assoc.* **83**(11), 615–624.

15. **Perry, J.** (1992). Basic functions. In *Normal and pathological function* (ed. J. Perry), pp. 19–47. Slack, Thorofare NJ31:

16. **Dananberg, H.J. and Guiliano, M.** (1999). Chronic lower back pain and its response to custom foot orthotic fabrication. *J. Am. Podiatr. Med. Assoc.* **89**(3), 109–117.

17. **Kirtley, C.** (2001). The importance of ankle push off power. *Br. J. Pod.* **4**(3), 80–83.

18. **Cornwall, T.G. and McPoil, M.W.** (1995). Footwear and foot orthotic effectiveness research: A new approach. *J. Orthop. Sports. Phys. Ther.* **21**, 337–44.

19. **Lafortune, M.A., Cavanagh, P.R., Sommer III, H.J. and Kalenak, A.** (1994). Foot inversion–eversion and knee kinematics during walking. *J. Orthop. Res.* **12**, 412–420.

20. **Eng, J.J. and Winter, D.A.** (1995). Kinetic analysis of the lower limbs during walking: what information can be gained from a three-dimensional model? *J. Biomech.* **28**(6), 753–758.

6

Specific soft tissue disorders

6.1 Acute neck pain and 'whiplash'

Donncha O'Gradaigh and Brian Hazleman

Introduction

Neck pain, though almost as common as low back pain and presenting the same difficulties in diagnosis and management, has received considerably less research attention, and the precise anatomical structures responsible and the most appropriate management remain unclear in most cases. This chapter will concentrate on conditions in which a rheumatologist's opinion is typically sought by general practitioners or others working in primary care, such as physiotherapists and sports physicians. Neck pain resulting from whiplash injuries is particularly relevant in this context. While various authors have suggested that whiplash-associated disorder is exclusively a somatization disorder, driven by psychosocial factors and compensation claims, the disorder is discussed here in the context of the available evidence in rheumatology and orthopaedic literature.

Descriptions of traumatic neck pain date back to accounts of 'railway spine' in the early nineteenth century. Undoubtedly, neck pain due to injury is not a new phenomenon, though the potential for traumatic and overuse injuries has increased since the industrial revolution and more recently with the advent of faster transport. The term 'whiplash' was first used in 1928 by M.E. Crowe, an American orthopaedic surgeon, to describe the mechanism of injury. A paper in the *Journal of the American Medical Association* in 1953 first increased awareness of the issue, as motor transport became more nearly universal. Interestingly, the incidence of whiplash increased in the 1970s with the introduction of compulsory seat-belts in cars, falling again as head-restraints were installed.

Definitions

Neck pain requires no definition. The duration of symptoms considered acute varies between studies, but is generally a period of less than 6 months. As pain in the arm (brachalgia) or shoulder may be cervical in origin, epidemiological studies often do not restrict their case definition to those with neck pain alone. Spondylosis refers to degenerative changes in the spine, while spondylitis should be reserved for conditions with a predominantly inflammatory component, such as ankylosing spondylitis. Spondylolysis describes a fracture of the pars intra-articularis. Definitions for the majority of the differential diagnoses suggested in Table 1 are self-evident. Distinctive clinical features are discussed in detail in the relevant sections.

The definition of 'whiplash' has undergone a number of revisions since Crowe's description of 'the manner in which the head is moved suddenly in acceleration–deceleration by an external force to produce a sprain in the neck'. A Task Force established to study this often contentious clinical syndrome offered a more lengthy definition, identifying 'whiplash injury' as the bony or soft-tissue injury caused by an acceleration–deceleration force, while 'whiplash-associated disorder' refers to a wide variety of clinical manifestations associated with such an injury.[1]

Table 1 Differential diagnosis of acute neck pain

Degenerative	Acute exacerbation of spondylosis
Discogenic	Acute pain with or without neurological features
Spondylitis	Spondarthropathies Ankylosing spondylitis Spondylitic psoriatic arthritis Rheumatoid arthritis (*NB* subluxation)
Infective	Osteomyelitis Soft-tissue (Lemiere's syndrome)
Trauma	Whiplash injury Spondylolysis Clay-shoveller's fracture (avulsion of spinous process C_7)
Tumours	Almost always metastatic
Vascular	Dissection of vertebral or carotid artery

Epidemiology

In a primary care survey, 12 per cent of women and 9 per cent of men reported neck pain at that time (point prevalence), while 34 and 28 per cent, respectively, reported experiencing neck pain at some time in the past. In another study, the life-time prevalence of neck or shoulder pain among a cohort aged over 29 years was 71 per cent. An annual incidence of between 12 and 34 per cent has been reported from a Scandinavian population. A clear relationship has been demonstrated between particular occupations and neck pain, manual workers having higher frequencies of neck pain than those in sedentary professions.[2] Worktime lost (which is comparable to that for low back pain in some industries) and high demands on therapists' and physicians' time have considerable cost implications—for example, the total cost of neck pain in the Netherlands in 1996 was estimated to be US $686 million (1 per cent of total health care expenditure).

Pain attributed to disc protrusion occurs with only one-quarter to one-half of the incidence of similar lesions in the lumbar spine.

Degenerative changes are almost inevitable with ageing, with 96 per cent of men and 84 per cent of women noted to have radiological changes by 65 years of age. Using more sensitive imaging such as magnetic resonance imaging (MRI), the incidence of such changes is even greater. However, there is a poor correlation between symptoms, imaging, and findings at surgery or autopsy.

Approximately 20 per cent of all road-traffic accidents (RTAs) involve rear-end collisions. Of those involved in RTAs, 30–60 per cent report neck pain and/or stiffness, amounting to one million cases annually in the United States. Women are affected twice as commonly as men. Of note, in a survey from Lithuania where there was (at that time) no experience of litigation following RTAs, the authors found a considerably lower incidence of cervical pain, with almost no reports of symptoms lasting more than 3 weeks.[3] Whiplash injury is also described in divers and among (military) pilots landing on aircraft carriers or experiencing high G-forces in high performance jet aircraft.

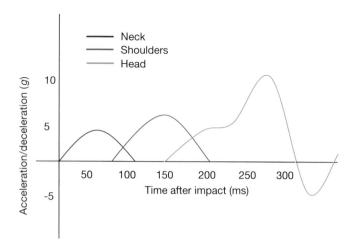

Fig. 1 Acceleration–deceleration of the neck, shoulders, and head after collision. Adapted from ref. 2

Whiplash injury and whiplash-associated-disorder

Clinical features

Neck pain is the essential feature of whiplash injury. This occurs in the first few hours after injury in only 25 per cent, while a further 25 per cent experience symptoms over 12 hours later. The remaining individuals do not report symptoms until at least 24 hours after injury. Pain is typically associated with stiffness and reduced range of movement in the neck, often exacerbated by painful spinal muscle spasms. Other features frequently described following a 'whiplash' type of injury include headache, myofascial pain referred to the neck, jaw, and shoulder, impaired memory, and neurological symptoms in the upper limb.

Pathogenesis

There is considerable debate about the nature of whiplash injury. Most commonly occurring in the setting of RTAs, similar presentations can follow diving and other accidents. The majority of studies are, however, based on RTA-associated whiplash injuries. Recent models, using electromyography (EMG) and cinematic techniques, have established the pattern of movement of the neck, shoulders, and head during the acceleration and deceleration that occur shortly after impact. Figure 1 illustrates that the earliest forward movement is of the neck, the head remaining fixed in space. Shortly afterwards, the shoulders also move forward. Because of the relatively greater inertia of the head, it only begins to move forwards some 150 ms after collision. The neck effectively acts as a lever, with the result that the head experiences a greater transmitted force and a greater reactive deceleration (the accelerating force is approximately $12g$ in a collision at 20 mph). Head restraints on the seats of vehicles prevent cervical hyperextension, and they reduced the incidence of whiplash injury by 15 per cent when introduced. However, restraints were incorrectly adjusted in 75 per cent of vehicles involved in an RTA in one study. The speed and direction of impact and the extent of damage to the vehicles involved have not been consistently correlated with the severity of whiplash injury symptoms.

The simplest model of whiplash assumes that the head, neck, and shoulders only move in one direction. However, if the head is turned or the impact is not from directly behind, a considerable rotational element further stresses the cervical structures. Bracing by the paraspinal muscles in response to impact takes 150–200 ms and occurs too slowly to protect the neck in an unexpected collision. This contrasts with deliberate head and neck impact, for example, in a rugby tackle or scrum, where whiplash-type injuries are rare.

The earliest descriptions of structural lesions were based on cadaveric studies or on animal models. Improvements in imaging have resulted in a greater appreciation of the range of structures that may be affected in whiplash injury. These are illustrated in Fig. 2. Using controlled nerve blocks, Lord and colleagues[4] implicated various injuries to the zygoapophyseal joints, particularly in more chronic cases. Others have found that soft tissue lesions involving ligamentous structures or paraspinal muscles are the most common of those illustrated. Fractures and disc injuries occur less frequently.

Contrasting the structures injured in direct trauma to the neck, a recent imaging study of a small number of cases found anterior disc injury occurred in 80 per cent of this group compared with 22 per cent of the whiplash-injured group, though disc herniation was evident in 60 and 44 per cent, respectively. Injury to the cervical cord was identified in all traumatic cases but did not occur in the whiplash group. In general, correlation between the structure injured and symptoms or outcome is poor. Similarly, effective management of whiplash injury does not appear to be influenced by detailed imaging.[5]

The extent to which psychological and emotional responses and prospects of lucrative litigation influence the severity and duration of symptoms is contentious. A psychological component may well be inevitable in a traumatic painful injury and should not be regarded as invalidating the patient's complaint. Personality and psychosocial parameters were not associated with outcome at 6-month follow-up, whereas more intense neck pain, cognitive impairment at time of injury, and increasing age were associated with a poorer outcome.[6] In contrast, an investigation of compensation claims found a higher recovery rate in those who successfully negotiated a claim within 6 months compared with a group whose claims remained unsettled at 18 months.[7] While confounding bias concerning the extent of injury cannot be excluded in this study, the Lithuanian experience mentioned above is of interest.[3]

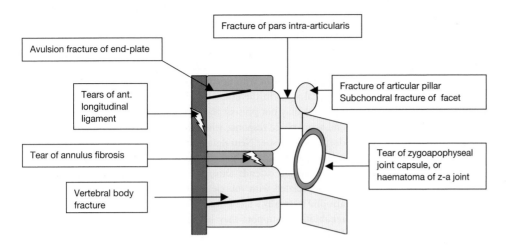

Fig. 2 Structures involved in various studies of whiplash injury.

Management

When first described, whiplash injury was considered to cause a sprain of cervical ligaments or a strain of paraspinal muscles. Appropriate management was therefore felt to be similar to that for other joint injuries—immobilization for a period of injury repair, followed by exercises to recover range of movement. The Quebec Task Force on Whiplash Associated Disorder[1] reported that 'most interventions have not been evaluated in a scientifically rigorous manner', and that those that had been 'show little evidence of efficacy'. This may partly be due to the natural history of whiplash injury, which is associated with spontaneous recovery in the majority. Therefore interventions may not appear to have a statistically significant benefit over control groups when the primary outcome is proportion improving rather than time to recovery. The past decade has seen increasing recognition that earlier mobilization of joint injuries promotes cartilage and/or ligament repair. The same principle has been investigated in the management of whiplash injury, achieving a more rapid return to a full and pain-free range of movement. The principles of management are to:

- relieve pain—from soft tissue injury, muscle spasm, or neurological referral
- recover range of movement
- prevent re-injury by strengthening stabilizer muscles.

Pain relief

A degree of soft tissue injury is likely in most cases of whiplash injury, and regular nonsteroidal anti-inflammatory drug (NSAID) treatment in the first 2 weeks is appropriate. Topical NSAIDs have not been studied, though the evidence in other settings would indicate that they offer no advantage. Additional analgesics, such as paracetemol or codeine-related compounds (e.g. codydramol, coproxamol, meptazinol), may be required. Muscle spasm can be effectively treated with low-dose (e.g. 2 mg three times daily) diazepam. Alternative antispasmodic drugs include cyclobenzapine, methacarbamol, or baclofen (unlicensed in whiplash injury). Treatment should be restricted to 1 week, being reviewed on an individual basis where symptoms persist. In their study that identified the zygapophyseal joints as the main

source of chronic neck pain, Lord et al.[4] found radiofrequency neurotomy to be of benefit.

Non-pharmacological treatment of pain has been achieved with soft cervical collars. However, the use of such collars, for so long the authentication of whiplash injury among litigants, is increasingly challenged by the studies of early mobilization and manipulative techniques. Effective analgesia has also been achieved in a trial of a cervical collar providing a pulsed low-energy electromagnetic field, and by short-wave diathermy and hydrotherapy outside of clinical trials. When a collar is prescribed, it should support the neck in a position of slight flexion. Regular periods out of the collar should be advised (e.g. 2 hrs on, 2 hrs off) within a few days of injury, and it should only be worn for *pain relief* thereafter—it is not necessary to wear a collar for recovery from whiplash injury. Acupuncture may be beneficial to relieve pain and stiffness, though myofascial triggering and local pain may prevent local points being used until the initial pain has subsided.

Mobilization/manipulation

The techniques described, usually compared to 'standard' treatment of a soft collar, have included traction, manipulation, or passive mobilization by a therapist and active exercises that may be supervised by a therapist or carried out by the patient at home after a short period of instruction. Bonk et al.[8] compared early mobilization with immobilization in a collar, noting that, while there were early benefits in range of movement and pain relief, there were no significant differences in outcome at 12 weeks. Rosenfeld et al.[9] found that active mobilization was only of benefit if commenced immediately after injury. If delayed for more than 2 weeks, there was no difference in outcome at 6-month follow-up. Techniques have not been directly compared and, because of differences in inclusion criteria, reported outcome measures, and in control interventions, it is not possible to recommend one approach over any other. A few general principles are noteworthy.

1. Exercises to gradually increase range of movement appear to be equally effective whether carried out under direct supervision or by the patient at home following a prescribed regime of exercises that are taught in a few sessions.

2. Such exercises should include all ranges of movement within the pain-free range and should also aim to strengthen the scalene, splenius, and sternocleidomastoid muscles.

3. Traction is particularly useful when there is radicular referral of pain.

4. Manipulation and mobilization techniques are contraindicated where there is evidence of vertebrobasilar arterial insufficiency, and are carried out within the pain-free range.

5. Local heat may be applied after mobilization for its analgesic properties and to prevent spasm in muscles that have been lengthened during treatment.

The complication rate for cervical spine manipulation is estimated to be between 5 and 10 cases per 10 million manipulations, including exacerbations of existing neurological deficits and cases of cerebrovascular events in the vertebrobasilar artery territory.

Outcome

The majority who fully recover from whiplash injury do so within 6 months of injury, and 60 per cent are free of symptoms by 4 weeks. Chronic symptoms, sometimes referred to as late whiplash syndrome, persist in approximately 25 per cent of cases, though in one study 40 per cent reported persistent symptoms after 15 years.[10] In such patients, the pattern and intensity of symptoms appear to remain static after about 2 years. Factors associated with poorer outcome are not well defined.[1] Though degenerative changes are almost universal by 65 years of age, one study has suggested that degenerative changes are accelerated by whiplash injury, affecting 39 per cent within 7 years of injury, compared with 6 per cent of matched controls.

Acute atraumatic neck pain

Clinical features and differential diagnosis

Neck pain may arise in the absence of trauma, most uncomplicated cases being associated with poor posture, anxiety and depression, neck strain, or occupational and sports injuries. Table 1 lists the differential diagnoses to be considered in more complex cases.

A careful history should identify pre-existing limitation in range of movement (e.g. difficulty reversing a car) or other, perhaps less severe, episodes of pain in the past. Discogenic neck pain is typically associated with referred pain into the arm (brachialgia), with or without paraesthesiae or other neurological manifestations, which typically do not conform to a dermatomal distribution. Motor weakness or reflex abnormalities occur about half as often as brachialgia or sensory disturbance. A disc lesion is further indicated by examination findings of asymmetry in the range of movement and more limitation of flexion than extension. Headaches are particularly common in those with upper cervical pathology. Pain from structures at these levels is often perceived in the distribution of the trigeminal nerve or at the back of the head, most probably mediated through the trigeminocervical nucleus in the upper cervical cord. Neurological presentations without pain should raise the possibility of cord lesions. Rheumatoid arthritis (RA) is a particular case, where atlanto-axial subluxation may occur spontaneously. A history of bilateral, progressive neurological symptoms in a patient with RA should be managed as a neurosurgical emergency. Transverse myelitis is a rare complication of systemic lupus erythematogus (SLE). It may occur at any spinal level, the patient describing back or neck pain associated with weakness. L'Hermitte's sign may be found (paraesthesia in the arms on neck flexion), though this is a non-specific test. Vascular abnormalities are suggested by the findings of a bruit with unequal pulses, typically associated with neurological signs in the cranial nerve distribution. Infective causes are rare, but may not present the expected pattern of fever, leucocytosis, and acute phase response when the infective focus is in bone, disc, or deeper soft tissue. Neuralgic amyotrophy is believed to follow viral infections though the patient frequently may not recall any illness. Pain classically extends across the shoulder and upper arm, and is initially associated with muscle weakness—though often quite marked, atrophy is usually a late feature. The condition is self-limiting, though rehabilitative support may be necessary to recover muscle strength. Metastatic disease involving cervical vertebrae is usually first suspected from imaging studies. Primary tumours causing neck pain are rare. Nasopharyngeal carcinoma is more common in Asian populations. Acute thyroiditis, myocardial ischaemia, and oesophageal complaints may all present with anterior neck pain. Musculoskeletal pain rarely radiates anterior to the sternomastoid muscle, and the absence of any associated loss of range of movement or pain on movement should alert the clinician to alternative pathology.

Investigation

Appropriate investigation should be directed at ruling out significant differential diagnoses or complications when clinically suspected—there is no 'routine' investigation of acute neck pain. Where exacerbation of previously documented degenerative spondylosis is the clinical diagnosis, further imaging is unhelpful.

Flexion and extension lateral cervical radiographs are often requested as a matter of course. However, the only indication for doing so is to investigate the presence of ligamentous instability, which is rare in the absence of trauma, most often occurring in rheumatoid patients. Indeed, one study found that one in three patients had too much pain and/or muscle spasm for adequate flexion/extension views to be obtained. More detailed imaging is indicated where this will influence management—this occurs most commonly when there are marked neurological features, or where such signs are intractable with conservative treatment. Magnetic resonance imaging is invaluable in assessing soft-tissue structures and in identifying intervertebral disc lesions. Imaging findings should, however, be correlated with the clinical impression as spurious lesions are increasingly common in older patients. Where bone pathology is suspected (e.g. on the basis of the plain film), an isotope bone scan may identify other sites of involvement, favouring metastatic disease over local pathology. Ultrasound assessment of vasculature may be indicated, offering some advantages over invasive techniques such as conventional or magnetic resonance angiography.

Management

In most cases, neck pain resolves spontaneously over several days to weeks. In one systematic review of the clinical course and prognosis of non-specific neck pain, a median of 46 per cent (range 22–79 per cent) of patients who had had symptoms for 6 months or more improved with treatment. Acute exacerbations of spondylosis and acute discogenic neck pain may be managed following similar principles to those discussed in the treatment of acute whiplash injuries, though restoration to a full range of movement may not be the aim in a =spondylotic patient. Home exercises have again been shown to be effective, as has postural advice and review of the working environment (see Chapter 6.13). Many physical modalities have been reported, often in small methodologically poor studies of non-specific neck pain, and sytematic reviews of their efficacy have been largely negative. Gross and colleagues[11] identified 13 randomized controlled trials involving a total of 760 patients and concluded there was no benefit from any of the following physical therapies: heat or cold; traction; electrotherapy; biofeedback; spray and stretch; acupuncture; or laser. Kjellman et al.[12] noted possible benefits from pulsed electromagnetic therapy and from active physiotherapy but not from traction, acupuncture, or other physical therapies.

Outcome

The rate of persistence of symptoms varies according to the underlying cause but ranges around 10 per cent.[13] The short-term outcome of acute exacerbations of degenerative spondylosis is good—over 90 per cent recover to the previous level of function and range of movement. However, further episodes almost invariably occur, though patients can learn techniques that reduce the frequency with which medication or other attention is sought. Discogenic presentations resolve with conservative management in over two-thirds of cases. As surgical intervention is rarely required as a first consideration, retrospective studies of outcome after surgery are biased by selection of more severe or complicated cases. Despite this, brachalgia, headache, and neurological manifestations are successfully treated in the few studies reported, but neck pain persists in approximately 25 per cent of these patients.

References

1. Spitzer, W.O., et al. (1995). Scientific monograph of the Quebec Task Force on whiplash associated disorder: redefining "whiplash" and its management. Spine 20 (suppl. 8), 1–73.

2. Holt, L. (1971). Frequency of symptoms for different age groups and professions. In Cervical pain (ed. C. Hirsch and Y. Zotterman), pp. 17–20. Pergamon Press, New York.

3. Schrader, H., et al. (1996). Natural evolution of late whiplash syndrome outside the medicolegal context. Lancet 347, 1207–1211.

4. Lord, S.M., Barnsley, L., Wallis, B.J., McDonald, G.J., and Bogdak, N. (1996). Percutaneous radiofrequency neurotomy for chronic cervical zygapophyseal-joint pain. N. Engl. J. Med. 335, 1721–1726.

5. Ronnen, H.R., et al. (1996). Acute whiplash injury: is there a role for MR imaging? A prospective study of 100 patients. Radiology 201, 93–96.

6. Radanov, B.P. and Sturzenneger, M. (1996). Predicting recovery from common whiplash. Eur. Neurol. 36, 48–51.

7. Barnsley, L., Lord, S., and Bogduk, N. (1998). The pathophysiology of whiplash. In Cervical Flexion – extension whiplash injuries. Spine State of the Art Reviews. vol 12. (ed. E.A. Malanga) pp. 209–242. Philadelphia.

8. Bonk, A.D., Ferrari, R., Giebel, G.D., Edelmann, M., and Huser, R. (2000). Prospective randomised controlled study of activity versus collar and the natural history of whiplash injury in Germany. J. Musculoskeletal Pain 8, 123–132.

9. Rosenfeld, M. et al. (2000). Early intervention in whiplash-associated disorder: a comparison of two treatment protocols. Spine 25, 1782–1787.

10. Squires, B., Gorgon, M.F., and Bannister, G.C. (1996). Soft-tissue injuries of the cervical spine: 15 years follow-up. J. Bone Joint Surg. (Br). 78, 955–957.

11. Gross, A.L., Aker, P.D., Goldsmith, C.H., and Pelos, P. (2000). Physical medicine modalities for mechanical neck disorders. Cochrane Database Syst. Rev. (2), CD000961.

12. Kjellman, G.V., Skugren, E.L., and Oberg, B.E. (1999). A critical analysis of randomised clinical trials on neck pain and treatment efficacy. A review of the literature. Scand. J. Rehabil. Med. 31, 139–152.

13. Mäkelä, M., Heliövaara, M., Sievers, K., Impivaara, O. et al. (1991). Prevalence, determinants and consequences of chronic neck pain in Finland. Am. J. Epidemiol. 134, 1356–1367.

6.2 Acute spinal pain

Jeremy Fairbank

Introduction

Back pain is so common as to be an almost universal affliction. Ennui or professed ignorance rapidly overwhelms all but a dedicated few of doctors when confronted with this complaint. However, it is a symptom that can be analysed by careful listening and a knowledge of the fascinating complexity of the spine and pain mechanisms. This chapter gives an account of 'acute' low back pain, although the definitions of 'acute' have been stretched, since many acute problems become chronic in this field. Back pain heads the list of condition-related health costs. In 1998 the estimated total health cost of back pain in the United Kingdom was £1632 million (of which a third was contributed by the patient) and employment-related costs were £10,668 million.[1] These costs relate to both acute and chronic back pain.

Acute spinal pain definitions

1. *Lumbago.* Traditional term for low back pain. Never properly defined.

2. *Low(er) back pain.* Usually in the region of the lumbar spine. May include buttock pain.

3. *Sciatica.* First citation by Shakespeare in *Timon of Athens* as a curse. Never properly defined since, and not for clinical use. Literally, 'hip pain'.

4. *Referred pain.* Phenomenon first identified by Kellgren.[2–4] Present throughout the spine, where pain is experienced distal from the site of stimulation. In the cervical and lumbar spine this is usually about two segments distal to the painful level. Figure 1 shows the pain patterns arising from segmental fractures or metastases. In the low lumbar spine, this means that pain spreads into the lower limbs. Usually this is the posterior thigh on one or both sides, but it may spread further when chronic or severe. It behaves like a 'thermometer' of pain severity and is frequently confused with root pain. It is synonymous with sclerodermal or myofascial pain. This type of pain can be generated by experimental stimulation of the apophyseal joints by hypertonic saline[5] and of the intervertebral disc by heat.[6] Pain arising in the hip is usually experienced in the groin or over the greater trochanter (rarely in the buttock), and may be referred into the anterior thigh or knee. This presents a well known diagnostic pitfall. About 5 per cent of back pain referrals in our unit have pain arising in the hip joint.

5. *Root pain.* Pain is experienced in the dermatomal distribution of a nerve root (see Fig. 2). L3 and L4 pains are usually experienced on the anterior thigh, and are exacerbated by the femoral stretch test. L5 pain is usually felt on the anterolateral aspect of the shin and dorsomedial foot. It is exacerbated by the sciatic stretch test. S1 pain

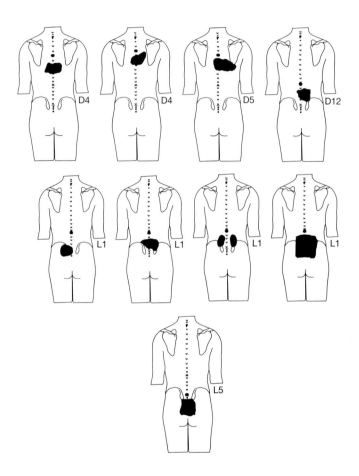

Fig. 1 Pain patterns arising from a single segment lesion (fracture or metastasis). (Taken from J.C.T. Fairbank (1981), MD (Cantab) thesis.)

is usually felt on the calf and lateral side and sole of the foot and exacerbated by the sciatic stretch test. Pain from more distal sacral nerve roots is experienced in the perineum, is more likely to be bilateral, and may be a warning of cauda equina compression. Note that root pain can be combined with referred pain as well as being confused with it. The dermatome charts look very neat and tidy, but remember their provenance (shingles, surgical section of a nerve root, disc prolapse, and microdissection). Remember too that there are anatomical variants (pre- and postfixation of the spine), which may mean that a clear-cut root level is not always established clinically. Standing, walking, and coughing often exacerbate root pain.

6. *Facet (or apophyseal) joints.* Paired synovial joints of varying size and orientation by level. Popular but often unconfirmed source of back and referred pain.

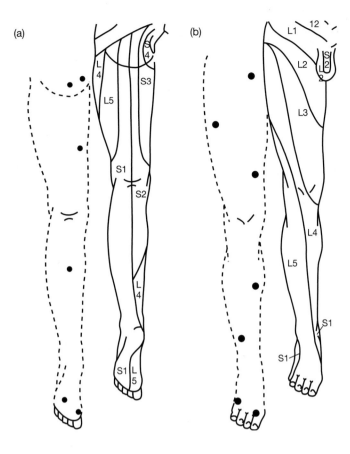

Fig. 2 (a) Posterior lower limb dermatome chart with advised areas in which to check sensation. (b) Anterior lower limb dermatome chart with advised areas to check sensation.

7. *Sacroiliac joints.* A paired, large and unique joint of the pelvic ring. Popularly attributed as a major source of back pain. This is only confirmed in a few cases.

8. *Neurogenic claudication* is back and leg pain exacerbated by standing and walking. Sitting or squatting down relieves it. Many patients find it easier to walk if they have something to lean on, such as a push chair or supermarket trolley. Many patients report that it is easier to use a bicycle than to walk.[7] Spinal stenosis was first described by Verbiest, who distinguished two types, developmental or acquired.[8] The term neurogenic claudication was coined by Blau and Logue.[9] Achondroplastic dwarfs commonly have developmental spinal stenosis. There is a normal distribution of lumbar spinal canal diameter in the population. Occasionally, those with very narrow canals may present as young adults with the symptom. More commonly, these individuals are vulnerable to secondary distortions of the vertebral canal by disc degeneration, osteophytes, and crumpling of the ligamentum flavum. Should a disc prolapse occur, it is much more likely to be symptomatic in individuals with a narrow canal.[10, 11] Symptoms may be uni- or bilateral. The former is more usually associated with stenosis of the 'lateral recess' or of the exit foramen. Bilateral symptoms may be due to central stenosis or to bilateral exit foraminal problems. More than one level may be involved.

9. *Chronic pain syndrome.* Whilst it is not directly in the remit of this chapter, all patients with chronic back pain have to start somewhere. It is not easy to predict which acute pain patient of today will become the chronic patient of tomorrow. Psychosocial factors are undoubtedly important, but they do not explain everything.[12, 13] Evidence for a reduced pain threshold has come from one recent study,[14] but this explains only 12 per cent of the variance.

Epidemiology

Much information has been gathered and the references given here should lead the interested back to other studies. I have quoted various sources, including a 1999 UK Department of Health survey,[15] a 1994 study from the University of York,[16] and the South Manchester Study.[13] All these surveys are poor at distinguishing one diagnostic group from another, not least because there is so little agreement as to classification.

It is generally agreed that the vast majority of early attacks of back pain are self-limiting. Fifty per cent have improved by 1 week and 90 per cent by 8 weeks. The rest (7–10 per cent) become chronic.[17] In a study from California, about half (49 per cent) of all episodes lasted 1 week or less, two-thirds of all episodes lasted 1 month or less, 84 per cent of episodes lasted 3 months or less, and 92 per cent of all episodes lasted 6 months or less.[18] The authors of this study concluded 'about 20–25 per cent of "non-elderly" adult Americans will have at least one episode of back pain care in a 3- or 5-year period. Over 70 per cent of these people will have only one episode during this time, and most of these episodes will be short lived (less than 1 month) and consist of a handful of practitioner visits . . . 5 per cent of persons had four or more episodes of back pain care during this time frame, and about 8 per cent of episodes lasted longer than 6 months or involved more than 20 practitioner visits'. There have been a number of studies to identify factors predicting chronicity. Factors that have been identified include high perceived disability at presentation (e.g. Oswestry Disability Index > 50 per cent), older age (e.g. > 45 years), abnormal gait, and a past history of taking time off work. These explain only a small part of this phenomenon (Dr Margareta Nordin, Presidential address, International Society for the Lumbar Spine, Adelaide 2000).

Prevalence, or the total number of cases at any one time, varies from 12 to 35 per cent between studies.[19] In one study, the 1-year prevalence of the general population reporting constant pain in last 12 months was 6 per cent.[16] The same report states a lifetime prevalence of back pain of 49–80 per cent.[16] The lifetime prevalence of 'sciatica' is 4–5 per cent.[19]

Back pain accounts for 13 per cent total sickness absence for all conditions in the United Kingdom Sickness and Invalidity benefit. Between 1986 and 1992 certified incapacity for back pain has increased from approximately 40–80 million working days (104 per cent increase compared with a 60 per cent increase for other conditions).[16] In the United States, episodes of disabling low back pain increased by 26 per cent between 1974 and 1978.[16]

Suggested factors to explain these increases include:

• prevailing socio-economic conditions (unemployment, workings of disability system)

• greater public awareness of back pain

• changes to increasing sedentary stressful lifestyle

• traditional medical management stressing rest and time off work.

Health costs

In 1998 the estimated health costs of back pain in the United Kingdom were £1632 million. The estimated work-related costs of back pain were £10,668 million.[1] Waddell reports an exponential rise in social security costs attributable to back pain. There is evidence that this rise has at least partially been contained by recent changes in the law in the United Kingdom.[20]

Occupational factors

Social class

Prevalence is increased in lower socio-economic classes. This is confounded by poor educational attainment, increased manual work, and smoking in these groups. This effect may be less obvious in men than women.[19]

Manual handling

Frequent bending and twisting may increase incidence up to six-fold.[19]

Exposure to vibration

Although vibration is commonly held to be implicated in low back pain,[21] this was not supported in a recent study.[22]

Smoking

There is some evidence to link smoking with back pain. It is dose-related and the incidence falls after stopping smoking. Smoking reduces the fusion rate in lumbar arthrodesis procedures.[23–30] In addition, candidates for spinal fusion are more likely to be smokers than age-matched controls.[31]

Driving

This is attributed to prolonged sitting and poor strength and endurance of trunk muscles.[26]

Clinical evaluation

Introduction

The history is the most important part of this process, and may take some time to gather. This is not always easy in a busy clinic. Low back pain is one of the most common presenting complaints in clinical practice. Back pain is sometimes the presenting complaint where there is serious underlying pathology. It may be difficult or impossible to distinguish these cases from the generality of back pain complaints. In general, history gives much more valuable information than the examination.[32]

The principal objectives of the clinician are: (1) to identify those patients with serious underlying pathology; and (2) to try to place the rest in clinical groups relevant to the available treatment options. Since the cause of the pain is not understood, both the diagnoses and explanations given to patients are inconsistent. This causes uncertainty and, in some cases, prolongation of symptoms. Generally, the treatment options are non-operative. Surgery has a definite role in the management of root pain, particularly in the presence of progressive neurological deficit or neurogenic claudication. The place of surgery in the

management of some cases of back and referred pain, usually when conservative treatment has failed, is both controversial and irrelevant to a chapter on acute back pain.

History

Diagnosis is made mainly on the basis of history, so time must be spent with the patient listening to their complaints. Proformas and computer-based interview systems may aid this process. Curiously, few studies have examined the reliability of the process of history-taking. The history may well not be as reliable as we might think it to be. For example, Biering-Sorenson and Hilden,[33] in a prospective study, found that only 85 per cent of patients with back pain could recall that they had an X-ray of their lumbar spine a year after the X-ray had been taken. We compared a structured history taken with the aid of a proforma from patients with low back pain with a history taken by computer-based questionnaire a week apart.[34] We had to use the verbal history as a baseline, and found a 95 per cent agreement between the two. It is commonplace for experienced doctors to obtain different histories from a patient on different occasions. As so much depends on the history, this is an area where more research is needed, and the clinician must always proceed with caution. Knowledge and experience help a clinician to ask the right questions, and it also helps to give the patient time to reply and to listen to what they are saying.

Age

Patients presenting with back pain who younger than 18 years or older than 60 should be reviewed with particular care. Symptomatic disc prolapse is uncommon in teenagers and unusual over the age of 60 years. Posterior annular tears usually occur under the age of 25 years following trauma (usually a severe axial and sometime rotatory injury to the lumbar spine). Neurogenic claudication is unusual below the age of 40, but can occur even in teenagers with developmental spinal stenosis. It is increasingly recognized in the post-retirement population, but there are no reliable data on prevalence available. Spondylolysis and spondylolisthesis may manifest themselves at any age, but they tend to cause back pain under the age of 40 years and neurogenic symptoms in older patients. Serious pathology (infections and tumours) presents in a larger proportion of patients outside this age range than within it. Vertebral crush fractures due to osteoporosis or metastases are common causes of back pain in the elderly.

Back pain in children

Back pain is common in children (between 7 and 40 per cent prevalence in cross-sectional series).[35–39] One longitudinal survey series concluded it had little to do with adult back pain.[40] Another carefully designed prospective study compared adolescents with and without back pain. They found that lack of exercise was frequent in the symptomatic group.[41] This confirmed a finding of our cross-sectional study.[37] The same investigator followed adolescents identified as having disc degeneration at the age of 14 and found that many of this selected population had become symptomatic by age 22.[42]

A brief account of other factors relating to back pain in children and adolescents follows and a detailed review can be found in Balagué *et al.*[39] Factors include age (it becomes more frequent with increasing age) and gender (it is slightly more common in females). Family history is relevant to disc herniation, spondylolysis, and non-specific back pain, and some early evidence implicates the vitamin D receptor gene.[43] Height and sitting height have been implicated in adolescent back pain in our study,[37] supported by references 41 and 44 but not supported by the earlier study in reference 45.

An audit of children referred with back pain to an orthopaedic surgeon found that up to 50 per cent had identifiable pathology to explain their symptoms.[46]

Pain

The clinician should be familiar with the concepts of referred pain, root pain, neurogenic claudication, and chronic pain syndrome—and the distinctions between them. The pain pattern, character, diurnal features, and exacerbating and relieving factors are all relevant. Severity can be assessed formally but an informal assessment is the normal process. The detection of exaggeration and illness behaviour is not easy, and many clinicians have been caught out by dismissing patients' symptoms of a serious underlying pathology as hysterical.

Red flags

The Royal College of General Practitioners has issued guidelines for possible serious spinal pathology, the so-called 'red flag' symptoms and signs (see Table 1).[47] These are based on opinion and observation.[48–50] In our experience these guidelines are by no means foolproof. Many patients with serious pathology fall within these categories, but a significant proportion do not. Constant vigilance for the unusual or unexplained is important. Screening with plain radiographs is unsatisfactory, and we recommend the use of magnetic resonance (MR) scanning when imaging patients with persisting unexplained symptoms. Radiologists have developed 'limited' scan protocols, which are useful in screening this group of patients.

Pain pattern

Pain from a specific level in the spine (e.g. a metastasis) is usually referred about two segments distal to its source in the cranial part of the spine (Fig. 1). The referral tends to be further from the source of the pain in the caudal part of the spine. This pain does not, in general, go to the front of the trunk or lower limb. Percussion or palpation of the spine may aid localization of the source level (although, curiously, pain from discitis, which is often severe and of fairly rapid onset, is not always exacerbated in this way).

Root pain is usually dermatomal, although there are significant individual variations. Historically, a variety of methods have been used to derive dermatome charts (see Fig. 2). Sometimes these can be

Table 1 Clinical guidelines for the management of acute low back pain

RCGP guidelines[47]
Presentation under age 20 or onset over 55
Non-mechanical pain
Thoracic pain
Past history—carcinoma, steroids, HIV
Unwell, weight loss
Widespread neurology
Structural deformity

confirmed by examination by light touch and pinprick testing. Referred pain is difficult, because it varies with sensitivity and is not associated with reliable clinical signs. It rarely radiates below the knee, unless the pain is severe or chronic.

Patients with neurogenic claudication have difficulty in defining the site and nature of their symptoms. Some deny that they experience pain at all, preferring such terms as 'heaviness'. The distribution of this pain is a poor guide as to which nerves are involved. Bilateral lower limb pain implies a central lesion. This may be central stenosis, a central disc prolapse, or a tumour affecting the cord, conus, or cauda equina.

The term myofascial pain describes a wide variety of musculoskeletal symptoms. These have characteristic pain patterns that may be small and localized. One such syndrome has trigger points over the posterior iliac crest and an associated pain pattern. These pains may respond to a local anaesthetic injection. Myofascial pain is dealt with in a detailed fashion in Chapter 6.11.

If a pain drawing is used to identify pain patterns, patients with excessive illness behaviour may be identified by the extent of their pain pattern and the graffiti that they add to the drawing. Pain drawings are simple and effective identifiers of these patients and may be used as an outcome measure.[51]

Pain arising in the hip joint is usually felt in the groin. It frequently radiates into the anterior thigh or knee. This pain is usually exacerbated by getting out of a chair as well as by walking, although, in the early stages of osteoarthritis of the hip, continued exercise can relieve pain after the initial painful movement. These symptoms can be fully evaluated by examining the hip. Gauvain's test, in which the extended leg is gently rolled by the examiner while the patient is lying and relaxed, produces either pain or involuntary ipsilateral abdominal contracture. Rotation in flexion or abduction may also reproduce hip pain.

Diurnal and longer-term fluctuations in back pain

Night pain can be a sinister symptom, and is one of the features of pain from fractures, metastases, and infections, especially if the pain is continuous in waking hours. Benign spinal tumours are notoriously difficult to diagnose. Consider them in patients with persisting night pain, especially when lying flat. They usually, but not always, have neurological signs. These signs include segmental alterations or deficits in sensation, absent abdominal reflexes, as well as the more familiar long tract signs. Scoliotics tend to have fatigue pain where the pain gets worse through the day. Ankylosing spondylitis is characterized by severe and prolonged morning stiffness (all patients with back pain report some morning stiffness to a greater or lesser extent).

Most patients' back pain is variable in its intensity, and in the duration and frequency of attacks. Patients with chronic back pain, particularly those in whom the pain itself has become a problem, complain of continuous symptoms and sleep disruption. Most, on direct questioning, admit sleeping several hours each night and concede that there are times when pain is not felt. In general, the pattern of periodicity is not of much help in diagnosing back pain syndromes, although it is of value in assessing disability. Many chronic sufferers of back pain describe their pain switching on and off for no obvious reason. They may seek medical advice because of a crescendo of frequency and duration of attacks of pain. The type 5 patient (see below) reports continuous and unremitting pain night and day.

Walking-related pain

Walking (and often just standing still) usually exacerbates root pain. Neurogenic claudication has a variable walking distance from day to day. The patient or spouse may notice a flexed posture during walking. Sometimes it is easier walking up hill. Riding a bicycle may not be painful, even when walking is severely restricted.[7] Many patients find it much easier to walk while pushing a supermarket trolley or wheeled-walker. This may reflect relief of pain and discomfort in the erector spinae muscles because of the flexed posture as much as any intrinsic pain due to the cauda equina compression. It is often not possible for these patients to 'walk through' the pain as vascular claudicants can. Neurogenic claudication may be distinguished from vascular claudication by the duration of recovery. Vascular claudicants usually can carry on walking after 1–3 min, whereas cauda equina claudication requires 5–20 min for recovery.[52]

Sitting-related pain

Many chronic back pain patients are intolerant of sitting, which may relate to raised intradisc pressure whilst sitting or during enforced and prolonged flexion of the spine.[53] Driving is a recognized risk factor for chronic back pain and intervertebral disc herniation. Sitting tends to relieve the pain of neurogenic claudication.

Gender

The overall incidence of back pain is similar in men and women. Disc degeneration and disc prolapse, lytic spondylolysis, and spondylolisthesis, are more common in males. Degenerative spondylolisthesis is more common in females.

Occupation

Heavy manual work is not as strong a factor as is often assumed. Manual handling may be related to an increased incidence of back pain. An outline is given in the 'Epidemiology' section of this chapter. Sitting and exposure to vibration is important,[21] and, on this basis, it is not surprising that driving is an important factor in the incidence of back pain. and of intervertebral disc prolapse. Coal miners are less likely to have an intervertebral disc prolapse but are more likely to develop disc degeneration at an earlier age than a control population of manual workers.[54] It is inevitable that, because of the difficulties that clinicians have in defining diagnostic groups, epidemiologists tend to lump all back pain syndromes together. Back pain undoubtedly presents more of a problem to members of social classes 4 and 5 because their work tends to be more physical, and social service payments depend on inability to work. The structure of workmen's compensation systems has a profound effect on the incidence and duration of back symptoms. The longer an individual is off work, the less likely he or she is to return to work. This finding seems to be less dependent on the welfare system. There are also strong confounding factors such as smoking and litigation following actual or perceived injury to the spine.[55]

Training in manual handling may be of importance in reducing symptoms in this group. There is some evidence that fitness programmes in the working environment can lead to significant falls in sickness absence for back pain and other conditions. There are some jobs at the extreme of the ergonomic envelope for spinal loads that may cause back problems, particularly if these involve lifting and twisting simultaneously. Rapid jerk lifts put much higher loads on the spine than slow gradual lifts.

Onset of symptoms

The nature of the original onset of symptoms, and how an attack starts is worth analysis. Type 1 pain (see below) usually starts acutely, usually whilst performing normal activities. Osteoporotic crush fractures usually precipitate acute pain if they are symptomatic (only about 25 per cent of osteoporotic crush fractures cause pain). Type 2 pain tends to begin insidiously at the start of an attack, although the sufferer may blame a particular episode for the pain. Frequently, patients will admit that there was no obvious precipitating factor to an attack. Disc prolapses almost always start with an insidious onset back pain followed at a later stage by root pain. The delay in onset of root pain varies from minutes to years. The appearance of the root pain may be accompanied by reduction or loss of the back pain.

There is the expectation amongst patients and their doctors that a precipitating cause for their back pain can always be found. Litigation may be a factor in this quest. In a study at the Canadian Back Institute, 70 per cent of 6000 non-compensation responders to a questionnaire were unable to identify a specific injury to account for the onset of their symptoms (Hamilton Hall, personal communication). There is no doubt that severe back symptoms can develop after an injury, and that the onset of symptoms may be delayed. The pathological basis for this observation comes from work in Adelaide on the consequences of a surgical injury to the annulus of a sheep's lumbar intervertebral disc. The initial wound heals rapidly, but degenerative changes invariably appear in the disc over the following year.[56] There is no evidence that this process causes pain to the sheep, and disc degeneration is often painless in humans. However, there is quite convincing evidence in the discography literature that an annular tear is often painful. Causation may be admitted if there is a delay between injury and symptom onset of up to 2 weeks. If the delay is longer than this, there must be convincing reasons for this such as an associated head injury, other injuries delaying the mobilization of the patient, or a spine fracture elsewhere in the spine masking the pain of the disc injury.

Other exacerbating and relieving factors

Changes in the weather or, more specifically, changes in barometric pressure often influence back pain. It is now widely accepted that coughing frequently exacerbates mechanical back pain with muscle spasm, as well as the more commonly recognized increase of dural and nerve root pain.

Pain type

The words used to describe back pain are often culturally determined. This means that many doctors discount the importance of the descriptive phrases. Some descriptive terms such as 'burning', 'pins and needles', or 'numbness', may be associated with radicular pain, whereas 'cramp' or 'ache' tend to relate to vascular or referred pain. Pain description is formalized in the McGill pain questionnaire, which uses precise descriptive terms to estimate the severity of pain.[57] In our own practice we have not found this technique helpful in assessing our patients. These terms may have some value in eliciting the source of pain in the individual, but they have resisted useful analysis.

Smoking

The role of smoking in the genesis of back pain is controversial. There is no consensus in the literature from epidemiological studies. There is a strong clinical impression that chronic back pain patients are heavy smokers, but the relationship has not yet been established. There are possible adverse effects on intervertebral disc nutrition. Smoking has been shown to be a risk factor in pseudo-arthrosis following spinal fusion.[23–30, 58, 59] Smoking is more common in a population of patients offered spinal fusion than in the general population.[31]

General medical questions

Some systemic conditions may present with back pain. Tuberculosis and other infections, metastases, lymphomas, pancreatitis, or a leaking aortic aneurysm can all cause pain in the back. Pain arising from metastases and from infection is frequently unremitting and may be worse at night. The patient should be asked about weight loss, eating habits, disturbances of digestion, bowel and bladder function, night sweats, drugs, and allergies. Diabetes mellitus, hypothyroidism, osteoporosis, osteomalacia and other metabolic bone diseases, psoriasis, and pregnancy may all be factors in the development of back pain. Extraforaminal root pain may be caused (rarely) by pressure, irritation, or invasion by a wide variety of agents, such as fibroids, other pelvic tumours, colonic malposition, psoas abscess, and the piriformis syndrome. Any patient with an unusual story should be listened to and examined with particular care.

Osteoporosis of the spine is common. There is no evidence to suggest that osteoporosis is intrinsically painful. It may well be associated with vertebral crush fractures. These fractures are common, and only about 25 per cent are symptomatic. The majority of cases are self-limiting, but a few can cause prolonged and severe symptoms. Management is discussed below.

Family history

Back pain is so common that a family history of back pain may be of little value. There is some evidence that intervertebral disc prolapse may run in families, particularly in adolescents and young adults. The evidence for familial spinal stenosis is tenuous. Intervertebral disc degeneration in adolescents is a risk factor for back pain,[42] and this might have genetic basis.

Psychological factors

Listening to the patient should be the most effective way of assessing the psychological component of a patient's history—the so-called 'yellow flags'. Unfortunately, even the most experienced clinician may be misled. Inconsistencies in the patient's history should be noted. The inappropriate symptoms and signs described by Waddell have some merit, Unfortunately, their reliability is not very good.[60] They have been misused in medicolegal practice, and the originators do not recommend them in this area.[61] They are not always good predictors of individual outcome.[62] These symptoms often resolve if the pain can be treated successfully.

The patient who gives a history full of psychogenic features may still have organic disease. Psychological questionnaires are widely used in the assessment of back pain patients. In the United Kingdom the DRAM is probably the most widely used. In the United States the MMPI is popular, but unwieldy. Studies have shown that outcomes are consistently worse in high scorers on these questionnaires. However, there is also evidence that high scorers on the DRAM questionnaire who do respond to treatment will record significant improvements in the DRAM score, suggesting that these responses are secondary to symptoms in at least some cases. Pain patterns may be a simple and effective alternative to these questionnaires.[63] Secondary gain through illness behaviour for economic or personal reasons is common. Illness behaviour also is manifest in individuals by their doctor's inability to cure their symptoms or to take them seriously. The structure of the social services payment system is an important factor in the rise in back pain symptoms in developed countries. Litigation over personal injury claims has long been recognized as having an important effect on treatment outcome and reported disability.

Assessment of impairment, disability, and handicap

Definitions are important here. The WHO (1980) defines disability as 'any restriction or lack of ability (resulting from an impairment) to perform an activity in the manner or within the range considered normal for a human being'. An impairment is 'any loss or abnormality of psychological, physiological, or anatomical structure or function'. Thus, back pain is an impairment that may cause disability. A handicap is 'a disadvantage for a given individual, resulting from an impairment or disability, that limits or prevents the fulfillment of a role (depending on age, sex and social and cultural factors) for that individual'. Again, back pain can be a potent source of handicap. Clearly, there are grey areas between these definitions, and assessment methods may cross between these groupings.

There are number of specific questionnaires designed to assess disability in back pain patients. In clinical practice the Roland–Morris questionnaire (especially in general practice) and the Oswestry Disability Index have emerged as front runners. The Shuttle Walking test shows promise as an 'objective' measure of disability and handicap.

Impairment measures often rely on range of movement of the lumbar spine. In clinical practice range of movement is a poor measure of impairment. Much work was done in this area by Professor Verna Wright's group in Leeds.[64] We have not found this approach useful as an outcome measure. I consider it to be an important part of the initial appraisal of a patient, but poor reliability limits its use. Complex and expensive equipment has been developed to assess muscle function in these patients, but these have not found favour in the United Kingdom. There are serious doubts concerning the value of this approach to patient assessment.

General health questionnaires assess disability and handicap, and allow cross-condition comparisons. SF-36 is widely accepted. The Euroquol is popular with health economists. Again there are many questionnaires, and fashions change rapidly in this area.

Specific and general outcome measures for back pain

Roland–Morris (R–M)

This was described and validated in general practice. It consists of 24 dichotomous questions and a linear analogue pain scale.[65]

Oswestry Disability Index (ODI)

The ODI has now been widely adopted in the spine literature since its description in 1980.[66] It was developed in a clinic where many chronic back pain patients attended. It was later modified by the MRC (version 2.0) which was a significant improvement. The ODI has been compared with Roland–Morris,[67] both of which had been modified for use on a computer. They correlate well with one another. The R–M scale is more sensitive for less severe symptoms, but is insensitive to change in the more severe spectrum of symptoms.[68] These instruments have been used to validate other scales, but no obvious improvement on them has emerged. A detailed review by Fairbank and Pynsent contains all the versions of ODI and its validation.[69]

Shuttle walking test

This was developed at Loughborough for the assessment of respiratory function.[70] It was developed for use in the fields of respiratory and cardiac medicine.[71–73] We have used it as an outcome measure for various randomized controlled trials of back pain treatments.[74–76] It has an application in the assessment of patients with neurogenic claudication.[77]

This test requires the patient to walk up and down a 10-m course identified at each end by two cones inset 0.5 m from each end to avoid the need for abrupt changes in direction. The explanation to the patient is standardized and played from a tape at the start of the test. Accuracy of the timed signal is assured by the inclusion on the tape recording of a calibration period of 1 min. The speed at which the patient walks is dictated by an audio signal played on the tape recorder. In the first minute the patient is required to walk up and down the walkway three times (amounting to distance of 30 m). The following minute requires the patient to walk faster and complete 40 m within the time dictated by the audio signal from the tape recorder. The distance is then increased each minute by 10 m, requiring incremental increases in walking speed until the end of the test (12 min in all). To assist the patient in establishing the routine of the test, the assessor walks alongside the patient for the first minute. No form of encouragement is permitted during the test. The patient has to reach the end of the walkway before a tone sounds. The observer counts the number of times the subject passes between the cones. Eventually, the subject cannot reach the other cone before the tone sounds. Even if the endpoint may be controversial on one pass, it rapidly becomes obvious in the next pass or two that it has been achieved. The endpoint of the test is determined either: (1) by the patient stopping because of increased pain or fatigue, or (2) by the operator, if the patient fails to complete a shuttle in the time allocated. This test has been shown to be sensitive to change in patients with chronic low back pain. This test will provide the main 'objective' test of function for patients in this study. A 50-m improvement (5 passes) is considered the minimal change of clinical significance following an intervention (this represents an improvement in speed *and* endurance). We have found that none of our patients selected for surgery for neurogenic claudication can manage more than 200 m, with a mean of only 70 m. A fit adult (mean age 64 years) can usually manage about 600 m on this test.

Examination

There are many accounts of how to examine the lumbar spine. The most important part of appraising the patient is from the history.

There are a few key points in examining a patient that I shall emphasize here. This is based on experience and a study we performed on the reliability of various physical signs.[60] The sequence is based on a series of positions. The patient should be fully undressed to their underclothes. Gowns are contraindicated, as in my experience they have led to important pathology being missed (e.g. a pelvic tumour so large that the contour of the body was obviously disturbed).

Standing

Have the patient point at the area where they are feeling their pain. If this is proximal to the lumbar sacral junction it may well be referred from higher up the spine.

Stand behind the patient and assess:

1. skin (e.g. midline hairy patches, scars, erythema ab igne, and café-au-lait spots);
2. shape of the trunk (e.g. postural asymmetry, rib hump, muscle spasm, tumours);
3. spine (sagittal and coronal alignment, kyphosis, lordosis, scoliosis);
4. sway (also Romberg's sign).

Ask the patient to bend forward and touch the toes if he or she is able. If you suspect a scoliosis, ask the patient to put the hand on his or her knees first, to assess the rib hump (if any). If the hump is on the right, the thoracic curve is convex to the right, and it should be described as such. Thoracolumbar and lumbar curves are best seen when fingertips are midshin or even at toe level. Again the side of the hump will give the direction of the curve. A 'sciatic' scoliosis seen when the patient is standing up normally corrects on forward bend. The degree of bend can be estimated as a percentage of total expected, measured with a tape measure (modified Schrober method),[78] a flexi-curve,[79] or a kyphometer.[80] You may see the trunk veer to one side or another. We found this an unreliable sign.[60] Patients with disc prolapses can sometimes have a surprisingly full forward bend. Side bending can also be assessed at this stage, and estimated or measured with a tape measure.[78] This is the time to assess simulated rotation by turning the pelvis. This is one of Waddell's signs,[81] but not in our experience very reliable.[60] S1 weakness is difficult assess when measuring resisted plantar flexion, so some advise getting the patient to stand on tiptoe on one leg. Unfortunately, this sign was also unreliable in our study. It may also be useful in detecting subtle disturbances of proprioception. Children with mild upper motor neuron problems cannot hop on one leg.

Sitting sideways on the couch, with the knees flexed over the side

I do not always do this, but it can be a time to check the knee and ankle reflexes if the patient finds it difficult to relax. It is a good position to assess 'real' trunk rotation for the Waddell tests. A version of the straight leg raise test can be assessed in this position by extending the knee, but I prefer not to do this (see discussion below).

Lying supine on the couch

Observe the patient's general agility. Inspect him/her for muscle wasting, skin marks, contractures, scars, etc. Feel to assess light touch in the lower limb dermatome areas. If in any doubt you should also assess pinprick sensation. I use the end of a partly unravelled paperclip for this—a disposable needle is too sharp. This examination should be extended up the trunk if you are suspicious of a spinal tumour. Check position sense at this stage if you think it may be abnormal by flexing and extending the great toe, holding its sides. This is the time to check the reflexes, while the patient is still relaxed: knee, ankle, plantar if you must, and abdominal reflexes if you suspect a tumour or if the patient has a scoliosis (absence of a reflex is seen in one or more abdominal quadrant). Reinforcement by clenching the teeth or the Jendrassic manoeuvre may be necessary. The ankle reflexes may also be checked when the patient is prone, if they have difficulty relaxing.

Assess *muscle power* next. This not easy in a patient in pain. I check in the following order: Great toe dorsiflexion (L5), foot dorsiflexion (L5 mainly), foot eversion (L5 mainly), foot plantar flexion (S1, S2—but not always easy to detect slight weakness), knee extension (L3,L4), knee flexion (L4,5;S1,2,3), Hip flexion (resisted straight leg raise) (L4,5;S1,2,3). All through this period assess tone and any spasticity.

The straight leg raise (SLR) test

This test has the highest predictive value for identifying root compression and predicting outcome of any part of the clinical examination. This can usually be done in all but the most distressed patients. It was reliable in our study, when the patient was examined in the way described here.[60] In principle, this test is easy to perform and to assess. Unfortunately, there are several ways of doing it, and so-called experts use all of them. A review of the history of this test will reveal why.[82, 83] Rather than reviewing these accounts, I shall explain my technique, with reasons.

I examine the symptomatic side first. This is the last examination with the patient supine. Experienced and 'professional' patients are used to this test being performed by slowly lifting the heel with the knee extended. This often leads to early overreaction and an inaccute assessment.

The knee and hip are flexed simultaneously, until the knee is in the chest, This will flex the hip fully and will at least flatten the lumbar lordosis, as in the Thomas test. This will reveal:

1. pain arising in the ipsilateral hip (and possibly knee), especially if the hip joint is rotated in flexion;

2. flexion deformities if any on the other side;

3. pain arising from flexion of the lumbar spine.

All of these findings can confuse the interpretation of the SLR test. This can usually be done in all but the most distressed patients.

1. The knee is *gently* extended, allowing the hip to extend, until the leg is straight in the full SLR position. Patients with genuine root pain may be positive at a very small angle, and this is extremely painful. Many other patients referred with reported limited SLR turn out to have no such thing when examined in this way. You will have to ask the patient where they are getting pain. Ideally this should be in the leg or thigh, but may be in the buttock or back.[84]

2. You may wish to confirm root pain by lowering the leg slightly and dorsiflexing the foot. Alternatively, the bowstring test may be used where the knee is slightly flexed, and the popliteal nerve is stretched by the pressure of the examiner's fingers.[85]

3. Cross-leg sensitivity is almost pathognomonic for a disc prolapse. This is when pain is induced in the opposite leg from the one examined.

Examination with the patient prone

Look for skin changes, erythema ab igne, hairy patches, or other midline abnormalities.

The femoral stretch test is in my experience useful for discerning patients with anterior thigh pain caused by root compression in the midlumbar spine. This includes patients with extraforaminal root compression at L4/5, which can cause considerable distress in the middle aged or older patient. Occasionally, you will see a cross-legged response from this test. I think this occurs when the nerve root is particularly sensitive. The test is performed by carefully flexing the knee to the maximum permitted by the patient.

Tenderness is surprisingly useful and reliable.[60] I start in the midline thoracic spine, and work distally. The tender level or levels usually reflects the symptomatic level. This should be related to the site where pain is felt identified during 'the standing up' part of the examination. Sometimes there is a tender spot on the iliac crest (iliac crest syndrome),[86] which is sometimes responsive to local anaesthetic/steroid injection.

The relative value of different clinical symptoms and signs in the evaluation of back pain

Differential diagnoses

A number of clinical and pathological classifications have been reported. A recent United Kingdom working group, CSAG, suggested a three-way classification for use in general practice based on the work of Waddell, to provide guidelines for specialist referral. He divides patients into 'simple', 'root pain', and 'serious pathology'. The problem with this scheme is that it does not identify patients with neurogenic claudication, and it labels all back pain patients as 'simple', which is often clinically inappropriate. In this book Fairbank and Hall's scheme is used. A version of this scheme has been validated, but few if any of its competitors have been.[87] Our scheme identifies the common diagnostic groups presenting to orthopaedic surgeons. Clinical classification is largely based on history. Examination is important, but provides only limited additional information. Plain radiographs have limited value, and should not be used for screening patients with back pain for serious pathology. Increasing use is made of magnetic resonance imaging (MRI) scanning in the routine investigation of patients with low back pain.

A classification of back pain

Type 1 (or 'simple' or 'non-specific' low back pain)

This is the common type of back pain. Attacks occur acutely, and often for no obvious reason. Patients and doctors will search for precipitating factors, although these are often everyday events or actions. The vast majority of attacks will settle within 6 weeks, and are generally handled in family practice, by physiotherapists, or by chiropractors and osteopaths. If the symptoms are prolonged or severe specialist advice is sought, depending on the structure and availability of services. The majority of pain is felt in the lumbar spine, but there may be referral to buttocks or thighs. Pain is rarely felt below the knee in this group. Pain tends to be worst sitting, and is often better with activity. Treatment is activity. Attacks are self-limiting, although they may be recurrent. Because attacks are relatively short, most interventions will show a good effect. Movement may be restricted and there are no abnormal neurological signs.

Type 2: chronic back pain

The interface between types 1 and 2 is indistinct. This group has chronic persistent symptoms that may recur. Often the onset is insidious or can be anticipated by the patient. The pain may be felt in the back or referred into the thigh or even further down the leg depending on severity—so-called thermometer pain. It tends to be unresponsive to simple physiotherapy. Again response may be seen to a wide variety of interventions. There is a trend towards managing these patients in specialized rehabilitation programmes. A small group of these patients may be suitable for spinal fusion/spinal stabilization. Usually there is restricted movement and localized spinal tenderness. There should be no abnormal neurological signs.

Type 3: root pain

These patients have back and leg pain in a dermatomal distribution. L5 can usually be distinguished from S1 in the distribution in the foot. L4 usually has a strong component of anterior thigh pain. In classical disc prolapse the back pain precedes the leg pain, which eventually predominates. It is not usually possible to distinguish lateral recess stenosis from disc herniation clinically. The straight leg raise is restricted and there may be motor deficits.

Type 4: neurogenic claudication

This group presents with walking-related back and leg pain. They are usually middle-aged or older, but it can occur in the young as well. These patients are intolerant of standing and walking and, usually, relieved by sitting, squatting, or lying. Often there are no neurological signs, or at least only ones that might be attributed to ageing.

Type 5: unclassifiable—includes tumour, infection, psychological back pain

These patients have symptoms that do not fit easily in other groups. Any patients with strange or persisting symptoms, rest pain, or night pain that cannot otherwise be explained fall into this group. On occasion, it is clinically impossible to distinguish those patients with serious pathology from those without. Serious pathology includes infection, fractures, and tumours (especially metastases).

Central disc prolapse

This is associated with severe back pain, often but not always bilateral, extending into the legs. The rate of onset varies considerably from acute to acute on chronic pain. There is usually but not always restriction in the straight leg raise test. Ankle reflexes are absent. There is altered or absent perianal sensation on one or both sides. There may well be lower limb weakness especially of plantar flexion. The patient has difficulty in standing straight. There may be disturbance of bladder or bowel function.

Disc space infection

Anecdotally, these seem to be becoming more common in the United Kingdom. This may reflect an increasing proportion of the elderly in the population and changes in the bacterial population. These patients will present with gradually increasing back pain with girdle or referred pain. The referred pain may predominate, so that chest or abdominal pain is the presenting feature. This is misleading and commonly diagnosis is delayed. There may be a history of urinary tract infection or other source of bacteraemia.

Investigation

Imaging

When it is available MR scanning is much the most useful investigation of low back pain. In the vast majority of cases of 'acute' low back pain no imaging is needed. It is necessary for cases falling into the type 3 and the type 5 groups. In general, no imaging is needed for the first 8 weeks, unless there are 'red flag' features, progressive neurology, or increasing pain. If there is a suspicion of spinal cord or cauda equina compression, then an emergency scan may be needed. MR is superior to other available modalities in diagnosing tumours, infections, and fractures.

Plain X-rays are really only helpful in assessing fracture. This diagnosis can usually be suspected from the history. X-rays carry poor specificity for infections and tumours, unless they are considerably advanced, and have no ability to detect disc prolapses.

Computerized tomography (CT) is helpful for delineating bony anatomy and can detect tumours and infection where there is bony destruction. CT scans can be used to detect disc prolapses. The problems with CT are, first, that it carries a significant radiation dose and, second, that it is impracticable to screen the whole lumbar spine. For these reasons I would not recommend CT as a primary investigation for low back pain.

Discography is not indicated for acute low back pain.

Facet blocks can be done under X-ray control for diagnostic and therapeutic indications. Rarely if ever are they indicated for the management of acute low back pain.

Blood tests

Tests for spondyloarthropathies are outside the scope of this chapter. Patients with suspected tumours and infections need a full blood count, sedimentation rate, and C-reactive protein measured. Those with suspected infection should have blood cultures. Serological tests for *Brucella* may be helpful.

Management

Type 1

This is generally self-limiting. Advice includes maintaining activity and avoiding bedrest. The points made below for type 2 back pain may also be relevant. The Back Book may be helpful. (HM Stationery Office, London.)

Type 2

Most patients referred to the hospital specialist will fall into this group. History and examination are important. Investigation depends on resources available and the preferred approach of the treating clinician. I prefer to have a limited MR scan on all patients except those with limited or short-lived symptoms.

The reasons in favour of scanning are these:

1. You can be sure that there is no serious pathology. Unfortunately, history and examination are not foolproof even in the most experienced hands.

2. The patient is confident that you 'know what the matter is'. My line is actually that in most cases we do *not* know what the matter is. It is likely that there are wear and tear changes in the discs that are seen in most adults. These changes are associated with back pain in some people, but that many have these changes without symptoms. I stress that muscle dysfunction is likely to be an important element in back pain. Exercises and physiotherapy and fitness programmes will help this, but will take time. I also say that whatever is done is unlikely to completely cure back pain, but that it will help to make it tolerable. I stress that the natural history is generally benign. Many patients have a view that they will be in a wheelchair before very long. I specifically discount this.

The reasons for not scanning are these:

1. You can find something 'wrong' on every scan performed.

2. These abnormalities may generate unnecessary alarm and despondency in the patient and precipitate ill-advised interventions or illness behaviour.

3. There are resource implications.

In my view alternative imaging is more misleading than MR is. It is possible to bring down the real costs of MR if limited scans are used and the unit is run efficiently.

There are many non-operative therapeutic interventions available. Many of these have been subjected to randomized controlled trials. I quote the meta-analysis of van Tulder *et al.*[88] to demonstrate the current level of evidence for these interventions. A Cochrane review of surgical intervention suggested that the there was poor evidence to support surgery for back pain.[89] It should certainly not be considered for the back pain patient.

Type 3

Many patients with root pain will recover within 6 weeks of onset. I encourage activity, but here the case against bed-rest is less strong. In some cases it may be appropriate for short periods. I discourage the 'strict' bed-rest regimes that many of us were trained to use. I think it quite reasonable for someone with severe sciatica to take to his or her bed several times a day, but they should be on the move between times. If the pain is severe and neurological signs are deteriorating, or if there is any other reason to suspect a central disc prolapse, then an MR scan is indicated without delay. Some patients have little or no evidence of root compression, and it is in these that I believe that epidural injections of steroids work best. The quality of evidence is not good in this area. The meta-analysis of Watts *et al.* is helpful to read for those interested.[90] It does not seem to make much difference by what route the epidural is given (caudal or interspinous). If there is significant root compromise clinically or radiologically then in my experience epidurals are less effective. We are still awaiting trials to resolve this area. It is very difficult to resolve the treatment effect in a condition where the natural history is towards resolution. There are wide variations in clinical practice.

Nerve root infiltration with local anaesthetic and steroid is an alternative to an epidural. A recent study of 160 patients found a beneficial effect of bipuvicaine/steroid (80 mg methyl prednisolone) over a injection of saline from the point of view of leg pain at 2 weeks, but the saline group was better at 3 months in terms of back pain. Both groups tended to improve with time. By 1 year, 18 in the steroid group and 15 in the saline group had had surgery.[91]

Natural history

Most patients with symptomatic disc prolapses get better. The most important study was completed by Weber in Oslo. He looked at a population of patients with disc prolapses. The most serious he operated on. The remainder he randomized to surgery or non-operative care. The surgical group showed a clear early advantage in pain relief. Four years post-intervention there was little to choose between the groups, and by 10 years the outcomes were identical. Recurrence rate varies from one study to another. My rule of thumb is 10 per cent recurrence in 10 years.

Surgical treatment

A Cochrane review of surgical intervention suggested that there was reasonable evidence to support surgery for disc prolapse.[89] The objective of surgery is to decompress a nerve root. This is usually achieved by removing the disc fragment or fragments. These may protrude from the disc, be extruded from it, or be sequestrated. It may be necessary to remove bone, ligamentum flavum, and joint capsule or even part of the facet joint to decompress fully the nerve root. The surgeon will also attempt to remove all loose fragments from the disc space to try to reduce the risk of recurrence. Some surgeons go to extreme lengths to remove endplate as well. There is no evidence that this practice is effective, and it may well increase postoperative back pain. The surgery itself may range from the very easy to challengingly difficult. As in many surgical procedures it is probably best (although difficult to prove) to find a surgeon who is operating on at least 20 discs each year. Many but not all surgeons use magnification (loupes or an operating microscope). There is doubt whether this affects outcome, but surgeons certainly find operation easier with good lighting and magnification. It also makes teaching the procedure easier.

Chemonucleolysis

This procedure dates back to the early 1960s. Lyman Smith first injected a purified extract of the papaya fruit into the intervertebral disc to treat intervertebral disc prolapse. It has been the subject of a series of randomized controlled trials. Its use has been fashionable in various countries at various times. It is fairly widely available in the United Kingdom. It is not now widely used in the United States. The main anxiety there is anaphylaxis. This is unusual in the United Kingdom, perhaps because meat tenderizer based on the same enzyme is not widely used. Chemonucleolysis is still popular in France. The most serious complication is transverse myelitis, which occurs in 1 : 18,000 to 1 : 25,000 cases (note that the risk of cauda equina damage is considerably higher in surgically treated cases (perhaps 1 : 1000).

Surgical treatment versus chemonucleolysis

I use both treatments in managing patients with disc prolapses when other interventions have failed. This means waiting 6 weeks as a minimum from the onset of symptoms. Often it is much longer. Chemonucleolysis is safer than surgery, but its success rate is less. I prefer to use chemonucleolysis in my younger patients (e.g. < 25 years), but there is evidence of efficacy in older patients as well. Sequestrated discs will not respond to chemonucleolysis.

Chemonucleolysis does generate a lot of back pain in the first 6 weeks (so does surgery, but patients find postsurgical back pain easier

Table 2 Risks and benefits of natural history or intervention in disc prolapse

	Natural history	Chemonucleolysis	Surgical discectomy
Relief of leg pain	90% in 4 years	70% in 6 weeks	90–95% in 6 weeks
Relief of back pain	30% in 4 years	30% in 6 weeks	30% in 6 weeks
Anaphylaxis		1%	
Serious neurological complication (cord or cauda equina)	The risk of a subsequent central disc prolapse (unknown)	1 in 18,000	? 1 in 1000
Nerve root complication	Unknown, but could occur	< 1%	1%
Infection	Very small	< 1%	1%
Deep vein thrombosis	Background risk	Background risk	Background risk
Haematoma	None	None	1%
Dural tear	None	Virtually none	1%
Arachnoiditis	None	None	< 0.1%
Recovery of preoperative foot drop	No data, but may well recover	No data	55/56 patients had neurological improvement. 36/56 had complete resolution[92]

to accept). This means there is not much to choose between the interventions in recovery time. The risk of recurrence is probably less with chemonucleolysis compared with surgery (which is about 10 per cent in 10 years). The size of the disc prolapse is irrelevant to outcome.

A risk/benefit equation

The figures given in Table 2 are my interpretation of various studies and my own experience, and are for guidance only. Other surgeons may disagree with this interpretation. They are figures I would use in obtaining a patient's consent. Some patients may well carry higher risks if they have pre-existing deficits or co-morbidity.

Type 4: neurogenic claudication

This is almost always a chronic presentation and outside the scope of this chapter.

Type 5 pain: Infection

Patients present with gradually increasing back pain with girdle or referred pain. These may predominate over the back pain, so that thoracic and upper lumbar disc space infections generate chest or abdominal pain. This causes diagnostic confusion to treating physicians. It is commonly some time before the correct diagnosis is made. The MR scan is much the best way of diagnosing the condition. It may also be detected on isotope scans. If advanced (> 4 weeks), there are plain X-ray changes with endplate destruction and disc space narrowing. Plain X-rays are often best imaging modality to monitor the evolution and response to treatment.

Treatment is by pain control with analgesics and, sometimes, extended splintage. A biopsy by fluoroscopy is essential (we avoid using CT-guided biopsy). This should be for both histology and culture. Most series report 70 per cent positive cultures. Blood cultures should also be done, and may sometimes identify the organism when

direct biopsy does not. Appropriate antibiotics should be started. We prefer to give at least 6 weeks of intravenous therapy followed by an oral regime.

Surgery is indicated if there is neurological involvement, an epidural abscess, an inconclusive biopsy, uncontrolled mechanical pain, or serious deformity. Normally we use an anterior (retroperitoneal or transthoracic) approach, but posterior approaches can be used in some cases. Sometimes metallic implants or bone grafts are needed to stabilize the spine. In this event antibiotic treatment is prolonged or indefinite.

Tumours

Metastases predominate in the spine. Surgery is indicated to obtain a biopsy, to decompress the cord or cauda equina, and to treat mechanical instability. If a percutaneous biopsy is successful and there is no neurological deficit, then radio- or chemotherapy will usually suffice. Surgery is worth considering if the prognosis is greater than 3 months, if there is pain uncontrolled by analgesics. Radiotherapy is ineffective in relieving cord compression, Surgeons are tending to use posterior stabilization methods where possible (as opposed to anterior surgery).

Fracture

The majority of osteoporotic crush fractures are either asymptomatic or the pain they generate is severe but short-lived. Simple analgesics and reassurance may well suffice. If the pain is severe consider using opiates, transcutaneous nerve stimulation, and external supports. Surgery is rarely indicated. There is interest and some evidence for the use of vertebroplasty.[93, 94] This involves the percutaneous injection of low-viscosity methyl methacrylate bone cement into the collapsed vertebral body. This method has been modified and probably improved by using a balloon tamp (kyphoplasty). A balloon is inserted in each pedicle of the collapsed vertebra and inflated. This can correct the kyphosis and creates a cavity within the vertebral body into which cement can be injected under fluoroscopic control. Currently this method is supported by observational studies only.[95]

Acute inflammatory disorders of the spine

These are outside the scope of this chapter.

References

1. Maniadakis, N. and Gray, A. (2000). The economic burden of back pain in the UK. *Pain* **84**, 95–103.

2. Kellgren, J. (1938). Observations on referred pain arising from muscle. *Clin. Sci.* **3**, 175–190.

3. Kellgren, J.H. (1939). On the distribution of pain arising from deep somatic structures with charges of segmental pain areas. *Clin. Sci.* **4**, 35–46.

4. Kellgren, J. (1941). Sciatica. *Lancet* **1**, 561–564.

5. McCall, I., Park, W., and O'Brien, J. (1979). Induced pain referral from posterior lumbar elements in normal subjects. *Spine* **4**, 441–446.

6. Derby, R., O'Neill, C., Berquam, J., and Vaughan, P. (2000). Mechanisms of leg pain in patients with intervertebral disc disorders. In *International Society for the Study of the Lumbar Spine*, Adelaide, 2000.

7. Dong, G. and Porter, R. (1989). Walking and cycling tests in neurogenic and intermittent claudication. *Spine* **14**, 965–969.

8. Verbiest, H. (1954). A radicular syndrome from developmental narrowing of the lumbar vertebral canal. *J. Bone Joint Surg. (Br.)* **36**, 230–237.

9. Blau, J. and Logue, V. (1961). Claudication of the cauda equina. An unusual syndrome resulting from central protrusion of a lumbar intervertebral disc. *Lancet* **1**, 1081–1086.

10. Porter, R.W., Hibbert, C.S., and Wellman, P. (1980). Backache and the lumbar spinal canal. *Spine* **5**, 99–105.

11. Porter, R.W., Hibbert, C.S., and Wicks, M. (1978). The spinal canal in symptomatic lumbar disc lesions. *J. Bone Joint Surg. (Br.)* **60B**, 485–487.

12. Jayson, M. (1997). Why does back pain become chronic? Chronic back pain is not the same as acute back pain lasting longer. *Br. Med. J.* **314**, 1639–1640.

13. Thomas, E., Silman A., Croft P., Papageorgiou, A., Jayson, M., and Macfarlane, G. (1999). Predicting who develops chronic low back pain in primary care: a prospective study. *Br. Med. J.* **318**, 1662–1667.

14. Clauw, D., Williams, D., Lauerman, W., Dahlman, M., Aslami, A., Nachemson, A., et al. (1999). Pain sensitivity as a correlate of clinical status in individuals with chronic low back pain. *Spine* **24**, 2035–2041.

15. Department of Health (1999). *The prevalence of back pain in Great Britain in 1998*. Stationery Office, London.

16. Klaber Moffett, J., Richardson, G., Sheldon, T., and Maynard, A. (1995). *Back pain: its management and cost to society*. Centre for Health Economics, York.

17. Dixon, A.S. (1973). Progress and problems in back pain research. *Rheumatol. Rehabil.* **12**, 165–175.

18. Shekelle, P., Markovich, M., and Louie, R. (1995). An epidemiologic study of episodes of back pain care. *Spine* **20**, 1668–1673.

19. Andersson, G. (1999). Epidemiological features of chronic low-back pain. *Lancet* **354**, 581–585.

20. Waddell, G. (1998). *The back pain revolution*. Churchill Livingstone, Edinburgh.

21. Pope, M.H., Wilder, D.G., and Frymoyer, J.W. (1980). Vibration as an aetiologic factor in low back pain. In *Proceedings of the Conference on Engineering Aspects of the Spine*. British Orthopaedic Association and the Institute of Engineers. Br. Orthop. Assoc. & Inst. Eng; 1980; U.K.

22. Drerup, B., Granitzka, M., Assheuer, J., and Zerlett, G. (1999). Assessment of disc injury in subjects exposed to long-term whole-body vibration. *Eur. Spine J.* **8**, 458–467.

23. Croft, P., Papageorgiou, A., Thomas, E., Macfarlane, G., and Silman, A. (1999). Short-term physical risk factors for new episodes of low back pain: prospective evidence from the South Manchester back pain study. *Spine* **24**, 1556–1561.

24. Deyo, R.A. and Bass, J.E. (1987). Lifestyle and low back pain: the influence of smoking, exercise and obesity. *Clin. Res.* **35**, 577.

25. Ducker, T.B. (1992). Cigarette smoking and the prevalence of spinal procedures. *J. Spinal Disord.* **5**(1), 135–136.

26. Kelsey, J., Githens, P., and O'Conner, T. (1984). Acute prolapsed intervertebral disc: an epidemiological study with special reference to driving automobiles and cigarette smoking. *Spine* **9**, 608–613.

27. Leboeuf-Yde, C., Kyvik, K., and Bruun, N. (1998). Low back pain and lifestyle: Part I: Smoking. Information from a population-based sample of 29424 twins. *Spine* **23**, 2207–2214.

28. Scott, S., Goldberg, M., Mayo, N., Stock, S., and Poitras, B. (1999). The association between cigarette smoking and back pain in adults. *Spine* **24**, 1090–1098.

29. Deyo, R.A. and Bass, J.E. (1989). Lifestyle and low back pain: the influence of smoking and obesity. *Spine* **14**, 501–506.

30. Ernst, E. (1993). Smoking: a cause of back trouble? *Br. J. Rheumatol.* **32**, 239–242.

31. Andersen, T., Christiansen, F., Laursen, M., Helmig, P., Hoy, K., Niedermann, B., et al. (2000). Candidates for spinal fusion smoke significantly more than the background population. Presented at International Society for the Study of the Lumbar Spine, Adelaide, 2000.

32. Vroomen, P., de Krom, M., Kester, A., Wilmink, J., and Knottnerus, J. (2000). Diagnostic value of history and physical examination in patients suspected of lumbosacral nerve compression—a primary care based study. Presented at International Society for the Study of the Lumbar Spine, Adelaide, 2000.

33. Biering-Sorenson, F. and Hilden, J. (1989). Reproducibility of the history of low back trouble. *Spine* **9**, 280–286.

34. Thomas, A., Fairbank, J., Pynsent, P., and Baker, D. (1989). A computer interview for patients with back pain—a validation study. *Spine* **14**, 844–846.

35. Salminen, J.J., Oksanen, A., Maki, P., Pentti, J., and Kujala, U.M. (1993). Leisure time physical activity in the young. Correlation with low-back pain, spinal mobility and trunk muscle strength in 15-year-old school children. *Int. J. Sports Med.* **14**(7), 406–410.

36. Sty, J.R., Wells, R.G., and Conway, J.J. (1993). Spine pain in children. *Semin. Nucl. Med.* **23**(4), 296–320.

37. Fairbank, J., Pynsent, P., Van Poortvleit, J., and Phillips, H. (1984). Influence of anthropometric factors and joint laxity in the incidence of adolescent back pain. *Spine* **9**, 461–464.

38. Taimela, S., Kujala, U., Salminen, J., and Viljanen, T. (1997). The prevalence of low back pain among children and adolescents: a nationwide, cohort-based questionnaire survey in Finland. *Spine* **22**, 1132–1136.

39. Balagué, F., Troussier, B., and Salminen, J. (1999). Non-specific low back pain in children and adolescents: risk factors. *Eur. Spine J.* **8**, 429–438.

40. Burton, A., Clarke, R., McClune, T., and Tillotson, K. (1996). The natural history of low back pain in adolescents. *Spine* **21**, 2323–2328.

41. Salminen, J.J., Erkintalo, M., Laine, M., and Pentti, J. (1995). Low back pain in the young: a prospective three-year follow-up study of subjects with and without low back pain. *Spine* **20**, 2101–2107.

42. Salminen, J., Erkintalo, M., Pentti, J., Oksanen, A., and Kormano, M. (1999). Recurrent low back pain and early disc degeneration in the young. *Spine* **24**(13), 1316–1321.

43. Videman, T., Leppavuori, J., Kaprio, J., Battie, M., Gibbons, L., Peltonen, L., et al. (1998). Intragenic polymorphisms of the vitamin D receptor gene associated with intervertebral disc degeneration. *Spine* **23**, 2477–2485.

44. Nissinen, M., Heliovaara, M., Seitsamo, J., Alaranta, H., and Poussa, M. (1994). Anthropometric measurements and the incidence of low back pain in a cohort of pubertal children. *Spine* **12**, 1367–1370.

45. Salminen, J., Maki, P., Oksanen, A., and Pentti, J. (1992). Spinal mobility and trunk muscle strength in 15-year-old school children with and without low back pain. *Spine* **17**, 405–411.

46. Burgoyne, W. and Edgar, M. (1998). Assessment of back pain in children. *Curr. Paediatr.* **8**, 173–179.

47. Waddell, G., Feder, G., McIntosh, A., Lewis, M., and Hutchinson, A. (1998). *Low back pain evidence review: clinical guidelines for the management of acute low back pain.* Royal College of General Practitioners, London.

48. Deyo, R., Rainville, J., and Kent, D. (1992). What can the history and physical examination tell us about low back pain? *J. Am. Med. Assoc.* **268**, 760–765.

49. van Tulder, M., Koes, B., and Boulter, L. (eds.) (1996). *Low back pain in primary care: effectiveness of diagnostic and therapeutic interventions.* Institute for Research in Extramural Medicine, Amsterdam.

50. Waddell, G. and Turk, D. (1992). Clinical assessment of low back pain. In *Handbook of pain assessment* (ed. D. Turk and R. Melzack), pp. 15–36. Guilford Press, New York.

51. Ohmeiss, D. (2000). Repeatability of pain drawings in a low back pain population. *Spine* **25**, 980–988.

52. Johansson, J.E., Barrington, T.W., and Ameli, M. (1982). Combined vascular and neurogenic claudication. *Spine* **7**, 150–158.

53. Nachemson, A. and Morris, J. (1964). *In vivo* measurements of intradiscal pressure. *J. Bone Joint Surg.* (*Am.*) **46A**, 1077–1092.

54. Porter, R.W. and Oakshott, G.H.L. (1988). Familial aspects of disc protrusion. *J. Orthop. Rheumatol.* **1**, 173–178.

55. Anderson, J.A.D. (1987). Back pain and occupation. In *The lumbar spine and back pain,* 3rd edn (ed. M. V. Jayson), pp. 16–37. Churchill Livingstone, Edinburgh.

56. Osti, O., Vernon-Roberts, B., Moore, R., and Fraser, R. (1992). Annular tears and disc degeneration in the lumbar spine. *J. Bone Joint Surg.* (*Br.*) **74B**, 678–682.

57. Melzack, R. (1975). The McGill pain questionnaire: major properties and scoring methods. *Pain* **1**, 277–299.

58. Hambly, M. and Mooney, V. (1992). Effect of smoking and pulsed electromagnetic fields on intradiscal pH in rabbits. *Spine* **17**, s83–s85.

59. Daftari, T., Whitesides, T., Heller, J., Goodrich, A., McCarey, B., and Hutton, W. (1994). Nicotine on the revascularisation of bone graft: an experimental study in rabbits. *Spine* **19**, 904–911.

60. McCombe, P., Fairbank, J., Cockersole, B., and Pynsent, P. (1989). Reproducibility of physical signs in low back pain. *Spine* **14**, 908–918.

61. Main, C. and Waddell, G. (1998). Spine update. Behavioral responses to examination: a reappraisal of the interpretation 'nonorganic signs'. *Spine* **23**, 2367–2371.

62. Bradish, C., Lloyd, G., Aldam, C., Albert, J., Dyson, P., Doxey, N., et al. (1988). Do non-organic signs help to predict the return of activity of patients with low-back pain? *Spine* **13**, 556–560.

63. Ohmeiss, D., Vanharanta, H., Estlander, A.-M., and Jamsen, A. (2000). The relationship of disability (Oswestry) and pain drawings to functional testing. *Eur. Spine J.* **9**, 208–212.

64. Helliwell, P., Moll, J., and Wright, V. (1992). Measurement of spinal movement and function. In *The lumbar spine and back pain* (ed. M.V. Jayson), pp. 173–205. Churchill Livingstone, Edinburgh.

65. Roland, M. and Morris, R. (1983). A study of the natural history of low back pain. Part 1: Development of a reliable and sensitive measure of disability in low-back pain. *Spine* **8**, 141–144.

66. Fairbank, J., Couper, J., Davies, J., and O'Brien, J. (1980). The Oswestry low back pain questionnaire. *Physiotherapy* **66**, 271–273.

67. Baker, D., Pynsent, P., and Fairbank, J. (1989). The Oswestry Disability Index revisited. In *Back pain: new approaches to rehabilitation and education* (ed. M. Roland and J. Jenner), pp. 174–186. Manchester University Press, Manchester.

68. Roland, M. and Fairbank, J. (2000). The Roland–Morris questionnaire and the Oswestry disability questionnaire. *Spine* **25**, 3115–3124.

69. Fairbank, J. and Pynsent, P. (2000). The Oswestry Disability Index. *Spine* **25**, 2940–2952.

70. Singh, S., Morgan, M., Scott, S., Walters, D., and Hardman, A. (1992). Development of a shuttle walking test of disability in patients with chronic airways obstruction. *Thorax* **47**, 1019–1024.

71. Keell, S., Chambers, J., Francis, D., Edwards, D., and Stables, R. (1998). Shuttle-walk test to assess chronic heart failure. *Lancet* **352**, 705.

72. Payne, G. and Skehan, J. (1996). Shuttle Walking Test: a new approach for evaluating the patient with pacemakers. *Heart* **75**, 414–418.

73. Ramsbottom, R., Brewer, J., and Williams, C. (1988). A progressive shuttle run test to estimate maximal oxygen uptake. *Br. J. Sports Med.* **22**, 141–144.

74. Frost, H., Lamb, S., Klaber Moffet, J., Fairbank, J., and Moser, J. (1998). A fitness programme for patients with chronic low back pain: two year follow up of a randomised controlled trial. *Pain* **75**, 273–279.

75. Frost, H., Klaber Moffett, J., Moser, J., and Fairbank, J. (1995). Randomised controlled trial for evaluation of fitness programme for patients with chronic low back pain. *Br. Med. J.* **310**, 151–154.

76. Frost, H., Fairbank, J., and MacDonald, J. (1997). Spine stabilisation trial. Implementation of a multicentre randomised controlled trial. *Physiotherapy* **83**, 645.

77. Pratt, R., Fairbank, J., and Virr, A. (2002). The reliability of the shuttle walking test, the Swiss Spinal Stenosis Score, and the Oswestry disability index in the assessment of patients with lumbar Spinal Stenosis. *Spine,* **27**, 84–91.

78. McRea, I. and Wright, V. (1969). Measurement of back movement. *Ann. Rheum. Dis.* **28**, 584.

79. Burton, A. (1986). Regional lumbar sagittal mobility; measurement by flexicurve. *Clin. Biomech.* **1**, 20–26.

80. Ohlen, G., Spangfort, E., and Tingvall, C. (1989). The measurement of spinal sagittal configuration and mobility with Debrunner's kyophometer. *Spine* **14**, 580–583.

81. Waddell, G., McCulloch, J.A., and Kummel, E. (1980). Nonorganic physical signs in low back pain. *Spine* **5**, 117–125.

82. Karbowski, K. and Radanov, B. (1995). Historical perspective: the history of the discovery of the sciatica stretching phenomenon. *Spine* **20**, 1315–1317.

83. Karbowski, K. and Dvorak, J. (1995). Historical perspective: description of variations of the sciatica stretch phenomenon. *Spine* **20**, 1525–1527.

84. Edgar, M.A. and Park, W.M. (1974). Induced pain patterns on passive straight-leg raising in lower lumbar disc protrusions. *J. Bone Joint Surg.* (*Br.*) **56B**, 658–667.

85. Troup, J.D.G. (1981). Straight leg raising (SLR) and the qualifying tests for increased root tension. *Spine* **6**, 526–527.

86. Fairbank, J.C.T. and O'Brien, J.P. (1983). Iliac crest syndrome: a treatable cause of back pain. *Spine* **8**, 220–224.

87. Wilson, L., Hall, H., McIntosh, G., and Melles, T. (1999). Intertester reliability of a low back pain classification system. *Spine* **24**, 248–254.

88. van Tulder, M., Koes, B., and Boulter, L. (1997). Conservative treatment of acute and chronic nonspecific low back pain: a systemic review of randomized controlled trials of the most common interventions. *Spine* **22**, 2128–2156.

89. Gibson, J., Grant, I., and Waddell, G. (1999). The Cochrane review of surgery for lumbar disc prolapse and degenerative lumbar spondylosis. *Spine* **24**, 1820–1832.

90. Watts, R. and Silagy, C. (1995). A meta-analysis on the efficacy of epidural corticosteroids in the treatment of sciatica. *Anaesth. Intens. Care* **23**, 564–569.

91. Karppinen, J., Malmivaara, A., Kurunlahti, M., Kyllonen, E., Pienimaki, T., Nieminen, P., et al. (2000). Treatment of sciatica—efficacy of nerve root infiltration. A randomized controlled trial. Presented at International Society for the Study of the Lumbar Spine, Adelaide, 2000.

92. Girardi, F., Parvataneni, H., Camissa, F., and Khan, S. (2000). Improvement of acute foot drop after lumbar surgery. Presented at International Society for the Study of the Lumbar Spine, Adelaide, 2000.

93. Levine, S.A., Perin, L.A., Hayes, O., and Hayes, W.S. (2000). An evidence-based evaluation of percutaneous vertebroplasty. *Manag. Care* **3**, 56–60.

94. Grados, F., Depriester, C., Cayrolle, G., Hardy, N., Deramond, H., and Fardellone, P. (2000). Long-term observations of vertebral osteoporotic fractures treated by percutaneous vertebroplasty. *Rheumatology* **39**, 1410–1414.

95. Lieberman, I.H., Dudeney, S., Reinhardt, M.-K., and Bell, G. (2001). Initial outcome and efficiency of 'kyphoplasty' in the treatment of painful osteoporotic vertebral compression fractures. *Spine* **26**, 1631–1638.

6.3 The shoulder

Cathy Speed

Introduction

Shoulder complaints cause significant pain and disability in the general population and represent a major burden upon the economy due to the cost of health care, lost earnings, and social security payments. Shoulder pain has a point prevalence of 7–21 per cent of adults in the community[1,2] and is the second most common acute musculoskeletal complaint presenting to primary care, with only back pain presenting more frequently. In the United Kingdom 1 per cent of adults over the age of 45 present to their general practitioner with a new episode of shoulder pain annually.[3]

While shoulder pain and dysfunction can have a significant impact on any individual, the consequences in older people are particularly significant and may be the determining factor that makes them socially dependent. The flexibility of the shoulder declines with age, due to the ageing process itself, to disuse, and/or to the presence of a local disorder. Greater shoulder flexibility is an independent determinant for independence in older populations.[4]

Shoulder complaints are poorly understood in relation to their epidemiology, impact upon the individual and society, appropriate management, and prognosis. Research has been limited by a lack of adequate randomization and blinding, the use of heterogeneous study populations, and a broad spectrum of treatment approaches, outcome measures, and follow-up intervals.[5, 6]

The vast majority of shoulder complaints are due to soft tissue lesions and, of these, rotator cuff disorders represent the largest diagnostic category. Many shoulder complaints are multifactorial in origin and articular and extraarticular disorders can coexist. Instability also plays a major role. The shoulder is the most mobile joint of the body, achieving this mobility at the expense of its stability. Loss of the fine balance between optimal mobility of the joint and its stability is a common, albeit frequently subtle, feature of shoulder complaints.

Functional anatomy

The shoulder 'joint' is better described as the shoulder 'complex', since it consists of a series of articulations: the glenohumeral, acromioclavicular, and sternoclavicular joints and the scapulothoracic articulation, where the scapula slides on the rib cage (Fig. 1). Further structures, the capsules, ligaments, muscles, tendons, bursae, and neurovascular elements, complete the framework of the shoulder complex (Figs 2–4). Many of these structures work in combination to achieve the remarkable range of mobility that is seen in this region, allowing the hand to be positioned in space to permit vital tasks to be performed. Such range of movement is particularly important to some sporting activities. Excessive mobility, however, can predispose to injury.

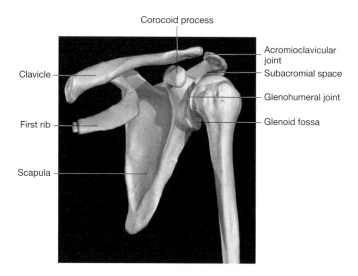

Fig. 1 The bony anatomy of the shoulder complex (anterior).

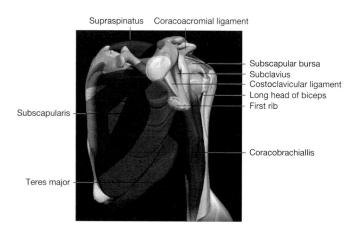

Fig. 2 Anatomy of the shoulder complex (anterior).

The mobility of the shoulder complex and in particular the glenohumeral joint (GHJ) is achieved through several interrelated factors.

1. Combinations of movements through the series of joints within the shoulder complex allow a greater range of movement to be achieved.

2. The articular surfaces of the glenohumeral joint are shallow and the area of bony congruity is small.

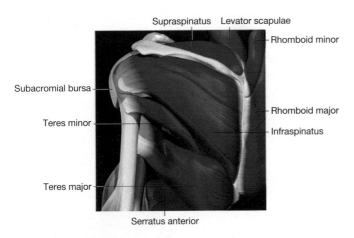

Fig. 3 Anatomy of the shoulder complex (posterior).

Table 1. Stability of the shoulder complex

Static stabilizers
Joint capsule
Glenohumeral and coracohumeral ligaments
Subscapularis
Slightly negative pressure within the joint
The glenoid labrum

Dynamic stabilizers
The muscles of the rotator cuff
Deltoid
Teres major

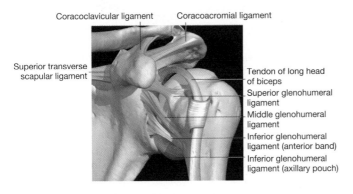

Fig. 4 The stability of the glenohumeral joint is aided by ligaments that behave as static stabilizers.

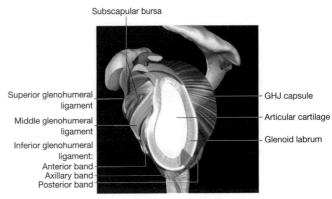

Fig. 5 The glenoid labrum contributes to stability by deepening the glenoid cavity.

3. Laxity of many surrounding soft tissue structures such as the joint capsule permits a wide range of motion.

Numerous characteristics of the GHJ contribute to its stability and can be divided into those that contribute to stability during movement (*dynamic stabilizers*) and those that also contribute at rest (*static stabilizers*) (Table 1). These are discussed further below.

Static Stabilizers

The proximal *humerus* consists of the surgical neck, so named as this is where fractures usually occur. Above this are the anatomical neck (which forms a space between the articular cartilage and ligament and tendon attachments) and the head. A ring, consisting of the greater and lesser tuberosities separated by the bicipital groove, provides attachments for muscles and ligaments (Fig. 4). The greater tuberosity receives insertions of the muscles of the rotator cuff (with the exception of infraspinatus), and acts as a pulley for the deltoid with elevation of the arm below 60°, helping to increase the lever arm of the supraspinatus.

The head of the humerus is spheroidal, is inclined superiorly, and sits slightly retroverted. A small area of the head articulates with the relatively shallow surface of the glenoid of the scapula. The humeral head is approximately two-thirds larger in diameter than the glenoid

fossa which, in combination with variations in glenoid morphology and the position of the scapula, may contribute to the inherent instability of the GHJ. Blood supply to the head of the humerus is via the circumflex humeral artery, branches of which enter the bone via the bicipital groove or one of the tubercles.

The *scapula* is composed of a flattened body with thickened processes where major muscles attach: the coracoid, acromion, spine of the scapula, and the glenoid. The lateral border and superior and inferior angles are also thickened for muscle attachments.

Soft tissue structures also contribute to the stability of the GHJ. The *coracohumeral and glenohumeral ligaments* are thickened folds of the joint capsule working to strengthen the anterior capsule and are important static stabilizers. The *glenoid labrum*, a fibrous rim that is thicker peripherally than centrally, deepens the glenoid cavity by up to 50 per cent. This increase in surface area for contact with the humeral head creates a buttress limiting humeral head translation and acts as an attachment for stabilizing glenohumeral (GH) ligaments. The labrum is weakest at the 4 o'clock position and may become detached (Fig. 5).

Dynamic stabilizers

Muscles act as the *dynamic stabilizers* of the GHJ. These can be divided into the outer sleeve of the deltoid and teres major and the inner sleeve, formed by the rotator cuff and long head of the biceps. The *deltoid*, supplied by the axillary nerve (C5), is composed of three portions: the anterior, middle, and posterior thirds. Loss of deltoid

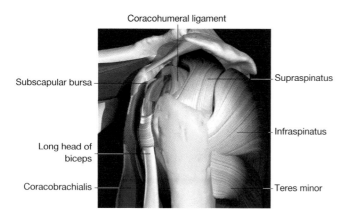

Fig. 6 Lateral view of the shoulder. The subacromial space and components of the rotator cuff.

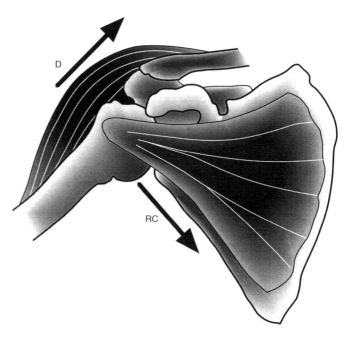

Fig. 7 The force–couple relationship between the deltoid (D) and cuff (RC) is fundamental to the stability of the shoulder.

function has a significant functional impact, as it is active in any form of elevation of the arm. It is assisted in the first 60° (and in particular the first 30°) of elevation of the arm by the rotator cuff, specifically the supraspinatus, as the deltoid has its shortest lever arm in this range.

The *rotator cuff* is a complex arrangement of four muscles, *the supraspinatus, infraspinatus, teres minor, and subscapularis*, which originate from the blade of the scapula and insert on to the humerus (Fig. 6). Although direct fibres from each rotator cuff tendon have specific sites of attachment, there is considerable interweaving of fibres between the musculotendinous units and with the articular capsule and ligaments. In addition, the coracohumeral ligament forms connections with the supraspinatus, subscapularis, superior gleno-humeral ligament, and glenohumeral joint capsule at the *rotator inter-val*, the region between the supraspinatus and subscapularis tendons, creating a thicker cuff in that area.

The primary roles of the rotator cuff are to contribute both to mobility and stability, restraining humeral head translation, limiting glenohumeral rotation, and controlling scapulohumeral rhythm and position. The muscles of the rotator cuff act synergistically to apply compressive and tensile forces to achieve stable and effective move-ment of the humeral head. The cuff acts to stabilize and depress the humeral head in the glenoid, counteracting the effect of the deltoid, which pulls the humeral head superiorly (Fig. 7). This force–couple relationship between the deltoid and cuff is fundamental to the under-standing of many shoulder disorders.

Subscapularis is the largest and most powerful of the rotator cuff muscles. It arises from the subscapular fossa and has tendinous inser-tions on to the lesser tuberosity, extends to form a sheath with the tendon of the long head of the biceps, and has more insertions along the surgical neck of the humerus. The tendon also interconnects with the tendon of supraspinatus and with the underlying periosteum. It works as an internal rotator of the GHJ and is also a passive stabilizer, since its upper region is rich with dense collagen fibres as it wraps around the humeral head.

Supraspinatus arises from the supraspinous fossa and runs through the supraspinatus outlet, composed of the acromion and acromioclav-iculan joint (ACJ) superiorly, coracoid base anteriorly, the spine of the scapula posteriorly, and the superior glenoid and humeral head super-iorly. It inserts on to the greater tuberosity, with interconnections with infraspinatus near its insertion and with the coracohumeral ligament at

the rotator interval. Active in all movements involving elevation, it cre-ates maximal effort in 30° of elevation. *Infraspinatus* arises from the scapular infraspinous fossa and inserts on the greater tuberosity, below the supraspinatus. *Teres minor* arises inferolateral to infraspinatus in the midlateral scapula, inserting below infraspinatus on the greater tuberosity. Both of these muscles act as external rotators, with infra-spinatus contributing 60 per cent and teres minor 40 per cent. The *long head of the biceps* (LHB) can be considered as the fifth tendon of the cuff, since its tendon is intimately associated with the cuff as it arises from the superoposterior glenoid labrum. It runs through the bicipital groove, which is roofed by the transverse humeral ligament. A sling of tendoligamentous structures at the entrance to the groove (the 'rotator interval sling') act to constrain the tendon within the groove. It contributes to dynamic stability and depression of the humeral head and functions as a flexor of the forearm in neutral and supination and contributes to flexion and abduction of the arm.

Other muscles contribute to scapulothoracic motion, including the trapezius, rhomboids, levator scapulae, serratus anterior, pectorals, teres major, and coracobrachialis (Fig. 8 and Table 2).

Other anatomical features of the shoulder complex

The *coracoid process* is easily palpable and is an important landmark, since neurovascular structures travel inferomedial to it. It serves as the origin of ligaments, the short head of the biceps, and coracobrachialis and the insertion of pectoralis minor (Figs 1, 2 and 4). Several anom-alies have been described; perhaps most importantly a coracoclavi-cular band or articulation is present in up to 1 per cent of the population.

The *acromion* has been the focus of much research, specifically in relation to the space below it (the subacromial space, or supraspinatus outlet) and the anatomical factors that reduce this space. Acromion

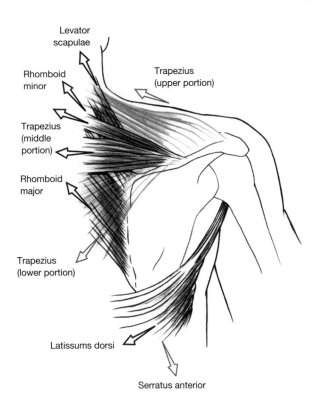

Fig. 8 Actions of scapulothoracic muscles are vital to normal shoulder movements.

Table 2 Muscles of the shoulder and scapulothoracic region act together in movement of the arm

Shoulder muscles	Scapular muscles
Flexion (main nerve roots: C5, C6)	
Flexors	Abductor
Anterior deltoid	Serratus anterior
Biceps	
Pectoralis major	
Corachobrachialis	
Lateral rotators	Lateral rotators
Infraspinatus	Serratus anterior
Teres minor	Trapezius
Posterior deltoid	
Abduction (main nerve roots: C5, C6)	
Abductors	Adductor
Deltoid	Trapezius (stabilizes scapula)
Supraspinatus	
Long head of biceps	
Lateral rotators	Lateral rotators
Infraspinatus	Trapezius
Teres minor	Serratus anterior
Posterior deltoid	
Extension (main nerve roots: C5–C8)	
Posterior deltoid	Adductors, medal rotators, elevators
Teres major	Rhomboids
Latissimus dorsi	Levator scapulae
Long head triceps	Pectoralis minor acts to tilt scapula anteriorly
Adduction (main nerve roots (C5–C8)	
Pectoralis major	Rhomboids
Teres major	Trapezius
Latissimus dorsi	
Long head triceps	

morphology, in particular its shape and angle, may be related to rotator cuff pathologies.[7] The coracoacromial ligament makes an important contribution to the roof of the subacromial space and anatomical variations of this ligament complex can reduce the size of the space. The *acromioclavicular joint* (ACJ) is formed by the outer end of the clavicle and the medial aspect of the acromial spine. A fibrous disc separates the articular surfaces and the joint is stabilized by thick ligaments and deltotrapezius thickening anterosuperiorly. Relatively little movement occurs at the ACJ but a small amount occurs with glenohumeral elevation and rotation, whilst the clavicle rotates upward on the sternum at the sternoclavicular joint. The ACJ is narrowed during adduction in the horizontal plane and in elevation above 90°. The posterior component of the joint narrows during extension in the horizontal plane. The morphology of the ACJ has also been divided into three types, vertical (type I), oblique (type II), and more horizontal than vertical (type III), with the former being associated with a greater incidence of ACJ osteoarthritis.[8]

The *sternoclavicular joint* (SCJ) is a synovial joint formed by articulation between the clavicle and sternum and first rib. It is an incongruent joint with only up to 50 per cent of the articular surfaces in contact, but an intraarticular disc converts the complex into a congruous unit, with additional stability conferred by surrounding ligamentous structures.

Bursae in the shoulder region are found, as in other regions, between tendon and bone, skin and bone, and near tendon insertions between muscle and bone, in order to reduce friction between structures. There are several important bursae in the shoulder complex. Clinically, the most important of these, the *subacromial* and *subdeltoid bursae*, frequently exist as one and may be best described as a space, with a capacity of up to 510 ml (Fig. 9). These bursae aid the free

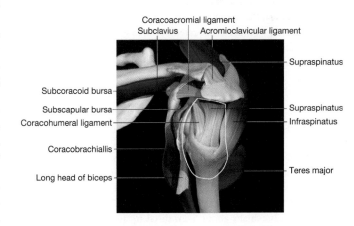

Fig. 9 The supraspinous outlet & subacromial space with the subacromial/subdeltoid bursa outlined.

movement of the rotator cuff beneath the acromion and do not communicate with the GH cavity in the healthy state. The subacromial bursa is attached to the undersurface of the coracoacromial ligament and the superior surface of the supraspinatus tendon. A sliding effect between the superior and inferior internal surfaces of the bursa occurs during abduction of the shoulder.

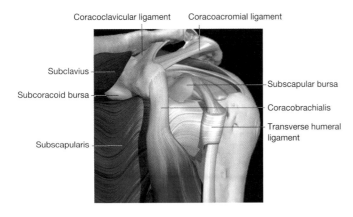

Fig. 10 Bursae of the anterior shoulder.

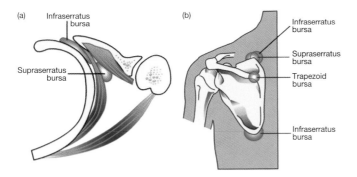

Fig. 11 (a and b) Anatomic and adventitious bursae may be found between tendinous insertions of many of the muscles of the shoulder complex.

The *subscapularis bursa* usually connects with the GHJ cavity and is found between the upper subscapularis and the neck of the glenoid (Fig 10). Further bursae are located between tendinous insertions of many of the muscles of the shoulder complex, between muscles such as teres major and latissimus dorsi, and beneath coracobrachialis (Fig. 11).

Nerves

Nerve trunks from the brachial plexus (C5–T1) pass under the clavicle, divide, and form the peripheral nerves of the arm (Table 3, Fig. 12). The *axillary nerve* (C5) runs with the axillary artery on subscapularis, inferior to the glenohumeral joint, and exits the quadrangular space with the posterior circumflex artery. It supplies deltoid and teres minor. The *musculocutaneous nerve* (C5–C7) runs obliquely to enter corachobrachialis about 5 cm distal to the coracoid process. It also supplies brachialis and biceps. The *suprascapular nerve* (C4–C6) travels posterolaterally beneath trapezius to the upper border of the scapula, medial to the coracoid process. It passes through the suprascapular notch beneath the transverse scapular ligament and supplies the spinati. The *radial nerve* (C5–C8), which supplies triceps, brachioradialis, and extensor carpi radialis longus, courses round the humerus in the spiral groove. It passes anterior to the lateral epicondyle and divides into the posterior interosseous and superficial branches in the antecubital fossa. The *ulnar nerve* (C8, T1) gives no branches above the elbow.

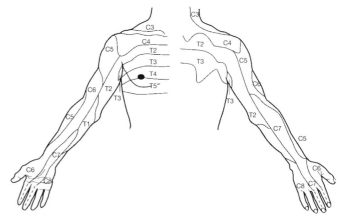

Fig. 12 Approximate dermatomes of the arm.

Clinical evaluation

History

Symptoms in the shoulder can arise due to intrinsic pathology or in relation to problems at distant sites. Since the differential diagnosis is wide and causation often multifactorial, it is important to obtain a through history (Tables 4 and 5).

Shoulder disorders can vary with respect to their nature and aetiology in different age groups. Hand dominance and occupational, sporting, social, medical, and family histories should all be taken into consideration in determining the aetiology of the complaint and its impact on the patient. The patient's expectations and the everyday demands that are imposed upon the upper limbs may influence approaches to management and compliance with therapy.

Uni/bilaterality of symptoms is often indicative of the underlying disorder. Polymyalgia rheumatica presents with bilateral symptoms, as can symptoms arising as a result of a mechanical neck disorder. Multidirectional instability is also commonly bilateral although other pathologies arising as a result may be unilateral, particularly affecting the dominant arm.

The primary symptom of most shoulder complaints is *pain*. A careful pain history is taken to determine the mode of onset, site, nature, radiation, associated symptoms, exacerbating and relieving features, and the presence of nocturnal symptoms.

The *mode of onset* should be established. Most shoulder disorders arise gradually and are associated with repetitive microtrauma (overuse) such as work with the arm in overhead or awkward positions. A history of trauma such as a fall on to the outstretched hand is often given in the acute cuff tear and is also frequently reported with an initial dislocation, but subsequent dislocations may occur with seemingly trivial incidents. ACJ sprains may be precipitated by a fall on to the tip of the shoulder, a fall on to the elbow, or an episode of heavy lifting. Rupture of the rotator cuff and/or tendon of LHB may appear to occur with minimal trauma, although there is frequently a preceding history of (often minor) shoulder pain. Some disorders arise spontaneously. Calcifying tendinitis and frozen shoulder can both have very sudden onsets, without any preceding symptoms.

The *site* of the pain is a useful indication of its source, although pain secondary to rotator cuff disease and GHJ and capsular disorders

Table 3 Motor supply of the arm

Nerve	Roots	Motor supply[a]	Quick motor test
Axillary	C5,6	Deltoid Teres minor	Shoulder abduction
Musculocutaneous	C5–C7	Corachobrachialis, brachialis, biceps	Flexion of supinated forearm
Suprascapular	C4–C6	Spinati	Supraspinatus test, external rotation of shoulder
Radial	C5–C8	Triceps, brachioradialis, ECR longus and brevis, supinator	Elbow extension, supination of extended forearm, wrist extension

Radial nerve branches:
    Posterior Interosseous
    Superficial radial
	C7, C8	Extensors of wrist/fingers
		
		—
			Wrist extension
			
			—

Ulnar	C8, T1	FCU, FDP of ring and little fingers, small muscles of hand except those supplied by median nerve	Abduction little and index fingers, adduction of thumb
Median	C7, C8, T1	Pronator teres, forearm flexors except those supplied by ulnar nerve, 1st and 2nd lumbricals, APB, opponens pollicis, FPB	Pronation of forearm; abduction, opposition of thumb
Median nerve branch: anterior interosseus nerve	C7, C8	FDP of index, middle fingers, FPL	Flexion distal phalanx of thumb, index finger

[a] ECR, Extensor carpi radialis; FCU, flexor carpi ulnaris; FDP, flexordigitorum profundus; FPL, flexor pollicis longus; APB, abductor policis brevis; FPB, flexor pollicis brevis.

Table 4 Differential diagnosis of general shoulder pain

Site	Lesions
Rotator cuff	Tendinosis, impingement Calcifying tendinitis Tear Global rupture
Tendon of long head of biceps	Tenosynovitis Subluxation/dislocation Tear/rupture
Capsule	Frozen shoulder
Joint complex and surrounding musculature	Glenohumeral instabilities, labral lesions
Bursae	Subacromial, subdeltoid, bursitis
Nerves	Lesions of axillary, suprascapular, long thoracic, radial, musculocutaneous nerves, brachial plexus, referred pain
Muscle	Myofascial pain syndromes
Joint	Glenohumeral arthritides
Others	Local destructive lesions

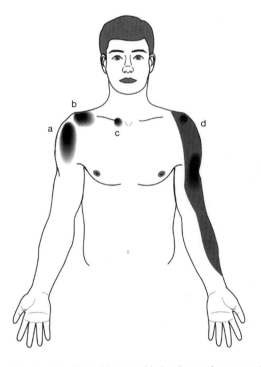

Fig. 13 Sites of shoulder pain: (a) glenohumeral rotator cuff or capsule; (b) ACJ; (c) sternoclavicular; (d) referred pain from the neck. The darker areas represent more intense pain.

have similar distributions (Fig. 13). Pain associated with glenohumeral instability may be felt anteriorly, posteriorly, or both. Acromioclavicular and sternoclavicular pain are usually well localized to the joint and the patient complaining of 'shoulder' pain that is arising from the neck frequently points to the upper trapezius as the site of their problem. Radiation of pain to the elbow and further distally is suggestive of referred pain from the neck or more peripheral neurological lesions. Additional neurological and neck symptoms should be sought. The *nature and timing* of the pain is also important.

Many shoulder complaints give rise to nocturnal pain, particularly when the complaint is severe. Pain that causes significant nocturnal disturbance, particularly when lying on the affected side, is characteristic of rotator cuff disorders. Pain that is constant, day and night, is typical of the frozen shoulder or underlying systemic disorders, which must always be excluded in presentations of shoulder pain. Pain that is worse with activity may represent an articular or

Table 5 Patient characteristics and symptoms in shoulder disorders[a]

Disorder	Age	Onset	Trauma	Night pain	Weakness	Associations
Rotator cuff tendinosis	Any	Acute/Chronic	+/—	+++	+/—	Instability in young Degeneration in older subjects Impingement
Calcific tendinitis	30–60 yrs	Acute	—	+++	—	? Cuff degeneration
Partial thickness rotator cuff tear	Acute:any. Chronic esp > 40 yrs	Acute/Chronic	May be trivial in older patients	+++	++	Instability and/or trauma in young Degeneration in older subjects
Full thickness rotator cuff tear	Esp > 40 yrs	Acute	Severe in young; trivial in older	+++	++++ (variable)	Degenerative cuff > 40 After dislocation > 40
Subacromial bursitis	Any	Acute/Chronic	+/—	+++	—	Impingement Cuff disease
GHJ instability	< 30 yrs	Episodic	+/—	—	In acute episodes	Rotator cuff pathologies Muscle imbalance Hypermobility Neurological symptoms in acute episodes
Labral tear	< 40 yrs	Acute	+	+/—	—	Instability; throwing sports
Rupture long head of biceps	> 40 yrs	Acute	+/—	+/—	+/—	Rotator cuff disease
Bicipital tendinitis	Young, sports	Acute/Chronic	—	+	—	Vast majority are associated with instability or rotator cuff disease
Frozen shoulder	40–70	Acute/subacute/chronic	+/—	+++	—	Diabetes, trauma, cardiothoracic disease
ACJ OA	> 30	Chronic	—	++	—	May cause cuff pathology
ACJ sprain	Any	Acute	++	++	—	Trauma
GHJ arthropathy	> 40	Chronic	—	+	—	—
Cervical spondylosis	> 35	Chronic	+/—	+/—	+	Neurological symptoms

[a] Note that all disorders can cause weakness in association with pain.

musculotendinous disorder. Pain associated with cervical spondylosis is often better at night once the patient gets their neck into a comfortable position, but referred or radicular pain is not. Neuropathic pain is typically constant, deep and burning in nature, and unaffected by movement.

Exacerbating and relieving features are also recorded. Pain with activities involving overhead work is suggestive of subacromial impingement or acromioclavicular pathology, usually osteoarthritis (OA). A painful arc may be described (Fig. 14). Coracoacromial impingement may be associated with pain when the arm is in the forward flexed position. Subscapularis lesions may present with pain when the arm is below shoulder height. Pain with carrying heavy objects is classically associated with ACJ sprains but can also occur with rotator cuff lesions or myofascial pain syndromes affecting the scapulothoracic musculature. In athletes, shooting pains radiating down the arm with paraesthesiae and temporary weakness of the arm immediately after releasing the ball with throwing or when serving or smashing in tennis is termed the 'dead arm syndrome' and suggests anterior or multidirectional glenohumeral instability with

brachial plexus traction during the activity. Pain that is unaffected by movement is often due to referred pain from extrinsic pathologies. An *activity history* may reveal a change in use of the affected limb prior to the onset of the complaint, such as a weekend spent gardening or performing DIY. In those who participate in sports involving throwing, swimming, racquet sports, etc, often seemingly minor changes in training or technique may be the culprit.

Clicking around the shoulder complex is a common symptom and is frequently longstanding in those who have congenitally lax joints. Clicking may also occur with rotator cuff tendinopathy, or tendinopathy, subluxation or dislocation of the biceps tendon. Clicking and clunking are also symptoms of labral lesions and of instabilities that, in the case of the acromioclavicular and sternoclavicular joints, are well localized compared to the more diffuse symptoms when the GHJ is involved. A *catching* sensation is frequently reported in rotator cuff/subacromial pathology. '*Crunching*' on movement can be associated with a variety of pathologies including OA of the acromioclavicular, glenohumeral, or sternoclavicular joints, rotator cuff pathologies, and subacromial bursitis.

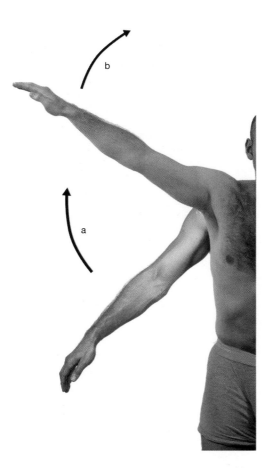

Fig. 14 A painful arc of abduction indicates (a) subacromial impingement or (b) acromioclavicular disorder.

Table 6 Causes of weakness of the shoulder

Pain
Rotator cuff tear
Global rupture of the rotator cuff
Neurological lesions—brachial neuritis, cervical root lesions, brachial plexus lesion, upper motor neuron lesion, peripheral nerve entrapment, multiple sclerosis
Muscular: muscular dystrophy, myopathy, muscle tear
Psychological

Enquiry about the presence of *systemic symptoms* is of paramount importance. Symptoms such as fever, weight loss, and anorexia may suggest sepsis, malignancy (e.g. primary lung, breast, gastrointestinal, or bone; myeloma; secondary deposits), or inflammatory arthritis. Polymyalgia rheumatica and calcifying tendinitis can present with systemic symptoms and shoulder pain and stiffness. The degree of *functional disability* may be assessed informally by determining the types and degree of activities affected and the number of days lost from work/play, or by the use of a formal evaluation. Some authors have simply measured range of motion but this is not a surrogate measure of function.

Development of a management regime for the complaint requires an assessment of the approaches taken and their effects to date. Medications, physiotherapy regimes, modalities, interventions of other health professionals including osteopaths, chiropractors, complementary therapists, etc. should all be listed.

Examination

Meticulous examination of the patient with a shoulder complaint can be very rewarding in reaching an accurate diagnosis (Table 7).

Inspection

Examination of the patient commences with observation of the patient as he/she enters the consulting room. When the shoulder is very painful, the patient may support the affected arm with the opposite hand and simple functional tasks such as removing a jacket are difficult. The adequately exposed patient should be inspected from the back, front, and side. Posture should be noted, as poor posture can contribute to shoulder pain and postural adjustments as a result of a local complaint are also common. It is normal to hold one shoulder (usually the non-dominant arm) higher than the other. Congenital deformities may predispose to shoulder problems and include a short neck (Klippel–feil Syndrome) and Sprengel shoulder (a congenitally high, poorly developed, and medially rotated scapula).

Inspection continues, starting at the SCJ and working laterally across the clavicle and chest wall to the ACJ, the acromion, the anterior GHJ, biceps, and deltoid, then moving posteriorly and working medially from the acromion, posterior deltoid, spinati, and other scapulothoracic musculature. The examiner is seeking evidence of muscle wasting or overdevelopment, soft tissue or bony deformity, and swelling, all of which may result in asymmetry. The presence of muscle fasciculation, scars, skin lesions (such as psoriasis), and discolouration should also be noted.

Any *previous history* of dislocations should be noted. The direction of the dislocation, its circumstances of onset (mechanism, degree of trauma, additional injuries) and details of subsequent episodes (including the frequency and ease of reduction), and symptoms of subluxation, rotator cuff tendinopathy, or any other lesion are all important. Patients may describe apprehension that their shoulder might sublux or dislocate with the arm in certain positions, for example in anterior GHJ instabilities when the arm is in external rotation in abduction. Determining whether recurrent dislocations are voluntary or involuntary is essential for planning appropriate management, although voluntary dislocators may deny that they perform such manoeuvres intentionally.

Weakness may be reported which may be true weakness, pain inhibition, or mechanical restriction. True weakness can result from a significant disruption to the gross structural integrity of tissues of the shoulder complex, usually in the form of a rotator cuff tear. Neurological lesions may also cause weakness (Table 6).

Swelling of joints of the shoulder complex can occur in relation to arthropathy, infection, or trauma. Swelling of the SCJ is a classical but frequently overlooked presenting feature of an inflammatory arthritis. An insidious onset of restriction or *stiffness* of the shoulder may be noted in relation to bony constraint such as in GHJ OA, soft tissue restriction such as frozen shoulder, or to pain in any local disorder of the shoulder complex. Stiffness may also have an acute onset in frozen shoulder, polymyalgia rheumatica, acute arthropathy, and after dislocations and fractures.

Table 7 Clinical signs in shoulder disorders

Disorder	Wasting	Painful arc	Active	Passive	Resisted tests	Impingement	Instability	Others
			Range of motion					
Rotator cuff tendinosis	+/−	+++[f]	Limited by pain only	Full[a]	Pain > weakness[b]	+++[f]	Younger patients	—
Calcific tendinitis	+/−	++	Limited by pain only	Full	Pain > weakness[b]	+/−	—	—
Partial tear rotator cuff	++	++	May be reduced	Full[a]	Pain & weakness[c]	++/−	—	—
Full thickness rotator cuff tear	++	+	↓	Full (↓ late)	Weakness ≫ pain	+/−	—	—
Subacromial bursitis	—	++	Limited by pain only	Full[a]	± Pain	++	—	—
GHJ instability	—	+/−	Normal	Normal	Normal	+/−	+++	Positive apprehension test(s)
Labral tear	—	+/−	Normal	Normal	Normal	+/−	++	—
Rupture long head of biceps	—	—	Normal	Full	Often normal; ± weakness of elbow, shoulder flexion, forearm supination only[d]	+/−[e]	—	Visible deformity
Bicipital tendinitis	—	—	Normal	Full	Pain on forward flexion straight arm	—	+/−	Provocation tests
Frozen shoulder	+/−	+(early)	Global ↓	Global ↓	Normal	+(early)	—	Medical conditions
Acromioclavicular OA	—	Superior arc	↓ Full elevation	May be ↓ full elevation	Normal	—	—	1. ± local deformity, tenderness+ 2. +ve ACJ stress test 3. X-ray changes
ACJ sprain	—	± Superior arc	± ↓ Full elevation	Full[a]	Normal	—	—	1. ± local deformity, tenderness++ 2. +ve ACJ stress test 3. +ve stress films
GHJ arthropathy	±	—	↓	↓	Normal	—	—	Radiological changes
Cervical Spondylosis	—	—	Normal	Normal	Normal	—	—	↓/painful neck movements

[a] May be limited by patient's pain.

[b] The planes in which pain and or weakness are noted indicate the portion(s) of the cuff involved.

[c] Pain and weakness may vary.

[d] Weakness of supination indicates rupture of radial (distal) insertion of biceps tendon: surgical intervention is necessary in such cases.

[e] May be present if concurrent rotator cuff tendinosis.

[f] Impingement is not always present in rotator cuff tendinosis.

Table 8 Causes of supraspinatus/infraspinatus wasting

Rotator cuff pathology (usually tear)

Myopathy

Disuse

Suprascapular nerve entrapment

C5 root entrapment

Table 9 Causes of winging of the scapula

Structural static winging
Deformity of the scapula, clavicle, thoracic spine, or ribs

Functional (dynamic) winging
Long thoracic nerve palsy
Spinal accessory nerve palsy
Rhomboid weakness
Multidirectional GHJ instability
Voluntary action
Painful shoulder with splinting of the GHJ and reversed scapulohumeral
   rhythm

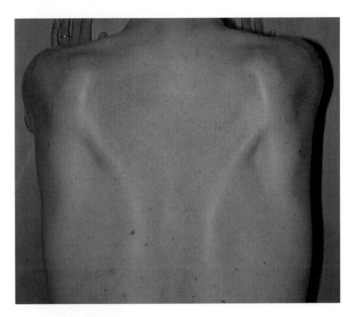

Fig. 15 Classical winging of the right scapula due to brachial neuritis.

SCJ prominence is associated with underlying inflammatory arthritis, OA, sepsis, or instability. Clavicular deformity is usually secondary to previous fracture or Paget's disease. ACJ prominence if bilateral may be normal but when unilateral suggests ACJ OA, previous dislocation or fracture or subcoracoid glenohumeral dislocation. A step deformity at the ACJ is indicative of an acromioclavicular sprain.

Muscles that can easily be inspected for wasting and asymmetry are the trapezius, paracervical, deltoid, biceps, supraspinatus, and infraspinatus muscles (Table 8). Abnormalities may be accentuated by the patients placing their hands on their hips and pressing hard against their hips. Atrophy of the upper trapezius is associated with spinal accessory nerve palsy and flattening of the deltoid may be seen with axillary nerve or C5 root pathology or after glenohumeral dislocation. The presence of *scapular winging* should be sought by standing behind the patient and asking him/her to push up against a wall. (Fig. 15). Classical winging occurs when the medial border of the scapula moves away from the posterior chest wall. Rotary winging occurs when the inferior angle of the scapula rotates further from the spine than the contralateral scapula (Table 9). Winging can be due to either structural or neuromuscular causes. *Structural winging* can occur as a result of deformities of the scapula itself or deformities of the clavicle, thoracic spine, or ribs; for example, thoracic scoliosis with a rotational element. The more commonly encountered form of scapular winging is that which is *functional*, where there is a lack of control of the scapula due to a neuromuscular defect or muscle imbalance.

Palpation

The supraclavicular fossa should be palpated for lymphadenopathy and other masses. Palpation of structures, starting at the SCJ and moving laterally along the clavicle to the ACJ, may help to identify the site of the primary complaint. Crepitus may be noted when there is localized OA or bursitis. Instability of the acromioclavicular or sternoclavicular joints may be detected through manual pressure. Further instability tests are described below ('Special tests'). Tender or trigger points may be evident, particularly in fibromyalgia or myofascial pain, respectively. Palpation of the tendon of the LHB may elicit tenderness in patients with rotator cuff and LHB disorders.

Movement

Evaluation of movement commences with inspection of the range, comfort, and rhythm of movement while the patient performs active movements and a useful screen can be performed by asking the patient to perform two composite movements as indicated in Fig. 16.1. Ability to perform both fully without pain excludes significant glenohumeral arthropathy, capsular pathology, and painful rotator cuff lesions. However, other lesions including intermittent problems such as instability are not ruled out.

Further active movement can be assessed, in particular, abduction, flexion, and adduction. Movement may be restricted due to pain or true restriction. Abnormal scapulohumeral rhythm is a commonly noted but non-specific indicator of a shoulder disorder. Normal scapulohumeral rhythm involves little or no movement of the scapula in the first 90° of abduction, as this is achieved through glenohumeral movement. The following 70° of abduction is achieved through scapular rotation and the final 20° through further movement at the GHJ. Any shoulder disorder can result in a loss of this normal pattern, with premature scapular rotation a particularly common feature.

Hitching of the shoulder is a common compensatory movement for a restricted or painful shoulder. A painful arc of abduction in midrange is typical of subacromial pathology and the pain is often eased with supination of the arm, which decreases impingement. In some cases a painful mid-arc is evident only on slowly lowering the arm from full abduction. A superior painful arc is found with acromioclavicular pathologies, in particular OA (Fig. 14).

Active range of movement can be compared with that of passive movement. Restriction of both is indicative of glenohumeral joint or

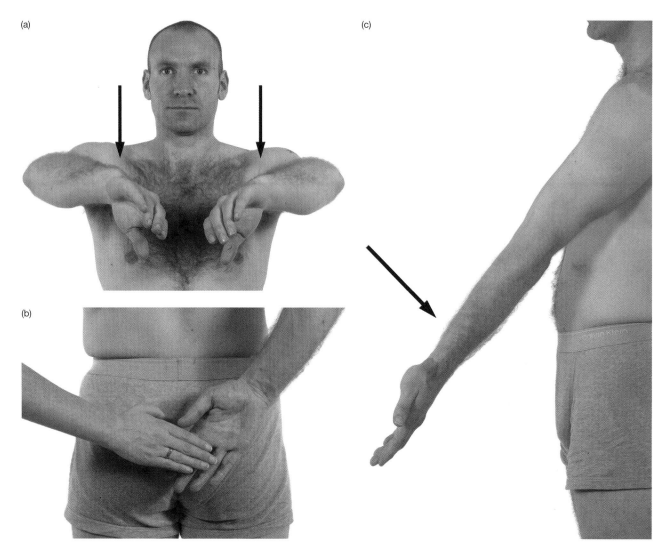

Fig. 16 Testing of the rotator cuff. The examiner applies resistence (indicated by arrows) which the patient resists. Pain and/or weakness indicate pathology. Supraspinatus (a) subscapularis (b) and long head biceps (c). Infraspinatus and teres minor are tested by resisted external rotation of the shoulder.

capsular pathology, whereas a good passive range of motion in the presence of active restriction indicates either a musculotendinous or neurological injury. Specific active movements are then tested against resistance provided by the examiner, who notes the presence of pain and weakness and whether the latter is out of proportion to the pain. The components of the rotator cuff can all be assessed (Fig. 16).

Special tests

Impingement can also be identified when there is pain on passive abduction and internal rotation of the shoulder (Fig. 17).

Glenohumeral instability. Several tests are helpful in the assessment of glenohumeral instability, as described in Fig. 18.

ACJ. Pathologies of the ACJ, in particular OA, can be identified through stressing the joint (Fig. 19).

Thoracic outlet syndrome. Stress manoeuvres in thoracic outlet syndrome are widely described but have limited utility. These are described in Fig 29. In these manoeuvres, the patient is seated and the examiner palpates the radial pulse of the affected arm, with a positive

test associated with a decrease in pulse volume and a reproduction of symptoms.

The cervical spine should also be assessed since it is a common source of shoulder pain. This includes evaluation of range of movement and the surrounding musculature. A full neurovascular assessment of the upper limbs should also be performed.

General shoulder pain

Rotator cuff tendinopathies

Classification

Rotator cuff disorders represent the most common complaint affecting the shoulder complex. Lesions can be classified as tendinopathies without tear (tendinosis), isolated tears, or global cuff ruptures. Calcifying tendinitis, a distinct subset, is a non-degenerative, self-limiting calcification of the cuff. With the advent of improved imaging techniques and arthroscopy, rotator cuff tears have been further

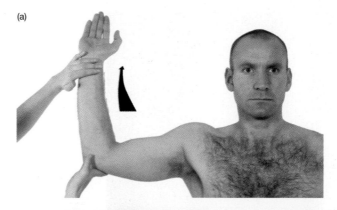

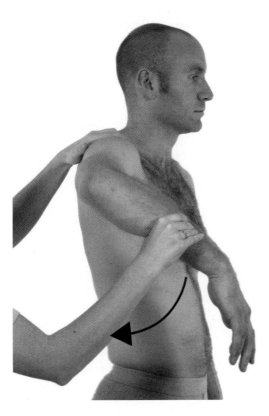

Fig. 17 A subacromial impingement test. Pain is reproduced with passive internal rotation of the abducted arm.

classified according to the tendon(s) of the cuff affected, whether they are partial or full thickness, their aetiology, duration, surface area, and additional pathologies. Partial tears may also be described according to their depth, their shape, and their site on the tendon surface (articular surface, bursal surface, intratendinous).[9–11] Other more elaborate systems appear to be of limited practical use. The relative importance of these descriptive features has yet to be determined. Some are only apparent at open operation, limiting their use in the normal clinical situation, whilst others depend upon knowledge of the exact moment of onset.

Rotator cuff tears are uncommon in those aged below 40 years, but degenerative changes are noted in up to 50 per cent of cadaveric studies in the elderly. Yamanaka and Fukuda reported on 249 cadaveric shoulders with an average age of 57.5 years, noting an incidence of full thickness tears of 7 per cent and partial thickness tears of 13 per cent, with intratendinous tears being at least twice as common as the others.[12] Rotator cuff tendon tears usually occur in the order supraspinatus (usually near its anterior insertion), infraspinatus, and subscapularis, with teres minor only rarely affected. The subscapularis tendon may tear first in an anterior dislocation of the glenohumeral joint.

Aetiology/pathogenesis

The pathogenesis of rotator cuff lesions is likely to be multifactorial. Avascularity has long been considered to play a central role, despite the demonstration by Moseley and Goldie in 1963 of a vascular supply to the cuff that is rich in anastamoses between tendinous and osseous vessels.[13] Furthermore, Rathbun and Macnab demonstrated that findings of avascularity of the cuff may have been positional, due to a

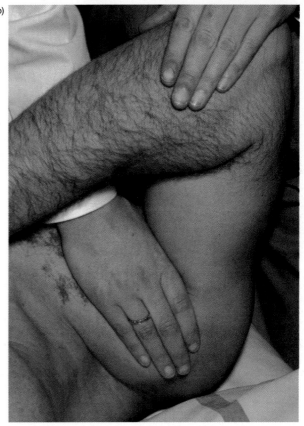

Fig. 18 Apprehension tests. Anterior glenohumeral instability can be assessed standing, sitting or supine (a). As the shoulder is moved passively into abduction and external rotation, the patient becomes apprehensive that the shoulder is going to dislocate anteriorly. Posterior instability can be assessed with the patient supine. The examiner forward flexes and medial rotates the shoulder and applies posterior force on the patient's elbow. The patient reports apprehension that the shoulder is going to dislocate posteriorly.

'wringing out' of the vessels with the arm in the adducted position.[14] Subsequent studies by others using laser Doppler demonstrated substantial flow in this area and in particular increased flow in the area of cuff tears.[15] It is therefore apparent that other factors play a significant role in the development of rotator cuff tendinopathies. These may include the presence of cytokines as a response to vibration and repetitive trauma, hypoxic reperfusion mechanisms, and the generation of free radicals, hyperthermia, a genetic predisposition, underlying

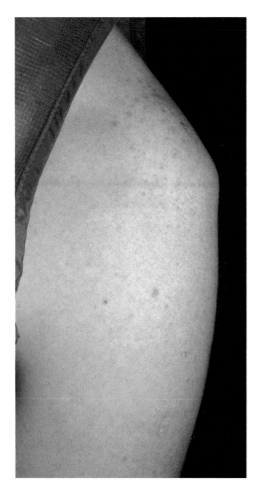

Table 10 Aetiology of rotator cuff tendinopathy

Extrinsic
Macrotrauma
Microtrauma
Foreign bodies
Corticosteroids

Intrinsic
Subacromial impingement:

    AC Joint OA
    AC Joint instability
    Thickened coracoacromial ligament
    Narrow subacromial space
    Type I or II acromial morphology
    Presence of os acromiale
    Low acromioscapular angle
    Thickening of rotator cuff tendon
    Calcification in subacromial space or cuff
    Neuromuscular dysfunction
        Scapulothoracic
        Scapulohumeral
    Posterior capsular tightness

Subcoracoid impingement
Internal impingement
Inflammatory arthritis
Diabetes
Hypothyroidism
Hyperparathyroidism
Amyloid
Chronic renal failure

Fig. 19 The inferior sulcus sign, indicating inferior laxity. Traction is being placed by the examiner on the arm, pulling the humerus inferiorly.

chronic disease such as diabetes mellitus, raised subacromial pressure with abduction of the shoulder, and mechanical trauma upon the cuff. *Impingement* of the rotator cuff, primarily upon the undersurface of the anterolateral acromion within the coracoacromial arch during elevation of the arm, has also long been considered to play a major role in injury to the tendons of the cuff. Other areas of impingement that have been implicated in rotator cuff lesions include internal impingement by the undersurface of cuff against the undersurface of glenoid rim (seen in throwing athletes) and impingement between the coracoid and the head of the humerus, particularly in forward flexion and internal rotation.

Subacromial impingement may be primary or may be secondary to numerous factors (Table 10), many of which cause narrowing of the coracoacromial arch, local friction to the rotator cuff, and/or migration of the humeral head, with resulting abutment on the cuff. Other shoulder pathologies may be present that cause shoulder and scapulothoracic dysfunction and impingement through weakness, pain, or muscle imbalance. Intrinsic changes within the tendon could themselves cause impingement through swelling or through scapulothoracic dysfunction due to pain.

Neer considered subacromial impingement to be the primary aetiological factor in rotator cuff lesions.[16] He proposed a natural history of initial oedema and haemorrhage of the tendon, followed by subacromial thickening, fibrosis, degeneration of the rotator cuff

tendon(s), formation of acromial spurs, and eventual tendon rupture. Whilst this description remains popular, the natural history of the condition has not been substantiated and mechanical impingement is not the only cause of rotator cuff lesions. Ogata and Uhtoff examined 76 cadavers, noting no correlation between rotator cuff tears and degenerative changes on the undersurface of the acromion.[17] With the further advancement of imaging and arthroscopic techniques there is now an opportunity to re-evaluate the natural history of the complaint.

As has been described, the GHJ is an inherently unstable joint. True instability of the joint occurs when there is abnormal translation of the humeral head within the glenoid fossa. Instability may take the form of dislocation, where there is complete loss of contact between articular surfaces, or subluxation when loss of contact between joint surfaces is incomplete. Subluxation can be subtle and may present as non-specific shoulder pain or with a rotator cuff tendinopathy. Detection of instability is vital to the appropriate management of the patient.

History

Rotator cuff disorders typically present with shoulder pain which is usually anterolateral but may be located posteriorly. Pain may be more severe with partial thickness cuff tears. A history of macro- or microtrauma may be given. Weakness secondary to a significant tear or more frequently simply due to pain may be reported. Nocturnal pain is frequently marked, particularly when lying on the affected side and pain is also usually exacerbated with activity, especially when working with the arm overhead. Lesions of subscapularis can cause pain with the arm below shoulder level. Symptoms suggestive of associated instability may be reported in younger and/or athletic individuals and those with a previous history of dislocation. These include clicking, clunking, or a 'dead arm', with sudden, transient numbness and weakness of the arm with throwing. Stiffness and/or restriction may be reported which may relate to pain and/or posterior capsular tightness. Crepitus may be noted by the patient with a thickened subacromial bursa.

Examination

Muscle atrophy may be noted particularly in the presence of a significant tendinopathy or longstanding rotator cuff tendon tear. Subacromial impingement may be demonstrated by the presence of painful arc of abduction (usually between 45° and 120°) and a positive impingement test. There is a full passive range of movement of the shoulder (if pain permits), with specific active movements limited by weakness if a significant tear is present. Pain on resisted testing of the rotator cuff in one or more planes indicates a tendinosis with an intact cuff, whilst significant weakness out of proportion to pain implies a tear is present. Associated features, such as acromioclavicular joint (ACJ) tenderness and deformity (indicative of possible OA) or glenohumeral instability may also be noted. A subacromial injection of local anaesthetic may help to differentiate impingement from other causes of shoulder pain, with improvement in pain and active and passive range of movement seen with impingement but not other disorders (Neer's test).[18] This test has not been validated against imaging or surgical findings.

Imaging the rotator cuff

Current guidelines for the use of imaging in rotator cuff disorders emphasize the importance of the roles of specialized investigations such as magnetic resonance imaging (MRI) and ultrasound (Table 11).[19] Plain radiographic examination is recommended if calcifying tendinitis is suspected, but plain radiography is not indicated routinely in early cases. However, plain X-rays may be an important diagnostic tool in other causes of shoulder pain such as metastatic disease.

In more advanced cases of rotator cuff tendinopathy the characteristic changes associated with chronic rotator cuff insufficiency may be seen, with subacromial sclerosis and osteophytes, greater tuberosity sclerosis and cystic changes, and reduced acromiohumeral distance. In massive rotator cuff tears, radiographs may reveal superior migration and/or deformity of the humeral head, with a sensitivity and specificity of 78 and 98 per cent respectively.[20]

MRI can help to confirm the diagnosis, to provide further insight into the nature of the lesion, to identify other lesions, and to provide information about surrounding structures. A high degree of correlation between histological changes within the supraspinatus tendon and modifications of its signal on MRI in a study of young cadaveric tendons has been demonstrated.[21] Calcifying lesions are not well demonstrated.

Standard imaging is performed in at least two planes, with a coronal oblique T2- or proton-density-weighted series aligned along the line of the supraspinatus tendon to visualize the supraspinatus and infraspinatus tendons, together with an axially acquired T1-weighted sequence to visualize subscapularis, long head of biceps, and teres minor. An additional sagittal T2-weighted sequence is sometimes added and provides additional information about the configuration of the acromion and ACJ in particular.

MRI has been particularly effective in the detection of full thickness rotator cuff tears (Fig. 20). In such cases, a continuous band of fluid that traverses the full thickness of the cuff, retraction of the tendon, and high signal intensity in the cuff on T2-weighted images are the most significant signs. The accuracy of diagnosis of rotator cuff tears using MRI is 90 per cent, having a sensitivity of 83 per cent[22] and a specificity of 78 per cent, with the accuracy for full thickness tears being superior to that of partial thickness lesions and tendinitis/tendinosis.[23] In partial thickness tears, fat-suppressed T2-weighted imaging may increase diagnostic accuracy. In addition, MR arthrography with gadolinium enhancement may help in the detection of articular sided partial thickness tears.

Ultrasound is highly operator-dependent, but has the advantage of being non-invasive, allows both shoulders to be examined and is

Table 11 Guidelines for radiological investigations in shoulder complaints (adapted from reference 19)

Complaint	Investigation	Comments
Painful shoulder	X-ray	Not indicated initially, unless calcifying tendinitis is suspected. Degenerative changes in the ACJ are common
Shoulder impingement	MRI	Impingement is a clinical diagnosis. Imaging is indicated if surgery is being considered, to define the anatomy
Shoulder impingement	Ultrasound	Allows dynamic imaging
Shoulder instability	CT arthrography MR arthrography	
Rotator cuff tear	Arthrography Ultrasound MRI	Choice of imaging modality is dependent upon local expertise.

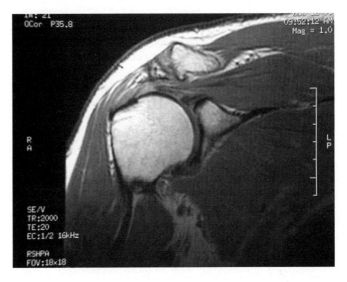

Fig. 20 T2 weighted MRI scan of the shoulder showing a full thickness rotator cuff tear and a degenerate AC joint with an inferior osteophyte.

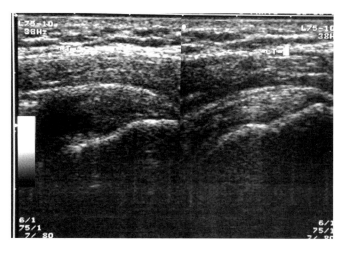

Fig. 21 Ultrasound of shoulders, showing right rotator cuff tendinosis. The cuff is swollen and shows areas of hypoechogenicity (left image), compared to the normal cuff of the left shoulder (right image).

rapid, inexpensive, and accessible. In a large study of 4588 shoulders, Hedtmann and Fett demonstrated an overall sensitivity of 91 per cent for partial-thickness and 97 per cent for full-thickness tears, with an overall false negative rate of less than 2 per cent and an accuracy of 95 per cent.[24] Farin *et al.*[25] found that the size of tears (partial and full thickness) could be established in 70 per cent of cases. Dynamic ultrasound may also confirm, but not exclude, impingement. Ultrasonographic evidence of fatty infiltration of disrupted muscles of the rotator cuff, which changes little after the repair of the tear, has been associated with the degree of tendon retraction and with severe functional impairment and recurrent tear after repair (Fig. 21). Such features may be play a role in the decision to intervene surgically.

Arthrography, has a reported accuracy of 82 per cent, with a sensitivity of 50 per cent and specificity of 96 per cent in the diagnosis of full thickness tears,[26] but it is difficult to localize the site and to quantify the size of the tear. It is not useful in the detection of intratendinous nor bursal surface tears. Resolution may be improved by using double contrast or single and double contrast arthrotomography. The latter has a sensitivity of 70 per cent in the diagnosis of partial thickness tears, although it can estimate the size in only 30 per cent of all tears. Arthrography and MRI have similar diagnostic and therapeutic impact,[26] although MRI is superior in providing information about surrounding structures, including acromial morphology and causes of impingement.

Subacromial *bursography*, in particular when coupled with helical computed tomography, has been used to assess the bursal side of the rotator cuff and may help in the diagnosis of bursal side lesions, which may be undetected by other imaging methods. Again, the accuracy and value of such a technique has not yet been established. *Diagnostic arthroscopy* has the advantage of allowing direct evaluation of the rotator cuff and has been a significant advance in particular in the identification of partial thickness tears and labral pathologies.

Management of tendinosis with an intact rotator cuff

Standard management of rotator cuff tendinosis commences with control of pain. Relative rest with avoidance of exacerbating activities,

regular applications of ice, heat packs to relieve muscle spasm, and the judicious use of a support are all frequently recommended. Nonsteroidal anti-inflammatory drugs (NSAIDs) and local modalities, including ultrasound, laser, and electromagnetic field therapy, may all assist with pain relief. Subacromial corticosteroid injections should be reserved for those individuals with persisting pain and where rehabilitation is limited. There is no evidence of benefit from intraarticular corticosteroids in rotator cuff tendinopathies.

Other treatments that have been advocated include local transdermal glyceryl trinitrate, intraarticular sympathetic block with guanethidine, transcutaneous nerve stimulation, and physiotherapy, although evidence for such approaches is limited.[5, 6]

Surgery is considered in the patient with a tendinosis who fails conservative measures when there are associated lesions such as those causing impingement. Subacromial decompression, resection of the distal clavicle, or excision/debridement of ACJ osteophyte(s) have all been advocated. Arthroscopic and open decompression appear to have similar long-term outcomes with reported success rates of 90 per cent (satisfactory or better improvement in pain and/or function).

Management of rotator cuff tears

Management of the patient with a rotator cuff tear is influenced by the age, activity level, expectations of the patient, the type and extent of the tear, its duration, mode of onset, and additional pathologies. Rotator cuff tears can be managed conservatively in the same manner as tendinosis. The use of corticosteroid injections in known tears is discouraged due to the possible deleterious effects of the corticosteroid on tendon, although they may be indicated in the older patient where function is very limited. There is much debate as to indications for surgery, the most appropriate surgical procedure, and the importance of the size and surface area of the tear in relation to the need for repair.

Surgical options include debridement, subacromial decompression and excision, and repair of the damaged tendon. In some patients who exhibit associated glenohumeral instability, a stabilization procedure may be considered. In full thickness tears, decompression and repair is the most common surgical approach, with up to 94 per cent reporting a 'satisfactory or better' outcome in a prospective uncontrolled study at 7.5 years follow-up.[27] Acute traumatic full thickness tears should be repaired early,[28,29] but patients with degenerative full thickness tears should be given a trial of conservative management of 4 months. Surgical intervention is considered if there is progression of symptoms and/or significant functional impairment. The outcome appears to be less satisfactory in older patients and those with large tears, poor active range of motion, or weakness preoperatively.

Surgery for the patient with a partial thickness tear is usually reserved for the patient who fails to respond to conservative measures. Debridement may be successful in younger patients, but decompression is usually necessary in older patients. Indications for excision and repair of the tendon have not been clearly defined, although surgery may be most appropriate for larger tears.

It has been reported that approximately 40 per cent of cases of articular surface partial thickness tears respond to conservative management, but that most cases of bursal side and intratendinous tears tend not to heal.[27, 30] Although imaging studies have shown that many partial tears commonly show progression with time, symptoms often improve in these patients. This emphasizes the difficulty with correlating clinical with imaging findings.

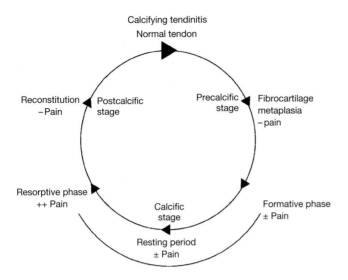

Fig. 22 Calcifying tendinitis.

Calcifying tendinitis

Calcifying tendinitis is a distinct and usually temporary clinical syndrome associated with the formation and resorption of calcific deposits within one or more portions of the tendinous portion of the rotator cuff. Although the disorder is considered to be relatively common, its true incidence is unknown. However, asymptomatic calcification within the cuff is frequently observed radiologically, with reported incidences of 2.7–20 per cent of adults. Calcifying tendinitis shows a relative female predominance and typically affects sedentary workers in the age range 30–50 years. The right shoulder is more commonly affected than the left and bilateral involvement has been described in up to 24 per cent.

Whilst several concepts have been proposed for calcifying tendinitis, the most popular is that of Uhtoff and colleagues, who describe the condition as consisting of three stages (Fig. 22).[31] During the first stage, the *precalcific phase*, fibrocartilaginous metaplasia occurs in the tendon of one or more of the components of the rotator cuff, affecting most commonly by far supraspinatus. The aetiology of such a transformation is unknown and no derangement of calcium or phosphate metabolism has been identified. This stage may be asymptomatic or a dull pain in the shoulder may be noted.

The second, *calcific stage* commences with the formative phase, involving formation and deposition of calcium within fibrocartilaginous areas of the tendon(s). During the resorptive phase of stage two these become surrounded by macrophages, fibroblasts, and multinucleate giant cells, forming a calcium granuloma. The resorptive phase is associated with the acute onset of constant, severe shoulder pain, which may be related to elevated intratendinous pressure. Should the deposits rupture into the subacromial bursa, an acute bursitis may occur but otherwise subacromial bursitis is unlikely to make a major contribution to symptoms. Eventually, stage 3 (the *post-calcific stage*) is reached, where following resorption of calcium the tendinous tissue is replaced by granulation tissue. In most cases, pain gradually resolves, although subacute flares may occur. From the clinical viewpoint, the resorptive phase of stage 2 is often described as the acute phase and other phases subacute or chronic. Other shoulder pathologies may also coexist with calcifying tendinitis (Table 12).

Table 12 Differential diagnosis of calcifying tendinitis

Other causes of radiological calcification
Glenohumeral arthropathy
Rotator cuff tear
Rotator cuff arthropathy
Milwaukee shoulder
Hyperparathyroidism
Subcutaneous calcification (infection, inflammation, ulceration)

Other causes of shoulder pain with systemic features
Sepsis
Crystal arthropathy
Other inflammatory arthropathies
Malignancy

History

The history is dependent upon the stage of presentation. Those who present in stage 1 typically complain of a nagging diffuse ache around the shoulder that may be associated with nocturnal disturbance. Patients presenting in stage 2 complain of severe shoulder pain and systemic symptoms including fever with leucocytosis, and an elevated erythrocyte sedimentation rate (ESR) may raise suspicion of sepsis, a crystal arthritis, or malignancy. A catching sensation and symptoms suggestive of impingement are frequently reported.

Examination

In the more acute stage, the patient may appear unwell and support and guard the affected arm, keeping the shoulder in internal rotation. Range of motion is limited in all planes by pain. A painful middle arc and a positive impingement sign are often noted. In more chronic cases wasting of the spinati may be evident.

Investigation

Investigations are performed to exclude other causes of shoulder pain with systemic symptoms. The ESR may be elevated and a leucocytosis may be evident. Plain radiography of the shoulder is performed, commencing with an anteroposterior view and if necessary internal and external rotation views to demonstrate calcification in the supraspinatus, infraspinatus, and subscapularis, respectively. Radiographic calcification in patients with calcifying tendinitis may appear as discrete deposits of uniform density in the formative phase, becoming fluffy with poorly defined margins in the acute stage (Fig. 23). Rupture into the bursa may be evident in the resorptive stage, during which both bursal and, more slowly, intratendinous calcification disappears. Coincidental calcification associated with articular degeneration may be distinguished from that of true calcifying tendinitis by its stippled pattern and location much nearer to the greater tuberosity. Other causes of radiographic calcification in the area of the GHJ include a rotator cuff tear, rotator cuff arthropathy, Milwaukee shoulder, and hyperparathyroidism. Further imaging in the form of MRI and ultrasound may be necessary if other pathologies are suspected. Ultrasound, but not MRI, is useful in demonstrating calcification.

Management

Treatment is dependent upon the stage of presentation. The initial focus is pain control. Rest and support of the affected arm, regular ice packs, analgesics, and/or NSAIDs may all provide some pain relief and reduce associated muscle spasm.

Physiotherapy commences with gentle mobilization of the joint and, when symptoms allow, the progressive introduction of stretching and range of motion exercises followed by a cuff-strengthening programme.

Ultrasound, both in the conventional form and high-energy ultrasound (extracorporeal shock wave therapy), has been demonstrated to be effective in reducing symptoms and calcification.[32, 33] Needling of the most symptomatic areas under fluoroscopic control has been recommended on the basis that it may relieve intratendinous pressure. Needling is followed by lavage and, in some cases, by injection of local anaesthetic and corticosteroid, although the latter is contentious as it may theoretically inhibit the progression of the condition to the resorptive phase through reduction of vascular proliferation and macrophage activity. The author reserves local corticosteroids for those patients who have subacute flares and/or impingement in the chronic stages. Surgical intervention is rarely indicated and is reserved for those with protracted symptoms, particularly in the

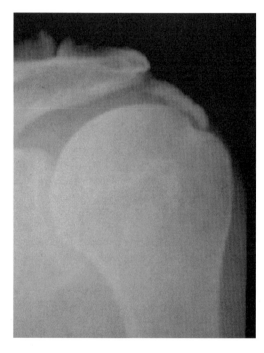

Fig. 23 Plain x-ray showing calcifying tendinitis of the shoulder.

formative phase. Theoretically the deposit should be easier to remove arthroscopically during the acute phase where the deposit is more liquid in consistency.

Complications of calcifying tendinitis include cuff tear, frozen shoulder, bicipital tendinopathy, and osseous penetration by calcium. Recurrence can also occur, although this is probably related to incomplete resolution of the initial episode.

Lesions of the tendon of the long head of the biceps (LHB)

As has been described, the tendon of the long head of the biceps (TLHB) is intimately associated with the rotator cuff, the labrum, and the rotator interval. It is not surprising then that lesions of the TLHB are commonly associated with pathologies at one or more of these sites. Biceps lesions include tendinopathy without significant tear ('tendinitis' or tenosynovitis), tear (partial/rupture), and instability within the bicipital groove (subluxation or dislocation). Habermayerr and Walch suggested a system of classification that helps to illustrate the numerous lesions with which LHB pathologies are associated (Table 13).[34] Damage to the TLHB at its origin (type I lesions) involves tearing of the biceps–labrum junction at the superior rim of the labrum. These lesions typically occur in throwing athletes and are described further in the section on glenohumeral instability (Fig. 24). A rotator interval lesion can be defined as a lesion of the intraarticular portion of the TLHB between the entrance to the bicipital groove and its origin on the superior glenoid, with no cuff pathology.

Biceps tendinosis/tenosynovitis

A primary isolated biceps tendinosis/tenosynovitis is a rare entity but is seen in swimmers, throwers, and weight-lifters, or after an episode of trauma or unaccustomed lifting. Rotational activities of the upper arm where there is extension of both elbow and shoulder, such as karate and table tennis or fast walking with hand weights, are also associated with bicipital pain. Anatomical variations such as a shallow bicipital groove or local osteophytes encroaching upon the bicipital groove and causing attrition, indirect or direct trauma, or fracture of the humeral tuberosities may all predispose to bicipital tendon lesions. Lapidus and Guidotti drew an analogy with deQuervain's tenosynovitis, suggesting that stenosis of the tendons with thickening of the transverse ligament and sheath occurs.[35] A proliferative tenosynovitis

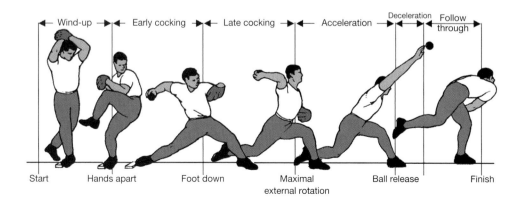

Fig. 24 Throwing sports vary in their techniques but most involve significant traction on the LHB and labrum. Many throwers also have lax shoulders, imposing greater demands on dynamic stabilizers.

Table 13 Classification of lesions of the tendon of long head of biceps (TLHB)

Origin of TLHB
Associated with SLAP lesions

Rotator interval lesions
Primary biceps tendinopathy
Isolated rupture
Subluxation
    Type I, superior
    Type II, at groove
    Type III, mal-/non-union of lesser tuberosity fracture

Associated with rotator cuff tear or severe tendinopathy
Tendinopathy
Dislocation
    Extraarticular with partial tear of subscapularis
    Extraarticular with intact subscapularis
    Intraarticular dislocation
Subluxation with cuff tear
Rupture with cuff tear

within the bicipital groove may also occur. However, impingement is the most common cause of LHB tendinopathy and signs of rotator cuff disease are frequently present.

Since bicipital tendinopathies have a varied aetiology and a range of associated lesions, a range of presentations can occur. Typically, LHB tendinosis/ tenosynovitis presents in young or middle-aged patients as anterior shoulder and upper arm pain radiating into the biceps muscle belly. It may also radiate proximally or present as impingement. Nocturnal symptoms are variable. The patient may give a history of performing the precipitating activities mentioned above or describe symptoms associated with other pathologies such as rotator cuff tendinosis. There may be a sensation of instability and, where subluxation is occurring, the patient may complain of snapping over the anterior shoulder. Ultrasound may demonstrate fluid in the tendon sheath.

There is tenderness over the bicipital groove, most easily found with the arm in 10° of internal rotation. This tenderness may reduce with further internal rotation of the arm (unlike subacromial impingement). Speed's test elicits pain (or weakness in tears). In isolated bicipital tendinopathy there is full range of movement, but in other cases limitation may occur due to other pathologies being present.

Management of tendinitis of the LHB is similar to that of rotator cuff tendinosis, with ice, analgesics, NSAIDs, and a graduated programme of rehabilitation forming the mainstays of therapy. A single local injection of short/moderate-acting corticosteroid into the sheath or joint may help to alleviate pain in more resistant cases. Where subacromial impingement is present, arthroscopic subacromial decompression may be necessary in resistant cases and is also useful to establish whether a cuff tear is present.

Biceps tendon subluxation

Subluxation and dislocation of the LHB tendon can occur due to trauma or repetitive microtrauma to the rotator interval sling, through active internal rotation of the arm. Biceps tendon subluxation has been classified into three types.[34, 36]

1. Superior (*type I*) subluxation occurs due to partial or complete tearing of the coracohumeral and superior glenohumeral ligaments, whilst the insertion of subscapularis remains intact. There is subluxation above the entrance to the bicipital groove. An articular surface partial tear of the tendon of supraspinatus may be associated.

2. *Type II* subluxation involves medial subluxation at the groove due to a tear of the outermost fibres of subscapularis, which usually anchors the TLHB.

3. *Type III* occurs secondary to fracture dislocation of the lesser tuberosity with malunion, resulting in loss of the bony restraint of the tendon. Subluxation of the TLHB frequently presents a diagnostic challenge. Patients may complain of painful clicking or snapping over the bicipital groove. Type III subluxation also is associated with pain on internal rotation. There is bicipital grove tenderness and pain on performing Speed's test. It is usually very difficult to feel subluxation of the TLHB. However, it may produce an audible snap or palpable click as the tendon subluxes when the patient slowly brings the arm from the passively fully abducted arm in external rotation. Dynamic ultrasound is helpful in confirming the diagnosis but arthroscopy may be necessary.

Chronic subluxation may lead to tendinopathy and tear due to attrition. Altered transmission of mechanical forces may also occur, resulting in a high incidence of degenerative changes in the anterosuperior portion of the labrum.

Dislocation of the tendon of the long head of the biceps

Dislocation of the TLHB predominantly occurs in men in their sixth decade and tends to involve the dominant arm. It can occur in association with rotator cuff disease or after chronic subluxation of the tendon, when the rotator interval sling and subscapularis tendon are torn. The tendon may intermittently dislocate with rotation of the arm or may be permanently displaced from the groove into either an extra- or intraarticular position.

The patient complains of shoulder pain and clicking. Signs of a rotator cuff tear are evident and the pain may be worse with flexion and rotation of the arm. There are no specific diagnostic tests but ultrasound, MRI and CT arthrography and arthroscopy are all sensitive in confirming the diagnosis.

Management of subluxation/dislocation

In the symptomatic patient or where the tendon is becoming compromised, arthroscopic or open surgical intervention should be considered. Approaches include reconstruction of the rotator interval sling and/or restoring the tendon to its groove. Other pathologies should be addressed and, where significant subacromial impingement is present, decompression is also performed.

Tears of the tendon of LHB

Tears of the tendon of LHB may be partial, complete, or may extend to a full rupture. Partial tears may occur in association with any of the causes of tendinitis, in particular, impingement, and may present with symptoms similar to those reported with tendinosis/tenosynovitis.

TLHB ruptures

Although certain factors such as osteophytes in the groove have been blamed for tendon ruptures, there is little evidence for this. Ruptures usually occur at the entrance to the bicipital groove, where the tendon is exposed to greatest mechanical stresses, resulting in chronic tenosynovitis and attrition. Mechanical impingement is the cause for most cases and additional cuff pathologies are usually present. It appears that the rupture itself may be due to increased stresses on the LHB by rotator cuff dysfunction and that impingement upon the TLHB is a secondary effect.

Lesions typically occur in the dominant arm of men over the age of 60 years and present with a 'Popeye' deformity of the upper arm, often with relatively little pain. There may be a prior history of shoulder or bicipital pain. Significant synovitis of the joint can occur and the remnant of the attachment of the tendon can become entrapped in the joint with a subsequent chondral lesion of the glenoid or humeral head. Whereas an isolated rupture of TLHB has only minor impact upon function, when combined with a rotator cuff tear the effects on upper limb strength are significant.

Management

Rupture of the TLHB can be managed symptomatically, with attention to rehabilitation of the cuff. In cases of painful rupture of the TLHB, a rotator cuff tear and/or SLAP (Superior Labral in the AnteroPosterior direction) lesion (see below) must be excluded and arthroscopy is useful in this situation. Tenodesis may be considered in the younger or more active patient and additional pathologies are managed as appropriate.

Glenohumeral instability

Glenohumeral instability is the inability to keep the humeral head centred in the glenoid fossa. It may take the form of dislocation when there is complete separation of the articular surfaces, or more commonly subluxation, involving excessive translation of the humeral head on the glenoid without separation of the articular surfaces. This may be subtle and easily missed by the unsuspecting clinician. Instability is also described according to its circumstances of onset, direction, degree, duration, uni-/bilaterality, and volition. Determination of these factors is important in planning appropriate management (Table 14).

Dislocations

Dislocations of the GHJ comprise 45 per cent of all dislocations. Almost 85 per cent of these are in the *anterior direction*. The most common type is subcoracoid, typically after trauma involving abduction, extension, and external rotation. More rare forms, usually in association with severe trauma, associated rotator cuff avulsion, and

fracture of the greater tuberosity, include subglenoid, subclavicular, intrathoracic, and retroperitoneal.

The patient usually holds the arm in slight abduction and external rotation. The humeral head may be palpable anteriorly. There is limited internal rotation and adduction. Neurovascular injuries are common and may also occur after reduction, so assessment prior to treatment is mandatory. The axillary nerve is the most commonly injured neural structure, although damage to the radial, musculocutaneous, median, ulnar, or entire brachial plexus may occur. Neuropraxias are the most common form of neurological injury—symptoms beyond 3 months have a poor prognosis for recovery. Vascular injury is indicated by a reduced or absent peripheral pulse, an expanding haematoma, pallor, or shock.

Avulsion of the anteroinferior glenohumeral ligaments and capsule from the glenoid rim represent a *Bankart lesion*, a common cause of recurrent instability after previous dislocation. A *Hill–Sachs lesion* often accompanies a Bankart lesion. This is a compression fracture of the posterior surface of the humeral head after impaction against the anterior glenoid rim (Fig. 25). Rotator cuff tears occur more commonly with increasing age of the patient, but may be difficult to detect in the acute presentation.

Posterior dislocations occur in relation to trauma but are also a feature of congenital laxity and multidirectional instability. Traumatic dislocations in relation to trauma are mostly subacromial or rarely subglenoid or subspinous and frequently are locked. All may arise due to axial loading of the adducted internally rotated arm or by violent muscle contraction such as during an epileptic seizure or an electric shock. Posterior dislocations are frequently missed, but are indicated by a hollow below the acromion, anterior deltoid flattening, and a palpable humeral head posteriorly. The patient holds the arm in adduction and/or internal rotation and there is a lack of active and passive external rotation. Sequelae include a fracture of the glenoid rim, proximal humerus, and a reverse Hill–Sachs lesion (a compression fracture of the humeral head). Rotator cuff and neurovascular damage are less commonly noted than with an anterior dislocation.

Inferior dislocations may be produced by a significant hyperabduction injury, which levers the humeral head inferiorly out of the glenoid, through abutment of the neck of the humerus against the acromion. Such dislocations are locked and, in contrast to posterior dislocations, they are easily identified. Avulsion of one or more portions of the rotator cuff, fracture of the greater tuberosity, and neurovascular damage

Table 14 Descriptive features of glenohumeral instability

Type	Subluxation/dislocation
Mode of onset	Traumatic/atraumatic
Duration	Acute/chronic
Side affected	Unilateral/bilateral
Direction	Unidirectional (anterior/posterior/inferior)/multidirectional
Volition	Voluntary/involuntary
Associated features	Congenital laxity/neuromuscular disorder/resulting pathologies (e.g. Bankart, Hill–Sachs lesions)

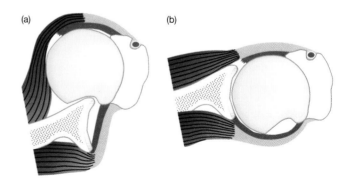

Fig. 25 A postero-lateral defect in the humeral head (Hill Sachs lesion) and an anterior capsulolabral tear (Bankarts lesion) commonly occur with anterior GHJ dislocation. (a) These persist after reduction of the dislocation. (b)

Table 15 Sequelae of acute dislocations

Site	Sequelae
Humerus	Anterior: posterolateral defect of the humeral head (Hill–Sachs lesion)
	Posterior: anteromedial compression fracture of the humeral head (reverse Hill–Sachs lesion)
	Fracture of greater tuberosity or more rarely surgical neck
Glenoid	Avulsion fracture of glenoid rim (Bankart lesion)
	Major fractures
Labrum	Tear
Capsule	Anterior calcification
Rotator cuff	Partial or complete tear
Neurological injuries	Most commonly axillary nerve or brachial plexus; other nerves of the upper arm can be affected.
Vascular injuries	Axillary artery

are all common. Superior dislocation is very rare and occurs after a major anterior and upward force on the adducted arm, with multiple injuries of surrounding structures (Table 15).

Investigations

Plain X-rays are performed in order to confirm a dislocation and to identify associated bony pathologies. Views in at least two planes are obtained, usually an anteroposterior (AP) view in the scapular plane (some recommend that this should be performed with the arm both in external and internal rotation) and a transthoracic lateral view. An axillary view is also helpful. Reliance only on AP views may result in a missed fracture. CT is useful in the detection of bony injuries and MRI in the evaluation of the integrity of the cuff.

Treatment

This involves early relocation after assessment and plain X-ray. Analgesics, muscle relaxants, and even a general anaesthetic may be necessary. Early reduction is important in order to minimize the effect on the joint and soft tissue structures. A variety of approaches for reduction are advocated and open reduction may be necessary. Neurovascular status and rotator cuff integrity should be assessed before and after reduction. The arm is then immobilized for 3–6 weeks in the younger patient, but for 1–3 weeks in older individuals as they are more prone to joint stiffness with prolonged immobilization. The position of the arm during this period is dependent upon the direction of the dislocation. After anterior dislocation the arm is maintained in adduction and internal rotation, and posterior dislocations are maintained in slight external rotation, abduction, and extension. Rehabilitation initially involves movement limited to 90° flexion and no external rotation, isometric strengthening of the rotator cuff and deltoid, and full range of motion of the elbow. A progressive cuff and scapular stabilizing programme is then commenced.

Recurrent instability

Recurrent glenohumeral instability may vary from repeated dislocations to subtle subluxation and can be broadly classified into two groups (TUBS and AMBRII), according to some of these features.[37] Although an oversimplification of the broad continuum of shoulder laxity, this classification provides a useful clinical approach to shoulder instability.

TUBS

Trauma to any part of the stabilizing complex may precipitate recurrent instability, which is typically reproduced by putting the arm into the position it was in when the trauma occurred. *T*rauma usually results in *u*nilateral instability and there is often other pathology, classically a *B*ankart lesion. Although such cases may respond to a rehabilitation programme, *s*urgery may be necessary. These lesions are therefore known as TUBS lesions.

The patient may present with an overt history of recurrent dislocation, with symptoms suggestive of subluxation, and apprehension that dislocation is about to occur with specific movements. Symptoms commonly occur with increasingly trivial provocation. Recurrent dislocation is particularly likely in the younger patient, with recurrence occurring in 80–90 per cent of patients below the age of 20 years, 40–65 per cent of those aged 20–40 years, and 0–15 per cent of those above the age of 40 years.[38] Recurrence in the younger age group is particularly common in sporting individuals and where additional pathologies are present, in particular labral, glenohumeral ligament, Bankart or Hill–Sachs lesions, or where there is weakness of subscapularis.

AMBRII

*A*traumatic cases (usually those with congenital laxity) typically demonstrate *m*ultidirectional instability that is *b*ilateral. Almost all respond to a *r*ehabilitation programme; the few who do not may be treated surgically by an *i*nferior capsular shift and repair of the rotator *i*nterval. These lesions are termed AMBRII.

Recurrent subluxation usually presents in the young patient in association with activities such as throwing, when there is pain, clicking, clunking, neurological symptoms, and a feeling of instability. Recognizing the AMBRII patient with symptoms of instability or who presents with rotator cuff tendinopathy or impingement is vital to appropriate management. A small proportion of the AMBRII group are voluntary habitual dislocators who sublux or dislocate the GHJ as a 'party trick' or in association with psychological disorders. Counselling of such patients is of primary importance.

A careful history is taken to document the mechanisms of injury, the degree of trauma involved, associated symptoms and previous injuries, and the degree of functional limitation. Examination includes an assessment for the presence of associated pathologies (such as tendinopathy and impingement), the degree of laxity of the shoulder compared to the unaffected side, response to apprehension stress tests, and for the presence of generalized joint laxity.

All individuals should be treated conservatively with an intensive rotator cuff and scapular stabilizing programme unless associated pathologies are present. Rehabilitation involves neuromuscular training of the muscles of the cuff, deltoid, scapular stabilizers, and pectoralis major. Much of the regime is initially low-intensity endurance exercise and this must be explained to the patient, particularly if the patient is an athlete who frequently prioritizes strength training for power. Those patients who are congenitally lax (AMBRII) often require lengthy rehabilitation and much encouragement.

Surgical management is considered in those with recurrent instability who fail to respond to an intensive programme and who continue to experience instability that is interfering with their activities. Surgery is discouraged in those who are habitual dislocators. A number of procedures have been described, involving repair of the anterior capsular mechanism and other stabilization procedures.

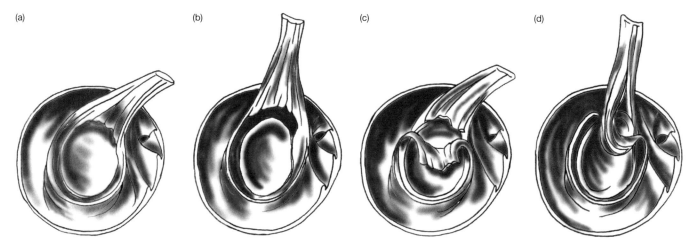

Fig. 26 SLAP lesions: (a) superior labral fraying; (b) labral amd LHB detachment from the glenoid rim; (c) bucket handle tearing of the labrum; (d) as (c) with extension into the LHB.

Labral pathologies

Injuries to the glenoid labrum are an increasingly recognized cause of persisting shoulder pain and instability. They typically occur after an episode of trauma where subluxation or dislocation has occurred but are also a feature of repetitive microtrauma, usually in throwers. Bankart and SLAP lesions are the most common forms of labral injuries. The aetiology of the Bankart lesion, involving detachment of the labrum and capsule from the rim of the glenoid in relation to anterior dislocation, has been described earlier.

The *SLAP lesion* involves a tear of the *superior labral* in the *antero-posterior* direction. This typically is seen in throwers, where there is traction on the tendon of LHB, which inserts at the superior labrum. Such lesions can also arise in relation to a variety of other activities, including a fall on to an outstretched arm with the shoulder in abduction and slight forward flexion, from acute traction or from an abduction–external rotation mechanism. Once a tear of the labrum has occurred, it may propagate anteriorly, posteriorly, or both. The resulting instability can lead to lesions of the rotator cuff and the LHB. Snyder *et al.* proposed a system of classification of SLAP lesions that includes such sequelae (Fig. 26).[39]

The patient may report non-specific, deep-seated shoulder pain and catching or popping with specific movements. Signs of associated LHB or rotator cuff pathologies may be noted and a SLAP test may be positive, but can be unreliable.

Investigations

Diagnosis of labral pathologies can be difficult. MR arthrography can demonstrate such pathologies, but many cases require diagnostic arthroscopy.

Management

Many cases may respond to conservative management including analgesia, modification of activities, and a stability programme. However, surgery may be necessary, either for diagnostic reasons or where conservative management fails. Resection or repair of torn labrum is performed and where necessary the shoulder is stabilized. Many individuals return to full activity after a postoperative rehabilitation programme.

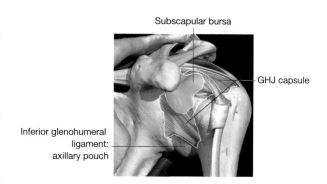

Fig. 27 The glenohumeral joint capsule.

Frozen shoulder

The painful stiff shoulder has long been an enigma in the broad spectrum of shoulder complaints, as illustrated by the many terms used to describe it, including periarthritis scapulohumerale, shoulder periarthritis, pericapsulitis, obliterative bursitis … the list continues. The term adhesive capsulitis, based upon findings of arthographic studies by Nevasier,[40] is the most popular alternative label for frozen shoulder (Fig. 27).

Epidemiology

The mean age of onset of frozen shoulder is during the sixth decade and the condition is rare before the age of 40. Women are more commonly affected than men and there is a slight tendency for the non-dominant arm to be affected. The incidence in the general population is approximately 2–3 per cent. There is no particular occupational association but certain conditions, including (often minor) trauma, may be associated (Tables 16 and 17). Such cases, where a recognized associated disorder is present, are termed secondary frozen shoulder. In diabetes mellitus the incidence may be as high as 35 per cent, with up to 42 per cent having bilateral involvement.

Pathophysiology

Arthroscopic studies have helped to define some of the processes that occur in at least a subset of patients presenting with a frozen

Table 16 Frozen shoulder: associated lesions

Primary
Idiopathic

Secondary
Shoulder trauma (including surgery)
Neurological lesions (e.g. hemiplegia)
Diabetes mellitus (types I and II)
Thyroid disease (hypo/hyper)
Cardiac disease/surgery
Pulmonary disorders

Table 17 Frozen shoulder: differential diagnosis

Rotator cuff tendinopathies

Impingement syndromes

Biceps Tendinitis

Polymyalgia rheumatica

Glenohumeral arthritides
  Osteoarthritis
  Rheumatoid arthritis
  Crystal arthopathies
  Sepsis
  Neuroarthropathy

ACJ osteoarthritis

Algodystrophy (shoulder–hand syndrome)

Neurological lesions:

  Nerve root lesions
  Brachial plexus lesions
  Pancoast's tumour
  Thoracic outlet syndrome
  Intradural lesions

Bone lesions
  Osteomyelitis
  Tumour (primary/secondary)

Referred pain
  Subdiaphragmatic lesions
  Thoracic lesions
  Phrenic nerve lesions
  Neck

Table 18 Stages of frozen shoulder

Stage	Arthroscopic findings	Shoulder movement
1	Fibrinous synovitis	Pain but minimal/no limitation of shoulder mobility
2	Acute proliferative synovitis with early adhesion formation particularly in dependent fold. Loss of normal interval between humeral head and glenoid	Pain. Severe global restriction
3	Synovitis lessens Capsular contraction develops Loss of axillary fold	Less pain. restriction.
4	Synovitis absent Capsular restriction and adhesions marked	Restriction

shoulder. Nevasier and Nevasier suggested four stages of involvement (Table 18).[41]

Histological and histochemical studies indicate that frozen shoulder is a cytokine-driven inflammatory process resulting in synovitis, fibroplasia, and capsular contracture. The specific cytokines involved have been identified and include platelet-derived growth factor (PDGF; which causes fibroblastic cell proliferation) and transforming growth factor-beta (TGF-β; which increases extracellular matrix in the development of capsular fibrosis). Findings seem to be associated with the chronicity of cases examined. After the initial acute inflammatory reactions, where chemotactic and cellular responses and synovitis occur, fibroplasia takes place and it is cases in the latter stage that seem to have been studied the most. Hence, although some studies have reported a normal synovial layer, the earlier synovitic stage may have been missed. Investigation within 3 months of the onset of symptoms

has demonstrated a non-specific synovitis which is negative for culture, crystals, and iron.[42] Lundberg interpreted the increase in the density of the capsular collagen, increases in sulfated glycosaminoglycans, and reduced amounts of glycoproteins as a repair reaction.[43] The condition has been likened to Dupytren's contracture.[44] The pathogenesis of frozen shoulder in diabetics may be related to the high blood glucose level but the mechanism, as in stiffness in other joints and in cheiroarthropathy, is not understood.

Systemic markers of inflammation (ESR, acute phase reactants), bone profiles, and immunoglobulins are normal in the frozen shoulder. No association has been demonstrated with smooth muscle, collagen, cartilage, complement, circulating immune complexes autoimmune factors, nor with immunoglobulin quantification and immunoelectrophoresis, lymphocyte transformability, nor DNA synthesis in response to antigens. Studies using *bone scintigraphy* in patients with frozen shoulder have reported an increase in uptake of [99mTc] relative to the opposite side.[45] However, there is no convincing evidence of an association between isotope uptake and likelihood of steroid responsiveness, disease severity, duration, or outcome.

Plain radiographs are normal or may show minor periarticular osteopenia or minor degenerative changes at the GH or AC joints on both the affected and unaffected sides. *The bone mineral density* of the affected humeral head may be significantly and irreversibly reduced, which does not appear to be associated with age or duration of the condition.

Characteristic features on *arthrography* (Table 19) are considered by some to be essential for the diagnosis of frozen shoulder (Fig. 28). However, some patients, particularly those with early disease (possibly the time at which interventions in the future may be most useful), will not show these changes. In addition, the clinical features and outcome have not been shown to differ between patients on the basis of their arthrograms. Arthrography is useful in helping to define those patients who have underlying rotator cuff tears, with up to 30 per cent of individuals showing free flow of contrast into the subacromial space prior to any joint manipulation. Binder *et al.*[46] noted a longer duration of symptoms in those patients with a normal arthrogram but no difference in severity of restriction and no difference in outcome. Normalization of arthrograms has been demonstrated in subjects who have recovered normal shoulder range.[47] *Dynamic ultrasonography* has been reported as a helpful form of imaging in the frozen shoulder.

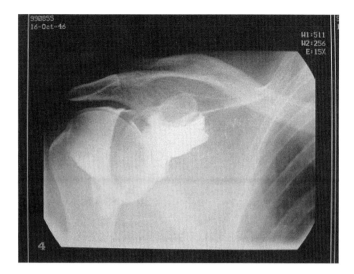

Fig. 28 An arthrogram of the shoulder showing a tight capsule (capsulitis).

Table 19 Arthrographic findings in some cases of frozen shoulder

Joint capacity < 10 cc, measured at the point when the contrast material re-enters the syringe when the examiner releases his/her grip

Obliteration of the axillary recess

Obliteration of the subscapular recess

Obliteration of the biceps tendon sheath

Others: reduced lymphatic drainage

Ryu *et al.* defined the sonographic criterion of adhesive capsulitis as the continuous limitation of the sliding movement of the supraspinatus tendon against the acromion of the scapula.[48] This characteristic showed a high sensitivity and specificity for the diagnosis of a frozen shoulder when compared to arthrographic criteria. However, dynamic ultrasound is usually currently utilized only to identify other pathology that may be present.

Clinical features

History

In the initial *painful phase*, there is an insidious onset of constant generalized shoulder pain, often described as a deep dull ache. Nocturnal pain is common, particularly when lying on the affected side. Restriction and functional limitation may also have been noted prior to presentation. Analgesics and NSAIDs usually provide little symptomatic relief. Symptoms suggestive of an associated disorder may be present (Table 16). In the *adhesive and resolution phases*, the pain eases and becomes more associated with movement than at night. Restriction often becomes the predominant complaint. Finally, gradual improvement in range is seen, but may not occur for months.

Examination

The diagnosis of frozen shoulder depends upon the demonstration of globally restricted range of active and passive range of movement of the shoulder without radiographic evidence of GHJ pathology. The arm may be held in adduction and internal rotation. Mild disuse-related wasting of the spinati and deltoid may be present. There is joint line tenderness and movements are mechanically restricted,

particularly in external rotation. A positive impingement sign may be found. Resisted testing is normal unless an associated disorder such as a rotator cuff tendinopathy is present.

Investigations

Frozen shoulder is a clinical diagnosis. Imaging findings have been discussed earlier.

Management

Frozen shoulder is frequently a lengthy condition and counselling the patient with respect to this and to the phases of the natural history of the complaint is important. Prophylaxis is recommended in those patients considered to be at risk of a frozen shoulder, with early active and passive range of motion exercises popularly employed. A wide variety of approaches to the treatment of the frozen shoulder has been advocated and the literature is abundant with papers on the subject. However, no conclusions can be drawn as to the efficacy of treatments for frozen shoulder. This may in part be related to poor study design and heterogeneous study populations or to true lack of effect. Many of the approaches are primarily anti-inflammatory. Their use may in theory be of greatest use in the initial painful phase of the complaint when inflammation is most significant.

The use of intraarticular injections relies on being able to access the GHJ space. Studies have shown this to be difficult even in shoulders that are not frozen and it would be expected to be even more difficult in the shoulder with a contracted capsule and small joint space. Although some studies have indicated that pain and range of motion may be improved with intraarticular corticosteroids, the evidence is limited and inconclusive. No change in the long-term rate or extent of recovery with this form of treatment has been demonstrated. Oral corticosteroids can improve pain, but do not alter the rate of recovery. Suprascapular nerve block can provide effective pain relief. Modalities and physiotherapy are commonly used, and it is rational to promote range of movement and cuff strengthening exercises in these patients to promote function. Distension of the joint may improve range of motion over the medium term. Manipulation under anaesthesia ruptures the inferior capsule close to the glenoid margin. It may also, however, rupture the insertion of subscapularis. Other potential complications of such a procedure include capsular haemorrhage, humeral fracture, and dislocation.

Other approaches to management include stellate ganglion blockade, joint irradiation, topical dimethyl sulfoxide, and magnetic necklace, although all are without conclusive evidence of benefit. It is no surprise that so many quote Voltaire, who advised 'to keep the patient occupied whilst the disease runs its inevitable course' in the management of the patient with the frozen shoulder.

Prognosis

Frozen shoulder is frequently a protracted condition, with the mean duration of symptoms reported to be 12–42 months. In most cases, symptoms do eventually settle but a detectable restriction in range of movement is usually present, although this is often not noted by the patient.

Patients with diabetes mellitus are known not only to have an increased incidence of frozen shoulder (and stiffness of other joints) but the condition is also frequently more severe and unremitting. Lesquesne *et al.* reported impaired glucose tolerance in 17 of 60 patients presenting with a painful stiff shoulder.[49] In such patients a more aggressive approach to management is advocated.

Neurological causes of shoulder pain

Axillary nerve lesions

The axillary nerve is closely related to the GHJ and supplies the deltoid and teres minor and provides cutaneous innervation to a small area over the lateral deltoid. It is commonly injured in dislocation of the GHJ by direct trauma and may also be entrapped in the quadrilateral space. The patient presents with shoulder and posterior axillary pain, deltoid wasting and weakness, and associated sensory loss. Electromyography (EMG) and nerve conduction studies confirm the lesion. Recovery can be lengthy and, although trick compensatory movements can be learned, deltoid weakness is commonly disabling. If no signs of improvement are noted at 4 months the nerve should be explored.

Brachial neuritis

Brachial neuritis is a term used to describe the sudden onset of weakness of some muscles supplied by the brachial plexus, with resulting painful dysaesthesias of the arm. The condition can occur after a viral infection (herpes zoster, Epstein–Barr), after immunizations, as part of an autoimmune disease, or as a result of mechanical trauma.

The patient reports a sudden onset of diffuse pain in the shoulder, upper arm, and occasionally the forearm. There is weakness and muscle wasting and variable sensory loss of the affected neuromuscular structures and winging is usually evident. EMG studies will confirm the diagnosis.

Treatment involves analgesia and amitryptiline or carbemazapine may be helpful. Some advocate the use of oral corticosteroids in the short term, providing there is no evidence of active infection. Rehabilitation is commenced early to prevent stiffness and to improve function, with range of motion exercises, progressive cuff and scapular stabilizing, and strength exercises.

Other peripheral nerve complaints

Long thoracic nerve palsy can occur as a brachial neuritis after compression due to prolonged recumbancy, such as when lying on an operating table or after local surgery to the breast. There is non-specific shoulder pain, difficulty elevating the arm, and winging.

The radial nerve may be injured in the axilla by trauma, inferior dislocation of the GHJ, local pressure such as under-arm crutches, or by pressure from leaning on the back of a chair. There is weakness of the extensor muscles of the arm, with the typical waiter's tip palsy being evident. Electrodiagnostic studies confirm the diagnosis. Removal of the precipitant cause and rehabilitation form the core management but recovery can be prolonged.

The musculocutaneous nerve (C5, 6) is rarely injured, but can be damaged when there is open trauma or after surgery for anterior GHJ instability. There is wasting of the flexor muscles of the upper arm, weakness of forearm supination, loss of the biceps reflex, and sensory loss over a small area on the lateral aspect of the forearm.

Thoracic outlet syndrome

This is a complex of symptoms that can arise as a result of compression of the neurovascular structures of the thoracic outlet, the brachial plexus, and subclavian artery. The term encompasses other entities, including 'hyperabduction', 'anterior scalene', and 'costoclavicular' syndromes. Local masses and anatomical variations are implicated including a high first or a cervical rib, fibrous bands, anomalies of the scalene muscle, or a transverse process of the seventh cervical vertebra.

Symptoms and signs are highly variable and are dependent upon the structures compressed. Neurogenic symptoms predominate and include dull ache in the entire upper limb, painful paraesthesiae, and weakness and wasting of the small muscles of the hand. Vascular symptoms, usually intermittent cyanosis but rarely trophic skin changes and digital ulceration, are also reported. Symptoms are often exacerbated when carrying heavy objects or when working with the arms in the overhead position, and clumsiness and fatigue may be noted in these positions.

As described earlier, numerous clinical tests have been proposed, but the accuracy of such tests is poor (Fig. 29). A bruit on auscultation may be noted. A chest X-ray allows evaluation of the outlet and will demonstrate the presence of a high first or cervical rib and local lung masses. A CT or MRI of the chest may also be helpful in identifying causative pathology and, where vascular symptoms predominate, angiography, Doppler studies, and venography may be considered necessary.

Treatment is dependent upon the cause. In most cases no cause is identified and physiotherapy in the form of range of motion and strengthening exercises of the cervical, scapulothoracic, and rotator cuff musculature is advocated. When present, excision of a cervical rib or fibrous band may be necessary in those with severe persisting symptoms.

Scapulothoracic and posterior shoulder pain

Scapulothoracic pain may arise due to neurological lesions, myofascial disorders, or bony injuries or may be referred from other sites. (Table 20). Myofascial disorders are discussed in Chapter 6.11 and bony injuries are beyond the scope of this text.

Suprascapular nerve lesions

The suprascapular nerve (C5,6) can be injured as a result of acute trauma to the shoulder complex and can be compressed by tight straps of a rucksack (backpacker's palsy), by a tight transverse scapular ligament, local synovitis (e.g. rheumatoid arthritis), or by a ganglion at the suprascapular notch (Fig. 30). The patient complains of posterior shoulder and scapular pain and there may be wasting of the spinati. Local anaesthetic infiltration into the suprascapular notch should abolish the pain. EMG and nerve conduction studies are necessary to confirm the diagnosis and MRI may be necessary to exclude local pathology. Treatment is dependent upon the cause. Local corticosteroid is unhelpful and surgical intervention may be necessary.

Snapping scapula

Snapping scapula is a syndrome of pain and/or palpable snapping at the medial edge of the scapula in association with scapulothoracic movement. It can occur spontaneously, after trauma, or after surgical procedures to the shoulder girdle. The reported incidence is variable. The snapping has been attributed to the presence of an exostosis on

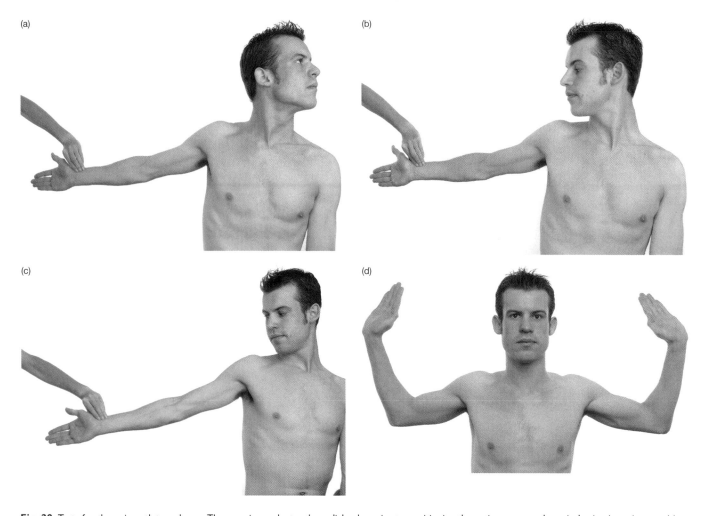

(a)   (b)

(c)   (d)

Fig. 29 Tests for thoracic outlet syndrome The examiner palpates the radial pulse prior to positioning the patients arm and cervical spine in various positions (such as those seen in Figs a-d). A positive test is associated with a decrease in the radial pulse volume and a reproduction of symptoms.

Table 20 Differential diagnosis of scapulothoracic pain

Local muscle injury

Myofascial pain syndrome

Subscapular bursitis

Snapping scapula

Suprascapular nerve palsy

Referred pain from cervical or thoracic spine

Bony injury, e.g. fracture or metastatic deposit in scapula

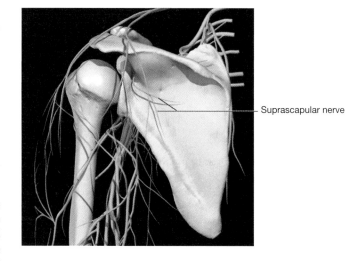

Suprascapular nerve

Fig. 30 The suprascapular nerve can be prone to compression near the suprascapular notch.

the undersurface of the vertebral angle of the scapula or local benign soft tissue tumour (elastofibroma dorsi), which rides across the rib cage.[50] The pain has been reported to be the result of inflamed bursae located between the scapula and adjacent thorax or over the scapular exostosis.[51] However, in many cases no cause is found and symptoms are commonly attributed to minor anatomical variations in the medial superior border and the inferior pole of the scapula and/or neuromuscular balance.

Symptoms usually respond to reassurance, analgesics, and physiotherapy, and surgery is usually not necessary. Where surgery has been performed, this has involved excision of the 2 cm of the medial scapular border or, where present, local exostosis. Three-dimensional CT is recommended as the main imaging modality in the evaluation of any patient with snapping scapula syndrome who is a candidate for surgical intervention.[52]

Localized shoulder pain

Acromioclavicular joint disorders

The ACJ is the sole site of articulation between the scapula and the clavicle. Injures to this joint may be described as scapuloclavicular injuries, since the term emphasizes the effects that such disorders can have upon the rest of the shoulder complex. ACJ disorders consist of ligamentous injuries and articular disorders. The latter are beyond the scope of this text.

Ligamentous injuries

The ACJ is stabilized by two major complexes—the acromioclavicular ligament, which confers horizontal stability, and the coracoclavicular ligaments, which provide vertical stability. Acromioclavicular *sprains and dislocations* form only a small fraction of shoulder complaints in the general population, but are common injuries in contact sporting activities and other forms of relative trauma. AC dislocations occur predominantly in males with a 5 : 1 male : female ratio and the vast majority occur in the second, third, and fourth decades of life.

ACJ ligament injuries, particularly those that are more severe, usually occur with direct trauma to the point of the shoulder. Indirect mechanisms such as downward traction or upward forces, particularly on the adducted arm, may also be involved. Such injuries can be graded according to either the severity of the ligamentous disruption or the structures involved (Fig. 31). Significant damage to the deltotrapezius unit, with detachment from the clavicle, is noted in types IV–VI and sometimes in type III. Type VI injuries are catastrophic usually with major neurovascular damage and are thus life-threatening.

History

A specific episode of trauma is frequently reported prior to the acute onset of characteristic ACJ pain, which is easily identified as the patient usually points to the ACJ as the site of pain. Local AC pain may also radiate to the upper arm. Pain can be severe even in low-grade AC injuries and is typically worse with certain movements, specifically lifting and pushing. Nocturnal pain is common with acute injuries. Symptoms of clicking and grinding may be reported and some patients have noted the development of a local deformity.

Examination

The patient may hold the arm in the adducted position, supported in slight elevation. In type I injuries, tenderness, swelling, and minor deformity may be noted. Deformity is more obvious in types III to VI. No instability is noted in type I injuries, but horizontal instability occurs in type II injuries. In higher grade injuries, both horizontal and vertical instability of the ACJ are present. In type III injuries it should be possible to reduce the dislocation clinically by downward pressure on the clavicle and upward pressure on the elbow. A dimple frequently overlies the outer end of the clavicle in the type IV injury, which increases on attempts to reduce the clavicle downwards. Multidirectional instability of the distal clavicle is clearly evident in the type V injury. In types III–VI, associated injuries should be sought,

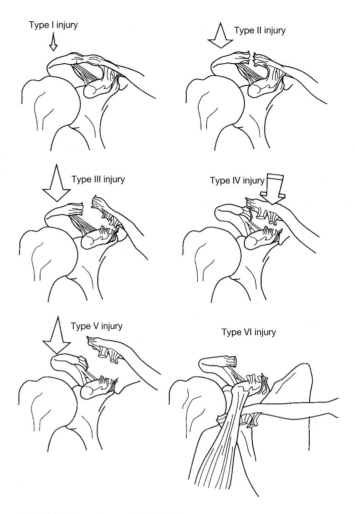

Fig. 31 The broad range of ACJ injuries.

including fracture of the clavicle and/or upper ribs, sternoclavicular joint dislocation, and brachial plexus traction injuries.

Imaging

Radiographic evaluation should include routine anteroposterior and axillary lateral views. Stress (weight-bearing) views in the same planes may be useful, particularly in the more subtle, low-grade injuries, in the detection and evaluation of instability. The injured and uninvolved sides are compared. Anteroposterior stress views are taken with the patient holding weights in the standard AP position. Lateral stress views involve the patient thrusting their shoulders forward, with the acromion displaced anteroinferiorly in the unstable ACJ (types III+). The placement of the acromion, the AC interval, and the size of the coracoclavicular space (with vertical instability suggested by widening of the latter) are all assessed in these stress views.

Management

Types I, II, and in some cases III are all managed conservatively. In low-grade injuries it is important to counsel the patient as it may take many months for symptoms to settle and minor deformity can cause unnecessary anxiety. Persistent pain with type I and II injuries is not uncommon and additional pathologies should be considered (Table 21). Relief of

Table 21 Additional pathologies and complications in ACJ ligament injuries

Torn, entrapped capsular ligaments

Loose articular cartilage

Detached intraarticular meniscus

Rotator cuff injury

Shoulder complex dysfunction, including impingement

Post-traumatic osteolysis of the clavicle

Frozen shoulder

Brachial plexus traction injury

Coracoclavicular ossification

Fractures

Dislocation of SCJ

Non union fracture of the coracoid process

Postoperative complications

ACJ osteoarthritis

pain may be achieved by the regular use of local ice packs, analgesics, and NSAIDs. Support of the injured arm using a sling may be useful in the acute stages until pain is controlled (typically for up to 2 weeks). Reduction of the subluxation in type II injuries has been advocated using manual mobilizations by a therapist or by a variety of braces, taping, supports, harnesses, and traction techniques. It may take many weeks of continuous pressure on the superior clavicle to allow reduction and healing. Alternatively, the subluxation may be ignored or, more eloquently, 'skilfully neglected'. When symptoms allow, range of motion exercises should be introduced early (weeks 0–3), beginning with gravity-dependent pendulum exercises, progressing to wall climbing, and then active function range of motion exercises. Thereafter, a progressive rehabilitation programme should be commenced, involving postural and neuromuscular co-ordination training and strengthening of the cuff and scapular stabilizers. Finally, provided that full pain-free mobility and control has been regained, return to sport-specific training can occur as appropriate (at 4–8 weeks). Heavy lifting and contact sports should be avoided for 12 weeks.

Excellent functional outcomes can be achieved by non-surgical management of many patients with type III injuries, but patients should be warned that deformity will persist. Surgical intervention may be necessary in those who fail conservative approaches, particularly in active patients and those involved in heavy manual work.

Operative management

Operative management may be recommended for many patients with type III injuries and for all types IV, V, or VI injuries. Some also recommend it for those with type II injuries who fail to settle with conservative approaches or those with demonstrable additional pathologies. In such patients, correction of the offending additional pathology, joint debridement, meniscectomy, and/or arthroplasty may be performed. Surgery for type III injuries may involve primary ACJ or coracoclavicular ligament fixation, excision of the distal clavicle, and/or dynamic muscle transfer, with such procedures being performed alone or in various combinations. Surgical approaches employed for the management of types IV–VI

injuries include open reduction, ligament reconstruction, excision of the distal end of the clavicle, dynamic muscle transfer, and ACJ stabilization.

Sternoclavicular disorders

Complaints arising from the SCJ are fortunately limited in number to primary articular disorders (osteoarthritis, inflammatory arthritis) and instability. Instability of the SCJ occurs in two forms, spontaneous or post-traumatic. Spontaneous instability usually occurs in the younger patient, may be bilateral, and occurs with minimal or no trauma. The patient notes a painful or painless clunking of the joint anteriorly or superiorly, which may be followed by swelling and local tenderness. Management is conservative and involves reassurance and advice to avoid precipitating activities. Surgical intervention is reserved for those with persisting and disabling symptoms but can be a major undertaking. A number of stabilization techniques have been described.

Traumatic instability of the SCJ occurs after dislocation, which accounts for 1 per cent of all dislocations of the shoulder girdle. Such injuries involve major trauma to the chest wall and, when in the anterior or superior directions, are easily diagnosed by the obvious deformity and can often be reduced by manual pressure. A posterior dislocation may be less evident and may result in airways obstruction—rapid reduction is required.

References

1. **Badley, E.M. and Tennant, A.** (1992). Changing profile of joint disorders with age: findings from a postal survey of the population of Calderdale, West Yorkshire, United Kingdom. *Ann. Rheum. Dis.* **51**(3), 366–371.

2. **Chard, M., Hazleman, R., Hazleman, B.L., King, R.H., and Reiss, B.B.** (1991). Shoulder disorders in the elderly: a community survey. *Arthritis Rheum.* **34**, 766–769.

3. Royal College of General Practitioners and Office of Population Censuses and Surveys, Department of Health and Social Security (1986). *Morbidity statistics from general practice. Third national study: socio-economic analyses*, series MB5, No. 2. HMSO, London.

4. **Cunningham, D.A., Paterson, D.H., Himann, J.E., and Rechnitzer, P.A.** (1993). Determinants of independence in the elderly. *Can. J. Appl. Physiol.* **18** (3), 243–254.

5. **Green, S., Buchbinder, R., Glazier, R., and Forbes, A.** (1998). Systematic review of randomised controlled trials of interventions for painful shoulder: selection criteria, outcome assessment and efficacy. *Br. Med. J.* **316**, 354–360.

6. **Speed, C.A. and Hazleman, B.L.** (2001). Shoulder pain. In *Clinical evidence*, Issue 6, pp. 945–960. BMJ Publishers, London.

7. **Bigliani, L.U., Morrison, D.S., and April, E.W.** (1986). The morphology of the acromion its relationship to rotator cuff tears. *Orthop. Trans.* **10**, 228.

8. **De Palma, A.F.** (1957). Degenerative changes in sternoclavicular and acromioclavicular joints in various decades. C.C. Thomas, Springfield, Illinois.

9. **Ciepiela, M.D. and Burkhead, W.Z.** (1996). Classification of rotator cuff tears. In *Rotator cuff disorders* (ed. W. Z. Burkhead, Jr), pp. 100–107 Williams and Wilkins, Baltimore.

10. **Patte, D.** (1990). Classification of rotator cuff lesions. *Clin. Orthop.* **254**, 81–86.

11. **Fukuda, H., Craig, E.V., Yamanaka, K., and Hamada, K.** (1996). Partial thickness cuff tears. In *Rotator cuff disorders* (ed. W. Z. Burkhead Jr), pp. 174–181. Williams and Wilkins, Baltimore.

12. Yamanaka, K. and Fukuda, H. (1981). Histological study of the supraspinatus tendon. *Shoulder Joint* **5**, 9.

13. Moseley, H.F. and Goldie, I.G. (1963). The arterial pattern of the rotator cuff of the shoulder. *J. Bone Joint Surg.* (Br.) **45**, 780–789.

14. Rathbun, J.B. and Macnab, I. (1970). The microvascular pattern of the rotator cuff. *J. Bone Joint Surg.* **52B**, 540–553.

15. Swiontkowski, M., Iannotti, J.P., Boulas, J.H., *et al.* (1990). *Intraoperative assessment of rotator cuff vascularity using laser doppler flowmetry*, pp. 208–212. Mosby Year Book, St Louis.

16. Neer, C.S. (1983). Impingement lesions. *Clin. Orthop.* **173**, 70–77.

17. Ogata, S. and Uhthoff, H.K. (1990). Acromial enthesopathy and rotator cuff tear. A radiologic and histologic postmortem investigation of the coracoacromial arch. *Clin. Orthop.* **254**, 39–48.

18. Neer, C.S. (1972). Anterior acromioplasty for the chronic impingement syndrome in the shoulder. A preliminary report. *J. Bone Joint Surg.* (Am.) **54**, 41–50.

19. Dixon, A. (ed.) (1998). Making the best use of a department of clinical radiology: guidelines for doctors, 4th edn. Royal College of Radiologists, London.

20. Kaneko, K., De-Mouy, E.H., and Brunet, M.E. (1995). Massive rotator cuff tears. Screening by routine radiographs. *Clin. Imaging* **19** (1), 8–11.

21. Miniaci, A. and Salonen, D. (1997). Rotator cuff evaluation: imaging and diagnosis. *Orthop. Clin. N. Am.* **28** (1), 43–58.

22. Imhoff, A.B. and Hodler, J. (1996). Correlation of MR imaging, CT arthrography, and arthroscopy of the shoulder. *Bull. Hosp. Joint Dis.* **54** (3), 146–152.

23. Seibold, C.J., Mallisee, T.A., Erickson, S.J., Boynton, M.D., Raasch, W.G., and Timins, M.E. (1999). Rotator cuff: evaluation with US and MR imaging. *Radiographics* **19** (3), 685–705.

24. Hedtmann, A. and Fett, H. (1995). Ultrasonography of the shoulder in subacromial syndromes with disorders and injuries of the rotator cuff. *Orthopade* **24** (6), 498–508.

25. Farin, P.U., Kaukanen, E., Jaroma, H., Vaatainen, U., Miettinen, H., and Soimakallio, S. (1996). Site and size of rotator-cuff tear. Findings at ultrasound, double-contrast arthrography, and computed tomography arthrography with surgical correlation. *Invest. Radiol.* **31** (7), 387–394.

26. Blanchard, T.K., Bearcroft, P.W., Constant, C.R., Griffin, D.R., and Dixon, A.K. (1999). Diagnostic and therapeutic impact of MRI and arthrography in the investigation of full-thickness rotator cuff tears. *Eur. Radiol.* **9** (4), 638–642.

27. Yamanaka, K. and Matsumoto, T. (1994). The joint side tear of the rotator cuff. A follow up study by arthrography. *Clin. Orthop.* **304**, 68–73.

28. Bassett, R.W. and Cofield, R.H. (1983). Acute tears of the rotator cuff. The timing of surgical repairs. *Clin. Orthop.* **175**, 18–24.

29. Arroyo, J.S., Hershon, S.J., and Bigliani, L.U. (1997). Special considerations in the athletic throwing shoulder. *Orthop. Clin. N. Am.* **28**, 69–78.

30. Breazeale, N.M. and Craig, E.V. (1997). Partial-thickness rotator cuff tears. Pathogenesis and treatment. *Orthop. Clin. N. Am.* **28** (2), 145–155.

31. Uhthoff, H.K. (1975). Calcifying tendinitis: an active cell-mediated calcification. *Virchows Arch.* [A] **366**, 51–58.

32. Loew, M., Daecke, W., Kusnierczak, D., Rahmanzadeh, M., and Ewerbeck, V. (1999). Shock-wave therapy is effective for chronic calcifying tendinitis of the shoulder. *J. Bone Joint Surg.* (Br.) **81** (5), 863–867.

33. Ebenbichler, G.R., Erdogmus, C.B., Resch, K.L., Funovics, M.A., Kainberger, F. *et al.* (1999). Ultrasound therapy for calcific tendinitis of the shoulder. *N. Engl. J. Med.* **340** (20), 1533–1538.

34. Habbermeyer, P. and Walch, G. (1996). The biceps tendon and rotator cuff disease. In *Rotator cuff disorders* (ed. W. Z. Burkhead, Jr), p. 142. Williams and Wilkins, Baltimore.

35. Lapidus, P.W. and Guidotti, F.P. (1957). Local injection of hydrocortisone in 495 orthopedic patients. *Ind. Med. Surg.* **26**, 234–244.

36. Walch, G. (1963). *La pathologie de la longue portion du biceps*. Conference d'Enseignement de la SOFCOT, Paris.

37. Thomas, S.C. and Matsen, F.A. (1989). An approach to the repair of avulsion of the glenohumeral ligaments in the management of traumatic anterior glenohumeral instability. *J. Bone Joint Surg.* (Am.) **71**, 506–513.

38. McLaughlin, H.L. and Cavallaro, W.U. (1950). Primary anterior dislocation of the shoulder. *Am. J. Surg.* **80**, 615–621.

39. Snyder, S.J., Karzel, R.P., Del Pizzo, W., *et al.* (1990). SLAP lesions of the shoulder. *Arthroscopy* **6**, 274–279.

40. Nevasier, J. (1945). Adhesive capsulitis of the shoulder: a study of the pathologic findings in periarthritis of the shoulder. *J. Bone Joint Surg.* **27**, 211–222.

41. Nevasier, R.J. and Nevasier, T.J. (1987). The frozen shoulder. Diagnosis and management. *Clin. Orthop. Rel. Res.* **223**, 59–64.

42. Nash, P. and Hazleman, B.L. (1989). Frozen shoulder. In The shoulder joint (ed. B.L. Hazleman and P.A. Dieppe). *Baillière's Clin. Rheumatol.* **3**, 551–566.

43. Lundberg, B. (1969). The frozen shoulder. *Acta Orthop. Scand.* Suppl. 119.

44. Bunker, T.D. and Anthony, P.P. (1995). The pathology of the frozen shoulder. A Dupytren-like disease. *J. Bone Joint Surg.* (Br.) **77**, 677–683.

45. Binder, A., Bulgen, D., and Hazleman, B. (1984). Frozen shoulder: an arthrographic and radionuclear scan assessment. *Ann. Rheum. Dis.* **43**, 361–364.

46. Binder, A., Bulgen, D., Hazleman, B., and Roberts, S. (1984). Frozen shoulder: a long term prospective study. *Ann. Rheum. Dis.* **43**, 361–364.

47. Reeves, B. (1966). Arthrographic changes in frozen and post traumatic stiff shoulders. *Proc. R. Soc. Med.* **59**, 827–830.

48. Ryu, K.N., Lee, S.W., Rhee, Y.G., and Lim, J.H. (1993). Adhesive capsulitis of the shoulder joint: usefulness of dynamic sonography. *J. Ultrasound Med.* **12**, 445–449.

49. Lesquesne, M., Dang, N., and Benasson, M. (1977). Increases association of diabetes mellitus with capsulitis of the shoulder and shoulder–hand syndrome. *Scand. J. Rheumatol.* **6**, 53–56.

50. Majo, J., Gracia, I., Doncel, A., Valera, M., Nunez, A., and Guix, M. (2001). Elastofibroma dorsi as a cause of shoulder pain or snapping scapula. *Clin. Orthop.* **388**, 200–204.

51. Carlson, H.L., Haig, A.J., and Stewart, D.C. (1997). Snapping scapula syndrome: three case reports and an analysis of the literature. *Arch. Phys. Med. Rehabil.* **78** (5), 506–511.

52. Mozes, G., Bickels, J., Ovadia, D., and Dekel, S. (1999). The use of three-dimensional computed tomography in evaluating snapping scapula syndrome. *Orthopedics* **22** (11), 1029–1033.

6.4 The elbow and forearm

Cathy Speed

Anatomy

Bones

The elbow is a compound synovial joint, composed of a complex of two closely related articulations between the humerus and both the ulna and radius. The superior radioulnar joint is continuous with these articulations and functionally forms part of the elbow complex. The capsule and joint cavity are continuous for all three joints.

The *humeroradial joint* is a hinge joint formed by articulation between the hemispherical humeral capitellum and the head of the radius. The *humeroulnar (trochlear) joint* is formed by the trochlea of the distal humerus and the trochlear notch of the ulna. This modified hinge joint permits 140–150° of flexion and extension, with an axis of movement that passes downward and medially. This results in the elbow travelling through an arc of movement, from valgus to varus during flexion. The carrying angle of the elbow, the valgus angle formed by the long axes of the upper arm and forearm when the arm is extended, is typically less than 5° in males and 5–10° in females. Most individuals can straighten their elbow completely (0° extension/flexion), but extension to 5° is normal particularly in young females.

The side to side joint movement necessary for supination and pronation exists due to incomplete contact between the trochlea and the medial and lateral aspects of the olecranon process in full extension and in full flexion, respectively. Approximately 5° of rotation also occurs at this joint during early flexion (medial rotation) and late flexion (lateral rotation). This subtle rotation may account for the osteophyte formation on the olecranon, typically seen in activities involving repetitive extension of the elbow, such as throwing.

The forearm can rotate through approximately 165° (80° pronation and 80–85° of supination), through movements at the radioulnar joints. The *superior radioulnar joint* is a uniaxial pivot joint. The head of the radius rotates with pronation and supination on the radial notch of the ulna and is held in position relative to the adjacent bones by the annular ligament. In the distal forearm the *inferior radioulnar joint*, formed by articulation between the head of the ulna and the ulnar notch of the radius, also allows supination and pronation.

Ligaments

The medial (ulnar) collateral ligament and the lateral (radial) collateral ligament support the humeroulnar and humeroradial joints, respectively (Fig. 2). Sixty-five per cent of the load to valgus strain is taken up by the *medial collateral ligament* (MCL), in particular by its anterior bundle. This arises from the inferior aspect of the medial epicondyle to insert on to the medial aspect of the coronoid process of the ulna. It divides into an anterior band (tight in extension and

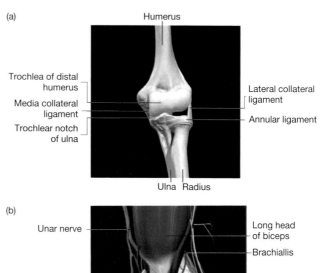

(a)

Humerus

Trochlea of distal humerus

Media collateral ligament

Trochlear notch of ulna

Lateral collateral ligament

Annular ligament

Ulna Radius

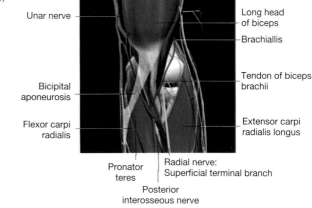

(b)

Unar nerve

Bicipital aponeurosis

Flexor carpi radialis

Pronator teres

Posterior interosseous nerve

Long head of biceps

Brachiallis

Tendon of biceps brachii

Extensor carpi radialis longus

Radial nerve: Superficial terminal branch

Fig. 1 The anterior elbow: (a) deep and (b) superficial structures.

therefore resistant to valgus strain in this position) and a posterior band (tight in flexion). The posterior bundle arises from the medial epicondyle to insert onto the medial olecranon. It is taut when the elbow is flexed more than 90°. The transverse bundle has no significant role in the stability of the elbow. The MCL and the flexor carpi ulnaris muscle form the *cubital tunnel*, through which travels the ulnar nerve.

The *lateral collateral ligament* (LCL) consists of four components that provide stability to the elbow against varus stress and, if compromised, can result in a loss of pronation and supination.

Muscles

Four groups of muscles act directly on the elbow: the flexors, flexor–pronators, extensors, and extensor–supinators (Figs 3 and 4). The *flexor group* is composed of the biceps brachii, brachioradialis, and brachialis. *Biceps brachii* acts as a primary elbow flexor when the elbow

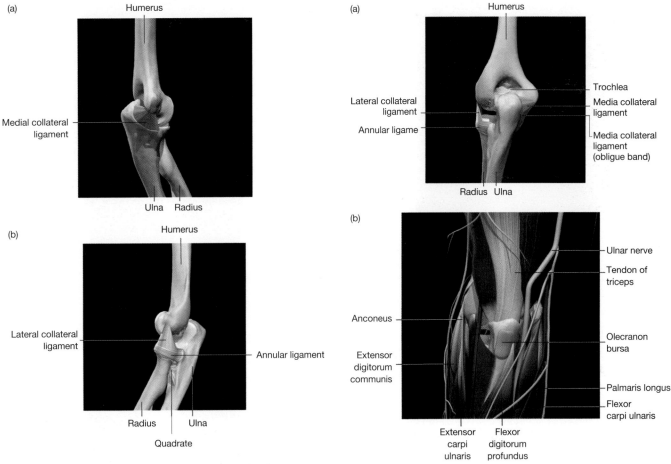

(a)

Humerus

Medial collateral ligament

Ulna   Radius

(b)

Humerus

Lateral collateral ligament

Annular ligament

Radius   Ulna

Quadrate

Fig. 2 (a) Medial and (b) lateral ligamentous anatomy of the elbow.

(a)

Humerus

Lateral collateral ligament

Annular ligame

Trochlea

Media collateral ligament

Media collateral ligament (obligue band)

Radius   Ulna

(b)

Ulnar nerve

Tendon of triceps

Anconeus

Olecranon bursa

Extensor digitorum communis

Palmaris longus

Flexor carpi ulnaris

Extensor carpi ulnaris

Flexor digitorum profundus

Fig. 4 The posterior elbow. (a) deep (b) superficial structures.

Long head of biceps

Brachialis

Medial collateral ligament (posterior band)

Tendon of biceps brachii

Olecranon bursa

Flexor digitorum profundus

Bicipital aponeurosis

Pronator teres

Flexor carpi radialis

Flexor carpi ulnaris

Flexor digitorum superficialis

Fig. 3 The medial elbow.

is supinated and aids in forearm supination when the elbow is flexed (Fig. 3). It has two origins: the long head arises from the superior glenoid tubercle at the superior rim of the glenoid fossa and the short head arises from the coracoid process. They insert on to the posterior aspect of the radial tuberosity and are innervated by the musculocutaneous nerve (C5, 6).

Brachioradialis functions primarily to flex the arm at the elbow. It originates from the lateral two-thirds of the lateral supracondylar ridge of the humerus and lateral intermuscular septum distal to the spiral groove, to insert on the lateral side of the styloid process of the radius. It is innervated by the radial nerve (C5, 6). *Brachialis* flexes the elbow in all positions of the forearm. It arises from the distal half of the anterior aspect of the humerus to insert on the ulnar tuberosity and coronoid process. It is innervated by the musculocutaneous nerve (C5, 6).

The *flexor–pronator group* consists of the pronator teres, flexor carpi radialis, palmaris longus, flexor carpi ulnaris (FCU), and flexor digitorum superficialis (FDS). All arise directly from, or in close proximity to, the medial epicondyle. The primary role of this group is flexion and pronation of the wrist and hand, while secondarily aiding elbow flexion. All are innervated by the median nerve (C6–8, T1), with the exception of flexor carpi ulnaris (ulnar nerve, C8, T1).

The *extensor group* is composed of the triceps and anconeus. The three heads of triceps arise from the proximal humerus and unite to form the two aponeuroses that join together to form the triceps tendon and insert on to the posterior surface of the olecranon and the deep fascia of the forearm (Fig. 4). Triceps is innervated by the radial nerve (C7, 8).

The *extensor–supinator group* (brachioradialis, extensor carpi radialis longus and brevis, supinator, extensor digitorum, extensor carpi ulnaris, and extensor digiti minimi) function primarily to extend and supinate the hand and wrist, while providing dynamic support for the

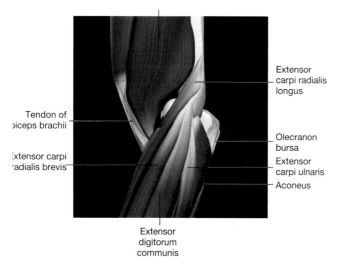

Fig. 5 The lateral elbow.

lateral elbow (Fig. 5). They originate at or near the lateral epicondyle and are innervated by the radial nerve (C5–8, T1).

Nerves

Four nerves are important in function of the elbow (see Table 3 of Chapter 6.3). The *musculocutaneous nerve* (C5–7) originates from the lateral cord of the brachial plexus, passes between biceps and brachialis muscles, and pierces the brachial fascia lateral to the biceps tendon, terminating as the lateral antebrachial cutaneous nerve.

The *median nerve* (C5–8, T1) originates from the lateral and medial cords of the brachial plexus, passes distally over the antero-medial aspect of the arm lateral to the brachial artery and then crosses the antecubital fossa to lie medial to the biceps tendon and brachial artery. It passes between the two heads of pronator teres and travels down the forearm beneath FDS. Anomalies in pronator teres may lead to median nerve compression at this site. The *anterior interosseous nerve* arises from the median nerve at the inferior border of pronator teres and travels along the interosseous membrane to innervate flexor pollicis longus and the lateral portion of FDP.

The *ulnar nerve* (C8, T1), arises from the medial cord of the brachial plexus, passes distally from the anterior to the posterior compartments of the upper arm through the arcade of Struther's, a fascial raphe between the medial head of triceps and the medial intermuscular septum (approximately 8 cm proximal to the medial epicondyle). It continues distally behind the medial epicondyle and through the cubital tunnel into the forearm. An articular branch and a branch to FCU arise at the elbow; there are no branches in the forearm.

The *radial nerve* (C6–8) arises from the posterior cord of the brachial plexus and travels down laterally in the spiral groove to pass anterior to the lateral epicondyle, posterior to brachioradialis and brachialis muscles. It then divides into posterior interosseous and superficial radial nerves at the antecubital fossa. The posterior interosseous nerve continues around the posterolateral aspect of the radius and passes between the two heads of the supinator muscle before dividing into terminal motor branches. The superficial branch continues distally to terminate in the hand (Figs 6 and 7).

Bursae

Many bursae have been reported to exist in the elbow region. There are three superficial bursae: the olecranon bursa and the medial and lateral epicondylar bursae. Only the former is a common site for pathology. Of several deep bursae, the most significant is the bicipital radial bursa. Intratendinous bursitis, located in the substance of the triceps tendon near its insertion, may occur with triceps tendinopathy.

The subcutaneous olecranon bursa is a superficial anatomical bursa, situated between the skin and the triceps tendon and olecranon (Fig. 8). The bursa is not present in young children but increases in size after the age of 7 years, with that on the dominant side usually being larger. The floor of the bursa adheres to the olecranon. In the healthy state no communication exists between the bursa and elbow joint.

Clinical evaluation

History

A careful history is obtained to determine the characteristics, mechanisms, severity, and functional consequences of the injury.

Onset

Was the onset of symptoms acute or insidious?

Mechanisms

How did the injury occur? A clear description of the mechanism of injury can indicate the anatomical structure(s) involved. In injuries without a clear acute episode, the patient may have his own views on contributing factors.

Symptoms

The duration and progression of symptoms can indicate the severity of the condition and help to plan management. Pain is the most common symptom and the characteristics should be determined, including its nature, site, radiation, temporal characteristics, and relieving and exacerbating factors. Other symptoms may include swelling, tingling, and numbness. The characteristics of these symptoms should be determined in a similar fashion to that used in taking a pain history. Symptoms in the proximal arm and neck should be specifically addressed, as symptoms may be referred. In those patients complaining of stiffness and restriction, the specific movements affected should be ascertained. Locking is suggestive of loose bodies within the joint complex.

The treatments used to date should be recorded and current and past medical history, including previous injuries to the affected arm and neck, are determined. Hand dominance and the functional impact of the injury in relation to the patient's occupation and activities may be significant. Such activities may also play a major role in the development and chronicity of the complaint.

Examination

Both of the arms and the neck should be adequately exposed and both arms should be visualized for comparison.

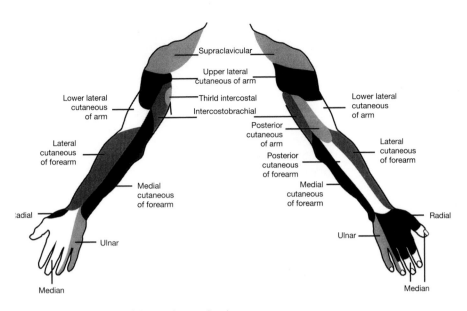

Fig. 6 Cutaneous supply of the arm by peripheral nerves.

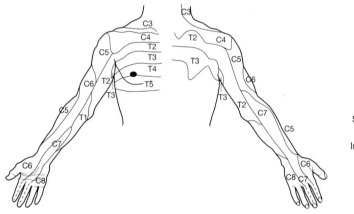

Fig. 7 Dermatomes of the arm.

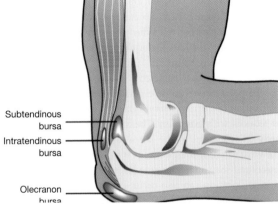

Fig. 8 Some bursae around the elbow.

Inspection

General

The general appearance of the arms, including soft tissue contour, evidence of wasting or asymmetry of muscle bulk, muscle fasciculation, scars, and swelling should be noted. Overdevelopment of the dominant arm is common in manual workers, throwers, and racquet sports players. Deformities and alignment should be evaluated. The carrying angle is evaluated with the arm extended. The antecubital fossa can be assessed anteriorly for swelling and soft tissue masses.

Inspection of the posterior aspect of the elbow allows the olecranon to be examined. Discrete bursal swelling at the olecranon or nodules more distally on the extensor surface of the forearm may be evident. Triceps tendon rupture may appear as an excessively bony prominence, with a gap just above the tip of the olecranon. When dislocation has occurred it is usually obvious, causing marked distortion of the bony contour, typically with a posteriorly prominent proximal ulna.

The lateral aspect of the elbow and forearm

If synovitis or a joint effusion is present, all three joints will be affected, since they are continuous. This is usually most evident in the triangular space between the lateral epicondyle, the head of the radius, and the tip of the olecranon. Swelling is also commonly evident on the posterior aspect. The patient usually holds the swollen elbow in the position of maximum volume, that is 70° flexion. There may be evidence of subcutaneous atrophy after repeated corticosteroid injections in the region of the lateral epicondyle in patients with chronic lateral elbow pain.

Palpation

Palpation of the bony landmarks is performed with the arm flexed at 90° and includes the medial and lateral epicondyles, the medial supracondylar line of the humerus (prominence can be associated with median nerve compression), the lateral supracondylar line of the

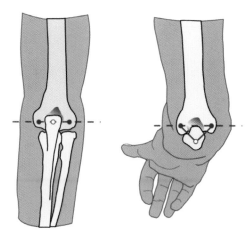

Fig. 9 The olecranon process and the medial and lateral epicondyles will normally form an isosceles triangle. When the arm is fully extended, these points form a straight line. Deformities of any of the involved bones results in loss of these features.

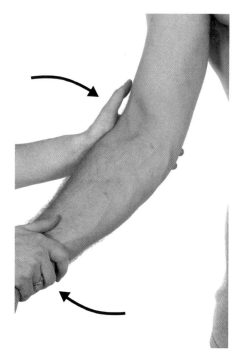

Fig. 10 Assessment of ligamentous stability of the elbow. Laxity is evaluated on applying valgus then varus stress on the elbow in slight flexion.

humerus, the olecranon, and ulnar border down to the ulnar styloid at the wrist.

In the normal position of function, with the elbow flexed to 90° and the forearm midway between supination and pronation, the olecranon process and the medial and lateral epicondyles will normally form an isosceles triangle (Fig. 9). When the arm is fully extended, these points form a straight line. Deformities of any of the involved bones result in loss of these features.

The *olecranon fossa* is best palpated with the elbow in less than 90° flexion, where the nerve can be evaluated for thickening. Where anterior subluxation of the ulnar nerve occurs, it may be evident with flexion and reduced with extension. The *radial head* can be palpated approximately 1 inch distal to the lateral epicondyle, just postero-medial to the wrist extensor muscle group. It can be felt with pronation and supination and may be tender after fracture or with synovitis or osteoarthritis. Dislocation can also occur. Palpation of several structures in the *cubital fossa* is possible. The *biceps tendon* is best identified from *brachioradialis* when the patient makes a fist of the supinated hand, places the hand under the edge of a table, and tries to lift it. Although the insertion is not palpable, the muscle belly and tendon are. The pulse of the *brachial artery* is easily felt and, directly medial to this, lies the *median nerve*. The *musculocutaneous nerve* that lies lateral to the biceps tendon is not palpable but is located deep under the brachioradialis, 2–5 cm above the elbow joint.

Posteriorly, the *olecranon bursa* may be enlarged, tender, and thick in a bursitis. The triceps tendon can be palpated at its insertion on the tip of the olecranon. *Rheumatoid nodules* may be evident on the extensor aspect of the forearm and must be differentiated form lipomata, ganglia, gouty tophi, and xanthomata.

Medially, the *ulnar nerve* can be palpated posterior to the medial epicondyle. The *flexor–pronator muscle group* may be tender at its origin with medial epicondylitis. The MCL cannot be palpated directly, but tenderness in this area, usually after a valgus strain, is indicative of an injury to this ligament.

Laterally, the LCL is not directly palpable but the area may be tender if injured, usually after varus stress. The *wrist extensors* are best assessed when the forearm is in neutral position and the wrist relaxed.

Local tenderness at or near the epicondyle is indicative of lateral epicondylitis although the differential diagnosis is wide (see below).

Movement

Passive and active range of motion and movement against resistance are evaluated. The latter is best assessed with the arm flexed to 90° and the elbow stabilized by one of the examiner's hands around the posterior aspect of the elbow, while the other hand grasps the distal forearm.

1. *Flexion*. Biceps is tested with the forearm supinated, brachialis with the forearm pronated, and brachioradialis with the forearm in mid-position.

2. *Supination and pronation*. The patient supinates from a pronated position against resistance and pronation is tested from a supinated position.

3. *Triceps* is tested against resistance from a position of full flexion.

4. *Neurovascular status* should also be assessed.

Special tests

Assessment of ligamentous stability is demonstrated in Fig. 10

The examiner notes (1) whether pain is provoked and (2) whether there is excessive laxity compared to the contralateral elbow. If laxity is noted, then the examiner must assess for the presence of a firm endpoint. Lack of a firm endpoint indicates total rupture.

Tests for lateral and medial epicondylitis

All tests for lateral and medial epicondylitis aim to reproduce pain at the lateral epicondyle. The test for lateral epicondylitis is as follows:

1. Extensor carpi radialis brevis (ECRB) is tested in two positions: Resisted wrist extension is tested with the forearm pronated and the elbow in two positions—first extended, then flexed to 90°.

2. Extensor digitorum communis (EDC) is tested when the patient extends elbow, pronates the forearm, and extends the fingers. The examiner applies downward force to the middle finger.

3. Passive movement of the elbow and forearm from full flexion and forearm supination to extension, forearm pronation, and wrist flexion reproduces pain if there is tightness of the extensor–supinator group (Fig. 11).

The tests for medial epicondylitis are as follows:

1. Resisted wrist flexion with the elbow flexed and forearm supinated reproduces medial elbow pain in medial epicondylitis.

2. Resisted forearm pronation with the forearm extended and in neutral rotation (shaking hands with the examiner) also reproduces pain.

3. Passive movement of the flexed pronated forearm into full flexion, supination with the wrist extended will reproduce pain if there is tightness in the flexor–pronator group.

Tests for neurological dysfunction

Tinel's test at the elbow is often used in suspected nerve compression. It is performed by tapping over the ulnar nerve in the ulnar groove. A positive sign is indicated by tingling in the ulnar distribution of the forearm and hand distal to the point of compression of the nerve. The most distal point at which abnormal sensation is felt is postulated to indicate the limit of nerve regeneration of the sensory fibres of a nerve. However, the test has a low level of sensitivity.

The elbow flexion test is similar to Phalen's test at the wrist. The patient sits with elbows flexed for up to 5 min. A positive test is indicated by tingling or paraesthesia in the ulnar nerve distribution of the forearm and hand and represents cubital tunnel syndrome. Like Tinel's test it has poor sensitivity and specificity.

Ulnar nerve instability can be demonstrated by repeated flexion/extension of the elbow, when the patient will complain of

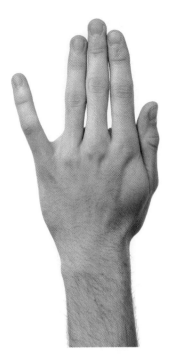

Fig. 12 Wartenberg's sign: inability to adduct the little finger indicates an ulnar nerve lesion.

tingling in the distribution of the nerve, pain at the medial elbow, and/or subluxation of the nerve may be detected.

In the test for *Wartenberg's sign* the patient sits with his/her hands resting on a table and the examiner passively spreads the fingers apart, instructing the patient to bring the fingers together. Inability to adduct the little finger indicates an ulnar nerve lesion (Fig. 12).

In the test for *pronator teres syndrome* the patient's elbow is extended from an initial position of 90° of flexion, while the examiner resists pronation of the forearm. A positive test is indicated by tingling or paraesthesia in the medial nerve distribution of the forearm and hand. Again, the sensitivity of this test is limited.

In the *pinch grip test* the patient attempts to pinch the tips of the index finger and thumb together. Normally, there should be tip-to-tip pinch. A pulp-to-pulp pinch indicates an anterior interosseous nerve lesion.

Reflexes and cutaneous sensation should also be evaluated and the remainder of the upper limb and neck examined as pain may be referred to the elbow from both proximal and distal sites.

Lateral elbow pain (Table 1)

Lateral epicondylitis

Lateral 'epicondylitis' is, in fact, a tendinopathy of the common extensor–supinator tendon rather than epicondylitis. It is characterized by lateral peri-epicondylar pain and tenderness that is exacerbated by gripping. In 1883, Major noted that this condition commonly affects tennis players, and the complaint subsequently became popularly known as tennis elbow.[1] Thirteen per cent of elite players and up to 50 per cent of non-elite tennis players have symptoms suggestive of lateral epicondylitis and approximately half of these have symptoms

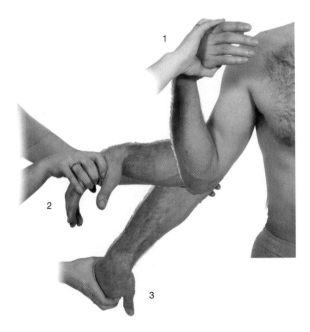

Fig. 11 With lateral epicondylitis, pain may be reproduced by passive extension of the elbow and flexion of the wrist.

Table 1 Differential diagnosis of lateral elbow pain

Lateral epicondylitis

Instability

Epicondylar apophysitis (adolescents)

Radiocapitellar bursitis

Forearm compartment syndrome

C6 root pathology

Radial nerve lesions

Radiohumeral joint pathology

    Osteochondritis dissecans

    Osteochondrosis of the radiocapitellar joint

    Instability of the radiocapitellar joint

Fracture/stress fracture

Synovitis of the radiohumeral head

Table 2 Issues relating to lateral epicondylitis in the tennis player

Technique

Bad technique (at risk)

Poor stroke mechanics

Poor body weight transfer

Power is generated by small muscles of forearm

Hits ball late

Off-centre impact

Elbow is ahead of ball at impact in serve and forehand

Over-pronation of the forearm during follow-through in backhand

Good technique (protective)

Swing comes from shoulder

Body weight is transferred through stroke

Power is generated by large muscles of upper arm, torso, and legs

Hits ball on sweet spot

Double-handed backhand may be protective

Equipment

Heavy or wet tennis balls

Racquet:

Grip size: too large/small

Weight: too heavy/too light

String type: large gauge absorbs less impact. Aim to use gauge of 1.3 mm or less

Sweet spot: Racquet head size: too small results in small sweet spot. Oversized heads increase the size of the sweet spot but if hit off centre the vibration is greater. Therefore choose moderate size

Note that any change in racquet tends to be beneficial

Training

Too much, too soon, too often

for an average duration of 2.5 years. Nevertheless, 95 per cent of cases occur in those who do not play tennis and it particularly affects those in manual occupations. The incidence of the complaint is equal among men and women, although in tennis players it may be more common in men. It particularly affects the age group spanning the fourth to the sixth decades, with those in the fifth decade four times more commonly affected than at other stages of this span.

Pathology

Degenerative microtears are found in the common extensor–supinator tendon, with the origin of ECRB most commonly affected. Anatomical studies have shown that the origin of ECRB and supinator share a common origin at the lateral epicondyle, joint capsule, and the orbicular ligament. Extensor carpi radialis longus (ECRL) arises from the epicondyle and more proximally from the lateral epicondylar ridge and EDC also takes part of its origin from the lateral epicondyle. All may be involved in the condition. The tears are likely to be due to repetitive mechanical overload. Typical microscopic features of surgical specimens include hyaline degeneration, fibroblastic and vascular proliferation, and a notable absence of any inflammatory component.[2] It is possible that the lack of an inflammatory component may lead to incomplete healing but it is important to note that such findings represent end-stage lesions and the characteristics of earlier lesions are not known.

History

The history is that of epicondylar pain and tenderness, worse with grip and resulting in functional difficulties. Such symptoms may be acute or insidious in onset. There is often a history of overuse, involving repetitive flexion–extension or pronation–supination activity and it is therefore no surprise that carpenters and builders are commonly affected. Among tennis players, the backhand appears to be the most commonly implicated stroke in the initiation of the complaint. Less skilled players with a faulty technique are most likely to sustain the injury (Table 2).

Equipment factors frequently play a role, and patient may give history of recent change in one or more aspects of equipment or there may be long-standing errors. These include the tennis racquet that is

too heavy or too light, a grip that is too big, string tension that is too tight, and the use of heavy or wet tennis balls.

Examination

There is usually tenderness over the ECRB origin at the lateral epicondyle, although the tenderness may be slightly more diffuse over the origins of EDC and/or ECRL. One or more provocation tests, as described earlier, may be positive.

Imaging

Imaging studies are not routinely performed. A 'gun-sight' oblique *plain radiograph* of the lateral epicondyle may show irregular punctate calcification in the region of the lateral epicondyle in chronic cases. *Ultrasound* features include decreased echogenicity, inhomogeneity, and thickening of the tendon. Rarely, a local fluid collection may be identified. In chronic cases there is often local calcification at the tendon insertion and irregularity of the bone surface. *Magnetic resonance imaging* (MRI) may demonstrate increased signal intensity of the

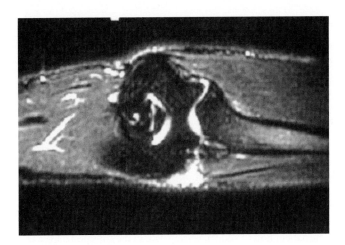

Fig. 13 T2-weighted MRI scan of the elbow showing increased signal intensity at the common extensor origin, indicative of lateral epicondylitis.

extensor tendons close to their insertion on the lateral epicondyle (Fig. 13). *Thermography* shows increased temperature at the site of the lesion.

Differential diagnosis

The differential diagnosis of lateral elbow pain is wide and there may be a tendency to overdiagnose lateral epicondylitis, as many of the other causes are not considered and there are few diagnostic clinical tests (Table 2).

Management

The treatment of lateral epicondylitis in the more acute stages involves relative rest, the use of ice (10–20 minutes every 2 hours in the acute stages), analgesia, and nonsteroidal anti-inflammatory drugs (NSAIDs) (topical NSAIDs are preferable).[3] The use of modalities such as ultrasound is of unproven benefit. In more chronic cases, transverse friction massage helps to break down scar tissue at the site. A compression strap or counterforce brace applied distal to the bulk of the extensor mass has been demonstrated to reduce muscle activity in EDC and ECRB on needle electromyographic (EMG) studies during isometric contraction of the wrist extensors in healthy subjects.[4] Such studies have not been performed in affected individuals and no definitive conclusions can be drawn concerning the effectiveness of these appliances for lateral epicondylitis.[5] If a brace is used, then it is tightened to a comfortable degree of tension with the forearm muscles relaxed, so that a maximum contraction is limited. Constant use of the brace is avoided as tightness of involved structures can occur. Those who benefit from its use may choose to wear it during times of significant use of the arm even after symptoms settle.

The use of corticosteroid injections may provide short-term pain relief, but there is no evidence of benefit over placebo in the longer term.[6] They should be limited to those patients with persisting disability despite the above measures and where rehabilitation is limited. The patient must be warned of the significant risk of subcutaneous atrophy, tendon rupture, and other standard risks, and informed consent must be obtained. A small volume of a short-acting corticosteroid such as hydrocortisone with 0.5–1 ml 1 per cent lignocaine is suitable. A positive response occurs when there is significant reduction in pain lasting for at least 6 weeks. Should symptoms recur, the injection may

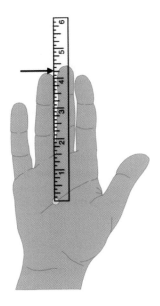

Fig. 14 Proper racquet handle size can be estimated by distance from mid-palmar crease to the ring finger.

be repeated at a minimum interval of 6 weeks, but the total number of injections should be limited to three. The injection should not be repeated if no response is seen with the first procedure. Dry needling and acupuncture both may provide pain relief and have fewer potential side-effects than local corticosteroid injections. Local injection is discussed in Chapter 5.3.

All of these approaches are used in order to allow rehabilitation to commence. Stretching of the forearm extensors and range of motion exercises at the elbow and wrist should start early. Progressive rehabilitation for strength and endurance of the forearm extensor–supinator group commences as soon as pain allows. The rate of progression is dependent upon the patient's symptoms and, if symptoms recur, the patient returns to a lower level of exercise. Ice may be necessary after early rehabilitation sessions to limit an excessive inflammatory response.

The most common cause for failure to respond to the above measures is failure to address the cause of the condition. This is particularly an issue in the manual worker who needs to continue to work, and may be an insurmountable problem. In tennis players, technique and equipment factors must be addressed. Proper racquet handle size can be estimated by distance from mid-palmar crease to the ring finger (Fig. 14). Evaluation of technique with the help of a coach may prove beneficial. Improvements may be noted by avoidance of the leading elbow during backhand, ensuring that the forearm is only partially pronated, the forward shoulder is lowered, and the trunk is leaning forward. The patient should also consider reducing string tension to 2–3 pounds less than the manufacturers' recommendations (i.e. 50–55 pounds), using slower, lighter tennis balls, and playing on slower courts.

Surgery should be reserved for those patients with disabling symptoms who fail to respond to all the above measures over the course of 1 year. Options include repair of the extensor origin after excision of the torn tendon and granulation tissue and local drilling of the subchondral bone of the lateral epicondyle with an aim to increasing blood supply. This can be performed under local or general anaesthesia. The elbow is placed in a posterior plaster splint for a week, then in a lighter splint for 2 weeks, with the elbow in 90° flexion and in neutral rotation.

Range of motion exercises are commenced thereafter, with a progressive strengthening regime. Light activities can be recommenced at 3 months, but the patient can expect to wear a counterforce brace initially.

Other surgical options include reduction of tension on the common extensor origin by fasciotomy, direct release of the extensor origin, or lengthening of the ECRB tendon distally. Fasciotomy and complete extensor tendon release can result in loss of strength and lengthening of ECRB distally appears to be effective only in the minority of cases. Whilst intraarticular procedures such as synovectomy and division of the orbicular ligament have been advocated, these seem inappropriate for an extraarticular condition. Some surgeons advocate decompression of the radial or posterior interosseous nerves on the basis that posterior interosseovs nerve entrapment is contributing to—or the primary cause of—chronic symptoms.

Radial nerve lesions

The radial nerve and its branches are vulnerable to compression at the elbow and forearm. Depending upon which portion of the nerve is affected symptoms may be motor (posterior interosseous nerve (PIN)), sensory (superficial radial nerve), or both. Posterior interosseous nerve entrapment occurs at five sites, but most commonly at the arcade of Frohse at the proximal edge of supinator. Nerve compression can also occur due to synovitis at the radiocapitellar joint, tumours, fractures, vascular anomalies, or other local masses. The superficial radial nerve can be entrapped alone or in combination with the posterior interosseous branch. The radial nerve can also be entrapped above the level of the elbow due to a lateral intermuscular septum, although this is rare.

History

The typical patient is one who performs repetitive rotary movements of the forearm, such as those involved in heavy manual labour (in particular, carpentry), or those performing sporting activities such as discus throwing and racquet sports. The primary symptom is aching pain in the belly of the extensor muscles, that is of insidious onset and worse with forearm pronation and wrist flexion. Pain may be more diffuse over the extensor aspect of the forearm and exacerbation after exertion and pain at night may be features. Such patients are those often considered to have a 'resistant tennis elbow'.

Examination

Examination reveals tenderness to palpation over the course of the PIN, deep to the extensor muscle belly, and just distal to the radial head. Pain may be reproduced with resisted extension of the middle finger with the elbow extended and on resisted supination of the extended forearm.

Investigations

EMG studies are frequently normal, although a decrease in motor conduction velocity in the radial nerve across the entrapment site and changes in the muscles innervated distal to the entrapment site may be noted.

Management

Management is symptomatic in mild cases, with stretching and activity modification. In resistant cases, exploration of the nerve is necessary. Procedures used in the treatment of lateral epicondylitis are often included.

Distal biceps tendinopathy

Tendinosis of the distal end of biceps brachii can occur with repetitive supination and pronation activities and can significantly affect function. Pain is felt in the antecubital fossa and local swelling and tenderness may be noted. Pain is worse with resisted supination. Management involves relative rest, ice, NSAIDs, and modification of activities. Failing to address the problem can result in rupture.

Rupture of the biceps insertion

Avulsion of the distal insertion of biceps accounts for 3–10 per cent of all biceps tendon ruptures and occurs in association with a single traumatic insult, usually with the elbow in 90° flexion. There is an increased incidence with anabolic steroid use.

The patient notes a sudden tearing pain in the antecubital fossa followed by a deep aching discomfort. There is bruising and considerable functional limitation with weakness of supination, and flexion and grip strength may also be reduced. The tendon is no longer palpable, having retracted into the forearm as a bulbous swelling. A palpable gap is present. A partial rupture of the tendon produces pain and local crepitus on supination and pronation. Treatment is early surgical repair.

Injury to the musculotendinous junction of biceps brachii and calcifying tendinitis of this unit are both rare.

Radial head bursitis

The deep bursa at the radial head can become inflamed with repetitive pronation/supination and may be confused with distal biceps tendinitis. There is local pain and tenderness in the antecubital fossa and there may be fullness or swelling in this area. Pain is worse with pronation. Treatment is symptomatic with modification of activities, ice, and NSAIDs.

Other causes of lateral elbow pain include articular disorders arthropathies, osteochondritis dissecans and osteochondrosis of the humeral capitellum, and radial head fractures. All are beyond the scope of this text. Referred pain from the neck is also a common and important cause of lateral elbow pain.

Forearm compartment syndrome

A compartment syndrome of the forearm can occur acutely after trauma or, less commonly, may present with chronic symptoms. The latter is extremely rare and presents with a history of exertional forearm pain such as performing manual work or lifting weights. Activities that involve elbow and wrist flexion may be particularly involved. Paraesthesiae in the forearm and hand may be reported. Symptoms gradually resolve with cessation of activity. Clinically, there may be little to find at rest, although the forearm is usually muscular. The diagnosis may be confirmed by intracompartmental pressure monitoring before and after exercise (normal range 0–8 mmHg), although diagnostic levels for forearm compartment syndrome have not been set. Treatment is fasciotomy.

Medial elbow

A range of disorders can result in medial elbow pain, as described in Table 3.

Table 3 Differential diagnosis of medial elbow pain

Medial epicondylitis

Medial apophysitis

Ulnar collateral ligament sprain/instability

Cervical spine radiculopathy

Ulnar neuropathy

Osteochondrosis/osteochondritis dissecans

Osteoarthritis

Fracture/stress fracture

Medial epicondylitis

Medial epicondylitis is not a true epicondylitis but rather an overuse injury of the common tendinous origin of the flexor–pronator muscle group. This injury commonly occurs as a result of repetitive flexion and pronation and, less commonly, with valgus stresses. Like its lateral counterpart, it is seen most commonly in manual workers, throwing and racquet sports, and in golfers ('golfer's elbow'). The condition is much less common than lateral epicondylitis and is frequently over-diagnosed.

History

It presents with an acute or insidious onset of aching pain at the medial elbow and proximal flexor musculature of the forearm. There may be weakness of grip, in particular in association with pain. Some patients report symptoms suggestive of an ulnar neuropathy with paraesthesiae in the ring and little fingers.

Examination

Decreased range of motion at the elbow may be noted, due to pain with stretching of the flexor–pronator group on full extension. There is tenderness at the medial epicondyle and symptoms are exacerbated by one or more of the provocation tests described earlier. The neck should be examined and other causes of medial elbow pain considered.

Investigations

Ultrasound will demonstrate features similar to those noted in lateral epicondylitis, specifically decreased echogenicity, inhomogeneity, thickening of the tendon and, more rarely, a local fluid collection may be identified. Local calcification within the tendon is seen in chronic cases.

Management

Medial epicondylitis is considered to be more resistant to treatment than lateral epicondylitis. This may be related to greater difficulty in avoiding stresses imposed on this area during daily activities, to characteristics of the tissue that make healing prolonged, or inaccuracy of diagnosis. The diagnosis should be questioned in any patient who fails to respond to standard treatment.

Management follows the same path as that described with lateral epicondylitis and includes relative rest, ice, analgesics, NSAIDs, and a reverse counterforce brace. Deep transverse friction massage is employed in chronic cases to break down scar tissue. All aim to allow the patient to commence rehabilitation, including early stretching of the wrist and elbow and a progressive strengthening regime of the wrist flexors and forearm pronators.

Return to activities can take place only when there is full pain-free range of movement and strength of grip and forearm pronation and wrist flexion have returned to at least 80 per cent of normal. Corticosteroid injections are used sparingly and are rarely necessary. Caution should be exercised with respect to the close proximity of the ulnar nerve.

Causative factors are addressed, including work habits, sporting technique, and equipment. Preventative measures also include adequate conditioning of the forearm, attention to sporting technique, and adequate warm-up, stretching, and cool down.

Surgical intervention is rarely required and is considered only in the most refractory of cases. Standard approaches include release of the tendinous origin of pronator teres and usually a portion of flexor carpi radialis (FCR), debridement and decompression of the ulnar nerve distal to the medial epicondyle. A rehabilitation regime is then commenced postoperatively and usually is continued for 6 months before a return to full activities. Complications of surgery include loss of full elbow extension (up to 5°) in 1 per cent of cases, superficial infection (in less than 1 per cent), and damage to the ulnar nerve and MCL.

Little leaguer's elbow

Little leaguer's elbow describes a spectrum of changes that can occur at the elbow of a young individual, in particular relation to throwing. The term refers to the group that this condition is seen in most commonly, that is young baseball pitchers (Fig. 16). These changes include a variable combination of a medial apophysitis, MCL injury and instability, and compressive changes at the radiocapitellar joint (Fig. 16).

Medial apophysitis is a true epicondylitis and occurs in the skeletally immature individual, when there is traction and inflammation of the growth plate at the medial epicondyle. It is seen in particular in children aged 10–14 years who are involved in throwing and racquet sports.

During throwing, repetitive forces secondary to contracture of the flexor–pronator origin at the medial epicondyle can lead to micro-injuries of the growth plate. In addition, repetitive valgus stress at the elbow leads to attenuation and microtears of the anterior bundle of the MCL (Fig. 17). This can progress to valgus instability of the elbow and subsequent compression of the radiocapitellar articulation laterally, with development of osteochondrosis. In some cases acute or repetitive traction on the MCL may lead to an avulsion injury at the apophysis.

History

The patient typically complains of an insidious onset of aching pain at the medial elbow on a background of the repetitive activities described above. Symptoms may be severe and nocturnal disturbance is common. Weakness of grip is commonly noted and there may be paraesthesiae in the distribution of the ulnar nerve.

Examination

Examination reveals swelling and tenderness at the medial epicondyle, and bruising and flexion contracture may be evident. Pain is exacerbated with passive extension of the elbow and wrist. If an avulsion

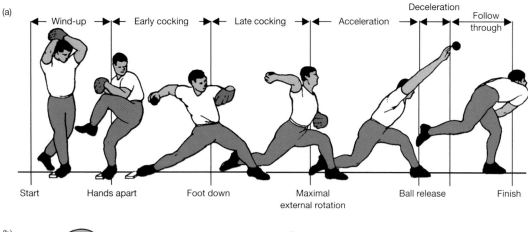

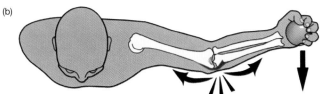

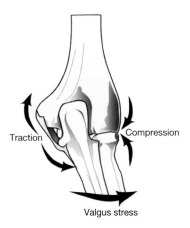

Fig. 15 (a and b) The baseball pitch. Note the valgus stress placed on the elbow in the late cocking phase.

Fig. 16 Little leaguer's elbow results from traction on the lateral elbow and compressive forces on the medial side.

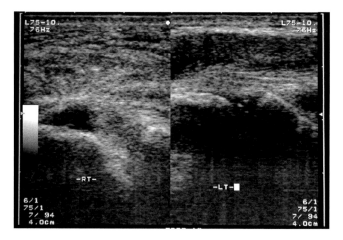

Fig. 17 Ultrasound showing a tear of the right common flexor tendon origin at the medial epicondyle.

injury at the epicondyle has occurred, then a fragment may be palpable. Stress testing may reveal medial instability. In those who have developed compressive changes, the lateral elbow may be tender, with pain exacerbated on movement and on compression of the joint.

Investigations

Plain X-rays may be normal or may show widening of the physis, fragmentation, or avulsion of the apophysis in comparison to the other side. Gravity valgus stress views may be necessary.

Management

Management in the form of relative rest from the causative activities, analgesics, ice, and gentle stretching is usually effective but healing can be prolonged and the patient, parent, and coach must be counselled with respect to this. Non-compliance may result in chronic apophysitis.

When avulsion has occurred, treatment is dependent upon the degree of displacement. Fragments that are rotated or more than 5 mm in diameter may require open reduction and fixation. Mild displacement is treated with immobilization for 2 weeks and then progressive rehabilitation.

Medial collateral ligament injury

Acute or chronic MCL injury in adults can occur due to repetitive valgus extension overload, most commonly seen in throwers or, less commonly, with direct trauma.

The throwing action involves specific phases, as described in Fig. 15. Medial valgus stress on the elbow, in particular during the acceleration phase of throwing, results in MCL instability and a wedging effect of the olecranon into the olecranon fossa with resulting formation of a posterior osteophyte. This in turn can irritate the ulnar nerve.

A history of medial elbow pain in a thrower should immediately raise suspicion of the condition. In the acute injury the patient typically reports a sudden onset of pain during throwing, with an associated 'pop' or 'snap'. In chronic cases, the patient reports progressive medial elbow pain that is functionally limiting and worse during the acceleration phase of throwing. The patient often adapts his/her throwing technique, usually to an earlier release, but this is less controlled.

Flexion contractures and cubitus valgus deformities are common in throwers. Swelling and local MCL tenderness and instability are present, particularly in the acute injury. Posteromedial osteophytes are occasionally palpable and posterior olecranon tenderness is worsened by bringing the arm into valgus and extension.

Investigations

Plain X-rays may be normal but in chronic cases commonly demonstrate ectopic bone formation in the MCL, posteromedial osteophyte formation at the olecranon and conoid tubercle and loose bodies. Stress films can help to confirm medial instability. MRI allows assessment of the MCL.

Management

The aims of treatment are to settle acute symptoms where present and to restore normal range of motion. Rest from exacerbating activities, ice, analgesics, and NSAIDs may all be helpful. Passive and active range of motion exercises are vital and commenced early, and a balanced strengthening regime commenced. When full range of motion is regained, then throwing activities can be resumed, with a programme of progressive velocity and endurance. Surgery is indicated in those who fail to respond, who have chronic instability and functional impairment. Excision of osteophytes and local debridement or a straight osteotomy, 1 cm proximal to the tip of the olecranon, are considered in those with impingement. When instability is a major feature, reconstruction using a tendon graft is recommended, although repair may be performed in the acute rupture.

Prevention of the condition is important through adequate conditioning, warm-up, stretching, and appropriate technique.

Ulnar neuropathy

The ulnar nerve is vulnerable to trauma, dislocation, and compression during its passage through the cubital tunnel posterior to the medial epicondyle. Individuals with shallow ulnar grooves within the tunnel, with hypermobility or laxity of the soft tissue constraints of the nerve in the tunnel, and those who perform repetitive throwing or flexion activities are particularly vulnerable to dislocation or subluxation of the nerve. Recurrent dislocation of the ulnar nerve is reported in 16 per cent of the normal population.[7] In any individual, the volume of the cubital tunnel decreases as the elbow is flexed, resulting in external compression of the ulnar nerve by boundaries of the tunnel, the MCL, and the arcuate ligament. The nerve itself is moved medially by the medial head of the triceps during elbow flexion. Scar tissue may tether the nerve and prevent this normal movement. Dislocation or subluxation is most likely during flexion activities and when this occurs the nerve is particularly at risk of direct trauma. It should be noted that ulnar nerve instability can be an incidental finding.

As has been described, the significant tensile forces at the medial elbow due to repetitive valgus stresses during throwing increase the possibility of a traction neuritis and this is particularly likely in individuals with MCL instability.

Other aetiological factors can lead to ulnar neuropathy at the elbow. The nerve can become compressed by hypertrophied forearm musculature, by the aponeurosis of flexor carpi ulnaris, a ganglion situated in the cubital tunnel, local bony anomalies, or by adhesions within the cubital tunnel.

History

There is deep aching pain at the medial elbow and proximal forearm, which may radiate proximally or distally and may be notable only during flexion and valgus stresses. Neurological disturbances including paraesthesia, dysaesthesia, and anaesthesia in the ulnar one and a half digits are usually experienced early in the condition. Whilst clumsiness is frequently reported, true motor weakness is rare since branches within the cubital tunnel to FCU and flexor digitorum profundus (FDP) are situated deep and therefore frequently spared. Those with recurrent dislocation or subluxation of the nerve, may report a popping or snapping sensation prior to the onset of pain and dysaesthesiae with elbow flexion and extension.

Examination

Valgus deformity of the elbow, a mild flexion contracture, and MCL instability may be present. Wasting of the small muscles of the hand and hypothenar eminence is a late finding. Soft tissue swelling at the ulnar groove, with tenderness and thickening of the nerve, may be evident. Those with ulnar nerve subluxation may be able to demonstrate the phenomenon and the examiner can frequently dislocate the nerve from the groove. Pressure or percussion may reproduce symptoms, but this is not a sensitive indication of pathology. Symptoms may also be reproduced on sustained elbow flexion (1 minute), particularly when the wrist is extended. Weakness of the small muscles of the hand may be evident. Sensory signs are frequently absent, but, in advanced cases, evaluation of the ulnar dorsal portion of the hand (supplied by the dorsal cutaneous branch of the ulnar nerve) and ulnar volar forearm (medial antebrachial cutaneous nerve) can indicate whether the nerve injury or compression is in the upper arm, the cubital tunnel, or at the wrist. A Martin Gruber anastamosis, where there is communication between the median and ulnar nerves in the forearm, occurs in 15 per cent of people and may confuse clinical findings.

Other causes of ulnar neuropathy should be considered (Table 4). The cervical spine should be examined and the patient evaluated for the presence of hypermobility syndrome.

Investigations

Nerve conduction studies classically show reduced conduction velocity across the site of compression compared to the unaffected arm. Although a decline of less than 25 per cent is considered normal, velocities that are reduced by more than 33 per cent are strongly suggestive of neuropathy.[8] Such findings must be considered in the clinical context and cannot be viewed in isolation. Provocative testing with the elbow in flexion is not usually performed due to difficulties in obtaining accurate measurements.

A *plain X-ray* of the elbow should be performed to identify associated bony abnormalities (in particular, osteophytes).

At the elbow

Fractures/dislocations

Progressive valgus deformity after ulnar collateral ligament injury or lateral epicondylar fracture

Pressure on the nerve at the ulnar groove

Entrapment between the two heads of flexor carpi ulnaris, distal to the medial epicondyle

At the wrist

Compression, e.g. fracture, osteoarthritis, compression against bicycle handlebars, tumours, haemorrhage

Mononeuritis multiplex

Diabetes, vasculitides, sarcoid, amyloid, rheumatoid arthritis, systemic lupus erythematosus, malignancy

Management

Ulnar neuropathies may be graded according to symptoms and clinical findings. These do not necessarily correlate with pre-treatment electrodiagnostic findings. Mild compression includes those with subjective sensory symptoms only. Moderate compression has additional weakness and wasting of the interossei and reduced sensation, and severe compression extends to include wasting of the adductor pollicis and hypothenar muscles and complete or partial anaesthesia of the ulnar-innervated portion of the hand.[9]

Non-operative management should be pursued in the first instance in most mild to moderate cases.[10] Those patients with only sensory symptoms in the absence of motor weakness or wasting are managed conservatively in the first instance. Stress on the ulnar nerve should be avoided by complete rest from exacerbating activities and the use of elbow pads. Splinting the elbow at 30° of flexion may provide symptomatic relief. Ice, NSAIDs, and simple analgesics may be tried but can frequently be unhelpful, whilst modalities are not indicated. Gentle range of motion exercises are commenced as soon as tolerated. Return to normal activities can commence after full strength is regained with a progressive strengthening regime of forearm musculature and correction of faulty technique where appropriate.

Prolonged symptom duration, motor and/or sensory deficit, and local joint pathology (especially MCL instability) are poor prognostic indicators. Half of the non-athletic population with mild compression will respond to conservative management. Excellent results in up to 90 per cent of patients are reported in both athletic and non-athletic patients with mild or moderate compression, with variable results reported in those in whom compression is severe.[10]

Surgery is considered in those patients who fail to resolve with conservative management, those with motor signs, and those with significant MCL instability. In such cases decompression may be suitable where there is localized compression of the nerve. Surgical options include cubital tunnel decompression or transposition of the nerve in those with nerve subluxation or valgus deformity of the elbow or those in whom decompression has failed. The nerve may be transposed anteriorly with a fascial sling or submuscularly. Medial epicondylectomy has also been advocated, but such a procedure may result in the creation of new sources of nerve pathology. It is recommended that at operation all potential sources of compression of the nerve are explored, even when a specific site of compression has been indicated by electrodiagnostic studies, since more than one site of compression can exist.[11]

Median nerve compression

Median nerve compression at the elbow or forearm can result in pronator or anterior interosseous syndromes.

The pronator syndrome

Median nerve compression at the elbow and proximal forearm, the *pronator syndrome*, results in vague aching pain at the proximal, volar surface of the forearm. There is often a history of repetitive strenuous use of the forearm. Rarely, there may be dysaesthesiae in the distribution of the median nerve in the hand.

Compression can occur at four sites that may indicate the specific site of compression. The ligament of Struthers, a band between the medial epicondyle and the supracondylar process, is commonly implicated and results in symptoms that are worse with flexion of the elbow against resistance between 120° and 135° flexion. Another fibrous band (the bicipital aponeurosis) can cause indentation of the pronator muscle mass below the medial epicondyle and symptoms are increased by active and passive forearm pronation. Compression can also occur within the pronator teres due to hypertrophy or tightness of the muscle, when symptoms are worse with resisted pronation of forearm with the wrist in flexion (to relax FDS). Direct pressure over the proximal portion of pronator teres approximately 4 cm distal to the antebrachial crease while exerting moderate resistance to pronation also reproduces the symptoms. Lastly, the nerve can be compressed under FDS, when symptoms are aggravated by resisted flexion of FDS of the middle finger and with passive stretching of finger and wrist flexors.

Tinel's test at possible sites of entrapment is an insensitive test. Weakness of median nerve-innervated muscles is uncommon but, when there is weakness of pinch grip, the condition should be differentiated from anterior interosseous syndrome.

Electrodiagnostic studies help to confirm median nerve latency but may not localize the lesion to the forearm, and exclusion of a carpal tunnel syndrome or double crush syndrome can be difficult.

Management includes passive stretching of the forearm musculature, passive stretching, NSAIDs, and elbow splinting in neutral rotation. Symptoms may take 2–3 months to improve. Surgical intervention involves exploration of the nerve from 5 cm proximal to the elbow and in the forearm at potential sites of compression.

Anterior interosseous syndrome

Compression of the anterior interosseous nerve results in a pure motor paralysis of flexor pollicis longus (FPL) and the index flexor digitorum profundus (FDP), often in combination with weakness of pronator quadratus. Those patients with a Martin Gruber anastomosis may experience weakness of the ulnar intrinsic muscles and/or weakness of flexor profundus to other fingers. This syndrome is described in individuals lifting heavy weights and where there is cumulative trauma. The patient reports a short episode of pain, which subsides to leave motor weakness. Examination will reveal weakness of pinch grip. After 2–3 weeks, EMG studies will show signs of denervation of affected muscles.

Management involves a course of NSAIDs and relative rest for 8–12 weeks. Those who remain symptomatic are considered for surgery, involving an approach similar to that for pronator syndrome.

Table 5 Differential diagnosis of posterior elbow pain

Triceps tendinopathies
Triceps avulsion
Traction apophysitis
Olecranon bursitis
C-spine radiculopathy
Fracture/stress fracture

Table 6 Causes of olecranon bursitis

Trauma (acute or chronic)
Sepsis
Metabolic/crystals
Inflammatory arthritis
Uraemia
Calcific deposits
Idiopathic

Posterior elbow pain

The differential diagnosis of posterior elbow pain is detailed in Table 5.

Triceps tendinopathies

Triceps tendinopathies, which include tendinosis and rupture, are rare.

Triceps tendinosis

Triceps tendinosis is an overuse injury associated with repetitive elbow extension, typically occurring in manual labour and in throwers. It is also associated with the presence of posterior osteophytes or loose bodies in the joint.

Patients present with posterior elbow pain, worse with elbow extension. Examination reveals tenderness at or just proximal to the tendon insertion and pain on resisted elbow extension. X-rays may confirm associated bony pathology. Ultrasound is useful in confirming the diagnosis.

Management is similar to that of lateral epicondylitis and surgical intervention is almost never necessary, although resection of a small part of the triceps insertion has been advocated.

Triceps rupture

Triceps rupture occurs much less commonly than that of other tendons such as the long head of biceps and the Achilles tendons. It typically occurs in men in the fourth and fifth decades. Right and left sides are equally affected and there appears to be no relation to hand dominance.

The mechanism of injury is usually a fall on to the outstretched hand, with sudden stress upon a contracted triceps. Rarely, the injury may arise after a direct blow to the tendon. As is the case with other tendons, spontaneous rupture with minimal trauma may also occur, usually on the background of a diseased (though frequently asymptomatic) tendon.

Rupture is usually an avulsion injury of the tendon at the tendo-osseous junction. Rupture at the musculotendinous junction occurs more rarely. Partial ruptures, usually in the central third of the tendon, can also occur. Other injuries may occur simultaneously, including fracture of the radial head. Anabolic steroid use and underlying systemic diseases that are associated with tendinosis should also be considered. The patient usually describes a mechanism of fall on to the outstretched hand, a direct blow, or more rarely a sudden tear or pop, with minimal trauma. Pain, swelling, and weakness of elbow extension result.

Investigations

In the majority of cases lateral *plain X-rays* show flecks of avulsed bone proximal to the olecranon. An additional fracture of the head of the radius should be excluded. *Ultrasound* will confirm tendon rupture.

Management

Conservative management is reserved for the frail patient, in particular when there is a partial tear and some elbow extension is still possible. Otherwise management is surgical. In the acute rupture, reattachment of the tendon is attempted. In the delayed presentation or in those with an underlying diseased tendon, reconstruction is considered. Results from surgery are reported to be good, with full restoration of strength and normal or near normal range of motion.

Olecranon bursitis (student's or miner's elbow)

Pathology affecting the superficial olecranon bursa is one of the most common sites of bursitis in the body. Bursitis may be acute or chronic, septic or aseptic. It occurs most commonly as a result of trauma in the form of a direct blow or repetitive friction. Septic bursitis can arise due to direct inoculation through local skin breaks that are often seemingly innocuous. Steroid injections precede infections in up to 10 per cent of cases. The most common causative organism is *Staphylococcus aureus* but group A beta-haemolytic *Streptococcus* and other *Staphylococci*, *Haemophillus influenzae*, *Pseudomonas*, and, in the immunocompromised patient, fungi, mycobacteria, or anaerobic bacteria may be involved. Bursitis in association with a crystal arthropathy is also common (Table 6).

History

The patient may give a history of direct trauma or repetitive microtrauma to the posterior aspect of the elbow. A history suggestive of other causes may also be reported and the possibility of sepsis must be addressed as a priority. The initial insult, where present, is followed by variable degrees of pain and swelling around the olecranon. Pain may be absent but can be particularly severe when crystals or sepsis are present. A history of a recent local steroid injection, fever and systemic upset, or coexistence of diabetes or immunosuppression should arouse suspicion of sepsis.

Examination

There is discrete swelling at the posterior elbow, representing thickened bursa or bursal fluid, or both. The overlying skin is inflamed in the acute and subacute cases and the skin should be closely examined for any sign of breakage. Inclusion nodules, consisting of fibrous tissue formed after significant inflammation within the bursa, may be palpable. A local effusion of the elbow may occasionally be present, particularly in inflammatory conditions, Those patients with a septic or crystal-induced bursitis may be systemically unwell with a fever and cellulites, and local lymphadenopathy may be noted where sepsis is present. Signs of associated conditions and sepsis elsewhere should be sought.

Investigations

Inflammatory markers (erythrocyte sedimentation rate (ESR), C-reactive protein (CRP)) and white cell count may be elevated in systemic sepsis and crystal-induced bursitis. Whenever there is suspicion of a septic bursitis, blood cultures and sterile aspiration of the bursal fluid with subsequent analysis by Gram stain and culture are essential. Bursal fluid can also be examined for crystals. X-rays are not performed routinely; calcification and olecranon spurs may also be evident although this may be coincidental.

Management

Most uncomplicated cases are managed symptomatically with regular ice, NSAIDs, and local protection by an elbow pad or dressing. Aspiration without injection can help to relieve pain and allows bursal fluid to be obtained for examination. Injection of corticosteroid (hydrocortisone 10 mg) may benefit persisting bursitis and is most useful when associated with an inflammatory arthritis/crystals. Injections are rarely necessary in post-traumatic bursitis and involve some risk of sepsis and local atrophy. Injections must not be performed if there is any suspicion of sepsis. Relative rest for 5 days after aspiration is recommended.

In those patients in whom sepsis is confirmed who are systemically well and with little cellulitis, aspiration of the bursa followed by oral broad-spectrum antibiotics (according to the initial Gram stain, but usually covering penicillin-resistant *Staphylococcus aureus*) is commenced, changing to the appropriate antibiotic according to the results of bursal fluid and blood culture and sensitivity tests. Progress should be monitored and intravenous antibiotics commenced in those who fail to respond and in those with systemic symptoms. Open drainage and lavage may be necessary, with the catheter left *in situ* until cultures from the tube are negative for 3 consecutive days. Antibiotics can then be administered by the oral route. There is no consensus on the appropriate duration of antibiotics in complicated and uncomplicated cases. In all cases splinting of the elbow, regular ice, and NSAIDs can provide symptomatic benefit.[12, 13]

In the acute posttraumatic bursitis, sterile aspiration of blood is indicated to provide symptomatic relief and should be followed by a compressive dressing, regular icing, and NSAIDs. Repeat aspiration may be necessary. Steroid injections have no role in the management of acute post-traumatic bursitis. Return to contact activities is permitted once the patient is asymptomatic but a protective elbow pad should be worn initially.

Chronic recurrent symptomatic bursitis can be managed surgically. This can involve simple debridement or excision of the bursa and/or a small amount of the underlying bone at the point of the olecranon. Drainage is continued for up to 2 days postoperatively and the elbow is splinted in 45–60° of flexion until the sutures are removed. Range of motion exercises are commenced early. Contact activities should be avoided for at least 6 weeks and an elbow pad worn for several months until all symptoms are settled. Individuals with a history of recurrent bursitis should be advised to wear elbow pads as a preventative measure.

References

1. Nirschl, R.P. (1974). The etiology and treatment of tennis elbow. *J. Sports Med. Phys. Fitness* **2**, 308–323.

2. Chard, M.D., Cawston, T.E., Riley, G.P., Gresham, G.A., and Hazleman, B.L. (1994). Rotator cuff degeneration and lateral epicondylitis: a comparative histological study. *Ann. Rheum. Dis.* **53** (1), 30–34.

3. Kamien, M. (1990). A rational management of tennis elbow. *J. Sports Med.* **9**, 173–191.

4. Snyder-Mackler, L. and Epler, M. (1989). Effect of standard and Aircast tennis elbow bands on integrated electromyography of forearm extensor musculature proximal to the bands. *Am. J. Sports Med.* **17** (2), 278–281.

5. Struijs, P.A.A., Smidt, N., Arola, H., *et al.* (2001). Orthotic devices for tennis elbow (Cochrane review). In *The cochrane library*, 2. Update Software, Oxford.

6. Hay, E.M., Paterson, S.M., Lewis, M., Hosie, G., and Croft, P. (1999). Pragmatic randomised controlled trial of local corticosteroid injection and naproxen for treatment of lateral epicondylitis of elbow in primary care. *Br. Med. J.* **319** (7215), 964–968.

7. Childress, H.M. (1975). Recurrent ulnar-nerve dislocation at the elbow. *Clin. Orthop.* **108**, 168–173.

8. Gilliatt, R.W. and Thomas, P.K. (1960). Changes in nerve conduction with ulnar nerve lesions at the elbow. *J. Neurol Neurosurg. Psychiatry* **23**, 312–320.

9. McGowan, A.J. (1950). The results of transposition of the ulnar nerves for traumatic ulnar neuritis. *J. Bone Joint Surg. (Br.)* **32**, 293–301.

10. Dellon, A.L., Hament, W., and Gittelshon, A. (1993). Nonoperative management of cubital tunnel syndrome: an 8-year prospective study. *Neurology* **43** (9), 1673–1677.

11. Kojima, T., Kurihara, K., and Nagano, T. (1979). A study on operative findings and pathogenic factors in ulnar neuropathy at the elbow. *Handchirurgie* **11** (2), 99–104.

12. Raddatz, D.A., Hoffman, G.S., and Franck, W.A. (1987). Septic bursitis: presentation, treatment and prognosis. *J. Rheumatol.* **14** (6), 1160–1163.

13. Smith, D.L., McAfee, J.H., Lucas, L.M., Kumar, K.L., and Romney, D.M. (1989). Treatment of nonseptic olecranon bursitis. A controlled, blinded prospective trial. *Arch. Intern. Med.* **149** (11), 2527–2530.

6.5 The wrist and hand

Seamus Dalton

Introduction

The anatomy of the wrist and hand is complex but it is this that provides the upper limb with its unique capacity for fine motor function and ability to obtain information from the surrounding environment. Not only is the hand our conduit for almost all upper limb function, but it also assists in communication and expression. The hand comprises 19 bones, 17 articulations, and 19 muscles, as well as the numerous tendons activated by muscles in the forearm. The risk of injury, both acute and overuse, is high. Many of these injuries resolve with no lasting loss of function but significant impairment may result from acute or chronic soft tissue disorders and early diagnosis is important. The aim of this chapter is to present the common and some of the more unusual soft tissue disorders of the wrist and hand. Fractures and dislocations are not discussed but the more common carpal instability patterns arising from ligamentous injuries are reviewed.

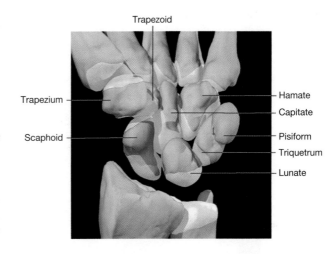

Fig. 1 The carpus.

Anatomy

The wrist is a complex multi-axial joint that connects the forearm to the hand. Its complexity lies in the number of bones and articulations with their array of interconnecting ligaments that makes understanding of the biomechanics of wrist function, let alone clinical assessment, difficult for most physicians.

The distal ends of the radius and ulna and connecting ligaments form the distal radioulnar joint and a concave articulation for the proximal row of carpal bones comprising the scaphoid, lunate, triquetrum, and pisiform. With the exception of the pisiform, the carpal bones are small, irregularly shaped ossicles with similar characteristics that are descriptively divided into a proximal and distal row. The mid-carpal joint lies between these rows and can be thought of as having a medial and lateral component. The distal row consists of the trapezium, trapezoid, capitate, and hamate with the palmar surfaces of the trapezoid and trapezium articulating with the scaphoid to form the lateral part of the mid-carpal joint, whilst the heads of the capitate and hamate are in contact with the concave surface of the proximal carpal bones to form the medial component.

The radiocarpal joint is an ellipsoidal articulation between the distal surface of the radius and the scaphoid, lunate, and triquetrum (Fig. 1). The distal ulna and pisiform do not form part of this joint but the triangular fibrocartilage complex (TFCC), which lies between the distal ulna and the carpus, forms the medial border of the radiocarpal joint.

Carpal bones

With the exception of the pisiform, the carpal bones are collectively described as having proximal, distal, medial, lateral, anterior (palmar), and posterior (dorsal) surfaces. The proximal and distal and, to a lesser extent, medial and lateral surfaces have articular cartilage covering but the anterior and posterior surfaces usually provide attachments for the ligaments and joint capsules. The scaphoid is the largest and most radial of the proximal carpal bones and it and its adjoining ligaments are especially vulnerable to injury with axial loading of the wrist and forearm.

Ligaments of the wrist

The capsular and ligamentous attachments of the wrist are too complex to describe in detail and for the clinician such analysis of the anatomy is unnecessary. The main structures are described here and some understanding of their relationship to wrist function and motion is essential in order to evaluate acute and chronic injuries to the wrist and hand, particularly those resulting in carpal instability (Fig. 2).

Intercarpal (interosseous) ligaments

The proximal carpal bones are joined by short thick interosseous ligaments that extend from the proximal articular surface of the lunate to the adjacent scaphoid and triquetrum. The distal row has three ligaments connecting the trapezium to the trapezoid, the trapezoid to the capitate, and the capitate to the hamate, with the latter being the strongest.

Dorsal radiocarpal ligament

This is formed by a thickening in the dorsal capsule which extends obliquely from the dorsal margin of the distal radius to the dorsum of the lunate and triquetrum. As the forearm pronates, this ligament passively pulls the carpus and hand to a position of pronation.

Palmar radiocarpal ligaments

These can be subdivided into the palmar radiocapite ligament (often described as a radioscaphocapite ligament), radiotriquetral ligament (which acts as a volar sling for the lunate), and the volar radioscapholunate ligament which must be disrupted before complete scapholunate dissociation can occur.

Radial collateral ligament

This ligament extends from the radial styloid process to the waist of the scaphoid and then on to the trapezium where it blends with the transverse carpal ligament and dorsal capsular ligament. It is crossed by the radial artery and only becomes taut at the extreme of ulnar deviation.

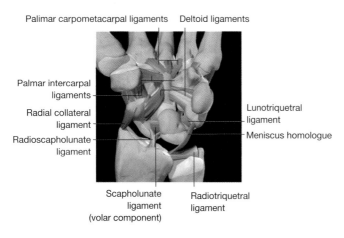

Fig. 2 The ligamentous structures of the carpus.

Ulnar collateral ligament

This ligament extends from the base and body of the ulnar styloid process and also from the border of the triangular fibrocartilage before narrowing and attaching to the pisiform, triquetrum, and transverse carpal ligament. It then extends distally to insert into the ulnar border of the hamate and base of the fifth metacarpal.

Triangular fibrocartilage complex (TFCC)

This is a homogeneous entity formed by multiple structures that include the triangular fibrocartilage and adjacent ulnocarpal meniscus (both of which attach to the dorsal ulnar corner of the radius), the ulnar collateral ligament, dorsal and volar radioulnar ligaments, and also the sheath of the extensor carpi ulnaris (ECU) tendon. It extends from the ulnar aspect of the radius to insert at the base of the ulnar styloid process and then continues distally where it joins the ulnar collateral ligament. It has ligamentous attachments to the triquetrum and lunate. Its dorsal attachments are weak whilst its volar attachments are strong and connect the palmar aspect of the ulnar carpus to the radius and not the ulna.

Flexor retinaculum and carpal tunnel

The flexor retinaculum or transverse carpal ligament is a strong fibrous ligament that extends from the pisiform and hook of the hamate medially to the tuberosities of the scaphoid and trapezium laterally. Its function is to hold the long flexor tendons in place during wrist flexion (Figs 3 and 4). It is under constant tension and therefore probably helps to maintain the carpal arch. The carpal tunnel is formed by the transverse carpal ligament (flexor retinaculum) and carpal bones and through it travel the four slips of the flexor digitorum profundus and the four slips of the flexor digitorum superficialis along with the flexor pollicis longus tendon which runs through the compartment with the median nerve (Fig. 5).

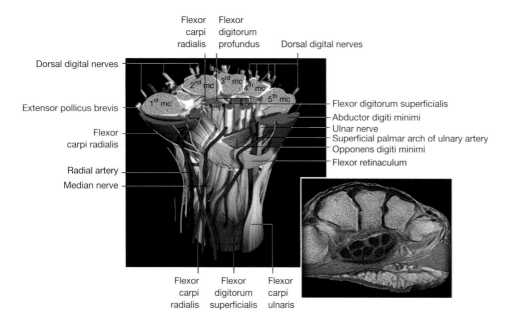

Fig. 3 Transverse section through the carpal tunnel.

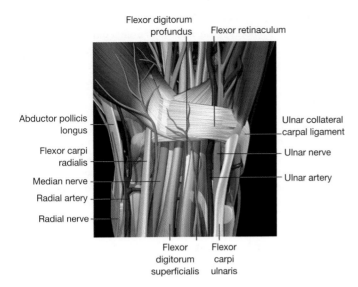

Fig. 4 The palmar aspect of the wrist.

Flexor digitorum profundus
Flexor retinaculum
Abductor pollicis longus
Flexor carpi radialis
Median nerve
Radial artery
Radial nerve
Ulnar collateral carpal ligament
Ulnar nerve
Ulnar artery
Flexor digitorum superficialis
Flexor carpi ulnaris

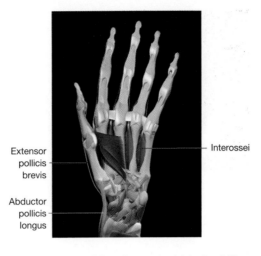

Fig. 6 Structures of the palmar aspect of the hand (1).

Extensor pollicis brevis
Abductor pollicis longus
Interossei

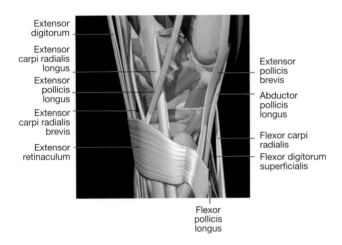

Fig. 5 The radial wrist.

Extensor digitorum
Extensor carpi radialis longus
Extensor pollicis longus
Extensor carpi radialis brevis
Extensor retinaculum
Extensor pollicis brevis
Abductor pollicis longus
Flexor carpi radialis
Flexor digitorum superficialis
Flexor pollicis longus

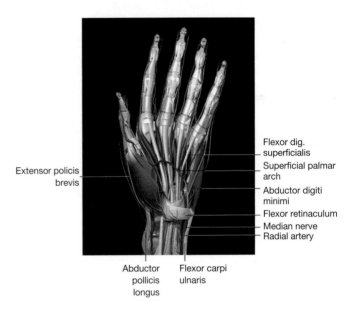

Fig. 7 Structures of the palmar aspect of the hand (2).

Extensor pollicis brevis
Flexor dig. superficialis
Superficial palmar arch
Abductor digiti minimi
Flexor retinaculum
Median nerve
Radial artery
Abductor pollicis longus
Flexor carpi ulnaris

Muscles and tendons

Broadly speaking, there are three groups of muscles that control the motor function of the hand (Figs 5 to 7). The intrinsic muscles, which include the thenar and hypothenar muscles, the palmar and dorsal interossei, and the lumbricals, control fine movements of the thumb and digits such as opposition and gripping. The tendons of the long flexor and extensor muscles of the forearm attach to the phalanges, metacarpals, and in some cases the carpal bones, and provide great strength for gripping as well as controlling gross movement of the wrist and hand. In addition, the tendons of the long and short flexors and extensors of the thumb and a long abductor pass across the wrist. Adequate knowledge of this anatomy is important if one is to be able to properly assess the wrist and hand and it is therefore the responsibility of every clinician to ensure that he or she has this knowledge.

Surface anatomy

A number of prominent bony landmarks and readily palpable tendons provides the clinician with an excellent template with which to assess the surface anatomy of the wrist and hand. For detailed examination of the wrist, it can be loosely divided into three dorsal and two palmar zones, which helps in the identification of anatomical structures and sites of pathology.[1]

Radial dorsal zone

This is bordered by the radial styloid process, the scaphoid and scaphotrapezial joint, the trapezium, the base of the first metacarpal, and first carpometacarpal joint. The soft tissues present in this zone include the abductor pollicis longus (APL) and extensor pollicis brevis (EPB) tendons and the extensor pollicis longus (EPL) tendon with the

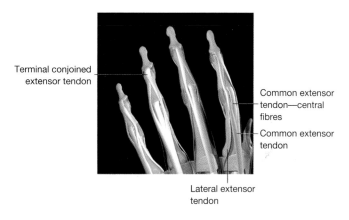

Terminal conjoined extensor tendon

Common extensor tendon—central fibres

Common extensor tendon

Lateral extensor tendon

Fig. 8 Extensor tendons of the fingers.

anatomical snuff box lying between the tendons of the first compartment (APL and EPB) and the EPL tendon.

Central dorsal zone

This is bordered by Lister's tubercle, the scapholunate joint, the lunate, capitate, the base of the second and third metacarpals, and the adjacent carpometacarpal joints. Soft tissues present in this zone include the distal attachments of the extensor carpi radialis brevis (ECRB) and extensor carpi radialis longus (ECRL) tendons along with the extensor digitorum communis tendons (Fig. 5).

Ulnar dorsal zone

This is bordered by the ulnar styloid, distal radioulnar joint, triquetrum, and hamate, and the base of the fourth and fifth metacarpals. Soft tissues present in this zone include the TFCC and the ECU tendon and sheath.

Radial volar zone

This is bordered by the scaphoid tuberosity, tubercle of the trapezium, the tendons of the flexor carpi radialis, palmaris longus, and long finger flexors, along with the median nerve.

Ulnar volar zone

This is bordered by the pisiform and hook of hamate with soft tissues present including the flexor carpi ulnaris (FCU) tendon and sheath and the ulnar nerve and artery.

Wrist motion

Wrist motion occurs in three planes: *sagittal* (flexion/extension); *frontal* (radial and ulnar deviation); and *transverse* (pronation and supination). True rotation does not occur but circumduction is possible through a combination of flexion, extension, and radial and ulnar deviation. The distal radioulnar joint allows 150° of rotation as the distal radius moves about the distal end of the ulna. Of extension 50–60 per cent of extension occurs at the radiocarpal joint and 40–50 per cent at the midcarpal joint. 40–50 per cent of flexion occurs at the radiocarpal joint and 50–60 per cent at the midcarpal joint.[2] This allows approximately 130° of total flexion/extension and 40° of radial/ulnar deviation.[3] Most activities of daily living require about 5° of flexion, 30° of extension, 10° of radial deviation, and 15° of ulnar

deviation. However, a functional range of motion probably requires 40° of flexion, 40° of extension, and 40° of frontal motion.

This wide range of motion is to a large extent dependent on the complex interosseous relationships in the wrist, and the range of ulnar and radial deviation is reduced when the arm is pronated and minimal when the wrist is fully flexed or extended. The main purpose of the ligaments is to provide stability in the frontal and sagittal planes and there is great potential for injury to these structures when force is applied to the wrist, as in falls on the outstretched arm. Of the axial load of the forearm, 20 per cent passes via the ulna, TFCC, and medial carpal bones with 80 per cent of the load being borne by the radius and lateral carpal bones.[4] Hence the high frequency of injury to the distal radius, scaphoid, and its ligamentous attachments.

Clinical evaluation

Proper evaluation of the wrist and hand requires a sound knowledge of basic and, more importantly, functional anatomy, particularly in the case of wrist injuries. Evaluation of the hand is relatively straightforward due to the excellent surface anatomy and fairly monoplanar motion in most joints of the hand. The structure of the wrist is more complex and physical examination more difficult.

History

The mechanism of injury, acute or overuse, and the position of the wrist at the time of the injury or when symptomatic need to be established. Knowledge of the anatomy and biomechanics of the wrist assists the examiner in determining the site of pain and anatomical structures involved. Most soft tissue disorders of the wrist and hand become readily apparent upon physical examination especially if swelling is present, the notable exception being injury to the intercarpal ligaments.

Careful questioning as to wrist position, direction and degree of load and stress applied, and functional limitation is needed. Dorsal and supination forces are likely to produce perilunate injuries, whilst palmar and pronation forces are likely to affect the ulnar side of the wrist. With chronic wrist pain it is necessary to determine the movements and activities that are painful, the presence of swelling, clicks, or clunks, stiffness or joint restriction, and the presence and distribution of any paraesthesia or numbness.

General questioning is needed to exclude other joint symptoms, gout, or other arthritides. The existence of diabetes, thyroid disease, neck pain, or other upper limb symptoms needs to be established, along with any history of previous injury. The presence of early morning stiffness, night pain, other systemic symptoms, and medication used should be noted.

Physical examination

Inspection

Look for deformities, that is, Dupuytren's contracture, previous fracture, congenital anomalies, and joint swelling or deformity related to an underlying arthropathy. In the acute injury there may be bruising, swelling, deformity, or an antalgic posture. In the chronic injury inspection should reveal the presence or absence of muscle wasting, skin colour or temperature changes, the presence of ganglia, and thickening or swelling of the tendon sheath.

Palpation

Palpation of the wrist and hand should clearly identify any joint synovitis, crepitus related to tenosynovitis, tendon nodules, and joint crepitations. The prominent bony landmarks should be palpated to elicit sites of tenderness and swelling. Typical landmarks on the dorsum of the wrist include the radial styloid process, Lister's tubercle, and the ulnar styloid process. On the palmar aspect of the wrist the bony landmarks are the pisiform, tubercle of the trapezius, hook of the hamate, and radial styloid process. Detailed examination of the wrist should incorporate a systematic palpation of the various anatomical zones. Tenderness at the anatomical snuff box may indicate a fracture or non-union of the scaphoid. Other clinical conditions typically associated with tenderness in the radial dorsal zone include de Quervain's tenosynovitis and arthritis of the carpometacarpal joint. Common clinical conditions associated with tenderness in the central dorsal zone include ganglia, scapholunate joint pathology, and extensor carpi radialis tendonitis. Disorders of the TFCC, extensor carpi ulnaris tendon, ulnar impingement, and distal radioulnar joint disease are usually associated with tenderness, clicking, or crepitus in the ulnar dorsal zone. In the radial volar zone tenderness may indicate carpometacarpal (CMC) joint disease with increased pain and crepitus elicited with passive rotation and axial compression of the joint. More superficial tenderness is found with inflammation of the flexor carpi radialis tendon. The median nerve lies deep within this zone under the flexor retinaculum but deep palpation or tapping over the nerve may provoke distal dysaesthesia in its distribution over the radial and palmar aspect of the hand (a positive Tinel's sign). In the ulnar volar zone the flexor carpi ulnaris tendon is easily palpated and Guyon's canal lies between the pisiform and the hook of the hamate (see 'Ulnar nerve lesions').

Range of motion

The range of motion of all joints should be tested noting the presence of joint restriction, pain, and crepitations. The absence of pain with full forced pronation and supination virtually eliminates the distal radioulnar joint and TFCC as potential sources for pain.

Special tests

Watson's test

This assesses scapholunate stability. The examiner grips the wrist with the thumb placed on the scaphoid tubercle and the fingers wrapping around the distal radius. The wrist is placed in ulnar deviation and the examining thumb applies pressure over the volar aspect of the scaphoid directing force dorsally whilst the wrist is deviated radially. If pain is felt as the wrist is deviated, this constitutes a positive test and, with an unstable scaphoid, a clunk may be felt or heard during this manoeuvre. Normally, the scaphoid flexes as the wrist is radially deviated but, with an unstable scaphoid, the volar pressure applied by the examiner's thumb prevents flexion of the scaphoid and forces the proximal pole of the scaphoid dorsally. This causes pain and often a palpable clunk but findings need to be compared with those from the opposite side.

Shear test

A number of tests have been described to demonstrate intercarpal instability such as Reagan's test of lunotriquetral shear.[5] This involves stabilizing the lunate with the thumb and index finger of one hand whilst attempting to displace the triquetrum and pisiform dorsally and then palmarly with the other hand. Excessive laxity associated with pain and crepitus represents a positive test.

Shuck test

In this test the wrist is held in flexion whilst the examiner resists active finger extension.[6] This loads the radiocarpal joint and is painful in a number of conditions, which include periscaphoid inflammation, radiocarpal or midcarpal instability, scaphoid rotatory instability, and Kienbock's disease.

Finkelstein's test

This is a test of de Quervain's tenosynovitis but can be positive in a normal wrist and therefore comparison with the opposite side needs to be made. In the test the wrist is forced into ulnar deviation along with adduction of the thumb. This tenses the tendons of the first compartment (APL and EPB).

Provocation tests for carpal tunnel syndrome

Phalen's test involves full passive flexion of the wrist for 15–60°. A positive test occurs when there is reproduction of numbness or paraesthesia in the distribution of the median nerve in the hand. With median nerve compression in the carpal tunnel, tapping over the transverse carpal ligament at the level of the proximal wrist flexion crease can elicit dysaesthesia in the distribution of the median nerve. This is deemed to be a positive Tinel's test or sign.

Radiographic investigation of the wrist and hand

Plain X-rays

Clearly, plain X-rays are important in demonstrating evidence of fracture, osseous pathology, or joint disease but are also important in the evaluation of underlying carpal instabilities. A routine series of plain X-rays should include a posteroanterior (PA), lateral, scaphoid ulnar deviated view, and also a clenched fist view. In some patients an additional carpal tunnel view or a 30° semi-supinated view to show the palmar aspect of the triquetrum, pisiform, and pisotriquetral joint may be required. This series of X-rays allows evaluation of ulnar variance, scapholunate angle, capitolunate angle, and radiolunate angle. It also allows assessment of radial inclination and palmar tilt.

A lateral X-ray also allows assessment of soft tissue swelling over the dorsum of the wrist along with the pronator fat plane over the ventral aspect.

The order of X-rays will obviously depend on the clinical condition being assessed and a basic series of four standard X-rays should suffice for most patients. However, when carpal instability is suspected, additional views are required. The scapholunate joint space is normally 1–2 mm in width and remains constant in ulnar or radial deviation of the wrist. Widening of the space beyond 3–4 mm suggests a scapholunate ligament tear or laxity and this widening of the scapholunate joint on plain X-ray is known as the 'Terry Thomas sign' (Fig. 9).

Arthrography

Radiographic dye can be injected into the distal radioulnar joint, radiocarpal joint, and midcarpal joint and may assist in the diagnosis of

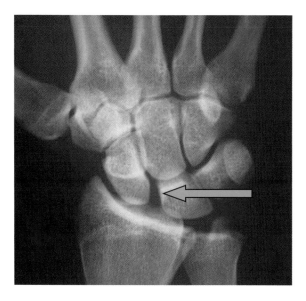

Fig. 9 The 'Terry Thomas Sign'.

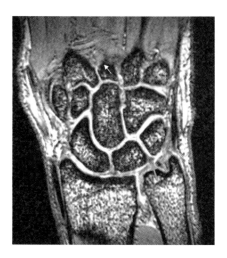

Fig. 10 T2-weighted MRI showing a TFCC tear.

intercarpal ligamentous pathologies. Usually these joints do not communicate and extravasation of contrast into the distal radioulnar joint after injection of the radiocarpal joint suggests a tear of the TFCC.

Extravasation of contrast into the midcarpal joint following injection of the radiocarpal joint suggests a tear of the scapholunate ligament, or lunotriquetral ligament, or the radial or ulnar joint capsule. However, arthrography has largely been superseded by more advanced imaging techniques such as magnetic resonance imaging (MRI) with or without gadolinium arthrography. Also, there are a number of normal anatomical variants making interpretation difficult.

Computerized tomography (CT) and MRI

CT scanning is usually not beneficial in the assessment of soft tissue disorders but MRI is particularly useful in the early diagnosis of avascular necrosis and, in conjunction with gadolinium arthrography, can assist in the diagnosis of carpal instabilities, tendon ruptures, and particularly tears of the TFCC (Fig. 10).

Bone scintigraphy

This can be useful in evaluating wrist injuries where missed fractures are suspected in the presence of normal X-rays. Occasionally spot views are needed. In synovitis, arthritis, and some other inflammatory disorders, increased isotope uptake is seen. Bone scanning is a useful screening investigation but has limited diagnostic value in the evaluation of soft tissue disorders.

Ultrasonography

Ultrasonography is a relatively cheap, available, and non-invasive means of investigating a wide range of soft tissue disorders of the wrist and hand. It is particularly useful in the assessment of tendon rupture, tenosynovitis, tendonitis, or soft tissue tumours, particularly ganglia. In skilled and experienced hands and with the newer generation scanners, small lesions such as ganglia and neuromas can be identified. Ultrasound also allows direct visualization and injection of tendon sheaths and the carpal tunnel, or aspiration and injection of ganglia.

Its role in the evaluation of carpal instability is limited but tears of the dorsal scapholunate ligament and some tears of the TFCC can be identified but, as with all musculoskeletal ultrasound, this investigation is very observer- and technology-dependent.

Tissue disorders of the wrist and hand

Soft tissue disorders of the wrist and hand can be loosely divided into three main categories: (1) local inflammatory, traumatic, or degenerative conditions affecting specific anatomical structures; (2) generalized regional pain disorders such as reflex sympathetic dystrophy (RSD) or repetitive strain injury (RSI); and (3) nerve lesions such as local entrapment neuropathies that need to be differentiated from peripheral neuropathies and cervical radiculopathy. Adequate history-taking should enable the clinician to make an early determination of which category the patient belongs to and the physical examination and subsequent investigation will provide a formal diagnosis.

Ligament injuries in the wrist

The distal radioulnar joint

The distal radioulnar (DRU) joint is inherently unstable and the soft tissue structures conferring stability on the joint consist of the joint capsule, the interosseous membrane, the TFCC, the pronator quadratus, and the forearm muscles. The primary function of the joint is rotation and, as the forearm pronates, as with power gripping there is shortening of the radius relative to the ulna thereby increasing the ulnar variance on radiography. This is associated with increased load across the TFCC. The precise role of the dorsal and palmar radioulnar ligaments in stabilizing the DRU joint is controversial, although both structures need to be intact to allow normal function of the joint through its full range of motion.

Volar dislocation of the joint typically results from a forced supination injury or direct blow to the dorsum of the forearm and often results in tearing of the TFCC. The patient presents with the arm locked in supination with prominence over the volar aspect of the joint. Following closed reduction the arm is immobilized in an above-elbow cast in a position of pronation for 4 weeks. Dorsal dislocation of the joint results from a hyperpronation injury and involves disruption of the dorsal radioulnar ligament of the TFCC and dorsal capsule of the DRU joint. The arm is locked in pronation and, following reduction, the arm is immobilized for 4 weeks in supination.

Chronic instability of the DRU joint gives rise to ulnar side wrist pain and is more common in the gymnastic population. Conservative treatment is usually recommended, especially in athletes, because of the loss of function resulting from surgery, which usually involves some form of distal ulnar excision.

Because of the wide variation in the extent of pathology in patients with DRU joint instability and injuries to the TFCC, treatment decisions are usually made on an individual basis. These injuries are classified as stable, partially unstable (subluxation), and unstable (dislocation) depending on the anatomical structures involved and clinical findings.

The triangular fibrocartilage complex (TFCC)

The TFCC acts as a major stabilizer of the DRU joint and ulnar carpus. It has been shown that the ulnar side of the wrist including the TFCC bears approximately 20 per cent of the load across the wrist. Gripping usually involves ulnar deviation and often pronation, especially in racquet sports and golf, and this repetitive activity can give rise to or aggravate TFCC injuries. Injury to the TFCC may be acute, typically involving an axial load with rotation as in a fall on to an outstretched hand or steering wheel impact injury, or the result of chronic repetitive loading as with chronic ulnar impingement or impaction. Chronic injuries are more common in people with ulnar neutral or positive variance, especially where repetitive pronation is involved.

TFCC tears may be traumatic or degenerative and can be further classified according to the anatomical site of the lesion. The most common type of tear involves the articular disc near the articular surface of the radius. The central portion of the disc is largely avascular so these tears usually do not heal. Undisplaced peripheral tears have a better chance of healing with rest and immobilization in a splint for 4–6 weeks in slight flexion and ulnar deviation. A gradual strengthening programme is then introduced.

Clinical evaluation requires a detailed history of the mechanism of injury, either acute or chronic. Usually the patient complains of pain on the ulnar side of the wrist aggravated by ulnar deviation and rotation. Patients may complain of clicking or locking of the wrist. Following acute injury there may be swelling and, if there has been injury to the ulnocarpal ligaments, there may be an ulnar sag deformity. There is usually some reduction in range of motion and grip strength. The site of maximal tenderness should correspond to the reported site of pain, which is usually just distal to the ulnar styloid between the FCU and ECU tendons. Differentiation from other causes of ulnar side wrist pain is important but can be difficult. Pain and clicking at the TFCC can be provoked with passive pronation, ulnar deviation, and axial compression of the wrist. TFCC lesions may be associated with instability or arthritis of the DRU joint and a 'shuck' test can be used to elicit increased translation of the DRU joint in cases of instability, or pain, crepitus, and limited forearm rotation may indicate DRU joint arthritis.

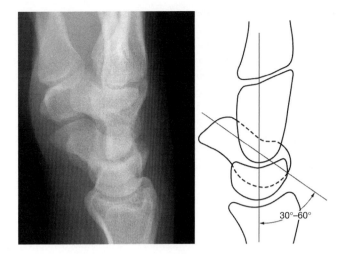

Fig. 11 The lateral X-ray can be particularly useful in assessment of ligamentous injuries to the carpus. The position of the lunate is evaluated and compared to the contralateral wrist. A scapholunate angle of 30–60° is generally accepted as normal and the capitolunate angle should be less than 30°.

Investigation

Standard X-rays are needed to look for ulnar variance and any evidence of degenerative arthritis in chronic cases. Arthrography, CT scanning, and MR can be helpful but none of these investigations have been found to have a level of sensitivity sufficient to replace arthroscopy as the gold standard for evaluation of TFCC pathology.

Treatment

For most patients with isolated tears of the TFCC a trial of immobilization in a splint for 4–6 weeks followed by taping and a strengthening exercise programme is a reasonable treatment of choice, but in more chronic cases and particularly in competitive athletes arthroscopic evaluation may be required. The surgical options include debridement of the tear and any associated chondromalacia of the ulna or lunate, repair of the TFCC tear, and ulnar shortening procedures, depending on the pathological findings and degree of ulnar variance.

Carpal instabilities

Because of the complexity of wrist kinematics much research has been devoted to the study of carpal instability patterns. Several kinematic models have been proposed to further our understanding of carpal pathomechanics. Whilst detailed analysis of these models is beyond the scope of this chapter, an appreciation of the pathology and clinical patterns of carpal instability is important for the clinician dealing with acute or chronic wrist pain. The traditional concept of the wrist as a link mechanism[7] has the radius, proximal carpal row, and distal carpal row as individual links that are stable in tension but collapse under axial compression. Another model describes the carpus in terms of a central (flexion–extension) column, a lateral (mobile) column, and a medial (rotation) column. Recent work refers to a perilunate pattern of injury and more recently midcarpal and proximal carpal instabilities have been described.[8]

Following injury, patients may develop instability patterns without symptoms but then this instability may progress to further ligamentous disruption and then go on to advanced degenerative joint disease. Instability patterns may be static, in which case there is intercarpal malalignment that can be identified on plain radiographs, or dynamic where there is abnormal intercarpal motion only seen on fluoroscopy or cineradiography CT or MRI. Five main static carpal instability patterns have been described. These include dorsiflexion instability (DISI, dorsal intercalated segmental instability), palmar flexion instability (VISI, ventral intercalated segmental instability), ulnar translocation, dorsal carpal subluxation, and palmar carpal subluxation. Various classifications of carpal instability patterns have been described.

Ligamentous injuries to the wrist, particularly the carpus, should be thought of as a spectrum of osseous and ligament damage. The position of the wrist at the time of injury, the magnitude and direction of forces applied to the wrist, and the biomechanical properties of the structures involved determine the extent and nature of the injury. As with the knee, there may be a progression of ligamentous disruption, which results in a wide spectrum of instability patterns, some of which can go undetected until the sequelae of chronic carpal instability (chronic pain, restricted motion, and posttraumatic arthritis) develop. Clinical evaluation can be very difficult and proper radiological investigation along with a high index of suspicion is usually the key to early diagnosis. A simple approach to the radiological evaluation of most major carpal instability patterns is to identify the lunate on the PA and lateral X-ray and to determine whether it is tilting ventrally or dorsally and whether it is displaced ulnarly, dorsally, or ventrally and then compare to the opposite wrist. Lateral X-rays are often more reliable. A scapholunate angle of 30–60° is generally accepted as normal and the capitolunate angle should be less than 30° (Fig. 11).

Scapholunate instability

More recently, this has been classified as one of the perilunate instabilities of the wrist. It is the most common of the carpal instabilities with a typical mechanism of injury being a fall on the outstretched hand with the wrist extended and an axial compression load applied to the base of the palm, particularly the hypothenar eminence. This forces the hand into extension and radial deviation thereby compressing the scaphoid and adjacent structures causing injury to the scapholunate ligament complex. The scapholunate ligament complex has three main components.

The dorsal scapholunate ligament and interosseous scapholunate ligament make up the intrinsic ligaments, whilst the extrinsic or palmar radiocarpal ligaments consist of the radioscaphocapitate (RSC), radioscapholunate (RSL), and radiolunotriquetral (RLT) ligaments. Injury to the short interosseous scapholunate ligament alone results in local tenderness and swelling in the anatomical snuff box but no definite instability and a negative radiographic investigation. If the dorsal scapholunate ligament is disrupted there is mild sub clinical rotatory subluxation of the scaphoid. Rupture of the palmar radiocarpal ligaments leads to complete subluxation of the scaphoid and static carpal instability which is usually identifiable on plain X-rays. The RSC ligament appears to be the critical palmar radiocarpal ligament and its disruption allows further rotatory subluxation of the scaphoid. It has been proposed that dynamic scapholunate dissociation occurs when the interosseous ligament and one of the other scapholunate ligaments is involved, but complete scapholunate dissociation only occurs if all three components are disrupted.[9]

This spectrum of injury accounts for the late presentation of many patients after an injury that has initially been diagnosed as a simple wrist sprain. Following undetected injury a pattern of dynamic scapholunate dissociation can progress to a static instability pattern as the palmar radiocarpal ligaments become lax with excessive loading following injury to the interosseous and dorsal scapholunate ligament.

Awareness and early recognition of injury to the scapholunate ligament complex is therefore important and should be suspected in any patient presenting with pain, tenderness, and swelling over the dorso-radial aspect of the wrist following a fall. The clinical presentation is similar to that of a subtle scaphoid fracture. Watson's test for scapholunate instability has been described but may be difficult to perform following acute injury and a scaphoid fracture needs to be excluded beforehand. Routine X-rays often do not reveal any abnormality and special views may be required.[10] Wrist arthrography and MRI may be inconclusive and arthroscopy may be needed to confirm the diagnosis in difficult cases.

Management Early diagnosis and treatment will give the best results and the optimal time for acute ligament repair is 3–5 weeks after injury, although some authors advocate soft tissue reconstruction much later than this.[11] The patient who has pain and swelling in the anatomical snuff box but negative X-rays, including stress views, may have an occult scaphoid fracture or rupture of the interosseous scapholunate ligament. Some authors advocate 3–6 weeks cast immobilization to allow the ligament injury to heal rather than adopting the standard protocol of either arranging a regional bone scan to exclude a scaphoid fracture or splinting the wrist for 10 days before arranging repeat X-rays and then immobilizing the wrist only if a fracture is identified. The next level of injury, where there is radiographic widening of the scapholunate joint on X-ray, warrants acute repair and internal fixation. In chronic cases that present more than 3 months after injury, monitoring of symptoms and avoidance of impaction stress activity is reasonable but, in those patients presenting with a chronically painful wrist and complete rotatory subluxation, ligamentous repair or stabilization is usually indicated. If left untreated, these patients develop progressive degenerative arthritis and may require limited arthrodesis of the carpal bones.

The arthritic changes usually develop in the radioscaphoid joint and progress to the capitolunate (mid-carpal) joint and this process is described as scapholunate dissociation with advanced collapse (SLAC) wrist. The radiolunate joint is usually spared.

Lunotriquetral instability

Lunotriquetral injuries are approximately one-sixth as common as scapholunate ligament injuries and are associated with ulnar plus variance.[12] They typically result from falls on to an outstretched hand with the forearm in pronation, with most lunotriquetral dissociations resulting from falls on to the hand with the wrist in an extended and ulnar-deviated position. Complete disruption of the lunotriquetral ligament leading to VISI is rare and most of these injuries lead to dynamic rather than static instability. Diagnosis can be difficult as signs are limited to point tenderness over the dorsum of the dorsoulnar carpus just distal to the TFCC, along with a number of specific provocation tests that have been described.[13] Also, the differential diagnosis of dorsoulnar and ulnocarpal wrist pain is fairly extensive.[14]

These injuries do not usually lead to progressive arthritis and, with proper immobilization, acute tears will heal in more than 80 per cent of cases.[15] Chronic pain due to lunotriquetral instability may respond to rest, nonsteroidal anti-inflammatory drugs (NSAIDS), or cortisone injection to the ulnocarpal joint. In some patients arthroscopic debridement of the ligament can be effective. Lunotriquetral arthrodesis has a high failure rate,[16, 17] and therefore ulnar shortening osteotomy is often performed for those patients with dynamic lunotriquetral instability (not VISI).

Ligamentous injuries and disorders of the hand and thumb

Hand

Injuries to the collateral ligaments and volar plates of the distal and proximal interphalangeal joints are common in sport and may be associated with fractures, joint dislocation, and varying degrees of joint instability. Recognition of the extent of injury is a priority as buddy taping and early mobilization is usually recommended for minor injuries whereas splinting or orthopaedic consultation may be needed for more significant injuries. Injury to the collateral ligaments of the metacarpophalangeal (MCP) joints of the finger is not common. The integrity of the ligaments should be tested in full flexion and complete rupture of the ligament is indicated by greater than 30° (gross instability) opening on stressing the joint and severe pain. This is best treated by surgery. Most injuries can be treated by buddy taping until pain-free and early mobilization, although the more severe injuries should be splinted in flexion for 3 weeks.

Thumb

Gamekeeper's thumb

Injury to the ulnar collateral ligament of the MCP joint of the thumb occurs when hyperabduction forces are applied to the thumb and is commonly seen following falls whilst skiing, as a result of tackles or falls in rugby or football, or in motor vehicle accidents when the thumb is forced against the steering wheel. The term 'gamekeeper's thumb' was coined in 1955 when Campbell described chronic laxity resulting from repeated stress applied to the ligament whilst extending the neck of rabbits. Proper evaluation of the acute injury is needed to minimize the risk of chronic laxity or instability that predispose to degenerative arthritis in the MCP joint of the thumb. When the ligament is ruptured, the MCP joint is unstable with pinch gripping giving rise to significant loss of hand function (Fig. 12).

A history of the mechanism of injury and the site of tenderness with pain on passive loading of the ligament confirms the diagnosis. An initial X-ray is recommended to look for an avulsion fracture at the distal end of the ligament before testing stability of the joint (Fig. 13). Stress radiographs may be useful but are usually not necessary, and some difficulties are encountered when trying to differentiate between complete and incomplete tears in some cases, although in one study of 60 cases the authors found a high correlation between preoperative stress evaluation of the joint and the presence of complete ligament disruption at surgery.[18] The role of arthrography is unclear but recently ultrasound has been found to be effective in the evaluation of these tears with 89 per cent specificity for displaced ulnar collateral injuries and 95 per cent specificity for non displaced injuries.[19–21] MRI can be useful but is usually not clinically indicated.[22] Complete tears can be associated with a Stener lesion

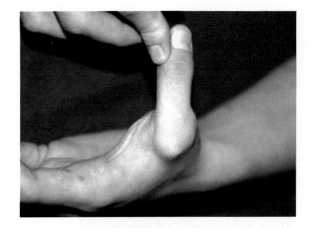

Fig. 12 Gamekeeper's thumb

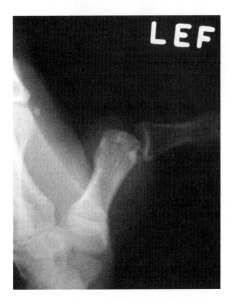

Fig. 13 X-ray of 'Gamekeeper's thumb'.

(interposition of the adductor aponeurosis between the torn ends of the ligament), which results in poor healing, residual laxity, and a poor result following non-operative treatment. This lesion has been variously reported in 14–83 per cent of patients with complete disruption of the ligament and therefore there is some justification for considering early operative intervention in those patients with complete tears.[18, 23]

If X-rays reveal an avulsion fragment with less than 2 mm displacement, the joint should be immobilized in a thumb spica cast for 4–6 weeks. If no fracture is seen, lateral stress testing of the ligament should be performed with the joint in full extension and 30° of flexion. The degree of acceptable laxity varies between authors but generally greater than 30° of instability (particularly with no firm endpoint) indicates complete disruption, which may be associated with volar subluxation of the proximal phalanx on a lateral X-ray. Acute partial ruptures can be treated with immobilization in a thumb spica cast for 4 weeks.[24] Complete tears are best treated surgically with 3 weeks in a postoperative spica cast and a further 3 weeks in a protective splint.

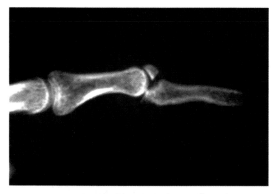

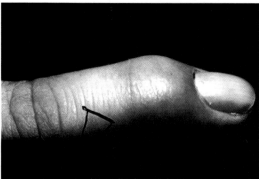

Fig. 14 Mallet finger

Patients with chronic instability of the ulnar collateral ligament of the thumb complain of weakness with pinch grip and grasping. X-rays are needed to look for evidence of secondary degenerative arthritis in the MCP joint and, if present, an arthrodesis may ultimately be required. If not, then a delayed ligament reconstruction can be considered.

Radial collateral ligament (RCL) of the thumb

Injuries to this ligament are reportedly less common and there are significant differences in anatomical configuration. Complete tears can be treated with immobilization in a thumb spica cast for 4–6 weeks but some authors recommend surgical repair for complete tears because of the high incidence of volar or ulnar subluxation of the proximal phalanx due to the unopposed pull of the adductor pollicis following complete disruption of the RCL.

Closed tendon injuries of the hand

Mallet finger

This describes disruption of the terminal extensor tendon at its insertion to the distal phalanx which is usually caused by a direct blow to the tip of the extended finger which produces forced flexion of the distal interphalangeal (DIP) joint (Fig. 14). It is probably the most common closed tendon injury in the sporting population and is typically associated with catching athletes. It may also result from a direct blow to the dorsum of the joint or even from a hyperextension injury. Unopposed flexion of the distal phalanx gives rise to the classical deformity.

Bony avulsion is often seen and may involve a significant portion of the articular surface or even volar subluxation of the distal phalanx.

Conservative and surgical management has been recommended by various authors but most cases can be treated conservatively if seen within 3 months of the injury.[25, 26] Splinting in full extension (not hyperextension) for 6 weeks is recommended for avulsion injuries, with 8 weeks splinting recommended for intratendinous ruptures. The proximal interphalangeal (PIP) joint should be left mobile. A gradual weaning period of 2 weeks with further splinting at night and removal of the splint several times a day to allow range of motion exercises is advisable. If, following complete removal of the splint, there is recurrence of the extensor lag then a further 6 weeks of splinting can be employed. Results are usually satisfactory, although a small residual extensor lag may remain. In younger patients a Salter Harris type IV fracture of the epiphysis needs to be excluded as open reduction may be required.

If left untreated a swan-neck deformity of the PIP joint can result from retraction of the extensor mechanism and increased pull in the intrinsic tendons and flexor digitorum profundus, particularly in hypermobile individuals.

Jersey finger

This describes avulsion of the flexor digitorum profundus (FDP) tendon from the distal phalanx of the finger. This is most commonly seen in young males involved in rugby or tackling sports and affects the ring finger in more than 75 per cent of cases.[26] Anatomical considerations appear to be responsible for the ring finger's increased susceptibility to this injury, although it has been described in all digits including the thumb.[27, 28] The injury occurs when the finger is forcibly extended during maximal contraction of the profundus muscle, for example when the tackling player's finger gets caught in an opponent's shorts or jersey. The injury may go undiagnosed because of lack of deformity, and the loss of active flexion at the DIP joint may be simply put down to local pain and swelling mistakenly attributed to ligament sprain. It is important to test for active flexion of the DIP joint and to localize the site of maximum tenderness in order to try and identify the distal end of the torn tendon, which may have retracted even as far as the palm. This injury has been classified into four types.[29, 30]

1. Type I avulsions involve retraction of the torn tendon into the palm with disruption of the blood supply to the tendon. Repair is needed within 7–10 days before the tendon becomes shrivelled and contracted.

2. In type II avulsions the torn tendon retracts to the level of the PIP joint and, occasionally, a small avulsed bony fragment is seen on X-ray. Early repair is recommended but delayed repair is usually possible.

3. Type III avulsion injuries occur when there is a large bony fragment that is caught by the A4 pulley. X-rays confirm the diagnosis and the treatment is open reduction and internal fixation of the avulsed fragment.

4. A rare type IV injury has been described in which there is a type III avulsion with simultaneous avulsion of the FDP tendon from the avulsed bony fragment.

In all types the injury is best treated early and surgically. If diagnosis is delayed there is often scarring in the tendon sheath and tendon retraction. Depending on the level of retraction, tendon reconstruction

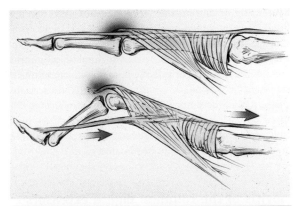

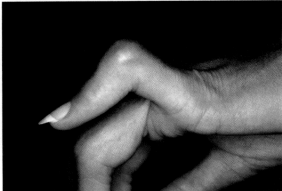

Fig. 15 Boutonniere deformity.

or arthrodesis of the DIP joint may be required. Tendon grafting is rarely employed.

Boutonniere deformity

A boutonniere deformity results from injury to the central slip of the extensor tendon at or near its insertion into the base of middle phalanx of the finger. It is usually caused by a direct blow to the dorsum of the proximal interphalangeal (PIP) joint or by sudden forceful flexion of the joint. The initial injury is often ignored due to a lack of swelling or loss of extension but, if unrecognized and left untreated, the central slip retracts and the lateral bands fall palmar to the axis of rotation at the PIP joint, causing them to act as flexors of the joint. As they retract proximally the DIP joint hyperextends and this produces the classical deformity, which is rarely seen acutely (Fig. 15). Deformity is also seen following unrecognized palmar dislocation of the PIP joint that has either reduced spontaneously or been reduced in the field of play. Following any injury to the PIP joint, disruption of the central slip needs to be considered. There is local tenderness often without any extension lag as, in an acute injury, the lateral bands can extend the PIP joint. Following acute injury the joint should be splinted in full extension whilst encouraging active flexion of the DIP joint. Splinting is usually needed for 4 weeks followed by periodic splinting for a further 2 weeks. Gentle active and passive range of motion exercises of the PIP joint are then introduced. Accidental flexion of the PIP joint must be avoided during the period of splinting. Bony avulsion of the middle phalanx may require internal fixation. In subacute cases where there has been a delay of several weeks before the diagnosis is made, there is likely to be an early boutonniere

deformity with developing contracture of the oblique retinacular ligament. Extension splinting is required for at least 8 weeks with serial casts if a contracture has developed.[26]

Management of the chronic boutonniere deformity is difficult because of secondary joint contractures. Even in these cases a trial of static and dynamic splinting is worthwhile because of the problems associated with surgical reconstruction. Surgical treatment should initially be directed to release of the contractures via capsulectomy followed by tendon reconstruction as a second procedure. In the more chronic stiff deformities, arthrodesis of the PIP joint may be needed. Surgery is usually reserved for those cases where there is good preservation of passive joint motion but more than 35–40° of extension lag. It is important to differentiate a true boutonniere deformity from the pseudoboutonniere deformity that results from a hyperextension injury to the PIP joint, which leads to a fixed flexion contracture of the joint with secondary mild hyperextension of the DIP joint. In these injuries passive extension of the joint is typically absent.

Injury to the extensor mechanism at the metacarpophalangeal joint

The extensor hood mechanism overlying the MCP joint is vulnerable to direct blows or sudden twisting injury. Subluxation/dislocation of the extensor tendon can occur, usually to the ulnar side. There is pain and swelling over the MCP joint, usually with an inability to fully extend the joint. Depending on the degree of swelling, the tendon may be palpated between the metacarpal heads and it may reduce with passive extension of the joint. If seen acutely, conservative treatment may be trialled with splint immobilization in extension for 4 weeks followed by dynamic extension splinting for a further 2–3 weeks. Surgery is usually required in the chronic symptomatic cases.

Boxer's knuckle describes an injury to the dorsal aspect of the MCP joint when X-rays are normal and there is no tendon subluxation.[31–33] There has usually been injury to the tendon itself, sagittal fibres, or the dorsal capsule. In one study of 27 surgical repairs the principal pathology was disruption of the extensor hood, usually with a tear of the sagittal band and subluxation or dislocation of the central tendon. Capsular tears noted in 19 cases were not repaired with no resulting functional deficit.[34] Chronic symptomatic cases don't usually settle with rest and splinting, and surgery may be required with repair of any identified tears.

Tendonitis and tenosynovitis of the wrist and hand

Tendonitis and overuse syndromes frequently affect the wrist and hand and are often the result of repetitive sporting or occupational activity. They may also present as part of a systemic inflammatory or connective tissue disorder such as rheumatoid arthritis.

De Quervain's tenosynovitis

The tendons of the EPB and APL usually pass through a single sheath at the radial aspect of the wrist. De Quervain's tenosynovitis of this common tendon sheath usually results from overuse of the wrist and hand and may be seen in clerical or manual workers or rowers. It has also been seen in association with rheumatoid arthritis, other inflammatory synovitides, psoriatic arthritis, and pregnancy. Repetitive radial and ulnar deviation of the wrist in conjunction with gripping leads to inflammation of the tendon sheath as it passes beneath the extensor retinaculum. Patients usually present with pain and tenderness that is felt with gripping and radial ulnar deviation. Usually the tendon sheath is tender and swollen and crepitus may be easily felt, but in many cases there is fibrous thickening of the tendon sheath resulting in stenosis and swelling and crepitus may not be present. The diagnosis can be easily made on clinical grounds with local tenderness, a positive Finkelstein's test, and exclusion of underlying joint pathology. The differential diagnosis includes osteochondritis of the carpometacarpal joint and intersection syndrome.

Diagnosis can be readily confirmed via ultrasonography which also allows accurate injection of cortisone into the tendon sheath. In early cases rest and topical or oral anti-inflammatories are usually effective. The wrist should be splinted in mild extension and radial deviation with the MCP joint of the thumb in slight extension. Gradual removal of the splint and modification of the aggravating activities can be effective if the diagnosis is made early. In chronic cases local corticosteroid injection can be very effective but in some cases, particularly those with stenosing tenosynovitis, decompression of the tendon compartment is often needed. Surgery is curative in most cases.

Intersection syndrome

This is an inflammatory condition that occurs at the intersection of the radial wrist extensors (ECRB and ECRL) and the tendons of the first dorsal compartment muscles (APL and ECB). It is seen as an overuse syndrome in rowers, weight-lifters, squash players, and in some occupations that involve repetitive wrist motion.

Clinical findings are pain and swelling approximately 5 cm proximal to the radiocarpal joint on the dorsal aspect of the distal forearm. In the more severe cases, palpable and occasionally audible crepitus occurs with movement of the wrist or thumb. Several pathophysiologies have been described, including the presence of an adventitial bursa beneath the APL and ECRB, tenosynovitis of the radial wrist extensors, and hypertrophy or degenerative changes in the APL and EPB muscle bellies leading to a localized compartment syndrome.

Conservative treatment is recommended initially with rest, the use of anti-inflammatory agents or medication, splinting, and possibly corticosteroid injection. An adequate trial of non-operative treatment is required but, if unsuccessful, surgical intervention should be considered. The surgery undertaken will depend on operative findings but probably involves exploration and decompression of the affected tendon sheaths. Modification of the aggravating activity is needed to prevent further injury.

Extensor pollicis longus tendonitis and tenosynovitis

The EPL tendon lies in the third dorsal compartment of the wrist and is susceptible to tenosynovitis as it passes around Lister's tubercle. This can be induced by any activity that requires repetitive thumb and wrist motion and it was first described in Prussian drummers. Diagnosis is fairly straightforward due to the superficial location of the EPL tendon with the classical findings of local tenderness, pain on passive stretching, and resisted contraction of the muscle. Initial treatment includes rest, anti-inflammatory measures, and splinting. Corticosteroid injection should be avoided if possible because of the theoretical risk of tendon damage or rupture in an area of compromised vascularity. In some patients there is an anatomical variant with extension of the EPL muscle belly into the third dorsal compartment, which may result in secondary tenosynovitis.[35] If conservative treatment fails, surgical decompression and transposition of the EPL tendon dorsal to the extensor retinaculum is effective. In those patients with a chronic degenerative tendonopathy, tendon rupture may occur and surgical repair is indicated in most cases.

Tenosynovitis of the common digital extensors

These tendons pass through the fourth dorsal compartment of the wrist and tenosynovitis may result from overuse but is more commonly seen in patients with a systemic inflammatory disease such as rheumatoid arthritis. Clinical signs are dorsal wrist pain with local swelling and tenderness but normal wrist motion. The usual conservative therapies are employed but symptoms are often slow to resolve and treatment may fail due to an anomalous muscle belly extending into the fourth dorsal compartment.[36] If conservative treatment fails after 8–12 weeks, surgical exploration and decompression should be considered.

Tenosynovitis of the extensor digiti minimi (EDM)

This tendon passes through the fifth dorsal compartment and stenosing tenosynovitis of the EDM has been described but usually follows trauma. An anomalous muscle belly may intrude into the fifth dorsal compartment and, in the majority of cases, multiple slips of the extensor digiti quinti minimi are found.[37, 38] Intracompartmental injection of local anaesthetic and corticosteroid along with splinting is recommended but surgical decompression may be required for chronic cases.

Extensor carpi ulnaris (ECU) tenosynovitis

The ECU tendon lies in the sixth dorsal compartment and may be subject to traumatic subluxation with the wrist forced into a position of supination, palmar flexion, and ulnar deviation—an example being the trailing hand following a baseball swing.[39] Because of swelling, subluxation of the tendon may be missed initially and, as with peroneal tendon subluxation/dislocation at the ankle, surgical stabilization is usually required. The ECU tendon sheath is the second most common site of stenosing tenosynovitis in the upper limb and ECU tendonitis is frequently found in sports where repetitive wrist motion is needed, such as rowing or squash. It can also be seen in association with pathology of the TFCC.

The mechanism of injury, whether it be acute or overuse, along with pain, local swelling, and tenderness over the dorsal aspect of the distal ulna, as well as pain on isometric loading of the ECU tendon, usually provides the diagnosis, which can be confirmed with ultrasonography which also allows accurate injection into the tendon sheath. Crepitus is uncommon and, if diagnosed early, ECU tenosynovitis and tendonitis usually respond to anti-inflammatory measures, splinting, and occasionally local injection.

Tendonitis of the flexor tendons at the wrist

Repetitive wrist motion can induce tenosynovitis or tendonitis of the flexor carpi radialis (FCR) or flexor carpi ulnaris (FCU) tendons, and repetitive gripping or finger flexion can result in tenosynovitis of the long flexors of the digits. Secondary tendonitis can also result from underlying arthritis, for example, scaphotrapezoid trapezial joint disease affecting the FCR tendon, or pisotriquetral arthritis leading to FCU tendonitis. Pain with resisted palmar flexion and either radial or ulnar deviation helps to confirm the diagnosis along with local tenderness. Differentiation from underlying joint synovitis or a volar carpal ganglion can be difficult in cases of FCR tendonitis and, in cases of longstanding joint synovitis, tendon rupture can occur.

Conservative treatment modalities are often effective. In cases of FCU tendonitis where there is underlying pisotriquetral instability or arthritis, excision of the pisiform has been recommended.[40]

Trigger finger

Tenosynovitis of the flexor tendons of the thumb or digits may initially present as a typical overuse strain with activity-related pain and tenderness and also pain with passive stretching or isometric contraction of the affected tendon. The pathology usually involves fibrosis and constriction of the sheath, which prevents normal gliding of the flexor tendon, and a painful nodule on the tendon often results.

The term 'trigger finger' refers to the mechanical catch as the nodule slides through the area of construction, often leading to locking with the finger in flexion as the nodule passes proximal to the first annular pulley overlying the MCP joint. Passive assisted extension of the digit is usually needed to straighten the digit and a palpable click is felt as the nodule passes under the pulley as the finger is extended. Isolated flexor tenosynovitis is simple to diagnose clinically, particularly once triggering has occurred.

Overuse from repetitive gripping activities is a common cause but flexor digital tenosynovitis is also seen with a number of systemic inflammatory disorders such as rheumatoid arthritis, psoriatic arthritis, diabetes mellitus, pigmented vilonodular synovitis, hyperthyroidism, sarcoid, and amyloidosis.

In early cases modified rest, heat, and NSAIDS with gentle exercises and extension splinting at night time may be effective, but often a local cortisone injection to the tendon nodule is needed and this has been shown to be effective in many cases. In chronic or recurrent cases where there is obvious triggering, surgical release of the fibrous annular pulley and sheath is usually required although a trial cortisone injection is worthwhile. An ultrasound-guided injection provides for more accurate placement of the needle into the tendon sheath.

Entrapment neuropathies of the wrist and hand

Carpal tunnel syndrome (median nerve lesion)

Swelling within the carpal tunnel can cause compression of the median nerve and resultant inflammation causes further nerve compression. This syndrome is associated with a number of medical conditions that should be suspected when symptoms are bilateral.

Acute injury to the median nerve following Colles' fracture is rare and compression of the nerve usually results from the progressive oedema and haematoma that develop subsequently. Delayed carpal tunnel syndrome can result from abundant callus formation and scarring with fracture healing and this is known as 'tardy median nerve palsy'. This can also result from carpal fracture or dislocation and Phalen reported similar numbers of carpal tunnel syndrome following carpal fractures and carpal injuries.[41]

Carpal tunnel syndrome is the most common entrapment neuropathy seen in the upper limb because of the susceptibility of the median nerve at the wrist to injury or compression with repetitive wrist flexion–extension. Some individuals, especially those with hereditary pressure sensitive neuropathy or tumunculous neuropathy (or a genetic expression of this), have a strong tendency to experience symptoms of median nerve compression when the wrist is held in a position of full flexion, particularly in bed. Repetitive occupational or sporting use leads to microtrauma and irritation that result in swelling in the tunnel and thence in median nerve compression. Essentially any disease or injury that leads to swelling within the tunnel or that causes distortion and deformation of the median nerve may lead to axonostenosis of the nerve.

Presenting symptoms are pain and paraesthesia in the palmar aspect of the wrist and hand that are typically worse at night and relieved by hanging the arm down or shaking the hand. Paraesthesia and numbness in varying degrees may occur without pain and usually affect the thumb, index and middle fingers, and the radial side of the ring finger. The motor branches of the median nerve distal to the carpal tunnel supply the abductor pollicis brevis, opponens pollicis, flexor pollicis brevis (superficial head), and usually the first and second lumbricals. In chronic cases there may be wasting of the thenar eminence and weakness of grip and pinch strength. Differentiation from other causes of wrist and hand paraesthesia can be difficult, especially in workers who present with diffuse upper limb symptoms. Carpal tunnel syndrome is often confused with brachalgia, thoracic outlet compression, and even cervical radiculopathy. Tinel's sign may be positive but not usually in early or mild cases and Phalen's test is more reliable. Neurological examination is needed to map out any sensory or motor dysfunction and confirmation should be made with electrophysiological studies. A positive study is associated with a delay in median nerve conduction velocity across the wrist with the delay in sensory conduction velocity usually becoming more prolonged before the onset of motor conduction delay. In severe cases an electromyogram (EMG) will show neuropathic changes but fibrillation potentials are rarely seen. However, it should be noted that 20 per cent of cases of clinically proven carpal tunnel syndrome have negative nerve conduction studies.[42] The patient should be assessed for any predisposing causes of carpal tunnel syndrome and radiological investigation is usually not needed unless there is a history of significant injury. The diagnosis is usually made clinically. Sometimes an overreliance on the results of nerve conduction studies precipitates a decision to proceed with surgical decompression on the basis of a mild sensory conduction delay at the wrist, sometimes leading to poor results following surgery. When the electrophysiological changes are unequivocal the decision is much more straightforward.

Initial treatment should include splinting in extension (cock-up splint) especially at night, and in equivocal cases a positive response to night splinting can be diagnostic. In cases where there is evidence of inflammation or swelling, NSAIDs should be used and in chronic cases cortisone injection into the carpal tunnel (preferably under ultrasound guidance) can be effective. In resistance or recurrent cases, or where there is evidence of a significant median nerve neuropraxia, surgical decompression is indicated.

Care should be taken when making this diagnosis in the presence of more proximal symptoms, particularly when electrophysiological studies are non-confirmatory. Often patients with regional pain syndromes may present with symptoms of pain or paraesthesia and, after a failed trial of conservative treatment, the clinician may proceed to surgical decompression at the wrist, often with disastrous consequences. This scenario is increasingly seen in workers' compensation cases.

Ulnar nerve lesion at the wrist

The ulnar nerve passes through Guyon's canal as it leaves the forearm to enter the palm. The canal is formed by the pisiform (medial border), hamate (lateral border), the volar carpal ligament, and dorsally by the retinacular ligament. At the distal end of the canal the nerve divides into two sensory branches and a deep motor branch. The superficial sensory branch supplies the ulnar one and a half digits and palm, while the deep motor branch innervates the hypothenar muscles, palmar and dorsal interossei, usually third and fourth lumbricals, the deep head of the flexor pollicis brevis, and the adductor pollicis brevis. Its superficial location makes the nerve vulnerable to blunt trauma or compression and the site of the lesion determines the clinical presentation. Compression syndromes of the ulnar nerve at the wrist can be classified accordingly.[43] Type I lesions occur proximal to Guyon's canal and therefore affect both motor and sensory function. Type II lesions involve the deep motor branch alone, whilst type III lesions only affect the superficial sensory branch. The most common cause of ulnar nerve compression neuropathy at the wrist is repetitive trauma leading to oedema and inflammation of tissues within the canal and compression of the deep terminal branch distal to the supply of the hypothenar muscles, which causes wasting and weakness of the intrinsics.

This compressive neuropathy can be found in cyclists (handlebar neuropathy) or racquet sports due to the impact of the racquet handle. In cycling prolonged hyperextension of the wrist may be partly responsible for this neuropathy. Less common causes include a ganglion cyst, fracture of the hook of hamate (seen in golfers), and ulnar artery thrombosis (hypothenar hammer syndrome), which need to be excluded by means of ultrasonography, X-rays, or angiography.[44]

Clinical findings may include local pain and tenderness over Guyon's canal, a positive Tinel's sign when the sensory branch is involved, and weakness and wasting of the muscles in the hand supplied by the ulnar nerve.

In cases of external compression neuropathy (as opposed to space-occupying lesions in Guyon's canal) elimination of external pressure and precipitating activity usually provides effective relief, particularly in acute cases. The usual gamut of rest, splinting, and NSAIDs can be trialled in more chronic cases. If symptoms do not improve in the presence of electrophysiological abnormalities, surgical decompression should be carried out to prevent permanent muscle atrophy and weakness. In sports or occupationally induced conditions, workplace modifications or alterations to technique will be needed.

Radial nerve lesion at the wrist

In the forearm the radial nerve divides into the posterior interosseous nerve and the superficial radial nerve which then passes distally to supply the dorsoradial aspect of the wrist and hand. It lies subcutaneously adjacent to the distal radius at the wrist but is not usually injured with distal radial fractures except by laceration. A neuropathy of the superficial radial nerve can result from direct blunt trauma to the dorsal and radial aspect of the wrist (such as the wearing of handcuffs) and rarely a neuropathy (Wartenberg's syndrome) occurs in sports that involve repeated pronation and supination of the wrist.[45] Patients complain of pain and/or paraesthesia over the dorsum of the thumb and radial portion of the hand and a positive Tinel's sign at the site of trauma or compression may be present. Treatment is almost always conservative.

Entrapment of the superficial radial nerve in the forearm may occur as it passes between the brachioradialis and extensor carpi radialis brevis and will result in similar symptoms. The absence of trauma to the wrist and the presence of a positive Tinel's sign in the proximal forearm confirm the diagnosis.

Digital neuropathy

Compression neuropathies of the digital nerves are rare but can result from chronic local pressure. One example is 'bowler's thumb' in which the gripping of a ten-pin bowling ball causes direct compression of the ulnar digital nerve of the thumb against the edge of the thumb hole.[46] This results in paraesthesia and pain along the ulnar border of the thumb.

Soft tissue tumours of the wrist and hand

Ganglia

Ganglia are localized cystic swellings containing gelatinous fluid that are usually tense but frequently painless. They always communicate with an adjacent tendon sheath or synovial joint capsule from which they are thought to originate. These are commonly found at the wrist and usually arise dorsally from the scapholunate joint. They may also arise from the second or third carpometacarpal joints where they can interfere with the tracking of the extensor tendon of the index finger, or they may coexist with a carpal boss.

The scapholunate ganglion is the most common soft tissue tumour of the hand. It can occur at any age but usually in the third to fifth decades, more commonly in women. The aetiology is debatable but probably involves remodelling of the fibrous capsule of the joint. Early on the ganglion wall is thin and ruptures easily, but with time it becomes thicker and more fibrous. Many ganglia disappear spontaneously and they are usually painless. However, they may become painful and rarely lead to nerve compression. One-third of patients have a history of trauma.

Most volar ganglia originate from the wrist joint capsule, often the trapezioscaphoid joint, and may lead to compression of the radial artery. They can also occur in the carpal tunnel, or Guyon's canal where they can compress the deep branch of the ulnar nerve. Small but very painful and tender ganglia may arise from the flexor aspect of the fingers. They may be treated by aspiration or rupture but there is a recurrence rate of approximately 50 per cent. The recurrence rate following injection of corticosteroid or a sclerosant (which is often best done under ultrasonographic control) is still on the order of 40–50 per cent. Even following surgical excision with removal of a portion of the joint capsule there is a 15 per cent risk of recurrence.[47] Usually surgery is not indicated unless symptoms are significant or where there is neurovascular compression.

Carpal boss

This is a bony prominence of unknown aetiology on the dorsal aspect of the second or third carpometacarpal joint. It occurs in early adulthood and is not usually painful. It appears to be the result of a build up of new bone on the metacarpal and carpal bones, possibly due to microtrauma-induced periostitis. There is no joint space narrowing or subchondral sclerosis on X-ray. It may be painful, particularly if associated with a ganglion or if there is focal tendonitis or calcification in the overlying extensor carpi radialis (ECR) tendon.

Other tumours

Lipomas are common in the hand and are usually found in the palm or at the thenar or hypothenar eminences. They may occur in the carpal tunnel and lipomas of the median nerve have been reported. Excision can be difficult when the lipoma extends along the tissue planes of the hand.

Giant cell tumours of the tendon sheath are more common in the hand than the wrist but can arise from the synovial tendon sheaths on the flexor or extensor aspect of the wrist. They typically present as slow-growing painless masses.

Cavernous and capillary haemangiomas commonly occur in the hand and wrist. Neurofibromas, neurolemomas, and glomus tumours have all been described. Malignant tumours are rare and usually metastases.

References

1. Brown, D.E. and Lichtman, D.M. (1998). Physical examination of the wrist. In *The wrist and its disorders* (ed. D.M. Lichtman), pp. 74–81. W.B. Saunders, Philadelphia.

2. Werner, S.L. and Plancher, K.D. (1998). Biomechanics of wrist injuries in sport. *Clin. Sports. Med.* **17**, 407–420.

3. Palmer, A.K., Werner, F.W., Murphy, D., *et al.* (1985). Functional wrist motion: a biomechanical study. *J. Hand Surg. (Am.)* **10A**, 39–46.

4. Werner, F.W., Palmer, A.K., Fortino, M.D., *et al.* (1992). Force transmission through the distal ulna: effect of ulnar variance, lunate fossa angulation, and radial and palmar tilt of the distal radius. *J. Hand Surg. (Am.)* **17A**, 423.

5. Reagan, D.S., Linscheid, R.L., and Dobyns, J.H. (1984). Lunotriquetral sprains. *J. Hand Surg. (Am.)* **9A**, 502–514.

6. Watson, H.K. and Weinzweig, J. (1997). Physical examination of the wrist. *Hand Clin.* **13**, 1.

7. Gilford, W.W., Bolton, R.M., and Lambrinudi, C. (1943). The mechanism of the wrist joint with special reference to fractures of the scaphoid. *Guy's Hosp. Rep.* **92**, 52–59.

8. Lichtman, D.M. and Martin, R.A. (1988). Introduction to the carpal instabilities. In *The wrist and its disorders* (ed. D.M. Lichtman), pp. 244–250. W.B. Saunders, Philadelphia.

9. Blatt, G. (1988). Scapholunate instability. In *The wrist and its disorders* (ed. D.M. Lichtman), pp. 251–273. W.B. Saunders, Philadelphia.

10. Nathan, R. and Blatt, G. (2000). Rotary subluxation of the scaphoid: revisited. *Hand Clin.* **16** (3), 417–431.

11. Lavernia, C.J., Cohen, M.S., and Taleisnik, J. (1992). Treatment of scapholunate dissociation by ligamentous repair and caopsulodesis. *J. Hand Surg. (Am.)* **17**, 354–359.

12. Trumble, T.E., Bour, C.J., Smith, R.J. *et al.* (1990). Intercarpal arthrodesis for static and dynamic palmar intercalated segment instability. *J. Hand Surg. (Am.)* **15**, 384–392.

13. Kleinman, W.B. (1985). The luno-triquetral shuck test. *Am. Soc. Surg. Hand Corr. News* **51**.

14. Taleisnik, J. (1987). Pain on the ulnar side of the wrist. *Hand Clin.* **3**, 51–68.

15. Cohen, M.S. (1998). Ligamentous injuries of the wrist in the athlete. *Clin. Sports Med.* **17** (3), 533–552.

16. Nelson, D.L., Manske, P.R., Pruitt, D.L., *et al.* (1993). Lunotriquetral arthrodesis. *J. Hand Surg. (Am.)* **18**, 1113–1120.

17. Sennwald, G.R., Fischer, M., and Mondi, P. (1995). Lunotriquetral arthrodesis. A controversial procedure. *J. Hand Surg. (Br.)* **20**, 755–760.

18. Melone, C.P., Beldner, S., and Basuk, R.S. (2000). Thumb collateral ligament injuries: an anatomic basis for treatment. *Hand Clin.* **16** (3), 345–357.

19. Hergan, K. and Mittler, C. (1995). Sonography of the injured ulnar collateral ligament of the thumb. *J. Bone Joint Surg. (Br.)* **77**, 77–83.

20. Bowers, W.H. and Hurst, L.C. (1977). Gamekeepers's thumb. Evaluation of arthrography and stress roentgenography. *J. Bone Joint Surg. (Am.)* **59**, 519–524.

21. O'Callaghan, B.I., Kohut, G., and Hoogewoud, H.M. (1994). Gamekeeper's thumb: identification of the Stener lesion with ultrasound. *Radiology* **192**, 447–480.

22. Spaeth, H.J., Abrams, R.A., Bock, G.W., *et al.* (1993). Gamekeeper's thumb: differentiation of non-displaced and displaced tears of the ulnar collateral ligament with MRI imaging. *Radiology* **188**, 553–556.

23. Diao, E. and Lintecum, N.D. (1996). Gamekeeper's thumb. *Curr. Opin. Orthop.* **7** (4), 10–16

24. Langford, S.A., Whitaker, J.H., and Toby, E.B. (1998). Thumb injuries in the athlete. *Clin. Sports Med.* **17** (3), 553–566.

25. Scott, S.C. (2000). Closed injuries to the extension mechanism of the digits. *Hand Clin.* **16** (3), 367–373.

26. Aronowitz, E.R. and Leddy, J.P. (1998). Closed tendon injuries of the hand and wrist in athletes. *Clin. Sports Med.* **17** (3), 449–467.

27. Gunter, G.S. (1960). Traumatic rupture of the insertion of flexor digitorum profundus. *Aust. NZ J. Surg.* **30**, 1.

28. Lunn, P.G. and Lamb, D.W. (1984). 'Rugby finger'—avulsion of profundus of ring finger. *J. Hand Surg. (Br.)* **9**, 69.

29. Leddy, J.P. (1985). Avulsions of the flexor digitorum profundus. *Hand Clin.* **1** (1), 77–83.

30. Stamos, B.D. and Leddy, J.P. (2000). Closed flexor tendon disruption in athletes. *Hand Clin.* **16** (3), 359–365.

31. Gladden, R.J. (1957). Boxer's knuckle. A preliminary report. *Am. J. Surg.* **93**, 388–397.

32. Posner, M.A. and Ambrose, L. (1989). Boxer's knuckle—dorsal capsular rupture of the metacarpophalangeal joint of a finger. *J. Hand Surg. (Am.)* **14A**, 229–235.

33. Koniuch, M.P., Peimer, C.A., VanGorder, T., *et al.* (1987). Closed crush injury of the metacarpophalangeal joint. *J. Hand Surg. (Am.)* **12A**, 750–757.

34. Hame, S.L. and Melone, C.P. (2000). Boxer's knuckle. Traumatic disruption of the extensor hood. *Hand Clin.* **16** (3), 375–380.

35. **Mogensen, B. and Mattson, H.** (1980). Stenosing tenovaginitis of the third compartment of the hand: case report. *Scand. J. Plast. Reconstr. Surg.* **14**, 127.

36. **Ritter, M. and Inglis, A.** (1969). The extensor indicis proprius syndrome. *J. Bone Joint Surg. (Am.)* **51**, 1645.

37. **Ambrose, J. and Goldstone, R.** (1975). Anomalous extensor digiti minimi proprius causing tunnel syndrome in the dorsal compartment. *J. Bone Joint Surg. (Am.)* **57**, 706–707.

38. **Schenck, R.R.** (1964). Variations of the extensor tendons of the finger. *J. Bone Joint Surg. (Am.)* **46**, 103–110.

39. **Fulcher, S.M., Kiefhaber, T.R., and Stern, P.J.** (1998). Upper extremity tendonitis and overuse syndromes in the athlete. *Clin. Sports Med.* **17**, 433–448.

40. **Palmieri, T.J.** (1982). Pisiform area pain—treatment by pisiform excision. *J. Hand Surg. (Am.)* **7**, 477–480.

41. **Phalen, G.S.** (1966). The carpal tunnel syndrome: seventeen years' experience in diagnosis and treatment of six hundred fifty-four hands. *J. Bone Joint Surg.* **48A**, 211–228.

42. **Gruetberry, A.B.** (1983). Carpal tunnel decompression in spite of normal electromyography. *J. Hand Surg.* **8**, 348–349.

43. **Shea, J.D. and McClain, E.F.** (1969). Ulnar nerve compression syndrome at and below the wrist. *J. Bone Joint Surg. (Am.)* **51**, 1095–1103.

44. **Nuber, G.W., McCarthy, W.J., Yao, J.S.,** *et al.* (1990). Arterial abnormalities of the hand in athletes. *Am. J. Sports Med.* **18**, 520–523.

45. **Dellon, A.L. and Mackinnon, S.E.** (1986). Radial sensory nerve entrapment in the forearm. *J. Hand Surg. (Am.)* **11**, 199–205.

46. **Howell, A.E. and Leach, R.E.** (1970). Bowler's thumb: perineural fibrosis of the digital nerve. *J. Bone Joint Surg. (Am.)* **52**, 379–381.

47. **Bogumill, G.P.** (1988). Tumors of the wrist. In *The wrist and its disorders* (ed. D.M. Lichtman), pp. 373–384. W.B. Saunders, Philadelphia.

6.6 The pelvis, hip, and thigh

Cathy Speed and Roger Hackney

Introduction

Pelvic pain arising from the groin, pelvis, and hip has a very wide differential diagnosis, crossing many clinical specialist boundaries (Table 1). Potential causes of groin and pelvic pain include disorders of the abdominal and pelvic organs, referred pain from the spine, neurological complaints, and localized articular and soft tissue complaints. Symptoms can be non-specific and diffuse and may have unusual patterns of referral.[1–4] It is not surprising then that making a diagnosis can be challenging and a multispeciality approach may be necessary.[5]

This chapter addresses musculoskeletal complaints of the hip, groin, and thigh and, in particular, those of soft tissues. It is important to emphasize that other causes of symptoms in this area must always be considered.

Functional anatomy

The pelvis serves as a midpoint for axial and rotary forces that are transmitted through the lumbosacral–pelvis–hip unit. The anatomy of the area is complex. The pelvis is a bony ring, comprising two paired inominate bones. Each of these is composed of three bones, the ileum, the ischium (Fig. 1) and the pubic bones, which join anteriorly at the symphysis pubis. Each component contributes to the acetabulum, which forms the deep socket for the hip joint. Stability across the hip joint is largely dependent upon the ligaments (especially the iliofemoral, pubofemoral, and ischiofemoral ligaments) that reinforce the capsule, extending in a spiral course from the acetabulum to the femur. All are tightened in internal rotation and are lax in external rotation. Normal hip motion allows 45° of external rotation, internal rotation and abduction, 20° of adduction, 135° of flexion, and 30° of extension. Considerable forces pass through the hip joint, both at rest and on weight-bearing, much of which must be dissipated through the muscular structures surrounding it. For example one-third of body weight passes through the hip on standing on two legs, 2.5 times body weight on standing on one leg, 3 times on walking up stairs, and 4.5 on running.

The pubic symphysis is a cartilaginous and mobile joint, with a hyaline cartilage surface to each side joined by thick fibrous bands. The joint is fibrous and does allow some movement in a vertical plane. Its nerve supply is from L1–2 and also S2–4 (via the genitofemoral and pudendal nerves).

The pelvis is joined to the sacrum of the spinal column via the sacroiliac joints. Each sacroiliac joint is fibrocartiliaginous in its upper third and synovial joint in the distal two-thirds, and supported by very thick intraarticular ligaments. The surfaces of the joint are highly irregular and reduce the scope for movement. The ligaments are highly important in the stability of the joint. Some rotational movement is possible.

The muscles arising from the pelvis move the hip and knee joints and support the spinal column. When the anatomy of the abdominal wall is considered, it is understandable that pain in the pelvic region

Table 1 Differential diagnosis of pain in the hip, groin, or thigh

Musculoskeletal causes

Musculotendinous
Adductor(s): muscle injury, tendinopathy
Psoas muscle and tendon: snapping psoas, bursitis
Trochanteric 'bursitis'
Hamstrings

Articular
Pubic symphysis: osteitis pubis, instability
Hip: arthritides, labral tears, loose bodies, subluxation, 'irritable hip'
Lumbar spine: 'mechanical' back pain, facet joint dysfunction/arthropathy, spondylolysis, intervertebral disc injury
Sacroiliac joint: sacroiliitis, instability/dysfunction

Neurological
Nerve entrapment: obturator, ilioinguinal, lateral cutaneous nerve of the thigh

Abdominal/urological causes
Hernia: clinical (inguinal, femoral), subclinical and 'sports hernia'
Intrapelvic genitourinary (including testicular) and gastrointestinal disorders

Gynaecological causes
Ovarian, uterine

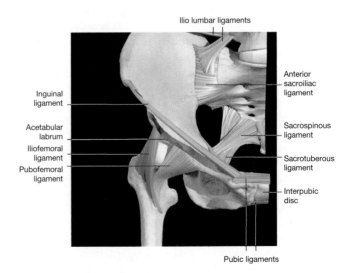

Fig. 1 Bony anatomy of the pelvis and hip.

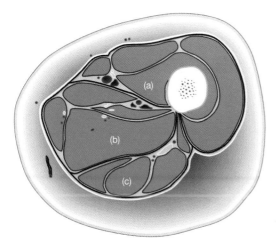

Fig. 2 Compartments of the thigh. (a) anterior; (b) medial; (c) posterior.

Table 2 Muscles of the gluteal region and thigh

Region	Muscles
Gluteal	Gluteals, piriformis, obturator internus, gemelli, quadratus femoris
Anterior thigh	Quadriceps, sartorius, pectineus, rectus femoris iliopsoas
Medial thigh	Adductors, obturator internus, gracilis
Posterior thigh	Biceps femoris, semimembranosis, semitendinosis

can arise from abdominal muscle pathology. Anteriorly, the abdominal wall has three layers of muscle which, from exterior to interior, are the external oblique, internal oblique, and transversus. On either side of the midline there is also the vertical, powerful rectus abdominus, arising from the symphysis and pubic crest to insert into the fifth to seventh costal cartilages and xiphoid. The external oblique arises from the lower eight ribs and fans to insert into the xiphoid, pubic tubercle, and the anterior half of the iliac crest. Internal oblique fibres run at right angles to the external oblique, arising with transversus from the lumbar fascia, the inguinal ligament, and anterior iliac crest, to insert into the lower three ribs, xiphoid, and symphysis. Transversus fibres also arise from the lower six costal cartilages and run horizontally forward to join the internal oblique to form a conjoined tendon that attaches to the inguinal ligament. The inguinal ligament is attached to the fascia lata of the thigh. There are two defects in the muscle layers in the inguinal region, the internal and external rings, allowing the passage of the ilioinguinal nerve and, in males, structures of the spermatic cord (in females, the round ligament of the uterus is found here). This is a potential area of weakness in males, where inguinal hernias can occur.

Movement between the spine and pelvis occurs with the help of the abdominal muscles. When the pelvis is fixed, the spine moves through actions of rectus abdominus, and obliques. The obliques laterally flex and rotate the trunk. Rectus abdominus flexes the trunk and stabilizes the pelvis.

Muscles of the gluteal region and the thigh work across the hip to flex, extend, abduct, adduct, and rotate the leg. The thigh is composed of three compartments—anterior, posterior, and lateral—separated by intermuscular septae and with the femur lying centrally (Fig. 2,

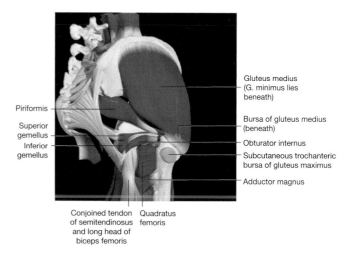

Fig. 3 The deep gluteal region: lateral view.

Table 3 Muscle actions at the hip

Movement	Muscles
Hip flexion	Strong: iliopsoas, rectus femoris Weak: adductor longus, gracilis sartorius, pectineus
Hip extension	Strong: gluteus maximus, adductor magnus (ischial portion) Weak: hamstrings gluteus medius, piriformis
Hip external rotation (hip and knee flexed)	Gluteus maximus and medius, obturators, quadratus femoris, gemelli, sartorius
Hip internal rotation	Adductors, gluteus medius and minimus, tensor fasciae latae, pectineus, gracilis
Hip adduction	Adductors
Hip abduction	Gluteus medius, gluteus minimus, tensor fasciae latae
Knee extension	Quadriceps
Knee flexion	Hamstrings
Motion of the pelvis at the hip	
Anterior pelvic tilt	Hip flexors, trunk extensors
Posterior pelvic tilt	Hip extensors, trunk flexors (rectus, obliques)
Lateral pelvic tilt	Contralateral hip abductors

Table 2). These muscles and several shorter muscles also help to control the stability of the pelvis and lower spine (Fig. 3). The significance of these shorter muscles in the prevention of low back and pelvic pain is becoming increasingly appreciated. Muscle actions at the pelvis and hip are described in Table 3.

The anterior compartment of the thigh

Muscles of the anterior compartment are sartorius, iliacus, psoas (iliopsoas), pectineus, and the quadriceps (Fig. 4). The *psoas* muscle is the largest in the body. It arises from the transverse processes of L1–5

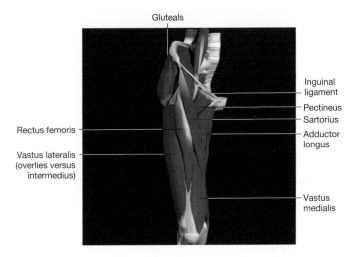

Fig. 4 The anterior thigh.

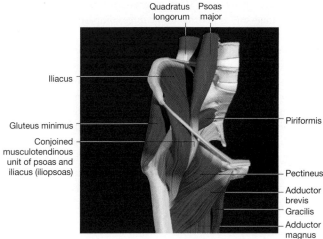

Fig. 5 Some important muscles of the pelvis and medial thigh.

and passes across the pelvis where it is joined by *iliacus*, which arises from the inner blade of the ileum. The '*iliopsoas*' then passes over the hip joint to insert into the lesser trochanter of the femur. The function of iliopsoas is to flex and internally rotate the leg when the hip is extended. When the hip is flexed, the psoas produces external rotation. The tendon of psoas flattens as it crosses the hip joint, separated from the hip joint by the psoas bursa.

Rectus femoris and the three *vasti* muscles (*vastus medialis, lateralis*, and *intermedius*) are the four muscles that form the *quadriceps* group, which are powerful extensors of the knee. The vasti arise from the femur. Rectus femoris has two heads of origin and crosses two joints (knee and hip). The straight (direct) head arises from the inferior superior iliac spine, and the reflected (indirect) head from the floor of the groove above the acetabulum. The fibres of rectus femoris blend with those of vastus intermedius to insert onto the superior pole of the patella. Vastus medialis is composed of two portions, vastus medialis obliquus (VMO) and vastus medialis longus. Fibres of VMO are at an angle of 30–45° from the long axis of the quadriceps group and prevent lateral subluxation of the patella. Vastus medialis and lateralis insert on to the medial and lateral aspects of the patella, respectively, and strengthen the capsule of the knee joint. Collectively, these tendons represent the quadriceps tendon, which encloses the patella as a sesamoid bone before inserting into the tibial tuberosity via the patella tendon. Expansions of the insertion are bound to the capsule and medial collateral ligament of the knee.

Sartorius, like rectus femoris, crosses both the hip and knee. It arises from the anterior superior iliac spine (ASIS) and inserts on to the medial tibia, forming part of *pes anserinus* (duck's foot). *Pectineus* arises from the pubis and inserts on to the pectineal line of the femur.

The medial compartment of the thigh

The medial compartment consists of the *adductors, gracilis*, and *obturator externus*. The adductor muscles (adductors magnus, longus, and brevis) and gracilis (another two-joint muscle) arise from pubic symphysis and rami to insert along the medial border of the femur, with gracilis forming part of the pes anserinus inserting on to the tibia. They produce hip adduction and, together with sartorius and tensor fascia lata, provide important control of the leg on the pelvis, which has been likened to three guide ropes (Fig. 5).

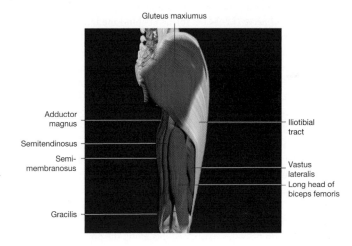

Fig. 6 The posterior hip and thigh.

The posterior compartment of the thigh

The *hamstring muscles* consist of the *semimembranosus, semitendinosus*, and *biceps femoris* and the *hamstrings portion of adductor magnus* (Fig. 6). They share a common origin on the ischial tuberosity, although semimembranous can arise as a separate slip in some individuals. Biceps femoris also has a short head, arising from the linea aspera of the femur. The two heads of the biceps femoris form a common tendon, inserting on to the head of the fibula, while semimembranosus and semitendinosus insert on to the proximal medial tibia, with the latter contributing to pes anserinus. The sciatic nerve runs vertically through the hamstring compartment.

Piriformis arises from the middle three sacral vertebrae, and extends medially between the anterior sacral foramina so that the sacral nerves and plexus lie upon the muscle. The superior gluteal nerve (L4, 5) and vessels pass over piriformis, and the sciatic nerve lies deep to the muscle, though it may pass through it. Piriformis passes laterally through the greater sciatic notch and crosses the buttock, behind the hip joint to the apex of the greater trochanter. The muscle acts as a stabilizer of the joint, abducts the flexed thigh, and laterally rotates the extended thigh.

The *iliotibial band (tract)* (ITB) represents the most lateral component of the thigh and is external to the three compartments. It is composed of thickened fascia, connecting the ilium with the lateral tibia, and arises from gluteus maximus and the *tensor fascia lata muscle* (TFL), which originates from the anterior iliac crest and lies over gluteus maximus. The deep fascia of TFL runs over the greater trochanter of the femur, separated by a bursa that in thin persons is quite superficial. During hip flexion the TFL pulls the ITB forward, while during extension it is pulled backward by gluteus maximus. The function of the TFL is to brace the iliotibial tract and abduct and medially rotate the thigh. The ITB has a stabilizing influence on the knee in flexion and extension. Often when standing upright the upward pull of the ITB is the most important factor keeping the knee extended; the quadriceps may be relaxed.

Nerve supply

The pelvis, hip, and thigh are supplied by the lumbosacral plexus via the femoral, obturator and sciatic nerves. The hip joint itself and its capsule receive sensory innervation from the femoral, obturator, superior gluteal, and sciatic nerves (Figs. 7 and 8).

The *femoral nerve* (L2–L4) is formed behind the bulk of the psoas muscle and runs down under the inguinal ligament in the femoral canal. In the femoral triangle it divides into a number of branches, both cutaneous and motor. The nerve supplies the quadriceps and pectineus muscles of the anterior thigh. Skin supplied exclusively by the femoral nerve includes the front and medial side of the thigh and, via the saphenous nerve branch, an area over the medial supply of the lower leg.

The *sciatic nerve* (L4–S3) emerges from the pelvis through the greater sciatic foramen deep to piriformis, then curves around midway between the greater trochanter of the femur and the ischial tuberosity under gluteus maximus. Behind the hip joint it supplies the long head of biceps femoris and, running over adductor magnus, supplies the hamstring muscles. In the proximal thigh it divides into the common peroneal and tibial nerves, to supply the hip flexors and muscles of the lower leg. It also provides sensory supply along the posterior thigh.

The *superior gluteal nerve* (L4,5) supplies gluteus medius and minimus and TFL. The *inferior gluteal nerve* (L5, S1) supplies gluteus maximus.

The obturator nerve (L2–4) is formed in the psoas muscle and descends within the muscle emerging from the medial border at the brim of the pelvis. The obturator nerve divides in the obturator notch into anterior and posterior divisions in the obturator foramen. The anterior division supplies the hip joint and adductor longus, brevis, and gracilis, with a sensory branch to the medial thigh. The posterior division supplies obturator internus and adductor magnus. The nerve supplies an area of skin along the middle of the medial thigh.

The *iliohypogastric nerve* (L1) pierces transversus abdominis near the iliac crest and dives into anterior and lateral cutaneous branches. Both pierce the oblique muscles and supply the skin over the inguinal canal.

The *ilioinguinal nerve* (L1) pierces transversus abdominis above the anterior part of the iliac crest. It passes through the internal oblique muscle and passes into the inguinal canal. The nerve leaves the canal through the superficial ring and supplies an area of skin over the medial thigh, and in the male the scrotum and root of the penis. The *genitofemoral nerve* (L1,2) also supplies part of the scrotal skin and the femoral triangle. The genital branch passes though the pelvis to emerge into the internal ring and pass along the inguinal canal. The femoral branch passes through the femoral sheath lateral to the femoral artery.

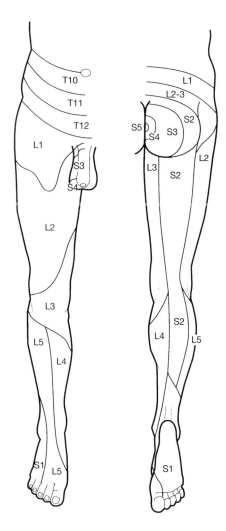

Fig. 7 Dermatomes of the leg.

The obliques and transversus are supplied by the lower six thoracic nerves and the iliohypogastric and ilioinguinal nerves. Rectus abdominus is supplied by T7–12.

Vascular supply

Vascular supply to the pelvis is through the internal and external iliac arteries and collateral circulation from the inferior aorta. The hip joint is supplied primarily by the femoral artery and its circumflex branches, with contributions from the artery of ligamentum teres, a branch of the obturator artery. The femoral artery gives rise to the profundus artery to supply the thigh.

Clinical evaluation

History

Symptoms relating to some soft tissue pathologies of the hip, thigh, and groin are often poorly localized, overlapping, and non-specific. This should not dissuade the physician from obtaining a very detailed history of the complaint, as it is nevertheless a vital step in reaching an accurate diagnosis and devising appropriate management strategies.

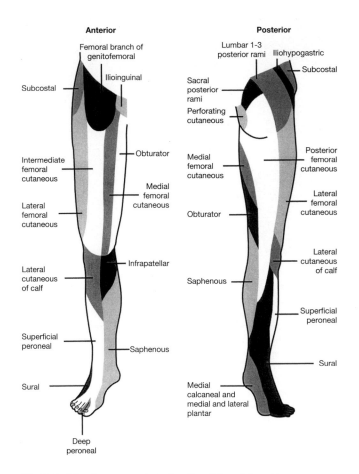

Fig. 8 Peripheral nerve supply to the skin of the pelvis and leg.

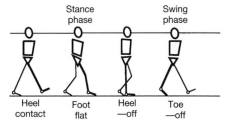

Fig. 9 Gait involves the stance phase (60% of the normal cycle) and the swing phase (40%). The hip is moved into extension during the stance phase and the abductors are critical in maintaining the single limb support phase. The hip moves into flexion during the swing phase, and the pelvis rotates approximately 40° anteriorly around the hip of the supported extremity.

Patients may present with an acute injury or, more commonly, with chronic symptoms. Frequently encountered symptoms include clicking, clunking, catching, a feeling of instability, restriction, limping, and falls. Nevertheless, the cardinal symptom, as with any soft tissue complaint, is pain. A thorough pain history should be obtained, starting with its nature, principal site(s), and radiation, and provoking and relieving factors. The mechanism of onset of the symptoms should be determined and may include trauma (e.g. a direct blow or twisting injury) or may be related to overuse. A full activity history is also obtained, including changes in the nature and intensity of activities preceding the onset. The timing of the symptoms and whether they are progressing or improving is also important.

Pain in the groin itself is representative of hip joint pathology, referred pain from the lumbar spine or sacroiliac joints, and pain from localized soft tissue disorders. Pain from herniae can radiate to the scrotum and this is particularly the case with the 'sports hernia'. Articular pain from the hip can radiate to the thigh, knee, and back. Lumbar and sacroiliac pain can also radiate to the buttock and typical sciatica can occur with a prolapsed disc or with piriformis syndrome. Exacerbating and relieving factors are noted. Pain worsened with coughing and straining is suggestive of herniae or spinal pathology. Specific movements may aggravate the condition through the range of motion required or due to impact.

The timing of the pain may be relevant. Early morning pain with stiffness that is worse with rest and lessened with activity is suggestive of an inflammatory process. Night pain may be reported. Pain may be localized and alter with sleeping position; for example, the lateral 'hip' pain of trochanteric bursitis is worse when lying on the affected side. Most complaints can cause pain on turning over in bed. Pain that is constant through the night regardless of position should raise the suspicion of articular pathology or serious underlying disease, including infection or malignancy. The presence of constitutional symptoms must be directly addressed as a priority.

A history of clicking or clunking when the hip is moved may be due to hip joint pathology, snapping hip syndrome, or a snapping trochanteric bursa. Hypermobile individuals with poor muscular control of the hip girdle also commonly report non-specific clunking.

Neurological symptoms such as tingling, burning, numbness, and weakness may indicate a peripheral nerve entrapment and the distribution of such symptoms should be ascertained. For example, obturator nerve entrapment can cause pain in the region of the adductor muscles, and sciatic pain may be induced by entrapment in the pelvis or buttock from an abnormal piriformis or hamstring muscle.

A full general medical history is taken, particularly assessing for symptoms of intrapelvic, gastrointestinal, and genitourinary disease to explore the possibility of pain from other than musculoskeletal sources. A history of groin or thigh pain in childhood or adolescence should provoke suspicion of Legg–Calve–Perthes disease, slipped capital femoral epiphysis, or apophysitis.

Previous injuries are noted. Recurrent injuries may be related to biomechanical aberrations such as a leg-length discrepancy or, in sportspeople, training or equipment errors.

Examination

Gait

Examination begins with a simple assessment of gait, which should involve pain-free, smooth movements with an even distribution of weight. In gait assessment, the patient should be watched walking from in front and behind. Walking involves two basic phases; the stance phase (60 per cent of the normal cycle) and the swing phase (40 per cent) (Fig. 9). The hip flexors and extensors work phasically in the initiation of gait: this includes eccentric work as the flexors slow and control extension and vice versa. The hip is moved into extension during the stance phase and the abductors are critical in maintaining the single limb support phase. The hip moves into flexion during the swing phase, and the pelvis rotates approximately 40° anteriorly around the hip of the supported extremity.

Loss of hip range of motion results in a compensatory increase in motion of the ipsilateral knee and contralateral hip and increased movement of the lumbar spine. Changes in gait as a result of abnormalities in the region of the hip include an increase in vertical motion of the body's centre of gravity, increased lateral shift of the trunk and pelvis, reduced stride length, and reduced rotation on the symptomatic hip. An *antalgic* gait due to localized pain involves a reduced stride length and a short stance phase, and the gait is slow and deliberate. An 'extensor lurch', due to a weak gluteus maximus, involves a thrust of the trunk backward at stance initiation to try to maintain hip extension and stability. An 'abductor lurch', due to a weak gluteus medius, is the typical *Trendelenburg gait*. The trunk lurches to the involved side to maintain stability by placing the centre of gravity over the affected hip. Bilateral gluteus medius weakness leads to a *waddling gait*. Leg-length inequality leads to a lateral shift to the opposite side and the pelvis tilts down towards the opposite side. Specific functions can then be evaluated, including squatting, hopping, and stair climbing, in order to reproduce symptoms.

Standing

The anterior and posterior superior superior iliac spines should be level with the contralateral side and skin creases symmetrical. Evidence of bruising, deformity, and discolouration should be sought. The spine is examined with the patient standing to assess posture, and the range and rhythm of lumbar movements and provocation of symptoms may indicate any abnormality that will require more detailed examination.

The *Trendelenburg test* evaluates the stability of the hip and the ability of the hip abductors to stabilize the pelvis on the femur. The patient stands on one limb—the pelvis on the opposite side normally should rise. If it drops, this normally indicates hip pathology and/or a weak gluteus medius on the weight-bearing leg.

The *sacroiliac joints* (SIJs) are difficult to assess, as pain reproduced by attempts to 'stress' the SIJs may be coming from other sites, in particular, the lumbar facet joints (Fig. 10).

Movement at the SIJs is very restricted, but does occur. The mobility of the sacroiliac joints can be measured with the patient standing or sitting, by comparing relative movement of the posterior superior iliac spine against the sacrum with finger palpation as the hip is flexed. In males, examination of the hernial orifices is performed with the patient standing and coughing.

Supine

With the patient supine, *leg-length discrepancy* (functional and apparent) can be assessed. The femoral triangle can be palpated. Next, *combined hip movements* are examined, with special attention paid to range of motion and reproduction of symptoms. Combined hip flexion, external rotation, abduction, and adduction are assessed. The capsular pattern of hip is flexion, abduction, and internal rotation but the order of restriction may vary. Combined flexion and internal rotation may reproduce hip joint pain, localized to the groin. Extension of the hip may be best assessed with the patient lying over the end of the couch with one leg flexed, knee to chest. A rectus femoris contracture is evident in this position (see Thomas's test, below) and can also be demonstrated in the prone position: when the affected knee is flexed,

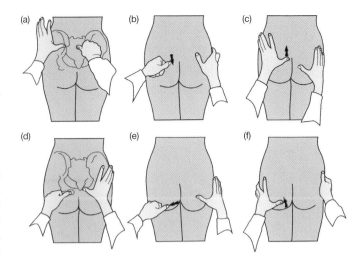

Fig. 10 Numerous tests to assess the SIJ have been proposed. Here the examiner evaluates for reduced movement relative to the contralateral side. Both the superior (a–c) and inferior (d–f) portions of the joint are evaluated. The examiner's left thumb is placed on the posterior superior iliac spine and the right thumb on a sacral process. The patient lifts the left leg. The examiner's left thumb may move downward (normal, b), or upward if it is fixed (c). For the lower portion of the joint, the left thumb is placed on the ischial tuberosity and the right thumb over the apex of the sacrum. Normally, lateral movement of the left thumb occurs when the patient's left leg is lifted (e), or upward when the joint is fixed (f).

the ipsilateral hip will spontaneously flex. Resisted testing of the musculotendinous structures of the region is then performed.

An iliopsoas lesion can be detected when the patient is lying supine, with the pelvis overlying the edge of the couch. The unaffected leg is flexed, knees to chest. The injured leg is extended, the examiner pushes the leg into further extension. This will reproduce the pain. Asking the patient to flex his hip against resistance makes the pain worse. The pain is aggravated by resisting flexion of the hip from a position of extension and external rotation. In the patient with a 'snapping hip', pain, clunking, clicking, or snapping may be experienced by the patient with active flexion of the hip and then moving it into abduction and external rotation followed by extension. This moves the psoas tendon over the front of the hip.

The *adductor stretch* is measured by bringing the feet together at the buttock and allowing the hips to abduct. Tenderness of the muscle belly and origin can be palpated, together with the pubic symphysis and tubercles in this position. Resisted adduction is assessed. *Hamstring stretch* can be assessed along with the straight leg raise. When a positive straight leg raise is noted, the knee is then passively flexed and further passive hip flexion is attempted. If none occurs, then the lesion causing the sciatica is in the buttock (e.g. abscess, neoplasm).

Attempts to stress the sacroiliac joints to reproduce symptoms can be made by 'springing' the pelvis, or by flexing the hip and knee and passively adducting the thigh across to the contralateral iliac fossa. *Gaenslen's test* is performed by flexing the hip of the unaffected side and hyperextending the other hip. Such tests are unfortunately non-specific.

The *hernial orifices* are palpated. In males invaginating the scrotum with a finger can be a reliable means of detecting a subtle inguinal hernia. Abdominal and pelvic examinations are performed as indicated.

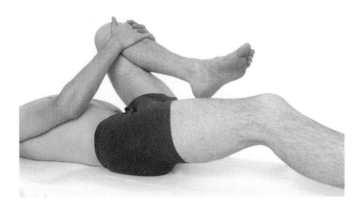

Fig. 11 Thomas' test assesses for hip flexion contracture. One of the patient's hips is flexed to flatten the lumbar spine. When the straight leg flexes on the table, a contracture is present in that hip. If performed with the knee at 90° over the edge of the table, extension of the knee indicates a probable rectus femoris contracture.

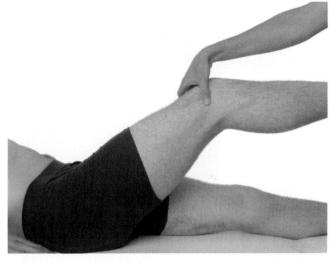

Fig. 13 The *Noble compression test* assesses for ITB friction syndrome at the knee.

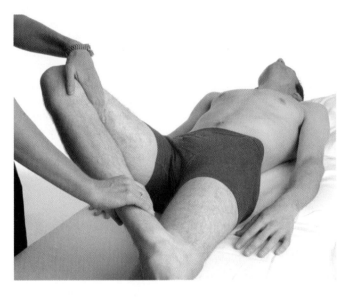

Fig. 12 The FABER test is a general test for hip, SIJ pathology, or iliopsoas spasm.

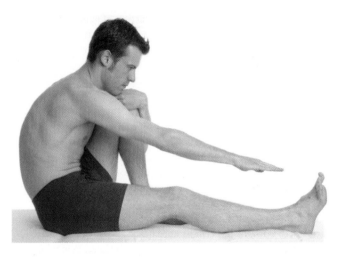

Fig. 14 A hamstrings contracture is evident when there is disparity between the fingers to toes stretch. Hamstrings flexibility should also be tested by passive extension of the leg in varying degrees of hip rotation.

Many additional tests assess for the presence of contraction of one or more structures of the region. *Thomas's test* evaluates for a hip joint or rectus femoris flexion contracture (Fig. 11). The patient lies supine and the examiner looks for excess lumbar lordosis, common when the hip flexors are tight. One hip is flexed to flatten the lumbar spine. In the absence of a flexion contracture, the other (tested) leg remains flat on the table, whereas it rises off the table when a contracture is present. A rectus femoris contracture is more likely if palpable tightness is noted.

To assess for an *abduction contracture*: the patient lies supine with the ASISs level. When a contracture is present, the affected leg makes more than a 90° angle with the line jointing the ASISs. Typically there is apparent leg discrepancy.

The *FABER (or Patrick's) test* assesses for hip or SIJ pathology and iliopsoas spasm (Fig. 12). The patient lies supine and the test leg is brought into *F*lexion, *AB*duction, and *E*xternal *R*otation, with the foot resting on the knee of the opposite leg. The test leg should fall into a position at least parallel to the opposite leg. Failure to do so implies pathology. The examiner may then stress the test leg further in the FABER position to attempt to reproduce the symptoms.

The *Noble compression test* assesses for ITB friction syndrome at the knee. The patient lies supine, flexes the knee to 90° with the hip in some flexion (Fig. 13). The patient extends the knee while the examiner applies pressure to the area 1–2 cm above the lateral femoral condyle. Symptoms are reproduced at this site when the knee is 30° from full extension.

A *hamstrings contracture* is evident when there is disparity between the finger to toes stretch, tested with the patient sitting, the legs extended, and the contralateral knee flexed to stabilize the pelvis (Fig. 14).

Lateral position

Further evaluation continues, with the patient lying on the unaffected side. The greater trochanter can be palpated by following the femur

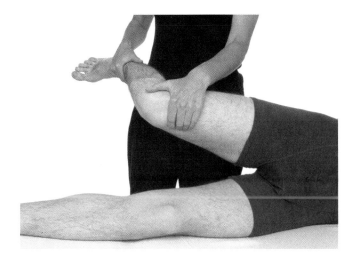

Fig. 15 Ober's test evaluates the flexibility of the iliotibial band. The ITB is tight if the patient's abducted and extended upper leg remains abducted when slowly released by the examiner.

proximally. Local tenderness and reproduction of pain in this area on adducting or flexing the hip may indicate a trochanteric bursitis, although hip joint pain can be referred to this area early in the history of degenerative change.

Ober's test for a tight ITB is performed with the affected leg uppermost (Fig. 15). The other leg is flexed at the hip and knee. The examiner then passively abducts and extends the upper leg with the knee extended, then slowly allows the upper leg to lower on to the couch. Ober initially described the test with the knee of the test leg flexed but gluteus medius, the main hip abductor, is tested with the leg in a few degrees of abduction. Pain may be reproduced. Failure to reach the couch indicates a tightness that may be the cause of ITB friction syndrome or trochanteric bursitis.

With the patient in the same position, the piriformis test can be performed. With the uppermost knee flexed and the hip flexed to 60°, the examiner applies downward pressure on the knee. Pain in the area of piriformis is reproduced if it is tight. Sciatica may be noted if piriformis is compressing the nerve.

Prone

The spine and sacroiliac joints can be palpated and the femoral stretch test is performed to assess for nerve entrapment. Gluteus maximus can be tested by resisted hip extension with the knee flexed (to relax the hamstrings). The ischiogluteal region (where a bursa is present) and the hamstring origin can be palpated for tenderness and the muscle group assessed by resisted knee flexion. Active external rotation of the leg during testing helps to isolate biceps femoris, while internal rotation helps to test semitendinosis and semimembranosis.

Investigation

Plain radiography

In acute injuries, plain radiography of the pelvis is required where significant trauma has occurred and where bony/articular damage is suspected. In children and adolescents, plain radiographs are warranted when there is a possibility of an avulsion injury. Oblique, anteroposterior (AP), and lateral views may be necessary. Plain radiographs of the pelvis

may also be indicated in chronic pain in the region, as the pubic symphysis, sacroiliac, and hip joints are all sources of symptoms. Osteoarthritis (OA) is surprisingly common in young sportsmen and women and should not be regarded solely as a complaint of the elderly. However, radiographic evidence of OA can be misleading in the interpretation of symptoms. Stork views with the patient standing on alternate legs are used to detect pubic symphysis instability. Radiological changes consistent with osteitis pubis are common in active asymptomatic males.

Isotope bone scanning

Bone scan can reflect the effects of pathological processes upon bone. Scan appearances are rarely specific to a given disorder, but certain patterns will reflect the type of process involved, particularly in the case of degenerative, inflammatory, infective, traumatic, and metastatic disease. Isotope scans are useful in demonstrating subtle avulsion injuries, stress fractures, and myositis ossificans.

Ultrasonography

Dynamic ultrasound is an invaluable tool in the evaluation of symptoms in the hip, groin, and thigh. Common clinical indications include assessment for masses, tendinopathies, bursitis, muscle contusions, tears, and ruptures. In 'snapping hip', dynamic evaluation also can demonstrate the iliopsoas tendon moving over the hip during movement, in association with the symptoms. The joint itself can be examined for synovitis, effusion, and loose bodies and subclinical herniae can also be demonstrated. Ultrasound is the initial investigation of choice for the evaluation of masses and fluid collections (with aspiration under guidance as necessary) and can demonstrate nerve lesions (schwannoma, neurofibroma, trauma). Testicular pathology and intrapelvic pathology can also be assessed using this imaging modality.

Computerized tomography (CT)

CT scanning is of more use in detecting bony pathology and with wider availability of magnetic resonance scanning is less often used for the investigation of soft tissues in the elective situation.

Magnetic resonance imaging (MRI)

MRI is very useful in detecting pathology within the pelvis and musculoskeletal components of the groin and pelvis (Fig. 16). Alterations in signal of musculotendinous units are, however, common in asymptomatic patients. MR arthrography can be useful in detecting intraarticular pathology of the hip joint, although arthroscopy is now superseding this. Gadolinium enhancement can reveal obscure pathology such as an obturator hernia and may also enhance other pathologies.

Hip arthroscopy

Hip arthroscopy is useful for the investigation of groin pain where articular pathologies are suspected, in particular where interventions can be performed simultaneously. It is technically demanding and requires the use of specialized equipment. As has been the case when other large joints are investigated with arthroscopic techniques, the preoperative diagnosis is often altered by the intraarticular findings. In one series of 328 patients who underwent hip arthroscopy, a preoperative diagnosis was reached in 174 patients (53 per cent), while the remaining 154 were diagnosed as having 'idiopathic hip pain'.[6, 7] In seven patients, access to the hip was inadequate. Arthroscopy

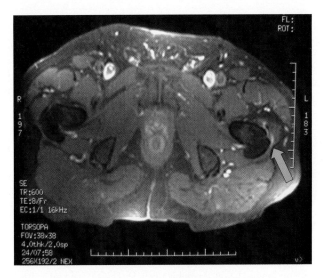

Fig. 16 T2 fast spin echo fat saturated MRI of the pelvis with gadolinium enhancement, showing a trochanteric bursitis/enthesophy.

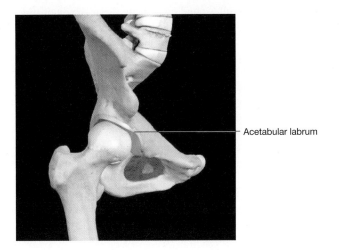

— Acetabular labrum

Fig. 17 The acetabular labrum.

altered the diagnosis in 176 hips (53 per cent). The new primary diagnoses were OA (75 patients), osteochondral defects (34), torn labra (23), synovitis (11), and loose bodies (9). In 172 hips (52 per cent) an operative procedure was undertaken. In the OA group the 70 procedures included 47 chondroplasties, 17 labrectomies, and six removals of loose bodies. In the remaining 84 patients (26 per cent), arthroscopy neither changed the diagnosis nor provided surgical treatment. Edwards *et al.* reported that hip arthroscopy is more reliable than MRI for the detection of chondral abnormalities, labral tears, and loose bodies. In their series, the most common new diagnoses made were of chondral lesions and labral tears (Fig. 17).[7]

Muscle injuries

Muscle strains

Muscle strains, where muscle fibres sustain damage due to indirect injury, are common injuries, particularly in the lower limb. Such

Table 4 Grading of muscle injuries (adapted from reference 8)

Grade of injury	Description	Clinical findings[a]
I	Microscopic damage to muscle or myotendinous unit	Pain on stretch and stress. Bruising may be evident. No/little effect on range of motion and function
II	Partial tear of muscle or myotendinous unit	Pain on stretch and stressing. A palpable gap and weakness may be evident. Decrease in range of motion and function
IIIA	Rupture of muscle or myotendinous unit	Obvious gap, significant decrease in range of motion and function
IIIB	Avulsion of tendon attachment to bone	

[a] Pain, tenderness, and bruising can be a feature of all.

Table 5 Avulsion injuries within the pelvic region

Site	Muscle
Anterior superior iliac spine	Sartorius
Anterior inferior iliac spine	Rectus femoris
Iliac crest	External oblique
Ischial tuberosity	Hamstrings
Lesser trochanter	Iliopsoas
Greater trochanter	Gluteus medius and minimus
Inferior pubic ramus	Gracilis

injuries usually occur at the myotendinous junction during eccentric contractions. Muscles at particular risk are those that have a relatively high percentage of type II (fast-twitch) muscle fibres, that frequently work eccentrically during fast movements, and that cross two joints (as they are susceptible to injury at both sites). O'Donoghue classified muscle strains into three groups, according to the extent of the injury (Table 4).[8]

Avulsion injuries typically occur in adolescents due to a sudden contraction of the muscle group across an open apophysis. The most commonly affected sites are the anterior superior and inferior iliac spines and the ischium (Table 5; Fig. 18).

The extent of symptoms and signs in muscle injuries is often indicative of the severity of the injury. The patient notes the acute onset of pain and, where significant injury has occurred, echymosis, swelling, and reduced function. Where a significant tear or rupture is experienced, there is a palpable lump and local defect in the muscle, representing the retracted muscle edge and the remaining gap.

Investigations are usually not necessary. However, bony avulsion fractures will be demonstrated on plain X-ray. In these cases care must be taken to compare with the unaffected side, as the injury may take the appearance of a widened physeal plate. Ultrasound and MRI can both demonstrate minor muscle strains, but are particularly useful in differentiation between grade II and III injuries. Ultrasound has the advantage of providing dynamic imaging, particularly useful in

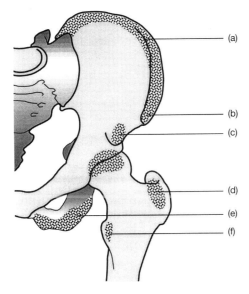

Fig. 18 Pelvic apophyses are sites of avulsion injuries in adolescents. (a) Iliac crest (external obliques); anterior superior iliac spine (sartorius); anterior inferior iliac spine (rectus femoris); (d) greater trochanter (gluteus maximus and medius) (e) ischial tuberosity (hamstrings); (f) lesser trochanter (iliopsoas).

chronic posterior thigh pain in the active individual. Fatty degeneration and fibrosis are common in chronic complete ruptures.

Treatment

The initial management of the acute muscle strain involves the RICE (rest, ice, compression, elevation) regime and analgesics. Ice massage is often very helpful but deep massage is avoided and other modalities are unproven. Passive and active range of motion exercises are encouraged and then a strengthening regime commencing with isometric work and progressing through concentric and eccentric contractions before sport-related activities are introduced. Correction of muscle imbalances, warm-up and stretching errors, and biomechanical and technical errors is vital. Return to sport occurs when these issues have been adequately addressed and at least 90 per cent of strength has been regained. It is rare for surgery to be necessary, even in grade III injuries.

Treatment of avulsion injuries also involves analgesia, protected weight-bearing, and progressive rehabilitation, and surgical intervention is rarely necessary.

Anterior hip and groin pain

Adductor injuries

Adductor injuries are common in the athletic population, particularly footballers and hurdlers, and may be related to an acute event or to chronic overuse. Injury may be localized to the musculotendinous junction, the muscle belly, or at the insertion on to the pubic tubercle, and the latter may be associated with osteitis pubis or symphysis instability. Muscle or musculotendinous injuries are graded in the same manner as other muscle injuries and usually involve adductor longus (Fig. 19).

In the acute injury, the typical mechanism is that of eccentric adductor contraction with the hip in abduction and external rotation, for example, a blocked kick in soccer. The pain, adductor spasm,

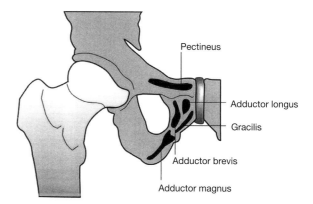

Fig. 19 Insertions of adductor muscles onto the pelvis.

tenderness, and (in the acute injury) swelling can be easily located to the adductor longus, below the pubic tubercle. There is pain on resisted adduction and, in some cases, flexion. Imaging studies are usually not necessary but may be indicated to exclude other causes of groin or thigh pain. In the suspected avulsion fracture, plain radiographs are necessary. MRI and ultrasound will demonstrate tendinopathies and muscle damage, but non-specific intratendinous alterations on imaging are common in the active asymptomatic patient.

Management

In the acute stage, the RICE regime is followed and then a strengthening and stretching programme commenced before sport-specific rehabilitation, as described earlier. Some recommend that acute muscle ruptures are surgically repaired, particularly in the athlete.[9] Chronic tendon injuries are treated similarly but progress may be slow and the patient must be counselled in relation to this in order to prevent premature return to sporting activities. A peritendinous cortisone injection near the insertion may help to reduce pain in resistant tendinopathies. Adductor longus tenotomy may also be considered in those with persisting localized pain,[10] followed by progressive rehabilitation. Although a decrease in muscle strength may result, this does not seem to be functionally relevant.

Pubic symphysis instability

Instability of the pubic symphysis can occur in females following childbirth when the ligamentous laxity induced in the ligaments of the pelvis at childbirth fails to repair—a phenomenon first recognized by Hippocrates. It also occurs in athletes (usually male) after several years of groin pain treated sufficiently to allow a return to sport but without adequate retraining or strengthening of the pelvic and other muscles controlling the symphysis. The patient presents with a nagging ache radiating from the midline down into the adductor region and the perineum. Walking and running exercise aggravates the pain, which persists with rest for some time. X-rays show signs of osteitis pubis. Stork views of the symphysis, performed standing on one leg and then the other, may reveal obvious instability across the symphysis. The normal displacement is <0.2 mm.

Management involves rehabilitation to regain muscle control with a core stability programme. The exercises are quite difficult to perform even without injury, and the re-training has to be given sufficient time, at least 3–6 months, to judge whether or not it is successful. In the female with instability post-childbirth, a sacroiliac belt and reassurance are particularly useful. A surgical fusion using autogenous bone graft and plate fixation can be effective,[11] but posterior pelvic instability with pain around the sacroiliac joints, occurring 1 and 5 years postoperatively, has been reported.[12]

Osteitis pubis

The term 'osteitis pubis' implies an inflammatory process affecting the pubic symphysis. However, inflammation of the symphysis is frequently not a histological finding in chronic symphysis pain and the term is more commonly used to describe radiological changes at the symphysis, including widening, demineralization, resorption, periosteal reaction, and sclerosis.[13] Such changes present a differential diagnosis that includes osteomyelitis, hyperparathyroidism, sarcoidosis, inflammatory arthritis, and haemachromatosis. In the absence of these disorders, biomechanical abnormalities are considered to be the cause, resulting in excessive movement across the joint. Such biomechanical aberrations may be associated with relative restriction in joints at other sites around the pelvis, resulting in increased stress at the symphysis. Changes are more common in soccer players and where there is cyclical loading such as in running, when compared with controls, but may be asymptomatic.

Pain ascribed to osteitis pubis is anterior midline, radiating bilaterally along the adductor muscles, and around into the perineum. There may be localized tenderness over the pubic symphysis in the early stages of the condition. In the early stages of osteitis pubis, pain may be bilateral, radiating to the adductor region. In this situation a flare can be seen on bone scan and MRI shows changes within the pubic rami. Secondly, when the condition reaches the stage where the pubic symphysis is frankly unstable, a midline pain or a dull nagging ache can become sufficiently severe to be disabling.

Where pain ascribed to osteitis pubis is present, the X-ray appearances of osteitis pubis can lag behind the clinical picture and may remain after the symptoms settle with conservative measures.[14] Le Jeune *et al.* investigated 32 cases of pubic pain with scintigraphy using technetium 99m and reported a closer relationship with the clinical course when the scan was positive, although they did not give the clinical history for their cases.[15] More recently, MRI scanning has shown changes of oedema within the pubic symphysis in patients with chronic groin pain.

Recommended treatment of osteitis pubis includes a long period of relative rest, analgesics, and an exercise regime to re-train the weakened pelvic musculature. A core stability programme to improve control of the pelvic muscles that control movement of the hip and lower spine, and to improve strength and control of the anterior abdominal wall is central to management, as with symphyseal instability. Symptoms may take 6–12 months or more to settle.

In recalcitrant cases, the use of steroid injection has been advocated. However, there is no convincing evidence that this is of any benefit and is more a reflection of the limited options available in a difficult condition.

Hernia

Inguinal hernia

A hernia is defined as the protrusion of a loop or knuckle of an organ through an abnormal opening. An *indirect* inguinal hernia leaves the abdomen at the internal ring and passes along the inguinal canal eventually leading to the scrotum. A direct inguinal hernia emerges between the inferior epigastric artery and the edge of the rectus muscle. The *direct* hernia is often simply a weakness wall of the posterior inguinal canal, formed by the internal oblique and transversalis abdominus muscles.

An inguinal hernia may cause pain as a presenting symptom. The patient complains of a dull nagging ache in the inguinal region, frequently prior to the swelling of the hernia becoming apparent (*subclinical hernia*). Interestingly, once the hernia appears the discomfort often subsides.

A hernia is detected by direct palpation over the inguinal canal and asking the patient to cough. A cough impulse is diagnostic. In males, the palpation is most accurately performed by invaginating the scrotum. A subclinical hernia can be identified using dynamic ultrasonography. Herniography is rarely used now as a result. The treatment is a surgical repair where symptoms warrant it.

Sports hernia (athletic pubalgia, Gilmore's groin)

The concept of the sports hernia, also known as athletic pubalgia, Gilmore's groin, and footballer's hernia, has been popularized in the last decade.[16–18] The condition is reported in males, in relation to a number of specific activities, especially soccer.

Aetiology

The condition is considered to be a generalized distension of the anterior abdominal wall with an incompetence of the posterior inguinal wall. Several theories of causation of sports hernia have been described.[19–23] According to one theory, a reduction in internal rotation of the hip joint produces a shearing force across the pubic symphysis from continued adductor pull.[20] Shearing across the pubic symphysis leads to stress on the inguinal wall musculature. The anatomical defects in the wall, that is, the inguinal rings, may account for the predominance of this condition in the male. The stretching of the conjoined tendon and transversalis with tearing of these structures from the inguinal ligament accounts for the pain.[21] An alternative theory is that it is simply a chronic stretching of the posterior inguinal wall due to the excess demands of sport.[22, 23] The condition is exceptionally rare amongst females, if it occurs at all.

History

The groin pain may be of gradual onset, or may develop after a sudden injury. The initial pain is often described as an ache or stiffness in the adductor region that develops after sport. Early symptoms include pain around the adductor muscles, across to the midline and the inguinal region and may spread laterally, proximally into the rectus muscles and distally into the perineum. There may be a history of cough impulse, and testicular pain is a feature in about 30 per cent of cases.

Examination

The findings on examination are also varied. Some clinical features are notably similar to those of osteitis pubis and symphysis instability. By definition, there is no palpable hernia.

There may be adductor spasm with tenderness around the belly and origin of the adductor longus. The ipsilateral pubic tubercle and the symphysis pubis and peripubic area are tender to palpation. There is pain with resisted hip adduction and with sit-ups. The inguinal rings and cough impulse must be assessed via the scrotum. The area around the enlarged external inguinal ring is tender. The midinguinal canal is the site of the worst discomfort and pain is aggravated by coughing, with the cough impulse felt over a wider area. The testes should be formally examined to exclude local pathology.

Investigations

Imaging studies are used primarily to exclude other pathologies. Plain X-rays may show changes consistent with osteitis pubis. MRI abnormalities are non-specific and common, and include changes consistent with osteitis and/or altered signal within structures of the abdominal wall (e.g. rectus abdominus), adductors, or the perineal region. Herniography shows a generalized distension of the anterior abdominal wall extending around to the perineum, indicating that the pathology is not related to the inguinal wall alone.[24] However it is not routinely used and clinical suspicion and direct visualization is the preferred approach.[25, 26]

Treatment

Conservative management includes a controlled progressive rehabilitation programme. This commences with relative rest and deep tissue massage, adding stretching exercises of the hip/thigh muscles and lumbar spine, performed 2–3 times daily. Light aerobic activity (e.g. static bicycling, aqua jogging, swimming) follows and then a progressive strengthening programme is introduced, targeting the abdominal muscles, hip flexors, and adductors. In the next stage, functional activities are included and, eventually, a graduated return to sport is attempted.

Typically, rest settles the pain, but it is reported to return rapidly on resuming sport. When patients fail to settle with conservative treatment, surgical repair should be considered, as excellent results are reported, with over 80 per cent returning to competition postoperatively.[27] Operative findings are a weakening and thinning of the conjoined tendon of transversalis and internal oblique muscles—the weakness amounts to a direct hernia. With a short duration of symptoms the defect seems to be more to the medial end of the inguinal canal. The repair tightens up the weaknesses, drawing down good tissue to strengthen the attenuated tissues. The surgical technique used does not seem to matter providing tension is restored to the muscles of the posterior wall of the inguinal canal. Laparoscopic repair has also been reported.[27] Postoperatively, a rehabilitation programme as described earlier is followed, with expected return to sporting activity at 6 weeks.

Snapping hip syndrome

A 'snapping hip' may arise as a result of a number of intra- and extraarticular pathologies (Table 6). The iliopsoas tendon and its underlying bursa is the most common source, due to tightness, tendinopathy, and/or bursitis, when the tendon glides over the lesser trochanter or iliopectineal eminence and snaps as it does so. Other causes of snapping hip include subluxation of the femoral head or flicking of the iliofemoral ligament over it, suction phenomena within the joint, and flicking of either the iliotibial band or tendon of gluteus maximus over the greater trochanter. Contributing factors are muscle imbalance and poor flexibility, biomechanical derangements, and training or technical errors.

Acute injury to the tendon or bursa can occur due to a direct blow or to overuse, particularly in runners, hurdlers, and soccer players.

Table 6 Causes of clicking or snapping hip

Extraarticular
Iliopsoas tightness, tendinopathy, or bursitis
Tight tensor fascia latae
Trochanteric bursitis
Piriformis syndrome
Articular
Loose bodies within the hip joint
Tear of the acetabular labrum
Subluxing hip joint

Iliopsoas bursitis is associated with a number of hip pathologies, including arthritides, sepsis, and osteonecrosis. Such complaints must always be considered in the patient with a bursitis.

History

Deep groin pain is reported, which is worse with activities, in particular, climbing stairs. Symptoms may also be aggravated by prolonged sitting, in particular, when a bursa is present. A 'click', 'clunk', or snapping sensation is felt deep in the groin when the leg is rotated and flexed, for example, as the trail leg crosses a hurdle. The clunk or snap can give rise to a deep ache. When sufficiently large, a bursitis may also present as a painful or painless inguinal mass, or with symptoms related to a compressive effect, such as femoral nerve irritation or femoral venous engorgement. A large bursa can even cause compression of the large bowel or bladder.

Examination

Localized tenderness over the iliopsoas tendon is present. A very large bursa may be palpable. Stretching the psoas tendon and stressing the musculotendinous unit through passive, active, and resisted movements of the hip can reproduce the pain felt by those suffering this injury and are used as a diagnostic tests, as described earlier.

Investigation

A plain radiograph is helpful in the initial evaluation to exclude other causes of groin pain, although articular disease and iliopsoas bursitis can coexist. MRI will image the soft tissue and bony structures more clearly, and is particularly useful when coexisting pathologies are likely. Dynamic ultrasonography is frequently diagnostic in a bursitis or tendinopathy. The bursa is typically heart-shaped or has an hourglass appearance in the transverse plane due to compression by the iliopsoas tendon. Concomitant effusion of the hip indicates communication between the joint and bursal space, and coexisting hip disease should be suspected. Although the frequency of the communication in the general population is in the region of 15 per cent, it is commonly noted in those with a bursitis and, in particular, with underlying hip disease, which is the primary pathology. The use of ultrasound also provides the opportunity for aspiration of the bursa under direct guidance. Aspiration is mandatory if sepsis is suspected and is also helpful in the relief of acute symptoms. Heterogeneity of iliopsoas fibres in the presence of a tendinopathy can also be demonstrated (Fig. 20).

Further investigations, including a white cell count, erythrocyte sedimentation rate (ESR), and uric acid and blood and bursal fluid cultures, are performed as appropriate.

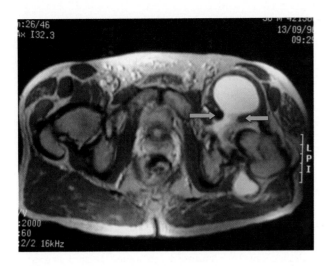

Fig. 20 T2-weighted spin echo MRI of the pelvis showing an iliopsoas bursa.

Treatment

Treatment of both tendinopathy and bursitis initially involves relative rest, nonsteroidal anti-inflammatory drugs (NSAIDs), and attention to the underlying cause(s) of the complaint (e.g. overuse, biomechanical abnormalities or primary hip disease). A stretching programme is usually very successful. The most common reason for failure of stretching is a poor stretching technique or poor compliance, which, when corrected, gives the desired result. In resistant iliopsoas tendinopathy, surgical division of the tendon may be considered.

In the most resistant cases of bursitis, a local corticosteroid injection (in the absence of sepsis) can be considered, but the physician must note the frequency of communication with the hip joint. When performed, injection under ultrasound guidance is the preferred option.

Calcific tendinitis of the hip

Calcification at the site of origin of one or more muscles of the thigh, most commonly the rectus femoris, gluteus maximus, or vastus lateralis, has been described, although it is a rare event. Acute groin pain and limitation of movement (due to pain), without a history of trauma, are presenting features. Management includes relative rest, analgesics or NSAIDs, ultrasound, shock wave therapy, and, if necessary, image-guided local corticosteroid injection.

Pain referred from the lumbar spine

Pain referred from the spine may cause groin pain. Asociated pathologies include 'mechanical' back pain, facet joint dysfunction/arthritis, lumbar root pain (e.g. from a prolapsed intervertebral disc), or a spondylolysis/lysthesis. Patients describe a poorly localized, diffuse pain in the anterior pelvis and thigh. Confusingly, there may be no back pain at all. The diagnosis is considered by excluding other causes of groin pain, closely scrutinizing the spine, and recognizing that the pattern of pain does not fit any of those described in this chapter.

Investigations

Investigations such as a plain radiograph and ultrasound may be necessary to exclude hip pathologies. Lumbar spine X-rays are not performed routinely, but, for example, where a spondyloslysis/lysthesis is suspected, oblique radiographs of the lumbar spine are necessary to demonstrate the defect of the pars interticularis. Bone scan, single-photon emission computerized tomography (SPECT) scan, or MRI will help determine whether the lesion (usually at L5) is active. A trial injection of local anaesthetic under X-ray control into the pars defect may trigger the patient's pain as the needle enters the pathological area—the pain is then relieved by the local anaesthetic. MRI scanning to assess for a prolapsed disc is performed if the clinical picture warrants it.

Treatment

Treatment of spinal conditions is addressed in other sections of this book. Treatment of spondylolysis initially involves relative rest and analgesics. A polypropylene brace may help to control symptoms. Recommendations for their use range from waking hours to 23 hours per day and from 3 to 6 months. If symptoms persist, then surgery (fusion/screw fixation) should be considered.

Ilioinguinal and genitofemoral nerve entrapment

Ilioinguinal and genitofemoral neuralgias are characterized by dysaethesiae and/or burning pain in the appropriate distribution of the nerve. Nerve injury or entrapment in the inguinal facia can occur after surgery (e.g. herniorrhaphy, appendicectomy, Caesarean section) and has also been described in systemic sclerosis. Local blockade of the ilioinguinal nerve or paravertebral blocks of L1 and L2 (genitofemoral nerve) can confirm the diagnosis. A tricyclic agent or carbemazepine may reduce symptoms but, if symptoms are severe, neurolysis may be indicated.[28, 29]

Hip joint pathology

The wide differential diagnosis of pain in the hip and groin includes articular diseases. These are briefly outlined here, but readers are referred to more extensive texts. Pain arising from the hip joint is a potent cause of pain arising from the groin anterior thigh and around the trochanteric bursa. Osteoarthritis is common and may cause pain.

Osteoarthritis of the hip joint

Although predominantly a disease of the elderly, OA is often missed as the cause of groin pain in younger people. Active individuals in particular can present with early disease, with symptoms interfering with—but not necessarily as a result of—their activities. There may be a history of hip problems as a child, such as Perthes disease and slipped upper femoral epiphysis. There is a history of a general aching in the groin, associated with weight-bearing and relieved by rest. As the degeneration progresses, stiffness and exacerbation of pain at the extremes of range of movement develop. Features such as night pain and profound restriction of range of motion occur relatively late in the progression of the condition.

A high association between labral lesions and adjacent acetabular chondral damage has been reported.[30] Arthroscopic and anatomical observations support the concept that labral disruption and degenerative joint disease frequently are part of a continuum of joint pathology.

Examination

The severely arthritic hip has a reduced range of motion in all planes. However, in early disease the limitation may be subtle. The first movements to be lost vary but tend to be those of combined flexion and external rotation, and abduction.

Investigation

The diagnosis is confirmed by plain X-ray. In early cases this will show changes that include increased subchondral sclerosis, slight reduction in joint space, and a flattening of the femoral head with curtain osteophytes. Subchondral cysts appear later. The findings may be quite subtle and need careful inspection. MRI scan is becoming increasingly accurate in examining the state of the articular surface and may reveal an early effusion. The most accurate investigation is hip arthroscopy.

Treatment

Treatment of early and moderate disease is symptomatic and includes counselling of the patient with respect to the nature of the condition, emphasizing a positive approach. Modification of activities may be necessary. Shock-absorbing insoles may be helpful to reduce impact associated with activities. Correction of a leg-length discrepancy and stretching and strengthening of the muscles of the hip girdle and thigh are very important as muscle weakness and imbalances are common. Analgesics or NSAIDs can be useful on an as-required basis but continuous or extensive use should be discouraged. Obese patients should be encouraged to lose weight. Coexisting soft tissue lesions such as trochanteric or psoas bursitis are relatively common and should be addressed. Glucosamine/chondroitin sulfate may be useful in slowing progression of early OA, although this is contentious. In the young patient with early/moderate disease, arthroscopy may be helpful in evaluating the joint surface for localized labral lesions and lavage.

Severe OA is often associated with constant pain, day and night. While all the measures described above should be pursued, surgery must be considered in such cases. Resurfacing techniques may be suitable in the younger patient without deformation of the femoral head. Otherwise, joint replacement is the intervention of choice.

Acetabular labral tears

The acetabular labrum is a thick rim of dense fibrous tissue that provides extra stability. The labrum can become degenerate and tear, producing a flap that can interfere with the joint giving a deep, painful clunk. This can occur in a wide range of activities. Some cases are idiopathic. Others are related to trauma.

Clinical examination is generally unhelpful, revealing an occasionally irritable hip joint, but there is no sensitive clinical test. X-ray may show lateral marginal sclerosis in longstanding cases.

MR arthrography of the hip is a minimally invasive diagnostic technique, which has been compared to the findings at subsequent operations.[31] In a study of individuals with groin pain, 22 subjects had a positive acetabular impingement test (pain in flexion and internal rotation) and 15 had radiological evidence of hip dysplasia.[31] In 21 of the patients, MR arthrography suggested either degeneration or a tear of the labrum or both. These findings were confirmed at operation in 18 patients, but there was no abnormality of the labrum in the other three. In two of the patients, MR arthrography erroneously suggested an intact labrum. Lesions of the superior labrum are most easily detectable and these may appear slightly larger on arthrography than at operation. Similar findings have been reported from investigating the technique when performed upon cadavers. A good correlation was found for large tears, less so for small tears and degeneration of the labrum.[32] Labral tears can be identified and trimmed arthroscopically.

Dislocation and subluxation of the hip joint

Dislocation generally requires a high degree of trauma, but subluxation has been described in adolescents with congenital hyperlaxity syndrome and, less commonly, in patients with significant neuromuscular impairment. Symptoms include a clunking, snapping, or popping felt in the groin followed by aching. This is rare and patients are generally aware of the nature of their underlying condition. Treatment generally involves reassurance and strength and stability exercises. Thermal capsular shrinkage of the hip may be considered.

Stress fractures of the pelvic bones

Although not soft tissue, stress fractures form an important part of the differential diagnosis of pain arising from the pelvis and groin. Stress fractures are a result of repetitive microtrauma which overcomes local healing mechanisms. They can arise due to overuse (fatigue fractures) or subnormal bone strength (insufficiency fracture). Pelvic stress fractures account for 1–2 per cent of stress fractures, but can be far more significant in terms of the harm they can cause. Fractures occur in the pubic rami or the proximal femur and, most seriously, the femoral neck.

The symptoms of a severe, deeply felt pain in the groin are of gradual onset. They follow an increase in training load for a sportsman or woman, and occasionally occur during a long-distance race, or with minimal or no trauma in an osteoporotic individual. Weight-bearing is painful, and pain occurs at rest and at night. A sudden worsening may indicate a completion of the fracture. With this story the patient must be investigated urgently and advised to rest the limb.

Investigations

The most common stress fracture of the pelvis involves the pubic rami. As with all stress fractures, the diagnosis can be made by plain X-ray after 3 weeks, but earlier by technetium bone scan or MRI scan.

Treatment

Stress fractures of the pubic rami can be treated with adequate rest in the expectation that they will heal without complication. Non-weight-bearing mobility with crutches while symptoms persist should be undertaken. Athletes can continue to exercise in non-weight-bearing sports when the stress fracture has settled sufficiently to allow walking.

Stress fractures of the femoral neck are seen on either the superior or inferior surfaces of the femoral neck. The biomechanics of the femoral neck produce compression on the inferior aspect and tension on the superior surface. With rest, compression fractures can be expected to heal. Tension fractures, however, will complete across the femoral neck if the patient continues to walk. This is an extremely serious situation as the fracture will not heal normally, and there is a risk that the femoral head will die. If the fracture is seen before completion, then prophylactic fixation is necessary. If the fracture completes, then reduction and fixation must be performed. However, in published series, no displaced fractures healed to produce a normal hip. In the worst case the patient requires joint replacement.

Anterior thigh pain

Injuries to the muscles of the thigh consist of contusions, delayed-onset muscle soreness, and strains (grades I–III). Such injuries are common: in an audit of injuries in professional football, thigh strains were the most commonly noted injury.[33]

Rectus femoris strains

Rectus femoris has two heads of origin—the reflected head arising just above the acetabulum and the straight head from the ASIS. It is the most superficial of the quadriceps muscles and is unprotected from injury relative to the other components of the quadriceps, particularly as it crosses two joints.

The mechanism of rectus femoris strain is that of forceful stretch of the muscle, as a result of resisted flexion of the hip and/or extension of the knee. This occurs with sudden acceleration, or a change in speed. Contributing factors include overload (e.g. weight-lifting), poor flexibility, lack of warm-up, and anabolic steroid intake.

Functional imbalance between quadriceps and hamstrings is also a major contributor. The normal quadriceps:hamstrings strength ratio is 3:2, but relative neglect of hamstrings strengthening commonly leads to ratios in the range of 5:1. The usual site of strain injuries is the myotendinous junction.

The patient presents with a history of acute thigh pain and reduced function and often a sensation of tearing during the acute event. The mechanisms described earlier are usually involved. There is usually swelling ecchymosis and a palpable lump or gap with significant injury may be particularly notable as the bruising begins to settle. Resisted knee flexion is painful and weak, particularly in hip extension if rectus femoris is involved. Investigations are not usually necessary. Ultrasound confirms significant injury, can exclude other causes of masses in the thigh, and provides an opportunity to perform ultrasound-guided aspiration of the haematoma.

Investigations

X-ray is necessary if a bony avulsion injury is suspected. MRI is indicated only when there is a diagnostic query.

Treatment

The usual RICE protocol is followed, with restricted range of motion, and then a progressive stretching and strengthening programme with correction of any functional imbalance of quadriceps/hamstrings. Grade I and II strains usually return to sport in 4–6 weeks, provided they have full pain-free range of motion and have regained nearly complete (90 per cent) strength. Grade III injuries also settle with this regime although they can take significantly longer to settle. Surgical reconstruction may be necessary in some.

Quadriceps haematoma

The quadriceps contusion is distinct from a strain and typically occurs as a result of a direct blow to the quadriceps muscle, causing a deep intra- or intermuscular haematoma. The injury can occur at any site involving the muscle or myptendinous unit, unlike the typical strain that affects the later. The English term for this is a 'dead leg' but it is referred to in the American literature as a 'Charley horse'.

Clinical features

There is pain and swelling, and a sympathetic knee effusion may appear in the first 48 h. Function, in particular, knee flexion, is reduced and rarely an acute compartment syndrome can develop with extensive haemorrhage. A dynamic ultrasound scan will reveal the extent and position of the bleeding. If there is extensive trauma, an X-ray to exclude a fractured femur is necessary.

Management

Initial management is ice packs, NSAIDs, and rest with the leg and hip in 30° flexion, mobilizing on crutches if necessary. If the patient can flex the knee to 90° degrees in 48 h, then the prognosis is good. Active knee range of motion exercises are commenced early. When pain-free knee flexion reaches 120°, functional rehabilitation including progressive strengthening is pursued. Return to sport is possible when pain-free range of motion reaches 90% of normal.[34] The main complications are myositis ossificans and failure to regain strength and flexibility, with a long-term reduction in function.

Myositis ossificans

Myositis ossificans occurs as a complication of a quadriceps contusion, when a deep haematoma that involves periosteum leads to ectopic ossification. The pathology is poorly understood and some individuals may be predisposed to the development of the condition. Risk factors have been identified and include previous quadriceps injury, prolonged restriction of knee flexion to <120°, and/or a delay in treatment.

Clinically, the patient with a quadriceps contusion fails to settle and reports ongoing anterior thigh pain and swelling, often with nocturnal disturbance. The differential diagnosis includes other causes of a mass in the thigh, in particular, tumour. The stages are described in Table 7. In spite of radiographic changes, some patients note little loss of function (Fig. 21).

Management

Management is symptomatic, with relative rest, analgesics, and graduated active range of motion exercises. Other therapies have been tried without success, including radiotherapy and bisphosphonates. Surgery to remove ectopic bone is rarely necessary and is relatively contraindicated for the first 6 months.[35]

Nerve entrapments

Femoral nerve entrapment

Femoral nerve entrapment is unusual compared with the more common sciatic nerve entrapment. Symptoms include anterior thigh pain with numbness and weakness of the quadriceps. The quadriceps reflex

Table 7 Radiographic staging of mysositis ossificans

Stage	Plain radiographic changes
I	X-ray normal. (Bone scan, ultrasound, MRI show periosteal reaction)
II	Sandstorm appearance usually around the mid-third of the femur
III A	Stalk: attachment to bone
III B	Periosteal: Continuity to underlying bone
III C	Broad-based: Projection into quadriceps with a radiolucent line separating it from the femur
IV	Resorption

(a)

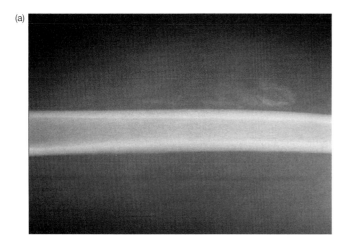

b)

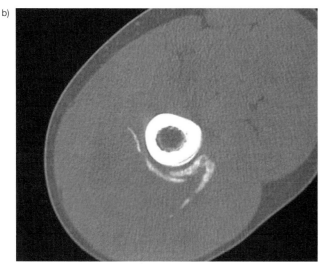

Fig. 21 (a) Plain X-ray and (b) CT of the thigh showing myositis ossificans.

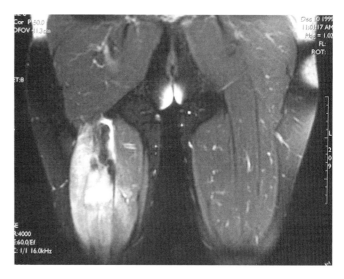

Fig. 22 T2 fast spin echo fat saturated MRI showing Grade III hamstrings injury.

jerk is reduced. The nerve roots are usually entrapped as they leave the spine, or rarely by a massive pelvic tumour.

Obturator nerve entrapment

Obturator nerve entrapment is not well recognized and is considered to be most commonly related to entrapment of the nerve within fascia as it leaves the pelvis. An obturator hernia is another possible cause, along with intrapelvic masses. The patient complains of pain and dysaesthesia in the medial thigh, together with weakness of the adductor group, worsened by activity. Specialized neurophysiological tests or nerve blockade are helpful in confirming the diagnosis. Surgical release of the fascia overlying the nerve in the obturator foramen will release the entrapment. Neurolysis along the length of the nerve from the obturator foramen to the fascia between pectineus and adductor longus is required to ensure release.[36]

Meralgia paraesthetica

Meralgia paraesthetica (Greek: *meros*, thigh; *algia*, pain) occurs when the lateral cutaneous nerve of the thigh (L2,3) becomes entrapped or irritated. The nerve is entirely sensory and supplies an area of skin over the lateral thigh. It runs along the lateral border of the psoas muscle and along the ilium, passing just medial to the ASIS. This is the most common site of entrapment, which may relate to direct trauma (including surgery in this region), pressure from tight-fitting clothes, weight gain, ascites, or pregnancy. The patient complains of a burning pain and dysaesthesiae in the distribution of the nerve. Symptoms may be exacerbated by activity, prolonged standing, or specific postures. Altered sensation of the affected skin is noted, and a Tinel's test at the site of entrapment may be positive. The diagnosis is usually clinical, although electrodiagnostic studies and nerve blockade with local anaesthetic can also be useful.

Treatment is to address the cause(s) and to control symptoms as necessary. NSAIDs may be helpful, as may local infiltration with corticosteroid and anaesthetic. In severe or intractable cases, surgical release of the nerve by a suprainguinal approach can be considered.[37]

Posterior hip, buttock, and thigh pain

Hamstring injuries

The hamstrings and, in particular, the biceps femoris are the most commonly injured muscle group in relation to sporting activities. The biceps femoris crosses two joints and is therefore more vulnerable to injury.

The medial hamstrings (semimembranosis and semitendinosis) are most likely to be injured during the swing phase of gait, whereas the lateral hamstrings (biceps femoris) are most vulnerable during take off, due to the heightened activity in these muscle groups during specific phases of gait.

Injuries include strains, avulsion injuries, and contusions and particularly occur in those sports that involve high-speed or ballistic movements: gymnastics, sprinting, hurdling, basketball, soccer, and rugby. Injury usually occurs when there has been a sudden hip flexion and knee extension. Poor flexibility, inadequate warm-up, muscle fatigue, muscle imbalance (medial hamstrings: lateral hamstrings, or hamstrings: quadriceps), leg-length discrepancy, and previous injury are all predisposing factors. Injury can occur within the muscle belly, at the myotendinous junction, or at the tendon insertion on the ischial tuberosity (Fig. 22).

The extent of symptoms and signs is indicative of the severity of the injury. Immediate pain in the posterior thigh with reduced function is noted at the onset, occasionally with a 'pop'. There is ecchymosis and swelling, muscle spasm, and, if rupture has occurred, a palpable lump and associated defect. Where the injury is chronic, symptoms present with a deep, dull ache in the thigh and occasionally the buttock. Symptoms are worse with passive or active stretching and frequently with prolonged sitting. Weakness is detectable where there is significant pain and/or disruption. Commonly, a loss of up to 20° of full knee extension in grade I injuries and >45° in grade III injuries is noted.

Treatment

Treatment is as described above. At least 90 per cent of strength should be achieved and the normal quadriceps:hamstrings strength ratio of 3:2 should be set as a goal before a return to sport is permitted. Ruptures can be managed conservatively, but can take 18 months and functional outcome may be poor. For this reason, some recommend early repair, particularly in proximal hamstring rupture in athletes.[38]

Hamstring insertion

Insertion injuries in the adult tend to involve chronic insertional tendinopathies or acute avulsion of the insertion from bone, whereas, in the child or adolescent with open growth plates, a bony avulsion injury should be suspected.

Bony avulsion injuries

There is pain, swelling, bruising, and a palpable defect. X-ray will show a displaced fragment where an acute avulsion injury has occurred. Management is as for grade III injuries. Non-displaced fractures can be treated with the leg in protected knee flexion for 6 weeks using a hip–knee–foot orthosis and monitoring to ensure there is no further displacement. Displaced avulsions can also be managed conservatively, but if significant, acute surgical reattachment may be necessary.

Other insertion injuries

These include chronic tendinopathies and apophysitis. The gradual onset of activity-related buttock pain in an active adolescent should raise the suspicion of ischial apophysitis, although, of course, other causes of such symptoms should be considered (Table 8). Treatment is relative rest, stretching, reassurance, and analgesia.

Table 8 Causes of posterior thigh and buttock pain

Musculotendinous injury
Hamstrings
Gluteals

Neurological
Piriformis or hamstrings syndrome
Mass compressing sciatic nerve
Referred pain from lumbar spine

Other
Referred from pelvic viscera
Sacroiliitis/sacroiliac dysfunction

Chronic tendinopathy affecting the hamstrings typically affects active adults. The differential diagnosis is wide and careful clinical evaluation is mandatory. The typical story is that of a gradual onset of dull ache in the buttock and/or posterior thigh in an active individual. There may be a history of an acute injury. Examination reveals a localized tenderness at the ischial tuberosity, pain on active and passive stretch, and, frequently, weakness of hamstrings function. Associated factors such as muscle imbalances and lumbar spine dysfunction should be actively sought and addressed in managing the condition, which includes the usual combination of stretching, avoidance of aggravating activities, anti-inflammatory approaches, progressive strengthening, and, *above all*, patience.

Piriformis and hamstring syndromes

The sciatic nerve can conceivably be compressed beneath the muscles under which it travels, in particular, the piriformis and hamstrings. The 'hamstring syndrome' occurs when the nerve is compressed beneath semitendinosis and biceps femoris, usually by a constricting band.[39] The pain is worst with a straight leg raise. Conservative treatment includes passive hamstring stretch, friction massage, and NSAID therapy. Surgical release has been reported as successful.[39]

Piriformis syndrome is considered present when there is sciatic nerve irritation, presumably by a tight piriformis. Robinson is credited with introducing the term and describing its six classic findings: (1) a history of trauma to the sacroiliac and gluteal regions; (2) pain in the region of the sacroiliac joint, greater sciatic notch, and piriformis muscle that usually extends down the limb and causes difficulty with walking; (3) acute exacerbation of pain caused by stooping or lifting (and moderate relief of pain by traction on the affected extremity with the patient in the supine position); (4) a palpable sausage-shaped mass, tender to palpation, over the piriformis muscle on the affected side; (5) a positive Lasègue sign; and (6) gluteal atrophy, depending on the duration of the condition.[40]

Conservative treatment includes gentle progressive passive stretching, and direct pressure over the muscle. Benson and Schutzer described 14 patients with an average age of 38 years who were managed with an operative release of the piriformis tendon and sciatic neurolysis.[41] All 14 patients had a history of a blow to the buttock, and all had pain in the buttock, intolerance to sitting, tenderness to palpation of the greater sciatic notch, and pain with flexion, adduction, and internal rotation of the hip. Eleven patients had severe radicular pain in the affected lower limb. All 14 patients failed to improve after a prolonged period of conservative treatment with non-steroidal medication or physical therapy, or both. Lasègue's sign is pain in the vicinity of the greater sciatic notch with extension of the knee with the hip flexed to 90° and tenderness to palpation of the greater sciatic notch. Pace and Nagle described a diagnostic manoeuvre that is now referred to as Pace's sign—pain and weakness in association with resisted abduction and external rotation of the affected thigh.[42]

Spinal referred pain

Spinal pain from many sources will refer to the buttock. The characteristic lumbar back pain spreads across the lower back and into the buttock and then into the back of the thigh. Facet joints, posterior longitudinal ligaments, dura, dorsal root ganglion, and myofascial structures are all recognized as pain-generating tissues. The intervertebral disc also has nociceptive fibres in the outer annulus and may give rise to pain in the distribution described. Examination of the spine aims to reveal signs to confirm the origin of the pain.

Ischial (ischiogluteal) bursitis

Ishcial bursitis can occur after a direct blow to the ischial tuberosity, resulting in localized pain and tenderness. Relative rest, ice, anti-inflammatories, and cushioning are usually effective but a local guided injection of corticosteroid may be necessary. Surgical excision of the bursa is rarely necessary.

Sacroiliac joint (SIJ) disorders

This joint is the subject of debate as to whether it is a cause of lower back and buttock pain in the absence of a true inflammatory sacroili-itis. The convention is that the joint is extremely stable due to its shape and surrounding ligamentous structures and considerable force is required to disrupt the strong, stable construction. Movements are small and complex and there is no single fixed axis of motion, with a combination of flexion/extension, translation, nutation, and rotation all contributing. The ilium glides up on the sacrum during extension with some of the bones anterosuperiorly and the reverse occurs in flexion. Such movements are very important. During gait the SIJs and ligaments absorb and dissipate stresses developed by twisting of the pelvis due to coupling of flexion of one hip and extension of the other. The results of loss of mobility are seen in ankylosing spondylitis, where stress fractures of the joint are seen.

Strain or dysfunction can arise in active individuals, such as the military population, presumably due to the stretching of these ligaments.[43] Potential mechanisms include a direct blow to the joint, forceful torsion of the pelvis when rising from the crouched position, or sudden strong contraction of the hamstrings and/or abdominal muscles. Many injuries considered initially to be sacroiliac strains are subsequently found to be due to other pathologies, and forces upon sacroiliac ligaments are more likely to result in injury to the lumbosacral ligaments.

Pain can be experienced in the buttock, groin, or thigh with activity and, in severe cases, at rest. Stress tests may exacerbate the pain (see examination section).

Investigation

X-rays of the SIJ are usually normal in the absence of an inflammatory process. Bone scans demonstrate sacroiliitis and stress fractures at the ridges of joint surfaces. Where sacroiliitis is demonstrated, the cause must be ascertained—most importantly, seronegative arthropathy or pyogenic infection.

Management

Manipulative therapists may be able to influence exercise-induced pain in the sacroiliac joint. Muscle imbalance affecting the muscles of the thigh and abdomen and coexisting abnormalities in the lumbar spine should be addressed. A sacroiliac belt can provide some symptomatic relief. Sacroiliitis as a part of an inflammatory arthritis should be treated with analgesics, anti-inflammatories, physiotherapy, other approaches indicated for the systemic condition and, where necessary, local corticosteroid injection under imaging.

Lateral hip and thigh pain

Trochanteric bursitis

The four trochanteric bursae are situated deep to the soft tissues at the lateral hip, protecting them from the bony surface of the greater trochanter. Three of these bursae are constant: the subgluteus minimus bursa lies slightly anterior to the superior surface of the greater trochanter while subgluteus medius and subgluteus maximus lie posterosuperior and lateral to the greater trochanter, respectively (Fig. 23). A fourth, unnamed, bursa is also frequently noted. The sub-gluteus maximus is the largest of the four, and the most commonly symptomatic. It is 2–4 cm in width and 4–6 cm in length and serves as a gliding mechanism to the tendon of gluteus maximus passing over the greater trochanter to insert on to the iliotibial band.

The aetiological and clinical features of trochanteric bursitis overlap with a stress enthesopathy of the insertion of gluteus medius and minimus. The condition is more common in females and is associated with direct trauma, when a blow to the area can cause a haemobursa. Most commonly, however, it is due to overuse. Associated factors include a leg length discrepancy, lumbar spine disease, and hip pathology, with limitation of internal rotation and reflex tightening of the external rotators. Unaccustomed activity and walking/running on a cambered road may also be reported and are typically associated with a tight iliotibial band.

Investigations

Plain radiography is unhelpful unless articular pathology is suspected, although irregularities of the greater trochanter or calcification within surrounding soft tissues (after trauma) or in the bursa may be noted. Ultrasound may demonstrate irregularities of the gluteal insertions or bursal enlargement, where the differential diagnosis is that of other causes of peritrochanteric fluid collections, namely haematoma, abcess, seroma, or necrotic tumour—all considerably more rare than bursitis.

MRI may demonstrate signal abnormalities in the gluteal tendons, iliotibial band/tensor fascia lata, or the bursae, especially with gadolinium enhancement.

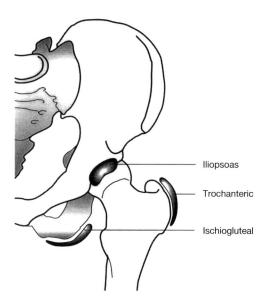

Fig. 23 Bursae around the pelvis.

Clinical features

Patients report deep aching at the lateral aspect of the hip and proximal lateral thigh, worsened with weight-bearing activities such as walking (particularly walking over uneven ground) and on inclines such as ascending stairs. A snapping, clicking, or clunking over the painful area may also be reported, due to thickened soft tissues flicking over the greater trochanter. Nocturnal pain when lying on the affected side is commonly noted.

Examination reveals localized tenderness over the greater trochanteric region. There is pain with local pressure during passive combined hip flexion and adduction and with resisted active abduction of the hip when lying on the opposite side. Gait abnormalities are common but may be cause or effect. Predisposing features include any cause of gait abnormality, including in particular leg-length discrepancy, a tight iliotibial band, coexisting lumbar spine and hip disorders, and other lower limb arthritis.

Treatment

Relative rest, NSAIDs, and stretching of the tensor fascia lata muscle and iliotibial tract are usually effective measures, providing causative factors are corrected. A heel raise may be necessary to correct a leg-length discrepancy. The efficacy of ultrasound and other modalities and massage are unproven.

Infiltration of local anaesthetic and corticosteroid into the bursal region can be highly effective. Surgery is the extreme last resort and is rarely indicated. A number of procedures have been described, including the release of the fascia lata, allowing the fascia to heal in a lengthened and tension-free position.

References

1. Clement, D.B., Taunton, J.E., and Smart, G.W. (1981). A survey of overuse running injuries. *Physician Sportsmed.* **9**, 47–58.

2. Gudas, C.J. (1980). Patterns of lower limb extremity in 224 runners. *Compr. Ther.* **6**, 50–59.

3. Renstrom, P.A. (1984). Swedish research in sports traumatology. *Chir. Orthop.* **191**, 144–158.

4. Muckle, D.S. (1982). Associated factors in recurrent groin and hamstring injuries. *Br. J. Sports Med.* **16**, 37–39.

5. Ekberg, O. (1988). Longstanding groin pain in athletes. A multidisciplinary approach. *Sports Med.* **6**, 56–61.

6. Baber, Y.F., Robinson, A.H.N., and Villar, R.N. (1999). Is diagnostic arthroscopy of the hip worthwhile? A prospective review of 328 adults investigated for hip pain. *J. Bone Joint Surg. (Br.)* **81B**, 600–603.

7. Edwards, D.J., Lomas, D., and Villar, R.N. (1995). Diagnosis of the painful hip by magnetic resonance imaging and arthroscopy. *J. Bone Joint Surg. (Br.)* **77B**, 374–376.

8. O'Donoghue, D.H. (ed.) (1984). *Treatment of injuries to athletes*, 4th edn. W.B. Saunders, Philadelphia.

9. Sangwan, S.S., Aditya, A., and Siwach, R.C. (1994). Isolated traumatic rupture of the adductor longus muscle. *Indian J. Med. Sci.* **48** (8), 186–187.

10. Akermark, C. and Johansson, C. (1992). Tenotomy of the adductor longus tendon in the treatment of chronic groin pain in athletes. *Am. J. Sports Med.* **20**, 640–643.

11. Williams, P., Thomas, D., and Downes, E. (2000). Osteitis pubis and instability of the pubic symphysis. When nonoperative measures fail. *Am. J. Sports Med.* **28**, 350–355.

12. Moore, R S., Stover, M.D., and Matta, J.M. (1998). Late posterior instability of the pelvis after resection of the symphysis pubis for the treatment of osteitis pubis. A report of two cases. *J. Bone Joint Surg. (Am.)* **80A**, 1043–1048.

13. Harris, N.H. and Murray, R.O. (1974). Lesions of the symphysis in athletes. *Br. Med. J.* **4**, 211–214.

14. Fricker, P., Taunton, J., and Ammann, W. (1991). Osteitis pubis in athletes: infection, inflammation or injury? *Sports Med.* **12**, 266–279.

15. Le Jeune, J.J., Rochcongar, P., Vazelle, F., *et al.* (1984). Pubic pain syndrome in sportsmen: comparison of radiographic and scintigraphic findings. *Eur. J. Nucl. Med.* **9**, 250–253.

16. Smedberg, S., Broome, A., Gullmo, A., and Roos, H. (1985). Herniography in athletes with groin pain. *Am. J. Surg.* **149**, 378–382.

17. Taylor, D.C., Meyers, W.C., Moylan, J.A., Lohnes, J., Bassett, F.H., and Garrett, W.E. (1991). Abdominal musculature abnormalities as a cause of groin pain in athletes. *Am. J. Sports Med.* **3**, 239–242.

18. Hackney, R.G. (1993). The sports hernia. *Br. J. Sports Med.* **27** (1), 58–61.

19. Lloyd-Smith, R., Bernard, A.M., Herry, J.Y., and Ramee, A. (1985). Survey of overuse and traumatic hip and pelvic injuries in athletes *Phys. Sports Med.* **10**, 131–141.

20. Williams, J.G.P. (1978). Limitation of hip joint movement as a factor in traumatic osteitis pubis. *Br. J. Sports Med.* **12** (3), 129–133.

21. Bowerman, J.W. (1977). *Radiology and injury in sport*, pp. 241–245. Appleton-Century-Crofts, New York.

22. Malycha, P. and Lovell, G. (1992). Inguinal surgery in athletes with chronic groin pain: the sportsman's hernia. *Aust. NZ Surg.* **62**, 123–125.

23. Polglase, A.L., Frydman, G.M., and Farmer, K.C. (1991). Inguinal surgery for debilitating groin pain in athletes. *Med. J. Aust.* **155**, 674–677.

24. Gullmo, A. (1980). Herniography, diagnosis of hernia in the groin and incompetence of the pouch of Douglas and pelvic floor. *Acta Radiol.* **361** (suppl.), 229–243.

25. Schilders, E. (2000). Groin injuries in athletes. *Curr. Orthop.* **14**, 218–423.

26. Simonet, W.T., Saylor, H.L., and Sim, L. (1995). Abdominal wall muscle tears in hockey players. *Int. J. Sports Med.* **16**, 126–128.

27. Ingoldby, C.J. (1997). Laparoscopic and conventional repair of groin disruption in sportsmen. *Br. J. Surg.* **84** (2), 213–215.

28. Harms, B.A., DeHaas, D.R., and Starling, J.R. (1984). Diagnosis and management of genitofemoral neuralgia. *Arch. Surg.* **119**, 339–341.

29. Starling, J.R., Harms, B.A., Schroeder, M.E., and Eichman, P.L. (1987). Diagnosis and treatment of genitofemoral and ilioinguinal entrapment neuralgia. *Surgery* **102**, 581–586.

30. McCarthy, J.C., Noble, P.C., Schuck, M.R., Wright, J., and Lee, J. (2001). The watershed labral lesion: its relationship to early arthritis of the hip. *J. Arthroplasty* **16** (8, suppl. 1), 81–87.

31. Leunig, M., Ungersböck, A., Ganz, R., Werlen, S., and Ito, K. (1997). Evaluation of the acetabular labrum by, MR arthrography. *J. Bone Joint Surg. (Br.)* **79B**, 230–234.

32. Plotz, G.M., Brossman, J., and Hassenpflug, J. (2000). Magnetic resonance arthrography of the acetabular labrum. Macroscopic and histological correlation in 20 cadavers. *J. Bone Joint Surg. (Br.)* **82B**, 426–432.

33. Hawkins, R.D., Hulse, M.A., Wilkinson, C., Hodson, A., and Gibson, M. (2001). The association football medical research programme: an audit of injuries in professional football. *Br. J. Sports Med.* **35** (1), 43–47.

34. Ryan, J.B., Wheeler, J.H., Hopkinson, W.J., *et al.* (1991). Quadriceps contusions: west point update. *Am. J. Sports Med.* **19**, 299–304.

35. Langeland, R.H. and Carangelo, R.T. (2000). Injuries to the thigh and groin. In *Principles and practice of orthopaedic sports medicine* (ed. W.E. Garrett, K.R. Speer, and D.T. Kirkendall), pp. 583–611. Williams and Wilkins, Philadephia.

36. Bradshaw, C., McCrory, P., Bell, S., and Brukner, P. (1997). Obturator nerve entrapment. A cause of groin pain in athletes. *Am. J. Sports Med.* **25** (3), 402–408.

37. Aldrich, E.F. and van den Heever, C.M. (1989). Suprainguinal ligament approach for surgical treatment of meralgia paraesthetica. *J. Neurosurg.* **70**, 492–494.

38. **Garret, W.E. Jr** (1996). Muscle strain injuries. *Am. J. Sports Med.* **24**, 52–58.

39. **Puranen, J. and Orava, S.** (1988). The hamstring syndrome. A new diagnosis of gluteal sciatic pain. *Am. J. Sports Med.* **16**, 517–521.

40. **Robinson, D.R.** (1947). Piriformis syndrome in relation to sciatic pain. *Am. J. Surg.* **73**, 355–358.

41. **Benson, E. and Schutzer, S.** (1999). Posttraumatic piriformis syndrome: diagnosis and results of operative treatment. *J. Bone Joint Surg. (Am.)* **81A**, 941–949.

42. **Pace, J.B. and Nagle, D.** (1976). Piriform syndrome. *Western J. Med.* **124**, 435–439.

43. **Chisin, R., Milgrom, C., Margulies, J., Giladi, M., Stein, M., Kashtan, H., and Atlan, H.** (1984). Unilateral sacroiliac overuse syndrome in military recruits. *Br. Med. J. Clin. Res.* **89**, 590–591.

6.7 The knee

David Perry

Introduction

The knee is the largest joint in the human body and in some lower mammals three distinct synovial cavities are found. The human joint has two tibiofemoral components and one patellofemoral, connected by the same synovial cavity. It is a modified hinge joint that also shows gliding and rotation of the articular surfaces on each other. As it is not constrained by the shape of its bones, it depends for stability on internal (cruciates and menisci) and external (capsule and capsular ligaments) soft tissues, supported by muscular function/co-ordination. However, the knee remains relatively unstable, being loaded in almost all activities by axial compression under the force of gravity and is therefore one of the most susceptible joints to soft tissue injury and osteochondral injury. Bone bruising or subchondral oedema shown by magnetic resonance imaging (MRI) scanning has only recently been recognized as a very common finding after injury reflecting the major loading forces through the knee, particularly in sport. It is one of the most common sites for osteochondritis dissecans, loose bodies, and synovial chondromatosis. In the seronegative spondarthritides, knee joint involvement is the most common isolated peripheral joint finding and symmetrical knee joint synovitis is common in rheumatoid arthritis. As it is the easiest joint to aspirate and a common target site for many arthropathies, including crystal synovitis, it is a frequent site for diagnostic aspiration.

Functional anatomy

Developmental anatomy

Studies of the fetal development of the knee show that by about 8 weeks it resembles that of the adult form, the patella becoming cartilaginous by 10 weeks. The cruciate ligaments and menisci develop *in situ* and are not therefore secondary capsular structures. They are lined by synovium, which in the fetus is a vascularized loose connective tissue covered by synovial cells of varied configuration. A fibrous capsule is present only in the posterior part of the joint and its appearance is so variable that it does not appear essential to the formation of intraarticular structures.

Development abnormality

The knee is commonly the site of abnormality in the disorders of epiphyseal growth. In the adolescent, ligamentous strength is effectively stronger than bone and therefore valgus/varus injuries (which in adults would be likely to cause ligamentous injury), in adolescence carry the risk of epiphyseal damage. If undetected, displacement occurs. This will lead to asymmetrical bone growth, particularly in the tibia, increasing the future risk of osteoarthritis. *Genu varum* or *valgum* will be found according to the main site of epiphyseal maldevelopment or injury. Genu varum is the most common finding in osteoarthritis because the load line of the knee is internal to the midline and genu valgum is the typical deformity of inflammatory joint disease, particularly rheumatoid arthritis.

Applied anatomy

As the knee is almost exclusively loaded in axial compression under the forces of gravity, it must combine the two opposed requirements of mobility and stability. As the femoral condyles glide and roll in the two concave curved gutters of the tibial and patellar surfaces, relative stability has to be achieved by a complex arrangement of ligaments, menisci, and tendons. The ligaments and menisci provide static stability and the muscles and tendons dynamic stability. In addition to the main function of flexion/extension, the knee allows not only gliding and rotation around a horizontal axis but also rotation though a vertical axis. In other words this allows internal and external rotation of the tibia, which is only possible because the anterior and posterior ends of the tibial condyles are flattened. The middle portion of the tibia forming the intercondylar spines acts as the central pivot, around which the movements of axial rotation occur.

Femoral condyles

The condyles are convex in both planes, the medial condyle extending a little more distally than the lateral. The tendency for the patella to slide laterally is reduced by the greater prominence of the lateral femoral condyle.

Tibial condyles

The tibial condyles are two curved gutters, flattened anteriorly and posteriorly, and the incongruity is corrected by medial and lateral menisci. During flexion and extension the tibia and patella act as a single structure in relation to the femur.

The menisci

The menisci or semilunar cartilages (Fig. 1) are crescent-shaped portions of fibrocartilage in the space between the femoral and tibial condyles. They each have an anterior and posterior horn and are triangular in cross-section. The anterior and posterior horns are anchored to the tibial condyles and correct the lack of congruence between the articular surface of tibia and femur, increasing the contact area, weight distribution, and shock absorption. It has been estimated that they transmit up to 70 per cent of body weight in extension through the lateral side and 50 per cent medially. Movement between the tibial surface and the menisci is limited by the *coronary ligaments*, connecting the outer border of the menisci with the tibial edge. The coronary ligament of the medial meniscus is shorter and stronger than that of

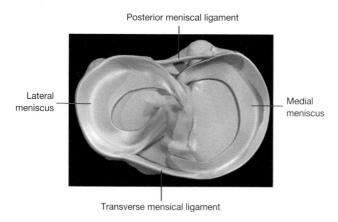

Fig. 1 Knee menisci.

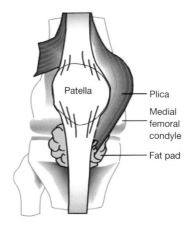

Fig. 2 The fat pad.

the lateral meniscus. The medial collateral ligament of the knee is attached by deep fibres to the outer border of the medial meniscus. There is no such connection between the lateral meniscus and the lateral collateral ligament.

The forces of injury (through sport particularly) and these anatomical attachments of the medial collateral ligament to the medial meniscus, which result in lesser mobility of the meniscus, are likely to explain the greater vulnerability of the medial meniscus to injury. The popliteus sends a fibrous band to the posterior border of the lateral meniscus and a few fibres of the semimembranosus tendon run to the posterior edge of the medial meniscus. The menisci do not have pain-sensitive structures, but the outer third does have some blood supply and therefore partial ability to heal if sutured early. The inner non-vascularized section receives nutrition through the synovial fluid and cannot be sutured.

Meniscal loading

The inner aspects of the menisci, attached by their horns to the tibial plateau, move with the tibia. During movement between tibia and femur, distortion of the menisci occurs with the body of the meniscus moving posteriorly in flexion and anteriorly in extension of the knee. In lateral rotation the menisci follow the movement of the femoral condyles, the lateral meniscus pushed forwards on the tibia and the medial meniscus pulled backwards. In medial rotation the medial meniscus is pressed forwards and the lateral meniscus backwards.

Capsule

The capsule is an ill-defined collection of fibrous sleeves mainly from tendons and their expansions. Only the synovial membrane is adherent to the peripheral surface of the menisci. The tibial attachment of the capsule is to the borders of the articular surfaces of the tibia, following its anteromedial and lateral margins. At the posterior border the synovial membrane follows the edges of the medial and lateral condyles forming a loop around the insertion of the anterior cruciate ligament. Anteriorly, the synovial membrane is indented by a large pad of adipose tissue called the infrapatellar fat pad (Fig. 2).

Anterosuperiorly, the capsule is attached proximal to the edge of the articular surface forming the suprapatellar pouch. On the lateral femoral condyle the attachment lies above the insertion of the popliteus tendon which therefore lies *intraarticularly* covered by the synovial membrane.

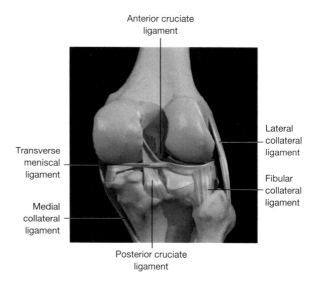

Fig. 3 The knee ligaments.

Posteriorly, the attachment follows the articular surfaces of the femoral condyle so that the attachment of the synovial membrane enters the intercondylar notch and forms a loop around the femoral insertions of the cruciate ligaments. The fused tendons of rectus femoris and vasti insert into the upper patella with superficial fibres continuing over the anterior patella into the ligamentum patellae. Thinner bands from the sides of the patella attach to the anterior border of each tibial condyle (medial and lateral patellar retinacula). Strong expansions of fascia lata lie more superficially (the iliotibial tract) and descend over the anterolateral knee to the lateral tibial condyle with a band to the lateral upper patella (superior patellar retinaculum).

Unlike other hinge joints the 'capsule' is continuous with the muscle above so that its tension can be modified in all positions.

Posterior capsule

Capsular fibres are attached to the femur above the condyle and to the intercondylar line vertically down to the upper tibia. Centrally they are strengthened by the oblique popliteal ligament. Inferolaterally they are strengthened by the arcuate popliteal ligament.

Medial capsule

These form the superficial collateral ligament, which is broad and flat and attaches to the medial epicondyle of the femur passing down and slightly anteriorly to the medial tibia. The superficial fibres attach below the tibial tubercle, deeper fibres to the medial meniscus.

Expansions of the semimembranosus tendon add considerable strength to the medial and posterior capsule.

Lateral capsule

The fibular collateral ligament is round and cord-like, separated from the lateral capsule and enclosed by an expansion of fascia lata splitting the tendon of biceps femoris.

The popliteus tendon lies between the lateral meniscus and capsule.

The lateral ligaments are most tightly stretched in extension and their lines of attachment prevent rotation of the tibia laterally or of the femur medially in extension. Rotation can therefore only be demonstrated in the flexed knee.

Stability of the knee

Medial stability

Extraarticular ligaments

The medial collateral ligament (MCL) is the *primary static stabilizer* of the medial side of the knee (Figs 3 and 4). It is the superficial component of the medial ligamentous complex, the deeper layers forming the capsular reinforcement.

The semimembranosus muscle acts as a *dynamic stabilizer*.

The MCL is a broad, flat, rather triangular band with a large femoral attachment to the posterior superior surface of the epicondyle. Its fibres run obliquely anteriorly and inferiorly to insert into the medial aspect of the tibia just behind the insertions of semitendinosus. The anterior fibres of the ligament are separated from the deeper capsular reinforcements. The anterior border of the ligament can therefore be palpated easily. The posterior fibres blend with the capsule and the medial border of the medial meniscus.

The MCL stabilizes the knee against valgus force and external rotation. *It slackens in flexion but the posterior fibres attached to the meniscus remain tight during flexion.*

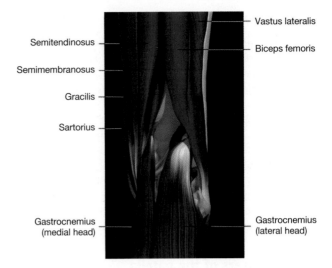

Fig. 5 The back of knee.

Lateral stability

The lateral fibular collateral ligament (Fig. 3) is a *static stabilizer* and biceps femoris with the iliotibial tract (Fig. 5) the *dynamic stabilizer*.

The lateral collateral ligament is phylogenetically the origin of peroneus longus and it extends from the lateral epicondyle of the femur to the head of the fibula. It splits the tendon of biceps femoris and is separated from the lateral meniscus by the tendon of popliteus. It is therefore important to note that the ligament lies completely free, separated from the capsule and the lateral meniscus. There is a small bursa between the lateral collateral ligament and popliteus tendon.

Intraarticular ligaments

These are named cruciates (Fig. 3) as they cross each other within the joint. They are covered by synovial membrane.

The anterior cruciate (ACL)

This extends obliquely upwards and posteriorly from the anterior intercondylar area of the tibia to attach to the medial aspect of the lateral femoral condyle. It therefore *prevents posterior displacement of the femur on the tibia*. It comprises three coiled bundles (anteromedial, intermediate, and anterolateral), which form a spiral from one insertion to the other. In extension the anterior bundle is taut and in flexion it is the posterior fibres, so that the anterior cruciate is tightest at the extremes of range of movement. The anterior cruciate prevents excessive rolling of the femoral condyles in flexion over the tibia which results in an anterior gliding of the femur. The anterior cruciate also prevents excessive tibial external rotation and varus.

The posterior cruciate ligament (PCL)

This is less oblique, shorter, and stronger. From its attachment in the posterior intercondylar area of the tibia it passes upwards and forwards, medial to the ACL, attaching to the lateral side of the medial femoral condyle. It prevents anterior displacement of the femur on the tibia, its strength is around double the anterior cruciate, and it is tightest in mid-flexion. In extension the PCL pulls on the femur causing posterior sliding and it also prevents anterior gliding of the femur during squatting. It resists hyperextension and has a role in the medial stability of the knee.

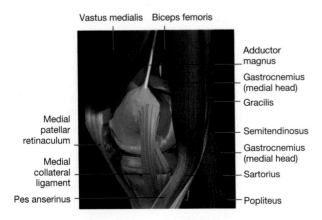

Fig. 4 The medial knee.

The patellofemoral joint

The triangular sesamoid patella is divided by a vertical median ridge on its articular surface between medial and lateral facets. The medial facet is convex, the lateral concave. The thickest articular cartilage, which may measure up to 5 mm in thickness, is present over the median ridge.

The contralateral surface of the femur has two trochlear facets, the lateral being larger and extending more proximally than the medial. The superior aspect of the lateral facet shows a smooth transition into the anterior femoral cortex, but the superior medial trochlear facet has a prominent bony and cartilagenous ridge (crescentic facet). The patella will tend to be displaced laterally during forced extension of the knee. This is counteracted by the buttress of the prominent lateral surface of the femur and the medial patellar stabilizers.

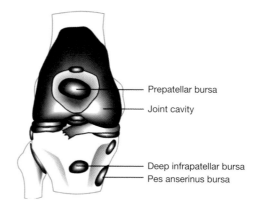

Fig. 6 The knee bursae.

Medial stabilizers of the patella

The static stabilizers on the medial side are the patellofemoral ligament superiorly and the meniscopatellar ligament inferiorly.

The dynamic stabilizers comprise the four components of the quadriceps muscle, with vastus medialis obliquus the most important component. The patellar ligament extends from the inferior portion of the patella to the tibial tubercle and has a slight lateral orientation (see Q-angle in the section on 'Patella tracking and abnormalities of patellar position').

Lateral stabilizers of the patella

The static lateral stabilizers are the patellofemoral ligament superiorly and the meniscopatellar ligament inferiorly, and the fascia lata to its attachment lateral to the patella. The static lateral stabilizers are stronger than the medial. Weakness in the stabilizers and abnormalities of patellar shape and tracking may all be components in patellofemoral symptoms.

Variations of patellar shape

Wiberg reported three major patellar variants:

1. type I, medial and lateral patella facets equal in size;

2. type II, the medial facet is slightly smaller than the lateral facet (most common type);

3. type III, the medial patella facet is smaller and there may be associated hypoplasia of the medial facet of the femur.

A flattened patella with one facet (alpine hunter's cap) is frequently associated with symptoms of instability.

A *bipartite patella* can be distinguished from a fracture radiologically by a clearly defined radiolucency with rounded margins separating the fragments with sclerosis of the margins. The lesions are usually bilateral and are seen in up to 1.5 per cent of knees. Following direct trauma they may become painful with inflammation of the fibrous union.

Patella tracking and abnormalities of patellar position

The screw-home mechanism of the knee occurs with external rotation of the tibia in the last 30 degrees of extension. This external rotation of the tibia produces the Q-angle, a valgus vector between the quadriceps

tendon and the patellar ligament. This valgus force carries the patella towards lateral displacement which must be resisted by the static and dynamic medial stabilizers and the bony architecture of the patellofemoral unit. As the knee flexes, the patella is drawn from its superolateral position on to the trochlear surface of the femur and gradually into the intercondylar notch. The patella facilitates knee extension by increasing the distance between the extensor mechanism and the axis of rotation of the femur. It also centralizes the action of the quadriceps muscle, allowing transmission of force around an angle during knee flexion with minimal friction effects.

Patellar plicae synoviales

Plicae synoviales are remnants of the embryological divisions within the knee (Fig. 2). The development of knee arthroscopy and, more recently, MRI scanning has shown that these bands are present in over 20 per cent of knees with medial plicae more common than lateral. Symptoms can develop after repetitive activities or direct injury, but it is essential before considering intervention to be sure that the symptoms do relate to the plica. At arthroscopy many plicae are probably excised unnecessarily.

Infrapatellar fat pad

The infrapatellar fat pad (Fig. 2) lies behind the patellar ligament. A portion of it is carried in between synovial folds and is frequently the site of hypertrophy. The synovial membrane, which covers the deep surface of the infrapatellar fat pad, leads to a triangular fold passing upwards and backwards to be attached by its apex to the anterior tip of the intercondylar fossa. The fold is called the infrapatellar synovial fold (ligamentum mucosum) and its free margins are known as the alar folds (ligamenta alaria).

When the knee joint is extended, the patella is drawn up by quadriceps contraction and the infrapatellar fat pad follows, thus preventing its impingement between tibia and femur. However, when the fat pad is hypertrophied or the quadriceps has lost its tone, the pad may not be drawn up sufficiently and may then be caught between the opposing articular surfaces. Repetitive impingement in this way may be associated with haemorrhage into the pad and further enlargement. Synovial folds and hypertrophy in association with generalized synovitis may also cause impingement.

Movement of the knee and patellar function (Table 1)

Extensor mechanism

The main extensor of the knee is the quadriceps femoris, one of the most powerful muscles in the body. It is formed by the rectus femoris, which spans both the knee and hip joint, and three vasti (medialis, intermedius, and lateralis), but these separate bellies have a common tendon that inserts into the anterior tibial tubercle. The patella, a triangular sesamoid bone, forms within the tendon so that there are tendon fibres all the way round the patellar edge. Therefore tenoperiosteal injury can occur at many sites although the inferior patellar pole is the most common. The infrapatellar fat pad can be seen on either side of the patellar ligament, as it lies posterior to the ligament separating this from the synovial membrane. The bursae associated with the extensor mechanism are discussed with the other bursae of the knee. The suprapatellar tendon is usually termed the quadriceps tendon and the inferior patellar tendon the patellar ligament, but the medial and lateral expansions blend with the patellar retinaculum (see 'Patellar plicae synoviales' above).

Patellar mechanism and abnormalities of patellar anatomy

The length of the patellar ligament is important as increase above the normal maximum relationship (patellar ligament 1.2 to patella length 1) further increases the risk of patellar subluxation. Abnormalities of patellar anatomy include:

- *patella alta* (high patella), with usually a small patella
- *patella baja* (low patella), seen with dysplasia or following quadriceps ligament injury.

Hyperextension of the knee is a common isolated finding in the knee, but may be part of a generalized hypermobility syndrome, for which the patient should be carefully examined particularly if involved in contact sport. Hyperextension associated with patella alta further increases the risk of subluxation and patellar injury.

As the rectus femoris crosses both the hip joint and the knee joint anterior to the flexion/extension axis to the hip, it acts as a hip flexor. As with other muscles that cross two joints (e.g. hamstrings), muscle tears appear to occur more frequently than in muscles crossing only one joint.

The vastus medialis obliquus (VMO) is the most important component of the quadriceps and contributes to medial stability of the patella and the 'screw-home' movement of the femur on the tibia in the last 10° of extension. Any injury to the knee joint produces inhibition of the quadriceps femoris, particularly in VMO, which rapidly loses bulk, tone, and control.

Some of the deeper fibres of vastus intermedius attach to the superior capsule of the knee joint preventing the suprapatellar pouch being trapped during knee movement. The tensor fasciae latae, through its attachment to the iliotibial tract, acts as a weak extensor of the knee when extended. In flexion greater than 30° the iliotibial tract causes weak knee flexion and external rotation. The main function of the iliotibial tract is *lateral stabilization of the knee*.

Knee flexion

Knee flexion is performed by the hamstrings (biceps femoris, semimembranosus, and semitendinosus) and the gastrocnemii.

1. The *biceps femoris*, through its insertion to the fibula head, fibular collateral ligament, iliotibial tract, and upper tibia and deep fascia of the calf, flexes the knee and provides lateral dynamic support.

2. *Semimembranosus*, by its insertion to the posterior and medial tibial condyle and posterior capsule, flexes the knee and gives posterior and medial stability. Its tendon extends across the posterior aspect from the medial tibial condyle upwards to the lateral femoral condyle as the *posterior oblique ligament*.

3. *Semitendinosus* joins the sartorius to insert into the upper and medial tibial shaft with gracilis ('pes anserinus' as the group of attachments looks like a goose's foot). There is an associated bursa.

Rotatory stability and rotation

Rotatory stability is achieved by the *popliteus*, which is a medial rotator of the tibia on the femur and protects the posterolateral portion of the lateral meniscus to which it attaches and therefore pulls back during knee flexion and medial rotation. Rotation is not possible in the fully extended stable knee but, as the knee flexes, *medial rotation* is performed by the sartorius, gracilis, semimembranosus, and semitendinosus. *Lateral rotation* is carried out by the biceps femoris and tensor fasciae latae.

The tibiofibular joint

The super tibiofibular joint is a plain joint with flat oval articular surfaces (facets) between the lateral condyle of the tibia and the fibula head. The *capsular ligament* attaches to the margins of the facets and

---

Table 1 Summary of knee muscle groups and innervation

Muscle groups	Peripheral nerve	Root level
Extension		
Quadriceps femoris	Femoral	L2, L3, L4
(Tensor fasciae latae)	Superior gluteal	L4, L5
Flexion		
With internal rotation		
Gracilis	Obturator	L2, L3, L4
Sartorius	Femoral	L2, L3
Semitendinosus	Tibial	L5, S1, S2
Semimembranosus	Tibial	L5, S1, S2
Popliteus	Tibial	L4, L5, S1
With external rotation		
Biceps femoris	Sciatic	L5, S1
Tensor fasciae latae	Superior gluteal	L4, L5, S1
Capsular control		
Medial: semimembranosus		
Lateral: popliteus		
Anterior: vastus intermedius		

is much thicker anteriorly. The synovial membrane of the joint may in some cases communicate with the knee joint through the popliteal bursa. The anterior ligament is two or three flat bands passing from the front of the fibula head obliquely upwards to the front of the lateral tibial condyle. The posterior ligament is a thick band from the back of the fibula head passing upwards obliquely to the posterior aspect of the lateral tibial condyle. Below the joint the shafts of the tibia and fibula are joined by the crural interosseous membrane. The *anterior tibial vessels* pass between the tibia and fibula through a gap in the upper interosseous membrane just below the fibular head.

The lateral popliteal nerve follows a line drawn from the apex of the popliteal fossa downwards and laterally along the medial side of the biceps tendon to the posterior head of the fibula. It can be rolled against the bone at this site. It then lies between the biceps femoris tendon and lateral head of gastrocnemius, winding around the fibular neck deep to peroneus longus, and then divides into musculocutaneous and anterior tibial nerves.

Popliteal fossa, nerves, and blood vessels

The popliteal fossa at the back of the knee joint (Fig. 5) is formed *superiorly* by biceps femoris laterally and semitendinosus and semimembranosus muscles medially. *Inferiorly*, the V-shape is formed by the heads of the gastrocnemii. The anterior floor of the fossa is the posterior capsule of the knee joint and popliteus. The deep popliteal fascia bounds it posteriorly. The fossa is crossed from above downwards by the tibial nerve (lateral), the popliteal vein and the popliteal artery (medial). The lateral popliteal (common peroneal) nerve descends along the inner border of the biceps. Posterior to the fibula head, the nerve splits into a deep branch, which curls around the head to enter the anterior compartment of the leg, and a superficial branch that supplies the peroneal muscles in the lateral compartment.

Vascular supply

The knee joint is supplied from branches of the popliteal, anterior tibial and a descending branch from the lateral circumflex femoral branch of the arteria profunda femoris (deep femoral artery).

Innervation and pain patterns of the knee

The knee joint is supplied by several branches of the femoral nerve, the common peroneal and tibial (sciatic). Innervation from the obturator nerve to the medial aspect of the knee explains the common referral pattern, particularly in children and the elderly, of pain from hip joint disease to the knee. Sportsmen with a rare obturator hernia also present with medial thigh and knee discomfort, sometimes with paraesthesiae.

The anterior aspect of the knee is represented by the second and third lumbar dermatomes. Therefore, where no clear cause for anterior knee pain can be found and particularly where the pain radiates upwards, the hip joint and lumbar spine must be examined carefully. Usually the patient will point to the suprapatellar area and the front of the thigh.

The skin over the posterior aspect of the knee is represented by the first and second sacral roots. Pain from the sacroiliac joint tends to refer posterolaterally to the thigh, but not as far as the back of the knee joint. Pain from the S1 and S2 roots tends to be ill defined in site and spreads upwards along the thigh or downwards into the calf. Lumbar disc compression of the S1 root or a narrowed lateral recess may just present with pain at the back of the knee. Tension tests or neurological findings should clarify the diagnosis. With discal protrusion the patient usually complains of increased pain on sitting and coughing, whereas with a narrow lateral recess, pain is usually present on walking and standing with bending relieving the pain.

Pain from localized knee lesions

Patients presenting with both localized intra-articular and extraarticular soft tissue lesions of the knee usually localize their pain very accurately.

Osteoarthritis, however, can refer down the leg and sometimes up into the thigh, but generally pain is well defined also. The pain of osteoarthritis is usually first noticed on exercise, but can initially be 'walked off'. The patient may also complain that the knee creaks or grates with episodes of swelling, particularly after unusual activity in a flexed position (e.g. squatting or kneeling). The swelling and a variable degree of inflammatory response in the synovium produces a stiff, tight feeling (inactivity stiffness, felt particularly at the back of the knee), but not the prolonged early morning stiffness of an inflammatory synovitis. Cartilage or bony fragments that separate into the joint may cause loose body locking. Pain from this may be very variable, because of changes in site of the loose fragment annd it may occasionally refer down the leg. Flexion deformity occurs due to protective hamstring spasm, and this may in time become a fixed flexion deformity.

In the later stages of osteoarthritis pain becomes more severe and constant often with progressive genu varum. The patient becomes unable to squat or kneel and has difficulty climbing stairs. Much of the early pain of osteoarthritis, however, is likely to be capsular and ligamentous and there are often tender ligamentous sites that may respond to injection.

Other pain patterns and associated symptoms

The causes of synovitis of the knee are dealt with in standard rheumatological texts. However, it is important to define, even in injury problems, whether there is associated or pre-existing synovitis. The patient will complain of pain and stiffness usually with marked morning symptoms. Tightness at the back of the knee may be very limiting, particularly if there is a palpable tense popliteal cyst. Flexion is often very restricted and extension difficult due to hamstring tightness. Flexion contracture will develop if the effects are not reduced by treatment of synovitis and, in some cases, splintage.

Localization of pain

As most soft tissue conditions outside the joint produce well localized pain it is important to recognize the site of pain, onset in relation to activity and, *on examination*, localized tenderness and pain on resisted activity or stretch. *Specific pain patterns* will be dealt with under the headings of individual disorders.

It is also important to recognize symptoms associated with intraarticular pathology such as locking and giving way which usually can be defined from extraarticular soft tissue problems.

Clinical evaluation

History of injury

Acute injury

It is important to define the history of the plane and forces of injury. The team doctor, coach, or physiotherapist may have observed the injury and be able to provide a clearer history if the patient cannot define this. At a sports event it is important to examine the injured knee immediately before protective spasm makes this impossible. Immediate swelling indicates haemarthrosis.

Chronic injury

The history of original injury must be sought and may be the main pointer to the likely damage in intraarticular lesions. However, a clear history of the onset of injury is often lacking in soft tissue problems. Therefore it is important to define factors such as overtraining, running on hard surfaces, loading, and biomechanical problems. An alternative pathology must be considered if the symptoms do not fit with a history of injury if present or the overloading stress does not fit with the pattern of injury seen. Sportsmen with inflammatory synovitis will often state that they have had an injury causing their problems, but by careful questioning it can usually be defined that no specific injury occurred at the time of onset of symptoms. *Spontaneous effusion of the knee even in sportsmen must be investigated to exclude a primary inflammatory cause.*

Haemarthrosis

Immediate swelling is noticed by the patient followed by rapid loss of knee movement. Taken with the history of injury, this requires urgent investigation—70 per cent of acute haemarthrosis in sport being due to cruciate ligament tear. Other causes are osteochondral injury; less commonly, peripheral meniscal tear and synovitis, including crystal synovitis. Therefore, when no history of injury has been defined, aspiration should include examination for cell count and urate or pyrophosphate crystals.

Giving way

It is important to define whether the patient is describing subluxation of the patella, when the patella slips temporarily over the condyle or a feeling of instability due to meniscal tear, usually noticed when changing direction suddenly. Major patellar instability is usually recognized by the patient because of the clear feeling of the patella relocating. Anterior cruciate instability, recognized by the patient and failing to be controlled by quadriceps/hamstring rehabilitation,[1] requires further orthopaedic referral.

Locking

Locking refers to the inability to fully extend the knee (blocked knee usually due to a meniscal tear). It should be noted that loss of hyperextension compared with the contralateral knee may also indicate a blocked knee even though extension is full.

Locking due to a loose body usually occurs suddenly in *midflexion* and prevents extension or flexion. A sudden intensity of pain with locking may cause the patient to fall and typically the site of pain is variable if the loose body moves within the joint. Recurrent episodes may lead to chronic effusion.

Examination of the knee

As with all lower limb joints, assessment should begin with observation of standing posture, gait, and leg length. Observe the alignment between the lower leg (tibia and fibula) and upper leg (femur).

Fixed flexion deformity

This is the clinical sign associated with loss of extension and the affected knee must be compared with the normal knee and the hip examined to exclude a primary hip flexion deformity, which will lead to knee flexion. Mild flexion deformity is frequently seen secondary to hamstring tightness, which may follow injury or spinal problems.

Genu varum

Genu varum refers to increased lateral curve to the leg occurring either in the tibia or tibiofemoral joint.

1. *Physiological tibial bowing* refers to minor bowing of the tibia, which is common before the age of 3 years and usually corrects with further growth.

2. *Pathological tibial bowing* can be due to a variety of pathologies, including childhood rickets, typically affecting the distal third, and fractures or osteomyelitis.

Congenital genu varum occurs because of abnormalities in epiphyseal growth. In *osteoarthritis*, genu varum develops when there is loss of the medial compartment cartilage and ligament laxity and in *avascular necrosis* it develops when there is collapse of the medial tibial condyle.

Genu valgum

Physiological genu valgum is usually bilateral and commonly resolves before the age of 7 years.

Unilateral pathological genu valgum may be due to trauma, infections, or congenital causes affecting epiphyseal growth.

Bilateral genu valgum is usually a result of inflammatory joint disease, for example, rheumatoid arthritis. This may be unilateral initially.

Genu recurvatum

This describes hyperextension of the knee beyond 10° and may be a part of a generalized hypermobility syndrome or have localized causes, including underdevelopment of the femoral condyles or relaxation of the posterior capsular structures and weakness in the calf and hamstring muscles. Genu recurvatum associated with a high patella (patella alta) increases the risk of patellar subluxation.

Muscle wasting

Observe the quadriceps muscle bulk and in particular the VMO, which tends to waste rapidly in any painful knee condition and may lead to secondary patellofemoral pain, which may confuse the history in terms of initial knee injury. Where there is marked wasting, exclude denervation due to root damage (positive femoral stretch test or reduction of knee jerk reflex) or primary muscle disease (myopathy or myositis) which is usually symmetrical. Myositis is usually associated with muscle tenderness, early morning stiffness, as well as proximal hip and shoulder girdle wasting. Look for *fasciculation* as a sign of denervation, particularly in diabetic amyotrophy. *Compare* muscle strength in quadriceps with that in hamstrings, as imbalance may be the cause of persistent symptoms, particularly in sportsmen, and it is important to achieve hamstring/quadriceps balance in rehabilitation after anterior cruciate ligament rupture.

A tape measure record of muscle wasting is rather poorly reproducible, but can be measured by taking a point between 6 and 10 cm marked above the superior patella pole on either side and then measuring the circumference on the two sides. Muscle bulk is often best assessed by looking from the foot end of the couch at the patient lying flat and relaxed and then asking for contraction.

Maximum calf circumference is more reproducible than thigh circumference and is perhaps of more value in defining venous calf distention or swelling following popliteal cyst rupture.

Swelling

Define whether this is generalized (e.g. effusion) or localized (e.g. meniscal or bursal).

Effusion

Look for filling in the parapatellar gutters, particularly medially, and suprapatellar pouch. Also examine for popliteal swelling, which is a common cause of posterior knee pain and may be intermittent.

A small effusion is best defined by the *bulge test*. Fluid is stroked down by the palm of the (right) hand from the medial joint line (begin at the tibial condyle) upwards into the suprapatellar pouch. The (left) hand is immediately placed across the upper medial suprapatellar region with the thumb resting on the patella thus controlling the fluid in the pouch and defining patellar movement. The fluid is then stroked down from the suprapatellar pouch by the back of the (right) hand running down the lateral jointline. A bulge of fluid seen at the medial patellar gutter confirms a small effusion. This must be defined from movement of the patella or soft tissues, controlled by the thumb resting on the patella.

A large effusion can be defined by cross-fluctuance, but the patella tap test is generally felt to be a rather inaccurate test and caution should be noted if there is patellar irritability, as this may cause severe pain. The 'balloon' sign is demonstrated by placing one hand over the suprapatellar pouch and with downward pressure on the patella with the other hand so that the fluid expands outwards against the examining hand.

Synovitis

This can be crudely assessed by feeling the thickness of tissue in the suprapatellar pouch below the main quadriceps bulk or by palpating swelling at the anterior jointline, which immediately reforms after pressure, although it should be noted that this is difficult to define where there is obesity.

Localized swelling

Define the following.

1. *Anatomical site.* Palpate the medial/lateral joint line to define meniscal cartilage cysts. Anterior bursae in relation to patella ligament.

2. *Size.* Meniscal cysts often range in size after activity and may be more easily visible in midflexion. Medial disappears in full is flexion (Pisani's sign, see p. 440).

3. *Consistency.* Meniscal cysts are often very firm.

4. *Reducibility.* Mobile loose bodies (mice) can be pushed back deeper into the joint.

5. *Tenderness.* Define if this reproduces the pain a patient recognizes.

6. *Transillumination.* Positive if cystic.

7. *Variability on joint movement.* See size.

8. *Communication with the knee joint or associated knee fluid.* Popliteal Baker's cyst.

9. *Pulsation* (examine for bruit). Particularly for posterior lesions.

Meniscal cysts

Observe whether the swelling is at the medial or lateral joint line, tracing a line from the midpatellar ligament. A cyst is usually quite tense and tender on local pressure. However, the swelling may be intermittent.

Bursae

There are many bursae of the knee (Fig. 6) but their individual presentation will be described as specific disorders in relation to the presentation of anterior, medial, lateral, or posterior knee pain.

Local tenderness

Define the site:

- bony
- soft tissue attachment to bone (enthesis) of tendon or ligament
- bursal
- joint line.

Define associated swelling and if any pain on resisted muscle action or stretch.

Movement and stability

Range of movement and stability should always be compared with that of the opposite knee. Note any loss of extension or hyperextension and flexion (see above).

Assess hamstring tightness (see Chapter 6.6), particularly for posterior pain and flexion deformity.

Test of medial stability (Fig. 7)

Valgus stress is applied with the knee in about 30° flexion. Minor symmetrical stretch is up to 5 mm separation. If laxity is found in full extension it indicates that a posterior cruciate tear is present as well.

Tests of medial ligament instability

Valgus force applied with the knee in flexion. If laxity is demonstrated in extension, it means that a posterior cruciate tear is present as well. Minor symmetrical stretch is normal with up to 5 mm of separation.

Following medial ligament tear the following patterns can be found.

1. Mild (first-degree). There is local tenderness and less than 5 mm separations (stable).

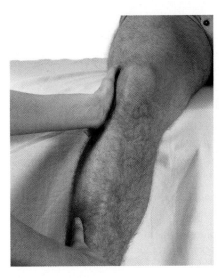

Fig. 7 Medial stability is assessed by application of valgus force in 30° flexion.

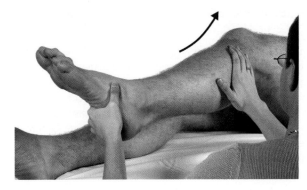

Fig. 9 The pivot shift test.

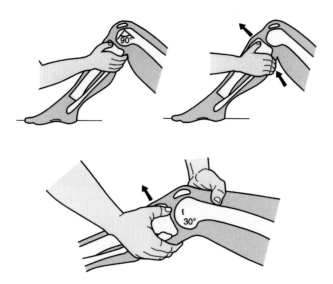

Fig. 8 The anterior drawer and Lachman's test evaluate the integrity of the anterior cruciate ligaments.

2. Moderate (second-degree). There is a moderate tear with marked local tenderness and between 5 and 10 mm separation.

3. Severe (third degree). There is more than 10 mm separation (unstable).

Tests of anterior stability (anterior cruciate ligament)

Lachman's test (Fig. 8)

This test is performed with the patient lying flat on their back with the knee flexed to 20–30°. The distal femur is grasped by the left hand on the lateral side to control just above the lateral femoral condyle. The examiner then uses the opposite hand to draw anteriorly the proximal tibia (Fig. 9). In acute rupture it may still be possible to elicit movement whereas the anterior drawer test is frequently inhibited by hamstring spasm.

Pivot shift test (Fig. 9)

This test recreates the instability and relocation of the tibia recognized by the patient as his feeling of instability.

The patient lies on his back with the hip flexed to about 45° with the knee in extension. With the foot in internal rotation, the lower leg is supported by the examiner while applying a valgus force as the knee is flexed from full extension. In anterior cruciate tear, as the tibia is subluxed on the femur, it jumps back into its correct position at about 30° of flexion and this is noticed by the examiner and the patient as a small jerk ('jerk' test).

Anterior drawer test (Fig. 8)

This is a less satisfactory test for anterior cruciate laxity, but may have to be used by those finding the Lachman test difficult to perform (hand size may make it difficult to provide sufficient purchase on large-limbed patients). With the knee in 90° of flexion, the examiner pulls forward with both hands on the upper posterior calf. Interpretation of the test is dependent on the position of the tibia in relation to the femur. In the neutral position, it tests the capsule and anterior cruciate.

With the tibia in internal rotation it tests the posterior cruciate. A pure anterior drawer movement in neutral with the knee at 90° and relaxed hamstrings is termed the *anterior drawer sign*. When the tibia is internally rotated, the posterior cruciate is tight so the anterior drawer movement cannot be achieved and therefore a positive anterior drawer test in internal rotation indicates a torn posterior cruciate ligament.

Anterior medial rotator instability indicates a tear of one or more of the medial compartment ligaments in association with anterior cruciate ligament tear increases the amount of subluxation of the medial tibial condyle. As the medial ligament is the second line of defence, in an isolated tear of the anterior cruciate the anterior drawer test will be negative.

Interpretation of the anterior drawer findings can be summarized as follows:

1. in internal rotation, torn posterior cruciate;

2. in neutral with equal tibial condyle movement, torn anterior cruciate with anteromedial/anterolateral laxity;

3. in neutral with lateral tibial condyle movement, anterolateral (accentuated by the anterior cruciate) instability;

4. in neutral with medial movement, anteromedial (accentuated by anterior cruciate) instability.

Tests of posterior stability (posterior cruciate ligament)

Posterior drawer test

With the knee in 90° of flexion, the alignment of the knee in relation to the femur is observed and compared with that of the opposite knee, to define if there is posterior subluxation of the tibia.

If there is subluxation, performing an anterior drawer test will now correct this position to normal (hence *posterior drawer sign*) thus distinguishing the signs from those of an anterior cruciate rupture. If the symptoms of pain and instability persist, urgent intervention has to be considered but initial rehabilitation to try and regain full range of movement and muscle function should be instituted.

Test of lateral tightness

Ober's test (See Chapter 6.6, Fig. 15)

This is a test of iliotibial band tightness and is usually positive in iliotibial band syndrome with a typical history.

The patient lies on his or her side and the lower hip is flexed to eliminate lordosis of the lumbar spine. The knee of the upper leg is flexed to 90° and the thigh is abducted and then extended. In a positive test, when the examiner's supporting hand is removed the hip remains abducted rather than dropping back towards the couch. The iliotibial band can often be palpated as a rigid band in the subcutaneous tissues below the iliac crest when tight.

When no abnormality can be defined within the knee, the history should be reviewed and further examination to exclude lumbar, hip, or other referred pain causing knee symptoms (see comments on pain referral patterns in section 'Innervation and pain patterns of the knee').

High tibial and femoral stress fractures can occasionally cause confusion in terms of knee symptoms, but usually the classical history is of crescendo bone pain increased with activity. The athlete's activity level gradually becomes reduced by the symptoms and there is usually well defined bony tenderness.

Anterior knee pain

Disorders of the patellofemoral joint and associated soft tissues are very common particularly in teenage girls, young women, and athletes.[2] As the spectrum of problems seen frequently reflects underlying anatomical and biomechanical factors, the anatomy of the patella must be considered an integral part of assessment and examination.

The Q-angle is a useful clinical assessment. When the Q-angle (normal about 14°), from a line from the tibial tubercle to the midpatella and a second line along the quadriceps muscle plane to anterior superior iliac spine, is 20° or more there is an increase in patellar instability and other patellofemoral problems. Increase in the Q-angle therefore results in a lateral vector to the extensor mechanism, tending to displace the patella laterally. The patella subluxes and may dislocate when a strong quadriceps contraction is combined with external rotation of the tibia, genu valgum, and slight knee flexion.

Recurrent patellar subluxation

Major

In major subluxation the patella tracks laterally over the femoral facet and returns to the patellofemoral groove with an audible snap at the beginning of knee flexion.

Minor

In minor subluxation the patella deviates laterally without the patient being aware of relocation, unless there is direct injury or valgus force producing complete dislocation.

Major traumatic dislocation

The *complications* of major traumatic dislocation are usually more severe than recurrent subluxation and include the following:

1. *tearing of the medial retinaculum*, through damage to the medial border of the patella or vastus medialis origin;

2. *tears of the medial capsule or cruciate ligaments and of the anterior horn of the medial meniscus*;

3. Major or recurrent injury may lead to chondromalacia patellae, osteochondritis dissecans, osteochondral fractures, loose bodies, and degenerative arthritis.

It is important therefore to try and counteract the lateral forces by patella taping (McConnell strapping), rehabilitation of VMO strength, and correction of hyperpronation in the feet, which will increase the valgus force particularly when running.

Patellofemoral pain syndrome

Anterior knee pain is a very common clinical problem and is usually associated with defined biomechanical factors and patellofemoral pain. A history of mild subluxation may also be noted and there may be frequent clicking or crepitus and pseudolocking.

Examination should focus on abnormalities of patellar anatomy, muscle function, and tender sites. Where no clear patellar history is found and clinical findings cannot explain anterior knee pain, other causes of pain including referred pain should be sought, rather than automatically labelling the patient as suffering from patellar pain syndrome.

Chondromalacia patellae

This is best limited to the description of patellofemoral changes seen at arthroscopy. It has been well reviewed and is beyond the scope of this text. It was initially described in 1928 by Allerman as posttraumatic change with episodes of crepitus and swelling, associated with softening and fissuring of the articular surface of the patella. It is therefore one of the causes of patellofemoral pain and can be classified according to grading of changes at arthroscopy and anatomical site. The MRI changes have been reviewed by Berquist.[3]

Other patellar lesions

Osteochondral fractures of the patella are common and often associated with patellar dislocation (up to 28 per cent in some series).

Avulsion fractures are also common and occur in the superior patellar pole, following enforced hyperflexion/hyperextension injury with traction of the quadriceps.

Inferior avulsion fractures may lead to secondary patella alta. Stress fractures of the patella have been reported in running and jumping sports and cricket particularly. They should be considered in the differential diagnosis of anterior knee pain, but are beyond the scope of this text.

Other causes of anterior knee pain

Patellar pole tendonitis/tendonosis

Symptomatic patellar pole tendonitis is more common at the inferior than proximal pole and is particularly associated with jumping sports (jumper's knee). Inferior pole tendonitis in adolescence is referred to as Sinding–Larsen–Johansson disease and probably reflects chondro-osseous failure, which may lead to calcification or ossification at the distal patellar pole. In adults, as the tendon tends to be weaker in comparison with adolescents (see above), there are variable degrees of patellar tendonosis, which usually appears to reflect repetitive micro-failure rather than major acute injury. Progressive degenerative change can lead to cystic change. There may be a component of inflammatory change in the early phase that could be considered a failure of normal healing process and may respond to local short-acting corticosteroid injection. However, in the later phases of tendonosis the dominant problem is breakdown and liquefaction, and in this situation corticosteroids have no part to play in management and may precipitate acute rupture. Adequate imaging is advised before corticosteroid injections are considered as this will define the extent of intratendinous degeneration.

Osgood–Schlatter disease (Fig. 10)

This is the most common extensor stress injury in adolescence and affects the inferior attachment of the patellar ligament to anterior tibial tubercle. This tuberosity normally fuses by age 13 in boys but earlier in girls, so that the condition tends to present at a younger age in girls. Clinical features of these conditions are outlined in Table 2 and include pain, swelling, and tenderness over the upper anterior tibia. A period of reduced activity and then rehabilitation with controlled stretching will see improvement in the condition.

Bursitis[4]

Prepatellar bursitis (carpetlayer's or housemaid's knee)

This bursa is present in about 90 per cent of the normal population. It is subcutaneous and anterior to the lower half of the patella and upper half of the patellar ligament. Following direct trauma or repetitive friction, for example, due to prolonged kneeling, a swelling may be noticed by the patient (Fig. 11). It is not usually painful, except on pressure, and the swelling is usually cool. In acute bursitis, other causes such as staphylococcal infection or gouty inflammation should be considered. Even in acute infective prepatellar bursitis, knee movement is usually well preserved with pain at the end range of movement

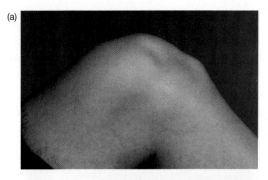
(a)

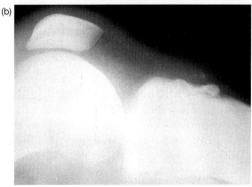
(b)

Fig. 10 (a and b) Osgood–Schlatter disease.

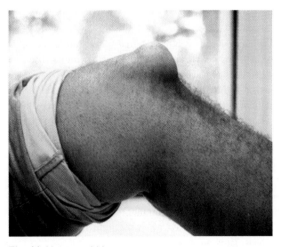

Fig. 11 Housemaids' knee.

Table 2 Common sites of traction apophysitis

Eponym	Site	Specific clinical features	Specific management features
Osgood–Schlatter	Tibial tubercle (patellar tendon)	Boys, esp. age 13–14 yrs Girls, esp. age 10–11 yrs Chronic condition may develop	Reduce activity initially Quadriceps strengthening and progressive stretching
Sinding–Larsen–Johansson	Inferior patellar pole (patellar tendon)	Tender inferior patellar pole and radiographic evidence of small inferior patellar avulsion	If acute usually requires immobilizing in cylinder cast

in flexion stretching the anterior soft tissues. It is essential when needle aspiration is performed that it is accurate and does *not* include aspiration of the knee joint as this could convert a relatively benign infective bursitis into deep-seated joint infection. In joint sepsis severe restriction and irritability of the joint is usually found.

Deep infrapatellar bursitis

This small bursa lies between the upper part of the tibial tubercle and the ligamentum patellae.[5] It is separated from the knee joint synovium by a fat pad. When it is inflamed, swelling can be noticed on either side of the patellar ligament insertion to the tibial tubercle. Infection is rare because this is a deeper bursa than the prepatellar bursa, but inflammation may follow direct trauma or repetitive pressure (prayer bursitis) or irritation from debris following previous Osgood–Schlatter disease.

The suprapatellar bursa of the knee *communicates* with the knee joint and will swell as part of joint effusion or synovitis.

Subcrural bursitis

The subcrural bursa, beneath the quadriceps tendon, usually *communicates* with the joint and therefore is affected by causes of joint swelling. Occasionally, it may be affected independently when separated from the joint and presents as a horseshoe swelling around the patella distended with fluid.

Other bursal swelling around the knee will be discussed in relation to the presentation of medial, lateral, or posterior knee pain.

Fat pad syndrome (Hoffa's disease)

When the infrapatellar fat pad is hypertrophied or the quadriceps has lost its tone, the fat pad may not be drawn up sufficiently and may trap between the articular surfaces.

Infrapatellar fat pad pain is often referred to as Hoffa's disease. It tends to occur in young people and may follow minor injury. The pain is only noticed when the knee is used and is situated directly behind the patellar tendon or slightly medially. The joint also tends to feel a little stiff and the patient may complain that the joint feels weak and liable to recurrent swelling. With increasing hypertrophy of the fat pad and trapping between the articular surfaces, a progressive limitation of extension occurs that makes the patient walk with a slightly flexed knee gait.

True locking does not occur, but at times the patient may complain of a feeling of giving way with a sharp stabbing pain. The fat pad on examination is usually enlarged with swelling on either side of the patellar tendon, but often more prominent medially. There is local tenderness that is often increased when the joint is fully extended. There may be associated quadriceps atrophy.

Treatment should include temporary restriction of full knee extension to reduce impingement and injection if there is significant hypertrophy particularly with synovial thickening. Occasionally, with persistent pain and swelling, the infrapatellar fat pad requires partial surgical excision.

Specific disorders causing medial knee symptoms

Extraarticular complaints

Referred pain

Referred pain from the hip or obturator hernia may spread to the medial aspect of the lower thigh and knee.

Bursitis

The sartorius, semimembranosus and semitendinosus attachments into the upper and medial tibial shaft resemble a goose's foot (pes anserinus) and the associated bursa may become inflamed because of direct trauma or repetitive rotation (e.g. breast-strokers knee). There is localized tenderness and occasionally swelling. Symptoms usually settle with restricted activity but occasionally bursal injection is necessary.

Articular soft tissue lesions

Medial patella and patellar retinacular pain has been dealt with above.

Medial plica syndrome

The *medial patella plica*, or medial shelf, appears to be the one most likely to cause clinical problems and was first described by Lino in 1939. It runs obliquely from the medial border of the knee joint downwards, inserting into the synovium and covering the medial infrapatellar fat pad.[6,7] During knee flexion, the plica glides over the medial condyle like a windscreen wiper. However, if the plica becomes thickened or inflamed due to trauma or synovitis, it may cause sudden pain as it is pinched between the patella and medial condyle of the femur. There may be pain and a feeling of a slight soft tissue block to full extension of the knee. A painful arc during flexion of the knee can occur if there is irregularity of the femoral condyle, for instance, due to osteochondral damage and a thickened plica riding over this area.

The plica can often be felt if the examiner rolls the medial capsule of the knee under the thumb or index finger with the knee flexed to about 45°. If this is painful and recognized by the patient as the pain previously felt, injection should be given. If the symptoms persist arthroscopic resection is occasionally indicated. Underlying synovitis of the knee joint may, however, be the associated cause and should be treated appropriately first. It should be stressed that the presence of a medial plica is a normal variant and, unless inflamed, with appropriate symptoms and clinical findings, arthroscopic resection should not be performed.

Medial collateral ligament bursitis

The medial collateral bursa lies under the MCL and is quite a common cause of localized knee pain, particularly in middle-aged female patients. It may also persist following trauma. There is localized pain that is worse during activity and eases with rest, but night pain may occasionally occur. Symptoms and signs of internal derangement must be excluded. Examination will show no joint abnormality, unless there is associated osteoarthritis. Extension should be normal, but flexion may be limited. There is a soft end feel, the limiting factor being pain. Valgus stress and rotation are usually painful. A swelling may be palpable under the medial ligament at the level of the joint line, which is often firm and may be confused with an osteophyte or medial meniscal cyst. Unlike a medial meniscal cyst, the swelling does not disappear during flexion and indeed may become firmer. Injection or deep friction may help but surgical intervention is rarely necessary.

Medial collateral ligament injury

The MCL prevents excessive valgus movement of the knee and its posterior fibres check external rotation at the tibia. The classical pattern of injury is marked valgus force on a semi-flexed and externally rotated knee. This is particularly seen in soccer when a player is tackled from the side or receives a direct blow on the outer side of his weight-bearing knee. The player may notice a crack and feel a sudden pain on the inner aspect of the knee. Typically the pain disappears quite quickly and in some cases it is possible to play on at a reduced level until the end of the game. Major symptoms tend to start after a few hours with increased swelling and local pain but the next day the player is often able to stand without support.

Examination

After major injury, the knee will be hot and swollen with a little loss of extension and flexion. By this stage it is impossible to perform ligamentous tests but the history is all important. Localized tenderness is usually found at the site of ligament injury. Midportion tears are the most common, but also the most serious as they may involve the deeply situated meniscotibial and meniscal femoral portions of the ligament. In a severe proximal tear X-rays should be performed to exclude an avulsion or bony fragment, particularly in adolescents, which requires surgical referral.

Natural history of MCL injury

The acute stage with knee joint swelling usually lasts about 2 weeks. Over the next 4–6 weeks the limitation of movement gradually reduces and the swelling decreases. However, local tenderness and sometimes warmth may persist medially. By 2–3 months the following three patterns should be defined.

1. Ligament is well healed with a strong non-adherent ligament.

2. The ligament is lengthened with laxity and potential symptoms of instability.

3. The ligament is adherent leaving the patient with chronic pain on activity.

Pellegrini–Stieda syndrome

Calcification of the MCL may occur, particularly at the proximal end after injury. At 4–6 weeks, instead of continuing improvement, the player complains of increasing limitation of flexion and pain together with a hard end feel. There may be tenderness and swelling at the proximal end of the medial lateral collateral ligament and X-rays show a linear shadow of calcification along the inner border of the medial femoral condyle. If recognized early and calcification defined by ultrasound before X-ray changes, there is anecdotal evidence that indomethacin or other anti-inflammatories may reduce the time course. However, once the calcification has developed, there may be a slow spontaneous recovery over 6 months to a year.

Treatment

Immediately after injury an ice compress, with protection from skin burning, should be applied to reduce inflammatory reaction. After severe injury immediate rest is advisable and non-weight-bearing with crutches. There must be no attempt particularly in the first week to straighten the knee into full flexion on weight-bearing as the MCL is taut in extension. Further stretching could worsen the injury. In the uncomplicated injury the player can usually return to sports after 6 weeks if there is full range of movement and ligamentum stress tests are negative. It is wise, however, to provide a protective knee brace for the first few weeks particularly if the player is involved in a contact sport.

If, unfortunately, the patient does not attend for medical attention until a chronic stage with probable adhesion or laxity, treatment must depend on the physical findings. If there is no instability, but pain, with some loss of range of movement implying adhesions, deep frictions may be helpful and physiotherapy to gradually restore full range of movement.

Surgical referral is indicated where there is major instability, particularly where an avulsion fracture is seen.

Medial coronary ligament injury

These injuries are probably poorly recognized, they may resemble a meniscal injury or a sprain of the medial collateral ligament.

Mechanism of injury

The classical mechanism of coronary ligament injury is felt to be a rotational strain in slight knee flexion, as with a medial meniscal injury. However, unlike in a meniscal injury, there is no history of locking of the knee after injury and the player can straighten the knee fully and may be able to continue playing. Pain tends to be noticed the day after injury, particularly on walking and there may be some knee swelling. Lateral rotation is painful but, unlike in an MCL injury, valgus force does not provoke pain. Anti-inflammatories and frictions to the medial coronary ligament with the knee flexed to over 100° may be beneficial. If activity is reduced, recovery usually occurs spontaneously within 2–3 months.

Medial meniscal injury

The medial meniscus is more commonly injured than the lateral, as it is much less mobile than the lateral meniscus (see 'Functional anatomy'). It is retained by the MCL and the medial coronary ligament, which attaches to the tibia.

Vertically torn meniscus (buckle-handle tear) is the most important and common injury and it typically occurs between the ages of 15 and 30.

Mechanism of injury

Typically, when a player attempts to kick a ball, the thigh rotates on a slightly flexed and weight-bearing knee, causing a rotational force of the femur on the static tibia and producing a shearing force through the meniscus. It should be noted that in normal flexion/extension the menisci move with the tibia to which they are attached, but during rotational movements they follow the femoral condyle. It is the combined movement with the forces involved, particularly in a contact sporting injury, that may prevent normal displacement of the meniscus, so that the meniscus shears between the tibia and femur. Previous anterior cruciate instability due to injury increases the risk of medial meniscal damage. At the time of injury the player usually notices agonizing localized pain on the inner aspect of the knee. The knee gives way and usually the player falls and rolls on the ground. On standing he is unable to straighten the knee, although flexion is usually retained initially. If examined forcibly initially, full extension may result in an audible click due to relocation of the torn segment, but the knee will become swollen following this. The knee may settle and the player may feel he has recovered but will tend to notice episodes of giving way on turning.

Blocked knee

Persistent loss of extension following injury (blocked knee) is a surgical emergency, because further force on a blocked knee may lead to an anterior cruciate rupture. The mechanical basis for the locking is that, in a normal knee, the collateral ligaments and posterior structures become taut during extension. The tibia and femur are strongly opposed so a displaced piece of cartilage cannot be accommodated. Sudden locking of the knee in partial flexion with immediate unlocking on manipulation is therefore typical of a bucket-handle tear.

Horizontal and posterior medial meniscal injury

These lesions are generally due to repetitive normal forces acting on a degenerative meniscus and are typically seen in the forty plus age group. They are usually posterior and are considered by some to be part of the normal ageing process. The history is usually less dramatic than a vertical tear, with a feeling of giving and with symptoms usually felt at the posteromedial aspect of the knee. Clicking may be noticed on kicking out, with a feeling that the knee unlocks. Slight rotation and flexion during weight-bearing may provoke a click that may be uncomfortable and is relieved immediately as the knee is straightening, for instance, getting out of a car. Examination may show slight joint swelling, but in chronic meniscal lesions swelling is often absent. Palpation along the joint line is very important and usually reveals a focal tenderness posteriorly. Rotational tests are now not generally recommended, as they may cause the knee to lock. Loss of extension and medial joint line pain and tenderness with a classical history is an indication for MRI scanning. The consensus view now of most orthopaedic surgeons is that arthroscopy is no longer a diagnostic examination alone and should rarely be performed if the MRI scan is negative.

Treatment

Persistent symptoms or a blocked knee, with positive MRI findings, are indications for arthroscopic partial meniscectomy.

Cysts of the medial meniscus

These are much less common than those of the lateral meniscus and usually reflect a partially torn meniscus displacing medially rather than into the joint. There is therefore a normal range of movement and tenderness or a palpable swelling on the medial joint line. Swelling is typically most prominent in about 30° of flexion and disappears on full flexion (Pisani's disappearing sign).

Treatment

It may be possible to aspirate fluid from the cyst with a large-bore needle and sometimes they appear to respond to intracystic steroids. If the cyst recurs and is symptomatic, arthroscopic excision may have to be considered.

Other disorders of the meniscus

Chondrocalcinosis in the medial meniscus is a common finding following major meniscal surgery. Deposition is also felt to be a normal component of the ageing process in some patients over the age of 60. There is increasing frequency on routine X-ray evidence with each decade. However, chondrocalcinosis seen without a history of trauma under the age of 50 usually indicates a metabolic disorder (Table 3) and needs to be fully investigated.

Table 3 Metabolic diseases predisposing to CPPD crystal deposition

Definite associations	Possible associations
Hyperparathyroidism	Gout
Haemochromatosis	Ochronosis
Hypophosphatasia	
Hypomagnesaemia	
Wilson's disease	

Changes to the structure of cartilage through deposition increase the risk of meniscal cleavage tear.

Other intraarticular causes of medial knee pain are beyond the scope of this text. It must be noted that MRI scanning has revealed frequent major bone bruising as a cause of medial pain, particularly after injury. Osteochondral damage associated with injury may be poorly recognized initially unless imaging is obtained and may present subsequently with locking or pain due to condylar damage.

Anterior cruciate ligament injury[1]

The history of presentation is as follows:

1. Acute injury—haemarthrosis

2. Instability. Knee instability occurs as a result of loss of static and dynamic function. Stability depends on the integrity of ligaments, congruency of joint surfaces with associated menisci, and well-balanced muscular control acting across the joint. Loss of proprioception and failure of rapid response to forces may be a major component of injury risk. The muscles and tendons should be considered the first line of defence to rapidly changing forces.

Mechanism of injury

Isolated tear of the ACL may occur following a hyperextension injury with medial rotation or deceleration with sudden change of direction. Chronic ACL deficiency appears to increase the risk of longitudinal meniscal tear, so combined lesions may be found where the initial cruciate tear is not recognized.

Symptoms

Immediate swelling after the injury indicates haemarthrosis. In less severe injury only a minor effusion may occur. Diagnostic aspiration should be performed and immediate repair of a complete cruciate tear is recommended by many. Where the patient presents with a preceding history of haemarthrosis and ACL injury, it is expected that clinical examination will reveal anterior instability, (see 'Tests of anterior stability').

Lateral causes of knee pain

Referred pain, lateral knee pain spreading down to the calf, frequently reflects L5 root symptomatology.

Lateral retinacular, coronary, or collateral ligament and meniscal causes are less frequent than equivalent lesions on the medial side. This is because the lateral ligament is separated from the lateral meniscus and the lateral meniscus is not tethered in the same way as the medial meniscus. Posterolateral pain, however, is quite common as a result of soft tissue injuries of the biceps femoris or the less commonly injured popliteus intraarticularly (see 'Functional anatomy') (Fig. 12).

Lateral collateral ligament injury

The lateral collateral ligament is very rarely sprained as it requires a severe varus movement on the outstretched knee. If injured, the immediate articular signs are less dramatic than in sprains of the medialcol lateral ligament because of the separation of the ligament from the joint. There is usually an acute stage for 2 weeks followed by gradual recovery as adhesions do not tend to occur.

Lateral meniscal injury

The most common congenital anomaly is the discoid lateral meniscus. The incidence in autopsy studies is up to 7 per cent but most do not appear to cause problems. The most common reason for problems appears to be the Wrisberg ligament type of discoid lateral meniscus. This type is described as lacking a posterior capsular attachment and presents in childhood with a snapping knee. The meniscus rolls up in front of the lateral compartment during flexion. During extension the meniscus becomes trapped anteriorly until it reduces suddenly with a dramatic audible snap. It usually presents in children or adolescents but other discoid lesions may present in adulthood with or without injury. A feeling of instability is less common than with medial lesions but the patient usually notices a posterior click confirmed on clinical examination as a palpable audible click causing major symptoms. Surgery is usually indicated.

Lateral meniscal tear in sportsmen without discoid meniscus may respond poorly to partial excision with persistent lateral pain and sometimes progressive lateral tibial condylar damage. Lateral meniscal cysts are palpable and should be injected rather than referred immediately for surgery because of the above problems.

Iliotibial band syndrome and bursitis

The iliotibial band is a thick extension of the fascia lata and inserts into the tibial tubercle of Gerdy. The band lies anterior to the flexion extension axis of the knee in extension, but posterior in flexion. The tensor fasciae latae acts through the band and it is therefore a weak external rotator and extensor of the knee (see 'Functional anatomy'). Lesions of the iliotibial band are common in long-distance runners (17 per cent of all knee symptomatology).

History of iliotibial band syndrome

The athlete typically notices lateral knee pain after about 7 miles, which forces him to stop, and gradually the mileage distance may decrease. The pain is more intense when the foot comes in contact with the ground during downhill running or rapid deceleration. When severe, the pain may develop on walking and an abnormal gait develops but this is uncommon. Examination reveals no abnormality of the joint but some discomfort when extension and lateral rotation are carried out against resistance. There may be a painful arc as the band slips over the lateral epicondyle at 30° of flexion. With a typical history but negative examination an iliotibial stress test should be performed. With the knee in 90° of flexion, pressure is applied at the ilio- tibial band over the lateral epicondyle and, as the knee is

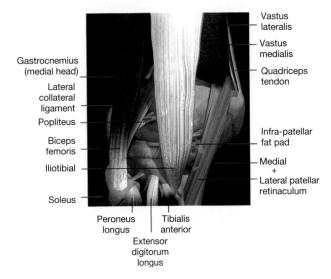

Fig. 12 The lateral knee.

gradually extended, the epicondylar area becomes painful at about 30° of flexion. Perform the Ober's test to assess tightness of the iliotibial band.

Iliotibial bursitis

This lies under the iliotibial band and acts as a cushion over the lateral epicondyle of the femur. It may become painful after direct trauma or repetitive irritation through long-distance running, cycling, or skiing. As with the iliotibial band syndrome, the patient complains of localized pain while walking or running and clinical examination reveals a painful arc at about 30° of flexion. It may be possible to feel a swelling between the condyle and the iliotibial band. The condition may coexist with a tight iliotibial band or may be isolated without discomfort on resisted extension and lateral rotation.

Treatment of the iliotibial band syndrome is to correct leg-length deformity, which might predispose to tightness of the iliotibial band, or camber running, where running on one side of the edge of the road produces an effective longer leg length on the outside leg because of the camber of the road. Biomechanical problems of the feet with asymmetrical gait may also predispose to iliotibial band syndrome. Where no such abnormalities can be found, the condition usually responds to reduced mileage and iliotibial band stretch programme. The bursa should be injected if symptoms fail to settle.

Pathologies of the popliteus musculotendinous unit

This is intraarticular (see 'Functional anatomy') and should be considered as the cause of pain when resisted flexion and internal rotation of the knee provoke symptoms at the lateral or posterolateral aspects of the knee. As the popliteus is an important active stabilizer of the lateral and posterolateral aspect of the knee joint, it explains the frequency of popliteal injury in long-distance runners and downhill skiers. The prevention of forward displacement is also a function of the posterior cruciate ligament as a passive stabilizer, so careful examination to differentiate is necessary. It may be possible to localize tenderness in the popliteus tendon or in the muscle belly. Tendinous lesions appear to respond well to injection. They are best confirmed by MRI scanning and injection performed with clear anatomical knowledge. Lesions of the muscle belly may respond to deep friction.

Disorders of the tibiofibular junction

Sprain of the upper tibiofibular ligament

This can develop after trauma to the ankle joint or as the result of repetitive strains. Laxity can be defined by pulling forwards on the back of the fibula. Contraction of the biceps pulls the fibula backwards on the tibia so resisted flexion and resisted external rotation hurt at the outer side of the knee. Findings can be differentiated between this and bicipital tendonitis, as in the latter there is no tenderness found over the insertion of the biceps. Tibiofibular ligament strain usually settles with rest but, if persistent, injection may be considered. Bicipital tendonitis similarly may require injection if persistent.

Lesions of the lateral popliteal nerve

Diffuse pain felt down the lateral aspect of the calf with or without paraesthesiae may be due to lateral popliteal nerve irritation. There may be a positive Tinel's test over the lateral popliteal nerve. There is occasional thickening or a defined band and, if symptoms are persistent with electrodiagnostic tests positive, exploration is indicated. In our experience symptoms appear to present in young adolescents in a growth spurt and they often have signs of dural tension. Careful spinal examination is essential before attributing symptoms to the lateral popliteal nerve only.

Causes of posterior knee pain

The most common causes of posterior knee pain are hamstring or gastrocnemius pain, popliteal cysts, and referred pain. Posterior cruciate instability only occurs after severe injury.

Popliteal cyst (Baker's cyst)

The posterior aspect of the knee joint is the weakest part and therefore a posterior cyst may develop, particularly with a large effusion that has already filled the suprapatellar pouch. The patient complains of a feeling of tightness behind the knee with some limitation of flexion but is not usually aware of the cyst.

Rupture of a popliteal cyst

The patient presents with a classical history of sudden upper calf pain (the patient may often feel they have been kicked in the calf) with reduction of pre-existing knee swelling followed by generalized calf swelling and there may be pitting oedema from the dorsum of foot to calf. The most important differential diagnosis is from deep vein thrombosis and sometimes, owing to secondary venous obstruction, a deep vein thrombosis can develop after cyst rupture. Patients with a popliteal cyst must be warned about this risk particularly if flying and prophylactic paediatric aspirin is generally indicated. Where rupture has occurred, a venogram is the investigation of choice as venous occlusion cannot be excluded. Treatment of a ruptured cyst is

treatment of the underlying cause. Aspiration and injection of the joint should be performed if there is a synovitis or management of an underlying mechanical cause within the knee causing recurrent effusion.

Semimembranous bursa

There are two posterior knee bursae, one between each of the heads of the gastrocnemii and the joint capsule. They often communicate with the joint.

The medial bursa (semimembranosus), lying between the medial head of gastrocnemius and the capsule, extends between gastrocnemius and semimembranosus. Enlargement of this bursa forms as a swelling in the linear aspect of the popliteal fossa and may follow repetitive knee flexion (gamekeeper's knee). It usually enlarges distally deep to the medial head of gastrocnemius and appears as an oval fluctuant swelling, limited laterally but less defined medially, in the popliteal space.

It tenses on extension and relaxes on flexion. If part of inflammatory joint disease it may respond to treatment of the underlying joint disease or injection. It must be distinguished from a Baker's cyst, which always communicates with the joint. If large and persistent, it will require surgical excision.

Popliteal bursa

This arises from the synovial membrane of the knee surrounding the popliteus tendon intraarticularly. When inflamed it sometimes can be seen as a rounded swelling behind the lateral condyle of the femur, deep to biceps femoris and the iliotibial band.

When inflamed it is usually seen as an overuse lesion and presents with pain on the posterolateral aspect of the knee. Examination of the knee is usually normal apart from resisted flexion reproducing the pain. Resisted external rotation may also be painful. Tenderness is found at the biceps tendon usually at the enthesis to the head of the fibula (see differentiation from tibiofibular joint injury). Treatment is by deep friction, muscle rehabilitation, and injection if persistent.

Posterior cruciate ligament injury

Posterior cruciate ligament (PCL) injury usually reflects major trauma. It may occur with severe hyperextension or during a car crash through 'dashboard injury' when the femur is forced forwards on the immobilized tibia. There is initially a marked traumatic arthritis with a posterior drawer test becoming more positive as the joint reaction settles.

Summary

The knee is the largest and most commonly injured joint in the human body. As it is a modified hinge joint, unconstrained by its bony surfaces, it is particularly prone to ligamentous, meniscal and osteochondral injuries. Anterior cruciate rupture is frequently misdiagnosed and chronic instability causes the risk of meniscal damage and progressive osteoarthritis. Most soft tissue conditions of the knee can be defined by careful history and examination, supplemented by soft tissue imaging where appropriate.

References

1. Wilk, K.E., Reinold, M.M., and Hooks, T.R. (2003). Recent advances in the rehabilitation of isolated and combined anterior cruciate ligament injuries. *Orthop. Clin. North Am.* **34**, 107–137.

2. Biedert, R.M., and Sanchis-Alfonso, V. (2002). Sources of anterior knee pain. *Clin. Sports Med.* **21**, 335–347.

3. Berquist, T.H. (2000). MRI of the *musculoskeletal system.* Lippincott Williams and Wilkins.

4. Dye, S.F., Campagna-Pinto, D., Dye, C.C., Shifflett, S., and Eiman, T. (2003). Soft-tissue anatomy anterior to the human patella. *J. Bone Joint Surg. Am.* **85**-A(6), 1012–1017.

5. LaPrade, R.F. (1998). The anatomy of the deep infrapatellar bursa of the knee. *Am. J. Sports Med.* **26** (1), 129–132.

6. Garcia-Valtuille, R., Abascal, F., Cerezal, L., Garcia-Valtuille, A., Pereda, T., Canga, A., and Cruz, A. (2002). Anatomy and MR imaging appearances of synovial plicae of the knee. *Radiographics.* **22** (4), 775–784.

7. Dupont, J.Y. (1997). Synovial plicae of the knee. Controversies and review. *Clin. Sports Med.* **16** (1), 87–122.

6.8 The lower leg

Cathy Speed and Graham Holloway

Anatomy

The bones of the leg, the tibia and fibula, articulate proximally at the proximal tibiofibular joint, which communicates with the knee joint. The joint is stabilized by surrounding ligaments, capsule, and the popliteal tendon and glides when the ankle comes into dorsiflexion. It dissipates tibial bending moments and torsional loads applied to the ankle and allows distal motion of the fibula with weight-bearing. The tibia and fibula are united in the midleg by the interosseous membrane and distally by the tibiofibular syndesmosis, a continuation of the interosseous membrane in combination with four ligaments at the distal aspect of the leg. The tibial tuberosity receives the patellar tendon.

The muscles of the leg are situated within four compartments, the anterior, lateral, and the superficial and deep posterior compartments (Fig. 1).

Anterior compartment

The muscles of the anterior compartment are tibialis anterior, extensor digitorum longus (EDL), peroneus tertius (actually a part of EDL), and extensor hallucis longus (EHL) (Fig. 2).

Tibialis anterior arises from the inferolateral surface of the tibial condyle, the upper two-thirds of the lateral surface of the tibia, and the interosseous membrane. In the upper part of the leg the muscle covers the anterior tibial vessels and the deep peroneal nerve, becoming tendinous in the lower third of the leg. The tendon passes under the extensor retinaculum in front of the ankle joint, travels across the medial side of the foot, and inserts on to the medial and plantar sides of the medial cuneiform and the base of the first metatarsal. It functions as the most important dorsiflexor of the foot and also assists in adduction and inversion of the foot.

EDL arises from the lateral side of the lateral tibial condyle, the proximal two-thirds of the anterior aspect of the fibula and the anterior intermuscular septum of the leg. It becomes tendinous proximal to the ankle, passing beneath the extensor retinaculum and inserting onto the middle and distal phalanges of the first four toes. EDL functions to dorsiflex the metatarsophalangeal joints (MTPJs), proximal interphalangeal joints (PIPJs), and distal interphalangeal joints (DIPJs) along with the intrinsic muscles. *Peroneus tertius* is actually a part of EDL which inserts on to the base of the fifth metatarsal.

EHL arises from the middle three-fifths of the anterior fibula (medial to the origin of EDL) and from the adjacent interosseous membrane. Its proximal half is covered by EDL and tibialis anterior. Its tendon passes beneath the extensor retinaculum to insert on to the distal (or in some, proximal) phalanx of the hallux. It functions as an extensor of the big toe and is also a weak supinator and dorsiflexor of the foot.

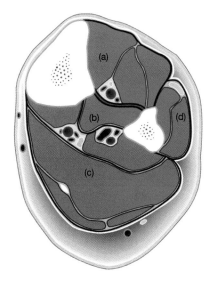

Fig. 1 Compartments of the lower leg. (a) anterior, (b) deep posterior, (c) superficial posterior, (d) lateral.

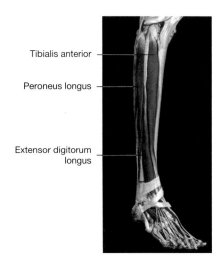

Fig. 2 The anterolateral leg. EHL arises deep to tibialis anterior and EDL.

The *saphenous nerve* is a sensory nerve, arising from the femoral nerve and enters the adductor canal. Here its two terminal branches arise and supply the anteromedial knee and medial leg.

Lateral compartment

The *peroneal muscles*, longus and brevis, represent the muscles of the lateral compartment of the leg. They are separated from the other compartments by intermuscular septae. *Peroneus longus* arises from the lateral aspect of the head and proximal two-thirds of the body of the fibula.

After passing around the lateral malleolus behind the tendon of peroneus brevis, the tendon of peroneus longus passes underneath the superior peroneal retinaculum to the cuboid notch, bends acutely medially, and travels to insert on to the medial cuneiform and base of the first metatarsal. Peroneus longus acts uniquely as a primary plantar flexor of the first ray and also acts as an accessory plantar flexor of the ankle and a weak evertor of the subtalar joint. *Peroneus brevis* arises from the lower two-thirds of the lateral fibula and adjacent intermuscular septae. The tendons of the two muscles share a common tendon sheath deep to the peroneal retinaculum behind the lateral malleolus, although they have their own sheaths further distally. Peroneus brevis inserts on to the styloid process of the fifth metatarsal. It is the strongest evertor of the subtalar joint and is a weak plantar flexor of the ankle. Both peroneii are also important in maintaining the longitudinal arch of the foot.

The *common peroneal nerve* leaves the lateral popliteal fossa, emerges from between the lateral head of gastrocnemius and biceps and winds around the neck of the fibula between the origins of peroneus longus. It then divides into superficial and deep branches. The *deep peroneal nerve* pierces the anterior intermuscular septum, passing into the anterior compartment of the leg, supplying its muscles, and entering the foot through the anterior tarsal tunnel. The *superficial peroneal nerve* passes between the peroneus longus muscle and the fibula to travel along the anterior intermuscular septum, supplying the peroneal muscles. It pierces the deep crural fascia approximately 10 cm above the lateral malleolus to divide into cutaneous branches.

The *anterior tibial artery* arises from the popliteal artery and enters the anterior compartment over the proximal interosseous membrane, descending to supply the muscles of the anterior compartment.

Superficial posterior compartment

The gastrocnemius, soleus, and plantaris muscles comprise the muscles of the superficial posterior compartment of the leg. The two heads of *gastrocnemius* muscle and the *soleus* muscle are collectively termed the *triceps surae* ('three-headed calf muscle'), which works as a prime mover and stabilizer of the rearfoot and is vital for propulsion.

The two heads of *gastrocnemius* arise from the posterior aspects of the femoral condyles and the posterior capsule of the knee. Bursae are situated deep to each head at its origin. The medial head is the larger of the two, whilst the lateral head has a bony sesamoid in approximately 11 per cent of individuals. The muscle becomes a broad tendinous sheet, the Achilles tendon, in the midleg (Fig. 4).

The *soleus* arises from the fibula and the posterior aspect of the tibia. It remains muscular deep to the Achilles tendon. The adherence of this muscular part of soleus is important to the vascularity of the gastrocnemius/Achilles tendon in its lowermost course. In the lower third of the leg the soleus muscle fibres are gradually replaced by tendon, blending with, and becoming part of, the Achilles tendon. When complete the inferior fibres of the Achilles tendon twist obliquely in their descent to their insertion on to the posterior aspect of the middle third of the calcaneus. Of the fibres, 13–52 per cent twist in an inferolateral direction around the long axis, with a degree of torsion of 11 to 65°. This torsion does not begin until the age of 10 years. The

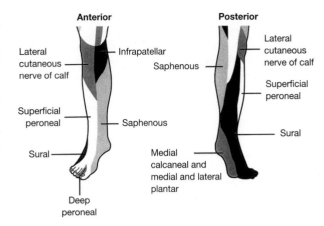

Fig. 3 Cutaneous supply of the lower leg.

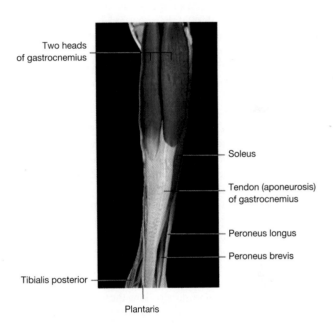

Fig. 4 The Achilles tendon is formed by the blending of the tendon of soleus with the overlying tendon of gastrocnemius.

course brings the fibres from the medial head of gastrocnemius to a more lateral position within the tendon at its insertion, and posterior fibres twist into a more lateral position. It may therefore affect any differential function of the two gastrocnemius heads at the foot. Localized torque stresses may result. Abnormal talocalcaneal motion places an uneven rotational force upon the fibres and this is the reason why hyperpronation, by increasing a strain on the medial fibres, is an aetiological factor in Achilles tendinopathies.

The Achilles tendon translates up to 4 times the power of other crural tendons and may regularly transmit 6–10 times the body weight during gait.[1] Forces of 12.5 times body weight have been recorded in the tendon when running at 6 m/s.[2] The strength of the tendon is related to its size, the gastrocnemius–soleus muscle mass, and to its having a long moment arm at the ankle. In comparison, all the other tendons acting on the ankle have short moment arms. Since the thickness of the Achilles tendon shows wide interindividual variation (up to 25 per cent), its strength is also highly variable.

The Achilles tendon is invested by a paratenon, which has no synovial component but which consists of loose elastic connective tissue that is able to stretch with movement of the tendon, allowing the tendon to glide freely.

The tendon derives much of its blood supply via the paratenon, as the musculotendinous and osseotendinous junctions are too distant to ensure adequate vascularization of this massive tendon. In a microangiographic study Lagergren and Lindholm demonstrated intratendinous vascular supply.[3] Carr and Norris subsequently showed that vascularity in the area 2–5 cm above the insertion is relatively poor.[4] This coincides with the area where most ruptures occur. Schmidt-Rohlfing *et al.* demonstrated that the area around the insertion site is also relatively hypovascular and may explain some of the pathologies seen at this site.[5]

Two bursae are associated with the Achilles tendon. The *retrocalcaneal bursa* is a horseshoe-shaped anatomical bursa and is located deeply between the upper third of the posterior surface of the calcaneus and the Achilles tendon. It is located where the tendon rubs against the posterior superior calcaneal process during ankle dorsiflexion. The bursa is filled with 1–1.5 ml of thick synovial fluid and has a synovial lining in the proximal portion, where it abuts against the Achilles fat pad.[6] The anterior bursal wall is composed of fibrocartilage laid over the calcaneus, while the posterior wall is indistinguishable from the epitenon of the Achilles tendon. Communication between the Achilles tendon at its insertion and the retrocalcaneal bursa has been demonstrated and is important when considering the impact that bursal injection may have upon the tendon proper.[7]

The second bursa commonly found in association with the Achilles tendon is the superficial or *subcutaneous calcaneal (retroachilles) bursa*, which is adventitious and develops as a result of local friction. In subcutaneous bursitis the tendon is rarely affected.

An *accessory* or *anomalous soleus muscle* is a rare variant, reported in less than 2 per cent of cases undergoing Achilles tendon surgery. There are two main types. The first and most common form is simply an extension of the muscle more distally along the tendon. The second variant is a separate insertion of soleus into the upper surface of the calcaneum via a separate tendon or insertion of the muscle directly without a tendinous component.

The *plantaris muscle*, which is absent in approximately 6 per cent of individuals, arises from the supracondylar line just above gastrocnemius. It has a short muscle belly, becoming tendinous whilst in the popliteal fossa and travelling down between gastrocnemius and soleus to emerge to insert just medial to the Achilles tendon. Like the palmaris longus muscle of the upper limb, it is a rudimentary muscle and is commonly used for tendon grafts.

Deep posterior compartment

The remaining foot and toe flexors lying deep to the gastrosoleus complex constitute the deep posterior compartment.

Flexor digitorum longus (FDL) arises from the posterior aspect of the midtibia, becomes tendinous in the lower leg, passes behind the medial malleolus, and enters the foot via the tarsal tunnel. The tendon then separates into each of its four tendons, which give origin to the lumbrical muscles and ultimately insert on to the base of the distal phalanx. FDL flexes the distal phalanges of the lateral four toes, assists in plantar flexion at the ankle, and helps to maintain the medial and longitudinal arches.

Flexor hallucis longus (FHL) arises on the posterior aspect of the fibula. Its tendon passes through the tarsal tunnel, gives off slips to the second and third toes, and then inserts into the base of the distal phalanx. FHL flexes the distal phalanx of the big toe, assists in plantar flexion at the ankle, and helps to maintain the medial arch. In the lower leg it is separated from the Achilles tendon by a fat-filled space and is in such close proximity that it can be used as a tendon graft for the Achilles.

Tibialis posterior (PT), the deepest muscle in the calf, arises from the posterior surface of the fibula, the medial posterior tibia, and the intermuscular septa. It becomes tendinous in the lower leg, lies immediately behind the medial malleolus, and enters the foot via the tarsal tunnel at the medial ankle. The tibialis posterior tendon crosses three joints along its course—the ankle, subtalar, and oblique midtarsal joints—causing specific actions at each joint it crosses, through the action of several bands. It works powerfully at the subtalar and midtarsal joints to invert the heel and supinate the foot. It also plantar flexes the foot at the ankle, plays an important role in maintaining the medial arch of the foot, and contributes to stability of the foot by its many bony attachments. It has been suggested that tibialis posterior occupies its own osteofascial compartment, distinct from the deep posterior compartment (the 'fifth compartment' of the lower leg).

Neurovascular supply of the posterior compartments

The leg is supplied by branches of the sciatic nerve, which divides into the common peroneal and tibial nerves in the popliteal fossa (Fig. 5). The tibial nerve (L4–S3) innervates the muscles of the superficial and deep posterior compartments (Fig. 5). It emerges from the popliteal fossa, passing down with the posterior tibial vessels on the tibialis posterior muscle and then on the posterior aspect of the tibia, to wind around the medial malleolus within the tarsal tunnel, terminating beneath the flexor retinaculum by dividing into the medial and lateral plantar nerves.

A branch of the tibial nerve, the medial sural nerve, is a cutaneous afferent nerve and originates from the tibial nerve, in the popliteal fossa, runs between the two heads of gastrocnemius, penetrates the superficial fascia at the junction of the upper two-thirds and lower one-third of the lateral leg, and joins with a branch of the lateral sural nerve in the lower leg to form the sural nerve. This then courses distally, providing sensation to the lateral aspect of the foot and ankle. It is in close proximity to the Achilles tendon, lying within 2 mm of the lateral border of the tendon at a level approximately 7 cm above the tip of the lateral malleolus (Fig. 5).

The posterior tibial vessels and their branches pass with the tibial nerve in the deep compartment, terminating distal to the flexor retinaculum by dividing into the medial and lateral plantar arteries.

Clinical evaluation

History

Many musculoskeletal complaints in the lower leg are activity related. Obtaining a thorough history is important in the clinical assessment of these disorders and will guide investigations since, in some complaints, there is little to find on examination at rest.

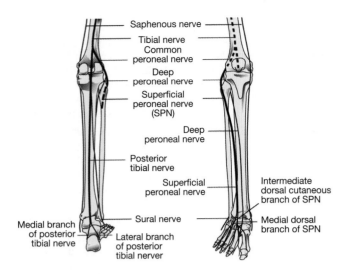

Fig. 5 Peripheral nerves of the lower leg.

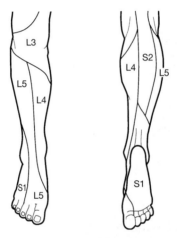

Fig. 6 Dermatomes of the lower leg.

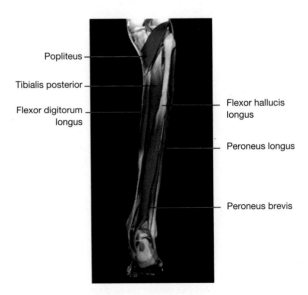

Fig. 7 The deep posterior and lateral leg.

Acute injuries are rare in comparison to those of gradual onset. The patient with a spontaneous Achilles tendon rupture usually reports a sensation of being kicked in the back of a leg, with difficulty in walking afterwards.

The duration of symptoms, nature of onset, relieving and exacerbating features, and progression should all be ascertained. Pain is the most common symptom and its site, nature, and radiation will help to define the site and nature of the injury. Nocturnal pain is suggestive of a neurogenic origin, bony damage, or an infective or malignant process. Start-up pain is typical of Achilles tendinosis.

The relation of the symptoms to activity is vital. Overuse injuries develop on the background of 'too much, too soon, too often'. Pain with stress fractures, medial tibial periostitis, and medial tibial stress syndrome is significantly worse with running or walking and pain at rest may occur. Symptoms with chronic compartment syndromes develop during specific modes of activity, are localized to one or more compartments, and settle quickly with rest.

Activities and hobbies are highly relevant, both in respect to their nature and any alteration prior to the onset of injury. Overuse is a common precipitant (Table 1). Surface and equipment factors should also be considered: has the patient been running on a hard concrete surface? What shoes does the patient wear? The use of orthotics should also be ascertained. Occupational factors, such as standing for long periods, may be relevant.

Swelling, creaking, and stiffness are common features of Achilles paratenonitis and tendinosis. Local swelling may also be reported with a stress fracture and swelling and tightness may occur in relation to a chronic compartment syndrome, settling with rest.

Table 1 Factors predisposing to overuse injuries (many apply to sport)

Extrinsic factors	Intrinsic factors
Training errors	Malalignment
Excessive volume	Pes planus
Excessive intensity	Pes cavus
Rapid increase	Rearfoot varus
Sudden change in pattern	Tibia vara
Inadequate recovery	Genu valgum
Faulty technique	Genu varum
Surface	Patella alta
Too hard	Femoral neck anteversion
Too soft	Tibial torsion
Cambered	Leg length discrepancy
Equipment (shoes)	Muscle weakness/imbalance
Inappropriate	Hypomobility/inflexibility
Worn out	General/local
Environment	Hypermobility
Too hot/cold/humid	Joint instability
Inadequate nutrition	Body composition
Psychological factors	

Vascular symptoms such as coldness, colour change, and numbness may indicate a vascular origin such as popliteal artery entrapment syndrome or a compartment syndrome, but medical causes such as peripheral vascular disease should also be considered, particularly in the older smoker and if symptoms are bilateral. Neurological symptoms raise the possibility of nerve entrapment, chronic compartment syndrome, or referred pain from the back. Bilateral symptoms increase the probability of the latter ('two legs equals one back').

Previous injuries should be noted, as this episode may be a recurrence or a 'second injury syndrome'. A medical history should also be recorded.

Examination

The lower leg is not examined in isolation but examination includes assessment of the entire lower limb and lumbar spine.

Inspection

Inspection begins with observation of the posture and attitude of the leg. Leg length (true and apparent) should be assessed as it can commonly cause lower leg complaints. Those with apparent (or functional) leg length discrepancies can be further assessed to evaluate the source of the problem. The patient stands in a relaxed position and the examiner palpates the anterior and posterior superior iliac spines (ASIS and PSIS, respectively), noting discrepancies in height. The patient is then positioned, standing, with the subtalar joints in a neutral position, with the toes pointing straight ahead. The examiner then palpates the ASIS and PSIS again. If the previously noted discrepancies remain, then the leg length discrepancy is due to changes at the pelvis and sacroiliac joints and these should be further examined. If the differences disappear, then the discrepancy is due to changes somewhere in the lower limb.

Many overuse conditions of the lower limbs are associated with biomechanical malalignments. Biomechanical aspects including femoral anteversion, tibial torsion, and the posture of the foot and ankle (Chapters 6.9 and 6.10) should be assessed. Tibial torsion is evaluated with the patient sitting with the knees over the end of the examination couch. The examiner places the thumb and index finger of one hand on the malleoli and then visualizes the axes of the knee and ankle. The lines usually form an angle of 12–18°, but internal torsion results in a reduction, and external torsion an increase, of this angle. Femoral anteversion can be assessed by asking the patient to lie flat with the knees still bent over the end of the couch. Passive rotation of the hips should be equal. An increase of internal rotation and decrease of external rotation indicate excess anteversion. An increase in external rotation and decrease in internal rotation indicate retroversion.

With the patient lying prone inspection continues for discolouration, local deformities, swelling, and calf asymmetry. A visible gap may be present after an Achilles tendon rupture.

Integrity of the Achilles tendon is first evaluated by assessing the 'angle of dangle' of the feet over the end of the examining couch. This is asymmetrical in an Achilles rupture, the foot hanging vertically since there is no plantar flexion from the normal gastrocnemius muscle tone (Fig. 9). Rupture is confirmed by no plantar flexion of the foot with squeezing the calf (Fig. 10).[8] It should be noted that this test can be insensitive, since the long extensors can perform this function. Many other tests have been suggested for Achilles tendon rupture but are no more sensitive.

Palpation

The entire tibial and fibula should be palpated to identify areas of tenderness. Percussion of these areas will exacerbate pain when stress fracture is present. The soft tissue attachments on the tibia are also palpated and the degree of tenderness compared to that of bone. This can help to identify whether pain is arising from bone or soft tissue. A palpable gap may be present after Achilles tendon rupture or after a gastrocnemius tear. Significant pain with squeezing the proximal or distal leg can indicate a syndesmosis injury. Neurovascular status is also assessed; Tinel's test should be performed over areas of suspected nerve entrapment.

Movement

Inability to perform a single heel raise test is indicative of Achilles tendon rupture, although pain may also be limiting factor. Flexibility of the calf musculature and hamstrings should be assessed; tightness of these structures can result in lower limb pain due to the biomechanical problems that result, including hyperpronation.

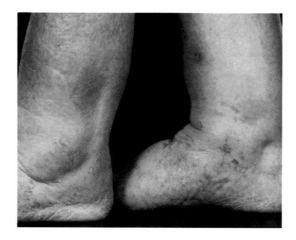

Fig. 8 The obvious gap indicates an Achilles tendon rupture, which in this patient occurred whilst on a fluoroquinolone antibiotic.

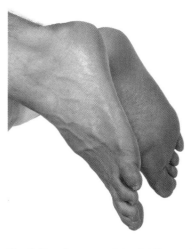

Fig. 9 Complete tears of the Achilles tendon can be diagnosed by assessing the 'angle of dangle' of the feet over the end of the examination couch.

Table 2 Causes of lower leg pain

Posterior

Chronic compartment syndrome

Gastrocnemius strain/tear

Popliteal artery entrapment syndrome

Muscle/fascial hernia(s)

Common peroneal nerve entrapment

Referred pain

  Nerve root compression

  Spinal stenosis

  Mechanical

Peripheral vascular disease

Anterior/anterolateral

Stress fractures

Medial tibial periostitis

Medial tibial stress syndrome

Muscle/fascial hernia(s)

Superficial peroneal nerve entrapment

Muscle strain, e.g. tibialis anterior

Tear of interosseous membrane

Syndesmosis injury

Tibiofibular synostosis (rare)

Others

Systemic disease: malignancy, myositis, inflammatory arthropathy

Cellulitis

DVT

Sepsis

Special tests

Many of the causes of lower limb pain are present only with exercise ('exertional lower leg pain'), and examination of the patient immediately after exacerbating activities, when symptoms are present, is usually necessary. In addition, compartment studies (described below) may be necessary.

Posterior leg pain

Achilles tendinopathies

The Achilles tendon is the largest and strongest tendon in the human body. As a consequence of its large size and immense functional demands, it is susceptible to a wide spectrum of acute and chronic injury along its entire length.

The nomenclature for conditions affecting the Achilles tendon is confusing and often misleading, not reflecting the underlying tendon disorders. Terms including tendinitis, tendinosis, tendinopathy, peritendinitis, paratenonitis, achyllodynia, degeneration, and insertitis

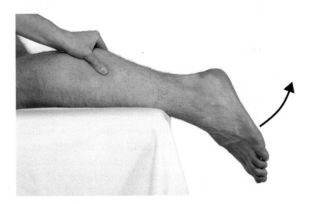

Fig. 10 Thomson's test. Achilles tendon rupture can be diagnosed if compression of the calf does not cause plantar flexion of the foot.

Table 3 Classification of Achilles tendon disorders

Term	Definition	Histology	Clinical[a]
Paratenonitis/tenosynovitis	Pathology of the paratenon/tendon sheath	Inflammatory cells in paratenon/tendon sheath	Swelling, pain, crepitus, local warmth, dysfunction
Tendinosis	Symptomatic intratendinous degeneration of the tendon	Fibre disarray, decreased cellularity, vascular ingrowth, calcification	Pain, fusiform swelling, palpable nodule
Enthesitis	Inflammatory/degenerative lesion of tendon insertion	Fibre disarray, decreased cellularity, vascular ingrowth, calcification	Localized pain, swelling, erythema, warmth, crepitus
Tear	Disruption of the structural integrity of the tendon	Significant fibre disruption, usually on background of tendinosis	Pain, weakness, palpable gap, poor response to therapy
Haglund's syndrome	Retrocalcaneal bursitis ± enthesitis in the presence of a prominence of the posterior superior portion of the calcaneum	Bursal inflammation, fibrosis, ± enthesitis	Localized pain, swelling, erythema, Haglund's deformity

a Swelling, warmth, and erythema can be minimal.

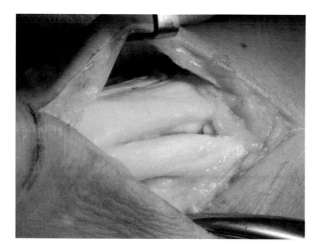

Fig. 11 A longitudinal tear of the Achilles tendon in a runner with chronic Achilles pain.

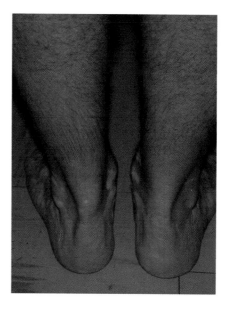

Fig. 12 Mild left Achilles tendinosis with fusiform swelling of the tendon.

are all often used interchangeably. Any classification scheme should be clinically useful aiding in treatment and should be as accurate as possible. A simple and clinically relevant classification encompassing the spectrum of injuries is described in Table 3.

Paratenonitis, tendinosis, and enthesitis

Most cases of Achilles paratenonitis and tendinosis are related to overuse, although there are some exceptions. Although 25–33 per cent of patients are reported to be not actively involved in sport,[9] occupational activities may be implicated in their development. Many of the studies on the incidence of injures have focused upon runners, where the incidence is reported to be 6.5–18 per cent[10, 11] with an incidence of 7–9 per cent in high-level runners. These studies have indicated that 55–65 per cent of lesions are peritendinous and 20–25 per cent are insertional. The vast majority (80 per cent) of those affected are men. There are no reports specifically addressing the relative risk in different sports and there appears to be significant variation between countries.[12–15]

A number of aetiological factors have been implicated in the development of Achilles tendon lesions. A common thread is one of repetitive impact loading and/or sudden acceleration (ruptures), associated with jumping. The left leg is more commonly affected, being more commonly the leg providing support and propulsion. Kvist observed one or more anatomical or biomechanical factors in 50 per cent of cases with Achilles tendinopathy.[13] Of 411 subjects, 21 per cent had calf muscle tightness, 17 per cent hyperpronation, and 15 per cent leg length inequality >1 cm.[16] However, there was no significant relationship demonstrated between these features and tendon rupture.

Oral fluoroquinolones are well recognized as a cause of Achilles tendinopathy and cause a florid inflammatory response (Fig. 8).[17, 18] This was first reported in 1983 with a single case report of bilateral Achilles 'tendinitis' during norfloxacin therapy for a urinary tract infection in a renal transplant patient. The first case report of associated Achilles tendon rupture was in 1991, in a patient on pefloxacin treatment. By 1992, 100 cases of tendon inflammation during fluoroquinolone therapy had been reported to French pharmacovigilance centres and pharmaceutical companies, including 27 cases of Achilles tendon ruptures. The average age of cases was 63 years (range, 25–84 years) and the mean time to symptom onset was 13 days (range, 1–90

days). Up to two-thirds of cases have other risk factors, including male gender, the use of systemic corticosteroid therapy, renal failure, and advanced age.[19] The adjusted relative risk (RR) of Achilles tendinopathy with fluoroquinolones was 3.7 (95 per cent, confidence interval (CI) 0.9–15.1) and 1.3 (95 per cent, CI 0.4–4.7) for other types of tendinopathy. Achilles tendinitis with ofloxacin had an RR of 10.1 (95 per cent, CI 2.2–46.0) and an excess risk of 15 cases per 100,000 exposure days.

The majority of cases involve the Achilles tendons. Fifty per cent of ruptures occur within 2 weeks of starting the fluoroquinolone, although it may occur after withdrawal of the drug.[20]

Hypercholesterolaemia plays a role in some cases. Both heterozygous familial type II hyperlipidaemia (where there is an increased total and low-density lipoprotein and a cholesterol level of 2–3 × normal) and mixed hypercholesterolaemia (increased cholesterol and triglycerides) are associated with tendon xanthomas and Achilles tendinopathy. Indeed, the musculoskeletal complaints may be the presenting features of these disorders.

Lipid storage diseases such as cerebrotendinous xanthomatosis, involving a primary defect in the synthesis of bile acids with associated elevated serum cholesterol, bile, and its precursors, may present with tendon xanthomas and/or tendinopathy, cataracts, progressive neurological dysfunction, arthralgias, and myalgias.

Haglund's syndrome

Haglund first described an exostosis of the lateral calcaneum in association with a retrocalcaneal bursitis in 1928. Haglund's syndrome is now commonly taken to represent this deformity with a retrocalcaneal bursitis, often with associated Achilles insertional tendinitis.

Ruptures

Rupture of the Achilles tendon is the most common form of spontaneous tendon rupture, affecting males more commonly than females, with studies indicating a relative frequency of 2 to 19 males for every

Table 4 Factors predisposing to Achilles tendinopathies in runners[a]

Extrinsic factors

Overtraining

Training type (e.g. too much heavy weight training)

Inappropriate surface

Poor footwear (too old, poor cushioning, high heel tab, wrong size)

Poor technique

Environment (too hot/too cold)

Iatrogenic: fluoroquinolones, corticosteroid injections

Anabolic steroid abuse

Intrinsic factors

Biomechanical malalignments including gait abnormalities (usually hyperpronation)

Stiff gastrocnemius–soleus complex, tight hamstrings

Leg-length discrepancy

Muscle imbalance

Hyper/hypomobile hindfoot

Haglund's deformity

Spondyloarthritides (enthesopathies)

[a] These factors apply to most soft tissue injuries in sport. Some can be extrapolated to the general population.

female affected.[21, 22] Ninety per cent of ruptures occur in relation to physical activity and the typical patient is the sedentary professional who participates in physical activities on the weekends (the 'weekend warrior').[23, 24] Twenty per cent are competitive athletes, who are usually younger than those recreational athletes affected.[14] Only 10 per cent of all those who rupture have had previous Achilles tendon symptoms, 30 per cent of whom are only mildly symptomatic.[13] The left leg is slightly more commonly affected than the right. Rupture most commonly occurs 3–6 cm above the insertion (83 per cent), whilst 12 per cent occur at the musculotendinous junction and 5 per cent at the insertion.[25] Simultaneous bilateral rupture is rare but successive ruptures are relatively more common.

Several studies suggest an increasing incidence of ruptures, possibly due to an increased participation of the public in sport and to increased rates of consultation and detection. The high incidence of spontaneous ruptures in the sedentary population compares with partial tears, where 76 per cent of those affected are reported to be competitive athletes.[25]

The hypothesis that rupture occurs in tendons where pre-existing degeneration is present is supported by angiographic, histological, and surgical evidence. Poor vascularity, trauma, genetic factors, muscle stiffness, and a relative weakening of the tendon are all considered to play a role in rupture and the degree of force required is often small.

Rarely, a direct contusion (such as that sustained by Achilles himself by the arrow from Paris's bow) can rupture the tendon. In these cases, the tendon is under high tension at impact. Other mechanisms are also described, including: (1) rupture with the thrust of the foot against the ground with simultaneous extension of knee, for example, when coming out of the starting blocks in a race; (2) sudden dorsiflexion of the ankle with the foot planted on the ground, for example, when stumbling into a hole; and (3) enforced dorsiflexion of the foot while it is in plantar flexion, for example, when falling from a height.

Kvist noted that the combination of a high longitudinal arch and an underpronating alignment of the ankle was significantly higher in patients with ruptures.[13] Although blood group O has been associated with Achilles rupture, further studies have refuted this.

Iatrogenic causes of Achilles tendon rupture must also be considered (Table 4). There are numerous uncontrolled case reports of Achilles rupture after *local corticosteroid injection* and there is evidence from animal studies of deleterious effects upon tendon. Crystals have been identified from tendon tissues 6 months post-injection,[26] with focal necrosis and foreign body formation around the crystals. In a review of the literature, Leppilahti and Orava found that Achilles rupture was reported to occur in a range of 0–8 per cent of cases after a corticosteroid injection for Achilles pain.[12] No rigorous studies have been performed.

The effects of *fluoroquinolones* have been described and tendon rupture may result. *Anabolic steroids* may also play a role in tendon rupture through a direct effect or as a result of increased muscular strength compared with that of the tendon.

Achilles tendinopathies
". . . this tendon, if bruised or cut, causes the most acute fevers, induces choking, deranges the mind and at length brings death . . ."
Hippocrates

History

Symptoms may vary from pain, stiffness, and severe inflammation to a minor ache, depending upon the specific disorder. Pain may be worst at the beginning of the day, with difficulty in putting the foot to the floor on getting out of bed. Precipitating factors must be sought, including activities, types of footwear, and trauma. In the sporting population a careful history must be taken of training patterns, surfaces, equipment use (including shoes), previous injuries, and additional training activities. In acute spontaneous ruptures the history of a loud bang and a feeling as if the patient has been kicked in the back of the leg, with subsequent difficulty in pushing off, is virtually diagnostic. However, pain may be absent and symptoms vague. Perhaps as a result, 25 per cent of Achilles tendon ruptures are missed at initial presentation to a physician. Partial tears of the Achilles tendon may occur as a result of a distinct episode or a series of episodes. The differential diagnosis of Achilles tendinopathy is summarized in Table 5.

In individuals with insertional tendinopathies, a systemic enquiry relating to the possibility of an associated spondyloarthritis is important (Table 6).

Examination

Paratenonitis, tendinosis and tears most commonly occur in the mid-third section of the tendon, where the area is relatively hypovascular. Local tenderness, inflammatory signs, and/or a palpable tendon nodule may be evident (Table 3). Stiffness of the gastrocnemius–soleus complex is common. The tendon may be swollen and generally tender with crepitus in acute paratenonitis.

In acute ruptures, swelling and bruising may be evident and, in the chronic ruptures, local thickening of the tendon and peritendinous tissues and muscle atrophy are commonly evident. Achilles tendon rupture can be detected using a variety of clinical tests,[8, 26–31] but the

Table 5 Differential diagnosis of Achilles tendinopathy

Calcaneal apophysitis

Sub- and retrocalcaneal bursitis

Posterior tibial stress syndrome

Peroneal and plantar flexor tendon problems

Plantar fasciitis

Stress fracture

Tarsal tunnel syndrome

Sural neuroma

Neuritis

Calcaneal periostitis

Gastrocnemius–soleus tears

Ankle ligament insertional tears

Bone anomalies—large os trigonum

Anomalous soleus muscle

Tumour

Os trigonum syndrome

Table 6 Enthesopathies: associated spondyloarthritides

Psoriatic arthritis

Reiter's syndrome/reactive arthropathy

Enteropathic arthritis (Crohn's disease, ulcerative colitis)

Ankylosing spondylitis

Seronegative enthesopathic arthropathy syndrome

Undifferentiated spondylitis

easiest is assessment of the 'angle of dangle' of the feet over the end of the examining couch. Rupture is confirmed by no plantar flexion of the foot with squeezing the calf.[8] The patient is unable to perform a single heel raise and a palpable gap may be present (Fig. 8).

Partial tears are often difficult to diagnose. Weakness of dorsiflexion and a failure to respond to conservative management should arouse suspicion but imaging is usually necessary.

Insertional tendinitis is commonly associated with a retrocalcaneal bursitis and a Haglund's deformity (an exostosis over the lateral aspect of the calcaneus caused by recurrent friction, particularly in association with a hypermobile rearfoot). Insertional tendinitis causes local tenderness, swelling, and hyperaemia at the insertion.

In retrocalcaneal bursitis, bursal swelling is often seen both sides of the Achilles tendon although it is not so obvious in chronic situations. In acute and subacute cases, there is painful swelling and occasionally hyperaemia of overlying skin in the posterosuperior corner of the calcaneus. Dorsiflexion of the foot is painful.

Predisposing anatomical factors should be sought (Table 4). Gait should be assessed for hyperpronation, leg-length discrepancy, and deformities. Footwear should always be closely examined, specifically inspecting the heel tabs, wear pattern of the sole (which may indicate a hyperpronatory gait), and overall condition and suitability for the purpose for which they are being worn.

Imaging of Achilles tendinopathies

Magnetic resonance imaging (MRI) and ultrasound are the two most useful approaches in imaging the Achilles tendon and surrounding features. Both can show areas of degeneration within the tendon (tendinosis) and areas of inflammation in either the tendon 'sheath' (paratenon) or the tendon itself (tendinitis). Retrocalcaneal and retroachilles bursae are also detected using these imaging modalities. The reported sensitivity to the detection of tears is variable but these techniques remain the best approach.

Plain X-rays may be helpful in the assessment of a Haglund's deformity, bony spurs associated with insertional tendon pain, and in excluding an os trigonum.

Management of Achilles tendinopathies

Paratenonitis, tendinosis, and enthesitis

Non-surgical management is appropriate for most cases, but the patient must be warned that progress may be very slow. As is the case with so many soft tissue injuries, controlling symptoms to allow rehabilitation to be performed is a central goal. In acute and subacute cases, the PRICES (protection, rest, ice, compression, elevation, and support) approach is appropriate. Rest is relative. Reducing the intensity, frequency, and duration of loading activities and cross training through the adoption of alternative modes of activity that do not stress the tendon (swimming, cycling) are encouraged. Whilst heel raises may be useful, they should not be worn constantly. In severe cases, functional casting or, rarely, the use of crutches may be necessary.

Cryotherapy in the form of ice, cold compresses or ice immersion is used to control pain, reduce muscle spasm, oedema, regional blood flow, and the metabolic demands of tissue, and thereby prevent further tissue damage. Cryotherapy can be used for up to 20 minutes at 1-hour intervals. To avoid cold injuries excessive compression should be avoided and the skin protected from direct contact.

Nonsteroidal anti-inflammatory drugs (NSAIDs) may provide pain relief and an earlier return to activities, but the patient should be warned of the masking of symptoms by NSAIDs. Topical NSAIDs are preferable, as high levels in the tendon can be achieved, they have the least risk of side-effects, and local massage of the drug into the tendon can in itself provide relief.[32]

In some European countries, local anticoagulant therapy is advocated for early management of acute paratenonitis, with the aim to reduce oedema, fibrin exudates, and resulting adhesions between tendon and peritendinous tissues.[13, 33] Convincing evidence for benefit is lacking and this approach is not widely advocated elsewhere.

Once the very acute symptoms have resolved, early stretching of the gastrocnemius and soleus muscles separately, in addition to attention to hamstring stretching, is very important. Heat may be useful later in providing analgesia, reducing muscle spasm, improving tissue extensibility, inducing vasodilatation, and to increase vascular permeability and metabolism. Warm whirlpools, warm packs, hot gels, contrast baths, paraffin wax, and infrared may all be used for this purpose.

Local modalities including ultrasound, deep heat, and laser may be useful. Massage, in particular deep transverse friction massage, often confers benefit, as does the use of a dorsiflexion night splint. Functional orthoses should be considered and gradual strength training of the lower leg musculature should be introduced once the patient is pain-free.

Glycosaminoglycan polysulfate (GAGPS) resembles the chemical composition of heparin and the proposed basis for its use is the reduction of fibrin deposition and thrombus formation and inhibition of collagen breakdown. Local injections of GAGPS are of unproven benefit and have potential side-effects including haemorrhage, thrombocytopenia, and hypersensitivity.[34] It is perhaps because of these side-effects that its use is not popular.

Attention to precipitating factors is very important. This may include altering the training in terms of intensity, types, and surfaces, addressing biomechanical issues and errors in technique, and changing equipment, particularly footwear, as discussed above. Heel tabs should be cut down to avoid impingement on the tendon.

In those cases where a fluoroquinolone is implicated, immediate withdrawal of the offending agent and treatment of the local disorder is necessary. In a study by Royer et al. 75 per cent of cases with fluoroquinolone-associated Achilles tendinosis had a favourable outcome with this strategy, with recovery of symptoms within 2 months.[35]

Where the tendinosis is associated with hyperlipidaemic states, hypolipidaemic therapy with a statin is indicated, with 63 per cent of cases showing significant improvement or resolution of symptoms with this approach.[36] Lipid storage diseases such as cerebrotendinous xanthomatosis are treated with chenodeoxycholic acid, although the effect on the tendon lesions is undocumented.

Appropriate rehabilitation is essential for a successful return to full activities. This includes stretching of the gastrocnemius–soleus complex and hamstrings and gradual strengthening of the calf musculature, including an eccentric muscle training programme. Return to activity should be gradual and closely monitored. The key to success is ensuring that the patient has a full understanding of the disorder and that the process of recovery may be a lengthy process.

Corticosteroid injections have no role to play, as they are usually ineffective and may weaken the tendon with resulting rupture.

Although most cases are managed conservatively, surgery may be considered in those individuals who remain significantly limited in spite of intensive rehabilitation for 12–18 months. Numerous surgical techniques, alone or in combination, have been advocated,[37] although none have been subjected to rigorous evaluation. Approaches include stripping of the paratenon, from the tendon proper, in particular in those patients with persisting paratenonitis where adhesions have developed. Tenotomy and excision and repair of areas of macroscopic tendinosis is also a widely applied technique. Percutaneous tenotomy with multiple longitudinal incisions of the area of maximal degeneration has also been proposed.[38]

There is a significant potential for complications of surgery in this area, and the reported incidence in such cases is up to 13 per cent.[9] Complications include poor wound healing, local nerve damage, infection, and failure of the repair.

Enthesitis and bursitis

Treatment approaches are similar to those detailed above, with the exception of the use of anticoagulant therapy. Relief of friction between the heel counter and the bursal projection through padding and the modification of the shape, height, and rigidity of the heel counter are all recommended. The height of the heel of the shoe influences symptoms: as the heel is raised, the angle of calcaneal inclination is decreased, bringing projection away from heel counter.

Although corticosteroid injections are recommended by some in the management of these lesions, they are usually not necessary and it is important to remember that the bursa frequently communicates with peritendinous tissue. In acute bursitis with intrabursal fluid, aspiration is performed. Haglund's syndrome may take many months to show signs of improvement with conservative measures.

Extracorporeal shock wave therapy (ESWT) can be useful in cases of calcific disorders or ossification of the Achilles tendon, which most commonly occurs at the insertion.

A seronegative arthropathy should be considered in those patients who have persisting insertional Achilles tendinopathy and/or retrocalcaneal bursitis. Patients with recalcitrant retrocalcaneal bursitis or Haglund's syndrome may be managed surgically, which may involve debridement or resection of the bursa or (as appropriate) excision of the posterior superior calcaneus (Haglund's deformity). Calcaneal osteotomy has also been advocated although it is considerably more invasive.

Rupture

Initial treatment of the acute Achilles tendon rupture involves the PRICES regime. The options are then early surgical repair and 6 weeks bracing or bracing for 8 weeks. Re-rupture rate is similar for both approaches but is variably reported to be 0–50 per cent. Early surgery results in less calf atrophy, greater range of motion, faster resumption of sporting activities, and fewer subjective complaints.[39] However, nonsurgical management is also acceptable, particularly where the patient is less active or not a good surgical candidate. Various techniques have been described, broadly categorized as primary repair or (less commonly) with augmentation using a gastrocnemius flap, plantaris tendon, fascial reinforcement, flexor hallucis longus, or artificial materials such as mesh.[40] An aggressive postoperative regimen is commonly followed, with early mobilization and commencement of rehabilitation. Complications of surgery in this region have been described above and occur at a similar rate to those in surgery for tendinosis.

Chronic tears

The neglected rupture should be treated surgically, as the functional results otherwise can be devastating. Primary repair may be attempted, but reconstruction using local tissue or FHL is more frequently necessary than in the acute rupture.

Partial tears

Partial Achilles tears are often classified as tendinosis and are managed in the same way. In the acute stage, management follows the PRICES regime for 4–7 days, with rest to prevent further tear and the use of a brace support. Surgery is rarely necessary but those who do not respond to conservative treatment, or those with substantial tears, can be managed with primary repair.

Gastrocnemius tear

A partial tear of the gastrocnemius ('tennis leg') usually occurs in the upper third of the muscle when it is overstretched, with the ankle in dorsiflexion and the knee in full extension. The patient notes acute searing pain preventing further activity. Extensive swelling and bruising develops quickly and may progress over the subsequent 48 h. A palpable defect may be present and there is weakness and pain with resisted ankle plantar flexion.

It is important to exclude a deep vein thrombosis and ultrasound/venography are frequently required. Ultrasound and MRI are both sensitive methods in the diagnosis of gastrocnemius tear. Inappropriate treatment with anticoagulants can lead to further bleeding into the muscle and precipitate an acute compartment syndrome. The latter can also occur in the absence of anticoagulation if the damage is extensive.

Management involves the PRICES support. Partial or non-weight-bearing for the first 2–3 days may be necessary. The patient is given a 0.5 inch heel lift for 2 weeks to ease the stretch on the injured muscle. Range of motion exercises are commenced early and gradual strengthening of the hamstrings and gastrocnemius–soleus complex introduced, when symptoms allow. Ballistic actions are avoided until full range of motion and strength are regained. A pre-exercise warm-up and stretching regime is introduced with the aim to prevent recurrence.

It may take 3 months or longer before a full return to activities is achieved, but the prognosis is excellent and surgical intervention is not usually necessary.

Effort-induced venous thrombosis

Although commonly noted in upper extremities, effort-induced venous thrombosis in the lower limb is less well recognized. An acute onset of pain in the calf after exercise is the predominant feature, although symptoms may be felt anteriorly. Examination reveals the typical signs of a deep venous thrombosis (DVT)—a tight tender and usually enlarged calf. An ultrasound and venogram are performed to confirm the diagnosis and treatment with anticoagulation is commenced immediately.

Anomalous soleus muscle

An anomalous soleus muscle can become painful, usually presenting between the ages of 9 and 27 years. Symptoms include pain and tenderness in front of the Achilles tendon and there is evidence of fullness or a bulbous mass at the medial or lateral side of the tendon. Various treatment recommendations exist: stretching, activity modification, a medial heel wedge, and orthotics should all be considered. Surgery in the form of fasciotomy or surgical excision is reserved for intractable cases.

Chronic exertional compartment syndromes (CECS)

Chronic compartment syndrome refers to calf muscle pain as a result of presumed relative ischaemia due to raised intracompartmental pressure during exercise. The raised intracompartmental pressure has been attributed to vascular factors, metabolic factors, and others, including fascial hypertrophy, muscular hypertrophy, and tissue oedema. Proposed mechanisms for the development of ischaemia as a result of raised compartment pressure include arterial spasm, obstruction of the microcirculation, arteriolar or venous collapse due to transmural pressure disturbances, or venous obstruction. The existence of tissue ischaemia in CECS has been questioned and alternative explanations for the pain have been proposed, including stimulation of sensory receptors in the periosteum due to elevated pressure or biochemical factors.

History

The patient typically reports dull aching pain and tightness in the lower leg with exercise. The symptoms typically commence at a defined point in the exercise session and may become progressively severe, frequently necessitating cessation of activity. The symptoms resolve with rest, only to recur when the activity recommences. In some cases there may be residual ache into the next day. The site of the pain varies according to the compartment(s) involved. Neurological symptoms may occur, varying according to the nerve(s) involved, but typically causing numbness and weakness. The most common is involvement of the anterior compartment, resulting in pain in the anterolateral aspect of the leg. Next most common is deep posterior compartment syndrome, when pain over the medial shin and/or distal posterior calf may spread to the medial foot. Superficial posterior compartment syndrome is uncommon, giving proximal calf pain. Isolated lateral compartment syndrome is rare; it is usually seen in the presence of an anterior compartment syndrome. It is common for more than one compartment to be affected and symptoms are commonly bilateral although they may be worse in one leg.

Examination

At rest, clinical examination is normal although the muscles in a compartment may feel rather tense. On standing there may be evidence of small muscle herniae. The patient must be examined when symptomatic, that is during and after the onset of symptoms with exercise. At this stage the compartment will be tense, firm, and painful to deep palpation and passive stretch. Neurological impairment may be evident. Anterior compartment syndrome results in deep peroneal nerve compression, with weakness of dorsiflexion, and altered sensation over the first web space. Lateral CECS causes superficial peroneal nerve impairment, with sensory signs over the lateral lower leg and dorsum of the foot and weakness of eversion. Deep posterior CECS can result in tibial nerve dysfunction, with sensory changes over the medial arch of the foot and/or cramping of the foot muscles. Distal pulses remain normal. The symptoms and signs will improve, usually over a short period of time during the assessment. Ankle reflexes may be diminished.

Muscle hernias are associated with CECS, particularly at the site where the superficial peroneal nerve exits the deep fascia at the lateral leg. Paraesthesia is common due to nerve entrapment at the site of the defect. Other causes of exertional lower limb pain must be considered during the evaluation.

Investigations: compartment pressure studies

The most useful investigation in suspected CECS is a compartment pressure study. Although high levels on compartment pressure measurements are considered to be necessary for the diagnosis of compartment syndromes, the apparatus, the methodologies used, and the specific compartment pressure levels for diagnosis of the complaint vary significantly. The accuracy, sensitivity, and specificity of compartment pressure studies are not known (Fig. 13).

Apparatuses have varied from needle manometers, side-ported needles, and simple needles to wick catheters, slit catheters, and using infusion or a non-infusion technique with an electronic transducer-tipped catheter.[41–43] Pressures can vary considerably with operator experience, apparatus, volume of instilled fluid, leg position, activity type, and the timing of measurement(s). Sejersted and Hargens pointed out that intramuscular pressure follows the law of Laplace, which means that it is determined by the tension of the muscle fibres, the recording depth and by fibre geometry (fibre curvature or pennation angle).[44] Such factors will also be sources of variation in the

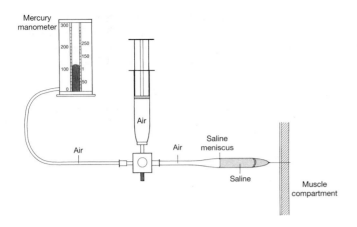

Fig. 13 Basic components of compartment pressure measurement: the Whiteside method.

Table 7 Diagnostic levels for chronic compartment syndrome

Authors (reference no.)	Criteria
Allen and Barnes (41)	Anterior compartment: > 15 mmHg
	Deep posterior compartment: > 40 mmHg
Bourne and Rorabeck (42)	Elevated post-exercise pressure and delay (> 5 min) in return to pre-exercise levels
Fronek et al. (43)	At least 10 mmHg at rest or at least 25 mmHg 5 min after exercise
Pedowitz et al. (44)	Appropriate clinical findings and at least one of:
	Pre-exercise pressure of > 15 mmHg
	1-min post-exercise pressure > 30 mmHg
	5-min post-exercise pressure > 20 mmHg
Rorabeck et al. (49)	Pressure > 15 mmHg at 15 min post-exercise

pressure level reading. The patient is tested during the activity that most usually exacerbates the symptoms, usually running, which is conveniently performed on a treadmill in a laboratory or clinic setting. Measurements are taken at rest and after exercise at specific stages, when symptoms are present, including during the recovery.

Willy et al.[45] performed a meta-analysis of 21 studies (1979–1998) measuring anterior intracompartmental pressures exercise. They evaluated the type of exercise, catheter technique, and the diagnostic criteria recommended. Their findings demonstrated that there has been no standardization concerning the type of muscular exertion (isometrics for 5–10 min, exercise on the treadmill between 3.2 and 12 km/h). In 8 of the 21 studies the results were attained through the unsuitable Wick-catheter-technique. There was little or no overlap in the use of suggested criteria for diagnosis between teams and there are considerable variations (by up to 500 per cent) regarding the recommended parameters. The authors concluded that no uniform recommendation for parameters of diagnostic relevance can be derived.

Positioning of the catheter is important although this is usually not a problem except in the tibialis posterior and deep posterior compartments. Melberg and Styf described some of the difficulties associated with pressure recording in the deep posterior compartment[46] and found that the result of pressure recording depends on which muscle in the deep posterior compartment is investigated and on the type of work performed. Ultrasound guidance also has the advantage of placement of the catheter tip into a specific muscle belly.

The patient with CECS may undergo a range of other investigations, usually to exclude other causes of exertional lower limb pain. Table 7 summarizes diagnostic levels used by various authors for chronic compartment syndrome.

Management

Treatment of chronic compartment syndrome is considered to be either restriction in activity or fasciotomy. Although the latter is claimed to be 'curative' in most cases, neither adequate follow-up studies nor randomized controlled trials have been performed

Although the standard surgery for exertional anterior compartment syndrome is subcutaneous fasciotomy of the anterior compartment through a short incision, some surgeons decompress the lateral compartment at the same time to prevent kinking or entrapment of

the superficial peroneal nerve as it exits the lateral compartment. Schepsis et al.[47] suggested that, when doing a fasciotomy for exertional anterior compartment syndrome alone, a lateral compartment release is not necessary.

Decompression of the superficial and deep posterior compartments may be done through a single long incision, protecting the saphenous nerve and long saphenous vein and its tributaries. Fasciotomy under direct vision is safer than blind subcutaneous fasciotomy.

Wallenstein[48] studied the results of fasciotomy of the affected muscle compartment in eight patients with chronic anterior-compartment syndrome and in nine patients with medial tibial syndrome (involvement of the deep posterior compartment), all of whom had pain with exercise. In the patients with chronic anterior-compartment syndrome, the preoperative intramuscular pressure in the anterior tibial compartment, as measured by the wick-catheter method, was increased 10 min after exercise to 52 ± 36 mmHg. After fasciotomy this pressure was significantly lowered to 4 ± 6 mmHg of ($p < 0.01$). In the patients with medial tibial syndrome, the preoperative intramuscular pressure in the deep posterior compartment was normal 10 minutes after exercise (8 ± 4 mmHg) and did not significantly change after the fasciotomy (5 ± 6 mmHg). The clinical results after fasciotomy were 'good' in both groups of patients. There was complete relief of pain in all of the patients with chronic anterior-compartment syndrome and in five of the nine patients with medial tibial syndrome. The other four patients considered their condition to be improved in spite of some remaining symptoms.

Rorabeck et al.[49] reported a higher likelihood of recurrence if the deep posterior compartment was involved. Micheli et al.[50] found a lower success rate with operative fasciotomy in young female athletes than those generally reported in studies that combine male and female patients. The reasons for this are unclear.

Christensen et al.[51] reported normalization of previously elevated compartment pressures in five active middle-aged men with chronic compartment syndrome after 2–3 weeks of diuretic therapy. Rorabeck et al.[49] noted poorer results in patients with deep posterior compartment syndromes and recommended that a formal release of the tibialis posterior at the time of decompression was performed—however, the results of this procedure were not given.

Closure of muscle herniae is contraindicated and may precipitate a compartment syndrome. Postoperatively, it is essential to commence an exercise programme after 24 hours to maintain muscle tone and bulk and to keep the fascia from healing without separation.

Popliteal artery entrapment syndrome

Vascular causes are an important cause of exercise-related leg pain but, with the exception of peripheral vascular disease, are rare. However, popliteal artery entrapment syndrome (PAES) is included in the differential diagnosis.

As the artery exits the popliteal fossa it can become entrapped by the gastrocnemius. Several anomalies have been described, most commonly an abnormal medial head of gastrocnemius, the accessory part of which may pass behind the popliteal artery. Other anomalies of the medial and lateral heads of gastrocnemius, accessory tendinous slips, and an abnormal plantaris muscle have also been implicated in this condition. The artery can also become entrapped at the adductor hiatus and isolated entrapment of the anterior tibial artery as it passes through the interosseous membrane can also occur.

History

The patient complains of an ill-defined deep ache in the calf and/or anterior aspect of the leg with exercise. The severity of symptoms is related to the intensity of the exercise and resolves with rest, typically more quickly than that of chronic compartment syndrome. In addition, unlike chronic compartment syndrome, the pain from PAES is unaffected by exercise the previous day. It should be noted that the conditions can coexist.

Examination

Examination of the patient at rest may reveal a popliteal artery bruit with active resisted plantar flexion or passive dorsiflexion with the knee in extension.

Investigations

Compartment studies are usually performed as clinical differentiation between the two syndromes is often difficult. Duplex ultrasonography of the arterial tree is performed with the ankle being actively and passively plantarflexed and dorsiflexed. If flow is reduced, digital subtraction angiography is done. MR angiography is probably the investigation of choice in the young adult with intermittent claudication. This may show displacement and compression of the popliteal artery on axial view.

If angiography shows no evidence of intramural vascular damage, simple division of constricting bands or muscles may be all that is necessary. Otherwise, the abnormal portion of the vessel is bypassed with a reversed vein graft, using the short saphenous vein.

Anterior leg pain

Stress fractures

Although not a soft tissue injury, stress fracture is vital to consider in the differential diagnosis of exertional lower limb pain and no apologies are offered for its inclusion here. A stress fracture can be defined as a partial or complete fracture of bone caused by an inability to withstand stress that is applied in a rhythmic repeated subthreshold manner. It is a reflection of a bone's inability to adequately remodel in response to mechanical stress placed upon it.

Stress fractures can be further classified as *fatigue fractures*, when due to overloading of normal bone, or *insufficiency fractures*, produced when physiological stress is applied to bone with reduced mechanical integrity. Fatigue stress fractures of the tibia and fibula usually occur in relation to running or marching and represent 45 per cent of all stress fractures seen in relation to sport. Since the tibia transmits approximately 83 per cent of body weight, it is the most common site for stress fractures in sport.

Stress fractures of the tibia and fibula can be further classified according to their site. Stress fractures of the tibia most commonly occur in the proximal or distal thirds of the posteromedial cortex. They may also be seen just distal to the tibial tuberosity in active young people. Those just below the tibial plateau may be clinically mistaken for pes anserinus bursitis or a medial collateral ligament (MCL) sprain. Most lesions occur at sites where bone is under compression stress, but they can also occur at sites of tension, such as the middle third of the tibia on the anterior cortex. Since the bone is under tension at this site, healing is more difficult, with significant risk of nonunion or full fracture. Such injuries must be monitored particularly carefully, as they are slower to heal and more likely to progress to a complete fracture. Aggressive management, including surgical intervention, may be necessary.

History

Symptoms usually commence after a change in the volume or intensity of activity, training techniques, equipment (footwear), or after another injury (Table 1). Menstrual irregularities are often associated with stress fractures in female athletes.

The patient reports a gradual onset of localized dull pain at the site of the injury, usually 2–6 weeks after an increase in training load. The pain is initially noted at a specific stage during exercise and, as symptoms progress, the pain occurs earlier during exercise, often leading to a restriction in the volume and/or intensity of the activity. Eventually, there is pain at rest, which may disturb the patient at night.

A detailed history is taken of training patterns, surfaces, equipment, technical alterations, diet, previous injuries, and, in females, a menstrual history. General health should also be evaluated in particular in relation to bone health.

Examination

There is local bony tenderness at the site of the stress fracture. Local swelling and warmth may be present and, in more chronic cases, periosteal thickening and/or callus may be palpable. Percussion both at and away from the site of the fracture reproduces the symptoms. Exacerbation of pain with the application of therapeutic ultrasound to the symptomatic area is a widely quoted but insensitive test. Intrinsic factors that may predispose the patient to developing a stress fracture must be considered and the patient evaluated appropriately.

Investigations

Plain X-rays have a low sensitivity for the detection of stress fractures and may be normal for up to 12 weeks. However, the specificity is high

Table 8 Imaging of stress reactions: grading system (52, 53)

Grade	Bone scan appearance	MRI appearance[a]
I	Small ill-defined cortical area of mild increased activity	Periosteal oedema: +/++ (T2-W) Marrow oedema: absent (T1-W, T2-W)
II	Better defined cortical area of moderately increased activity	Periosteal oedema: ++/+++ (T2-W) Marrow oedema: present (T2-W)
III	Wide to fusiform cortical-medullary area of highly increased activity	Periosteal oedema: ++/+++ (T2-W) Marrow oedema: present (T1-W, T2-W)
IV	Transcortical area of increased activity	Periosteal oedema: ++/+++ (T2-W) Marrow oedema: present (T1-W, T2-W) Fracture line clearly visible

[a] +, Mild; ++, moderate; +++, severe. T1-W, T2-W: T1- or T2-weighted images, respectively.

when changes are evident. Periosteal reaction is the first sign, followed by cortical lucency as osteoclastic resorption occurs. The healing stress fracture will demonstrate thick periosteal new bone formation, endosteal thickening, and cortical hypertrophy. Demonstration of a fracture line is variable. Similar findings may be noted in an osteoid osteoma, osteomyelitis, osteogenic sarcoma, exostoses, or tumours that result in periosteal reaction, peripheral bone reaction, or destruction and Paget's disease.

A triple phase isotope bone scan is the current investigation of choice in the early detection of a stress fracture.[52, 53] It is highly (virtually 100 per cent) sensitive, with all phases of the triple phase scan being abnormal within 2 days of onset of the lesion, demonstrating an increased uptake of radionuclide. A grading system has been developed, based upon the degree and pattern of tracer uptake (Table 8). The system reflects a continuum of changes, from the early 'pre-fracture' bone strain, through stress reaction, to stress fracture. Bone strain and stress reactions can be apparent on scintigrams in the absence of symptoms, as a reflection of bone remodelling in response to mechanical stress. Only a percentage of cases will progress to develop a stress fracture. The fusiform appearance of an established stress fracture differs significantly from the more diffuse linear uptake seen in medial tibial periostitis.

As healing of the stress fracture progresses, the first (angiogram) phase and subsequently the blood pool images become normal. Delayed images remain abnormal for at least 3–6 (and often up to 12) months. A false-positive rate of 10–20 per cent is reported, and is due to accelerated bone remodelling. Positive scans are also seen at the epiphyses of adolescents.

MRI is being increasingly used in the investigation of the suspected stress fracture and may soon supersede the use of isotope bone scanning for this purpose, having the advantage of lack of radiation exposure, faster imaging time, and demonstration of surrounding anatomy. A combination of T1-weighted sequences that optimize anatomical detail and a sequence that depicts bone oedema (such as short T1 inversion recovery (STIR), fat-suppressed proton density, and T2-weighted fast-spin echo sequences) are required.

Computerized tomography (CT) can help to differentiate between conditions that can mimic stress fractures, such as osteoid osteoma as described earlier. This mode of imaging is also helpful in demonstrating a fracture line as evidence of stress fracture, as opposed to a stress reaction.

Management

Management is dependent upon the location and severity of the lesion and is based upon reducing the stress at the affected site to allow healing to occur. Relative rest by the reduction of loading activities is the cornerstone of management in most cases. Cross-training allows fitness to be maintained to a large extent through activities that involve little or no loading, such as swimming, water running, indoor rowing, and cycling. Strength training can be continued provided that excessive loading of the affected area is avoided.

In the early stages, ice packs, analgesics or NSAIDs, and interferential electrical stimulation may provide symptomatic relief. The use of a pneumatic brace (Air-Stirrup leg brace) may also help to relieve symptoms and has been shown to reduce the time taken to return to activity and probably works through unloading the tibia by compressing the lower leg, redistributing the forces (including to surrounding soft tissue), and decreasing the amount of tibia bowing. Modification of risk factors is vital to the prevention of recurrence. Progressive activity is strictly regulated, as indicated by a sample programme, given in Table 9. When the patient resumes full training it is important to ensure that adequate recovery sessions are scheduled between periods of heavy training and that all training errors have been corrected.

Stress fractures of the anterior cortex of the midshaft of the tibia are prone to non-union, delayed union, and complete fracture. If the patient presents late, then a plain radiograph may demonstrate the 'dreaded black line', due to bony resorption and indicative of non-union. Isotope bone scan at that late stage may show no abnormality. Management involves avoidance of aggravating load-bearing, use of a long pneumatic leg brace (Aircast), and close monitoring, both clinical and radiographic, to ensure healing is taking place. The mean time to heal is 9 months. Failure to show signs of healing after 4–6 months is an indication for surgical intervention.

Medial malleolar stress fractures are also prone to delayed or non-union. They extend from the tibial plafond proximally in an oblique direction. They are inherently unstable and may require extensive period of casting. Early internal fixation with screws has been advocated.

Table 9 Typical training programme for the athlete with a stress fracture[a]

Stage	Instructions
1	Non-weight-bearing (NWB) until pain-free. NWB exercise daily in a pool and with light weights
2	Progress to partial weight-bearing until pain-free
3	Progress to full weight-bearing (walking)
4	When pain-free, run at 50 per cent pace according to following schedule

	Day 1 (min)	Day 2 (min)	Day 3 (min)	Day 4 (min)	Day 5 (min)	Day 6 (min)	Day 7 (min)
Week 1	3	0	3	0	3	0	6
Week 2	0	6	0	6	0	9	0
Week 3	9	0	9	0	12	0	12
Week 4+	Etc., until 15 min, on alternate days is reached. Then increase to 75 per cent pace over 2–3 weeks. Then return to full pace and gradually introduce short runs on rest days. Then resume full training.						

[a] If pain is experienced, go back one stage.

Fibular stress fractures are usually found just proximal to the tibiofibular syndesmosis, where stress is particularly concentrated during muscle contraction. Less commonly, stress fractures can occur anywhere on the neck of the fibula.

Medial tibial periostitis

Several anatomical structures have been proposed to cause traction of the periosteal–fascial junction at the posteromedial tibial border, resulting in medial tibial periostitis.[54] Soleus is the most likely to be involved, since it partially attaches medially to the investing fascia. FDL and the deep crural fascia have also been implicated. The role that tibialis posterior plays is controversial. In an anatomic dissection study, Saxena *et al.* demonstrated that the origin of the tibialis posterior does include a portion of the lower third of the tibia.[55] The mean distance from tibialis posterior's origin to the medial malleolus was only 7.77 cm. In addition, to further explain lower leg pain, the authors investigated the crossing point of tibialis posterior and FDL. A mean distance for this to occur in the same 10 specimens was 8.16 cm proximal to the medial malleolus. These findings may imply that these structures play a role in medial tibial periostitis and medial tibial stress syndrome. The most accepted theory on the aetiology of the condition is that, in some athletes when running, an excessive degree or velocity of pronation increases the eccentric stress on supporting musculature, in particular, the soleus. The velocity of pronation may be a more important factor than the actual degree. Stiffness of the gastrocnemius–soleus musculature may also be a contributing factor.

Training errors are reported as aetiological factors in 60 per cent of those who develop the condition. Usually, there is an abrupt increase in the frequency, duration, or intensity of training. Training on hard surfaces, hill training, and inappropriate footwear, with inadequate cushioning and/or support, are also common associated factors. The relevance of physical conditioning to the complaint is unclear.

It has been postulated that those patients who develop the condition acutely after a sudden exposure to high-intensity training (such as in the military) may progress to develop a stress fracture. This is considerably less likely in those with chronic symptoms.

History

The patient complains of dull pain along the posteromedial border of the distal two-thirds of the tibia in association with weight-bearing activity. Symptoms usually commence after a change in one or more of the typical extrinsic factors or may be associated with various intrinsic characteristics associated with overuse injuries. Symptoms appear initially in the early phase of exercise but may disappear if exercise continues, only to return towards the end of the session. At this stage there is no pain at rest. As the condition progresses, symptoms occur earlier in the activity session and, when severe, can be present during daily activities and finally will disturb the patient at rest.

Examination

The patient should be evaluated for deformities of the leg, foot, and ankle, and limb alignment should be assessed. There is diffuse tenderness along the posteromedial border of the distal two-thirds of the tibia, more marked on the bone than adjacent soft tissue. Local oedema and warmth may be noted. Stretching of the soleus may exacerbate the symptoms. Passive and active movements of the ankle and foot are pain-free and normal. Pain will also be exacerbated by progressive loading of the plantar flexor musculature, through forced passive dorsiflexion, active plantarflexion against resistance, two-leg standing toe raises, two-leg standing jumps, and maximal stress with one-legged jumps. The condition must be differentiated from other causes of lower limb pain. Percussion of the tibia should not cause a local increase in pain and no callus should be palpable. Neurovascular examination is normal.

Gait analysis, looking in particular at rearfoot motion is also performed, in particular to assess the degree of pronation.

Investigation

Plain radiographs are almost always normal. In chronic severe cases there may be evidence of periosteal reaction, with new bone formation and cortical hypertrophy at the site of symptoms. The investigation of choice is a triple phase isotope bone scan, which will demonstrate diffusely increased uptake on the posteromedial border of the tibia in the delayed phase of the scan. This differs from the more intense focal uptake seen in tibial stress fractures. Medial and lateral views may help to localize the uptake better. Tomographic bone scans and single-photon emission computerized tomography (SPECT) may help to identify difficult lesions, although this is rarely necessary.

MRI may demonstrate periosteal fluid or bone marrow oedema in chronic cases or alteration adjacent to the insertion of the plantar flexor muscles in more acute cases. The sensitivity of MRI in this condition has yet to be established.

Management

No intervention will be successful without identification and correction of the underlying causes (Table 2).

Relative rest varies according to the severity of the symptoms and may involve simply reducing the intensity or volume of training to total avoidance of load-bearing activities. Cross-training such as cycling, swimming, and water running in an aqua vest, is helpful in maintaining cardiovascular fitness and muscle strength. Ice in the form of cold compresses and ice massage, local massage, NSAIDs, acupuncture, and stretching are useful. Muscle imbalances should be corrected. Orthoses are often useful in this condition. A medial heel post is used in those with hyperpronation, while a medial forefoot post may help in those with forefoot varus. Heel pads and cushioned insoles may provide shock absorbency. Cushioned, supportive footwear should be recommended, avoiding shoes with a wide heel, which can increase the velocity of foot pronation through heel strike.

When the patient is pain-free, progressive weight-bearing conditioning commences, supplemented by calf muscle stretching muscle balance work. Generally, the volume can be increased by 10 per cent per week, providing the patient remains pain-free. Should symptoms recur, then the patient should rest until pain-free for several days and then recommence the programme at a lower level. Ice massage after exercise sessions may help to reduce a reaction. Rehabilitation may be lengthy, and the most common cause of recurrence of symptoms is a premature return to activities. Surgery may be considered in those who fail conservative management and may involve fasciotomy of the posteromedial superficial and deep fascia of the tibia. Some advocate denervation by cauterization of the periosteum along the entire posteromedial border of the tibia, in order to achieve scarring and reattachment of the periosteum to underlying bone. Return to light loading activities is then permitted after 4–6 weeks of rest.

Medial tibial stress syndrome (MTSS)

MTSS is a term used by some to describe medial tibial periostitis. We use it as a diagnosis of exclusion, reserved for patients with exertional lower limb pain, in whom all investigations are normal. MTSS and medial periostitis are probably part of a continuum, from strain of the muscles that cause the traction periostitis to true periostitis. Aetiology and history are the same as described for periostitis, while tenderness may be located to the soft tissue structures adjacent to the bone rather than the bone itself. Investigations are normal. Management of the condition is the same as that for medial tibial periostitis.

Tibiofibular synostosis

Ossification of the interosseous membrane is very rare. It can be congenital or acquired and may be proximal, distal, or diaphyseal. Congenital forms may present in adolescence. Acquired synostosis occurs in relation to repetitive microtrauma or to a single injury, in particular, an ankle sprain, where there is tearing of the anterior and posterior tibiofibular ligaments and the lower third of the interosseous membrane. Bone develops from either side as a flat exostosis or across the interosseous membrane, creating a synostosis. Certain individuals appear to be predisposed to this condition, although the specific factors involved are undetermined.

The patient presents with a history of 'spasm' in the anterior leg, worse with weight-bearing and with movement of the ankle. Symptoms suggestive of ankle instability may be present. There is tenderness over the synostosis and limitation of motion of the ankle, especially dorsiflexion.

A plain X-ray may be normal during the early stages of synostosis formation. An isotope bone scan will show diffuse uptake in the area of the synostosis if the process is active. Later the bone scan is cold, but radiographic changes are apparent.

Treatment involves treating the initial injury (usually ankle sprain), modification of activities, and rehabilitation, initially focusing upon flexibility and proprioception and then a progressive strengthening programme. Further management is dependent upon symptomatology as the long-term effects on ankle biomechanics are unclear. Where the patient remains symptomatic, surgery may be necessary, but it is very invasive, involving excision of the synostosis. Recurrence is common.

Nerve entrapment syndromes

Nerve entrapment syndromes in the leg may give rise to pain and sensorimotor symptoms that may be present only during activity. Deep burning pain may be accompanied by shooting pains in the distribution of the nerve. Symptoms can be non-specific and there is considerable interindividual variation.

When taking a *history*, the location and nature of the pain and associated neurological symptoms should be sought. A history of back pain and the existence of any 'red flags' that may indicate a serious underlying disorder should be specifically sought (Table 10).

Examination aims to identify the peripheral nerve involved and to exclude other causes of lower limb pain that may mimic nerve entrapment (Table 11). Neurological symptoms may arise in relation of other complaints affecting the lower leg, such as compartment syndromes.

Investigations. Electrodiagnostic tests in the lower limb are used to confirm nerve entrapment but they are often less definitive than those in the upper limb, for a number of reasons, which are summarized in

Table 10 Red flags in lower limb neurological symptoms

Systemic symptoms: fever, night sweats, weight loss, anorexia
Night/rest pain
Bladder/bowel dysfunction
Claudicant limb/buttock pain
Bilateral involvement

Table 12. It is vital to ensure the clinical features are consistent with the electrophysiological findings. Nevertheless, they are useful, nerve conduction studies may demonstrate a conduction block where localized entrapment is present and, where the lesion is severe or chronic, there may be evidence of denervation.

Abolition of symptoms after infiltration at the site of entrapment with local anaesthetic also helps to confirm the diagnosis.

Common peroneal nerve (CPN)

The CPN is vulnerable to injury and compression at the neck of the fibula, for example, by a tight leg cast. In addition, activities that cause repetitive pronation and inversion (machine operators, running) may cause traction injuries of the nerve. Compartment syndromes result in dysfunction of the CPN or, more typically, its superficial (anterior compartment) or deep (deep posterior compartment) branches.

Superficial peroneal nerve (SPN)

The SPN is more vulnerable to injury than the deep branch. It can be entrapped or compressed as it exits the crural fascia approximately 10 cm proximal to the lateral malleolus, to divide into its cutaneous branches. Compression by local masses such as a ganglion or lipoma or by callus formation from a previous fracture of the fibula and traction on the nerve by repeated ankle sprains can all occur. There is pain and sensory changes at the cutaneous distribution of the nerve brought on by exercise. These may be clinically evident with resisted dorsiflexion and eversion, and with passive plantar flexion and inversion of the foot. Even normal increases in compartment pressures can cause impingement of the nerve against the edge of a fascial defect. The SPN is also vulnerable where its terminal branches cross the anterior ankle subcutaneously, particularly when shoe laces are too tight.

Electrodiagnostic studies may be necessary to exclude an L5 radiculopathy.

Table 11 Causes of neurogenic lower limb weakness other than nerve entrapments (56)

Neurogenic
Diabetic amyotrophy
Root or lumbar plexus lesion
Motor neuron disease
Myopathic
Inflammatory myopathies
Endocrine, toxic, drug-induced myopathies
Muscle dystrophies
Myotonic dystrophy
Acid maltase deficiency
Benign congenital myopathies
Neuromuscular blocking disorders
Myasthenic syndromes
Demyelinating polyneuropathy

Treatment

Fascial defects must not be closed as this can precipitate an acute compartment syndrome. Conservative management involves appropriate rehabilitation of ankle sprains, including peroneal muscle strengthening and proprioceptive training, a medial heel wedge to reduce the traction on the nerve. A tricyclic agent may help to reduce neuralgia. Fascial release and/or neurolysis is the preferred option when surgery is considered.

Deep peroneal nerve (DPN)

The DPN can be compressed with an acute anterior compartment syndrome and where an anterior tarsal tunnel syndrome (TTS) is present or where there are anterior osteophytes on the anterior aspect of the ankle causing nerve irritation. In the latter two cases, the symptoms are localized to the foot with numbness confined to the dorsum of the first web space. In 22 per cent of individuals, extensor digitorum brevis is innervated by an accessory DPN and therefore weakness may not be present.

In anterior TTS, symptoms may respond to modification of activities and correction of equipment and/or biomechanical factors and padding to protect against further nerve compression. When conservative measures fail or where a compartment syndrome exists, surgery may be necessary to decompress the nerve and deal with any underlying problems such as removing anterior osteophytes.

The sural nerve

Sural nerve entrapment is relatively uncommon, but the nerve may be compressed or entrapped by local mass lesions such as a ganglion, scar tissue, thrombophlebitis, or tight boots or leg casts, or it may be traumatized at surgery. Repeated inversion sprains of the ankle may lead to traction scarring and entrapment. Treatment involves correction of causative factors, footwear modification, protective padding, ankle rehabilitation and, where necessary, excision of scar tissue or a ganglion where these are implicated in the symptoms.

The saphenous nerve

The saphenous nerve may be injured in the adductor canal in the thigh by trauma, or at the knee, usually relating to surgery. It has also been

Table 12 Limitations to electrodiagnostic studies in the lower limb (adapted from reference 57)

Protocols have a wider range on normal values
Peripheral neuropathy preferentially affects the lower limbs which may confound results
Oedema plays a greater role in impeding the recording of wave forms
Temperature is more variable
The plane of the foot is different from that of the leg, affecting distance measurements
False-positive needle electromyographic findings are possible for intrinsic muscles of the foot
Electrodiagnostic findings are more variable and changes follow a less orderly progression than, e.g. CTS

suggested that repeated knee flexion may stretch the nerve. The patient reports claudicant medial lower leg pain. Where the site of entrapment is in the thigh, pain is exacerbated by compression of the nerve in the medial thigh and altered sensation in the cutaneous distribution of the nerve is present. Treatment is symptomatic and may involve the use of a tricyclic agent or, in severe cases, neurolysis.

Tibial nerve entrapment

The tibial nerve may be entrapped in the popliteal fossa by a local mass such as a Baker's cyst, ganglion, or a popliteal artery aneurysm, but injuries or entrapments affecting this nerve are rare. In contrast, its continuation as the posterior tibial nerve can become entrapped at the ankle in the tarsal tunnel (Chapter 6.9).

References

1. Scott, S.H. and Winter, D.A. (1990). Internal forces of chronic running injury sites. *Med. Sci. Sports Exerc.* **22**, 357–369.

2. Komi, P.V., Fukashiro, S., and Jarvinen, M. (1992). Biomechanical loading of Achilles tendon during normal locomotion. *Clin. Sports Med.* **11** (3), 521–531.

3. Lagergren, C. and Lindholm, A. (1958). Vascular distribution in the Achilles tendon. An angiographic and microangiographic study. *Acta Chir. Scand.* **116**, 491–495.

4. Carr, A.J. and Norris, S.H. (1989). The blood supply of the calcaneal tendon. *J. Bone Joint Surg. (Br.)* **71** (1), 100–101.

5. Schmidt-Rohlfing, B., Graf, J., Schneider, U., and Niethard, F.U. (1992). The blood supply of the Achilles tendon. *Int. Orthop.* **16** (1), 29–31.

6. Canoso, J.J., Wohlgethan, J.R., Newberg, A.H., and Goldsmith, M.R. (1989). Aspiration of the retrocalcaneal bursa. *Ann. Rheum. Dis.* **43** (2), 308–312.

7. Frey, C., Rosenberg, Z., Shereff, M.J., and Kim, H. (1992). The retrocalcaneal bursa: anatomy and bursography. *Foot Ankle* **13** (4), 203–207.

8. Thompson, T.C. and Doherty, J.H. (1962). Spontaneous rupture of tendon of Achilles; a new clinical diagnostic test. *J. Trauma* **2**, 126–129.

9. Rolf, C. and Movin, T. (1997). Etiology, histopathology, and outcome of surgery in achillodynia. *Foot Ankle Int.* **18** (9), 565–569.

10. Clement, D.B., Taunton, J.E., and Smart, G.W. (1984). Achilles tendinitis and peritendinitis: etiology and treatment. *Am. J. Sports Med.* **12** (3), 179–184.

11. Krissoff, W.B. and Ferris, W.D. (1979). Runner's injuries. *Physician Sports Med.* **7** (12), 55–64.

12. Leppilahti, J. and Orava, S. (1998). Total Achilles tendon rupture. A review. *Sports Med.* **25** (2), 79–100.

13. Kvist, M. (1991). Achilles tendon injuries in athletes. *Ann. Chir. Gynaecol.* **80** (2), 188–201.

14. Kvist, M. (1994). Achilles tendon injuries in athletes. *Sports Med.* **18** (3), 173–201.

15. Leppilahti, J., Orava, S., Karpakka, J., and Takala, T. (1991). Overuse injuries of the Achilles tendon. *Ann. Chir. Gynaecol.* **80** (2), 202–207.

16. Leppilahti, J., Korpelainen, R., Karpakka, J., Kvist, M., and Orava, S. (1998). Ruptures of the Achilles tendon: relationship to inequality in length of legs and to patterns in the foot and ankle. *Foot Ankle Int.* **19** (10), 683–687.

17. McGarvey, W.C., Singh, D., and Trevino, S.G. (1996). Partial Achilles tendon ruptures associated with fluoroquinolone antibiotics: a case report and literature review. *Foot Ankle Int.* **17** (8), 496–498.

18. Movin, T., Gad, A., Guntner, P., Foldhazy, Z., and Rolf, C. (1997). Pathology of the Achilles tendon in association with ciprofloxacin treatment. *Foot Ankle Int.* **18** (5), 297–299.

19. Szarfman, A., Chen, M., and Blum, M.D. (1995). More on fluoroquinolone antibiotics and tendon rupture. *N. Engl. J. Med.* **332** (3), 193.

20. van der Linden, P.D., van Puijenbroek, E.P., Feenstra, J., Veld, B.A., Sturkenboom, M.C., Herings, R.M., Leufkens, H.G., and Stricker, B.H., (2001). Tendon disorders attributed to fluoroquinolones: a study on 42 spontaneous reports in the period 1988 to 1998. *Arthritis Rheum.* **45** (3), 235–239.

21. Carden, D.G., Noble, J., Chalmers, J., Lunn, P., and Ellis, J. (1987). Rupture of the calcaneal tendon. The early and late management. *J. Bone Joint Surg. (Br.)* **69** (3), 416–420.

22. Zollinger, H., Rodriguez, M., and Genoni, M. (1983). Atiopathegenese und Diagnostik der Achillessehnenrupturen im Sport. In *Sportverletzungen und Sportschaden*. G. Thieme, Stuttgart. (ed. G. Chapchal), pp. 78–79.

23. Trepman, E. and Yodlowski, M.L. (1996). Occupational disorders of the foot and ankle. *Orthop. Clin. North Am.* **27** (4), 815–829.

24. Leppilahti, J., Forsman, K., Puranen, J., and Orava, S. (1998). Outcome and prognostic factors of achilles rupture repair using a new scoring method. *Clin. Orthop.* **346**, 152–161.

25. Josza, L., Kvist, M., Balint, B.J., Reffy, A., Jarvinen, M., Lehto, M., and Barzo, M. (1989). The role of recreational sports activity in Achilles tendon rupture. A clinical, pathoanatomical and sociological study of 992 cases. *Am. J. Sports Med.* **17**, 338–343.

26. Tomassi, F.J. (1992). Current diagnostic and radiographic assessment of tendo Achillis rupture. *J. Am. Podiatr. Med. Assoc.* **82**, 375–379.

27. O'Brien, T. (1984). The needle test for complete rupture of the Achilles tendon. *J. Bone Joint Surg. (Am.)* **66**, 1099–1101.

28. Hattrup, S.J. and Johnson, K.A. (1985). A review of ruptures of the Achilles tendon. *Foot Ankle* **6** (1), 34–38.

29. Copeland, S.A. (1990). Rupture of the Achilles tendon: a new clinical test. *Ann. R. Coll. Surg. Engl.* **72** (4), 270–271.

30. Davies, M.S., Peereboom, J., and Saxby T. (1998). Hyperdorsiflexion sign in tears of the tendo Achilles. *Foot Ankle Int.* **19** (9), 647.

31. Cyriax, J. (1982). *Textbook of orthopaedic medicine*, Vol. 1: *Diagnosis of soft tissue lesions*, 8th edn., pp. 421–422. Bailliere Tindall, London.

32. Rolf, C., Movin, T., Engstrom, B., Jacobs, L.D., Beauchard, C., and Le Liboux A. (1997). An open, randomized study of ketoprofen in patients in surgery for Achilles or patellar tendinopathy. *J. Rheumatol.* **24** (8), 1595–1598.

33. Allenmark, C. (1992). Partial Achilles tendon tears. *Clin. Sports Med.* **11** (4), 759–769.

34. Sundqvist, H., Forsskahl, B., and Kvist M. (1987). A promising novel therapy for Achilles peritendinitis: double-blind comparison of glycosaminoglycan polysulfate and high-dose indomethacin. *Int. J. Sports Med.* **8** (4), 298–303.

35. Royer, R.J., Pierfitte, C., and Netter P. (1994). Features of tendon disorders with fluoroquinolones. *Therapie* **49** (1), 75–76.

36. Klemp, P., Halland, A.M., Majoos, F.L., and Steyn, K. (1993). Musculoskeletal manifestations in hyperlipidaemia: a controlled study. *Ann. Rheum. Dis.* **52** (1), 44–48.

37. Alfredson, H. and Lorentzon, R. (2000). Chronic Achilles tendinosis. Recommendations for treatment and prevention. *Sports Med.* **29** (2), 136–146.

38. Maffulli, N., Testa, V., Capasso, G., *et al.* (1997). Results of percutaneous longitudinal tenotomy for Achilles tendinopathy in middle- and long-distance runners. *Am. J. Sports Med.* **25**, 835–840.

39. Cetti, R., Christensen, S.E., Ejsted, R., Jensen, N.M., and Jorgensen, U. (1993). Operative versus nonoperative treatment of Achilles tendon rupture. A prospective randomized study and review of the literature. *Am. J. Sports Med.* **21** (6), 791–799.

40. Popovic, N. and Lemaire, R. (1999). Diagnosis and treatment of acute ruptures of the Achilles tendon. Current concepts review. *Acta Orthop. Belg.* **65**, 458–471.

41. Allen, M.J. and Barnes, M.R. (1986). Exercise pain in the lower leg. Chronic compartment syndrome and medial tibial syndrome. *J. Bone Joint Surg. (Br.)* **68** (5), 818–823.

42. Bourne, R.B. and Rorabeck, C.H. (1989). Compartment syndromes of the lower leg. *Clin. Orthop.* **240**, 97–104.

43. Fronek, J., Mubarak, S.J., Hargens, A.R., Lee, Y.F., Gershuni, D.H., Garfin, S.R., and Akeson, W.H. (1987). Management of chronic exertional anterior compartment syndrome of the lower extremity. *Clin. Orthop.* **220**, 217–227.

44. Pedowitz, R.A., Hargens, A.R., Mubarak, S.J., and Gershuni, D.H. (1990). Modified criteria for the objective diagnosis of chronic compartment syndrome of the leg. *Am. J. Sports Med.* **18** (1), 35–40.

45. Wiley, J.P., Doyle, D.L., and Taunton, J.E. (1987). A primary care perspective of chronic compartment syndrome of the leg. *Physician Sports Med.* **15**, 111–120.

46. Melberg, P. and Styf, J. (1989). Posteromedial pain in the lower leg. *Am. J. Sports Med.* **17**, 747–750.

47. Schepsis, A., Martini, A.D., and Corbett, M. (1993). Surgical management of exertional compartment syndrome of the lower leg. *Am. J. Sports Med.* **21**, 811–817.

48. Wallenstein, R. (1983). Results of fasciotomy in patients with medial tibial syndrome or anterior compartment syndrme. *J. Bone Joint Surg.* **65A**, 1252–1255.

49. Rorabeck, C.H., Fowler, P.J., and Nott, L. (1988). The results of fasciotomy in the management of chronic exertional compartment syndrome. *Am. J. Sports Med.* **16**, 224–227.

50. Micheli, L.J., Solomon, R., Solomon, J., Plasschaert, V.F., and Mitchell, R. (1999). Surgical treatment for chronic lower-leg compartment syndrome in young female athletes. *Am. J. Sports Med.* **27** (2), 197–201.

51. Christensen, J.T., Eklof, B., and Wulff, K. (1983). The chronic compartment syndrome and response to diuretic treatment. *Acta Chir. Scand.* **149** (3), 249–252.

52. Zwas, S.T., Elkanovitch, R., and Frank, G. (1987). Interpretation and classification of bone scinitgraphic findings in stress fractures. *J. Nucl. Med.* **28**, 452–457.

53. Boam, W.D., Miser, W.F., Delaplain, C.B., Gayle, E.L., and Macdonald, D.C. (1996). Comparison of ultrasound examination with bone scintiscan in the diagnosis of stress fractures. *J. Am. Board Fam. Pract.* **9**, 414–417.

54. Kortebein, P.M., Kaufman, K.R., Basford, J.R., and Stuart, M.J. (2000). Medial tibial stress syndrome. *Med. Sci. Sports Exerc.* **32** (3), S27–S33.

55. Saxena, A., O'Brien, T., and Bunce, D. (1990). Anatomic dissection of the tibialis posterior muscle and its correlation to medial tibial stress syndrome. *J. Foot Surg.* **29** (2), 105–108.

56. McCrory, P. (2000). Exercise-related leg pain: neurological perspective. *Med. Sci. Sports Exerc.* **32**, S11–S14.

57. Glennon, T.P. (2000). Electrodiagnosis of nerve entrapment syndromes that produce symptoms in the foot and ankle. In *Foot and ankle disorders* (ed. M.S. Myerson), p. 801. W.B. Saunders, Philadelphia.

6.9 The ankle

Cathy Speed and Andrew Robinson

Introduction

Soft tissue injuries of the ankle are among the most common soft tissue injuries and their consequences are frequently underestimated. The numerous ligamentous bands, the 11 major tendons that cross the joint, and other local soft tissue structures are prone to both acute and overuse injuries due to the significant forces imposed upon the region. The stability of the ankle joint is vital to normal function but is frequently compromised through injury.

Functional anatomy

The ankle (talocrural) joint, is a synovial hinge joint made up of three bones, the tibia, fibula, and talus (Fig. 1). This forms a mortise, allowing primarily dorsiflexion and plantar flexion. The ankle and foot articulate but have separate functions. The ankle functions to transmit weight-bearing forces from the body to the foot and its motion and biomechanics are closely linked to that of the hindfoot.

Bony anatomy

The *talus* is the central component not only of the ankle, but also of the hindfoot (Fig. 2). It is almost entirely covered in cartilage and can be divided into the body, head, and neck. The body of the talus forms the distal part of the ankle joint, sitting within the ankle mortise and articulating with the malleoli medially and laterally. Superiorly, the saddle-shaped surface of the body (the *dome*), articulates with the flat surface of the distal tibia (the *tibial plafond*). The tibial plafond covers

approximately 60 per cent of the talar dome at any one time. The distal tibia forms the medial malleolus, which is short and allows inversion of the subtalar joint. The tibialis posterior, flexor digitorum longus, and flexor hallucis longus tendons of the posterior compartment pass behind the medial malleolus en route to their insertions in the foot. The lateral malleolus is formed by the distal fibula, which extends distally and more posteriorly than the medial malleolus. The peroneal tendons pass around the lateral malleolus. The talar dome is not a cylinder, but is a truncated section of a cone—a 'frustrum'. The talus is wider anteriorly and is shaped to resist transverse motion. The joint is most stable with the foot in dorsiflexion—in this position there is also greater tension across the distal *tibiofibular syndesmosis*. The syndesmosis is composed of the anterior, posterior, and interosseous tibiofibular ligaments and the latter is in continuity with the interosseous membrane. This ligament complex increases ankle stability against torsional and angular stresses.

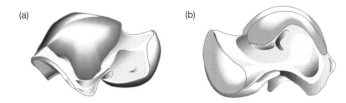

Fig. 2 The lateral (a) and medial (b) talus is shaped to promote both mobility and stability of the ankle and hindfoot. The talar dome in particular is covered by cartilage.

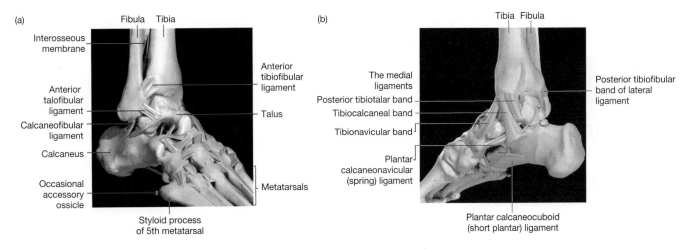

Fig. 1 Bony and ligamentous structures of the ankle: (a) lateral and (b) medial.

Soft tissue anatomy

The ankle is stabilized by bony, tendinous, and ligamentous structures. All can be damaged, although the lateral ligamentous structures are the most frequently injured, due to the relative instability of the ankle in inversion.

Retinacula

Five retinacular bands formed by the deep fascia of the leg surround the ankle and are attached to bone. They serve to protect and guide the tendons and neurovascular bundles. Many of the tendons lie within defined compartments, where they are invested within a synovial sheath. The inferior extensor retinaculum is a retention system, which prevents bow-stringing of the tendons that run beneath it (namely, the long extensors of the toes, and tibialis anterior). It is Y-shaped, originates from the sinus tarsi laterally, and inserts medially on to the medial malleolus (superomedial band) and the navicular and medial cuneiform (inferomedial band).

Ligaments

The *medial*, or *deltoid, ligament* is a large and strong ligament, which is rarely injured. It consists of a superficial and a deep component. The superficial component originates on the medial malleolus, and has a continuous fan-shaped insertion along the sustentaculum tali to the navicular. The deep component inserts on to the talus.

The *lateral ligament complex* of the ankle consists of three anatomically distinct ligamentous bands, namely, from anterior to posterior, the anterior talofibular, calcaneofibular, and posterior talofibular ligaments (Fig. 1a). The *anterior talofibular ligament* (ATFL) runs parallel to the long axis of the foot from the anterior lateral malleolus to the talar neck. It consists of three bands that restrict anterior displacement and internal rotation of the talus. It is also a weak stabilizer of the ankle against inversion stresses and is the most vulnerable of the three lateral ligaments, being the first to tear in the typical inversion injury.

The *calcaneofibular ligament* (CFL), unlike the other ankle ligaments, is anatomically distinct from the ankle capsule. It crosses both the ankle and the subtalar joints, runs deep to (and partly in continuation with) the peroneal tendon sheaths, and inserts on to the calcaneus. This close relationship with the peroneal tendon sheaths explains the significant incidence of peroneal tendon injury in association with CFL tear.

Table 1 Ligaments of the ankle

Ligament	Primary function
Anterior talofibular	Limits anterior talar displacement
Calcaneofibular	Limits inversion of calcaneus
Posterior talofibular	Limits posterior talar displacement
Deltoid	Supports ankle, subtalar, and midtarsal joints; limits abduction and eversion of ankle and subtalar joint; limits talar pronation, eversion, and anterior displacement

The *posterior talofibular ligament* (PTFL) is both the strongest and the smallest of the three lateral ligaments of the ankle and lies parallel to the subtalar joint. It runs from the posteromedial aspect of the lateral malleolus to the lateral talar tubercle. It acts as a restraint to posterior dislocation of the talus but is not stressed during physiological ankle movements. It also restricts external rotation of the talus in the neutral or dorsiflexed position.

The orientation of the ankle ligaments varies with the position of the foot, such that with the foot in neutral the ATFL and CFL both support the joint, whereas in plantar flexion the ATFL acts almost in isolation to stabilize the ankle against inversion. In dorsiflexion the CFL is the principal stabilizer of the ankle (Table 1).

In addition to the medial and lateral ligaments of the ankle, stability is conferred to the mortise through the peroneal muscles, the syndesmosis, and joint congruity. The *peroneal muscles (peroneus longus and brevis)* are important dynamic stabilzers of the ankle joint. The muscles contract in a reflex response to proprioceptive input from the ligaments and capsule, working to counteract the effect of tibialis posterior, which plantar flexes and inverts the foot. The peronei originate in the lateral compartment of the leg, with peroneus longus becoming tendinous in the mid-leg and receiving muscle fibres until 3–5 cm proximal to the lateral malleolus (Fig. 3). Peroneus brevis becomes tendinous 2–3 cm proximal to the lateral malleolus, lying initially deep to peroneus longus then anterior. At the level of the lateral malleolus the brevis comes to lie superior to the longus tendon. The tendons curve behind the malleolus. In 82 per cent of people, the posterior aspect of the fibula has a sulcus; in the other 18 per cent the fibula is either smooth or convex.[1] The groove is deepened by a fibrocartilage ridge and the peroneal tendons are secured by a retaining band to prevent their dislocation or subluxation. The most important part of this retinaculum is its superior portion (the superior peroneal retinaculum, SPR), which not only restrains the peroneal tendons but can also act as an accessory CFL. The peroneal tendons run in separate sheaths proximal to the malleoli but the sheaths unite to form a common sheath in the retromalleolar region, which subsequently bifurcates at the level of the peroneal tubercle.

Neurovascular supply

The sciatic nerve innervates the ankle and foot via the tibial (medial and lateral plantar nerves), common peroneal (deep and superficial branches), and sural nerves. The exception is the saphenous nerve, a branch of the femoral nerve. Motor and sensory supply are described in Fig. 4 and Table 2.

The *sural nerve*, a branch of the tibial nerve, arises in the posterior superior popliteal fossa and passes down the posterior calf, piercing

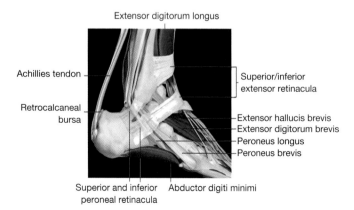

Fig. 3 The lateral ankle.

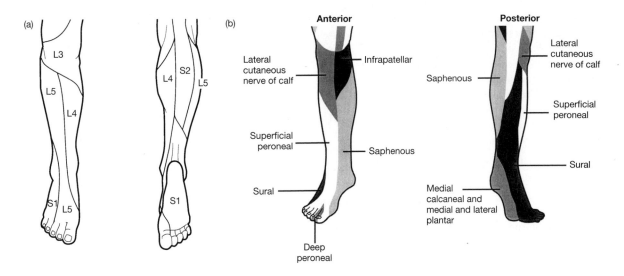

Fig. 4 Dermatomes and peripheral nerves around the ankle.

Table 2 Movements and innervation of the ankle and subtalar joint

Muscles involved[a]	Innervation	Nerve roots
Plantar flexion of ankle		
Gastrocnemius, soleus, FHL, FDL	Tibial nerve	S1–S3
Tibialis posterior	Tibial nerve	L4–L5
Peroneus longus and brevis	Superficial peroneal nerve	L5, S1–S2
Dorsiflexion of ankle		
Tibialis anterior	Deep peroneal nerve	L4–L5
EDL, EHL	Deep peroneal nerve	L5–S1
Inversion		
Tibialis posterior	Tibial nerve	L4–L5
FDL, FHL	Tibial nerve	L5–S1
Tibialis anterior	Deep peroneal nerve	L4–L5
EHL	Deep peroneal nerve	L5–S1
Eversion		
Peronei	Superficial peroneal nerve	L5, S1–S2
EDL	Deep peroneal nerve	L5–S1

[a] FHL, Flexor hallucis longus; FDL, flexor digitorum longus; EDL, extensor digitorum longus; EHL, extensor hallucis longus.

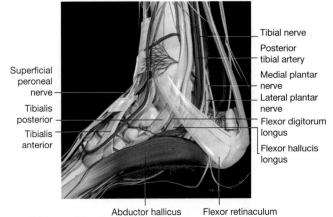

Fig. 5 The medial ankle.

the deep fascia in the mid calf. The nerve runs behind and below the tip of the lateral malleolus and forms the cutaneous supply to the inferior part of the lateral malleolus and lateral foot.

The *superficial peroneal nerve* pierces the fascia to become subcutaneous 10–15 cm above the ankle and provides sensory innervation to the anterolateral ankle and foot.

Medial ankle (Fig. 5)

The main ligamentous structure of the medial ankle is the deltoid ligament, one of the strongest soft tissues complexes in the body, which confers significant stability against talar eversion and rotation. It consists of five bands that can be divided into superficial and deep components that provide significant resistance to eversion stress than to inversion.

The *flexor retinaculum* attaches to the medial malleolus and medial surface of the calcaneal process to form the *tarsal tunnel*. This tunnel is formed by the medial wall of the calcaneus, the talus, the tibia and medial malleolus, and the flexor retinaculum. The latter attaches proximally to the posterior distal medial malleolus and fans out to attach to the sheaths of the structures within the tarsal tunnel. The retinaculum restrains the tendons of the three muscles of the deep compartment of the leg as they pass posteromedially to the ankle joint and into the plantar compartments of the foot. These structures lie superficial to the deltoid ligament and form an arc at the medial malleolus, from anteromedial to deep posterolateral in the order: tibialis posterior, flexor digitorum longus, the posterior tibial artery and veins, the tibial nerve and its medial calcaneal branch, and flexor hallucis longus. The tibialis posterior and flexor digitorum tendons have their own retinacular compartments at the medial malleolus.

The *posterior tibial tendon* (PTT) passes inferior to the spring ligament, where a fibrocartilaginous or bony sesamoid may be located. The tendon crosses three joints along its course—the ankle, subtalar, and oblique midtarsal joints—causing specific actions at each joint it crosses, through the action of several bands. Tibialis posterior works powerfully at the subtalar and midtarsal joints to invert the heel and supinate the foot. It also plantar flexes the foot at the ankle, plays an important role in maintaining the medial arch of the foot, and contributes to the stability of the foot by its many bony attachments:

1. The anterior band inserts on to the navicular tuberosity, the medial cuneiform, and the inferior capsule of medial navicular–cuneiform joint;

2. The middle component travels more deeply and inserts distally on to the second and third cuneiforms, the cuboid, and the bases of the middle three metatarsals;

3. The posterior band inserts on to the anterior sustentaculum tali.

Having passed medial to the edge of the sustentaculum tali, *flexor digitorum longus* (FDL) passes into the central compartment of the foot to insert as four slips on to the base of the distal phalanx of each of the lateral four toes. FDL flexes the distal phalanges of the lateral four toes, assists in plantar flexion at the ankle, and helps to maintain the medial and longitudinal arches.

Flexor hallucis longus (FHL) has a rather deviated course from its origin, since it arises on the posterior aspect of the fibula, is laterally placed in the tarsal tunnel, and inserts into the base of the distal phalanx. FHL assists in plantar flexion at the ankle, flexes the distal phalanx of the big toe, and helps to maintain the medial arch.

The *tibial nerve* is a terminal branch of the sciatic nerve. It gives a branch, the medial calcaneal nerve, 2–7 cm above the medial malleolus, and then bifurcates within (or occasionally proximal to) the tarsal tunnel to form the medial and lateral plantar nerves. The medial plantar nerve can occasionally arise from the lateral plantar nerve.

The *medial calcaneal nerve* travels anterior to the Achilles tendon and enters the foot via the tarsal tunnel. It divides into anterior and lateral plantar branches, which innervate the sole and the medial aspect of the foot. The *saphenous nerve* arises from the femoral nerve and innervates the ankle, medial malleolus, and medial border of the foot.

The *posterior tibial artery*, arising from the popliteal artery, passes behind the medial malleolus, where it is easily palpated. Through its medial and lateral plantar branches it contributes with dorsalis pedis to provide vascular supply to the foot. The *peroneal artery* arises from the posterior tibial artery in the lower leg and divides into branches that supply the ankle.

Anterior foot and ankle

The tendons of tibialis anterior, extensor hallucis longus, extensor digitorum longus, and peroneus tertius (a part of extensor digitorum longus (EDL)) all pass to the foot on the anterior aspect of the ankle. The tendons pass under the inferior extensor retinaculum. Tibialis anterior functions to dorsiflex the ankle and invert the foot. It also actively supports the medial arch.

The branches of the *superficial peroneal nerve* pass in the subcutaneous tissue of the skin across the front of the ankle, in a variable distribution. These branches supply sensory innervation to the dorsum of the foot. The *deep peroneal nerve* travels with the anterior tibial artery under the inferior extensor retinaculum and lies lateral to the dorsalis pedis artery between extensor hallucis longus (EHL) and EDL on the dorsum of the foot, between the first and second rays. It provides sensory supply to the first web space through its medial branch, while its lateral branch innervates extensor digitorum brevis (EDB) and provides sensory supply to the midtarsal joints and forefoot.

The *anterior tibial artery* can be palpated medial to EHL at the anterior ankle. As it passes below the extensor retinaculum it becomes the dorsalis pedis artery and then lies lateral to EHL. It gives branches to the ankle, sinus tarsi, and the dorsum of the foot.

Posterior ankle

The *Achilles tendon* passes posterior to the ankle joint to insert on to the calcaneal tuberosity. Its anatomical features were described in Chapter 6.8. An accessory ossicle, the *os trigonum*, articulates with the posterior talar process and is present in 6–8 per cent of the population.

Clinical evaluation

History

Patients with ankle problems may present after an acute injury or with chronic symptoms. Even minor complaints involving the foot and ankle can lead to protracted pain due to the constant forces of weight-bearing. An initiating event is frequently recalled and a detailed history of this episode should be taken. Common ankle symptoms are pain, giving way/repeated inversion injuries, swelling, clicking, popping and locking. The timing and mechanism of the onset of such symptoms should be ascertained.

The nature, intensity, and distribution of *pain*, exacerbating and relieving features, and the presence of nocturnal pain help to determine the structures involved and the severity of the complaint (see Table 3 in Chapter 4.1).

Events immediately after the initial injury are important. *Inability to weight-bear* immediately after an injury suggests fracture or major soft tissue damage. The timing of onset of *swelling* is ascertained: significant swelling occurring immediately after injury is suggestive of significant damage to soft tissue or articular structures. Swelling may also be reported in chronic injuries.

Giving way of the ankle is typically caused by either primary ligamentous instability or to pain leading to the sensation of giving way via a pain reflex. *Popping, snapping*, or *tearing* is indicative of ligament, tendon, or cartilage damage. *Locking* of the ankle joint is a characteristic feature of loose bodies within the joint. *Stiffness* is common after an acute injury. Chronic stiffness also occurs with a soft tissue injury and degenerative articular complaints. Significant morning stiffness is characteristic of inflammatory joint disease.

Specific details of the previous treatments, their timing, compliance, and their effects should also be obtained. These include the use of supports, taping, insoles, and orthotics. Finally, a general medical history should be established, including a history of diabetes mellitus, inflammatory arthropathy, psoriasis, gout, and poliomyelitis. Low back disorders may present with foot and ankle complaints.

Examination

Evaluation of the ankle may be limited in the acute stage after injury due to pain and swelling. In such situations it may be necessary to review the patient after a period of conservative management of the acute injury, with rest, ice and elevation. The old maxim of 'look, feel, move' is followed.

Inspection

Gait and the use of walking aids, supports, and taping are assessed as the patient enters the room. Inspection of the ankle commences with the patient standing, as the ability to weight-bear and the presence of deformities can be noted. Heel alignment should be carefully assessed. The normal heel lies in slight valgus. Excessive valgus is seen in the flatfoot (pes planus), characterized by hindfoot valgus, forefoot abduction, forefoot supination, and loss of arch height. Conversely, pes cavus presents with heel varus, cavus, and forefoot valgus. Forefoot valgus describes the first ray being more plantarly displaced than the lateral rays. The toes are also clawed. The presence of heel varus is an important factor in lateral ankle ligament instability. If a deformity is present, it should be determined whether the deformity is correctable or not. Where surgery becomes necessary, a correctable deformity can be treated with soft tissue surgery, whereas a fixed, or non-correctable deformity requires bony surgery.

The patient is then asked to lie supine and the site and extent of any pain, swelling, deformity, and discoloration are noted. Swelling may be due to a soft tissue injury or ankle effusion. The degree of swelling over the first 24 h after a lateral ligament sprain indicates the degree of the injury. Bruising usually occurs distal to the site of injury: if seen proximal to the lateral ligament after sprain, more extensive injury should be expected. If the patient has difficulty describing the site of pain, it is useful to ask them to point, with a single finger, to the location. If there is more than one site of pain it is worth asking them to quantitate the severity of the pain in each location. For example, the patient is told that 'if the pain is 100 in the worst area, what is the severity of the pain at point 2?'

Palpation

Palpation for, and localization of, tenderness is very important in the foot and ankle, where there are so many structures in close proximity. Placement of the thumb on the most anterior portion of the lateral malleolus and passive plantar flexion of the patient's foot allows the anterolateral portion of the talar dome to become palpable as it rotates out from under the ankle mortise. The sinus tarsi can be palpated in the depression one fingerbreadth inferior and one fingerbreadth anterior to the lateral malleolus. The medial and lateral ligaments of the ankle, the syndesmosis, and tibiofibular ligaments should also be palpated. A neurovascular assessment is performed, in addition to Tinel's test if nerve entrapment is suspected.

Movement

Active and passive range of motion are assessed. Reproduction of pain with particular movements may be a helpful marker of injury. For example, pain with extreme dorsiflexion may indicate a syndesmosis tear or talar dome injury, while posterior ankle pain with plantar flexion indicates impingement. Movement against resistance should also be assessed to evaluate musculotendinous structures crossing the ankle (Table 2). When assessing the ankle joint, particular attention should also be taken of subtalar movement. Repeated ankle sprains are associated with tarsal coalition, which limits subtalar mobility.

Special tests

Assessment of the lateral ankle ligament complex

Assessment of ankle stability involves evaluation of *functional* and *mechanical stability*. Evaluation of functional stability commences with the assessment of proprioception. The patient is asked to balance firstly on the unaffected foot, and then on the affected foot, firstly with their eyes open and then closed. The ability to balance is noted and the left and right sides compared. With lesser degrees of injury, more difficult tasks may be set, including balancing on tiptoes and/or on an unstable surface such as a wobble board.

Mechanical stability of the ankle can be evaluated using the anterior drawer and talar tilt tests. In the *anterior drawer test*, the patient lies supine and relaxed with the knee in approximately 60° of flexion to relieve tension in the gastrocnemius. The examiner stabilizes the tibia and fibula, holds the foot in 20° of plantar flexion, and draws the talus forward in the ankle mortise. The examiner subjectively assesses whether there is excessive translation and, if so, whether there is a firm endpoint. A visible dimpling on the anterolateral side of the ankle (the 'suction' sign) helps to confirm excessive translation. Excessive translation and the absence of a firm endpoint indicates rupture of the ATFL. If a firm endpoint is present, the positive drawer may be due to ligamentous laxity, in which case the finding is noted bilaterally (Fig. 6).

The *talar tilt test* assesses the integrity of the CFL when the ankle is in neutral or slight dorsiflexion, but also assesses the ATFL if the ankle is in plantar flexion (Fig. 16). Alternatively, with the patient supine and the knee flexed to 90° to relax the gastrocnemius–soleus complex, the examiner stabilizes the tibia with one hand and applies an inversion stress at the heel with the other hand. The talar tilt, the angle between the talar dome and tibial plafond, is evaluated and compared with that on the unaffected side. An excessive tilt indicates CFL and/or ATFL tear, depending upon the position of testing. In experienced hands the anterior drawer test is a more reliable indicator of ATFL rupture than talar tilt.

Assessment of the tibiofibular syndesmosis

The syndesmosis is assessed by the *squeeze test*, which is performed by compressing the fibula and the tibia together at the midtibia. The test is considered positive when compression reproduces pain over the syndesmosis. Pain is exacerbated by lateral rotation of the foot with the knee flexed to 90°.

Assessment of the peroneal tendons

Reproduction of symptoms with resisted dorsiflexion and eversion indicates peroneal tendon pathology. The peroneal tendons may sublux or dislocate. This can often be directly observed.

Assessment of the tibialis posterior tendon

This is important in assessment of the ankle as it is a common site of pathology.

1. The *single heel raise test*. The patient is viewed from behind and raises the unaffected foot off the ground and is then asked to rise up on tiptoe 4–5 times. The patient is allowed to balance with one finger on a surface in front of him/her, but should be told *not* to

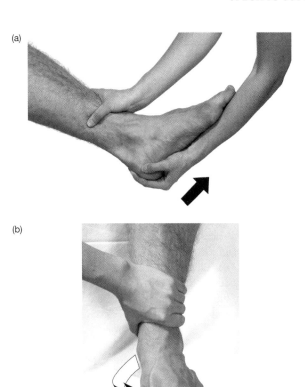

Fig. 6 (a) Anterior drawer and (b) talar tilt tests.

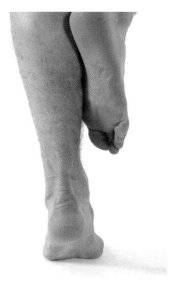

Fig. 7 Single heel raise test. The examiner takes note of (a) the ability to perform a single heel raise; (b) provocation of pain; (c) heel inversion during heel raise; and (d) fatiguability with repetition. The two feet are compared.

Imaging

Plain radiographs

The standard series is the weight-bearing antero posterior (AP), mortise, and lateral views, although there is an argument that the AP view adds little to the mortise view, particularly in acute fracture.[3] To obtain a mortise view the foot is internally rotated so that the transmalleolar axis is perpendicular to the X-ray beam. This allows clear visualization of the medial and lateral joint space, distal fibula, and lateral talar dome. In the fracture patient, talar shift is also apparent. The lateral view helps to demonstrate tibiotalar congruity and bony causes of posterior impingement. A lateral view in plantar flexion will demonstrate impingement caused by a prominent lateral posterior process or os trigonum. Weight-bearing radiographs also allow assessment of joint space narrowing and talar tilt in cases of chronic lateral ligament instability.

Ultrasound and magnetic resonance imaging (MRI)

MRI scanning has advanced both the understanding and diagnosis of soft tissue and bony pathology around the ankle. Whilst it has been reported that MRI scanning showed a 95 per cent sensitivity, and 100 per cent specificity for posterior tibial tendon tears,[4] others have shown that MRI is less accurate (66 per cent) than ultrasonography (94 per cent) when both were compared to the intraoperative findings.[5] The disadvantage of ultrasound is that it does not image the bony structures and is operator-dependent. In summary, careful clinical examination with appropriate imaging is the best practice.

Lateral ankle pain (Table 3)

Acute lateral ankle sprain

Lateral ankle sprains represent one of the most common soft tissue injuries, with a conservative estimate of 5000 such injuries occurring

assist the raise using this finger. The examiner, viewing from behind, takes note of: (1) the ability to perform a single heel raise; (2) whether there is pain in so doing; (3) whether the heel inverts normally during heel raise; and (4) fatiguability with repetition. The test is repeated for the affected foot and the two sides compared. Weakness, fatiguability, pain, and lack of heel inversion with heel raise are all signs of posterior tibial tendon disease. Patients with marked weakness and/or pain from other causes, such as tarsometatarsal arthritis, are often unable to perform this test (Fig. 7).

2. The *first metatarsal rise sign* is reported to be a sensitive sign of PTT dysfunction. The patient stands and the heel of the affected foot is passively placed into varus, or the tibia is externally rotated, which also brings the heel into varus. The head of the first metatarsal rises in PTT dysfunction but remains on the ground in the normal foot.[2]

3. The '*too many toes*' sign refers to the number of toes visible from behind the patient and represents forefoot abduction. The normal number is 1–3 toes, but the sign is much more helpful in unilateral involvement, and comparison of the two sides is important.

Assessment of the *Achilles tendon* was described in Chapter 6.8.

Table 3 Causes of lateral ankle pain

Lateral ligament sprain/rupture
Sinus tarsi syndrome
Peroneal tendinopathy or instability

Impingement
  Synovial
  Bony osteophyte 'footballer's ankle'

Fibular stress fracture, fracture, or avulsion injury
Superficial peroneal nerve lesion
Tumour
Referred pain

in the United Kingdom and 23,000 in the United States every day.[6] Of ankle injuries 75 per cent are sprains,[7] which constitute 7–10 per cent of all attendances to hospital casualty departments.[8] Overall, it is the most common injury in sports—25 per cent of injuries in running and jumping sports are lateral ankle sprains. Such injuries can lead to significant long term sequelae with conservative estimates of recurrent instability or prolonged disability occurring in 25–40 per cent.

Mechanism

Lateral ankle sprains usually occur during plantar flexion, adduction, and inversion, as this is the position of least stability of the lateral ankle ligament complex. Partial tears and complete ruptures of the lateral ligaments usually occur in the mid-substance of the tissue, with only 15 per cent of ruptures occurring at the insertion, with or without a bony avulsion. Since the ATFL is the primary lateral stabilizer of the ankle in the position of injury, it is usually the first part of the ligament complex to be injured. As the severity of the stress increases, injuries to the CFL, joint capsule, and PTFL follow sequentially. Rarely, a pure inversion injury can occur with the ankle in a neutral position. Here the CFL is particularly at risk, although the other two lateral ligaments are frequently involved.

If the inversion is severe, the ligaments of the syndesmosis may be injured. These injuries usually occur with severe external rotation and/or dorsiflexion, since the anterior dome of the talus is wider than its posterior portion, resulting in the tibia and fibula being pushed apart with dorsiflexion. Of all ankle sprains, 65 per cent of injuries involve the ATFL, 20 per cent the ATFL and CFL, 10 per cent also involve the anterior inferior tibiofibular ligament, and only 3 per cent the medial (deltoid) ligament. The PTFL is involved only rarely.[9] It plays no role in ankle stability until the ATFL and CFL are both torn.

In the skeletally immature, since ligaments are stronger than bone, the incidence of fractures is higher. In addition, a number of conditions can present as an ankle 'sprain' in children. When any child presents with ankle pain, it is particularly important to exclude systemic and other more serious causes, such as infection, tumour, fracture, and referred pain.

Classification

Lateral ligament injuries may be classified according to the degree of tissue disruption, but the resulting morbidity does not necessarily correlate with the extent of tissue damage: even mild sprains can lead to long-term disability if not correctly managed. A clinically useful approach to grading is described in Table 4.

History

The history is important in determining the severity of the injury and the structures involved. It is also important to ascertain whether this is the first injury, or not. The mechanism may be clearly described and may indicate the specific ligaments involved. However, in repeated sprains the mechanism may be unclear and the degree of trauma trivial.

In the acute inversion sprain, the patient typically reports the onset of lateral ankle pain, and may be unable to continue playing. The degree of swelling, its timing, and its progress is indicative of the severity of the injury. Significant haemarthrosis can occur with severe injuries. The onset of swelling is associated with increasing pain and stiffness and skin discolouration gradually develops over the following 24 h, mostly at and distal to the injury. Patients may report symptoms suggestive of functional or mechanical instability of the ankle, with the ankle giving way on weight-bearing.

The presence of a sensation of popping, snapping, or tearing at the time of injury may indicate ligament rupture or associated peroneal tendon injury. True inability to weight-bear immediately after the injury should raise the suspicion of underlying bony injury or other significant pathology (Table 5). Details should be obtained of any previous injury to either the foot or ankle, all footwear and ankle supports used, and any specific treatments used and their effects. A sporting and occupational history should also be taken.

Inversion sprains of the ankle may result in persisting pain and instability (Table 6). Instability may be due to true mechanical instability after ligament rupture, or to loss of proprioception and

Table 4 Grading of lateral ankle sprain

Grade	Description[a]
1	Partial or complete rupture of ATFL
2	Partial or complete rupture of CFL along with ATFL
3	Injury to all three ligaments
Instability	None/functional/mechanical/both

[a] ATFL, Anterior talofibular ligament; CFL, calcaneo fibular ligament.

Table 5 The Ottawa ankle rules: when to use ankle or foot radiography (reference 10)

Ankle (inversion) injury
Standard radiograph of the ankle is indicated if the patient has pain near the malleoli and one or more of the following:
Age ≥ 55 years
Inability to weight-bear
Bone tenderness at the posterior edge or tip of either malleolus

Foot injury
Standard radiograph of the foot is indicated if the patient has pain in the midfoot and one or more of the following:
Bone tenderness at the navicular, cuboid, or base of the fifth metatarsal
Inability to weight-bear

Table 6 Causes of persisting pain after ankle sprain (modified from reference 4)

Articular injury
Chondral/osteochondral fracture
Meniscoid lesion

Bony injury
Fibula

Nerve injury
Superficial peroneal/posterior tibial/sural

Tendon injury
Tibialis posterior (tear, tendinosis)
Peroneal (subluxation/dislocation/tear/tendinosis)

Ligament injury
Mechanical instability due to lateral ligament damage
Syndesmosis/subtalar joint

Impingement
Anterior osteophyte/anteroinferior tibiofibular ligament

Miscellaneous
Failure to regain normal motion (tight Achilles tendon)
Proprioceptive deficit with repetitive sprains (functional instability)

Table 7 Anatomical variations that may predispose to ankle sprain

Proprioceptive deficiency

Peroneal muscular weakness

Peroneal tendon pathology

Varus tibial plafond (radiographic)

Varus hindfoot

Posteriorly positioned fibula

neuromuscular control (functional instability). These forms of instability may occur alone or in combination. Many patients with functional instability have a subjective feeling of instability without the ankle actually moving beyond the normal physiological range.

Examination

Examination is performed to evaluate the nature and extent of the injury and to identify additional pathologies. Examination of the normal ankle will establish the anatomy, function, and stability of the unaffected side.

Examination commences with inspection for the degree of swelling, discolouration, deformity, and the ability to weight-bear. This is followed by gentle palpation of those anatomical areas that may be involved, namely the ATFL, CFL, PTFL, malleoli, the peroneal tendons, fifth metatarsal, and syndesmosis. If syndesmotic tenderness is present then palpation of the proximal fibula will determine the likelihood of a high fibular (Maisonneuve) fracture. The presence of a palpable defect in the lateral ligaments should also be noted.

Range of movement is usually limited at this stage due to swelling. Mechanical stability should be assessed using the anterior drawer and talar tilt tests. In many cases these cannot be performed in the acute stage, due to swelling, pain, and spasm. In the acute setting it may be better to delay definitive examination for up to 5 days, as previous to this the swelling and tenderness tend to be diffuse, making accurate diagnosis impossible. Should this be the case, then the degree of swelling should be regarded as evidence that rupture of at least one ligament has occurred. The patient should be managed accordingly and reassessed when the swelling and pain have subsided. Similarly, it is difficult to test proprioception and functional stability at this stage. The importance of examination should not be underestimated. The specificity and sensitivity of delayed physical examination for the presence or absence of a lesion of an ankle ligament have been found to be 84 and 96 per cent, respectively.[11] Delayed physical

examination gives information of diagnostic quality that is equal to that of arthrography and causes little discomfort to the patient. The two most important factors are the presence of a haematoma over the ATFL and the presence of a positive anterior draw sign.[11]

The presence of a syndesmosis injury is indicated by tenderness over the distal tibia and fibula, a positive squeeze test, and pain on dorsiflexion and external rotation of the foot. The peroneal tendons should be tested against resisted eversion in dorsiflexion to exclude subluxation, dislocation, or significant weakness. Where possible, the patient should also be evaluated for additional specific anatomical variations that may predispose to ankle sprain (Table 7).

Imaging

Plain radiographs may be indicated in some cases (Table 5). These should include AP, lateral, and mortise views.

Stress radiographs are controversial. The talar tilt angle is determined from a mortise view, with the ankle in forced inversion. Different authors recommend different positions for both the position of the knee (flexed or extended) and ankle (dorsiflexion, neutral, and plantar flexion). The authors use 15° as the upper limit of normal for the talar tilt angle. It should be noted, however, that Rubin and Whitten showed that 5 per cent of normal ankles had a talar tilt angle greater than 15°.[12] The radiological anterior drawer test also exhibits variability. The authors use a value of greater than 5 mm of anterior translation as an indication of ATFL rupture. Nevertheless, in the majority of cases stress radiographs offer little that a thorough clinical examination does not.

MRI scanning has supplanted computerized tomography (CT), peroneal tenography, and arthrography in imaging the acute injury, as it also allows evaluation of the ligaments and other structures.[13] However, as the indications for acute surgical repair are infrequent, and in the chronic injury interpretation of the MRI scan is more difficult, the role of MRI has yet to be fully evaluated.

Isotope bone scanning may be useful if a stress fracture is suspected, but will also show increased uptake in an osteochondral fracture, an inflammatory arthritis, and osteomyelitis.

Ultrasound is used mainly in the examination for the presence of peroneal tendon tears, which may occur after inversion sprain.

Treatment

Early diagnosis and aggressive functional rehabilitation are the vital components of management of acute ankle sprains, allowing most patients to return to work and sports. It is assumed that the prognosis for untreated ankle fractures is good. However, patients who are treated functionally do better than those who are not treated at all, or those who are immobilized for 6 weeks. Most consider that surgery is not necessary in the acute setting, unless there is associated pathology such as peroneal tendon injury or an osteochondral fracture. However, Pickenburg *et al.* in a meta-analysis showed that operative treatment with postoperative functional rehabilitation leads to better results than simple functional treatment. This is a controversial view and it should be noted that the results of operative treatment are similar, whether surgery is undertaken early or late.[14]

In the acute injury the PRICES approach is utilized, with the aim of limiting excessive swelling and controlling pain (Table 8). The use of nonsteroidal anti-inflammatory drugs (NSAIDs) may assist in controlling these features. Modalities such as ultrasound and interferential are of unproven benefit. A pneumatic walking boot or ankle brace is helpful in limiting excessive swelling, easing pain, and promoting mobilization. These can be removed to allow application of ice compresses and massage, for 15 min every 2 h. Use of crutches in the first 24–48 h may be necessary but the patient should be encouraged to mobilize as soon as possible. Range of motion exercises are started immediately and peroneal and posterior tibial strengthening exercises can be commenced as soon as symptoms allow. Once the patient can walk comfortably, the strengthening exercises can be progressively

Table 8 The PRICES regime in acute soft tissue injuries

Protect

Relative Rest

Ice

Compression

Elevation

Support

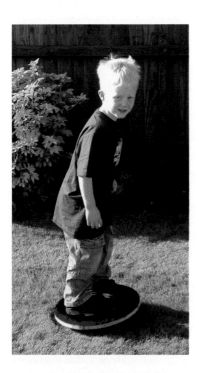

Fig. 8 The wobble board—important to ankle rehabilitation, as well as a potential source of entertainment.

increased and proprioceptive training commences. This begins with simple exercises performed on the floor, progressing to more difficult balancing tasks and the use of a wobble board (Fig. 8). Functional activities are also commenced at this stage and depend upon the activity levels of the patient. They begin with heel and toe raises, then jogging slowly in a straight line, and are followed by progressively more difficult activities at variable speeds and directions and skipping. The use of ice after rehabilitation sessions helps to limit swelling and pain induced in the region of the recently injured tissues.

The use of taping or custom made supports such as the Aircast brace has been shown to be beneficial in returning patients to activity, due to improved proprioceptive feedback. However, such approaches are not a substitute for proprioceptive training. Supports have the benefit over taping, which may stretch with activity, although the latter has the advantage of allowing a 'custom fit'.

Return to sports should occur only when the patient can perform all of the complex actions that their chosen sports involve without provoking any symptoms, although in the out-patient setting the ability to hop on a single foot is a good indicator of recovery sufficient to start to return to sport. Recovery can take 3 months or longer.

Despite the work of Pickenburg *et al.*, the vast majority of patients with an acute ankle sprain are treated non-surgically. *Surgery* is indicated in the presence of associated pathologies, such as an osteochondral lesion, and in those with a diastasis of the tibiofibular joint (see below). Leach and Schepsis also recommended repair in athletes with disruption of both the ATFL and the CFL, a clinical anterior draw, or talar tilt of more than 10°.[15] The presence of specific predisposing anatomical features, particularly a varus hindfoot, should be identified prior to surgical intervention as the outcome to surgery is often poor in such cases, unless the heel varus is treated.[15]

The surgical repair consists of direct suture, or bony reattachment of the damaged ligaments, with repair of the anterior capsule. Postoperatively the patient is placed in a cast for 3–4 weeks. This is then changed to an ankle brace and functional rehabilitation commenced, increasing as tolerated. The brace is worn for sports for 6 months.

Chronic ankle instability

Chronic symptoms after an ankle sprain occur in up to 40 per cent of individuals. The causes are numerous and evaluation requires careful examination and often further imaging with radiographs, bone scanning, and MRI as appropriate. It should be determined whether the patient's principal complaint is one of pain or instability, and the relationship between the two. If the primary complaint is of pain, the cause of the pain should be determined (osteochondral lesion, anterior impingement, meniscoid lesion, etc.). In those patients with chronic instability, examination and imaging should be undertaken as outlined above.

Ankle instability after lateral ligament sprain is common and debilitating. The patient commonly complains of recurrent inversion sprains or 'giving way' of the ankle, usually with minimal or no trauma. Walking on uneven ground is often difficult. Non-specific pain is also commonly reported. Examination of the patient follows the same pathway as that for an acute ankle sprain. Mechanical and functional stability should be assessed and compared to that of the other (unaffected) side. Associated underlying pathologies should be sought. In many cases, rehabilitation has been inadequate and the patient should undergo a trial period of appropriate rehabilitation, with the emphasis being placed on peroneal tendon strengthening exercises and proprioceptive training. The indications for surgery are persisting symptomatic instability in a patient who has failed non-operative treatment.

Surgical treatment of the instability may involve arthroscopic or open intraarticular surgery. Kibler showed that 83 per cent of patients exhibited intraarticular pathology.[16] This included anterolateral soft tissue lesions (26 per cent), tibial/talar osteophytes (26 per cent), meniscoid lesions (15 per cent), chondral lesions (13 per cent), and loose bodies (13 per cent). Taga *et al.* showed that 29 per cent of acute and 95 per cent of chronically injured ankles had chondral lesions.[17]

Surgical techniques for reconstruction of chronic lateral ankle ligament instability are numerous, but can be divided into two principal groups: (1) the 'anatomical' techniques, such as a Broström procedure, or (2) tenodesis operations such as the Chrisman–Snook procedure. The Broström procedure consists of imbricating the ligaments to try to re-establish their pre-injury length and tension. The repair is then reinforced by reflecting the extensor retinaculum over the reconstructed ATFL. There are numerous eponymously named tenodesis procedures. Currently, those based upon the Chrisman–Snook procedure are favoured, as these clinically reconstruct both the ATFL and CFL. The tenodesis procedures utilize one-half of the peroneus brevis tendon.

The concerns with tenodesis operations are various. Firstly, the use of one of the dynamic stabilizers of the ankle as a reconstruction seems undesirable and, secondly, the tenodesis is a more extensive procedure and may lead to stiffness of the subtalar joint. However, paradoxically, stabilizing the subtalar joint may be advantageous, as subtalar instability is a difficult diagnosis to make, and use of the tenodesis treats instability of both joints. There is also evidence that tenodesis operations lead to greater stiffness, and have more complications.[18] Nevertheless, the success rates of both the anatomical and tenodesis procedures are high. Hamilton *et al.* reported 96 per cent excellent or good results after Bostrom repair,[19] and Nimon *et al.* reported 97.7 per cent of patients satisfied after an Evans procedure.[20] In a comparative study by Henrikus *et al.*, both the Chrisman–Snook and modified Broström repairs provided greater than 80 per cent excellent or good stability, although the Broström group had fewer complications and better scores.[21] The non-anatomical repairs seem to lead to inferior results in terms of functional and mechanical stability as well as overall satisfaction at long-term follow-up.[22]

Osteochondral lesions

Osteochondritis dissecans, or osteochondral defects (OCD), affect the talar dome (Fig. 9). The exact aetiology is uncertain, but trauma certainly plays a role. The lesions are found on both the medial and lateral side of the talus, in a ratio of 2:1.[23] The medial lesions are typically posterior and the lateral are anterior. Further description of these lesions may be found in orthopaedic texts.

Anterolateral ankle pain

As opposed to anteromedial and anterocentral ankle pain, which are most commonly caused by bony impingement (footballer's ankle), anterolateral ankle pain is most often due to *soft tissue impingement*. Syndesmosis injuries can also cause pain anterolaterally.

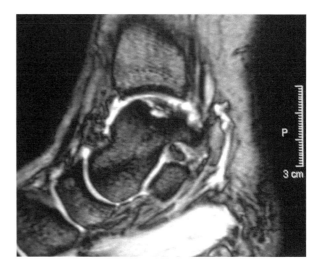

Fig. 9 A talar dome defect.

There are two different anterolateral soft tissue lesions. An abnormal distal slip of the anterior tibiofibular ligament can impinge on the talus; this is known as 'Basset's ligament'. The second is a build-up of impinging synovial tissue, often with hyaline degenerative cartilage, which is also known as the 'meniscoid' lesion. Both lesions can be treated by arthroscopic debridement. Ferkel *et al.* reported 85 per cent good or excellent results after such treatment.[24] Ferkel *et al.* do not consider that patients with instability of the ankle have anterolateral impingement, although Kim and Ha recently described 94 per cent good and excellent results following resection of the anterolateral soft tissue lesion, even in patients who had demonstrable instability, as long as the patients had been functionally stable for 6 months.[25] Kim and Ha also found that five of six patients with a symptomatic Basset's ligament had associated synovial proliferation.

Syndesmosis injuries

Syndesmosis injuries can also cause anterolateral ankle pain and are discussed further below.

Peroneal tendinopathies

Peroneus longus and brevis work as important dynamic stabilizers of the ankle. Contraction of the peroneal muscles in an attempt to stabilize the ankle at the moment of injury can result in a spectrum of injuries to one or both tendons, including tenosynovitis, tendinosis, longitudinal tear, rupture, subluxation, and dislocations. Such lesions are frequently overlooked but should be considered in any patient with lateral ankle pain. Peroneal tendon injuries can occur independently of an overt ankle injury.

Most peroneal pathologies present with a variable combination of lateral ankle pain, swelling, and instability. Pain is frequently worse with walking on uneven surfaces. Symptoms are often mistakenly attributed to a 'simple' ankle sprain, since this is an aetiological factor in many cases. Pathology affecting the peroneus longus is rare, as the peroneus longus lies posterior to peroneus brevis and is thus more protected at the fibular level. Most of the clinical problems are related to the peroneus brevis and peroneal instability. Peroneus longus pathology is more often related to the peroneal tubercle or the os peroneum, and is described further in Chapter 6.10.

Tenosynovitis

Tenosynovitis of the peroneal tendons can occur at three sites: in the peroneal sulcus posterior to the lateral malleolus, at the peroneal trochlea, and at the plantar surface of the cuboid. Pathologies at the latter two sites are discussed in Chapter 6.10. Peroneal tenosynovitis around the lateral malleolus is often associated with peroneal tendon instability. Krause and Brodsky reported that the most reliable clinical sign of peroneal tendon tears is swelling, and they considered chronic subluxation to be the cause of the tears in 90 per cent of their cases.[26] Tenosynovitis can develop following a direct blow to the lateral malleolus or after an ankle sprain. Some patients present with peroneal tenosynovitis as a manifestation of an inflammatory arthropathy. The patient presents with swelling, localized tenderness, and crepitus over the peroneal tendons. Pain is exacerbated on passive stretch, by forced plantar flexion and inversion, and on active contraction against resistance. An antalgic gait may be noted. Differentiation between peroneus brevis and longus involvement is based upon the site of pain. The specific movements affected may also be an indicator. Pain with eversion and with restricted plantar flexion of the first ray indicates peroneus longus involvement, whereas pain only with resisted eversion occurs with peroneus brevis lesions. The diagnosis may be confirmed where necessary by ultrasound or MRI.

Treatment involves relative rest, NSAIDs, ice and ice massage, and the use of a lateral heel wedge. Exacerbating activities, such as walking on uneven surfaces or up and down ladders, are avoided. The use of local corticosteroids is inappropriate. Rehabilitation exercises commence early, with a flexibility programme and a gradual strengthening and ankle stability programme.

In those with persisting symptoms, a trial of a rocker bottom walking boot or casting in non-weight-bearing is appropriate. Should these approaches fail, then surgical exploration should be considered. Exposure of the tendons at the level of the distal fibula involves division of the superior peroneal retinaculum. This should be repaired to avoid postoperative subluxation. Indeed, at the time of surgery a careful assessment for peroneal instability should be made, as Krause and Brodsky noted that in only 40 per cent of their cases was the instability documented preoperatively.[26] Peroneal instability is discussed below. Assessment of the peroneal tubercle and an os peroneum should be considered, although this is discussed in Chapter 6.10.

Tendinosis and longitudinal tears

The clinical features of peroneal tendon tears are similar to those of tenosynovitis. There may be associated lateral ankle instability. Tenderness and swelling are usually well localized to the retromalleolar groove. A snapping sensation may be elicited with active eversion, although this is most commonly noted if the tendons are dislocating or subluxing (see below).

Chronic peroneus brevis tendon tears are frequently overlooked or misdiagnosed. Indeed, many seem to be asymptomatic. Degenerative tears in peroneus brevis are reported with an incidence of 11.3–20.6 per cent in cadaveric studies. Sammarco and DiRaimondo reported longitudinal splits in peroneus brevis in 23 per cent of 47 patients undergoing lateral ankle ligament reconstruction.[27] Tears of the peroneus longus are, on the other hand, rare. Longitudinal

tears, or splits, of the peroneal tendons can occur in relation to an acute inversion injury, chronic lateral ankle laxity, intratendinous degenerative change, or after a calcaneal fracture. Mechanical wear in the retromalleolar groove is considered to play a major role in the development of degenerative change and it is at this site that most lesions occur. Local compression of peroneus brevis within the groove, eversion of the foot, subluxation of the peroneal tendons, laxity or rupture of the SPR, and a sharp posterior fibular edge all may contribute to this mechanical wear.[28] Krause and Brodsky related 90 per cent of their series of peroneus brevis tears to instability at the level of the superior peroneal retinaculum and only 40 per cent of their patients had clinically demonstrable peroneal instability.[26]

Tears can also occur after a calcaneal fracture, when splits in the tendon occur secondary to impingement of the peroneal tendons between the fibula and the displaced calcaneal wall.

Investigation

Ultrasound and MRI are both sensitive methods of detecting the presence of longitudinal tears and tendinosis of the peroneal tendons, although as many as 27 per cent of tears can be missed on MRI scanning.[26]

Management

Whilst non-operative treatment with orthoses, walking casts, and NSAIDs can be tried, such measures are frequently ineffective. At surgery any instability should be addressed (see below). Longitudinal tearing and splaying out of the peroneus brevis tendon is most commonly seen intraoperatively. The options for repair include primary suture, tubulization of a splayed out tendon, excision of the damaged tendon, or tendon transfer. Krause and Brodsky advocated resection of the damaged tendon, and repair, with or without tubulization, when less than 50 per cent of the tendon was involved.[26] If more than 50 per cent of the diameter of the tendon is involved, excision of the damaged portion of the tendon and a peroneus brevis to longus tenodesis is performed. The occasional cases where both the tendons are extensively damaged or where there is even complete rupture are more difficult to treat. The options include mobilization and direct repair, interposition grafting (e.g. with the plantaris tendon), or tenodesis to the lateral wall of the calcaneus. Following surgery the recovery is prolonged, but the majority of patients achieve good to excellent function.

Subluxation and dislocation

The peroneal tendons are normally stabilized by three mechanisms. The tendons run in the peroneal groove, which is deepened by a fibrocartilaginous ridge. The SPR then forms the major restraint to tendon subluxation. Shallowness of the fibular groove or the fibrocartilaginous rim, overcrowding of the peroneal tunnel by a low-lying peroneus brevis muscle belly, or the presence of a peroneal quartus tendon are all associated with peroneal instabilities. When injured, the SPR is avulsed from the fibula. The fibrocartilaginous ridge, with or without a bony flake may also be avulsed.

Subluxation and dislocation of the peroneal tendons was first described by Monteggia in a dancer in 1803.[29] The patients are often initially diagnosed as having sustained a lateral ankle ligament complex injury. Unfortunately, a delay in diagnosis is common. Subluxation usually involves anterior subluxation of the peroneus longus over the inferior surface of the distal fibula. Less commonly, both peroneus longus and brevis may sublux. Occasionally, the

Table 9 Mechanisms of peroneal tendon subluxation/dislocation

Inversion ankle sprain, particularly recurrent sprains

Reflex contraction of the peroneals with either sudden
forceful passive dorsiflexion or plantar flexion of the inverted foot

Significant trauma such as ankle dislocation, fracture

Snow/water skiers: the ski is edged into snow while making a turn

Direct trauma

tendons dislocate and cannot be relocated in the groove. Longitudinal tears of the tendon(s) may also occur. During contraction, the tendon of peroneus longus is forced anteriorly against that of peroneus brevis, which may splay along the posterior border of the fibula. Partial subluxation of peroneus brevis over the edge of a sharp posterior border of the fibula will cause further tearing. There are several potential mechanisms, as described in Table 9, although in some patients there is no obvious precipitant.

The patient typically complains of lateral ankle pain and a snapping sensation. There may be functional and/or mechanical instability of the ankle. Swelling is the most reliable clinical sign. A snap may have been noted during the acute injury and walking is often difficult early after the initial injury. Subluxation of one or both of the peroneal tendons can be elicited by resisted dorsiflexion and eversion, or circumduction of the ankle. In a minority of cases the tendon(s) will be permanently dislocated.

Investigation

Subluxation of the peroneal tendons is a dynamic complaint and a clinical diagnosis. Static investigations may be unhelpful. However, plain AP, lateral, and mortise radiographs of the ankle are helpful in excluding other causes for pain and may reveal a fleck of bone avulsed from the posterolateral fibula, which is pathognomonic of peroneal tendon dislocation. MRI may help to identify anatomical anomalies associated with tendon subluxation, to confirm the location of the tendons, and to assess the integrity of the retinacula. It will also help to detect other causes of lateral ankle sprain. Ultrasound is a dynamic examination and may demonstrate subluxation of the tendons out of the fibular groove. It is also a sensitive method of evaluating the tendon for tears, tendinosis, and tenosynovitis.

Management

Acute peroneal tendon dislocations can be managed conservatively in a below-knee moulded cast, commencing with a 3-week period of cast immobilization with the ankle held in plantar flexion and inversion for 3 weeks then in the neutral position for the second 3 weeks. The success rate of non-operative treatment is approximately 50 per cent, with some authors reporting up to 74 per cent of patients requiring later surgery.[30] Success rates of this level in a young, sporting population may be considered unacceptable where surgery has a high success rate.

After cast immobilization, a progressive rehabilitation programme is commenced, beginning with gentle range of motion exercises and stretching and the gradual introduction of a strengthening programme. Ankle stability exercises are introduced when symptoms permit.

There are numerous operations described for peroneal tendon instability.[30] These can be divided into five basic groups. These are:

(1) direct SPR repair; (2) SPR reconstruction using tendon graft; (3) bone block procedures to produce a bony barrier to dislocation; (4) retromalleolar sulcus-deepening procedures; and (5) re-routing the tendons under the calcaneofibular ligament. For primary procedures we prefer to use a direct repair of the SPR, imbricating the SPR and securing it with stitches placed through drill holes in the fibula. If the retromalleolar sulcus is shallow, then the groove is deepened, attempting to maintain the integrity of the base of the groove where the tendons run. This is achieved by elevating the floor of the groove, removing the cancellous bone from the fibula, and then replacing the periosteal flap in its deepened position. Occasionally, further stabilization is required, in which case the tendons are re-routed under the peroneal tendons. Any tendon pathology is treated as outlined above.

Posterior ankle pain

Posterior ankle pain can be classified according to whether it is medial or lateral (Table 10).

Posterior impingement syndrome

The posterior impingement syndrome occurs when there is impingement between the posterior tibial joint surface and the talus and/or calcaneum. It can occur due to an acute plantar flexion injury or secondary to overuse in activities involving repetitive plantar flexion of the ankle. It is most commonly seen in dancers because of the extremes of plantar flexion at the ankle (Fig. 10).

The posterior talus has medial and lateral processes, in between which runs the FHL tendon. In 2.7–7.7 per cent of people there is an os trigonum.[31] This may represent an accessory ossicle, or an

Table 10 Causes of posterior ankle pain

Posteromedial	Posterolateral
FHL tendinitis	Os trigonum impingement
Posteromedial coalition	Fracture of posterior talar process
Tibialis posterior tendinitis	Peroneal tendinitis
Soleus syndrome	Pseudomeniscus syndrome

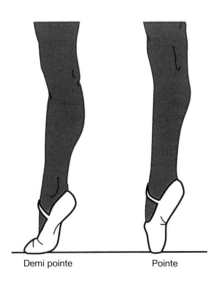

Demi pointe   Pointe

Fig. 10 Demi pointe and en pointe positions in ballet.

un-united fracture of the lateral process of the talus. Those with an unusually large lateral talar tubercle (Stieda's or trigonal process) may also develop this condition. Symptoms in both groups typically commence after a lateral ankle sprain. Other causes of posterior impingement include soft issue entrapment (e.g. a synovial plica or pseudomeniscus), ankle instability, and degenerative joint disease with impingement by osteophytes.

The patient typically complains of posterolateral ankle pain. There may be a history of swelling and catching. Dancers frequently try to compensate for the loss of plantar flexion by placing the foot in an improper position, usually having a more inverted posture en pointe ('sickling'). This results in an increased load on the ATFL and hence a higher risk of lateral sprain. Other compensatory postures can lead to more diffuse lower leg, foot, and ankle complaints. On examination there is tenderness on deep palpation behind the fibula. Pain is exacerbated by extreme passive plantar flexion and by resisted plantar flexion or dorsiflexion of the great toe. Infiltration with local anaesthetic may confirm the diagnosis.

Management

Relative rest and modification of activities, ice massage, NSAIDS and a local corticosteroid injection may be effective in reducing symptoms. A 4–6-week period of casting may be required. A progressive strength training programme is commenced when symptoms permit and technical factors should be addressed in dancers. Taping can help to prevent excessive plantar flexion when the patient returns to activities.

Surgery is considered in those with intractable symptoms. The os trigonum can be excised through a lateral, medial, or arthroscopic approach. The advantage of the medial approach is that it allows the FHL tendon to be decompressed. The disadvantage is that great care has to be taken to protect the neurovascular structures, in particular, the calcaneal branches of the posterior tibial nerve. Return to dancing after surgery is slow and Hamilton found that the time to full recovery was 3–8 months after surgery.[32] With arthroscopic excision, Marumoto et al. found that all patients achieved their maximum recovery by 3 months.[33]

Nerve injury and entrapment

Lateral ankle and foot pain can commonly arise due to nerve injury or entrapment. Traction injuries to the sural, superficial peroneal, or common peroneal nerves are common after inversion sprain, although frequently overlooked. Neuropraxia (where the axons are not disrupted) and axonotmesis (where they are) can result in burning pain, paraesthesia, dysaesthesia, anaesthesia, shooting pains in the distribution of the affected nerve, and motor weakness. Symptoms can intensify during reinnervation. Specific features are dependent upon the nerve affected and the level of injury. A Tinel's test may be positive local to a site of entrapment. Resolution of symptoms with infiltration with local anaesthetic can help to confirm the diagnosis, as can electrodiagnostic tests. Imaging may be necessary to determine the cause of entrapment where this is suspected.

Management includes treatment of the associated injury, as reduction in local swelling may improve neurological symptoms. Support of the affected limb, for example, in a boot walker, may be necessary, and in cases where foot drop has developed a night splint in the form of an ankle foot orthosis can help to prevent gastrocnemius–soleus contractures. Neuralgic pain may respond to measures such as a transcutaneous

Table 11 Causes of sural and superficial peroneal nerve injuries

Trauma

Macrotrauma, including surgery, ankle sprain (traction), myositis ossificans, fractures (sural: fifth metatarsal, cuboid, calcaneus; both: fibula), microtrauma (overuse)

Compression

Intrinsic: by fascia at the nerve pierces crural fascia, by enlarged/scarred Achilles or peroneal tendons, anomalous bands, bony ridge, venous insufficiency, ganglion, neuroma, connective tissue disease, enlarged peroneal tubercle (sural nerve)

Extrinsic: by tight stockings or boots

electrical nerve stimulation (TENS) unit, a tricyclic agent, or gabapentin. Neurapraxia usually settles after 2–3 months but, where axonotmesis has occurred, recovery commonly can take 6 months to a year.

Lateral ankle pain may also arise from other forms of injury or entrapment of the superficial peroneal and sural nerves in the leg (Table 11). The superficial peroneal nerve is vulnerable to direct trauma at its origin from the common peroneal nerve at the proximal fibula and is liable to become entrapped or traumatized as it exits the through the deep fascia in the distal leg. If non-operative treatments fail, the occasional patient requires surgical decompression of the nerve and limited fasciotomy.

Anterior ankle pain (Table 12)

Tibialis anterior tendinopathy

Tibialis anterior provides 80 per cent of the power of dorsiflexion of the ankle. It works eccentrically after heel strike to control deceleration of the foot to the floor and then concentrically after toe off to assist in clearance and ankle dorsiflexion. The tendon is covered in a sheath from 5 cm above the superior extensor retinaculum to the proximal portion of the inferior extensor retinaculum.

Tenosynovitis

Tenosynovitis (or paratenonitis) is seen in those individuals who run or walk down hill. It is also seen in skiers and skaters when poorly fitting boots or skates cause compression. The patient reports pain and swelling over the anterior ankle and difficulty walking up and down inclines. There is evidence of swelling over the anterior ankle and resisted dorsiflexion of the ankle is painful.

Management involves avoidance of inappropriate footwear, use of local padding and appropriate lacing, anti-inflammatories, and ice and relative rest. A graduated exercise programme can then be commenced.

Tendinosis and rupture

Tendinosis is very rarely symptomatic until an acute rupture of the tendon occurs. This is typically seen in men over the age of 60 years. Spontaneous rupture can occur in diabetes, after a local corticosteroid injection or in those on long-term systemic corticosteroids, and in those with inflammatory arthropathies such as rheumatoid arthritis and gout. Rupture is also associated with the presence of an exostosis on the dorsum of the ankle.

Table 12 Causes of anterior ankle pain

Syndesmosis injury

Impingement syndrome 'footballer's ankle'

Anterior tibial tendinopathy

Extensor hallucis longus tendinopathy

Lateral or medial instability

Talar dome injury

Tibial plafond injury

Ganglia

Referred pain

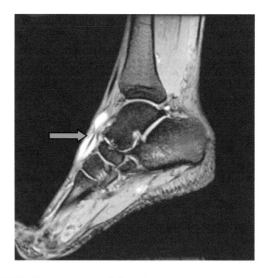

Fig. 11 MRI showing extensor hallucis longus tenosynovitis.

There may be a history of a sudden contraction against a plantar flexed ankle, but in many cases there may be no obvious precipitant. The patient may report local pain and swelling or simply notice functional difficulty with dorsiflexion of the foot. The usual site of rupture is 1.5–3 cm above the insertion of the tendon but rupture can also occur anywhere, including at the musculotendinous junction. Gait is abnormal with slapping or dragging of the foot and there is eversion of the foot with attempted ankle dorsiflexion due to action of the extensors. There may be local swelling on the dorsum of the ankle, a visible and palpable gap, and weakness of ankle dorsiflexion with the toes plantar flexed (which prevents action of the EDL).

Management is dependent upon the age and expectations of the patient. Older or more frail patients may prefer functional bracing to surgery. Plattner and Mann reported good results with non-operative treatment.[34] In the younger patient, treatment should be operative with either direct repair or, if there is a defect between the two ends, an FHL transfer or a sliding graft of the tibialis anterior tendon.

Extensor tendinopathies

The mechanisms of development of tenosynovitis of the extensor tendons of the foot and ankle tenosynovitis are similar to those involved in the development of tenosynovitis of tibialis anterior.

Extensor digitorum longus (EDL) tendinopathies

Patients present with pain and swelling over the anterior ankle joint, just lateral to EHL. There is pain on resisted testing of extension of the lateral four toes. When rupture has occurred, there may be local swelling and an inability to extend the second to fifth toes. Unlike ruptures of tibialis anterior, rupture of EDL is usually due to a laceration. Rarely, insertional avulsions and closed ruptures may occur, usually in association with trauma or tight footwear or systemic causes as listed above.

Extensor hallucis longus (EHL) tendinopathies

EHL tenosynovitis presents with pain and swelling over the tendon at the ankle joint. There is tenderness, crepitus, and pain on resisted extension of the hallux. Lacerations or blunt trauma are the usual source of tendon rupture, with resulting pain swelling and inability to extend the hallux (Fig. 11).

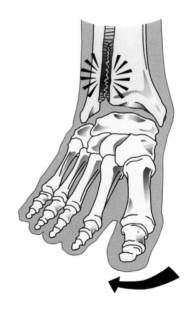

Fig. 12 Syndesmosis tears usually occur with very severe external rotation and/or dorsiflexion of the ankle.

Management of tenosynovitis of the extensor tendons

Lacerations and ruptures near the ankle are usually repaired, with end-to-end suture or tendon transfer. Those more distal to the metatarsophalangeal joint (MTPJ) may be treated non-operatively because of the extensor hood, which prevents retraction.

Syndesmosis injuries

Often termed 'high ankle sprains', syndesmosis injuries can occur with or without a lateral ankle sprain (Fig. 12). Such injuries result in significant pain and dysfunction and are one of the most important causes of chronic pain after an ankle sprain. Injuries to the syndesmosis are reported to occur in 10 per cent of all ankle sprains, being particularly common in collision sports. Syndesmosis injuries vary from sprain to rupture of the syndesmosis. They may involve any or all of the three components of the syndesomsis—the anterior and posterior inferior tibiofibular ligaments and the interosseous membrane. Rupture of the syndesmosis, resulting in diastasis of the tibia and fibula, is fortunately a rare injury, requiring a violent force. However, less extensive syndesmotic injuries can occur with comparatively minor trauma and may be missed without maintaining a high index of suspicion.

Syndesmosis sprains can be associated with lateral ankle sprains, occurring after a plantar flexion and inversion injury. Nevertheless, the more severe injuries to the syndesmosis occur with dorsiflexion and external rotation of the foot on the leg, for example, in pivoting, cutting, or if someone falls on the individual from behind. The torque of external rotation can sequentially tear the ATFL, syndesmosis, posterior tibiofibular ligament, and interosseous membrane and may result in a high fibular (Maissoneuve) fracture. Disruption of the peroneal artery can occur, resulting in an acute compartment syndrome. Since injuries to the syndesmosis usually involve significant trauma, avulsion fractures of the medial malleolus or injuries to the medial ligament of the ankle are commonly seen. A pure abduction injury affecting only the syndesmosis is rare. Severe eversion injuries are rare but can tear the deltoid ligament and disrupt the syndesmosis and interosseous membrane, with resulting distal tibiofibular diastatsis. The distal fibula often fractures before the syndesmosis is completely torn. The most frequent mechanism occurs when the athlete has the weight-bearing foot planted and slightly pronated and is struck on the lateral aspect of the leg with the foot fixed. Deltoid ligament injury can also occur in association with a fracture of the proximal or distal fibula.

Injuries are classed as either acute or chronic. Within this classification they can then be divided into simple sprains, syndesmotic injuries that are only unstable on stress testing, and frank diastasis.

Examination

Examination will reveal swelling and discrete tenderness over the anterior tibiofibular ligament. There may be associated tenderness over the deltoid ligament. The squeeze test, where the tibia and fibula are compressed above the syndesmosis, should be performed and may reproduce the pain. Abduction and external rotation stress may also reproduce the pain. The medial side and the entire length of the fibula should be examined for tenderness.

Investigation

A plain AP radiograph of the lower leg and lateral and mortise views of the ankle should be obtained: an increased tibiofibular space may be evident. Harper and Keller defined the typical radiographic relationship between the tibia and fibula as being: (1) at least 6 mm of tibiofibular clear space; (2) at least 6 mm of overlap of the tibia and fibula at the incisura; and (3) at least 1 mm of overlap between tibia and fibula on the mortise view.[35] Plain X-rays may be normal and stress views in external rotation and abduction, CT, MRI, or bone scan may be necessary to confirm the diagnosis. Calcification or synostosis of the tibia and fibula may be noted on X-ray in chronic injuries.

Management

Sprains of the syndesmosis usually respond to a programme of RICE (rest, ice, compression, elevation), splinting, and a 3-week period of non-weight bearing, followed by mobilization in a stirrup brace or taping. A rehabilitation programme similar to that for lateral ligament sprain is instituted, although progress is usually slower. A 1 cm heel lift may provide some symptomatic benefit, preventing the anterior talus from irritating the mortise during gait. Injuries that are only unstable on stress testing can either be treated by a period of 4–6 weeks non-weight-bearing followed by weight-bearing, or surgically. Frank diastasis requires surgical stabilization, by transfibular screw fixation 1 cm above the syndesmosis. This is followed by 6 weeks non-weight-bearing with early range of motion exercises after the first 3 weeks. This is followed by mobilization in a walking cast. There is great debate regarding removal of the screw, but most surgeons remove the diastasis screw at 8–12 weeks.

Delayed diagnosis of a diastasis leads to the rapid onset of degenerate change. As long as the arthritic change is not too advanced, surgical debridement and delayed fixation should be considered. Ogilvie-Harris and Reed reported good results 2 years after injury using arthroscopic debridement.[36]

Chronic syndesmosis injuries can be complicated by interosseous ligament ossification, at times with heterotopic bone formation. Fortunately, this bone does not usually limit tibiofibular motion. Tibiofibular synostosis does occur and leads to mortise restriction and anterior ankle pain with dorsiflexion.

Medial ankle pain (Table 13)

Posterior tibial tendinopathies (PTT)

Posterior tibial tendon (PTT) disorders represent a commonly neglected cause of posteromedial ankle and foot pain, with significant consequences in the form of the development of a progressive flatfoot deformity. Amongst other functions, the PTT is a powerful dynamic stabilizer of the hindfoot against eversion, prevents valgus deformity, and is under considerable stress during gait just after heel strike. The PTT brings the hindfoot from loaded eversion into increasing inversion, maximizing the mechanical advantage of the more laterally placed Achilles tendon as the patient rises on to the forefoot. The tendon also maintains midtarsal and forefoot stability through its attachments. The large mechanical stresses applied, its relative hypovascularity, and constriction beneath the flexor retinaculum make the PTT particularly vulnerable in its course from the medial malleolus to its insertion on the navicular tuberosity (Fig. 5).

Numerous associations with PTT disease have been reported (Table 14).

The consequences of PTT disorders involve not only the PTT but also the capsule and ligamentous structures of the hindfoot and midfoot (Table 15). The spectrum of disorders that can affect the PTT include dysfunction, tenosynovitis, tendinosis, dislocation, tears, and rupture. The short excursion of the tendon enhances its function. Since the main effect of PTT disease is tendon elongation, the hallmark of

Table 13 Causes of medial ankle pain

Posterior tibial tendinopathy
Flexor hallucis tendinopathy
Tarsal tunnel syndrome
Deltoid ligament injury
Referred pain

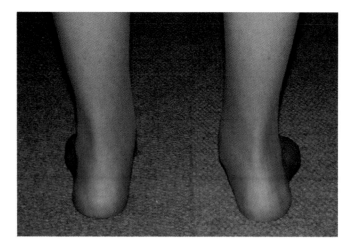

Fig. 13 The rheumatoid foot: posterior tendon disease and valgus deformity predisposes to tarsal tunnel syndrome.

Table 14 Predisposing factors to posterior tibial tendon disorders

Extrinsic factors	Intrinsic factors
Overuse	Hereditary factors
Running sports that require a sudden shorter change in direction	Leg length discrepancy (excessive stress on shorter leg)
Training errors such as camber running	Hyperpronation
Trauma	Tight gastrocnemius–soleus copmlex
	Hypertension
	Diabetes
	Inflammatory arthritis
	Obesity

PTT disease is the adult-acquired flatfoot, in which the medial longitudinal arch collapses, the heel goes into valgus, and the forefoot abducts and becomes supinated (varus). As the disease progresses the spring ligament stretches and eventually degenerate change in the joints occurs. Classification systems have been proposed, based on either clinical findings, duration of symptoms, or imaging characteristics. Johnson and Strom classified PTT disorders in three stages, according to clinical and pathological findings.[37] Myerson later added a fourth stage[38] and we have further adapted this, as shown in Table 15.

History

PTT insufficiency is most common in middle-aged women. Most patients present with posteromedial ankle pain and swelling. A gradual flattening of the foot through loss of the longitudinal arch may have been noted. Progressive fatigue with exercise, weakness, and pain on pushing off or standing on tiptoe may also be reported. With late-stage disease symptoms are associated with degenerative joint disease affecting predominantly the ankle and subtalar joints. Disorders are often missed in their early stages and consequently patients may present with irreversible deformities.

Examination

Clinical signs vary according to the stage of disease, but posteromedial ankle tenderness is invariably present. Swelling is variable. Progressive flattening of the foot with hindfoot valgus eventually occurs which becomes fixed in later stages of the disease along with degenerative changes of the ankle joint. The single heel raise test elicits pain and fatiguability in early disease, and with progressive disease (late stage 2 and stage 3) the heel fails to invert and, finally, heel raise becomes impossible. Resisted inversion of the foot in plantar flexion (to isolate the PTT) elicits pain and weakness. Observing the foot from behind the hindfoot valgus and abduction of the forefoot lead to the 'too many toes' sign, where the number of toes observed is increased on the

Table 15 Posterior tibial tendon disorders (adapted from references 37 and 38)

Stage	Pathology	Signs
1A	Tendon normal length Mild tendinosis/tenosynovitis	No deformity The gastrocnemius–soleus complex is often tight Pain with resisted testing of PTT; single heel raise usually normal but painful Tenderness and swelling along course of tendon
2	Tendinosis of tendon with stretching out of tendon	Correctable valgus hindfoot, abduction of the forefoot, forefoot varus Tenderness, swelling along tendon 'Too many toes' sign and pain with resisted testing Abnormal single heel raise (weak, lack of inversion)
3	Progressive tendinosis and degenerative articular pathology in the foot	The deformities listed above become fixed Poor/absent single heel raise Lateral ankle pain may arise due to impingement
4	Progression of (3), with joint pathology now involving the ankle	As 3 Ankle deformity (valgus talar tilt with lateral tibiotalar degeneration)

affected side. In late-stage disease there may be lateral pain secondary to impingement between the lateral calcaneus and the fibula, with entrapment of the interposed peroneal tendons.

Differential diagnosis

The differential diagnosis is that of any other cause of posteromedial ankle pain and of adult-acquired flatfoot.

Imaging

Weight-bearing AP and lateral radiographs are helpful in assessing PTT insufficiency. They should be inspected for subtalar and mid-tarsal degenerate change. The AP radiograph should be inspected as to degree of uncovering of the talar head by the navicular and the presence or absence of degenerate change. On the lateral view, there is a collapse of the medial longitudinal arch, and talonavicular and navicular cuneiform sagging may be apparent. If pathology involving an accessory navicular is suspected, a reversed oblique radiograph should be obtained. If stage 4 disease is suspected, a standing mortise view of the ankle should be obtained.

MRI has been shown to be sensitive to intratendinous change within the PTT, and may be predictive of clinical outcome (Fig. 14).[39] MRI has the advantage of providing more information about the state of the surrounding soft tissue structures. Associated features such as thickening of the anterior portion of the flexor retinaculum, attrition of the plantar calcaneonavicular ligament, hypertrophy of the navicular tubercle, and the presence of an accessory navicular may all be demonstrated. Nevertheless, ultrasound has been shown to be more accurate than MRI (94 versus 65 per cent) in the evaluation of the PTT.[40] In many cases surgical decision-making is based upon clinical findings and not the special investigations.

Management

The aims of treatment are to control the symptoms and to prevent progression. Management is dependent upon the stage of the dysfunction and the characteristics and expectations of the patient. Conservative measures include the use of a below-knee walking cast

for 4–6 weeks, the use of a medial longitudinal arch support and, in stage 3 disease where the deformity is uncorrectable, a cushioned non-corrective total contact insole is indicated. In late stage 2 disease an ankle foot orthosis can be used. Simultaneous anti-inflammatory approaches such as ice and NSAIDs may also be of use. In the subacute or chronic stages a custom orthotic or ankle foot orthosis work to provide arch support and correct the flexible component of the deformity. Physical therapy—including calf muscle and Achilles stretching and progressive strengthening of tibialis posterior—is vital.

Surgical management is utilized when conservative measures have failed. There is a view that tenosynovectomy may prevent the progression of stage 1 to 2 disease, and that tendon transfer for stage 2 disease is often preferable to arthrodesis for stage 3 disease.

Surgical options are as follows. Stage 1 disease is treated with tenosynovectomy.[41] Stage 2 disease is treated with a tendon transfer, supplemented with a bony procedure. The spring ligament should also be repaired. The FDL tendon or the tibialis anterior tendon is used as the transfer. The bony procedure used is either a medial displacement calcaneal osteotomy, or a calcaneocuboid fusion, with a bone graft inserted to lengthen the lateral column. Simple tendon transfer does not lead to correction of the medial longitudinal arch.[41] Stage 3 disease is salvaged with a subtalar or triple fusion, if non-operative treatment fails. Stage 4 disease can be managed by an ankle foot orthosis. Failing this transcalcaneal nail (subtalar and ankle) or pantalar arthrodesis is undertaken. These are salvage procedures for the low-demand patient.

Flexor hallucis longus (FHL) tendinopathy

The FHL functions to plantar flex the interphalangeal joint of the hallux and to dynamically stabilize the first MTPJ (and hence the whole forefoot) (Fig. 15). It is prone to injury at extremes of ankle plantar flexion and MTP dorsiflexion. The spectrum of disorders of the FHL include tenosynovitis, tendinosis, tear and rupture of the tendon.

FHL tenosynovitis is the commonest problem and can occur at three sites, which from proximal to distal are: at the posterior ankle where it enters the fibro-osseous tunnel between the talar tuberosities; behind the flexor retinaculum and, lastly, between the sesamoids. It is a rare condition, although it can occur in runners, spring board divers and, most commonly, dancers. The patient typically complains of posteromedial as opposed to posterolateral ankle pain with an os

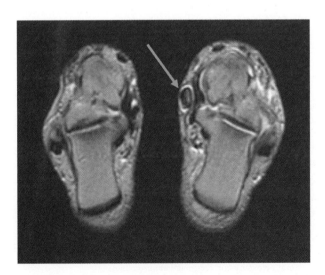

Fig. 14 MRI of the ankle, showing tenosynovytis of the posterior tibial tendon behind the medial malleolus.

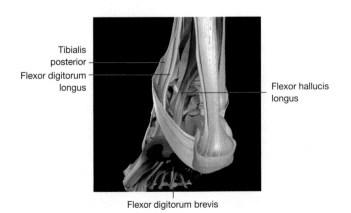

Tibialis posterior
Flexor digitorum longus
Flexor hallucis longus
Flexor digitorum brevis

Fig. 15 Flexor hallucis longus: 'The beef of the heel'.

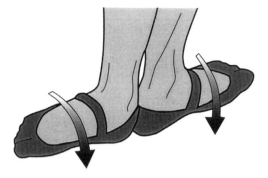

Fig. 16 FHL Tenosynovitis in dancers is exacerbated by forcing the turn out position, in addition to movements on to the ball of the foot (demi pointe) and onto the tip of the toe (pointe), and by the hyperplantarflexion of the relevé.

trigonum, and swelling. In dancers the pain is exacerbated by forcing the turn-out position, movements on to the ball of the foot (demi pointe) and on to the tip of the toe (pointe), and by the hyperplantarflexion of the relevé (Fig. 16). The condition can be associated with poor technique, excessive turn-out at the hip so that the dancer is not centred over the feet, weakness and inadequate flexibility of the other soft tissue structures of the lower leg and foot, hard surfaces, excessive training, and poorly fitting and inappropriate shoes.

Clinical features are posteromedial ankle pain, crepitus, swelling, and tenderness along the course of the tendon pain with motion of the hallux exacerbated by the specific movements mentioned above. There is pain with passive, active, and resisted movements of the toe. When the site of the condition is more distal, the tenderness is local to that site.

Stenosing tenosynovitis can also occur at any of the three sites and is associated with triggering that is difficult to localize, although a palpable nodule and the site of a sensation of popping or snapping felt by the patient may act as a guide.

Management

FHL tenosynovitis in the acute phase is treated by relative rest, anti-inflammatory approaches, and addressing the associated causes, including dancing/sporting technique where relevant. If dancing is to be continued, then the en pointe position should be avoided. In more chronic cases the dancer must be counselled that recovery can be prolonged. A short period of immobilization of 2–3 weeks in a brace may be necessary. There is no role for the use of local corticosteroids in this condition.

Surgery is undertaken if conservative measures fail. A medial incision is used to decompress the tendon, and to release any triggering caused by nodules on the tendon. Surgery is often combined with os trigonum excision (see above).

Ruptures of FHL can occur at any of the sites listed above as a result of tendinosis, mechanical irritation, secondary to longitudinal tears, or due to direct lacerations. Surgical repair is recommended, although rupture of the FHL tendon proximal to its connection with FDL in the foot may result in only minimal pain and functional limitation, although the tendon may retract 5–7 cm into the calf.

Flexor digitorum longus (FDL) tendinopathies

Flexor digitorum longus tendinopathies are much less common then those affecting FHL, but rarely tenosynovitis or tendinosis may be seen, particularly in dancers. Lesions occur at two sites: under the flexor retinaculum at the posteromedial ankle; and at the level of the plantar plate. Patients present with symptoms similar to these of FHL tenosynovitis but, clinically, pain is worsened on resisted flexion of the toes. Treatment is similar to that used in FHL complaints.

Most tears or ruptures of the FDL are due to a laceration and require primary repair.

Tarsal tunnel syndrome (TTS)

Tarsal tunnel syndrome refers to entrapment primarily of the posterior tibial (PT) nerve within, proximal to, or distal to the flexor retinaculum or within the abductor hiatus. During its course the PT nerve gives sensory calcaneal branches and then medial and lateral plantar branches that have sensory and motor components. TTS can be subdivided into proximal TTS, representing entrapment of the PT nerve, and distal TTS, where the medial and/or lateral plantar nerves are involved. TTS has to be differentiated from 'high tarsal tunnel syndrome', where the tibial nerve is entrapped in the leg by a band of tight gastrocnemius fascia. Symptoms are similar except that tenderness is maximal in the lower calf.

A number of factors within and outside of the tarsal tunnel can be involved (Table 16). Excessive subtalar pronation frequently plays a major role and is often associated with hindfoot valgus and forefoot varus, with stretching of the tibial nerve. Additional stretching of the flexor retinaculum and abductor hallucis muscle causes further compression of the nerve and branches within the abductor hiatus. Other pathologies associated with hyperpronation, such as posterior tibial tendinitis, can also contribute to nerve compression. Synovitis associated with inflammatory arthropathy and other systemic disorders are commonly associated with tarsal tunnel syndrome and should be considered in any patient with TTS.

Table 16 Aetiology of tarsal tunnel syndrome

Intrinsic factors

Soft tissue masses (ganglia, lipomas, neurilemomas, neurofibromas, synovial sarcomas)
Inflammatory arthritis (synovitis)
Tenosynovitis (FHL, tibialis posterior)
Scar tissue (previous surgery or trauma)
Venous insufficiency leading to local varicosities
Presence of accessory musculature
Posterior tibial artery aneurysm

Extrinsic factors
Biomechanics: excessive subtalar pronation (hindfoot valgus, forefoot varus)
Systemic disease—diabetes, hypothyroidism
Trauma (blunt trauma, fracture of ankle mortise, talus, or calcaneus, iatrogenic)
Structural deformity and congenital abnormalities such as tarsal coalition
Scar tissue (previous surgery or trauma)

Symptoms

Diagnosis is often difficult as symptoms and clinical signs are variable and electrodiagnostic tests have limitations (see below). The presentation varies according to the cause and site of entrapment. A burning ache or pain around the medial ankle and/or foot is commonly reported, with shooting pains into the plantar aspect of the foot. Paraesthesiae/dysaesthesiae in the same distribution and cramp in the foot are also common. Depending on the cause, symptoms may be worse with weight-bearing or with the activity of an inflammatory arthropathy. Removal of tight footwear and rest may help.

Examination

Local oedema over the medial ankle, synovitis, and/or an ankle effusion may be present in those with an underlying systemic cause. Tenderness is noted on palpation over the tarsal tunnel and, more notably, proximal and distal to the site of compression (the Valleix phenomenon). Pain and paraesthesiae radiating proximally or distally on percussion over the tunnel (Tinel's sign) suggest proximal tarsal tunnel syndrome. Deep compression over the tunnel may also reproduce symptoms. Exacerbation of symptoms with forced pronation of the foot may be noted. There may be a decrease in two-point discrimination between involved and uninvolved extremities. Late findings include loss of sensation along the medial and/or lateral plantar nerves and atrophy of intrinsic muscles of the foot, resulting in hammer toe deformities. If symptoms are related to activity it is necessary to examine the patient after a period of weight-bearing and/or performing the activity associated with the onset of symptoms. Patients with hyperpronation have increased tibial nerve tension during eversion, dorsiflexion, and cyclic loading with increased internal rotation.

Investigations

Considerable controversy exists in relation to the use of *electrodiagnostic studies* in TTS. They may be helpful but have limitations and do not distinguish between proximal and distal entrapment. Sensory conduction tests have a reported sensitivity of 65–90.5 per cent. Mixed nerve conduction tests appear to have similar levels of sensitivity. Motor conduction tests have a reported sensitivity of 54 per cent, possibly due to alterations in motor conduction occurring later in the disorder and to difficulties with defining the precise onset of evoked muscle action potential during the test.[42] Limitations in the sensitivities of electrodiagnostic tests may also be related to difficulties in locating the precise site for nerve testing. Those patients with biomechanical causes of TTS and who have symptoms only when weight-bearing may have normal studies at rest. Electrodiagnostic tests in the form of sensory and mixed nerve conduction studies performed under controlled conditions are useful in the diagnosis of TTS, in particular, when asymmetric values between the affected and unaffected sides are noted. It is possible to differentiate between high TTS and TTS using electrodiagnostic approaches.

MRI is helpful in evaluating the musculotendinous and vascular structures in the tarsal tunnel and will demonstrate any local space-occupying lesions. *Gait analysis* can identify biomechanical factors that may be playing a role in the complaint.

Management

Successful outcome is dependent upon identification of the underlying aetiology of the condition. The patient should have a trial of NSAIDs and topical applications may provide relief. Regular icing may provide benefit and relative rest is important. Short-term use of orthoses to counteract hindfoot valgus are frequently helpful in alleviating symptoms and may also be used in the longer term to correct associated biomechanical factors. Casting for a 3–6-week period may be necessary if symptoms are severe. In those with an underlying inflammatory arthritis, an injection of local anaesthetic and corticosteroid into the tarsal tunnel should be considered. Local corticosteroid injections are rarely necessary in patients with local tenosynovitis. Other measures should be applied intensively. Where appropriate, physiotherapy may include massage to break down local scar tissue and to mobilize the nerve as well as stretching and appropriate strengthening exercises where biomechanical factors are involved.

Failure of conservative management is an indication for surgical intervention. Surgical decompression is through division of the flexor retinaculum. The nerve is carefully dissected out. Any prominent leashes of venous vessels are ligated and divided. Great care is taken to dissect out the calcaneal branches, medial and lateral plantar nerves, and also the nerve to abductor digiti quinti minimi (Baxter's nerve), which is the first branch of the lateral plantar nerve. Cimino reviewed the literature and found that, after such a release, 69 per cent of patients had a good result, 22 per cent of patients were improved, and 7 per cent had poor results.[43] Patients with a biomechanical cause for their TTS respond poorly to decompressive surgery.

Medial ankle sprain

The medial (deltoid) ligament of the ankle is the largest and strongest ligament of the ankle and is injured where there is significant eversion or abduction force. Such injuries constitute only 5–6 per cent of ankle sprains. The majority of these injuries are associated with other injuries, and isolated medial ligament injuries are rare.[44] The patient presents with severe medial ankle pain after an episode of trauma, and acute eversion or abduction of the foot and ankle may be described. These injuries may be overlooked due to the presence of other injuries such as a syndesmosis and/or high fibular fracture. Examination reveals swelling, discolouration, local tenderness, and pain with eversion of the foot. Other pathologies should be sought, including damage to the syndesmosis, tibia and fibula, other ligaments, PTT, spring ligament, and neurovascular structures. Plain radiographs are usually necessary to exclude bony injury.

Management of an isolated sprain involves relative rest, ice, NSAIDs, and use of an Aircast brace. In cases where other pathologies such as fracture or syndesmosis disruption are present, surgery is necessary. However, even if the deltoid ligament is ruptured it is treated conservatively, unless it is caught within the joint, and requires open removal to allow reduction. Rarely, chronic medial ankle instability can result from a neglected medial ligament sprain. The patient complains of persisting medial ankle pain and there is progressive ankle and subtalar valgus and development of an adult-acquired flatfoot. Associated problems, including PTT and spring ligament dysfunction, can be present.

Stress radiographs may show valgus instability, and MRI can help to make the diagnosis. However, this is usually a difficult diagnosis to make.

Treatment is with supportive treatment, including physiotherapy, orthoses, and an ankle brace. If these measures fail, surgery can be undertaken with either direct repair of the ligament to the medial malleolus, or utilization of a half of the FDL tendon as a deltoid ligament reconstruction.

References

1. Edwards, M.E. (1928). The relations of the peroneal tendons to the fibula, calcaneus and cuboideum. *Am. J. Anat.* **421**, 213.

2. Hintermann, B. and Gachter, A. (1996). The first metatarsal raise sign: a simple, sensitive sign of tibialis posterior tendon dysfunction. *Foot Ankle Int.* **17**, 236–241.

3. Brage, M.E., Rockett, M., Vraney, R., *et al.* (1998). Ankle fracture classification: a comparison of reliability of three X-ray views versus two. *Foot Ankle Int.* **19**, 555–562.

4. Rosenberg, Z.S., Cheung, Y., Jahss, M.H., Noto, A.M., Norman, A., and Leeds, N.E. (1988). Rupture of posterior tibial tendon: CT and MR imaging with surgical correlation. *Radiology* **169**, 229–235.

5. Rockett, M., Waitches, G., Sudakoff, G., and Brage, M. (1998). Use of ultrasongraphy versus magnetic resonance imaging for tendon abnormalities. *Foot Ankle Int.* **19**, 604–612.

6. Brooks, S.C., Potter, B.T., and Rainey, J.B. (1981). Inversion injuries of the ankle: clinical assessment and radiographic review. *Br. Med. J.* **282**, 607–608.

7. Garrick, J.G. (1977). The frequency of injury, mechanism of injury and epidemiology of ankle sprains. *Am. J. Sports Med.* **5**, 241–242.

8. Viljakka, T. and Rokkanen, P. (1983). The treatment of ankle sprain by bandaging and antiphlogistic drugs. *Ann. Chir. Gynaecol.* **72**, 66–70.

9. Broström, L. (1964). Anatomic lesions in recent sprains. *Acta Chir. Scand.* **128**, 483–495.

10. Stiell, I.G., McDowell, I., Nair, R.C., Aeta, H.C., Greenberg, G., *et al.* (1993). Decision rules for the use of radiography in acute ankle injuries. Refinement and prospective validation. *J. Am. Med. Assoc.* **269**, 1127–1132.

11. Van Dijk, C.N., Lim, I.S.L., Bossuyt, P.M.M., and Marti, R.K.J. (1996). J Physical examination is sufficient for the diagnosis of sprained ankles. *J. Bone Joint Surg. (Br.)* **78B**, 958–962.

12. Rubin, G. and Whitten, M. (1961). The talar tilt angle and the fibular collateral ligament: a method for the determination of talar tilt. *J. Bone Joint Surg.* **42A**, 311–326.

13. De Simoni, C., Wetz, H.H., Zanetti, M., *et al.* (1996). Clinical examination and magnetic resonance imaging in the assessment of ankle sprains treated with an orthosis. *Foot Ankle Int.* **17**, 177–182.

14. Pickenburg, A.C.M., Van Dijk, C.N., Bossuyt, P.M.M., and Marti, R.K. (2000). Treatment of ruptures of the lateral ankle ligaments: a meta-analysis. *J. Bone Joint Surg. (Am.)* **82A**, 761–772.

15. Leach, R.E. and Schepsis, A.A. (1990). Acute injuries to ligaments of the ankle. In *Surgery of the musculoskeletal system*, vol. 4, 2nd edn (ed. C.M. Evarts), pp. 3887–3913. Churchill Livingstone, New York.

16. Kibler, W.B. (1996). Arthroscopic findings in ankle ligament reconstruction. *Clin. Sports Med.* **15**, 799–804.

17. Taga, I., Shino, K., Inoue, M., *et al.* (1993). Articular cartilage lesions in ankles with lateral ankle ligament injury: an arthroscopic study. *Am. J. Sports Med.* **21**, 120–127.

18. Hennrikus, W.L., Mapes, R.C., Lyons, P.M., and Lapoint, J.M. (1996). Outcomes of the Chrisman–Snook and modified Broström procedures for chronic lateral ankle instability: a prospective randomised comparison. *Am. J. Sports Med.* **24**, 400–404.

19. Hamilton, W.G., Thompson, F.M., Snow, S.W. (1993). The modified Broström procedure for lateral ankle instability. *Foot Ankle* **14**, 1–7.

20. Nimon, G.A., Dobson, P.J., Angel, K.R., Lewis, P.L., and Stevenson, T.M. (2001). A long term review of a modified Evans procedure: a 5 to 15 year follow up of 111 ankles. *J. Bone Joint Surg. (Br.)* **83B**, 14–18.

21. Hennrikus, W.L., Mapes, R.C., Lyons, P.M., and Lapoint, J.M. (1996). Outcomes of the Chrisman–Snook and modified Broström procedures for chronic lateral ankle instability: a prospective randomised comparison. *Am. J. Sports Med.* **24**, 400–404.

22. Krips, R., van Dijk, V., Halasi, T., *et al.* (2001). Long-term outcome of anatomical versus tenodesis for the reconstruction of chronic anterolateral instability of the ankle joint. *Foot Ankle Int.* **22**, 415–421.

23. Berndt, A.L. and Hardy, M. (1959). Transchondral fractures (osteochondritis dissecans) of the talus. *J. Bone Joint Surg.* **41A**, 988–1018.

24. Ferkel, R.D., Karzel, R.P., Del Pizzo, W., Friedman, M.J., and Fischer, S.P. (1991) Arthroscopic debridement of anterolateral ankle impingement. *Am. J. Sports Med.* **19**, 440–446.

25. Kim, S.-H. and Ha, K.-I. (2000). Arthroscopic treatment for impingement of the anterolateral soft tissue of the ankle. *J. Bone Joint Surg. (Br.)* **82B**, 1019–1021.

26. Krause, J.O. and Brodsky, J.W. (1998). Peroneal tendon tears: pathophysiology, surgical reconstruction and clinical results. *Foot Ankle Int.* **19**, 271–279.

27. Sammarco, G.J. and DiRaimondo, C.V. (1989). Chronic peroneus brevis lesions. *Foot Ankle* **9**, 163.

28. Sobel, M., DiCarlo, E., Bohne, W., *et al.* (1991). Longitudinal splitting of the peroneus brevis tendon: an anatomic and histologic study of cadaveric material. *Foot Ankle* **12**, 165.

29. Monteggia, G.S. (1803). *Institutzini Chirurgiche*, Parte Secondu. Milan.

30. Escalas, F., Figueras, J., and Merino, J. (1980). Dislocation of the peroneal tendons: long-term results of surgical treatment. *J. Bone Joint Surg.* **62A**, 451–453.

31. Sarrafian, S.K. (1983). *Anatomy of the foot and ankle*, 2nd edn, pp. 18, 52–53, 94. J.B. Lippincott, Philadelphia.

32. Hamilton, W.G. (1982). Stenosing tenosynovitis of the flexor hallucis longus tendon and posterior impingement upon the os trigonum in ballet dancers. *Foot Ankle* **3**, 74–80.

33. Marumoto, J.M. and Ferkel, R.D. (1997). Arthroscopic excision of the os trigonum: a new technique with preliminary clinical results. *Foot Ankle Int.* **18**, 777–784.

34. Plattner, P. and Mann, R.A. (1993). In *Surgery of the foot and ankle*, 6th edn (ed. R.A. Mann and M. Coughlin), p. 805. C.V. Mosby, St Louis.

35. Harper, M.C. and Keller, T.S. (1989). A radiographic evaluation of the tibiofibular syndesmosis. *Foot Ankle* **10**, 156.

36. Ogilvie-Harris, D.J. and Reed, S.C. (1994). Disruption of the ankle syndesmosis: diagnosis and treatment by arthroscopic surgery. *Arthroscopy* **10**, 561–568.

37. Johnson, K. and Strom, D. (1989). Tibialis posterior tendon dysfunction. *Clin. Orthop.* **239**, 196.

38. Myerson, M.S. (1996). Adult acquired flatfoot deformity. *J. Bone Joint Surg. (Am.)* **78**, 780.

39. Conti, S., Michelson, J., and Jahss, M. (1992). Clinical significance of magnetic resonance imaging in preoperative planning for reconstruction of posterior tibial tendon ruptures. *Foot Ankle Int.* **13**, 208–214.

40. Teasdall, R.D. and Johnson, K.A. (1994). Surgical treatment of stage I posterior tibial tendon dysfunction. *Foot Ankle Intl.* **15**, 646–648.

41. Mann, R.A. and Thompson, F. (1985). Rupture of the posterior tibial tendon causing flat foot: surgical treatment. *J. Bone Joint Surg.* **67A**, 556–561.

42. Johnson, E.W. and Ortiz, P.R. (1996). Electrodiagnosis of the tarsal tunnel syndrome. *Arch. Phys. Med. Rehabil.* **47**, 776–780.

43. Cimino, W.R. (1990). Tarsal tunnel syndrome: a review of the literature. *Foot Ankle* **11**, 47–52.

44. Clanton, T.O. (1999). Athletic injuries to the soft tissues of the foot and ankle. In *Surgery of the foot and ankle*, 7th edn (ed. M.Y. Coughlin and R.A. Mann), p. 1126. Mosby, St Louis.

6.10 The foot

Cathy Speed and Andrew Robinson

Anatomy

The anatomy of the foot is closely linked to its diverse functions, in particular, support, stability, flexibility, propulsion, acceleration, deceleration, and the provision of sensory information. This is achieved through a series of arches and chains formed by bones and soft tissues. These allow the foot to transform from a rigid and stable unit to a flexible system. The foot can be divided into three regions: the hindfoot; midfoot; and forefoot (Fig. 1). Inevitably, the function of each region is affected by the others.

Bony anatomy

The hindfoot

The hindfoot is composed of the two largest bones in the foot, the talus and calcaneus, along with their attachments. These two bones transmit the entire body weight to the floor.

The *talus* forms three main articulations: the talocrural (ankle), talocalcaneal (subtalar) and talonavicular joints. The talus is divided into the body, neck, and head. The head of the talus can be located in the depression midway between the medial malleolus and the tuberosity of the navicular.

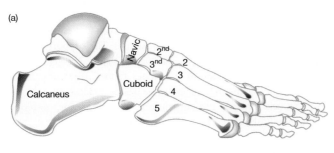

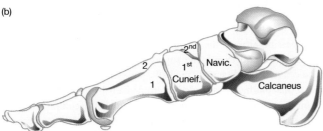

Fig. 1 Bony anatomy of the foot. (a) Choparts joint is formed by the navicular medially and the cuboid laterally articulating on the calcaneus and head of the talus. (b) Lisfranc's joint is formed by articulation of the three metatarsal bases with the three cuneiforms and the cuboid.

The talus has no musculotendinous attachments, but the body and neck of the talus provide attachments for the ligaments and fascia of the ankle and hindfoot. The posterior process of the body of the talus consists of two tubercles, separated by a central groove. The tendon of flexor hallucis longus (FHL) runs in this groove. The lateral tubercle is usually the larger and is particularly vulnerable to fracture due to its position. When it is abnormally large it is known as Stieda's process. The os trigonum is an accessory ossicle that is associated with the posterolateral tubercle in 2.7–7.7 per cent of individuals.[1] It is more often bilateral than not.

Small bones are usually reliant on blood supply from muscles attaching to them. As the talus does not have this opportunity, it receives its blood supply from branches of the posterior tibial, dorsalis pedis, and peroneal arteries. The vascular supply of the talus is easily compromised.

The *sinus tarsi* and *tarsal canal* are found between the talus and calcaneus. The canal separates the middle and posterior facets of the calcaneus. The sinus tarsi is clinically the more important, being a frequent source of symptoms. The sinus lies anterior to the posterior facet of the calcaneus, and gives attachment to a number of structures, namely the extensor digitorum brevis (EDB), the intermediate and medial roots of the extensor retinaculum, the cervical, calcaneonavicular, and calcaneocuboid ligaments. The structures of the sinus tarsi are taut in inversion.

The *calcaneus*, the largest bone in the foot, consists mainly of cancellous bone and has a rich blood supply. Articulations are formed with the talus in the hindfoot, and the navicular and cuboid in the midfoot to form the subtalar and midtarsal joints. It is at these sites that inversion and eversion of the foot takes place.

The posterior section of the calcaneus can be divided into superior, central, and inferior thirds. The Achilles tendon inserts into the central third, with plantaris inserting on its medial aspect. The lengthened posterior section of the calcaneus between the posterior facet and the insertion of the Achilles tendon increases the moment arm of the tendon at the ankle joint, resulting in increased mechanical efficiency. The development of the bone at the Achilles insertion is important in withstanding the large forces being applied by the gastrocnemius–soleus complex.

The superior portion of the calcaneus slopes away from the Achilles tendon, forming a space that is occupied by the retrocalcaneal bursa. The inferior third of the calcaneus forms a tuberosity, the calcaneal process, that divides inferiorly to form the medial and lateral calcaneal processes. These provide attachments for the deep plantar fascia and the first layer of intrinsic plantar muscles. The larger, medial process is a common site for heel spur formation.

The sustentaculum tali, projecting medially from the calcaneus approximately 2.5 cm below the tip of the medial malleolus, is a shelf-like process that 'sustains' the head of the talus at the medial junction of the subtalar and midtarsal joints. Important structures pass close to this shelf. The tendon of tibialis posterior courses above the sustentaculum towards its navicular insertion, the tendon of FHL travels within an osseofibrous tunnel below the sustentaculum, while the tendon of flexor digitorum longus (FDL) passes around its medial edge. Unlike its medial surface, the lateral surface of the calcaneus is flat, with the exception of a small tuberosity—the peroneal tubercle. The peroneus brevis passes above, and the peroneus longus below the tubercle.

The plantar ligaments also make a major contribution to stabilization of the medial longitudinal arch. The long and short plantar ligaments are thick, with strong, longitudinally oriented fibres. The *short plantar (plantar calcaneocuboid) ligament* attaches to the anterior tubercle on the plantar surface of the calcaneus and helps to maintain the position of the calcaneus and to support the midtarsal joint inferiorly. Two other ligaments, the *spring (plantar calcaneonavicular)* and the *long plantar ligaments* also contribute. The former runs medial to the short plantar ligament, from the anterior edge of the sustentaculum tali and inserts broadly on to the navicular. The long plantar ligament forms a thick band superficial to the short plantar ligament and lateral longitudinal arch and inserts into the inferior surface of the calcaneus, the cuboid, and the bases of the metatarsals.

When loaded in gait, the calcaneus and these attached soft tissues provide elastic recoil in the arch system.

The midfoot

The *navicular, cuboid,* and *three cuneiforms* represent the bones of the midfoot. The *tarsal navicular* (scaphoid) is the keystone above the longitudinal arch of the foot (Fig. 2) The midfoot articulates with the hindfoot through the midtarsal, or *Chopart's joint* and with the forefoot through the tarsometatarsal, or *Lisfranc's joint.*

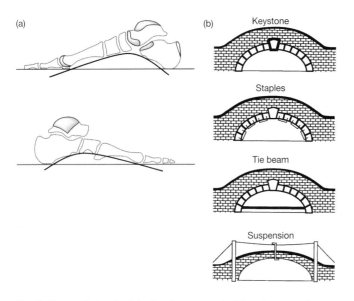

Fig. 2 The medical arch of the foot is composed of the calcaneus, talus, navicular, three cuneiforms, and the first three metatarsals. The lateral longitudinal arch is composed of the calcaneus, cuboid, and the 4th and 5th metatarsals. The transverse arch (not shown) is composed of the metatarsal bases, the cuboid and three cuneiforms. All arches are supported by similar mechanisms that are used in bridge construction.

The medially placed navicular tuberosity receives the insertion of the posterior tibial tendon and can be palpated two fingerbreadths in a distal and plantar direction from the medial malleolus. The blood supply to the navicular is through dorsal, plantar, and tuberosity vessels. The accessory navicular (os tibiale) is found on the postero-medial aspect of the navicular, and is incorporated into the insertional fibres of the tibialis posterior tendon. The frequency is reported as between 2 and 11 per cent.

The *cuboid* articulates with the calcaneus proximally, the fourth and fifth metatarsals distally, and the lateral cuneiform and navicular medially. It has a groove on its inferior surface for the tendon of peroneus longus.

The *three cuneiforms* articulate with the first three metatarsals distally. The intermediate cuneiform is recessed in comparison to its medial and lateral counterparts. Consequently, the second metatarsal is mortised between the first and third metatarsals, giving an extra element of bony stability to Lisfranc's joint.

The forefoot

The forefoot begins distal to the tarsometatarsal joint and includes the ball of the foot and the toes. The toes have three phalanges, with the exception of the big toe, which has two. The five metatarsals articulate with the proximal phalanges, with the second ray acting as the stiffest portion of the foot. The base of the fifth metatarsal has a palpable styloid at its base where the tendon of peroneus brevis inserts.

Accessory ossicles and *sesamoids* are commonly found in the foot. The sesamoid complex under the head of the first metatarsal is constant and receives contributions from seven muscles. Sesamoids can also be found in the metatarsophalangeal (MTP) and interphalangeal (IP) joints. Ossicles can be found, among other places, at the posterolateral aspect of the talus (os trigonum), in the tibialis posterior tendon (the accessory navicular), and the base of the fifth metatarsal (os Vesalianum).

The arches of the foot

The foot, being a segmented structure, can support weight only if it exists as one or more arches. There are three such arches, the medial and lateral longitudinal and transverse arches. The support of these arches can be described using the analogy of a stone bridge, which is dependent upon the shape of the stones (bones), the connections between them (ligaments), the use of tie beams (plantar aponeurosis, flexor hallucis longus), and suspension (tibialis anterior, posterior, and the peroneals) (Fig. 2).

Soft tissue anatomy

The lateral foot

After passing around the lateral malleolus, the tendon of *peroneus longus* passes underneath the superior peroneal retinaculum to the cuboid notch, bends acutely medially, passes under the inferior peroneal retinaculum, and is guided inferomedially by the peroneal tubercle on the calcaneus (Fig. 3). It exits from this retinaculum and turns again to enter the plantar tunnel under the cuboid and fifth metatarsal within a groove on the cuboid tuberosity. In approximately 5 per cent of individuals there is a sesamoid bone within the peroneus longus tendon, which can be a site of pathology. The tendon then inserts into the medial cuneiform and base of the first metatarsal. The sheath of peroneus longus terminates within the cuboid notch but it receives a

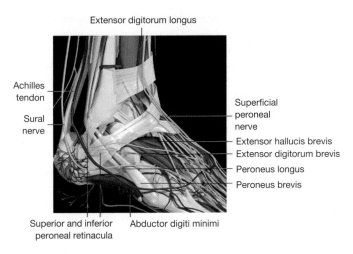

Fig. 3 The lateral foot and ankle.

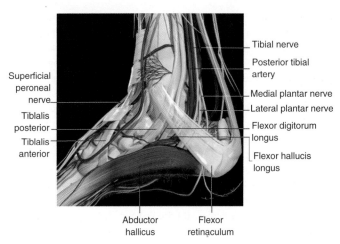

Fig. 4 The posteromedial foot and ankle.

second sheath in the sole of the foot extending medially from notch to insertion. These two sheaths of peroneus longus rarely communicate with each other. The primary function of peroneus longus is to act as a primary plantar flexor of the first ray. This is a unique function and cannot be substituted by other muscles. It also acts as an accessory plantar flexor of the ankle and a weak evertor of the subtalar joint.

Peroneus brevis emerges from the inferior fibular retinaculum to pass to its broad insertion on the styloid process of the fifth metatarsal. It is the strongest evertor of the subtalar joint and is a weak plantar flexor of the ankle. Both peroneii are important in maintaining the longitudinal arch of the foot.

The sheath of peroneus brevis extends to within 2 cm of its insertion on the base of the fifth metatarsal.

The anomalous peroneus quartus muscle is present in 13–22 per cent of the population. Its origin, insertion, and size vary greatly. It runs behind the lateral malleolus and may insert on to an often enlarged peroneal tubercle (most commonly), the cuboid tuberosity, or the tendon of peroneus longus. It may be associated with attrition of the peroneus brevis, due to the presence of an enlarged peroneal tubercle.[2]

Medial foot and ankle

Posterior tibial tendon (PTT)

The PTT originates from the upper two-thirds of the tibia, intermuscular septum, and fibula (Fig. 4). It passes behind the medial malleolus, and inferior to the spring ligament, where a fibrocartilaginous or bony sesamoid may be located. The insertion of the PTT is complex. The anterior component of the insertion is to the tuberosity of the navicular, but other insertions are to the bones of the tarsometatarsal joint, and also to the sustentaculum tali.

The tendon crosses three joints along its course—the ankle, subtalar, and oblique midtarsal joints, causing specific actions at each joint it crosses. The PTT works powerfully at the subtalar and midtarsal joints to invert the heel and supinate the foot. It also plantar flexes the foot at the ankle, plays an important role in maintaining the medial arch of the foot, and contributes to the stability of the foot by its many bony attachments.

Flexor digitorum longus (FDL)

Having passed medial to the edge of the sustentaculum tali, the FDL passes deep to abductor hallucis and into the central compartment of the foot, crossing the tendon of FHL, from which it receives a strong slip. It is here that it also receives the insertion of the quadratus plantae muscle. The tendon then separates into each of its four tendons, which give origin to the lumbrical muscles. Each tendon enters the fibrous sheathes of the lateral four toes, perforates the corresponding tendon of flexor digitorum brevis (FDB), and inserts on to the base of the distal phalanx. FDL flexes the distal phalanges of the lateral four toes, assists in plantar flexion at the ankle, and helps to maintain the medial and longitudinal arches.

Flexor hallucis longus (FHL)

The FHL has a rather deviated course from its origin. It arises on the posterior aspect of the fibula, is laterally placed in the tarsal tunnel, and inserts in the medial foot. The FHL may have a muscle belly that extends as far as the talar tubercles through which the tendon passes. It is separated from the Achilles tendon by a fat-filled space. The close proximity of these tendons is one reason for the use of the FHL as a tendon graft for the Achilles, just as the close proximity of the FDL is taken advantage of in surgery for tibialis posterior lesions. The tendon of FHL travels below the sustentaculum tali into the medial compartment of the foot, deep to the FDL. It enters the fibrous sheath of the big toe and inserts into the base of the distal phalanx. FHL flexes the distal phalanx of the big toe, assists in plantar flexion at the ankle, and helps to maintain the medial arch.

Anterior foot and ankle

The tendon of tibialis anterior (TA), the long extensors, and peroneus tertius all pass into the foot on the anterior aspect of the ankle. Medially, TA emerges from beneath the inferior extensor retinaculum to insert into the medial edge of the foot at the first metatarsal base and the first cuneiform. It functions to dorsiflex the ankle and invert the foot. It also actively supports the medial arch.

Extensor hallucis longus (EHL) exits the inferior extensor retinaculum medial to the dorsalis pedis artery, and the deep peroneal nerve, and travels to insert on to the distal phalanx of the hallux. Insertion onto the proximal phalanx occurs in approximately 50 per cent of people.

Extensor digitorum longus (EDL) splits into 4 slips that pass dorsally to form the extensor hood of the first four metatarsophalangeal joint (MTPJs). Each tendon divides into three slips, the central portion inserting on to the base of the middle phalanx, the slip on the tibial side having a lumbrical insertion, and the extensor hood inserting on to the distal phalanx. EDL functions to dorsiflex the MTPJs, proximal interphalangeal joint (PIPJs), and distal interphalangeal joint (DIPJs) along with the intrinsic muscles.

Peroneus tertius is actually a part of EDL, which inserts on to the base of the fifth metatarsal.

The *anterior tarsal tunnel* is a narrow space between the fascia overlying the talus and navicular and the Y-shaped inferior extensor retinaculum. The deep peroneal nerve passes through this space deep to EHL and EDL and divides into medial and lateral plantar branches proximal to the head of the talus.

The muscles of the plantar aspect of the foot can be further divided into four layers, described by their position in relation to the sole (Table 1 and Fig. 5). The muscles of the first layer all arise from the calcaneus and insert on to the proximal phalanges. They play a major role in maintaining the longitudinal arch. FDB forms four tendons that pierce the fibro-osseous tunnel beneath the metatarsals and divide into two portions, allowing the tendons of FDL to pass between them.

The muscles of the second layer control toe motion. The quadratus plantae muscle inserts on to each of the tendons of the FDL. There are four lumbricals, each a short muscle arising from the segmented tendons of FDL and inserting on to the medial aspect of the extensor hood with the interosseous muscles.

The third layer of muscles is related to the big and little toes. Flexor hallucis brevis (FHB) functions to stabilize and flex the first MTPJ. Adductor hallucis functions to flex and adduct the hallux. Flexor digiti minimi helps to stabilize the fifth toe.

The fourth layer consists of the interosseous muscles: four plantar interossei and three dorsal, named according to their function in relation to the second metatarsal. Those moving the toes toward the longitudinal axis of the second metatarsal are adductors; those moving the toes away from the axis are abductors. Two additional tendons are included in the fourth layer; those of tibialis posterior and peroneus longus.

Other soft tissue structures of the foot are the plantar fascia and heel pad. *The plantar heel pad* cushions the foot with each heel strike. It consists of U-shaped, fat-filled tissue septae which are reinforced by elastic tissue. Spirals of fibrous fascia are anchored to one another, the calcaneus, and the skin.

Plantar aponeurosis (plantar fascia; Fig. 5)

The deep fascia of the foot is thickened to form the flexor retinaculum and the plantar aponeurosis. The function of the latter is to assist in the maintenance of the arches of the foot, to give firm attachments to the skin, and to prevent damage to the underlying structures of the foot. It forms a triangular sheet that is thick centrally and thinner in its medial and lateral parts. It is attached to the medial and lateral tubercles of the calcaneus. Its base divides at the bases of the toes into five slips, each of which divides further into two bands, one passing to the skin and the other passing deeply to the toe. Here each deep band divides further into two bands that diverge around the flexor tendons and finally fuse with the fibrous flexor sheath and the deep transverse ligaments. The medial and lateral borders of the thick central aponeurosis are continuous with the thinner deep fascia covering the abductors of the big and little toes. Fibrous septa pass from these borders into the sole to create three muscle compartments for the muscles of the first plantar layer, all of which arise from the medial calcaneal process.

The connections between the calcaneus, the ligaments, and the skin allow the plantar aponeurosis to work as a *windlass mechanism* (Fig. 6). This is a stabilizing mechanism such that, when the toes are dorsiflexed as in the last part of stance just prior to toe off, the aponeurosis is pulled distally and tightens. This stabilizes the bones of the foot and, as a consequence, the foot functions as a unit.

There is continuity between the deep fascia of the foot and that surrounding the ankle and between the deep plantar fascia and the Achilles tendon.

Table 1 The muscles of the plantar aspect of the foot

Muscles[a]	Functions
Layer 1	
Abductor hallucis	Flexion, abduction big toe, braces medial arch
Flexor digitorum brevis	Flexes lateral four toes, braces both longitudinal arches
Abductor digiti minimi	Flexion, abduction fifth toe, braces lateral arch
Layer 2	
Four lumbricals (and FDL, FHL)	Toe extension at interphalangeal joints
Layer 3	
Flexor hallucis brevis	Stabilize and flex first metatarsophalangeal joint, support medial arch
Adductor hallucis	Flexion, adduction hallux
Flexor digiti minimi	Stabilises fifth toe
Layer 4	
Interossei (and peroneus longus, tibialis posterior)	Abduction, adduction of toes

[a] FDL, Flexor digitorum longus; FHL, flexor hallucis longus.

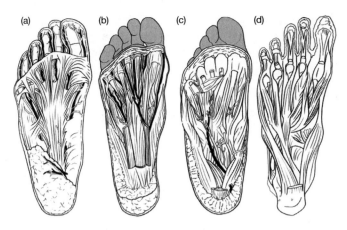

Fig. 5. The sole of the foot is composed of layers of soft tissue structures, from the thick superficial plantar aponeurosis (a); to that 1st (b), 2nd (c) and deep 3rd & 4th (d) layers of muscles. See also Table 1.

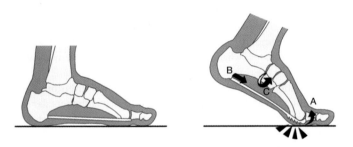

Fig. 6. The windlass mechanism. When the toes are dorsiflexed just prior to toe-off, the aponeurosis is pulled tight, stabilising the arches of the foot and allowing its many structures to work as a functional unit.

Table 2 Some intrinsic and extrinsic risk factors for the development of an overuse injury of the foot

Extrinsic factors	Intrinsic factors
Overuse (too much, too soon, too often, too intense)	Hypermobility/hypomobility
	Weakness/easy fatiguability
Equipment: inappropriate footwear	Leg length discrepancy
Surface: too hard/too soft	Leg/heel/forefoot malalignment
Technique: technical errors in running	Coexisting disease (e.g. diabetes, rheumatoid arthritis

of the foot giving off the first plantar metatarsal artery before joining with the plantar arch.

Clinical evaluation

Without treatment, even minor complaints involving the foot can lead to protracted pain due to the constant forces of weight-bearing. The foot is a common site for overuse injuries and patients frequently present at a late stage. In evaluating the individual with a foot injury, it is helpful to consider intrinsic and extrinsic risk factors (Table 2).

History

There are two principal modes of presentation of foot problems: pain and deformity. Other methods of presentation include stiffness, and instability. In clinical practice, the area of pain and the nature of any deformity help in establishing the diagnosis.

The foot is a complex arrangement of structures and initial evaluation aims to precisely localize symptoms. Referred pain must always be considered. The unilaterality or bilaterality of symptoms can be a useful clue and should raise the suspicion of referred pain from the spine—'two legs equals one back'.

Pain may occur in association with swelling, clicking, creaking, and popping. There may be symptoms in the ankle or a history of ankle injury (Chapter 6.9). The nature, intensity, and distribution of pain should all be determined (see Table 3 in Chapter 4.1). Exacerbating and relieving features, in particular the relationship of pain to activity, should be determined, since the severity of soft tissue injuries can be graded according to the timing of their pain. Nocturnal pain is suggestive of a significant soft tissue injury and neurogenic pain can signify an infective or a malignant process. Episodic burning pain radiating distally through the foot suggests a neurogenic origin.

The timing and mechanism of onset of symptoms should be ascertained to define whether the condition is acute, acute-on-chronic, or a chronic overuse injury. A history of previous local or distant injury may be relevant as the resulting alteration in gait may result in further injury (second injury syndrome). Many injuries are insidious in onset without a clear mechanism. Progression or alteration of symptoms with time should be determined.

Recording of events immediately after an acute injury can indicate the extent of the injury—ability to weight-bear, timing, site and progression of swelling, and the presence of deformity are all relevant.

Neurovascular anatomy

The sciatic nerve supplies the majority of the innervation of the foot through the tibial, common peroneal (deep and superficial branches), and sural nerves (the main sensory supply). The exception is the saphenous nerve, which arises from the femoral nerve and supplies sensory innervation to the ankle, medial malleolus, and medial border of the foot.

The S1 dermatome supplies the lateral ankle and lateral border of the foot including the fourth and fifth toes and the entire sole of the foot with the exception of the great toe (L5). L5 also supplies the medial aspect of the dorsum of the foot and the first to third toes. The medial ankle is supplied by the L4 dermatome.

Vascular supply

Arterial supply to the foot arises from branches of the popliteal artery. The posterior tibial artery divides into the medial and lateral plantar arteries after passing behind the medial malleolus. The lateral branch is larger and curves medially at the base of the fifth metatarsal to form the plantar arch. This anastomoses with the dorsalis pedis artery at the proximal end of the first intermetatarsal space, giving plantar digital arteries along its course. The medial plantar artery supplies the medial side of the big toe. The anterior tibial artery becomes the dorsalis pedis artery on the anterior aspect of the ankle, giving branches to the ankle, sinus tarsi, and the dorsum of the foot. It passes into the plantar aspect

Table 3 Associations of pes cavus (reference 3)

Neuromuscular—muscle disease

Muscular dystrophy

Neuromuscular—peripheral nerve/spinal root

Hereditary sensorimotor neuropathy type 1

Spinal dysraphism

Intraspinal tumour

Neuromuscular—anterior horn cell

Poliomyelitis

Spinal dysraphism

Diastematomyelia

Syringomyelia

Spinal cord tumours

Spinal muscular atrophy

Neuromuscular—central nervous disease

Friedrich's ataxia

Cerebellar disease

Congenital

Idiopathic

Congenital talipes equino varus

Arthrogryposis

Traumatic

Compartment syndrome sequelae

Malunion of fracture foot

Stiffness is common after an acute injury, or with chronic soft tissue complaints and degenerative articular complaints. Significant morning stiffness of 15 minutes or more is characteristic of inflammatory joint disease and the patient should be questioned about other articular and systemic symptoms in relation to this possibility. Vascular symptoms include pain, coldness, colour change, and numbness. These may be reported in patients with claudication, Raynaud's phenomenon, or arterial entrapment. Where vascular symptoms are present, the uni/bilaterality of symptoms should be determined and the presence of predisposing factors such as smoking and diabetes should be established.

Specific details of the treatment approaches used, their timing, compliance, and their effects should be obtained.

Many foot and ankle injuries are activity-related. In sporting individuals a full training history should be obtained, including the specific activities involved, the intensity, frequency, and duration of training sessions, and details of warm-up, stretching, and cool-down periods. Any change in the training pattern prior to the injury may be important. Attention should also be given to equipment used—in particular footwear. The types, use pattern, and age of footwear and use of socks should be ascertained. Use of supports, taping, insoles, and orthotics should be defined. Other aspects of the sport such as technique (e.g. in dancers) and additional activities involved should be addressed.

Occupation may play an important role in the development and persistence of symptoms. In particular, standing for long periods, significant weight-bearing activity, and the use of specific footwear should be considered. Some repetitive tasks are also common at work, such as the use of a pedal in the operation of machines. In some instances an ergonomic evaluation may be necessary.

A medical history should be established, specifically enquiring regarding diabetes mellitus, psoriasis, inflammatory arthritis, gout, poliomyelitis, and low back complaints.

Examination

Inspection: deviations and deformities of the foot and ankle

Posture

In the foot, combined, triplanar motion in several joints is often described by a single term.

Pronation of the foot involves eversion of the heel, abduction of the forefoot, medial rotation of the leg relative to the foot, and dorsiflexion of the subtalar and midtarsal joints. Greater subtalar motion is present in the pronated than in the supinated foot. The foot is naturally pronated in infancy, becoming more supinated as the arches form.

Hyperpronation during propulsion is common and can result in premature fatigue of the leg muscles since more muscle work is required to maintain stability during gait. Callus formation, plantar fasciitis, arch problems, and joint subluxations are seen. Hyperpronation can also cause strain on the medial knee structures and may also inhibit normal motion of the sacroiliac joint of the trailing leg and cause low back pain. This occurs due to the spine leaning towards the side of the trailing leg with lack of smooth transfer of weight to the leading leg. An abductory twist at toe-off may be seen in the hyperpronator, when the foot pivots on the lateral metatarsal head(s) while the rearfoot swings inward toward the midline.

Supination of the foot involves a combination of inversion of the heel, adduction at the forefoot, and plantar flexion at the subtalar and midtarsal joints. The leg is laterally rotated relative to the foot. The supinated foot is more rigid.

The relationship of the hindfoot to the forefoot

Assessment of the foot when the subtalar joint is in neutral position allows identification of structural variations. The terminology describing hindfoot–forefoot relationships is complex and confusing. In assessment of these relationships the hindfoot is evaluated first (Fig. 7).

Hindfoot valgus

This involves angulation of the calcaneus away from the midline. Heel valgus is associated with the flatfoot. The forefoot balances heel valgus by 'supinating' into forefoot varus, where the fifth ray is more plantar flexed than the first.

Hindfoot varus

The involves calcaneal angulation towards the midline, and is seen in pes cavus, or the 'cavo-varus foot'. The forefoot compensates for hindfoot varus by 'pronating' into forefoot valgus, where the first ray is more plantar flexed than the fifth. Failure to compensate leads to excessive weight-bearing on the fifth metatarsal head. These forefoot deviations can be assessed when the hindfoot is brought into neutral.

Pes cavus

Pes cavus is defined as a foot with an elevated longitudinal arch. Not only are there many causes and associations (Table 3), but the spectrum of deformity is broad. Brewerton *et al.* in their series found neurological abnormalities in 66 per cent, of which the most common abnormality was Charcot–Marie–Tooth disease, or type 1 hereditary sensorimotor neuropathy.[4] Thus careful neurological evaluation is mandatory in this group of patients.

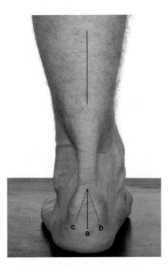

Fig. 7 Alignment of leg and heel. (a) Neutral, (b) varus, and (c) valgus.

Clinically, pes cavus presents with a varus heel, a high arch, excessive plantar flexion of the metatarsals, and clawing of the toes. The patients present with a painful foot that fatigues quickly. They may complain of lateral ankle ligament instability due to the varus heel. The claw toes can be painful and metatarsalgia (particularly under the fifth toe) is often a problem.

Pes planus (flat foot)

All infants have flat-feet up to approximately the age of 2 years, due to the presence of a fat pad and incomplete formation of the arches. In the adult there is a permanent structural deformity, leading to alterations in the tarsal bones and talonavicular joints. The medial longitudinal arch is reduced so that, on standing, its border comes into contact with the ground. The calcaneus is in valgus, whereas the forefoot is pronated. Unfortunately, the natural history of the flat-foot is unknown. However, Harris and Beath reviewed 3600 men and did not find that the lack of a medial longitudinal arch was associated with symptoms.[5]

Therefore, the majority of children, who will have a flexible and painless flat-foot, and their parents can be reassured that, whilst the foot is flat, this should not lead to symptoms in the future. Furthermore, there is little substantive evidence to show that shoe modification or orthotic treatment alters the natural history of the flatness of the foot.

There are, however, a small number of patients who require further advice, investigation, and even treatment. These patients can usually be detected clinically, and it is the patient with painful or non-flexible or asymmetrical pes planus who merits further investigation. The differential diagnosis is shown in Table 4.

The toes

Hallux valgus is a deformity of the first MTPJ, involving a valgus and rotational deviation of the hallux. The first metatarsal head becomes prominent medially.

A *bunion* is formed by the combination of a callus that develops over the medial side of the head of the metatarsal, a thickened bursa, and an exostosis.

Table 4 Differential diagnosis of the flat-foot (after reference 6)

Congenital
Asymptomatic flexible
Symptomatic flexible
Rigid associated with tarsal coalition
Accessory navicular
Congenital deformity residual (club foot, vertical talus)
Joint laxity (Ehler–Danlos, Marfan's syndrome)

Acquired
Posterior tibial tendon dysfunction
Arthritis (talonavicular, tarsometatarsal joint, rheumatoid arthritis)
Traumatic (calcaneal, midfoot, tarso-metatarsal fracture, spring ligament injury)
Charcot foot (diabetes mellitus)
Neuromuscular (poliomyelitis, cerebral palsy)
Tumour

The normal range of motion at the first MTPJ is 65–75° dorsiflexion and >20° of plantar flexion. *Hallux rigidus* is a clinical diagnosis and occurs when there is limited dorsiflexion (extension) of the big toe. It is often bilateral and can be functional (where dorsiflexion of the first MTPJ is limited only when the foot is loaded) or structural, where limitation occurs in both the loaded or unloaded foot (see below). Considerable confusion exists regarding the terminology for lesser toe deformities. The simplest is a *mallet toe*, in which there is a flexion deformity of the DIPJ. A *hammer toe* consists of a flexion contracture of the DIPJ and PIPJ. The most complex, and most common to require treatment, is a *claw toe*, which is the same as a hammer toe, but with a hyperextension deformity of the MTPJ.

Prominent areas of bone, often with overlying callus, are found at sites of irritation secondary to trauma, overuse, or pressure. An excessively prominent superior calcaneal process is known as a '*Haglund deformity*' or '*pump bump*'.

Further inspection and palpation

Observation of the patient as he or she enters the consulting room is helpful, since his or her attitude, comfort, and use of walking aid(s) is noted. Then, with the patient adequately exposed, the lower legs and feet are inspected and compared firstly on weight-bearing and then when non-weight-bearing, from the sides, front, and from behind. Leg length discrepancy and other asymmetries of the lower limbs should be noted. The presence of deformities, skin lesions, scars, callosities, swelling, bruising, and local and proximal muscle bulk are noted. The toenails should also be examined for evidence of fungal infections, psoriatic changes, traumatic lesions, etc. The position of the pelvis, spine, and trunk should also be evaluated. For example, lateral or medial rotation of the hip or trunk can elevate or flatten the medial longitudinal arch of the opposite foot.

In weight-bearing the talus is considered to be fixed and compensation for structural and functional abnormalities can be seen, which does not occur when non-weight-bearing. The posture of the foot (neutral, supinated, or pronated) should be noted.

Footprint patterns, help to demonstrate the shape of the foot and can easily be obtained by sprinkling talcum powder on the patient's moist feet and asking them to stand on some coloured paper (Fig. 8).

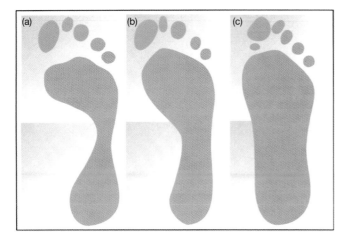

Fig. 8 Footprints: (a) Pes Cavus; (b) normal; (c) Pes Planus.

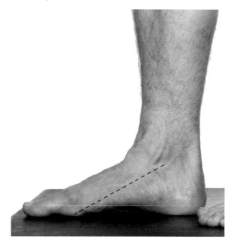

Fig. 9 The Feiss line.

The longitudinal arches are most easily seen in the medial view. The medial arch should be higher than the lateral. There are many useful methods of evaluating the arches further. The *Feiss line* is a line joining the apex of the medial malleolus and the plantar aspect of the first MTPJ, drawn when the patient is non-weight-bearing. The patient then stands and the navicular tuberosity is located, which should be on or close to the line. The patient has a first-degree flatfoot if the tuberosity falls one-third of the distance to the floor, a second-degree flat-foot if two-thirds towards the floor, and third-degree if it touches the floor (Fig. 9).

The mobility of a flat-foot can be assessed when the patient moves from a normal stance to tip toes. When performing this movement the heel should invert, the longitudinal arch should become visible, and the leg should externally rotate. Failure of this mechanism can be the result of tibialis posterior tendon dysfunction, arthritis of the mid- or hindfoot, or congenital abnormalities such as a vertical talus or a tarsal coalition. The 'too many toes' sign refers to the number of toes visible from behind the patient and represents forefoot abduction. The normal number is 1–3 toes, but the sign is particularly helpful in unilateral involvement, when the two sides should be compared.

The sole of the foot is examined for calluses, plantar fibromatosis, and also to localize any areas of tenderness. If the Achilles tendon is symptomatic it may be easier to examine the patient prone.

Evaluation of the foot when the subtalar joint is in a neutral position allows assessment of the relationship between the forefoot and hindfoot. With the knee flexed, and the leg and foot dangling over the side of the couch, the heel is aligned with the longitudinal axis of he leg. The forefoot is then taken in the other hand. The thumb is then placed over the talonavicular joint. The forefoot is then moved to find the position where this joint is reduced, or maximally covered. This is the *subtalar neutral position*. The relative positions of the fore- and hindfeet are then observed (Fig. 10).

Leg–heel alignment is assessed by placing a mark over the calcaneus in the midline at the Achilles insertion with another placed 1 cm below this. A line is drawn connecting the two. A second line connects two points on the lower leg in the midline. With the foot in subtalar neutral the relationship between the two lines is examined. A normal alignment is seen when the lines are parallel or in 2–8° of varus. Less than this indicates hindfoot varus (inversion), whilst more than this indicates hindfoot valgus (eversion) (Fig. 7).

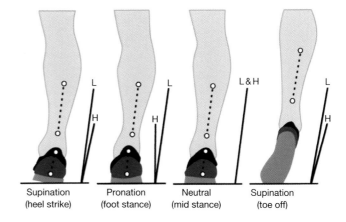

| Supination (heel strike) | Pronation (foot stance) | Neutral (mid stance) | Supination (toe off) |

Fig. 10 Changes in the leg (L) heel (H) alignment during running.

Forefoot–heel alignment is assessed with the patient supine and the feet over the edge of the table. The foot is maintained in the subtalar neutral position and the relationship between the vertical axis of the heel and the plane of the metatarsal heads is noted. Normally, the plane is perpendicular to the vertical axis. If the medial side of the foot is raised, the patient has forefoot varus and if the lateral side is raised, there is forefoot valgus.

Tibial torsion was described in Chapter 6.8. It is assessed in the sitting position with the patient's knees over the edge of the couch. The examiner visualizes the axis of the knee and the ankle. There is normally 12–18° of external rotation.

The patient remains in the supine position to allow further inspection and palpation of all aspects of the foot and ankle for sites of specific bony or soft tissue tenderness, swelling, and deformity. As a general rule it is advisable to palpate areas of least tenderness first, progressing towards more painful sites. The sinus tarsi can be palpated in the depression one fingerbreadth inferior and one fingerbreadth anterior to the lateral malleolus.

Movement

Passive, active, and resisted movements should be evaluated, observing for range of motion, reported pain, weakness, and reproduction of subluxation or dislocation of soft tissue structures, in particular the peroneal tendons. Muscles of the foot, their action, and innervation are detailed in Table 5.

Pain on resisted testing is indicative of musculotendinous pathology of one or more of the units responsible for that movement. The site of the pathology may be further defined by the notable presence of swelling within a tendon sheath or tenderness at, for example, the tendon insertion. Pain may also arise during a resisted movement due to significant intraarticular pathology. Weakness out of proportion to pain indicates rupture or a significant tear of a musculotendinous structure.

Special tests

The *single heel raise test* evaluates the posterior tibial tendon and was described in Chapter 6.9. The *first metatarsal rise sign* and the '*too many toes*' sign were also described in Chapter 6.9. Assessment of the Achilles tendon was described in Chapter 6.8.

Pain on direct compression of the calcaneum between the examiner's palms is indicative of a calcaneal stress fracture (the *calcaneal squeeze test*).

Neurovascular status should be assessed, including assessment for nerve entrapment. Percussion over the posterior tibial nerve as it travels behind the medial malleolus, and the anterior tibial branch of the deep peroneal nerve as it crosses the front of the ankle is performed. Reproduction of tingling, paraesthesia, or pain distally indicates a positive test and implies nerve entrapment or irritation. Similar percussion tests over other peripheral nerves is performed as appropriate.

Further examination of the patient during gait is vital to evaluate functional status. Gait analysis was described in the Chapter 5.8. Foot and ankle pain may be referred from more proximal structures or may be the result of altered biomechanics due to a primary condition more proximally.

Imaging

Plain radiographs

Plain radiographs may be imprecise due to subject variation in stance and weight distribution, which may alter during an examination. There are also interindividual variations in bony relationships and interobserver reliability.

In our practice we find weight-bearing views are more representative. A standing anteroposterior (AP) and lateral, with an oblique view are routinely obtained. AP views provide good views of the forefoot, midfoot, and midtarsal joint. An AP view with 15° of angulation in the sagittal plane gives better visualization of the tarso-metatarsal joints. The lateral view shows the posterior facet of the subtalar joint, the talonavicular joint, and the first metatarsal–cuneiform articulation.

Specialized views may be required in specific conditions. For example, the sesamoid view in sesamoid disease, the reversed, or medial oblique, in the presence of an accessory navicular, axial views of the calcaneus, and Broden's views of the subtalar joint.

In the paediatric patient, since many bones may not be completely ossified, computerized tomography (CT) or magnetic resonance imaging (MRI) may be needed to provide additional information to assist in the management of congenital and acquired lesions in the foot.[7]

Other imaging modalities

CT scanning and MRI are both well established in the investigation of pain in the foot. CT is primarily used for bony lesions, whilst MRI

Table 5 Lower extremity nerve function: preliminary checklist

| | Sciatic (L4–S2) | | | | | | Gluteal | | |
| | Peroneal | | Posterior tibial (L5–S2) | | | | | | |
	Deep (L4–S1)	Superficial (L5–S1)		Medial plantar (S1, S2)	Lateral plantar (S1, S2)	Femoral (L1–L3)	Obturator (L2–L4)	Superior (L4–S1)	Inferior (L5–S2)
Hip						Flexion	Adduction	Abduction, medial rotation	Extension, lateral rotation
Knee		Flexion				Extension			
Ankle/subtalar joint	Dorsiflexion	Foot eversion	Plantar flexion, foot inversion						
Toes	Extension great toe	Extensor digitorum brevis	Flexion	Toe flexion; abduction, great toe	Abduction, adduction				
Sensory	First web space, dorsum of foot	Dorsum of foot (excluding first web space)	—	Great toe	Small toe	Anterior thigh, medial calf	Medial thigh	—	—

provides significant anatomical detail for the evaluation of the osseous and soft tissue structures of the foot and ankle.[8] MR arthrography can be used for staging and detecting osteochondritis dissecans of the talus, anterolateral soft tissue impingement, and chronic lateral ankle instability.[9]

Isotope bone scanning remains the investigation of choice when a stress fracture is suspected. Dynamic ultrasonography is a quick, relatively inexpensive imaging modality that is suited for the assessment of tendons, soft tissue masses, and suspected foreign bodies.[10] Although perhaps less useful than at other sites, it has superseded isotope scanning in the imaging of proximal plantar fasciitis.

As ever, careful clinical examination with appropriate imaging is the best practice.

Lateral foot pain (Table 6)

Peroneal tendinopathies

The peroneal muscles are the primary evertors of the foot, assist in plantar flexion, and are important dynamic stabilizers of the ankle. Injuries to either of these tendons is largely a result of the degree of stress to which they are exposed in addition to the winding course that they follow. In the foot, tenosynovitis, tendinosis, longitudinal tear, rupture, and avulsion occur. These pathologies, in addition to subluxation and dislocations, can occur at the lateral ankle, as was detailed in Chapter 6.9.

Peroneal pathologies in the foot may present with clicking, palpable dislocation, pain, and swelling, which are exacerbated by walking on uneven surfaces. A history of overuse may be given or there may be a history of acute or chronic trauma, usually in the form of an inversion sprain of the ankle.

Tenosynovitis

Tenosynovitis of the peroneal tendons is associated with peroneal tendon subluxation, hypertrophy of the peroneal tubercle, or with an os peroneum. In some cases the tenosynovitis is stenosing in nature, due to the circuitous course that these tendons follow. The occasional patient has an inflammatory arthropathy. Tenosynovitis may progress on to peroneal tendon tears, which are dealt with in the next section.

The typical presentation is with pain over the peroneal tendons, worsening with exercise. Swelling, localized tenderness, and crepitus over the peroneal tendons may be present. Pain is exacerbated on passive stretch, by forced plantar flexion and inversion, and also by active

Table 6 Causes of lateral foot pain

Peroneal tendinopathy

Symptomatic os peroneum

Ankle instability

Stress fracture of fifth metatarsal

Avulsion injury at fifth metatarsal

Cuboid instability

Bunionette

Sural nerve injury

Referred pain (S1)

contraction against resistance. An antalgic gait may be noted. Differentiation between peroneus brevis and longus involvement is based upon the site of pain. The specific movements affected may also be an indicator. Pain with eversion and with restricted plantar flexion of the first ray, indicates peroneus longus involvement, whereas isolated pain with resisted eversion occurs with peroneus brevis lesions. Tenosynovitis and tears of peroneus brevis may be insertional and a stress fracture of the base of the fifth metatarsal must be excluded. Similarly, an avulsion fracture of the fifth metatarsal can occur after lateral ankle sprain.

Treatment of peroneal tenosynovitis depends on the cause, and hence the location. Peroneal tendon instability was described in Chapter 5.9. The os peroneum syndrome is dealt with below.

Generally, non-operative treatment involves relative rest non-steroidal anti-inflammatory drugs (NSAIDs), and ice. The use of a lateral heel wedge may be helpful. Exacerbating activities, such as walking on uneven surfaces or up and down ladders, are avoided. The use of local corticosteroids is inappropriate. As symptoms settle, a gradual strengthening programme of the peroneals commences.

In those with persisting symptoms a trial of a rocker bottom walking boot or even a non-weight-bearing cast is appropriate. If non-operative treatment fails, surgery should be considered. The tendons are exposed, and any constriction of the sheath released. An os peroneum or hypertrophied peroneal trochlea should be resected if it is considered to be the cause of the symptoms. Any tears in the tendons are repaired (see below).

Tears and rupture of the peroneii in the foot

Tears of the peroneal tendons may either involve the peroneus brevis, longus, or both tendons. As with tenosynovitis there are three classical (and different) clinical pictures. These pictures are anatomically distinct, and occur at the level of the lateral malleolus, at the peroneal tubercle, and os peroneum. The first group principally affects the brevis tendon, the other two the longus tendon. Obviously, some tears do not conform to any of the classical pictures, and spontaneous ruptures are described in diabetes and rheumatoid arthritis, as well as in fit athletic individuals.

Peroneal tenosynovitis around the lateral malleolus is often associated with peroneal tendon instability. Krause and Brodsky[11] reported that the most reliable clinical sign of peroneal tendon tears was swelling, and they considered chronic subluxation to be the cause of the tears in 90 per cent of their cases. Tears in this area are more thoroughly dealt with in Chapter 6.9, but more commonly involve the peroneus brevis than the longus.

Longitudinal tears of peroneus brevis can also occur in the foot at its insertion. It can be difficult to differentiate this from an insertion tendinosis. A tear should be suspected in those cases that fail to settle with conservative measures.

The peroneus longus is guided towards the cuboid by the peroneal tubercle in up to 44 per cent of individuals. An enlarged peroneal tubercle is associated with attrition of the longus tendon.

The os peroneum lies within the substance of the peroneus longus tendon, at the level of the cuboid. The os may separate or be fractured in an acute ankle sprain. The os peroneum complex can also be injured by direct trauma. This results in either tenosynovitis, a partial tear, complete rupture, or simply chronic pain at the os peroneum.

Examination frequently reveals tenderness along the course of peroneus longus distal to the fibula, pain, and weakness with resisted plantar flexion of the first ray and with active eversion. Patients may report a sensation of walking on a pebble—presumably due to malalignment of the os peroneum on the cuboid.

Plain radiographs (oblique views) may demonstrate disruption of the os peroneum. Axial CT is useful in assessing the peroneal tubercle and os peroneum—cuboid articulation. MRI, ultrasound, and bone scanning all have a role in the evaluation of disease in this area.

Management

Conservative management has little role to play in these injuries, although a trial of cast immobilization and orthotics may be attempted. Sobel *et al.* found that cast immobilization was only effective in 20 per cent of patients with chronic peroneus longus symptoms.[12] Krause and Brodsky considered the treatment of peroneus brevis tears to be primarily surgical, to address the underlying instability.[11]

Surgical treatment needs to address both the underlying pathology and the tendon tear. In the case of peroneal tendon instability the superior peroneal retinaculum is repaired. The peroneal tubercle is resected or smoothed and, if there is a symptomatic os peroneum, this is excised. If there is proliferative tenosynovium this is excised, and any constrictions in the sheath are released.

Repair of the tendon can take several forms. Krause and Brodsky recommended resection of the damaged portion if it consisted of less than 50 per cent of the tendon diameter.[11] If more than 50 per cent of the tendon is involved, in the more proximal regions a tenodesis between the longus and brevis tendons can be undertaken. In some cases the tendon is flattened out, in which case it is tubulized. In cases where the tendon has ruptured, either a direct repair or a tendon graft may be required to salvage the situation.

Following surgery a period in cast is required. Postoperatively the recovery is slow, but good to excellent in the majority of patients.

Sinus tarsi syndrome

Sinus tarsi syndrome presents with pain over the sinus tarsi, usually as a result of trauma. Most patients give a history of at least one inversion sprain, although the syndrome may occur in individuals with arthritides, pes planus, pes cavus, and chronic subtalar instability.[13] The syndrome was first described by O'Connor.[14] and is thought to be caused by scarring and impingement of the soft tissues of the sinus tarsi. There may be additional synovitis of the subtalar joint.

The patient complains of lateral ankle and/or foot pain, which is worse with walking on uneven surfaces or simply with standing. Examination reveals tenderness in the sinus tarsi. The ankle is usually not unstable. Symptoms are relieved temporarily with a local anaesthetic injection into the sinus tarsi.

Management

A local corticosteroid injection may be effective, but if this fails surgical management is indicated. O'Connor treated approximately one-third of his patients surgically with resection of the fat pad and the superficial ligamentous floor, with all patients noting that their symptoms were improved after surgery.

More recently, Frey *et al.* reported 94 per cent good and excellent results following subtalar arthroscopy and debridement.[15] Interestingly they found that following arthroscopy, the diagnosis was altered in every case. The majority of patients had interosseous ligament tears, but arthrofibrosis and subtalar degeneration were also seen.

Sural nerve entrapment

Sural nerve entrapment or injury can occur at any point along its course (Table 7). The nerve may be entrapped as it exits the deep fascia of the middle and distal thirds of the leg, at the ankle or on the dorsolateral aspect of the foot. Iatrogenic sources represent the most common cause (Figs 11 and 12).

Symptoms are dependent upon the site of entrapment, but the patient usually reports burning pain and numbness along the lateral border of the foot. Symptoms may be worse with walking and wearing boots. There is often a history of ankle instability or a sprain.

Examination may reveal a positive Tinel's sign at the site of entrapment and evidence of the underlying cause (Table 7). Relief of pain with infiltration with a small amount of local anaesthetic at the suspected site of entrapment confirms the diagnosis.

Plain radiography, ultrasound, and MRI may all assist in determining the cause of the compression and excluding other pathologies in the differential diagnosis.

Table 7 Causes of sural nerve entrapment or injury

Trauma

Macrotrauma including surgery, ankle sprain, fractures of the fifth
  metatarsal, cuboid, calcaneus, fibula

Microtrauma (overuse)

Compression

Intrinsic: by enlarged or scarred achilles or peroneal tendons, anomalous
  bands, bony ridge, enlarged peroneal tubercle, venous insufficiency,
  ganglion, neuroma, connective tissue disease.

Extrinsic: by tight stockings or boots

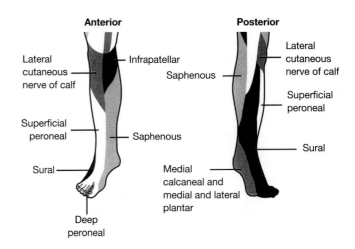

Fig. 11 Cutaneous supply of the lower leg and foot.

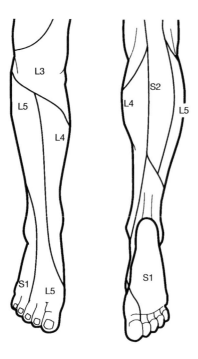

Fig. 12 Dermatomes of the lower leg and foot.

Cuboid instability

Also known as cuboid syndrome or calcaneocuboid subluxation, cuboid instability is a cause of ill-defined pain on the lateral border of the foot and lateral plantar surface beneath the cuboid. This is most commonly seen in dancers and others with a hypermobile foot. The pain may arise due to synovial impingement between the fourth and fifth metatarsal bases and the cuboid or between the cuboid and calcaneum. There is tenderness on deep palpation of the cuboid and variably of the base of the fifth metatarsal. It is important to exclude a stress fracture of the fifth metatarsal (or rarely the cuboid). Imaging studies are normal. Management involves manipulation of the cuboid, which typically resolves the pain. Orthotics with some lateral posting may be helpful, although recurrence and the need for further manipulation are common.

Central and lateral forefoot pain

FDL tendinopathies are rare and most injuries to the FDL are due to a laceration and require primary repair. However, tenosynovitis or tendinosis may be seen in dancers at two sites: under the flexor retinaculum and at level of the plantar plate. Treatment is relative rest with avoidance of exacerbating activities, local regular icing, NSAIDs, and support.

Medial foot pain (Tables 8 and 9)

Posterior tibial and flexor hallucis longus tendinopathies were described in Chapter 6.9 as common causes of posteromedial ankle pain. Typically symptoms also arise in the midfoot and, in the case of the FHL, under the hallux.

Posterior tibial tendinopathies were described in Chapter 6.9. PTT dysfunction typically causes posteromedial ankle pain, but symptoms may also be noted in the medial arch. In addition, an insertional tendinopathy of the PTT may occur.

The painful accessory navicular

An accessory navicular is a congenital variant, where the navicular tuberosity develops from a secondary centre of ossification. It is seen in 2–14 per cent of the population and can cause medial foot pain. Patients usual present in early adolescence.

If the complaint is of an asymptomatic bump, the patient can be reassured and discharged. Alternatively, the patient may present with pain, and some experience progressive flattening of the arch, due to PTT dysfunction, in which case treatment is required. Radiographs may confirm the diagnosis, although in some cases bone scanning, CT, or MRI may be necessary.

Management

Treatment is initially with a medial longitudinal arch support or a cast, relative rest, and analgesics. Progress may be slow. As pain settles a gradual strengthening regime can be commenced. In some cases this approach is not successful, and operative intervention may be considered.[16] There are two operative approaches, either simple excision of the accessory navicular or reattachment and advancement of the PTT (the Kidner procedure). The results of excision or PTT

Management

Management involves correction, where possible, of the underlying cause(s). NSAIDs, relative rest, ankle support, and massage are commonly recommended but symptoms are often resistant to simple measures. A trial of a tricyclic agent may be necessary. Surgical intervention is indicated where other measures have failed. The site of compression is identified preoperatively and the nerve is released. Any bony prominence is smoothed off.

Superficial peroneal nerve injury

Superficial peroneal nerve entrapment occurs at one of two sites. Proximally the nerve can be trapped at its origin from the common peroneal nerve at the neck of the fibula. Distal entrapment occurs where the nerve pierces the deep fascia, approximately 10 to 12 cm above the tip of the lateral malleolus, to become superficial and divide into its medial and lateral branches. Typically the superficial nerve is injured as a result of traction during an inversion sprain or due to local trauma.

The patient presents with typical symptoms of nerve compression: burning pain, numbness, tingling, and dysaesthesiae in the distribution of the nerve and its branches. There is local tenderness at the site of compression and there may be a positive Tinel's test. Of patients 60 per cent have a palpable deficit. Local nerve block is also helpful in making the diagnosis.

Peroneal strengthening exercises, NSAIDs, strapping of the ankle, and, if necessary, a local injection should be used prior to considering surgery. Surgery is performed by releasing any constriction of the nerve by the fascia. There may be muscle herniation, in which case a wider fascial release is required to free the nerve.

Table 8 Causes of medial foot pain

Posterior tibial tendinopathy
Symptomatic accessory navicular
Flexor hallucis longus tendinopathy
Tarsal tunnel syndrome
Disorder of lateral plantar nerve or its first branch
Talonavicular arthritis
Navicular stress fracture
Tarsometatarsal arthritis
First ray instability

Great toe
Turf toe
Hallux rigidus
Hallux valgus
Sesamoiditis
Toe nail problems

Table 9 Causes of pain in the sole of the foot: midfoot pain

Mid-substance plantar fasciitis
Plantar fibromatosis
FHL tendinopathy
Spring ligament injury
Peroneus longus or brevis tendinitis ± avulsion fracture of fifth
  metatarsal base
Cuboid instability
Tarsometatarsal (Lisfranc's) joint sprains
Tarsal stress fracture/fracture
Neurological: tarsal tunnel syndrome, sural nerve, common or superficial
  peroneal nerve lesions
Referred pain: root lesions

Table 10 Causes of forefoot pain

Metatarsalgia
Metatarsal stress fracture
Synovitis of the metatarsophalangeal joints
Freiberg's disease
Interdigital neuritis/neuromata
Flexor or extensor tendinopathies
Hammer toe
Turf toe
Hallux valgus
Hallux rigidus
Lesser toe deformity
Sesamoiditis
Tarsal tunnel syndrome
Referred pain

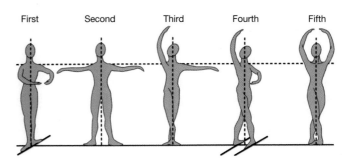

Fig. 13 The five basic positions of classical ballet.

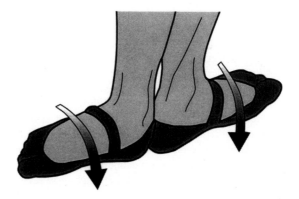

Fig. 14. Rolling in is a common error in technique that results in a number of injuries in classical dance, including those affecting the foot.

advancement are both good, with the majority of patients having good or excellent results. Theoretically, however, the Kidner procedure has the advantage of advancing the PTT, and thus reinforcing the spring ligament, and also of supporting the sagging talonavicular joint.[17]

Medial forefoot pain (Table 10)

FHL tendinopathy

FHL tendon disorders most commonly occur at the entrance to the fibro-osseous tunnel, at the level of the sustentaculum tali. This causes posteromedial ankle pain and crepitus, as described in Chapter 6.9. In the foot, FHL tenosynoviits can occur at the level of the sesamoid complex. Typically occurring in dancers, it is also seen in runners, jumpers, and spring board divers. As in the ankle, tenosynovitis is the most common form of FHL tendinopathy in the foot and may be stenosing in nature. It causes swelling, crepitus, and triggering beneath the first MTPJ. In dancers, symptoms are worse with movements on to the ball of the foot (demi-pointe) and on to the tip of the toe (pointe), by the hyperplantarflexion of the relevé.

FHL tendinopathy is associated with overuse, hard surfaces, inappropriate footwear, poor technique, and excessive turn-out at the hip so that the dancer is not centred over the feet (Figs 13 and 14). Weakness and inadequate flexibility of the other soft tissue structures of the lower leg and foot also contribute.

Examination findings include local tenderness and crepitus along the course of the tendon and at the sesamoid complex. In stenosing tenosynovitis (trigger toe), triggering may be described but difficult to localize, although a palpable nodule and the site of a sensation of popping or snapping felt by the patient may act as a guide. Symptoms are exacerbated by the movement of the hallux. There is pain with passive, active, and resisted movements of the toe.

Trigger toe, which can be mistaken for a functional hallux rigidus, is associated with an inability to extend the big toe at the metatarsal and interphalangeal joints, usually after forcible flexion of the FHL. The toe can be flexed with ease with the foot in a neutral position but, when the foot is plantar flexed, flexion at the first MTP is not possible. Release of the toe is achieved by gentle passive extension of the toe.

Tears of FHL in the foot are less common than tenosynovitis and are usually due to direct trauma, in particular a laceration.

Management

In the acute phase, FHL tenosynovitis is treated by relative rest with avoidance of exacerbating activities, local regular icing and NSAIDs, and the use of an orthotic. The underlying cause must be addressed and the patient advised that recovery may be slow.

When conservative treatment fails, surgical treatment should be considered. This consists of release of the FHL tendon through a posteromedial incision. Some authors advocate performing this surgery under local anaesthetic, so that the patient can move the toe during surgery to help determine the location of the entrapment. If the entrapment is associated with posterior impingement, this is addressed through the same incision. If the entrapment occurs in the mid- or forefoot, the tendon is released in the respective areas.

Sesamoid injuries

The sesamoid complex of the hallux works to give FHL a mechanical advantage and considerable forces are transmitted through it. Injuries to the complex are often grouped under the term 'sesamoiditis'. Although most are not soft tissue complaints, they represent an important differential diagnosis of medial forefoot pain and are thus included here.

Turf toe

The term 'turf toe' is often used to describe injuries of the first MTPJ. It was initially described by Bowers and Martin as a dorsiflexion and eversion or inversion injury to the first MTPJ, resulting in a ligamentous sprain of the sesamoid complex.[18] The name arises from the high incidence of these injuries in American football, probably as a result of the introduction of hard playing surfaces and a change in footwear from stiff-soled cleats to more flexible footwear. The condition is also seen in other sports such as soccer, basketball, and track events, along with the occasional episode in the non-sporting individual. Where an additional axial load was present at the time of injury, additional cartilaginous lesions, fractures, or diastasis of a bipartite sesamoid may be present. Sprains have been classified according to their severity (Table 11). Great toe dislocations share a similar mechanism of injury and the classification can be extended to include dislocations, although these severe injuries are beyond the scope of this text.

The patient usually presents with a clear description of the mechanism of injury, usually involving aggressive push-off and/or pivoting (Fig. 15). There is swelling and tenderness at the first MTPJ, worse with movement, particularly on extension of the joint. Stress testing, where possible, will determine the degree of the injury. Additional injuries, in particular a fracture or dislocation of the sesamoid, should be excluded by an AP X-ray, compared with the opposite side. Proximal migration of the sesamoids indicates plantar plate avulsion, confirmed by a lack of movement of the sesamoids from neutral to dorsiflexion on a stress dorsiflexion view.

Management

If plain radiographs are normal, the patient is managed conservatively, with rest in a walking boot for 3 weeks, ice massage, and NSAIDs, until the swelling subsides. Pain and swelling may take many weeks to

Table 11 Classification of turf toe (reference 19).

Grade	Description
I	Stretching of capsuloligamentous complex
II	Tear of capsuloligamentous complex
III	Tear of capsuloligamentous complex with articular injury

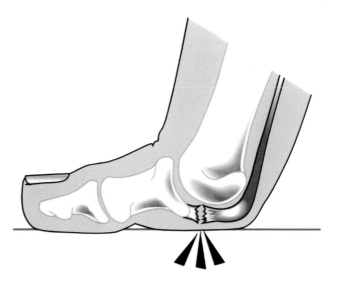

Fig. 15 Turf toe.

settle. When symptoms permit the patient may return to normal activities (including sports) with supportive taping of the hallux in slight plantar flexion and advice to wear stiff supportive shoes.

A total contact functional orthosis with a Morton's extension may be necessary long-term (Fig. 16). Surgery is indicated in those patients with a grade III sprain where there are chondral flaps or loose bodies in the joint. This surgery can be performed either open or closed. If a fracture dislocation has occurred, surgical reduction or surgical repair of the sesamoid complex is more commonly indicated.

Sesamoiditis

The aetiology of sesamoid pain can be divided into two groups. Firstly, there is a group of well characterized diseases causing pain, these include degenerate and inflammatory arthritis, infection, and prominence-causing plantar keratoses. The second group consists of diseases where there is a debate as to nomenclature and pathology. This group includes: sesamoiditis, avascular necrosis, congenital partitism, stress fracture, chondromalacia, and osteochondritis of the sesamoid. The clinical presentation of all of these conditions is identical: *pain*. As the disease progresses the surrounding structures, in particular the FHL, become inflamed and associated pain and dysfunction results. Sesamoiditis is associated with forefoot valgus, rigid pes cavus, and the existence of a multipartite sesamoid.

Plain radiographs (AP, oblique, lateral, and axial views) may be necessary to determine if the sesamoid is partite or fractured: a partite sesamoid is regular, with smooth borders and with little separation. Diastasis of a partite sesamoid can be demonstrated by a stress view with the hallux dorsiflexed. In the early stages bone scanning is often positive, even if the radiographs are normal.

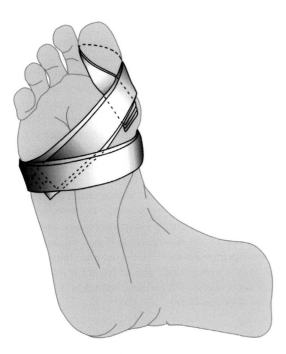

Fig. 16 Taping for turf toe.

Histological examination of sesamoiditis reveals a non-united fracture to be the underlying pathology in the majority of the cases. Avascular necrosis appears to be secondary to the fracture, rather than vice versa.

Management of sesamoiditis is relative rest with activity modification. A change in footwear to cushioned supportive shoes with lower heels, a total contact orthosis with metatarsal relief, regular ice and NSAIDs, and a 6-week period of non-weight-bearing in a cast may be necessary. Surgery is indicated if symptoms persist for longer than 6 months.

Hallux valgus

Hallux valgus causes forefoot symptoms in a number of ways, there may be pain over the 'bunion' area, pain in the second MTPJ secondary to synovitis, clawing of the lesser toes, or Morton's neuromas.

Initial treatment should concentrate on avoidance of those activities exacerbating the symptoms, anti-inflammatory medication, and shoe modification. An orthosis, to be fitted within shoes, should also be considered. A soft medial longitudinal arch support is often helpful. In the presence of lesser toe involvement, metatarsal padding may be required.

Surgical correction is successful in the majority of individuals in the general population. However, in the athlete or dancer, surgery needs to be approached with great caution. Mann has shown that, using proximal crescentic osteotomy, the satisfaction rate was 93 per cent. But postoperatively the range of dorsiflexion was only 55°, only 59 per cent could wear any shoe that they desired, and only 39 per cent believed that they could perform more activities on their feet than they could preoperatively.[16] In our opinion it is sensible to delay hallux valgus corrective surgery until the symptoms begin to threaten the individual's level of performance in sport, or dance.

There are over 100 described procedures for hallux valgus. Discussion of the merits of the individual procedures is beyond the scope of this text.

Table 12 Causes of pain in the sole of the foot: plantar heel pain

Proximal plantar fasciitis

Plantar fascial rupture

Heel bruise syndrome

Heel pad atrophy

Plantar fibromatosis

Nerve lesion

    Tarsal tunnel syndrome

    Disorder of lateral plantar nerve or its first branch (Entrapment/ irritation/neuroma)

    Postoperative neuroma of medial calcaneal sensory nerves

Calcaneal stress fracture

Tumour

Medial calacaneal nerve entrapment

Table 13 Causes of posterior heel pain

Achilles tendinopathies

Retro-achilles bursitis

Retrocalcaneal bursitis

Posterior impingement

Referred pain

Pain related to Haglund deformity

Bony injuries: talar dome, os trigonum, and calcaneal fractures/stress fractures

Plantar heel pain

The causes of plantar heel pain (Table 12) are diverse and differentiation between the individual causes is difficult. A thorough medical history and clinical evaluation is necessary to identify the specific condition involved. The specific site of the pain and its characteristics help to narrow down the diagnostic possibilities. The causes of posterior heel pain are given in Table 13.

Proximal plantar fasciitis

Aetiology

During the gait cycle, the MTPJs dorsiflex and the windlass mechanism of the plantar fascia tightens and raises the longitudinal arch. Repetitive traction can occur at the insertion of the plantar fascia, leading to microtears at the insertion. Biopsy studies have indicated that these microtears, which may have an inflammatory component in the early stages, progress to show degenerate changes later. Traction at the insertion of the FDB muscle leads to the formation of calcaneal spurs over time. 'Spurs' are seen in 50 per cent of patients with plantar fasciitis. Such spurs are therefore not the cause but are the effect of the same mechanism that can lead to plantar fasciitis. Spurs are also seen in 16 per cent of the asymptomatic population. Only 10 per cent of individuals with spurs have plantar heel pain.

Proximal plantar fasciitis is especially common in the fifth decade and in those who are overweight. Females are twice as commonly affected as males. Other aetiological features may be identified, including prolonged standing or walking (hence 'policeman's heel'), overuse, a recent increase in activity and/or footwear, direct trauma, or as part of a seronegative arthropathy.

History and examination

The history is of acute or chronic plantar heel pain. Start-up pain is typical, due to tightening of the plantar fascia with rest, particularly overnight. The pain is also worse with prolonged standing and towards the end of the day. Radiation and neuritic pain are unusual.

Examination reveals point tenderness at the medial calcaneal tuberosity, with less marked tenderness 1–2 cm distally. Swelling is absent. Pain on passive dorsiflexion of the toes may be present if the plantar fascia is particularly tight, although this is uncommon. Associated gastrocnemus-soleus tightness should be examined for, as this can slow response to treatment. It is important to consider associations such as seronegative arthritis and other causes of plantar heel pain (Table 13).

The diagnosis is made on the clinical features and further imaging is usually not necessary. Routine X-rays are not warranted. A delayed techetium-99 bone scan will show localized uptake at medial calcaneal insertion (compared with the diffuse uptake shown with a calcaneal stress fracture). MRI will show thickening and signal alterations at the plantar fascial origin.[20] Typical findings on ultrasonography are an increased thickness loss of distinction and reduced echogenicity of the plantar fascia.[21]

Management

Most patients settle with non-operative management, but progress may be slow. The cause must be addressed and weight loss and modification of activity levels are usually necessary. In the sports person, reducing training volume, in particular the intensity of exercise, and reducing high impact through running on softer surfaces and resorting to swimming and cycling are beneficial. Care must be taken to avoid a compensatory injury through alteration of gait due to pain.

The use of anti-inflammatory approaches including NSAIDs and regular ice massage are recommended but of variable benefit. Provision of supportive, cushioned footwear, heel inserts, and in some cases orthoses may all provide symptomatic benefit. Dorsiflexion night splints can help to prevent excessive tightening of the plantar fascia overnight. Stretching of the plantar fascia and calf muscles and a programme of strengthening for the intrinsic muscles of the foot should be commenced early.

In chronic resistant cases where the above measures over 8–12 weeks have not been effective and where rehabilitation is inhibited by pain, then a local corticosteroid injection is indicated. Care must be taken to inject deep, close to the medial calcaneal tuberosity, avoiding damage to the heel pad. Injudicious placement of injection, use of long-acting preparations, and multiple injection can all lead to fat pad atrophy.

In resistant cases, a course of treatment with extracorporeal shock wave therapy (ESWT) may help to reduce symptoms. There is little evidence for benefit from the use of other modalities such as conventional therapeutic ultrasound, phonophoresis, iontophoresis, and laser, both in early and late plantar fasciitis.[22] As a final resort before considering surgery, a period of cast immobilization for 3–6 weeks may be attempted.

Surgery

Approximately 95 per cent of patients resolve their plantar fasciitis after a period of 12–18 months without operative treatment.[22, 23] This leaves a small number of patients with recalcitrant but significant symptoms. Many surgical procedures are described. These range from percutaneous release, to endoscopic release, to open procedures. The structures that are treated surgically include release of the plantar fascia, excision of the calcaneal 'spur', release of the first branch of the lateral plantar nerve to abductor digiti quinti minimi (Baxter's nerve), and release of the tarsal tunnel. As entrapment of Baxter's nerve is difficult to diagnose clinically, and is said to cause heel pain in 20 per cent of cases,[24] we prefer to perform a partial plantar fascial release and release of Baxter's nerve using an open technique. The reported success rate of such an approach is that 76 per cent of patients have only mild or no pain postoperatively. However, only 49 per cent of patients are totally satisfied with the outcome.[25] However, when the degree of disability of the patient with resistant plantar fasciitis is considered, complete plantar fascia release, and proximal, as well as distal tarsal tunnel release may all be considered.

Plantar fascial rupture

Acute plantar fascial rupture is a relatively rare condition, presenting with the acute onset of proximal heel pain and, in some cases, more diffuse symptoms in the lateral or medial midfoot. The mechanism of injury may be by acute hyperextension of the midfoot as a result of the foot becoming jammed in a pothole when walking or running. More commonly, however, there is no specific incident involved. Plantar fascial rupture may occur after a steroid injection for plantar fasciitis. Typically the patient notices an improvement after injection and then a sudden return of pain, which may be of a different nature to that of their original complaint.

On examination there is often local bruising, tenderness at the medial calcaneal tubercle, and a palpable defect. The fascia may be tender more distally and there is diminished tension in the plantar fascia with windlass stretch testing.

Management involves the use of NSAIDs and regular ice, supportive shoes with a medial longitudinal arch support, and, if necessary, a non-weight-bearing cast for 4–8 weeks. Symptoms usually resolve over the course of 6–8 weeks,[26] although recovery time can be significantly longer in those who have ruptured after a steroid injection.[27]

Heel fat pad pain

Pain may arise directly from the fat pad in a number of circumstances.

Heel fat pad atrophy

This typically occurs in the elderly patient, particularly if overweight, who reports heel pain when walking on hard surfaces or wearing hard shoes. Unlike other causes of heel pain the overlying skin may be inflamed. The fat pad is thin and prominent calcaneal tubercles are easily palpable. Maximal tenderness is located in the central weight-bearing portion of pad.

Management includes the use of analgesics, including NSAIDs and ice, particularly after activity. Heel cups are usually more useful than in proximal plantar fasciitis. A shock-absorbing insert may also be beneficial and a slight heel elevation may help through shifting the weight anteriorly. High impact activities should be avoided and the obese patient should be instructed to lose weight. There is no place for the use of corticosteroids or surgical intervention.

Painful heel fat pad syndrome

This can also occur in patients without obvious fat pad atrophy, typically in the obese or after high impact. With the exception of thinning of the pad, the clinical features and management are similar to those with fat pad atrophy.

Piezogenic papules

Piezogenic papules may also cause heel pain. These present as white, subcutaneous papules, which form with the coalescence of the fat chambers, associated with degenerative changes in the dermis of the heel pad. The papules develop and appear with weight-bearing. In the majority of cases they are painless, and the patient can be reassured. In rare cases they become painful. It is not clear why they are painful, although it has been suggested that herniation of subcutaneous fat through defects in the dermis may lead to areas of ischaemia. Management is symptomatic—a heel cup or orthosis may be effective.

Separation of the heel fat pad

Separation of the heel fat pad from its anchor on the plantar aspect of the calcaneus can occur after significant trauma to the region. A cyst forms between the calcaneus and the fat pad—the pad becomes painful and is freely mobile. MRI scanning is diagnostic. Treatment involves aspiration of the cyst and then immobilization in a non-weight-bearing cast. On occasion surgical resection of the cyst and several millimetres of calcaneus is required. Postoperatively a firm dressing is applied. The aim of surgery is to allow the heel pad to reattach.

Nerve entrapment

Proximal or distal tarsal tunnel syndrome

Proximal or distal tarsal tunnel syndrome (entrapment of the first branch of the lateral plantar nerve) may cause intractable heel pain or more diffuse symptoms as described above. Entrapment or irritation of the *first branch of the lateral plantar nerve* is a commonly cited cause of heel pain. The nerve is typically trapped by a well-developed abductor hallucis and is said to be a factor in 20 per cent of cases of heel pain.[28] It is particularly common in those athletes whose sport involves substantial activity on their toes, such as sprinters, dancers, figure skaters, and gymnasts.

The nerve is also vulnerable at the medial calcaneal tuberosity. Local inflammation, swelling, fibrosis, and spur formation in and around the FDB brevis muscle can lead to compression of the nerve against the long plantar ligament. It is therefore possible that proximal plantar fasciitis can lead to nerve entrapment.

The diagnosis is clinical. Symptoms are those of burning or sharp pain in the heel, which may radiate distally into the lateral foot. Pain is noted particularly after prolonged weight-bearing and towards the end of the day, in comparison to the typical morning start-up pain of proximal plantar fasciitis. Tenderness is maximal where the nerve is compressed between the deep taut fascia of abductor hallucis muscle and the medial caudal margin of the quadratus plantae muscle. As described above there may also be features suggestive of proximal plantar fasciitis. Although weakness of abductor digiti minimi is reported, this muscle is not present in all individuals and is therefore

not a helpful clinical sign. There is no sensory deficit and paraesthesiae with palpation or percussion is a rare feature.

With the refinement of electrodiagnostic techniques, detection of isolated entrapment of nerves such as the lateral plantar nerve and its branches is possible. Nerve conduction velocities are diminished and there may be prolonged distal motor latencies.

Management is fortunately similar to that of proximal plantar fasciitis and most cases will settle with such conservative measures. Hyperpronators often benefit from a medial longitudinal arch support. A tricyclic agent such as amitryptiline can be effective in symptom control. The surgical approach is discussed fully under the section dealing with proximal plantar fasciitis.

Medial calcaneal nerve entrapment

Injury or entrapment of the medial calcaneal nerve, a sensory nerve, can result in burning, stabbing, itching, or tingling around the medial plantar heel, particularly after a period of weight-bearing. Causes include trauma, including that after injection and surgery for proximal plantar fasciitis, a congenital accessory abductor hallucis muscle, overuse, hyperpronation, and compression by local lesions such as a rheumatoid nodule.

Electrodiagnostic studies may be helpful in demonstrating delayed conduction velocity through the nerve.

Management is similar to that used for proximal plantar fasciitis and lateral plantar nerve entrapment. The underlying cause(s) are addressed. In the acute phase, a trial of a NSAIDs and strapping to support the plantar aponeurosis is recommended. Stretching of the gastrocnemius–soleus complex and plantar fascia, control of hyperpronation by the use of orthoses and/or a tricyclic agent may be necessary. Surgical intervention is reported as being successful in the resistant case.[29]

Other causes of plantar heel pain must always be considered. A *glomus tumour* is occasionally found in the heel and is exquisitely painful. Management is surgical removal. *Calcaneal injuries*, in particular stress fractures, are part of the differential diagnosis, particularly in the runner. A positive calcaneal squeeze test is an indication to obtain an isotope bone scan or (in those with chronic symptoms) a plain radiograph.

Arch pain

Distal plantar fasciitis

Distal plantar fasciitis is rare in comparison to proximal plantar fasciitis, but is still a significant source of foot pain. It presents with pain located in the midportion of the plantar fascia, usually of gradual onset. It particularly occurs in individuals with pes planus or pes cavus, as more stress is transmitted through the midportion of the plantar fascia. It is also seen in sprinters and middle distance runners who run on their toes.

The main differential diagnoses are FHL tenosynovitis and plantar fibromatosis, but careful palpation of the structures involved and resisted testing of FHL will help to differentiate between the conditions.

Distal plantar fasciitis is often more resistant to treatment than is the proximal condition. Management involves the standard strategy of pain relief (simple analgesics and/or NSAIDs), relative rest, activity modification, appropriate footwear, and regular ice massage.

Stretching of the plantar fascia and calf muscles is recommended, although the plantar fascia itself is usually not as tight as those with proximal plantar fasciitis. Although a medial longitudinal arch support is usually not tolerated as it irritates the affected tissue, a medial heel wedge may be useful. Circumferential taping of the midfoot using 1 inch tape over a non-adhesive elastic wrap may be tolerated and provides short-term relief. The patient can be taught to apply the taping themselves.

Surgery is occasionally indicated in those patients who do not settle with non-operative treatment, and in this case a simple partial plantar fascial release is undertaken.

Plantar fibromatosis

Plantar fibromatosis is a common benign condition of unknown origin, in which there is nodular proliferation of the medial border of the plantar fascia. Patients present with painful nodules on the plantar aspect of the foot during weight-bearing. The nodules are usually located on the medial side, just proximal to the first MTPJ. Nodules are usually multiple and less than 2 cm in diameter. Management is symptomatic and reassurance is given. Surgical resection is required in rare instances. In those cases requiring surgery an aggressive approach is recommended.[29] Aluisio et al. found that subtotal fasciectomy, as opposed to local excision, or wide local excision, led to a lower incidence of recurrence.[30] With such a surgical approach 86 per cent of patients are satisfied.[29, 30]

Isolated entrapment of the medial plantar nerve can also occur at the navicular tuberosity and lead to symptoms mimicking distal plantar fasciitis.

References

1. Sarrafian, S.K. (1983). *Anatomy of the foot and ankle*, 2nd edn, pp. 52–53. J.B. Lippincott, Philadelphia.
2. Sobel, M., Levy, M., and Bohne, W. (1990). Congenital variations of the peroneus quartus muscle, an anatomic study. *Foot Ankle* **11**, 81–89.
3. Ibrahim, K. (1990). Pes cavus. In Evarts CM (ed). *Surgery of the musculoskeletal system*, 2nd edn (ed. C.M. Evants). Churchill Livingstone, New York.
4. Brewerton, D.A., Sandifer, P.H., and Sweetnam, D.R. (1963). Idiopathic pes cavus: an investigation into its aetiology. *Br. Med. J.* **2**, 659.
5. Harris, R.I. and Beath, T. (1947). Army foot survey: an investigation of the foot ailments of Canadian soldiers. *Ottawa Nat. Res. Council* **1**, 52.
6. Mann, R.A., Rudicel, S., and Graves, S.C. (1992). Hallux valgus repair utilizing a distal soft tissue procedure, and proximal metatarsal osteotomy: a long term follow up. *J. Bone Joint Surg.* **74**, 124–129.
7. Harty, M.P. (2001). Imaging of pediatric foot disorders. *Radiol. Clin. N. Am.* **39** (4), 733–748.
8. Timins, M.E. (2000). MR imaging of the foot and ankle. *Foot Ankle Clin.* **5** (1), 83–101.
9. Trnka, H.J., Ivanic, G., and Trattnig, S. (2000). Arthrography of the foot and ankle. Ankle and subtalar joint. *Foot Ankle Clin.* **5**, 49–62.
10. Erickson, S.J. (2000). Sonography of the foot and ankle. *Foot Ankle Clin.* **5**, 29–48.
11. Krause, J.O. and Brodsky, J.W. (1998). Peroneal tendon tears: pathophysiology, surgical reconstruction and clinical results. *Foot Ankle Int.* **19**, 271–279.
12. Sobel, M., Pavlov, H., Geppert, M., *et al.* (1994). Painful os peroneum syndrome: a spectrum of conditions responsible for lateral foot pain. *Foot Ankle* **15**, 112–124.
13. Taillard, W., Meyer, J.M., Garcia, J., and Blanc, Y. (1981). The sinus tarsi syndrome. *Int. Orthop.* **5**, 117–130.
14. O'Connor, D. (1958). Sinus tarsi syndrome: a clinical entity. *J. Bone Joint Surg.* **40A**, 720.
15. Frey, C., Feder, K.S., and DiGiovanni, C. (1991). Arthroscopic evaluation of the subtalar joint: does sinus tarsi syndrome exist? *Foot Ankle Int.* **20**, 185–191.
16. Grogan, D., Gasser, S., and Ogden, J. (1989). The painful accessory navicular: a clinical and histopathological study. *Foot Ankle* **10**, 164–169.
17. Chater, E.H. (1962). Foot pain and the accessory navicular *Irish J. Med. Sci.* 442–471.
18. Bowers, K.D. and Martin, R.B. (1976). Turf toe: a shoe-surface related football injury. *Med. Sci. Sports Exerc.* **8**, 81.
19. Trevino, S.G. (2000). Disorders of the hallucal sesamoids. In *Foot and ankle disorders* (ed. M.S. Myerson), p. 384. W.B. Saunders, Philadelphia.
20. Berkowitz, J.F., Kier, R., and Rudicel, S. (1991). Plantar fasciitis: MR imaging. *Radiology* **179**, 665–667.
21. Kane, D., Greaney, T., Shanahan, M., Duffy, G., Bresnihan, B. *et al.* (2001). The role of ultrasonography in the diagnosis and management of idiopathic plantar fasciitis. *Rheumatology* **40**, 1002–1008.
22. Crawford, F. (2001). Plantar heel pain (including plantar fasciitis). *Clin. Evidence* **6**, 918–926.
23. Sammaro, G.J. and Helfrey, R.B. (1996). Surgical treatment of recalcitrant plantar fasciitis. *Foot Ankle Int.* **17**, 520–526.
24. Baxter, D.E. and Pfeffer, G.B. (1992). Treatment of chronic heel pain by surgical release of the first branch of the lateral plantar nerve. *Clin. Orthop.* **279**, 229–236.
25. Davies, M.S., Weiss, G.A., and Saxby, T.S. (1999). Plantar fasciitis: How successful is surgical intervention? *Foot Ankle Int.* **20**, 803–807.
26. Ahstrom, J.P. Jr. (1988). Spontaneous rupture of the plantarfascia. *Am. J. Sports Med.* **16**, 306–307.
27. Acevado, J.I. and Beskin, J.L. (1998). Complications of plantar fascial rupture associated with steroid injection. *Foot Ankle Int.* **19**, 91–97.
28. Henricson, A.S. and Westlin, N.E. (1984). Chronic calcaneal pain in athletes: entrapment of the calcaneal nerve? *Am. J. Sports Med.* **12** (2), 152–154.
29. Sammarco, G.J. and Mangone, P.G. (2000). Classification and treatment of plantar fibromatosis. *Foot Ankle Int.* **21**, 563–569.
30. Aluisio, F.V., Mair, S.D., and Hall, R.L. (1996). Plantar fibromatosis: treatment of primary and recurrent lesions and factors associated with recurrence. *Foot Ankle Int.* **17**, 672–678.

6.11 Fibromyalgia and myofascial pain and chronic fatigue syndromes

Donncha O'Gradaigh and Brian Hazleman

Introduction

Patients with these conditions have diffuse symptoms and a paucity of clinical signs. Their presentations vary considerably, though common factors identify distinct patterns. Despite a number of theories to explain the disorders, management remains largely empirical, comprising physical, medical, and alternative approaches. Opponents of these terms argue that such labelling of 'non-diseases' legitimizes patients' illness behaviour, creating a population of 'worried well' with the attendant adverse social and psychological consequences observed with the Australian experience of the diagnosis 'repetitive strain injury'. The counterargument is that a positive diagnosis (e.g. fibromyalgia) relieves the anxiety and frustration of many years of unhelpful investigations and treatment (the average duration of symptoms before diagnosis of fibromyalgia is 5 years). This also provides the basis to recommend positive coping strategies, activity rather than inactivity, work modification rather than cessation. The absence of an accepted pathogenesis or of physical and laboratory abnormalities does not negate the considerable physical and emotional suffering of these patients, and the entities described here are useful descriptors that facilitate patient understanding and provide a framework for a constructive approach to improving the patients' well-being.

Historical perspective

Over 250 years ago, an illness characterized by 'listlessness, great lassitude and weariness all over the body... [and] little flying pains' was described by Sir Richard Manningham as the 'febricula' (little fever). An association with life stresses and preponderance in women of the upper classes was noted. Beard recorded a similar description in 1869 in the absence of fever and coined the term 'neurasthenia'. In 1841, Valleix described tender points at widespread anatomically discrete points, and called this 'fibrositis'. A number of apparent epidemics of neurasthenic symptoms were reported throughout the late eighteenth and nineteenth centuries, resulting in numerous eponyms and synonymous terms. A conference in 1978 to address 'epidemic neuromyasthenia' and its related conditions led to the term myalgic encephalomyelitis. In the 1950s, a distinction was noted between those with diffuse muscular aching and a group with triggering of painful muscular spasms on palpation. Simons and Travell described this as a myofascial pain syndrome. In the past decade, two consensus conferences have led to the definitions of fibromyalgia and chronic fatigue syndrome below.

Definitions

Under the auspices of the American College of Rheumatology, a group of experts with a particular interest in the symptom complex variously described as fibrositis, interstitial myofibrosis etc. agreed a two-step classification (Table 1) and adopted the term fibromyalgia (FM).[1] These criteria were primarily devised for epidemiological and other research purposes, but have come to be used in clinical practice as a diagnostic classification. A 3-month history of widespread pain is required, involving left and right sides of the body at sites above and below the waist, and including axial locations. A physical examination is then carried out to identify tenderness at the points illustrated in Fig. 1. Criticism of these criteria has centred on the reproducibility of such tenderness and variation in the degree of pressure applied. However, following a training period, its proponents have demonstrated a high level of within- and between-examiner reproducibility. As a rough guide, the points are palpated with the thumb with sufficient pressure applied to blanch the distal portion of the thumbnail.

Chronic fatigue syndrome (CFS) replaces 'post-viral' and 'post Epstein–Barr virus' fatigue syndromes, and is the preferred term to describe myalgic encephalomyelitis and the synonyms that preceded it (such as Royal Free Disease, Iceland Disease, and the somewhat cynical 'yuppie flu'). Criteria have been proposed by the Centers for Disease Control and Prevention (Table 2).[2] It is important to reiterate that these criteria formally require the exclusion, on history, examination, and laboratory investigation, of possible alternative explanations for these symptoms. In contrast, fibromyalgia does not

Table 1 The 1990 American College of Rheumatology criteria for the classification of fibromyalgia[1]

1. History of widespread pain, present in all of the following sites:

   left and right sides of the body; above and below the waist; axial pain

   and

2. The presence of pain in 11 of the following 18 bilateral tender points on digital palpation (approximate force of 4 kg; must elicit the subjective sensation of pain):

   occiput (insertion of suboccipital muscles)

   lower cervical (anterior aspects of intertransverse spaces C_{5-7})

   midpoint of upper border of trapezius

   origin of supraspinatus (above and near medial border of spine of scapula)

   second chostochondral junctions

   2 cm distal to lateral epicondyles (elbow)

   upper outer quadrant of gluteal muscles (buttock), in anterior fold of muscle

   posterior to the prominence of the greater trochanter

   medial fat pad of knee (proximal to joint line)

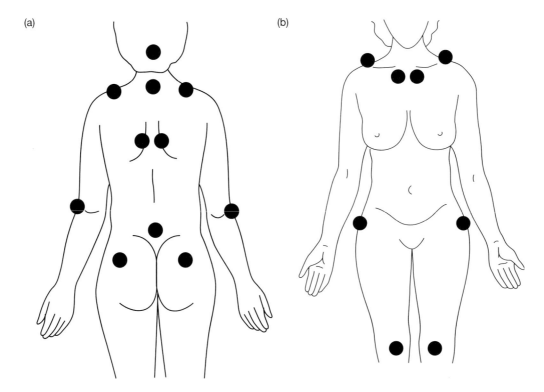

Fig. 1 (a and b) The tender points of fibromylagia.

Table 2 Centers for Disease Control and Prevention (revised) definition of chronic fatigue syndrome[2]

Chronic fatigue syndrome

(a) Clinically evaluated[a] and unexplained, persistent or relapsing fatigue of at least 6 months duration, that is

    of new/definite onset (i.e. not lifelong)

    not the result of ongoing exertion

    is not substantially relieved by rest

    results in substantial reduction in previous levels of occupational, educational, social, or personal activities

and

(b) Four or more of the following symptoms concurrently present for more than 6 months:

    impaired memory or concentration

    sore throat

    tender cervical or axillary lymph nodes

    muscle pain

    multiple joint pain

    new headaches

    unrefreshing sleep

    post-exertion malaise

Idiopathic fatigue syndrome—fatigue of at least 6 months duration that does not meet the definition (above) of chronic fatigue syndrome

[a] See text for recommended minimum clinical evaluation of fatigue.

require such exclusion, and can coexist with other conditions (see detailed discussion below). While the cause of CFS is unknown (i.e. 'idiopathic'), the term 'idiopathic chronic fatigue' has confusingly been reserved for those with unexplained fatigue that does not fulfil the criteria in Table 2.

Myofascial pain syndrome (MPS) has not been the subject of such detailed criteria or classification. Two characteristic features help distinguish it from similar presentations. MPS symptoms are typically regional, for example, involving the neck, shoulder, and upper arm on one side. The second characteristic is the presence of a myofascial trigger point. This is a hyperirritable point associated with a hypersensitive nodule in a taut band of skeletal muscle. The point is painful on compression and can give rise to referred pain, tenderness, and motor dysfunction (such as an involuntary muscular twitch). The patterns of pain referral do not conform to dermatomal distributions (such as trigeminal neuralgia) or to an extrasegmental pattern (as in sciatica). Table 3 lists some of the atypical referral patterns noted.[3]

There are similarities between some of these presentations and chronic upper limb pain described elsewhere. These include a predominance among women (at least for FM and CFS), overlap in the theories of pathogenesis, and similar management strategies. This range of conditions might more accurately be considered as a spectrum of possible presentations among a susceptible group of individuals.[4]

Epidemiology

FM is the most common generalized soft tissue diagnosis in rheumatology clinics.[5] In a population survey in the United States, about

Table 3 Location of referred pain associated with common trigger points in myofascial pain syndrome (adapted from reference 3)

Muscle	Referred pain	Associated features
Upper trapezius	Back of neck, temporal region	—
Sternal head of sterno cleidomastoid (SCM)	Occiput, cheek, periorbital	May mimic sinus pain
Clavicular head of SCM	Across forehead, in/behind ear	—
Temporalis, masseter	Teeth, jaw	—
Serratus anterior	Side of chest, border of scapula	Shortness of breath
Levator scapulae	Base of neck	Anxiety/depression may follow whiplash
Supraspinatus	Middle deltoid to elbow	Mimics cervical radiculopathy
Infraspinatus	Shoulder joint, upper arm	Mimics cervical radiculopathy
Quatratus lumborum	Lower back	—
Quadriceps	Kneecap, anterior thigh	—
Gastrocnemius	Over calf to instep	—
Soleus	Heel, ipsilateral sacroiliac joint	—

2 per cent of the general population had fibromyalgia, ranging from 0.5 per cent among males to 3.4 per cent in females. The incidence increased with age from 1 per cent in 18–29-year-old women to a peak of 7 per cent among women 60–79 years of age. Figures from Dutch and Norwegian studies are comparable. Such studies include those with fibromyalgic symptoms superimposed upon another conditions, of which systemic lupus erythematosus (10–40% having both diagnoses) and osteoarthritis (10–30%) are the most common. Children are also affected by FM. An incidence of 1.2 per cent was recorded in Mexico and 1.3 per cent were affected in a Finnish case-finding study. However, an Israeli study reported a much higher incidence of 6 per cent. Veterans of the First Gulf War appear disproportionately affected—in one cohort, 65 per cent reported widespread pain and fatigue, and one in three were diagnosed with FM. (Of interest, one of the 'epidemics' of neuromyasthenia concerned a military barracks in Switzerland in 1939.)

Fatigue is a common complaint in the population, affecting 2 per cent of those attending primary care physicians. Only one in ten of these fulfilled the diagnostic criteria for CFS. A lower incidence (1/1000) was found in a survey by Irish general practitioners, but a study of nurses reported a ten-fold higher frequency (1088 cases in 100,000). The incidence is higher in lower income groups, and the male:female ratio is 2:1.

Myofascial pain most commonly occurs among people with other painful conditions, such as osteoarthritis or cervical spondylosis. In one such group, 31 per cent had characteristic trigger points. Temporomandibular MPS occurred in 42 per cent of a group with CFS and/or FM. Of patients referred to a dental clinic for chronic head and neck pain, 55 per cent had active myofascial trigger points accounting for their pain.[6] Women present more frequently with MPS, though it has not been established whether the incidence of MPS is in fact any higher than in men. All ages are affected, but most present in the middle years (30–60 years of age).

Fibromyalgia

Clinical features

Fatigue and widespread pain are the dominant features of fibromyalgia. Sleep is commonly disturbed, the patient feeling exhausted on waking. Early morning stiffness is also commonly described (over 75 per cent in one study). A subjective sensation of joint swelling is often reported, but the distinction from inflammatory joint disease is straightforward as there are no objective signs of inflammation. Nondermatomal paraesthesiae and Raynaud's-like symptoms (rarely accompanied by the colour changes of true Raynaud's phenomenon) also occur. FM is 'associated' (i.e. occurs in the same group of the population) with irritable bowel syndrome, headaches (including typical migraine), and the female urethral syndrome.

In one study, males appeared to have more pain, fatigue, and stiffness than women matched for age and educational standard. A higher proportion of men also reported sleep disturbance and irritable bowel symptoms, but paraesthesia and headache were less frequent. Using a dolorimeter, women experienced more pain on palpation of tender points.

While the positions in Fig. 1 are the standard points palpated to confirm a diagnosis of FM, tenderness is frequently more widespread ('control points' tender in 63 per cent of cases). This should not exclude the diagnosis of FM if this impression is otherwise appropriate. Patients may also describe pain on palpation at sites that were not included in their history. Typically, the patient will continue to report pain long after the examination has been completed.

A characteristic feature of FM in both men and women is the severe disability reported. In one study, 31 per cent reported themselves 'totally disabled', and 26 per cent received partial or total disability compensation. Psychological and cognitive function may be impaired in FM, and most report significant stressors in the period preceding their symptoms. In the absence of abnormal physical findings, this has led some critics to consider FM a somatization disorder in people with a psychologically inappropriate response to stress. However, as discussed later, stress is also associated with physiological responses that some believe to be pathogenic.

The symptoms experienced by children are broadly similar. Psychological stresses are frequent before the onset of symptoms, particularly in adolescents. Sleep disturbance is less common than in adults, and the mean number of tender points over a series of visits is typically less than in adults. Some have suggested, therefore, that the classification criteria (requiring 11/18 tender points) should be modified for children.

The prognosis in typical FM is guarded. In a specialist clinic in the United States, 57 per cent of adults reported their condition as 'poor' or 'fair' after 5 years. However, continued attendance at a specialist clinic is likely to have a selection bias towards those with more intractable disease (and might even result in a poorer outcome). In a more representative population, 36 per cent reported resolution of symptoms after 2 years. Greater severity and duration of symptoms before first intervention are the most significant predictors of a poor outcome. The prognosis in children is considerably better. For example, only 25 per cent remained symptomatic at 1-year follow-up in the Finnish study. Relapse is rare in those who recover.

Pathogenesis

The cause of FM is unknown. Initially, fibrous bands were noted on muscle biopsy, leading to the term fibrositis. A fibrosing process is now in doubt, though reference to it remains in the term FM. Current concepts focus on the importance of changes in sleep pattern, on neuropeptides, and on the hypothalamic–pituitary–adrenal axis.

Muscle changes

Findings have included ragged red fibres (normally associated with mitochondrial myopathies) and hypoxic changes. Compared with normal controls, a statistically significant difference was not found. Others reported band-like structures around glycerinated muscle fibres (the so-called 'rubber-band' morphology). Reduced high-energy phosphates have been inconsistently reported by ^{31}P magnetic resonance imaging. Olsen and Park[7] proposed a capillary endothelial lesion resulting in muscle ischaemia and membrane damage with consequent fluxes of potassium and calcium further impairing muscle activity and stimulating pain pathways. These changes are not specific to FM, and it is unclear whether they are causative or the result of disuse.

Sleep disturbances

Normal sleep cycles between rapid-eye-movement (REM) and non-REM sleep, with characteristic electroencephalograph (EEG) patterns. The α-wave of the waking state disappears during phase I of non-REM sleep, to be gradually replaced by δ-waves in stages III and IV. Intrusion of α-waves during non-REM sleep (called α-wave intrusion or δ-wave sleep interruption) is associated with FM,[8] and some (though not all) studies have found that deliberate interruption of non-REM sleep in healthy volunteers results in FM symptoms. While sleep disturbance is reported in 60–90 per cent of people with FM, it is non-specific as it also occurs in depression and following head trauma. Causitive theories include the observation that growth hormone is secreted during δ-wave sleep (interruption therefore

causing reduced levels) or that low levels of serotonin are implicated in both allowing δ-wave sleep interruption and inducing FM symptoms. However, it remains disputed whether the sleep-wave disturbance associated with FM is a primary abnormality (causing the features of FM), or is secondary to sleep disruption by pain.

Peptides and hormones

Insulin-like growth factor (IGF)-1 (also called somatomedin C) levels reflect growth hormone secretion and are reduced in FM and in CFS. However, the mechanism by which this observation might be associated with FM remains unclear. Serotonin has an important role in the modulation of pain. In patients with FM, levels are reduced, together with increased receptor density and impaired transportation of tryptophan, the amino-acid required for its synthesis. However, treatment with serotonin reuptake inhibitors or with high doses of tryptophan has been disappointing, suggesting a more complex interaction between serotonin and other factors.

Cerebrospinal fluid levels of norepinephrine are reduced, while substance P is increased. The former may explain autonomic disturbances in FM and CFS (e.g. orthostatic hypotension, abnormal heart rate, and blood pressure responses to exercise), while the latter, together with evidence of impaired blood flow in the caudate and thalamic pain centres, implies abnormal pain signal modulation.

The hypothalamic–pituitary–adrenal (HPA) axis

In the physiological response to stress, the hypothalamus secretes corticotrophin-releasing hormone (CRH), which acts on the anterior pituitary to produce adreno-corticotrophic hormone (ACTH), which in turn activates cortisol release from the adrenal gland. The serum cortisol level has a diurnal variation, being highest in the early morning and lowest in late evening. In studies in FM (reviewed in reference 9), 24-h urinary cortisol is reduced. There is usually a blunted cortisol response to exercise or to insulin-induced hypoglycaemia, though contrary findings have also been reported. Others have shown increased cortisol response to low doses of ACTH but a blunted response to higher doses. Suggested mechanisms include hypersensitivity to negative feedback or altered regulation of receptor responses at the hypothalamic and/or pituitary level. Differences in ACTH and cortisol responses to stress are implicated in the distinction between FM and CFS, these differences in turn being attributed by some authors to levels of arginine vasopressin (AVP), a hypothalamic peptide that acts with CRH in the stimulation of ACTH release. Compared with controls, AVP is increased in FM whereas it is reduced in CFS. Supporting theories of HPA dysfunction, similarities are noted between FM and symptoms of acute steroid withdrawal, while others have found that the prevalence of FM in women correlates with their level of dihydroepiandrosterone (DHEA; which roughly reflects HPA axis activity). However, corticosteroid therapy is clinically ineffective in CFS or FM (though correction of cortisol levels is noted).

In summary, there is no convincing theory to date for the pathogenesis of FM, and rationally based therapeutic strategies have generally been disappointing. A central, stress-related, disturbance of pain and sleep/wakefulness regulation involving complex interactions between neural and endocrine pathways seems the most plausible. In the meantime, the concept of fibromyalgia is a useful one, allowing many unnecessary investigations to be avoided and appropriate treatment advice to be given.

Management

Three critical elements of FM management are:

- the patient's understanding of FM
- constant review of medication use
- involvement of a multi-disciplinary team.

Explaining FM to a patient can be difficult. Patients typically have high scores on anxiety and depression questionnaires, and there may be considerable resistance to the idea of a clinical diagnosis being made without further intensive investigation. The concept that severe pain and disability are not associated with tissue damage is also difficult to explain. Disturbance of sleep, perhaps as a result of stress, with alterations in muscle's endurance and increased levels of 'pain chemicals' include the dominant symptoms and reasonably reflect current paradigms. This also introduces the various possible modalities of treatment in a way the patient can comprehend, encouraging their active participation and reducing the likelihood of self-medication, etc. As many patients have suffered disappointment with treatment and ongoing pain and exhaustion, they may find it hard to believe they can improve and need much encouragement from doctor and therapists. If the patient has specific fears (cancer being common), these should be identified and resolved early. It is useful to acknowledge the influence of psychological factors, though it is also important to point out, particularly if antidepressants are used (see below), that the diagnosis of FM is a musculoskeletal, not a psychiatric diagnosis. It is important to bear in mind that patients increasingly consider information from the internet or other sources in their decisions about the medical information they receive.

Pharmacological management

'Antidepressants'

The association of low levels of serotonin or norepinephrine with FM led to trials of the antidepressants. However, they are not used for their antidepressant properties in this context (a point that ought to be explained to patients who often resist psychotropic medication). Amitriptyline is the most frequently used, in doses of 10–50 mg, usually taken at night. Early morning drowsiness may be overcome by taking the drug earlier in the evening. Not all symptoms respond equally—improvements are seen in the fibromyalgia impact questionnaire (FIQ), sleep, pain, and patient's global assessment, but fatigue and the number of tender points are not reduced. While about 25–30 per cent report improvement within 1 month, attenuation of response is also noted after 3–6 months of therapy. Therefore, it is important to consider withdrawal of treatment for a period (about 4 weeks) if there has been a good response. Anticholinergic side-effects are more troublesome at higher (antidepressant) doses with little evidence of greater efficacy.

Cyclobenzaprine is a tricyclic compound that does not have antidepressant properties but does have similar anti-cholinergic side-effects to those of amitriptyline. Used in doses up to 40 mg/day, this has also been effective in studies in FM. Venlafaxine is a non-tricyclic antidepressant that has proven effective in an open-label trial. A significant placebo response has been noted in some FM trials, and open-label studies should be interpreted with caution.

Selective serotonin reuptake inhibitors have been associated with fewer side-effects. However, citalopram and fluoxetine were not effective for FM when used alone. The combination of 25 mg amitriptyline with 20 mg fluoxetine was superior to either drug used alone (for example, 63 per cent had a 25 per cent improvement in the FIQ).[10]

With respect to theories of low serotonin levels, high-dose supplementation of tryptophan (100 mg tds for a month) was effective for pain, stiffness, and fatigue. Conversely, calcitonin, which is another serotonin precursor (used for pain relief in reflex sympathetic dystrophy and osteoporotic vertebral fractures), was ineffective in a FM study.

Analgesics

Conventional analgesics are not usually effective in this condition, and nonsteroidal anti-inflammatory drugs (NSAIDs) are unhelpful. Tramadol is believed to act on opioid, serotoninergic, and adrenergic pathways, and is therefore the preferred choice of opioid-type analgesic in FM. Used orally, significant improvements in pain are reported, with fewer withdrawals due to lack of efficacy compared with placebo. Parenteral tramadol has also been shown to be effective. However, oral treatment should be considered in the first instance. Other opioid analgesics may be used in FM. Concerns about addiction may be raised, though it is generally held that, when correctly used in the treatment of pain, dependence is rarely encountered. However, it should be borne in mind that FM requiring opioid analgesia is unlikely to remit, and such treatment is therefore likely to continue indefinitely.

Lidocaine (lignocaine) may be used for injection of tender points. This has provided short-term relief (over 2 weeks, considerably longer than the half-life of the drug itself), though these injections are more effective in MPS. Of interest, dry needling of tender points has been shown to release similar levels of enkephalins as saline or lidocaine injections. Whether this accounts for the analgesic effect is debated (and is of relevance in discussions of acupuncture analgesia in FM and other contexts).

Other agents

Daily injections of growth hormone for 9 months resulted in a statistically significant improvement in the FIQ and pain (improvements in the placebo group were not statistically significant). This treatment is, however, impractical as a standard approach for FM, and the study only included those women with low IGF-1 levels (pituitary disease having been excluded).

Benzodiazepines have considerable risks of dependence and of seizures on withdrawal. Alprazolam, with or without ibuprofen, had equivocal results when compared against a significant placebo response. The only other studied benzodiazepine was also combined with a NSAID (temoxicam)—again, the placebo response was considerable and no significant treatment benefit was observed.

S-adenosyl methionine is available as an over-the-counter supplement in the United States, but requires a prescription in most European countries. It has been shown to be effective for relief of pain and tender point count.

Non-pharmacological interventions—the multidisciplinary team

As described earlier, current understanding of FM implicates biological pathways that may be influenced by these pharmacological interventions, but is likely to also involve muscular fatiguability and psychological responses to stress. Thus an approach that involves clinical psychologists and occupational and physical therapists is appropriate.

FM patients frequently use complementary medicine (91 per cent in one survey). As interactions have been reported in some instances (Committee for the Safety of Medicines), familiarity with the available range is useful. Devil's claw and meadowsweet are the most commonly used for 'arthritis', and appear to have anti-inflammatory properties (meadowsweet contains salicylic glycosides, similar to aspirin). Rhus-tox and St. John's wort are commonly included in pain and sleep remedies.

Acupuncture is the most thoroughly investigated of the alternative approaches in FM. In a detailed consensus review, the National Institute of Health in the US found sufficient evidence to support the role of acupuncture in FM 'as an adjunct treatment or an acceptable alternative or [part of] a comprehensive management program'.[11] A systematic review found seven studies, of which three were randomized controlled trials and a further three were prospective cohort studies. While only one was considered of high methodological quality, the criteria used are difficult to apply to acupuncture studies (blinding, particularly). In one study, acupuncture with electrical stimulation of the needles was effective. In another study, the combination of acupuncture with a tricyclic-related antidepressant (mianserin) showed greater improvement over baseline compared with either alone—however, direct comparisons were not made between groups. Moreover, the relapse rate at 6 months was 14 per cent in the acupuncture group, compared with 20 per cent in the mianserin group, whereas no patients who had combination therapy relapsed during this time. Acupuncture typically does require 'booster' treatments, and two cohort studies suggest this is an effective approach. However, pain may be increased as a result of needle insertion.

Cognitive–behavioural therapy, biofeedback, and exercise

In a systematic review and meta-analysis of randomized controlled trials of cognitive and behavioural therapy for chronic pain (including FM and MPS), tender point number, FIQ, and pain improved in each study.[12] Relaxation therapy, meditation, and understanding and management of pain are among the techniques used, largely by occupational therapists. Biofeedback may be combined with cognitive–behavioural therapy. Electromyographic analysis is used in physiotherapist-led retraining of muscle balance, and may also be used as part of an aerobic training programme. Compared with controls, almost 90 per cent of FM patients were found to have below-average aerobic exercise capacity. While it is unclear whether this is a pathogenic factor or a consequence of disuse, exercise does appear to have benefits in pain and tender points, though many patients struggle to persevere with an aerobic fitness training programme.

Chronic fatigue syndrome

Clinical features

The clinical features are dominated by the experience of fatigue (Table 2). This is not qualitatively different from tiredness experienced in numerous other settings, and the physician must therefore ensure that the initial evaluation is thorough. The recommended clinical evaluation prescribed in the Centres for Disease Control definition includes:

1. a detailed medical history and examination;
2. a mental status assessment;
3. a minimum laboratory screening to include:

(a) full blood count (including differential white cell count);

(b) erythrocyte sedimentation rate (ESR);

(c) serum alanine aminotransferase, albumin, and total protein; calcium, phosphorus, and alkaline phosphatase; urea, sodium, potassium, creatinine; glucose; thyroid-stimulatory hormone (TSH);

(d) urinalysis.

These investigations should be regarded as a minimum. Additional investigations prompted by the clinical history might include an anti-nuclear antibodies (ANA) or more specific auto-antibodies, particularly anti-Ro or -La (fatigue being a dominant feature of Sjögren's syndrome). As discussed in the pathogenesis section, a viral aetiology has not been identified for CFS, and the term 'post-viral' should be avoided. A screen for the more common viruses will probably have been carried out at an earlier stage (bearing in mind that 6 months must have elapsed before a diagnosis of CFS can be considered). The herpes family of viruses are the most commonly associated with a prolonged illness. Epstein–Barr virus (Paul–Bunnel test) and cytomegalovirus should specifically be ruled out. The European variety of Lyme disease rarely presents in this way, though a prolonged fatiguing illness has been associated with the North American form: a history of recent travel should be obtained, bearing in mind that the initial tick-bite is rarely recalled.

A sore throat and lymphadenopathy are two specific features that distinguish CFS from FM. Other aspects, such as muscular pain, headaches, and unrefreshing sleep, clearly overlap with FM. Indeed, many authors believe these to be alternative presentations of the same illness,[4] and the approach to management contains many of the same principles. Thus it is more important to identify the individual patient's main difficulties and rule out alternative diagnoses than to attempt to place the patient into a definite category.

Pathogenesis

Many of the observations on which pathogenic theories are based predate the clinical definitions now used. Therefore, the detailed discussion of pathogenesis described in the section on FM applies also to CFS (with the possible exception of the muscle biopsy findings).

Regarding the HPA axis, subtle differences identified in some studies between CFS and FM may explain the alternative clinical presentations. There is reduced diurnal variation in serum cortisol levels and reduced overall cortisol in about one-third of patients.[9, 13] ACTH and CRH in the CSF are normal, but this is regarded as being inappropriate in the face of reduced serum cortisol. A contradictory finding, however, is that the adrenal response to low doses of exogenous ACTH is increased, suggesting an altered 'set-point' in receptor regulation. Levels of AVP (a hypothalamic hormone stored in the posterior pituitary that influences ACTH release) are reduced in CFS compared with controls (in contrast to FM in which AVP is increased).

A viral aetiology has been considered for many years in the pathogenesis of CFS. Indeed, 'epidemic encephalomyelitis' was once felt to be a new variant of poliomyelitis. Similarities to infectious mononucleosis led others to believe CFS was a prolonged form of the same illness, while others have reported associations with echoviruses and others. However, none has been consistently implicated. Other names for CFS have included reference to chronic immunodeficiency. There is no evidence of a true impairment or deficiency of the immune system, though some have pointed to increased expression of major histocompatibility complex (MHC) antigens and prolonged T-cell activation as evidence of immune dysregulation, attributed to slow-virus-like infections.

Neuroimaging techniques to study brain metabolism have suggested that brainstem hypometabolism is a diagnostic feature of CFS. This in turn has been associated with autonomic dysfunction, though abnormalities of both parasympathetic and sympathetic systems are inconsistent in studies.

Management

Many of the points made regarding the management of FM are also relevant to CFS. The comprehensive history, examination, and laboratory evaluation should be set in the context of CFS being a valid differential diagnosis, not a last resort in the event of tests being normal or negative. The physician should ensure that the patient has a clear understanding of CFS and of the rationale for various treatment options.

Involvement of a clinical psychologist or a psychiatrist may meet with considerable resistance. However, a mental state examination by a non-expert may miss subtle signs, and any suggestion of psychological disturbance should be actively pursued.

Pharmacological options

Of the options described for FM, amitriptyline and other antidepressants are the most useful in CFS.

Both hydrocortisone (predominantly glucocorticoid action) and fludrocortisone (a mineralocorticod) have been used in CFS. Fludrocortisone (0.1–0.2 mg/day) had no benefits in a double-blind, cross-over study. Hydrocortisone (25 mg/day) has been associated with relief of symptoms, but concerns of adrenal suppression preclude its long-term use.

Eight of twenty-six patients responded to nicotinamide (required in the synthesis of adenosine triphosphate (ATP)), compared with two of twenty-six placebo-treated controls.

Non-pharmacological treatment

Studies are again limited, the best results coming from studies of hypnotherapy, biofeedback, cognitive-behaviour therapy, with mixed results from acupuncture and exercise.

Despite the lack of evidence-based treatment approaches to CFS, the outcome is somewhat better than for age-matched individuals with FM. Having had a variety of treatments in a multidisciplinary approach, 62 per cent had returned to gainful employment with a further 28 per cent functioning at an equivalent level. Twelve per cent reported ongoing disability.

Myofascial pain syndrome

Clinical features

Unlike FM, the pain experienced in MPS is usually localized to a region. Fatigue is not a common feature, and MPS is not typically associated with headaches, irritable bowel syndrome, etc. Both of these observations have set MPS somewhat apart from FM and CFS in terms of pathogenesis and treatment. However, it is likely that the nociceptive response that results in point tenderness (in FM) may also be responsible for contraction within the palpable muscular band (in MPS). There are no longitudinal studies to determine if a subset of patients with MPS develop more classical FM.

Palpation for trigger points should be carried out by rolling the fingers firmly across the point, looking for both the presence of a palpable band within the muscle and for the twitch response. This occurs when the palpating fingers are snapped across the taut band of an active trigger point, eliciting a local muscular twitch that may be visible in superficial muscles or felt by the examining fingers. Points tend to be located along the longitudinal axis of a particular muscle or group of muscles, and are reproducible within and between patients. The pattern of referral of pain in response to such a trigger is described in Table 3. The pain is typically deep-seated, dull, and aching, and may be constant (active trigger points) or may only be felt in response to trigger point palpation (latent points). Palpation of active trigger points may also result in pain at secondary 'satellite' points within the referral area. Autonomic disturbance has also been reported, in particular, reduced skin temperature in the painful region.

Pathogenesis

MPS may occur in the setting of other painful conditions. For example, tension headaches are associated with temporalis, suboccipital, and cervical trigger points, while scalene and pectoralis muscles may have trigger points in thoracic outlet syndrome. The mechanism by which a painful condition results in triggering is unknown. Overtraining in athletes, and particularly overuse injuries, have also been associated with (latent) trigger points. Poor posture or workplace design, muscle imbalance, and fatigue of secondary (stabilizer) muscles have also been implicated (see Chapter 6.13). Muscular tension induced by psychological stress may also be contributory. Others have suggested deficiencies in B-group vitamins, though this has not been supported in trials.

Treatment

Needling of trigger points is the mainstay of MPS management.[3, 14] However, this is most effective where the underlying factors mentioned above are also addressed. They should not be used in the acute setting, as increased pain may result. It appears that the substance injected is less important than the technique used, as dry needling has also been shown to be effective—however, use of local anaesthetic reduces the pain of injections. Injection of corticosteroid does not appear to have any benefit. The needle should be inserted at the most tender point. This may elicit a trigger response, confirming the appropriate placement of the needle.

Stretch-and-spray techniques were first described by the authors that first described MPS.[15] The principle is based upon stretching the taut muscle fibres and maintaining the restored muscle fibre length with passive and active exercises. The spray of local anaesthetic is applied across the painful area a few times before stretching the involved muscles. Active movements are then continued for 10–20 minutes. Treatment may continue daily for 2–3 weeks. However, improvement is usually rapidly apparent. Therefore if there is no noticeable change after a few treatments, underlying factors (including pyschological aspects) must be re-evaluated.

Electrical nerve and/or muscle stimulation by needle electrodes has also been studied. While nerve stimulation appeared to offer greater pain relief, muscle tightness was relieved more effectively by muscle stimulation.

A programme of muscle retraining, correcting imbalance, and increasing endurance should be an integral part of treating MPS. Maintaining a full range of stretching in the affected muscles reduces the likelihood of trigger-point recurrence. While medication (particularly NSAIDs, analgesics, and occasionally tricyclics (as in FM, above)) may be useful during trigger-point treatment, they should not be continued once triggering is resolved.

Conclusion

Fibromyalgia and myofascial pain are among the most common soft-tissue presentations to the rheumatologist. Both conditions may coexist with other conditions, and these diagnoses should be considered, particularly when pain appears unresponsive to conventional treatment, or when disability appears disproportionate to the degree of visible injury. Chronic fatigue syndrome may also present with muscular pain, but should only be considered as a diagnosis by exclusion. While numerous theories have been proposed to explain these disorders, therapeutic options remain empirically based, and each patient should be treated in a holistic and individualized manner.

References

1. Wolfe, F., Smythe, H.A., Yunus, M.B., Bennett, R.M., Bombardier, C., Goldenberg, D.L., et al. (1990). The American College of Rheumatology 1990 criteria for the classification of fibromyalgia report of the multicenter criteria committee. *Arthritis Rheum.* **33**, 160–172.

2. Fukuda, K., Straus, S.E., Hickie, I., et al. (1994). Chronic fatigue syndrome: a comprehensive approach to its definition and study. *Ann. Intern. Med.* **121**, 953–959.

3. Fomby, E.W. and Mellion, M.B. (1997). Identifying and treating myofascial pain syndrome. *Phys. Sports Med.* **25**, 67–75.

4. Wessley, S., Nimnuan, C., and Sharpe, M. (1999). Functional somatic syndromes: one or many? *Lancet* **354**, 936–939.

5. Goldenberg, D.L. (1999). Fibromyalgia syndrome a decade later: what have we learned? *Arch. Intern. Med.* **159**, 777–785.

6. Fricton, J.R., Kreonnig, R., Haley, D., and Siegert, R. (1985). Myofascial pain syndrome of the head and neck: a review. *Oral Surg. Oral Med. Oral Pathol.* **60**, 615–623.

7. Olsen, N.J. and Park, J.H. (1998). Skeletal muscle abnormalities in patients with fibromyalgia. *Am. J. Med. Sci.* **315**, 351–358.

8. Moldofsky, H. (1989). Sleep disturbance and fibrositis syndrome. *Rheum. Dis. Clin. N. Am.* **15**, 91–103.

9. Parker, A.J.R., Wessley, S., and Cleare, A.J. (2001). The neuroendocrinology of chronic fatigue syndrome and fibromyalgia. *Psychol. Med.* **31**, 1331–1345.

10. Goldenberg, D., Mayskiy, M., Mossey, C., Ruthazer, R., and Schmid, C. (1996). A randomised double blind crossover trial of fluoxetine and amitriptyline in the treatment of fibromyalgia. *Arthritis Rheum* **39**, 1852–1859.

11. NIH Consensus Conference (1998). Acupuncture. *J. Am. Med. Assoc.* **280**, 1518–1524.

12. Morley, S., Eccleston, C., and Williams, A. (1999). A systematic review and meta-analysis of randomised controlled trials of cognitive-behaviour therapy and behaviour therapy for chronic pain in adults excluding headaches. *Pain* **80**, 1–13.

13. Demitrack, M.A. and Croffard, L.J. (1998). Evidence for and pathophysiologic implications of hypothalamic–pituitary–adrenal axis dysregulation in fibromyalgia and chronic fatigue syndrome. *Ann. NY Acad. Sci.* **840**, 684–697.

14. Gunn, C.C., Milbrandt, W.E., Little, A.S., et al. (1980). Dry needling of muscle motor points for chronic low back pain: a randomized clinical trial with long-term follow-up. *Spine* **5**, 279–291.

15. Simons, D.G. and Travell, J.G. (1983). Myofascial origins of low back pain: 1: principles of diagnosis and treatment. *Postgrad. Med.* **73**, 66–73.

16. Buskila, D. (2000). Fibromyalgia, chronic fatigue syndrome and myofascial pain syndrome. *Curr. Opin. Rheumatol.* **12**, 113–123.

17. Ernst, E. and White, A. (eds) (1999). *Acupuncture—a scientific appraisal.* Butterworth-Heinemann, Oxford, UK.

18. Leventhal, L.J. (1999). Management of fibromyalgia. *Ann. Int. Med.* **131**, 850–858.

6.12 Myofascial pain syndromes

Mike Cummings

Introduction

Somatic pain is likely to be the most prevalent cause of pain in the general population—it is certainly a common reason for extended absence from work. The prime environmental aetiological factors are probably degeneration and abuse of the musculoskeletal system, and it should be no surprise that the areas which suffer most are those exposed to the greatest loads and activity over time—the articular surfaces of weight-bearing joints and the postural muscles of the limb girdles and axial skeleton. A recent epidemiological study, performed on a random sample of 5036 patients from the Grampian region of Scotland, indicated that half the population suffered chronic pain, and the most common sources were arthritis and back pain.[1] A prior study, which investigated the frequency of musculoskeletal disorders in a similar population, found that the most common site of pain was back (23 per cent; 95 per cent confidence interval (CI) 21–25), followed by knee (19 per cent; 95 per cent CI 18–21), and shoulder (16 per cent; 95 per cent CI 14–17).[2] Whilst the pain and dysfunction from degeneration of joints has been the focus of much research, and medical and surgical intervention, pain derived from skeletal muscle has remained an interest for only the minority of clinicians and researchers. There are likely to be a number of reasons for this.

1. Pain derived from skeletal muscle has not been perceived as clinically important. This may be because the pain is often diffuse, difficult to localize, and referred some distance from its source, although these characteristics of muscle pain were clearly demonstrated in 1938.[3]

2. There has been no objectively identifiable pathology related to the clinically identified sites of origin of this pain, at least not until very recently.[4]

3. Different investigators around the globe have independently identified palpable bands and points of tenderness in skeletal muscle, and they have described their findings in a variety of ways. This has resulted in considerable confusion and a lack of credibility within the general medical community. Such terms as 'muscle callouses',[5] 'muscular rheumatism',[6] 'myitis chronica rheumatica',[7] 'myogeloses',[8] and 'muscle hardenings'[9] were the forerunners to the term 'fibrositis', which was first introduced by Gowers in 1904.[10] The latter term has survived in common use until surprisingly recently, considering that inflammation of connective tissue has never been consistently and reliably demonstrated in biopsy studies.[11]

Having noted the pain referral patterns described by some of his patients with tender muscle nodules, Kellgren investigated the pain referral patterns produced by injecting hypertonic saline into the muscles and other soft tissues of experimental subjects and, in true scientific spirit, subjected himself to many such procedures. In muscle he found that pain was more diffuse than in other soft tissues and that, as the stimulus intensified, the pain pattern could spread over a wide area. Kellgren and his peers concluded that the distributions were generally segmental, but recognized that the pain must have a 'common path' in the central nervous system when several spinal segments were included.[3] Investigation of muscle pain syndromes continued independently on three separate continents following Kellgren's work. Formerly from Poland, Good (Gutstein) continued his work in England. He described the patient's pain reaction, which was later termed the 'jump sign', and he felt that the process responsible for 'myalgic spots' was a local constriction of blood vessels due to overactivity of the sympathetic nerves supplying them.[12] The Australian, Michael Kelly, evolved the concept that 'fibrositis' was a functional neurological disturbance due to a local rheumatic process, with little or no local pathology, and a central nervous system reflex disturbance causing the referred pain.[13] Travell, an American physician, devoted her career to the study of what she termed 'myofascial trigger points'. She initially emphasized the importance of the referral pattern from the trigger point, and postulated that any fibroblastic proliferation was secondary to a functional disorder, with pathological changes occurring only if the condition existed for a long time. She went on to develop the concept that the self-sustaining characteristic of trigger points depended on a feedback mechanism between the trigger point and the central nervous system.[14] Latterly she collaborated with Simons to produce a very comprehensive manual—*The trigger point manual*—covering the field of what are now popularly termed myofascial pain syndromes.[11, 15]

Whilst in modern times the medical profession has been slow to accept the importance of pain derived from skeletal muscle, therapists have devoted their careers to treating such pain throughout recorded history. In the East, acupuncture points were described, many of which were located within skeletal muscle. In clinical circumstances, some were referred to as 'Ah Shi' points; named after the exclamation of the patient, 'Oh yes!', when the points were palpated. Trigger points, described independently in the West some 2000 years later, have been shown to correlate anatomically and clinically with classically described acupuncture points in 71 per cent of cases (see Fig. 1 as an example).[16] Indeed, it has been suggested that acupuncture developed as a progression of empirical therapies initially aimed at the treatment of skeletal muscle pain, or more specifically, myofascial pain.[17]

Definitions

The term myofascial pain syndrome is used in two ways. In this chapter it is used as a specific term to describe a clinical syndrome encompassing sensory, motor, and autonomic symptoms caused by one or more myofascial trigger points in a specified skeletal muscle or skeletal muscle group. It is used by some in a more general sense to refer to any regional pain syndrome of soft tissue origin.

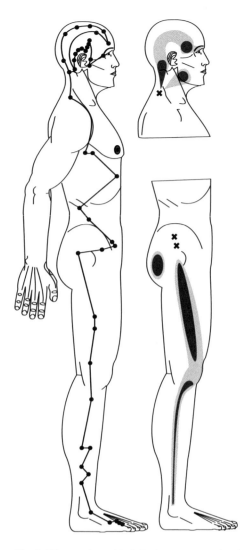

Fig. 1 Trigger points with their characteristic referral patterns are often coincident with classical acupuncture points and meridian paths. The meridian illustrated is the Gallbladder meridian, and the trigger points are in trapezius and gluteus minimus.

Janet Travell was the musculoskeletal physician who introduced the term 'myofascial trigger point' to describe the palpable source of these ubiquitous regional pain syndromes related to skeletal muscle.[18] In the latest edition of 'The trigger point manual', Simons et al. define the myofascial trigger point as follows:[4]

A hyperirritable spot in skeletal muscle that is associated with a hypersensitive palpable nodule in a taut band. The spot is painful on compression and can give rise to characteristic referred pain, referred tenderness, motor dysfunction, and autonomic phenomena.

The trigger point (TrP) is further defined by type.

1. An *active* TrP causes a clinical pain complaint.

2. A *latent* TrP does not cause spontaneous pain, but is painful on compression and causes some restriction of movement.

3. A *primary* TrP is activated directly by some form of mechanical trauma to the skeletal muscle in which it occurs.

4. A *central* TrP is closely associated with dysfunctional motor end-plates and is located near the centre of the muscle fibre.

5. An *attachment* TrP occurs at the muscle attachment to tendon or bone, and identifies the enthesopathy created by tension in a muscle band resulting from a central TrP.

6. An *associated* TrP occurs concurrently with a TrP in another muscle. One may have induced the other, or both may have been set up by the same mechanical or neurological stressor.

7. A *key* TrP is responsible for activating one or more satellite TrPs.

8. A *satellite* TrP is a central TrP induced through a neural or mechanical mechanism by the activity of a key TrP, or by some other somatic or visceral pathology. Satellite TrPs are prone to develop within the pain reference zone of the key TrP, within the zone of pain referred from a visceral disease, or in muscles affected by the mechanical dysfunction associated with the key TrP or other somatic pathology, in particular, degenerative joint disease.

These further definitions are based on those proposed by Simons et al.,[4] although the wording varies in places.

Prevalence

Myofascial trigger points are recognized by many clinicians to be one of the most common causes of pain and dysfunction in the musculoskeletal system. They have been detected in the shoulder girdle musculature in nearly half of a group of young, asymptomatic military personnel[19] and with a similar prevalence in the masticatory muscles of a group of unselected student nurses.[19] Active trigger points, those causing spontaneous pain, have been diagnosed as the primary source of pain in 74 per cent of 96 patients seen by a neurologist in a community pain medical centre,[20] and in 85 per cent of 283 consecutive admissions to a comprehensive pain centre.[21] Of 164 patients referred to a dental clinic for chronic head and neck pain, 55 per cent were found to have active myofascial trigger points as the cause of their pain,[22] as were 30 per cent of those presenting with pain to a university primary care internal medicine group practice from a consecutive series of 172 patients.[23] A recent study of musculoskeletal disorders in villagers from rural Thailand has demonstrated myofascial pain as the primary diagnosis in 36 per cent of 431 subjects with pain during the previous 7 days.[24]

Clinical features in general

Patient history

Pain

This is by far the most common presenting complaint. Typically, the pain is described as deep, aching, and poorly localized. It is usually restricted to one quadrant of the body, although complex patterns from multiple TrPs may give a wider distribution. It is important to determine the precise nature and pattern of the pain, as would be done when taking a standard medical history. Paraesthesia is not uncommon in association with the pain, and often confirms in the patient's mind the false impression that they have a 'trapped nerve'. Symptoms are generally exacerbated by activity. However, some light exercise involving gentle stretch of the affected muscle may relieve the aching.

Some patients will find a tender point in muscle, particularly if the TrP is in an accessible site, and a few will describe some sort of technique they have developed to relieve the pain, which usually involves the application of pressure to the TrP.

Dysfunction

TrPs may be responsible for minor autonomic dysfunction, such as excessive lacrimation or regional pilomotor activity. TrPs appear to affect proprioceptive function. In the cervical musculature, in particular sternomastoid, this may be responsible for dysequilibrium, even to the extent that the patient may describe true vertigo. In the limb musculature this may result in distorted weight perception. Motor dysfunction includes restricted range, weakness, reduced co-ordination, and spasm in other muscles.

Sleep

Myofascial pain may disturb sleep but, more importantly, sleep position often aggravates TrP activity by allowing affected muscles to shorten.

Age

TrPs occur in all age groups but present most commonly in the middle years. The muscles of young active people are probably more resistant to injury, and faster to repair, so less likely to develop or sustain active TrPs. By comparison, the musculoskeletal system of the middle-aged adult is becoming increasingly degenerate, less resilient, and slower to heal. In general, the middle-aged are less active, but engage in unaccustomed bouts of physical activity. They tend to suffer most with the pain of active TrPs. Latent TrPs can be found in the majority of elderly people, causing stiffness and reduced active range of movement, but this age group presents less frequently with the pain of active TrPs.

Sex

Women seem to present more frequently with myofascial pain than men. It has not been established whether myofascial pain is more common in women, or whether they are more likely to present with this type of pain. It is certainly true that phenotypic differences can influence biomechanical loading and, for the same mass, women tend to have wider hips and narrower shoulders than men. Biological factors such as these may be important, but socio-economic differences in terms of working environments may also have an influence. For example, a higher proportion of the male workforce perform physically strenuous jobs, and it has been noted that these individuals suffer less from myofascial pain than sedentary workers.

Examination findings

Tender point

This is the key feature of a TrP, although it is clearly not exclusive to TrPs. A tender point is usually a discrete area in the soma that, when pressure is applied to it, produces more pain than its immediate surroundings. In a clinical setting, pressure is usually applied with the fingertips on to the surface of the body. The pressure is transmitted through a range of soft tissues that are compressed between the examiner's fingertips and an unyielding surface beneath. The latter is often bone, but may be a soft tissue layer under tension. Hopefully, it is not the examination couch! There are a number of sites on the human body that appear to be tender because of inconsistency in the unyielding surface beneath. Pressure applied to these areas is concentrated over a small volume of soft tissue, rather than distributed more widely and evenly to the surroundings. Thus consistent extrinsic pressure, whether applied with fingertips or an algometer, generates greater pressure within the soft tissues at these sites than is produced in their surroundings, giving a false impression of tenderness. Therefore, it is always worth comparing tenderness at the site of a suspected TrP, with the same anatomical site on the asymptomatic side of the body. In the myofascial pain syndrome, active TrPs are rarely symmetrical, as opposed to fibromyalgia, in which tender points are widespread and often symmetrical.

When trying to determine the tissue that is tender, it can be useful to stretch the muscle layer whilst palpating, or to get the patient to perform an isometric contraction whilst putting pressure over the tender point. Both of these techniques tend to increase the relative pressure in the muscle layer, and therefore have some discriminative value.

Taut band

The taut band associated with a TrP is palpated by drawing the fingertips of the examining hand forward and back perpendicular to the fibres of the relevant muscle. The muscle should be placed on a slight stretch, and the skin and subcutaneous tissues are moved with the fingertips as the muscle fibres are palpated. Some superficial muscles can be palpated between finger and thumb in a pincer grip, and the taut band is felt as the fibres are allowed to slip between the palpating digits. The latter technique often requires the relevant muscle to be slackened off.

Pain

As an active TrP is palpated, the patient will often exclaim 'that's it', or give a similar verbal indication that they recognize the pain. The pain is usually sufficient to cause the patient to give an involuntary jerk, withdrawing slightly from the palpating fingers. This is referred to as the 'jump sign'. It is very important to ask the patient if it is their usual pain that is generated by applying pressure to the TrP, and ask them to indicate the pattern of pain produced. The pain referral patterns produced by TrPs in skeletal muscle are frequently characteristic of the specific muscle and, with experience, the musculoskeletal specialist can determine the most likely muscles involved from the history alone, so that detailed examination can be targeted to the relevant areas.

Local twitch response

When the palpating fingers are snapped across the taut band of an active TrP, there is often a detectable contraction of the band. This local twitch can be visible if the muscle is superficial, or may be felt by the examiner. The local twitch response (LTR) is more frequently encountered when directly needling the TrP.

Other examination findings

TrPs invariably cause shortening of the affected muscle, and may cause a reduction in power without muscle atrophy. Muscle shortening results in decreased range of movement (ROM) of the associated joint or joints. This can be a very helpful sign, but its usefulness is determined by how easy it is to measure the relevant ROM in a clinical setting. Assessment of power is generally not useful in deter-mining the presence of TrPs. However, the manoeuvre used to test power, resisted muscle contraction, often causes pain if the muscle tested is harbouring an active TrP, especially if the resistance is applied with the muscle in a shortened position.

Reliability of clinical diagnosis

There have been several studies testing the interobserver reliability of examining for TrPs. Those using untrained examiners failed to demonstrate reliability.[25, 26] A further study using trained examiners gave a marginal result.[27] The most recent study, using experienced clinicians, demonstrated reliability in its second phase after the examiners underwent a 3-hour period of training.[28] The following clinical features tested are placed in order of overall interrater reliability:

1. tender point;

2. pain recognition;

3. taut band;

4. referred pain;

5. LTR.

Simons et al. recommend that the minimum acceptable criteria for diagnosing a myofascial TrP are the combination of spot tenderness in a palpable band of skeletal muscle and subject recognition of the pain, but he admits that palpation of a taut band is conditional on the acces-sibility of the muscle.[4]

Special investigations

Algometry

A number of devices have been used in an attempt to objectively meas-ure the relationship between applied pressure and pain produced at TrP sites. The most popular to date has been the spring-loaded pressure algometer. Whilst this device gives an accurate reading of the pressure applied over its footplate, how and where the pressure is applied is determined by the operator and is thus subject to some degree of variation. The pressure transmission characteristics of the tissues, as discussed above, is another variable factor. The pressure algometer has been used in experimental and clinical studies (see below). However, it has not been found to be suitable as a diag-nostic investigation for TrPs.

Needle electromyography (EMG)

This technique has been used to study muscle and nerve activity for many years. There is currently considerable interest in its application to the study of TrPs, but not as a diagnostic technique. There is a discussion of recent findings below.

Surface EMG

Several aspects of muscle dysfunction associated with TrPs have been demonstrated using surface EMG measurements: increased respons-iveness; inappropriate co-activation; delayed relaxation;[29] and decreased endurance.[30] Referred dysfunction in the form of muscle spasm with pain has been implied from a reduction in EMG activity and resolution of pain in the ipsilateral masseter, following injection

of trapezius TrPs in an open and uncontrolled study of 20 subjects.[31] It has been suggested that bilateral surface EMG monitoring may be useful in the rehabilitation of patients with myofascial pain syn-drome,[29] but it seems unlikely that this technique will have an applica-tion in its diagnosis.

Thermography

Thermography has been used to study TrPs in both humans[32–39] and animals (von Schweinitz, personal communication 1998). However, the research to date does not support any clear conclusions about its value as a diagnostic technique. There is a discussion of thermography research below.

Ultrasound

Gerwin and Duranleau have reported identifying the twitch of a TrP using high-resolution ultrasound imaging.[40] However, the use of imaging alone, without looking for LTRs, did not prove useful in dif-ferentiating clinically apparent, active TrPs from contralateral asymp-tomatic muscle in 11 subjects with unilateral myofascial pain.[41] The value of this technique in the assessment and treatment of TrPs is yet to be determined.

Pathophysiology

Sensory phenomena

Pain

Tenderness has been investigated using pressure algometry, and several studies have demonstrated that this is a reliable tool for assess-ing TrP sensitivity.[42–44] One study examined pressure pain thresh-old, referred pain threshold, and pain tolerance at three different sites in the extensor digitorum muscle: over the TrP itself (active $n = 15$, latent $n = 24$); over another site within the same taut band; and over a normal area within the same muscle.[45] It was found that the pres-sure required to produce referred pain was more highly correlated with the pressure pain threshold in cases with active TrPs ($r = 0.88$) than in cases with latent TrPs ($r = 0.62$). Also, the difference between the pressure pain threshold and the referred pain threshold was much less for the active TrP cases. Referred pain was produced by pres-sure over each of the active TrPs but over only 46.8 per cent of the latent TrPs. Pressure over the taut band also produced referred pain in every case associated with an active TrP, but in only 36.2 per cent of the cases associated with a latent TrP. Even pressure over normal muscle produced referred pain in some cases—specifically, in 68 per cent of the cases with active TrPs and in 23.4 per cent of those with latent TrPs.

Another study investigated the nociceptive process in the myofas-cial pain of 40 cases of chronic tension-type headaches compared with 40 healthy controls.[46] The relationship between the pressure applied over a TrP and the associated pain was found to be linear, that is, incre-ments in pressure were proportional to the resulting increments in pain. Over normal muscle the relationship was found to be non-linear. Typically increments in pressure over normal muscle do not cause pain until a threshold is reached, beyond which pain increases dispro-portionately. The authors postulate that myofascial pain is mediated by low-threshold mechanosensitive afferents projecting to sensitized dorsal horn neurons.

Temperature

Thermograms can be recorded using liquid crystal films, which make direct contact with the surface under analysis, or by infrared radiometry, which measures emission of electromagnetic radiation in the infrared band of the spectrum. The latter method appears to be the most convenient and reliable in a clinical setting and has been used by a number of investigators to study TrPs.[32–39] This thermographic technique measures skin surface temperature to a depth of only a few millimetres. The temperature at the skin surface is regulated by the circulation, which is in turn controlled by the autonomic nervous system. There is evidence that TrP activity is also regulated to a degree by sympathetic tone,[47–49] so it is reasonable to hypothesize that thermographic imaging may be useful in the detection or analysis of TrPs. The most consistent finding seems to be an area of hyperthermia over the TrP.[32–36] However, this phenomenon is not specific to the TrP and seems to occur just as often in subjects without TrPs.[50] Whilst an area of hyperthermia is clearly not a discriminating sign, hypothermia over the area of pain referral from an active TrP after pressure is applied to the TrP appears to be a more promising indication.[36] Unfortunately, this has only been tested in 11 subjects with trapezius TrPs and healthy controls, and it is possible that a similar sympathetically mediated vasoconstriction would occur with pressure over other tender tissues that are not TrPs.

Motor phenomena

Whilst taut bands have been detected in muscle for a very long time,[5] the orthodox medical world has shown some reluctance to believe in the existence of TrPs. This has been fuelled in part by an inability to demonstrate histologically a pathological process. It is only relatively recently that a pathophysiological marker, in the form of spontaneous needle EMG activity, has been identified within a 1–2 mm nidus of a TrP.[51] Spikes (100–600 μV, biphasic, initially negative) and continuous low-amplitude action potentials (10–80 μV) were recorded in the vicinity of an active TrP, but only the continuous low-amplitude action potentials could be recorded from latent TrPs. Several investigators have found similar findings. However, there is controversy over the likely site of origin of this electrical activity. Hubbard and Berkoff postulated that the source was intrafusal fibres within the muscle spindle,[51] but, more recently, Hong and Simons have put forward a strong argument in favour of dysfunctional motor endplates.[52] It is unfortunate that this type of electrical activity is not specific to TrPs, and can be demonstrated in the endplate zone outside a TrP, although it has not been demonstrated outside the endplate zone.[4]

Spontaneous electrical activity (SEA)—referring to the continuous low-amplitude action potentials—has been shown to vary significantly in amplitude between symptomatic (patients suffering from tension headaches and fibromyalgia) and control subjects.[51] In normal subjects with latent TrPs, SEA recorded from the upper trapezius has been shown to increase dramatically in amplitude as a result of psychological stress alone,[47] and phentolamine, an α-adrenergic blocker, appears to diminish the amplitude and frequency of spikes recorded from TrPs in humans[53] and in a rabbit model.[54]

The LTR has been studied electrophysiologically in both man and the rabbit model.[52] The muscle contraction of an LTR appears to occur only within the taut band, and the latency of the contraction following direct mechanical stimulation of the TrP is consistent with a polysynaptic reflex. LTRs can be abolished by a local anaesthetic block or by transection of the innervating nerve, and are diminished following cord transection, although they recover almost completely after the period of spinal shock.[52]

Histopathology

Simons et al.[4] suggest that highly contracted portions of muscle fibres, which they call 'contraction knots', may be a specific histological marker for the TrP (see schematic representation in Fig. 2). They were first described in 1951 in biopsies of 'Muskelhärten' (muscle indurations)[55] and again in 1960 in biopsies from similar sites in patients described as having fibrositis.[56] In 1976 TrP criteria were used to investigate canine muscle, and sites that were clinically equivalent to TrPs in humans were examined histologically.[57] Muscle cross-sections revealed some darkly staining, large, round fibres. The equivalent longitudinal appearance showed central bulges within some muscle fibres where there was a highly contracted portion. Either side of this bulge the fibre was narrow and elongated to compensate for the central 'knot' of contracted sarcomeres. More recently, these histological findings have been confirmed, and further elaborated with the use of electron microscopy, on biopsies of human gluteus medius TrPs from fresh cadavers.[58]

Since the demonstration of SEA from TrPs, Simons has proposed that the contraction knot is likely to be the source of this activity.[59] He cites experimental research on mammalian skeletal muscle[60] and the microscopic appearance of a contraction knot in canine gracilis muscle[57] to support his contention that the contraction knots observed in TrP biopsies occur at the site of the motor endplate. He adds further support to this suggestion by observing that the longitudinal dimension of these knots is similar to the length of a motor endplate.

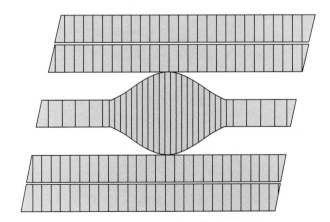

Fig. 2 This is a schematic diagram of a contraction knot in a muscle fibre between normal muscle fibres. The striations are representative of the contractile elements (sarcomeres). The fusiform swelling of the contraction knot may contain 100 maximally contracted sarcomeres, and either side of this, within the same fibre, the sarcomeres are elongated to compensate.

Aetiology

Empirical

Travell and Simons put forward three aetiological factors responsible for the development of primary TrPs:[15] acute physical overload; overwork fatigue; and chilling. They also describe TrPs developing secondary to some other pathological process or event. Their assertions are supported only by empirical evidence, and how such factors may cause the development of TrPs is the subject of much speculation.

In the second edition of *The trigger point manual*,[4] Simons *et al.* avoid listing chilling as a direct aetiological factor, and add radiculopathy and gross trauma. Gunn was the first to suggest that radiculopathy may be the cause of TrPs,[61] and Chu has performed some clinical research suggesting a relationship between the two.[62,63] However, the latter research is of low methodological quality, and Gunn's hypothesis relating clinically undetectable radiculopathy to supersensitivity in muscle tissue is not convincing.[64]

Pathogenesis of the TrP

Simons considers that the taut band is the major precursor for TrPs, based on clinical observation that taut bands occur very commonly in asymptomatic individuals within the population.[65] He has proposed that taut bands may form as a result of excessive intracellular Ca^{2+} release from the sarcoplasmic reticulum in certain fibres exposed to trauma or abnormal stress. Excessive Ca^{2+} release causes uncontrolled shortening of the fibres, and thus increased metabolism within them. Sustained contraction impairs local circulation, and this exacerbates the accumulation of products of metabolism, resulting in an energy crisis. The Ca^{2+} pump that returns Ca^{2+} to the sarcoplasmic reticulum requires adenosine triphosphate (ATP), and is more sensitive to low ATP levels than the contractile mechanism. If the energy crisis is sufficient to impair uptake of Ca^{2+} into the sarcoplasmic reticulum, contractile activity would be sustained, thus completing a 'vicious cycle', and resulting in taut band formation. Simons goes on to propose that individuals prone to developing taut bands are more likely to develop active TrPs within those bands as a result of psychological or biomechanical stresses, perhaps combined with a genetic predisposition towards TrP development.[52]

Overview of aetiology for clinical application

The following represents the author's view of the aetiology of TrPs, based on study of empirical and research data:

- degeneration
- abuse
- central sensitization
- genetic predisposition
- environmental factors.

Degeneration

Latent TrPs can be detected in about 50 per cent of young adults, and the incidence is thought to increase with age. In the author's experience it is exceedingly uncommon to find a middle-aged individual who does not have palpable taut bands in key areas of their musculature. These key areas seem to correspond to sites of biomechanical disadvantage for the biped—in particular, the antigravity muscles of the shoulder girdle and the hip girdle are affected.

Abuse

This refers to physical abuse of one's own musculoskeletal system, whether from poor posture or excessive activity. Psychological stress may also be included under this heading. One of the physiological effects of stress is an increase in muscle tension mediated through sympathetic innervation of the muscle spindle or influence at the motor endplate. If this tension persists for a sufficient length of time, it may result in the formation of TrPs in pre-existing taut bands.

Central sensitization

TrPs may form in pre-existing taut bands as a result of sensitization of sensory pathways within the central nervous system. Segmental dorsal horn sensitization, or 'wind-up' can occur with chronic C-fibre input, for example, from visceral pathology. The resultant influence on the soma may be to activate TrPs in susceptible areas of the same segment. It is possible that this is mediated through increased secretory activity in small-diameter muscle afferents, referred to by some as neurogenic inflammation, resulting in sensitization of motor endplates in the vicinity. If these motor endplates are chronically bathed in an excess of activating neurochemicals, they may become dysfunctional, with the result that TrPs are set up *de novo* or latent TrPs activated. Such sensitization of neural structures seems a more likely explanation of the development of satellite TrPs than Gunn's hypothesis of undetectable radiculopathy resulting in denervation supersensitivity. A plausible alternative to afferent secretion influencing endplate function as the mechanism for development of satellite TrPs would be segmental activation of sympathetic fibres. This localized sympathetic activity could increase muscle tension, either via the muscle spindles or by a direct influence on the motor endplate.

Fibromyalgia may be an example of a process of sensitization occurring over the whole of the soma, with generalized lowering of sensory thresholds and activation of numerous TrPs at sites of pre-existing taut bands. This would be consistent with the often symmetrical pattern of tender points and the more reluctant response shown by patients with fibromyalgia to sensory stimulation in the form of dry needling. It has been demonstrated by Hong and Hsueh that injection of TrPs in patients with fibromyalgia results in significantly greater posttreatment soreness than in patients with simple myofascial pain syndrome.[66]

Genetic predisposition

It is likely that the specific make-up of the individual's musculoskeletal and nervous systems predisposes that individual, to a greater or lesser extent, to the formation of taut bands and subsequently TrPs. The individual's phenotype can certainly influence the degree and distribution of biomechanical stress to different areas of the body. The work performed by the hip abductors during locomotion, for example, is directly related to the width of the pelvis. This is likely to be one of the key reasons that woman present more frequently than men with hip girdle pain related to TrPs in gluteus medius and gluteus minimus.

Environmental factors

There are many environmental factors that could theoretically influence the development of TrPs. A sedentary occupation appears to be a risk factor. Travell and Simons[15] report that chilling of muscle can influence the generation of TrPs. They also report a number of potential influences from drugs and the diet.

Clinical examples of myofascial pain syndromes

The following clinical examples describe the main features of a small selection of the common myofascial pain syndromes. For a more detailed description of these and many other myofascial pain syndromes the reader is referred to the two volumes of *The trigger point manual* by Travell and Simons.[4, 15] In the figures that illustrate the sites and typical pain referral patterns of these TrPs, the site is marked with an 'X' on the relevant muscle and the typical pain referral pattern is coloured in two shades of red—the dark red areas represent the most common areas of referred pain. The pain patterns are merely representative of a typical clinical case and may vary considerably from this in some individuals.

Trapezius

Upper fibres

This is probably the muscle most frequently affected by TrPs. Latent TrPs have been identified in the upper free border of trapezius in nearly 50 per cent of young healthy adults,[19] and the author has rarely found an individual over the age of 30 who does not have taut bands palpable in trapezius. TrPs in the upper free border are easily accessible to the examiner, and pressure over them almost invariably refers pain up the posterolateral aspect of the neck to the mastoid process (Fig. 3(a), (b)). In some individuals the pain referral extends to the temporal region, and can also be felt behind the orbit. Occasionally, pain is referred to the angle of the jaw. This wider referral to the head and face is associated with the more anteriorly placed TrP (Fig. 3(a)).

Satellite TrPs can be set up in the posterior cervical musculature, particularly semispinalis capitis, and in temporalis and masseter. Overlapping patterns of pain referral can produce a variety of presentations of headache or facial pain, so trapezius should always be examined in case it harbours the key TrP.

The upper fibres of trapezius are particularly prone to chronic overuse because they oppose the effect of gravity on the shoulder girdle. Whilst the fibres attaching to the lateral third of the clavicle are almost horizontal, contraction results in rotation of the clavicle around the sternoclavicular joint, with the overall effect of elevating the shoulder. Thus tasks that involve sustained shoulder elevation can result in the development of TrPs in this area of the muscle. Acute trauma to the neck, for example, in a car accident, is another potential cause. Indeed it would be unusual to find a case of cervical strain injury following a car accident in which there were no TrPs in trapezius.

The upper fibres of trapezius seem to be particularly prone to the effects of psychological stress. SEA recorded from latent TrPs in the upper free border of trapezius has been shown to increase significantly during psychological stress in a controlled experiment.[47]

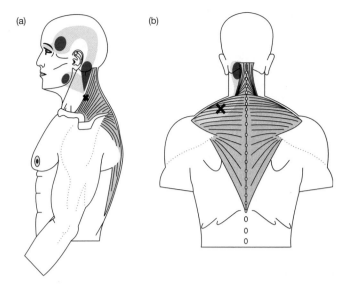

Fig. 3 (a) Central TrP in the upper free border of trapezius with its typical pain referral pattern. The dark red areas represent the most common areas of referred pain. (b) Central TrP in the upper fibres of trapezius, just posterior to that shown in (a), with its typical pain referral pattern. Note that TrPs in this area tend not to refer pain beyond the mastoid region.

Furthermore, patients with anxiety almost invariably have bilateral and symmetrical TrPs in this area of the muscle, but, in these patients, physical treatments alone cannot be expected to have sustained effects.

There are several ways to position the patient for examination of the upper fibres of trapezius. The author finds the most convenient approach is from behind the patient, with the patient seated on a height-adjustable examination couch. The upper free border of the muscle can be grasped in a pincer grip by the thumb and middle finger of the examiner's hand. The fibres are allowed to slip between the thumb and fingertip as the examiner's hand is moved slightly up and forward. The patient will jerk involuntarily as an active TrP is put under sudden pressure on slipping between the examiner's thumb and finger tip. The other method of examining these fibres is to use flat palpation perpendicular to the fibre direction with the fibres on slight stretch. The latter is achieved by slight flexion of the patient's head, full lateral flexion to the contralateral side, and rotation to the ipsilateral side.

The restriction of movement that is most clinically apparent, resulting from TrPs in the upper fibres of trapezius, is rotation of the head. Sometimes there is no restriction but, if there is significant shortening of a taut band within the upper fibres, neck rotation is restricted more towards the affected side than away from it. If this restriction is caused purely by a TrP in trapezius, inactivation of the TrP should result in an immediate restoration of the full range of rotation.

Lower and middle fibres

The lower border of trapezius is another common site for a central TrP, and it is often overlooked clinically. Pain can be referred widely over the trapezius from this site, although it tends to concentrate in the high cervical paraspinal area, the adjacent mastoid area, and the acromium (Fig. 4). Travell and Simons describe referred tenderness from TrPs in the lower border of trapezius to the suprascapular

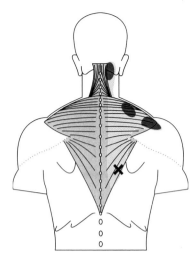

Fig. 4 Central TrP in the lower fibres of trapezius with pain referral widely over the muscle, concentrating in the high cervical paraspinal area, the adjacenet mastoid area, and the acromium. The area within the pain referral pattern which is coloured in an intermediate shade of red represents the site of referred tenderness, as described by Travel and Simons (4).

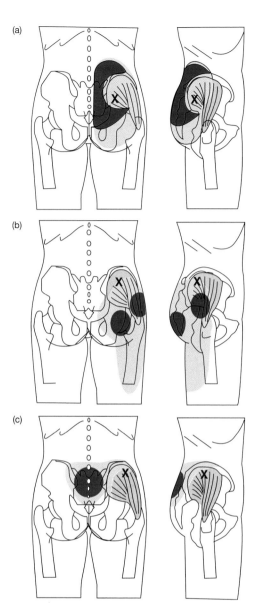

Fig. 5 (a)–(c) Three sites in gluteus medius where TrPs are commonly found and the typical pain referral patterns associated with each Trp.

region—not to be confused with satellite TrPs that can develop or be activated at the same site.[15] The former referred tenderness is described as diffuse, and should easily be distinguishable from the focal tenderness associated with a satellite TrP. The middle fibres of trapezius are less frequently the site of primary TrPs and, as a rule, the pain produced by them is fairly local.

The middle fibres are examined with flat palpation from behind the seated patient. A degree of stretch is achieved by asking the patient to slouch with the arms allowed to dangle over the edge of the couch between the legs, but without leading forwards. The position is one of full lumbar and thoracic flexion with almost full protraction of the scapulae. A similar approach is used to examine the lower fibres: starting from the position just described, the trunk is rotated 30–45° to the contralateral side, and the ipsilateral arm is allowed to hang over the contralateral leg. If more stretch is required, the patient can be asked to point the elbow of the ipsilateral arm directly forwards. This action increases protraction and elevation of the ipsilateral scapula. The examiner must remember that the lowermost fibres of trapezius are angled downwards from the spine of the scapula to the spinous process of T12, and the examining fingertips must be moved perpendicular to this line, that is, towards and away from the contralateral shoulder. If the examiner palpates along the line of the fibres, the lower edge of rhomboid major will be felt instead—another site that commonly harbours TrPs.

Gluteus medius and minimus

These short powerful muscles have extensive attachments to the outer surface of the ilium, and below they attach to the external surface of the greater trochanter. They are the key abductors of the hip whose prime function is to support the pelvis when the body weight is transferred on to the ipsilateral leg. TrPs in these muscles are often the cause of hip girdle pain, ipsilateral low back pain, and pain that radiates down the leg (Figs 5 and 6). Myofascial pain from such TrPs is frequently misdiagnosed as L5 or S1 radiculopathy, zygapophyseal

joint arthrosis, sacroiliac joint dysfunction or disease, or trochanteric bursitis.

TrPs can be activated in these muscles by direct trauma, prolonged or unaccustomed locomotor activity, particularly if it involves side to side movements (such as in tennis and other racket sports), and weight-bearing on one leg for an extended time. Injection into the muscle has also been cited as a cause of TrP activation, especially if the injected substance is irritating to the tissues.[15] Uncorrected leg length inequality can be an important factor in the development and persistence of these TrPs, and should always be considered in any musculoskeletal assessment of the lower limb or spine. Another important developmental variation which can predispose to TrPs in these muscles is a long second toe and short first toe, as described by Morton.[67]

These muscles are examined with the patient side-lying on an examination couch. The lower leg is flexed slightly at the hip and the

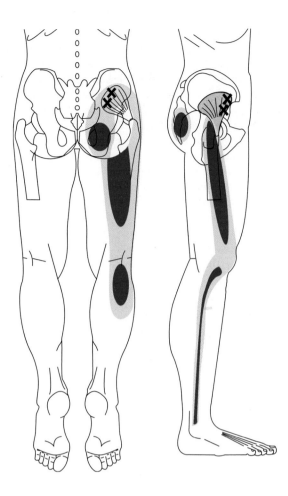

the piriformis. In this position the nerve lies between the body of the muscle and the bony anterior rim of the foramen. In the most frequent anatomical variant from this arrangement, which occurs in about 10 per cent of cases, the peroneal division of the sciatic nerve pierces the body of the muscle. In either of these arrangements it appears possible for the muscle to cause nerve compression. Any circumstance

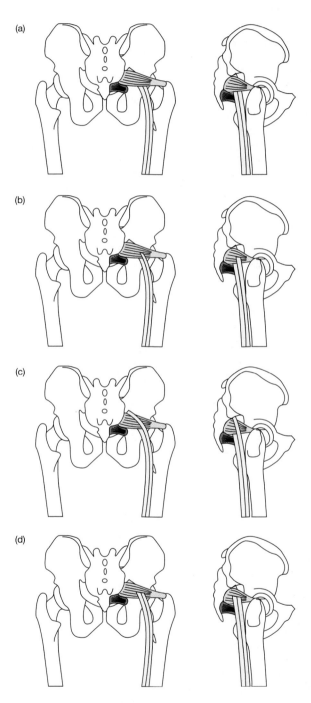

Fig. 6 The sites in gluteus minimus where TrPs are commonly found and the typical pain referral patterns associated with each TrP.

knee allowing the upper leg to drop directly behind it. The knee of the upper leg is flexed slightly to allow it to rest on the examination couch, increasing the angle of adduction of the limb and stretching the abductor muscles being examined. The examiner must palpate firmly into the tissue that lies in a fan shape from the greater trochanter to the iliac crest, remembering to run the fingertips perpendicular to the fibre orientation. To achieve adequate tension in the most posterior fibres of gluteus medius, the positions of the patient's knees are swapped so that the upper knee lies in front of the lower knee, with the upper leg flexed to about 45° at the hip. A latent TrP is almost invariably present in the posterior half of the gluteus medius, so the examiner should always be sure to compare the tenderness on the opposite side.

Piriformis

Piriformis is one of the short lateral rotators of the thigh. It has been the subject of much discussion and controversy for at least the last 60 years, and there is even a syndrome named after it. Its function is probably less important than its anatomical position. Attaching medially to the anterior surface of the sacrum and laterally in a rounded tendon to the upper medial surface of the greater trochanter, its body fills the greater sciatic foramen. The sciatic nerve also exits the pelvis via the greater sciatic foramen, usually passing anterior and inferior to

Fig. 7 The four reported anatomical variants in the relationship of the two divisions of the sciatic nerve and the piriformis. (a) The usual pattern with both divisions passing anterior to the muscle. (b) The peroeal division piercing the muscle (approximately 10% of cases). (c) The peroneal division passing superior and posterior to the muscle (approximately 1% of cases). (d) Divisions piercing the muscle (approximately 1% of cases).

that causes increased tension or bulk of the muscle may exacerbate or initiate symptoms of nerve compression, depending on the relative size of the muscle in relation to the foramen. Figure 7 illustrates four of the six reported anatomical variants in the relationship of the two divisions of the sciatic nerve and the piriformis.

Fröhlich and Fröhlich found latent TrPs in piriformis in 5 per cent of 100 healthy subjects, and in 49 per cent of 97 patients presenting with lumbogluteal pain.[68] Active piriformis TrPs were found in 21 per cent of the patient group. The usual pain pattern seen with such TrPs is intense local pain in the buttock or just below the sacroiliac region, and diffuse less intense pain over the whole of the buttock and upper two-thirds of the posterior thigh (Fig. 8). In the author's experience, the symptoms of nerve entrapment related to piriformis TrPs are referred pain and paraesthesia to the lateral surface of the lower leg, without obvious muscle weakness or loss of reflexes.

Piriformis is examined with the patient side-lying on an examination couch, and the upper leg is flexed to 90° at the hip and the knee so that the upper knee comes to rest on the couch. An imaginary line from the greater trochanter to the sacral hiatus corresponds with the lower margin of the piriformis. On deep palpation, usually with both thumbs, the muscle can be felt as a band of tissue running above and parallel to the line just described. Pressure over a point approximately one-third of the way along the muscle from the greater trochanter will be painful. This may be a latent TrP. If pressure reproduces the patient's pain, it is likely to be an active TrP. If there are symptoms suggestive of nerve entrapment, these may be made worse by such pressure, or by further stretching the muscle. The latter is achieved by rolling the patient's pelvis away from the upper knee and pressing the knee back down towards the couch, that is, increasing adduction of the upper leg at the hip. If the patient's symptoms have not been brought on by the above manoeuvres, the patient can be asked to lift the upper knee against resistance. Digital pressure can be added over the piriformis, and the upper leg allowed to abduct to the limit of movement or until the symptoms are reproduced. This movement allows piriformis to shorten under load, thus increasing the volume it occupies in the greater sciatic foramen.

Management

There are many different therapies applied to the treatment of myofascial pain throughout the world. They are categorized below under the headings of 'needling therapies' and 'non-needling therapies', but equally the titles 'invasive therapies' and 'non-invasive therapies' could be used.

Needling therapies

Needling of TrPs is one of the most common treatments for myofascial pain in global terms. This is because of the use of acupuncture in the East. Acupuncture is also popular in the West, but not on such a scale, and is sometimes referred to as dry needling. Wet needling, or injection therapy, is perhaps more commonly applied in the West, with a variety of injected substances, from the relatively innocuous physiological saline to the toxin derived from *Clostridium botulinum*. Acupuncture and TrP injections are discussed in Chapter 5.4.

Non-needling therapies

There is a great variety of these non-invasive therapies. The most commonly applied in clinical practice are probably physical treatments. Whilst they are given many different titles, most involve the application of some form of mechanical pressure to the TrP or stretch of the affected muscle, or both. Travell and Simons developed the technique of 'stretch and spray'.[15] This involves the use of a vapocoolant spray applied in a defined pattern just prior to stretching the involved muscle. The sudden sensory stimulus of the spray acts as a distraction and reduces the discomfort from stretching a muscle shortened by a TrP. Various other techniques are described to enhance stretching. Post-isometric relaxation[69] and reciprocal inhibition[4] involve voluntary muscle contraction by the patient of the target muscle or its antagonists, respectively. Accessory techniques, including phased respiration and eye movements, can also be used to augment stretching. Pressure has been applied to TrPs in the form of ischaemic compression, shiatsu, acupressure, pressure release, and many forms of massage. Simons *et al.* give a comprehensive account of reported therapies applied to TrPs in the second edition of *The trigger point manual.*[4]

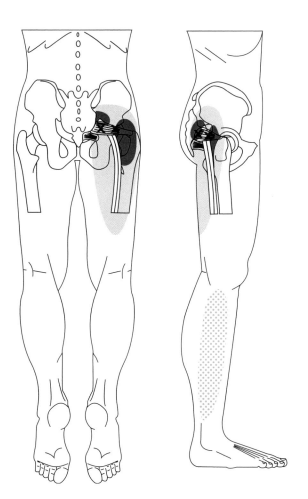

Fig. 8 Two TrP sites in the piriformis muscle with the typical pain referral patterns. This figure also illustrates one possible variation of nerve entrapment with paraesthesia on the lateral aspect of the lower limb. The latter would be consistent with irritation of the peroneal division of the sciatic nerve.

Despite the prevalent use of physical therapies in the treatment of myofascial pain, surprisingly few of them have been subjected to controlled clinical trials. In five patients with bilateral active TrPs in trapezius, Jaeger and Reeves randomly selected the side for treatment with stretch and spray, and demonstrated a significant reduction in TrP sensitivity (pressure pain threshold measured with an algometer) compared with that on the untreated side.[70] Pain scores decreased significantly but did not correlate with TrP sensitivity. This was the only controlled trial the author could find testing stretch in the treatment of myofascial pain. Gam *et al.* performed a randomized controlled trial comparing ultrasound, massage, and exercise with sham-ultrasound, massage, and exercise with a no-treatment control group in a population of patients with TrPs of the neck and shoulders.[71] Ultrasound was shown to be ineffective. Both active treatment groups improved significantly compared to the control, but the latter was inadequate to conclude that massage and exercise had a specific effect.

TrPs have become a popular target for enthusiasts of low-level laser therapy (LLLT). Several randomized controlled trials have been reported, and positive results[72–74] have exceeded the negative.[75] A systematic review published in 1992 concluded that 'laser therapy appears to have a substantial specific therapeutic effect'.[76] However, a plausible mechanism is still lacking as there is no sensory stimulation perceived from active LLLT and the photon beam has very limited penetrance. Moreover, experimental work by Lundeberg and colleagues has demonstrated that this type of laser stimulus has no demonstrable effect on nerve tissue.[77,78]

Transcutaneous electrical stimulation of various sorts has been tested on TrPs. Graff-Radford *et al.* tested four modes of transcutaneous electrical nerve stimulation (TENS) and a no-stimulation control on 60 patients with myofascial pain. High-intensity TENS was effective in reducing myofascial pain but not TrP sensitivity. In light of this it is not surprising that, in a trial 9 years later of subthreshold TENS applied to patients with myofascial pain and dysfunction of the masticatory system, the active intervention proved no better than the sham.[79] Electrical stimulation over TrPs with a pocket-sized stimulator has been shown to increase pain threshold algometer readings over the treated points compared with a no treatment control,[80] but whether this would correlate to clinically significant symptom relief has not been established. Furthermore, Jaeger and Reeves have indicated that there may be no correlation between pain reduction and TrP sensitivity.[70] Hsueh *et al.* compared electrical nerve stimulation (ENS), using a standard TENS machine set at 60 Hz, with electrical muscle stimulation (EMS) at 10 Hz.[81] The latter, but not the former, was sufficient to induce muscle contraction. A third group received a sham control. Sixty patients were randomized to the three groups. ENS proved more effective for pain relief, but EMS resulted in a greater improvement in range of movement.

Treatments that have been shown to be ineffective include sphenopalatine ganglion block for myofascial pain of the head and neck,[82,83] occlusal splints for myofascial pain of the jaw muscles,[84] and oral sumatriptan for myofascial pain of the temporal muscles.[85] Low-dose clonazepam proved superior to placebo in the treatment of myofascial pain related to temporomandibular joint dysfunction,[86] but benzodiazepines are not suitable for lengthy treatment because of the risk of dependence.

More unusual treatments involve mud baths and magnetic fields. According to a randomized controlled trial by Pratsel *et al.*, mud baths containing sulfur compounds reduce the sensitivity of TrPs compared to those that do not contain sulfur compounds.[87] Pain scores in postpolio patients reduced significantly as a result of the application of 300–500 Gauss magnetic devices to their 'pain trigger points', compared with the use of placebo devices.[88]

To finish on a specific area—myofascial pain syndrome of the peroneus longus responded significantly better to dynamic insoles compared with simple correction of leg length inequality with heel lifts.[89]

Prognosis

Despite the lack of convincing evidence of specific efficacy for any of the therapies regularly applied to TrPs, the empirical experience of clinicians treating myofascial pain is very positive. Simple clinical audit suggests that the majority of people get better with dry needling[90] and the same probably applies to the popular non-needling physical therapies. As a general rule, myofascial pain syndromes that have been present for 6 months or less appear to be curable, but those that have been present longer or that have followed a chronic relapsing course can only be treated symptomatically, with a latent tendency to relapse remaining (White, personal communication 1994).

TrPs may appear to move during treatment. This is likely to be an apparent movement rather than actual movement of a specific TrP, and can occur as a result of treatment of a series of satellite TrPs. If the key TrP is identified and treated in the first instance, this apparent movement is unlikely to occur.

If there is not a rapid initial response to treatment, after say two or three sessions, the therapist must consider the possibilities that:

1. the key TrP has not be correctly identified and treated;

2. the diagnosis of MPS is incorrect;

3. there are factors causing persistence of the treated TrP that have been overlooked.

The last is the most likely cause of treatment failure if initial assessment has been performed by an experienced clinician. Persistent biomechanical stress is likely to be the most prevalent factor, but psychological stress with increased muscle tension, particularly affecting the neck and shoulders, is also very common. Less common factors include borderline hypothyroidism[91] and a host of other endocrine, metabolic, and nutritional inadequacies. Whilst these factors have been suggested by empirical observation and remain to be validated, a working knowledge of the most common is essential to clinicians treating myofascial pain, and Simons *et al.*'s detailed account of 'perpetuating factors' is recommended.[4]

Caution

In the author's perception there appears to be a number of conditions that fall into the grey area between the clear-cut myofascial pain syndrome affecting a single muscle and the widespread involvement of the soma in fibromyalgia. A typical presentation has features of both, and often appears to be a more complex version of the former. Usually limited to a single quadrant of the body, unlike fibromyalgia, there is a generalized tenderness of soft tissue compared with that on the unaffected side. This might represent a myofascial pain syndrome with an abnormal degree of central sensitization in the affected segments on one side of the spinal cord. Whatever the pathogenesis, these conditions are difficult to treat, and direct somatic stimulation of the tender points or TrPs should be avoided, at least initially.

Summary

Myofascial pain syndromes are a prevalent source of regional pain and dysfunction. They appear to respond well to therapies targeted at the key TrPs, although there is a lack of rigorous evidence confirming specific efficacy of the most popular therapies. The common manifestations can be identified and treated with limited training, but the more complex and esoteric presentations require detailed knowledge of functional anatomy and factors that perpetuate the condition.

References

1. **Elliott, A.M., Smith, B.H., Penny, K.I., Smith, W.C., and Chambers, W.A.** (1999). The epidemiology of chronic pain in the community. *Lancet* **354** (9186), 1248–1252.

2. **Urwin, M., Symmons, D., Allison, T., Brammah, T., Busby, H., Roxby, M.,** *et al.* (1998). Estimating the burden of musculoskeletal disorders in the community: the comparative prevalence of symptoms at different anatomical sites, and the relation to social deprivation [see comments]. *Ann. Rheum. Dis.* **57** (11), 649–655.

3. **Kellgren, J.H.** (1938). Observations on referred pain arising from muscle. *Clin. Sci.* **3**, 175–190.

4. **Simons, D.G., Travell, J.G., and Simons, P.T.** (1999). *Travell and Simons' myofascial pain and dysfunction. The trigger point manual*, Vol. 1. *Upper half of body*, 2nd edn. Williams and Wilkins, Baltimore.

5. **Froriep, R.** (1843). *Ein Beitrag zur Pathologie und Therapie des Rheumatismus*. Weimar.

6. **Virchow, R.** (1852). Ueber parenchymatösa Entzündung. *Arch. Path. Anat.* **4**, 261–279.

7. **Helleday, U.** (1876). Om myitis chronica (rheumatica). Et bidrag till dess diagnostik och behandling. *Nord. Med. Arch.* **8**, Art. 8.

8. **Schade, H.** (1921). Untersuchungen in der Erkältungstrage: III. Uber den Rheumatismus, insbesonderedn Muskelrheumatismus (Myogelosis). *Müench. Med. Wochenschr.* **68**, 95–99.

9. **Lange, F. and Eversbusch, G.** (1921). Die Bedeutung der Muskelhärten für die allgemeine Praxis. *Müench. Med. Wochenschr.* **68**, 418–420.

10. **Gowers, W.R.** (1904). Lumbago: its lessons and analogues. *Br. Med. J.* **1**, 117–121.

11. **Travell, J.G. and Simons, D.G.** (1983). *Myofascial pain and dysfunction. The trigger point manual*, Vol. 1. *The upper extremities*, 1st edn. Williams and Wilkins, Baltimore.

12. **Good, M.G.** (1951). Objective diagnosis and curability of nonarticular rheumatism. *Br. J. Phys. Med.* **14**, 1–7.

13. **Kelly, M.** (1945). The nature of fibrositis: 1. The myalgic lesion and its secondary effects: a reflex theory. *Ann. Rheum. Dis.* **5**, 1–7.

14. **Travell, J.** (1976). Myofascial trigger points: clinical view. In *Advances in pain research and therapy*, Vol. 1. (ed. J.J. Bonica and D. Albe-Fessand), pp. 919–926. Raven Press, New York.

15. **Travell, J.G. and Simons, D.G.** (1992). *Myofascial pain and dysfunction. The trigger point manual*, Vol. 2. *The lower extremities*, 1st edn. Williams and Wilkins, Baltimore.

16. **Melzack, R., Stillwell, D.M., and Fox, E.J.** (1977). Trigger points and acupuncture points for pain: correlations and implications. *Pain* **3** (1), 3–23.

17. **Filshie, J. and Cummings, T.M.** (1999). Western medical acupuncture. In *Acupuncture—a scientific appraisal* (ed. E. Ernst and A.R. White), pp. 31–59. Butterworth Heinemann, Oxford.

18. **Travell, J. and Rinzler, S.H.** (1952). The myofascial genesis of pain. *Postgrad. Med.* **11**, 425–434.

19. **Sola, A.E., Rodenberger, M.L., and Gettys, B.B.** (1955). Incidence of hypersensitive areas in posterior shoulder muscles. *Am. J. Phys. Med.* **3**, 585–590.

20. **Gerwin, R.D.** (1995). A study of 96 subjects examined both for fibromyalgia and myofascial pain [abstract]. *J. Musculoskel. Pain* **3** (suppl. 1), 121.

21. **Fishbain, D.A., Goldberg, M., Meagher, B.R., Steele, R., and Rosomoff, H.** (1986). Male and female chronic pain patients categorized by DSM-III psychiatric diagnostic criteria. *Pain* **26** (2), 181–197.

22. **Fricton, J.R., Kroening, R., Haley, D., and Siegert, R.** (1985). Myofascial pain syndrome of the head and neck: a review of clinical characteristics of 164 patients. *Oral Surg. Oral Med. Oral Pathol.* **60** (6), 615–623.

23. **Skootsky, S.A., Jaeger, B., and Oye, R.K.** (1989). Prevalence of myofascial pain in general internal medicine practice. *West. J. Med.* **151** (2), 157–160.

24. **Chaiamnuay, P., Darmawan, J., Muirden, K.D., and Assawatanabodee, P.** (1998). Epidemiology of rheumatic disease in rural Thailand: a WHO-ILAR COPCORD study. Community Oriented Programme for the Control of Rheumatic Disease. *J. Rheumatol.* **25** (7), 1382–1387.

25. **Wolfe, F., Simons, D.G., Fricton, J., Bennett, R.M., Goldenberg, D.L., Gerwin, R.,** *et al.* (1992). The fibromyalgia and myofascial pain syndromes: a preliminary study of tender points and trigger points in persons with fibromyalgia, myofascial pain syndrome and no disease. *J. Rheumatol.* **19** (6), 944–951.

26. **Nice, D.A., Riddle, D.L., Lamb, R.L., Mayhew, T.P., and Rucker, K.** (1992). Intertester reliability of judgments of the presence of trigger points in patients with low back pain. *Arch. Phys. Med. Rehabil.* **73** (10), 893–898.

27. **Njoo, K.H. and Van der Does, E.** (1994). The occurrence and inter-rater reliability of myofascial trigger points in the quadratus lumborum and gluteus medius: a prospective study in non-specific low back pain patients and controls in general practice. *Pain* **58** (3), 317–323.

28. **Gerwin, R.D., Shannon, S., Hong, C.Z., Hubbard, D., and Gevirtz, R.** (1997). Interrater reliability in myofascial trigger point examination. *Pain* **69** (1–2), 65–73.

29. **Donaldson, C.C., Nelson, D.V., and Schulz, R.** (1998). Disinhibition in the gamma motoneuron circuitry: a neglected mechanism for understanding myofascial pain syndromes? *Appl. Psychophysiol. Biofeedback* **23** (1), 43–57.

30. **Hagberg, M. and Kvarnstrom, S.** (1984). Muscular endurance and electromyographic fatigue in myofascial shoulder pain. *Arch. Phys. Med. Rehabil.* **65** (9), 522–525.

31. **Carlson, C.R., Okeson, J.P., Falace, D.A., Nitz, A.J., and Lindroth, J.E.** (1993). Reduction of pain and E.M.G activity in the masseter region by trapezius trigger point injection. *Pain* **55** (3), 397–400.

32. **Diakow, P.R.** (1988). Thermographic imaging of myofascial trigger points. *J. Manipulative Physiol. Ther.* **11** (2), 114–117.

33. **Diakow, P.R.** (1992). Differentiation of active and latent trigger points by thermography. *J. Manipulative Physiol. Ther.* **15** (7), 439–441.

34. **Fischer, A.A. and Chang, C.H.** (1986). Temperature and pressure threshold measurements in trigger points. *Thermology* **1**, 212–215.

35. **Fischer, A.A.** (1988). Documentation of myofascial trigger points. *Arch. Phys. Med. Rehabil.* **69** (4), 286–291.

36. **Kruse, R.A., Jr and Christiansen, J.A.** (1992). Thermographic imaging of myofascial trigger points: a follow-up study. *Arch. Phys. Med. Rehabil.* **73** (9), 819–823.

37. **Swerdlow, B. and Dieter, J.N.I.** (1992). An evaluation of the sensitivity and specificity of medical thermography for the documentation of myofascial trigger points. *Pain* **48** (2), 205–213.

38. **Scudds, R.A., Heck, C., Delaney, G.,** *et al.* (1995). A comparison of referred pain, resting skin temperature and other signs in fibromyalgia (FM) and myofascial pain syndrome (MPS). *J. Musculoskel. Pain* **3** (suppl. 1), 97.

39. Scudds, R.A., Landry, M., Birmingham, T., *et al.* (1995). The frequency of referred signs from muscle pressure in normal healthy subjects [abstract]. *J. Musculoskel. Pain* **3** [suppl. 1], 99.

40. Gerwin, R.D. and Duranleau, D. (1997). Ultrasound identification of the myofacial trigger point [letter]. *Muscle Nerve* **20** (6), 767–768.

41. Lewis, J. and Tehan, P. (1999). A blinded pilot study investigating the use of diagnostic ultrasound for detecting active myofascial trigger points. *Pain* **79** (1), 39–44.

42. Reeves, J.L., Jaeger, B., and Graff-Radford, S.B. (1986). Reliability of the pressure algometer as a measure of myofascial trigger point sensitivity. *Pain* **24** (3), 313–321.

43. Delaney, G.A. and McKee, A.C. (1993). Inter- and intra-rater reliability of the pressure threshold meter in measurement of myofascial trigger point sensitivity. *Am. J. Phys. Med. Rehabil.* **72** (3), 136–139.

44. Bendtsen, L., Jensen, R., Jensen, N.K., and Olesen, J. (1994). Muscle palpation with controlled finger pressure: new equipment for the study of tender myofascial tissues. *Pain* **59** (2), 235–239.

45. Hong, C.-Z., Chen, Y.-N., Twehous, D., and Hong, D.H. (1996). Pressure threshold for referred pain by compression on the trigger point and adjacent areas. *J. Musculoskel. Pain* **4** (3), 61–79.

46. Bendtsen, L., Jensen, R., and Olesen, J. (1996). Qualitatively altered nociception in chronic myofascial pain. *Pain* **65** (2–3), 259–264.

47. McNulty, W.H., Gevirtz, R.N., Hubbard, D.R., and Berkoff, G.M. (1994). Needle electromyographic evaluation of trigger point response to a psychological stressor. *Psychophysiology* **31** (3), 313–316.

48. Lewis, C., Gevirtz, R., and Hubbard, D. (1994). Needle trigger point and surface frontal EMG measurements of psychophysiological responses in tension-type headache patients. *Biofeedback Self Regul.* **19** (3), 274–275.

49. Chen, J.T., Chen, S.M., Kuan, T.S., Chung, K.C., and Hong, C.Z. (1998). Phentolamine effect on the spontaneous electrical activity of active loci in a myofascial trigger spot of rabbit skeletal muscle. *Arch. Phys. Med. Rehabil.* **79** (7), 790–794.

50. Swerdlow, B. and Dieter, J.N. (1992). An evaluation of the sensitivity and specificity of medical thermography for the documentation of myofascial trigger points. *Pain* **48** (2), 205–213.

51. Hubbard, D.R. and Berkoff, G.M. (1993). Myofascial trigger points show spontaneous needle EMG activity. *Spine* **18** (13), 1803–1807.

52. Hong, C.Z. and Simons, D.G. (1998). Pathophysiologic and electrophysiologic mechanisms of myofascial trigger points. *Arch. Phys. Med. Rehabil.* **79** (7), 863–872.

53. Hubbard, D.R. (1996). Chronic and recurrent muscle pain: pathophysiology and treatment, and review of pharmacologic studies. *J. Musculoskel. Pain* **4** (1–2), 123–143.

54. Hong, C.Z., Chen, J.T., Chen, S.M., and Kuan, T.S. (1997). Myofascial trigger point is related to sympathetic activity [abstract]. *Am. J. Phys. Med. Rehabil.* **76**, 169.

55. Glogowski, G. and Wallraff, J. (1951). Ein Beitrag zur Klinik und Histologie der Muskelhärten (Myogelosen). *Z. Orthop.* **80**, 237–268.

56. Miehlke, K., Schulze, G., and Eger, W. (1960). Klinische und experimentelle Untersuchungen zum Fibrositissyndrom. *Z. Rheumaforsch* **19**, 310–330.

57. Simons, D.G. and Stolov, W.C. (1976). Microscopic features and transient contraction of of palpable bands in canine muscle. *Am. J. Phys. Med.* **55**, 65–88.

58. Reitinger, A., Radner, H., Tilscher, H., *et al.* (1996). Morphologische Untersuchung an Triggerpunkten [Morphologic study of trigger points]. *Manuelle Medizin* **34**, 256–262.

59. Simons, D.G. (1999). Diagnostic criteria of myofascial pain caused by trigger points. *J. Musculoskel. Pain* **7** (1–2), 111–120.

60. Leonard, J.P. and Salpeter, M.M. (1979). Agonist-induced myopathy at the neuromuscular junction is mediated by calcium. *J. Cell Biol.* **82** (3), 811–819.

61. Gunn, C.C. (1980). "Prespondylosis" and some pain syndromes following denervation supersensitivity. *Spine* **5** (2), 185–192.

62. Chu, J. (1995). Dry needling (intramuscular stimulation) in myofascial pain related to lumbosacral radiculopathy. *Eur. J. Phys. Med. Rehabil.* **5** (4), 106–121.

63. *Chu, J.* (1997). Does EMG (dry needling) reduce myofascial pain symptoms due to cervical nerve root irritation? *Electromyogr. Clin. Neurophysiol.* **37** (5), 259–272.

64. Gunn, C.C. (1989). *Treating myofascial pain, intramuscular stimulation (IMS) for myofascial pain syndromes of neuropathic origin.* University of Washington, Seattle.

65. Simons, D.G. (1996). Clinical and etiological update of myofascial pain from trigger points. *J. Musculoskel. Pain* **4** (1–2), 93–121.

66. Hong, C.Z. and Hsueh, T.C. (1996). Difference in pain relief after trigger point injections in myofascial pain patients with and without fibromyalgia [see comments]. *Arch. Phys. Med. Rehabil.* **77** (11), 1161–1166.

67. Morton, D.J. (1935). *The human foot. Its evolution, physiology and functional disorders.* Columbia University Press, New York.

68. Fröhlich, D. and Fröhlich, R. (1995). Das piriformissyndrom: eine häufige Differentialdiagnosedes lumboglutäälen Schmerzes [Piriformis syndrome: a frequent item in the differential diagnosis of lumbogluteal pain]. *Manuelle Medizin* **33**, 7–10.

69. Lewit, K. and Simons, D.G. (1984). Myofascial pain: relief by postisometric relaxation. *Arch. Phys. Med. Rehabil.* **65** (8), 452–456.

70. Jaeger, B. and Reeves, J.L. (1986). Quantification of changes in myofascial trigger point sensitivity with the pressure algometer following passive stretch. *Pain* **27** (2), 203–210.

71. Gam, A.N., Warming, S., Larsen, L.H., Jensen, B., Hoydalsmo, O., Allon, I., *et al.* (1998). Treatment of myofascial trigger-points with ultrasound combined with massage and exercise—a randomised controlled trial. *Pain* **77** (1), 73–79.

72. Ceccherelli, F., Altafini, L., Lo, C.G., Avila, A., Ambrosio, F., and Giron, G.P. (1989). Diode laser in cervical myofascial pain: a double-blind study versus placebo. *Clin. J. Pain* **5** (4), 301–304.

73. Snyder-Mackler, L., Barry, A.J., Perkins, A.I., and Soucek, M.D. (1989). Effects of helium–neon laser irradiation on skin resistance and pain in patients with trigger points in the neck or back. *Phys. Ther.* **69** (5), 336–341.

74. Snyder-Mackler, L., Bork, C., Bourbon, B., and Trumbore, D. (1986). Effect of helium–neon laser on musculoskeletal trigger points. *Phys. Ther.* **66** (7), 1087–1090.

75. Thorsen, H., Gam, A.N., Svensson, B.H., Jess, M., Jensen, M.K., Piculell, I., *et al.* (1992). Low level laser therapy for myofascial pain in the neck and shoulder girdle. A double-blind, cross-over study. *Scand. J. Rheumatol.* **21** (3), 139–141.

76. Beckerman, H., de Bie, R.A., Bouter, L.M., De Cuyper, H.J., and Oostendorp, R.A. (1992). The efficacy of laser therapy for musculoskeletal and skin disorders: a criteria-based meta-analysis of randomized clinical trials. *Phys. Ther.* **72** (7), 483–491.

77. Lundeberg, T. and Zhou, J. (1988). Low power laser irradiation does not affect the generation of signals in a sensory receptor. *Am. J. Chin. Med.* **16** (3–4), 87–91.

78. Lundeberg, T., Hode, L., and Zhou, J. (1988). Effect of low power laser irradiation on nociceptive cells in Hirudo medicinalis. *Acupunct. Electrother. Res.* **13** (2–3), 99–104.

79. Kruger, L.R., van der Linden, W.J., and Cleaton-Jones, P.E. (1998). Transcutaneous electrical nerve stimulation in the treatment of myofascial pain dysfunction. *S. Afr. J. Surg.* **36** (1), 35–38.

80. Airaksinen, O. and Pontinen, P.J. (1992). Effects of the electrical stimulation of myofascial trigger points with tension headache. *Acupunct. Electrother. Res.* **17** (4), 285–290.

81. Hsueh, T.C., Cheng, P.T., Kuan, T.S., and Hong, C.Z. (1997). The immediate effectiveness of electrical nerve stimulation and electrical muscle stimulation on myofascial trigger points. *Am. J. Phys. Med. Rehabil.* **76** (6), 471–476.

82. Scudds, R.A., Janzen, V., Delaney, G., Heck, C., McCain, G.A., Russell, A.L., *et al.* (1995). The use of topical 4% lidocaine in spheno-palatine ganglion

blocks for the treatment of chronic muscle pain syndromes: a randomized, controlled trial. *Pain* **62** (1), 69–77.

83. **Ferrante, F.M., Kaufman, A.G., Dunbar, S.A., Cain, C.F., and Cherukuri, S.** (1998). Sphenopalatine ganglion block for the treatment of myofascial pain of the head, neck, and shoulders. *Reg. Anesth. Pain. Med.* **23** (1), 30–36.

84. **Dao, T.T., Lavigne, G.J., Charbonneau, A., Feine, J.S., and Lund, J.P.** (1994). The efficacy of oral splints in the treatment of myofascial pain of the jaw muscles: a controlled clinical trial. *Pain* **56** (1), 85–94.

85. **Dao, T.T., Lund, J.P., Remillard, G., and Lavigne, G.J.** (1995). Is myofascial pain of the temporal muscles relieved by oral sumatriptan? A crossover pilot study. *Pain* **62** (2), 241–244.

86. **Harkins, S., Linford, J., Cohen, J., Kramer, T., and Cueva, L.** (1991). Administration of clonazepam in the treatment of TMD and associated myofascial pain: a double-blind pilot study. *J. Craniomandib. Disord.* **5** (3), 179–186.

87. **Pratsel, H.G., Eigner, U.M., Weinert, D., and Limbach, B.** (1992). [The analgesic efficacy of sulfur mud baths in treating rheumatic diseases of the soft tissues. A study using the double-blind control method]. *Vopr. Kurortol. Fizioter. Lech. Fiz. Kult.* **3**, 37–41.

88. **Vallbona, C., Hazlewood, C.F., and Jurida, G.** (1997). Response of pain to static magnetic fields in postpolio patients: a double-blind pilot study. *Arch. Phys. Med. Rehabil.* **78** (11), 1200–1203.

89. **Saggini, R., Giamberardino, M.A., Gatteschi, L., and Vecchiet, L.** (1996). Myofascial pain syndrome of the peroneus longus: biomechanical approach. *Clin. J. Pain* **12** (1), 30–37.

90. **Cummings, T.M.** (1996). A computerised audit of acupuncture in two populations: civilian and forces. *Acupunct. Med.* **14** (1), 37–39.

91. **Sonkin, L.S.** (1997). Therapeutic trials with thyroid hormones in chemically euthyroid patients with myofascial pain and complaints suggesting mild thyroid insufficiency. *J. Back Musculoskel. Rehabil.* **8** (2), 165–171.

6.13 Work-related upper limb pain

Donncha O'Gradaigh and Brian Hazleman

Introduction

Work-related musculoskeletal disorders comprise a heterogeneous group of conditions whose natural history is for the most part poorly understood. A variety of terms have been used in different ways. For some, 'work-related upper limb disorders', 'cumulative trauma disorders', and 'repetitive strain disorders' are synonymous and describe a range of conditions—some well defined, others less so—arising or appearing to arise from frequent overuse at work. For others, repetitive strain injury (RSI) refers to a particular diagnosis made by exclusion: chronic upper limb pain ascribed to overuse at work for which no clinical diagnosis can be made. The apparently simple question, 'which musculoskeletal problems are work-related', has proved difficult to answer. Study data are weakened by cross-sectional designs and by selection bias. In addition, it is necessary to distinguish between work that 'causes' a condition and activities that aggravate it. Here, we assess the epidemiology of the various disorders, their natural history, and factors peculiar to the working environment.

Historical perspective

Efforts to associate upper limb symptoms with occupational causes are not new. Cramp among goldsmiths was described in 1473, and Paracelsus noted the hand symptoms of miners a century later. Virchow reported musicians' cramp, milkmaids' cramp, and shoemakers' cramp. Ramazzini's description in 1713 of neck and shoulder pain in writers is regarded as the first comprehensive overview of such problems. A significant development was the addition in 1908 of telegraphist's cramp to the schedule of compensatable illnesses under the British Workmen's Compensation Act. The proportion of workers reporting such symptoms increased to 60 per cent over the next 4–5 years. Shortly afterwards, it was concluded that the cramp was due to a 'nervous breakdown', after which the incidence declined. In the early 1980s, 34 per cent of all telephonists working with Telecom Australia reported upper limb pain attributed to repetitive trauma at work, and the term 'repetitive strain injury' (RSI) was first coined. The rapid increase in incidence that followed was described as an 'industrial epidemic'. Cleland[1] described the condition as a model of social iatrogenesis, in that advice and expectations focused on pain in the workplace led to minor discomfort becoming a protracted and disabling condition. As studies failed to confirm any pathological changes, critics dismissed the condition as psychosomatic. However, a declining incidence in Australia also coincided with improvements in work practices, and with abandoning the use of the term RSI. Most recently, Judge Prosser in 1993 in the United Kingdom determined from the evidence presented to him that RSI 'did not exist as a separate medical condition'. Against this background we must consider the possibility that well-established entities such as carpal tunnel syndrome arise from work activities, and whether there is a condition of work-related chronic upper-limb pain in which no alternative clinical diagnosis can be made.

Epidemiology

Estimates of the size of the problem vary depending on case definition and the source of the statistics. In general, there are data on the prevalence and incidence of conditions in the community, and on how these conditions vary by age and sex. Many studies also describe associations with work, though most are cross-sectional in design, which does not permit the true sequelae of events to be observed and cannot therefore examine cause and effect. Both cross-sectional and case-control studies are also vulnerable to selection bias. For example, if the worst affected patients are unable to work, a cross-section of those in employment will tend to underestimate the prevalence. In contrast, a case-control design may select those with more severe presentations, or controls may have a subclinical degree of the condition, diminishing the apparent influence of the factor under investigation.

Using a broad classification of upper limb pain, community-based surveys reported an incidence of 25 new cases per 1000 person years, increasing between 25 and 45 years of age.[2] Lifetime prevalence as high as 60 per cent has been reported. However, such figures mask a wide variation, from 2 per cent for epicondylitis among workers to 20 per cent for shoulder complaints in a 31–74-year-old cohort (Table 1). The entity of 'chronic upper limb pain' not fulfilling more specific diagnostic criteria was typically excluded from these surveys.

Studies of work-related chronic upper limb pain are strongly influenced by the definition selected, reflecting contrasting medical and legal attitudes. Since the peak annual incidence of around 50 cases per 1000 workers, rates as low as 1 per cent have been reported (though this study specifically excluded carpal tunnel syndrome which is among the most frequently diagnosed disorders). Prevalence figures are similarly variable. In a recent report,[4] the US Department of Labor estimated that 15–20 per cent of Americans had ongoing upper limb symptoms, and that, by the year 2000, 50 per cent of the entire workforce would have had occupational injuries (not restricted to work-related upper limb pain). No social or professional group has been spared, though the self-employed are not usually affected, and low-paid, monotonous jobs predominate.

Clinical and pathological features

Table 2 illustrates the criteria proposed by an international expert panel for the diagnosis of a number of upper limb disorders. Of note,

Table 1 Point-prevalence studies of regional pain disorders in the neck and upper limb (from reference 3)

Disorder	Age group	Prevalence (%)	Study population
Shoulder pain	31–74	20	Community
	Working age	13	Aeroengineering factory
Elbow pain	Working age	11–13	Aeroengineering factory
Epicondylitis	Working age	2	Aeroengineering factory
	31–74	2.5	Community
Tenosynovitis	33–39	3.5	Textile workers
Carpal tunnel syndrome	25–74 (male)	0.6	Community
	25–74 (female)	8	Community
Neck pain	25–74	10	Community
	Working age	10	Aeroengineering factory

Table 2 Proposed diagnostic criteria for upper limb disorders (see reference 5 and evaluation in reference 6)

Disorder	Criteria
Rotator cuff tendinitis	History of pain in the deltoid region *and* pain on resisted active shoulder movements (abduction, external and internal rotation)
Shoulder capsulitis	History of pain in the deltoid area *and* equal restriction of active and passive shoulder movement affecting external rotation > abduction > internal rotation
Bicipital tendinitis	History of anterior shoulder pain *and* pain on resisted active shoulder flexion or supination of the arm
Lateral epicondylitis	Epicondylar pain *and* tenderness *and* pain on resisted wrist extension
Medial epicondylitis	Epicondylar pain *and* tenderness *and* pain on resisted wrist flexion
De Quervain's disease	Pain over radial styloid *and* tenderness over first extensor compartment and *either* pain on resisted thumb extension *or* positive Finkelstein's test[a]
Wrist tenosynovitis	Pain on movement localized to tendon sheaths of the wrist *and* reproduction of the pain by resisted active wrist movement(s)
Carpal tunnel syndrome	Pain *or* paraesthesiae *or* sensory loss in the median nerve distribution *and ONE of* positive Tinel's test,[b] positive Phalen's test,[c] nocturnal exacerbation of symptoms, motor loss and wasting of abductor pollicis brevis, abnormal nerve conduction studies
Non-specific diffuse forearm pain	Pain in the forearm in the absence of specific diagnosis (above or other) (may include loss of function, allodynia, tenderness, weakness, cramp, slowing of fine movements)

[a] Pain on ulnar deviation of the wrist with the thumb straight, adducted against the border of the index finger; a variation of Finkelstein's test describes the thumb flexed and enclosed in the palm by the fingers.

[b] Pain or paraesthesia in the median nerve distribution on percussion over the nerve at the carpal tunnel.

[c] Pain or paraesthesia on maximal passive wrist flexion (elbows on table, forearms up) for 60 seconds.

each is associated with definitive objective clinical signs and neither requires the condition to be attributed to a repetitive activity nor to the person's occupation. These disorders can be broadly grouped according to the pathological site of injury.

In *tenosynovitis*, there is inflammation of the synovium within a tendon sheath. While the term tenosynovitis, colloquially called 'teno', is widely used for any hand pain associated with work, this is inaccurate as the term should not be used when synovium is normal, and a causative association between occupation and true tenosynovitis is rarely noted. Neither has a correlation with overuse in other settings been established, though, undoubtedly, those with tenosynovitis will find repetitive use of the affected limb painful.

In contrast, most consider peritendonitis to be related to overuse (in sports or in occupational settings). Almost a century ago, von Frisch found oedema with congestion of the peritendinous tissues, mainly at the musculotendinous junction, and this is associated with crepitus on palpation of the moving tendon.

The terms *tendinitis* and *tendinosis* are often used interchangeably in the literature. The former term should be reserved for acute lesions, in which there is an inflammatory infiltrate, the latter term denoting a chronic state where myxoid degeneration of the substance of the tendon is the dominant pathological picture. A mild chronic inflammatory exudate is sometimes seen. Increasingly, these changes are believed to accumulate as a result of repeated microtrauma, possibly mediated by release of interleukin-1β (IL-1β) and tumor necrosis factor-α (TNFα) from inflammatory cells during acute exacerbations. Of interest, a tendon's tolerance to deformation by a load (elasticity) appears to be reduced in women, (in whom these conditions are generally more common) though explanations relating this to oestrogen levels are contested.[7]

Stenosing tenovaginitis is the preferred term for de Quervain's disease. There is increased vascularity and cellular infiltration resulting in fibrous thickening of the sheath(s) enclosing the tendons of abductor pollicis longus and/or extensor pollicis brevis (they may run in a common sheath or in two separate structures) and in the overlying extensor retinaculum. There is inflammatory proliferation of the epitendon and expansion of part of the tendon to form a nodule where the tendon passes into the narrowed sheath. This condition is characterized by pain on movement, particularly grasping and pinching, localized to the radial aspect of the wrist. This can occur on returning to work after a prolonged absence or, less commonly, may follow a change to unfamiliar work requiring rapid movements (discussed later).

Lateral epicondylitis is believed to arise principally from overexertion of the finger and wrist extensors. There is often a history of unaccustomed, repetitive use involving hand dorsiflexion. The pathological lesion remains uncertain, but is thought to involve tears in the tenoperiosteal junction of the common extensor origin at the lateral humeral epicondyle. Medial epicondylitis, though less common, is believed to result from similar mechanisms involving the finger and wrist flexors and their origin at the medial epicondyle.

Dupuytren's contracture affects up to a quarter of all male pensioners. The palmar fascia becomes thickened and contracted. Thomas and Clarke[8] found that Dupuytren's contracture was twice as common in 500 men with vibration-induced white finger compared with controls, and there are many other reports associating this disorder with working conditions.[9]

Carpal tunnel syndrome (CTS) is often ascribed to inflammation of the flexor tendons in the carpal tunnel resulting in compression of the median nerve. However, the association of CTS with a number of conditions such as pregnancy, diabetes, hypothyroidism, or rheumatoid arthritis suggests that pathogenic mechanisms may vary. Case-control studies have identified associations with activities in which the wrist is repeatedly flexed or extended, and with use of vibrating tools.

Muscular symptoms have been studied less extensively. Increases in serum creatinine kinase were found in a study of volunteers who experienced neck or shoulder pain following repetitive shoulder flexion exercises. A cross-sectional study[10] found abnormalities on biopsy of the first dorsal interosseus muscle, particularly noting a higher proportion of type 1 muscle fibres in cases versus controls and hypertrophy of all fibre types. Mitochondrial abnormalities were noted in both cases and controls. These findings were more marked in those with more severe symptoms but, as this is a cross-sectional study, it is not clear whether this correlation is causative or is a secondary effect of disuse.

Hand and arm problems in musicians

Musicians are prone to a variety of problems in the upper limb that produce significant disability—these include overuse syndromes, entrapment neuropathies, and focal dystonias. The diagnosis can be difficult as symptoms may be mild and occur only on playing. Episodes may be triggered by increased playing time and changes in repertoire, technique, or instrument. Problems occur in musicians of all ages and levels of skill. The weight of wind instruments frequently leads to pain in the first web space. In contrast, percussionists have a low prevalence of regional pain syndrome, possibly as their playing is more intermittent.

In reviewing several series of musculoskeletal injuries, Hoppmann and Patrone[11] reported that, of 178 injured musicians, 62 per cent had overuse syndromes, 18 per cent had nerve entrapment thoracic outlet syndrome, and 10 per cent had problems of motor control. Some of the musculoskeletal problems in musicians are listed in Table 3.

Diagnosis and management are helped by a detailed understanding of the instrument used and the specific dynamics of music making. Treatment must take into account the specific injury and the instrument played. Table 4 lists some of the treatments that are generally applicable. Greater consideration is being given to the ergonomics of playing music, technique being assessed as a significant risk factor.

Table 3 Musculoskeletal problems in musicians

Overuse injury
Tenosynovitis (specific sites)
Non-specific diffuse forearm pain
Entrapment neuropathies
Focal dystonia
Thoracic outlet syndrome
Hypermobility syndrome
Osteoarthritis

Table 4 Treatment of musculoskeletal injuries in musicians

Rest periods during practice
Correct posture
Consider muscle tone/movements that aggravate symptoms
Splints, exercise, adaptive devices
Relaxation/biofeedback techniques
NSAIDs/local steroid injections
Surgical treatment of nerve entrapment

Chronic upper limb pain

There remains a group of patients with arm pain that lacks the specific features or localizing signs of these named conditions. In the absence of an anatomical or pathological diagnosis, various terms have been used, of which *chronic upper limb pain* is currently preferred and is used throughout this chapter. Pain is the principal feature (Table 5) and may be associated with inability to perform routine work or household tasks. There may have been an ache in the arm, shoulder, or neck for some weeks before presentation, or symptoms may follow a specific soft-tissue injury. Pain may fluctuate with activity, emotional stress, or temperature changes. Up to 20 per cent develop more generalized pain involving the lower back, buttocks, or legs.

Generalized fatigue is common, and patients report disturbance of their usual sleep pattern with frequent waking and feeling tired in the morning. In addition, the patient describes dysaesthesia in the hand, poor grip strength, and may report a sensation of swelling though objective evidence is typically absent.

Vasomotor changes may be apparent in the forearm. Altered pain threshold such as tender points may be noted (typically in the first web space of the hand). There is no evidence of synovitis, tenosynovitis, or neurological abnormalities.

The RSI Advisory Committee to the Department of Industrial Relations in New South Wales, Australia, proposed the following staging of the disorder.

Stage 1: Weeks to months of aching or weakness without physical signs, occurring during work activity, improving with time off work. This stage is reversible.

Stage 2: Persisting for months; onset of symptoms is more rapid, with difficulty remaining at work. Physical signs (tenderness, etc.) may be present. Treatment is more difficult at this stage.

Stage 3: Symptoms present at rest; sleep and non-occupational activities disrupted; unable to carry out light duties. Prognosis for recovery is poor.

Aetiology

In the absence of recognized pathological processes or injury, a number of theories have been proposed to explain chronic upper limb pain. These include ideas based on dynamic or vascular aspects of muscle function, or on a neurogenic model. These will be discussed first, before considering occupational factors that have been implicated in the aetiology of work-related upper-limb pain.

Table 5 Features of chronic upper limb pain

Chronic pain in one or both hands, arms, neck, or chest wall

Affecting activities (often repetitive) requiring controlled posture

Inability to achieve previous level of work or leisure performance

Variable subjective hand, forearm, or upper arm swelling

Poor grip strength, taut proximal muscles

Poor sleep pattern, often with mood changes

Mild vasomotor features

Psychological factors often contributory

The vascular hypothesis

This theory[12] is based on observations that, at low loads, diastolic rather than mean blood pressure determines muscle perfusion. During prolonged eccentric contraction without variation in muscle fibre length, muscle oedema develops. Even at 10 per cent of maximum voluntary contraction, pressures of 40–60 mmHg have been recorded in the flexor compartment of the forearm. Pressures of over 30 mmHg maintained for 8 hours or more have been shown to result in muscle necrosis, potentially mediated by free radicals and cytosolic free calcium (which is normally returned to the sarcoplasmic reticulum but requires up to 30 per cent of available energy for this active transportation). A variation of the vascular hypothesis has been proposed by researchers who noted reduced resting and post-exercise diameter of the radial artery in individuals with diffuse forearm pain. This group also had a reduced brachial artery response to ischaemia. This has been related to inhibition of endothelial nitric oxide synthetase, though the cause of such inhibition remains obscure. Neither mechanism explains the abnormalities in tendons or their synovial sheaths identified in some conditions.

Cinderella fibres

Here, it is believed that only a proportion of muscle fibres is recruited throughout the duration of low-load isometric activities.[13] However, these fibres are also required for higher load concentric and eccentric contraction, and so are never rested—hence the term 'Cinderella fibres'. Through poorly understood mechanisms, these fibres then induce pain that is initially relieved by rest but progressively appears within a shorter time at work. An important implication of this theory is that the person's activities both in and outside of work contribute to the condition. Thus, resting only from work may not correct the problem. As with the vascular hypothesis, this model also concentrates on the muscular symptoms characteristic of the diffuse upper limb pain pattern without signs, and does not satisfactorily explain other upper limb disorders associated with repetitive use.

The neurogenic hypothesis

In this model, perineural inflammation is caused by a minor injury or trauma during activity.[14] Fibrous connective tissue forms between the nerve and the surrounding structures, tethering the nerve and limiting its movement during activity. Joints maintained at the end of range stretch the nerve as it is unable to glide normally (termed adverse neural tension), causing pain and occasionally paraesthesiae. There is reduced tolerance in the nerve to compression injury, both at sites of tethering and at distal (e.g. hand) and proximal sites (e.g. at the neck and shoulder). This is reflected in the diffuse muscular tenderness (hyperalgesia) and allodynia (pain from innocuous stimuli) experienced by these patients. The conductive function of the nerve at rest is minimally impaired or even normal, explaining the normal nerve conduction studies, that are often observed.

Occupational factors

As described earlier, chronic upper limb pain disorders have almost exclusively been associated with repetitive strain in the workplace—overuse injuries in athletes have many similarities but are not normally considered in this group. The relative contribution of occupational factors, the individual's anthropomorphic measures, and psychological factors is controversial.

The relation between carpal tunnel syndrome and work has been studied extensively. Using an electrophysiological definition of CTS, Gerr and Letz[15] found that 81.5 per cent of the variation in incidence in an industrial workforce could be attributed to body-mass index, age, and the ratio of wrist width to depth. In contrast only 8.3 per cent of variation was attributable to work factors. However, another group used an 'attributable fraction' (calculated as [odds ratio−1]/[odds ratio]), noting that workload factors accounted for 50–90 per cent of cases of CTS.

Viikari-Juntura[16] reviewed the effects of age, gender, and four work-related factors on common upper limb disorders (Table 6). Increasing age was only associated with rotator cuff tendonitis, while gender had no clear association. The female : male ratio varies from 16 : 1 for carpal tunnel syndrome (more women affected) to equal proportions being affected at other sites.[7] It remains unclear whether gender is a true aetiological factor or reflects the predominance of females in at-risk occupations. In the Australian National Occupational Health and Safety Commission's report,[17] production workers and clerical workers were considered at high risk of chronic upper limb pain (referred to in the report as repetitive strain injury). However, there were also high numbers of cases among labourers, tradesmen, farmers, and fishermen.

Work conditions implicated in upper limb pain disorders include the use of tools, particularly vibrating machinery, and the design of the workstation, particularly the posture of the neck and shoulder in carrying out the task. The force required, the repetitiveness of the task, and the duration for which the activity is continued without interruption have also been implicated (see Table 6). The combined number of repetitions and force generated varies considerably for different tasks. In one study, cases and controls were assessed during externally rated keyboarding tasks. Both groups generated 4–5 times the force required to activate the keys, but this force was greater in affected individuals. Conversely, the workers with the lowest rates of repetitive strain injury during the Australian 'epidemic' were those with the highest keystroke rates. Force was not assessed in this particular study, though it is notable that the group with the highest rates of RSI was telephone operators, where little force is required.

Static forces in muscles (especially in eccentric contraction) may be important contributory factors. High-precision, low-load activities (such as those of keyboard operators) require the wrist to be held in a fixed position as a stable platform for finger flexion operating the keys. Electromyography studies have demonstrated that fatigue occurs most commonly in muscles that do not vary in length over a prolonged period, whereas muscles in which contraction length and/or velocity varies rarely fatigue with low loads. Extreme angles of joints (corresponding to extremes of muscle contraction or extension) are also frequently associated with risk of symptoms.

Posture during activities has also been implicated in neck and shoulder pain. Typically, seated operators maintain a forward flexed attitude, with the shoulder flexed and abducted to elevate the forearm to the required operating height. The muscles involved are primary global mobilizers, mostly comprising fast-twitch fibres that produce high torque but fatigue rapidly. As the activity continues, these muscles tire and become weaker. Smaller, secondary stabilizer muscles then have to increase tone, resulting in painful cramping and stiffness. These muscles are unable to sustain the activity, reflecting the characteristic reduction in the time to symptom onset in later stages of chronic upper limb pain.

It has been said that two features unique to humans are their hands and the psyche. Psychological factors are notoriously difficult to assess and are particularly contentious in work-related upper limb pain (see 'Historical perspective', above). Compensation fraud has further obscured psychological influences on symptoms. Recently, Worker's Compensation adjusters in the United States reported that 19 per cent of claims were fraudulent.[18] Most people use their hands at work, and bring their psychological responses to stress, pain, and the working environment with them. While workplace stressors are felt to be significantly greater now than in the past, studies comparing self-assessment of stress at work by RSI cases and their asymptomatic colleagues found no difference in perceived stress levels. There are undoubtedly important interactions between disease, illness behaviour, and the ability or otherwise to continue in employment. However, it is important to bear in mind that the stressors influencing a person's symptoms may be located outside the working environment.

Management

The management of upper limb pain disorders is largely based on empirical evidence. Clinical trials have been small, varying in case definitions used and in duration of follow-up. Treatment paradigms

Table 6 Factors associated with the most common upper limb disorders (adapted from reference 16 and other data)[a]

Diagnosis	Rotator cuff tendonitis	Lateral epicondylitis	Extensor tenosynovitis	Carpal tunnel syndrome
Key movement	Shoulder abduction in flexion	Gripping with twist	Gripping or keying	Grip in non-neutral position; Vibrating tools
Associated with				
Age	Increases with age	?	Younger patients	?
Gender	+/−	+/−	+/−	+ (female)
Force of activity	+/−	+	+	+
Repetitions	+	+/−	+	+
Vibrations	−	?	?	++
Combinations	+	+	++	++

[a] ? Insufficient evidence; +, positive association; − no association; +/− conflicting studies.

for the more clearly defined conditions (such as epicondylitis or carpal tunnel sydrome) are generally supported by more robust trial evidence. Many alternative treatments have also been proposed though few have been formally validated.

A thorough review of the individual's circumstances is important, and should include:

1. previous occupations—were repetitive tasks involved? Were there symptoms?;

2. duration of work/task before onset of symptoms;

3. anatomical description of symptoms and progression;

4. work schedules and pacing, incentives for overtime;

5. experience of symptoms outside of work, e.g. during sports, domestic chores;

6. period from onset of symptoms to first seeking advice—from whom?;

7. previous interventions and response—involvement of employer/occupational health staff.

Underlying conditions should specifically be sought (such as hypothyroidism, acromegaly, other infiltrative diseases, vasculitis). In addition to occupational factors, often readily volunteered, domestic difficulties, psychological stresses, and sleep pattern are relevant. This ensures an empathic response to the patient's symptoms and concerns about their workplace, while ensuring that underlying factors that might impair a successful outcome are identified.

A careful physical examination includes passive and resisted tests to identify localizing signs. This can also determine the degree of available movement, grip, etc. Dynamometers (to assess grip strength) have been devised that are reliable in detecting those who fail to make a genuine maximal effort on testing.

A detailed assessment of the individual's workstation, equipment and environment (lighting, noise, temperature) may not be possible or practical, but should be considered in difficult cases where litigation is being considered or where symptoms have returned after successful treatment. Identifying modifiable factors in the workplace without implying liability may be difficult, but is an essential component of secondary prevention.

Investigations may be undertaken if there is a high clinical suspicion of localized pathology. However, undirected negative investigations are wasteful and counterproductive as they may give the impression that an injury has not been found, rather than reassuring the patient that there has been no tissue damage. High-resolution ultrasound and magnetic resonance imaging (MRI) are the most sensitive when indicated; the former has the advantage of allowing dynamic testing.

Tenosynovitis, tendinitis, epicondylitis, bursitis

In the acute setting, these lesions respond to rest of the affected part. Splinting is appropriate, provided the patient has a clear understanding that this is a short-term measure before beginning rehabilitative therapy—otherwise, muscle atrophy may ensue. Corticosteroid injections are the mainstay of treatment, although randomized controlled trials do not support their use in every setting. Overall, injection was effective in 84 per cent of mixed upper limb disorders, compared with 66 per cent for splinting. Hydrocortisone is recommended for soft-tissue lesions, as long-acting steroids such as methylprednisolone may lead to soft tissue atrophy and disfiguring skin lesions, particularly with superficial injections (e.g. epicondylar injection). Injection into the substance of a tendon must be avoided, as there are concerns that steroid is harmful. (While cases of tendon rupture following injection are reported, studies have also suggested that rupture will only occur in an already degenerate tendon and that intrasubstance injection into a normal tendon requires a very high pressure, thus being easily recognized). Lignocaine is added to relieve the discomfort of injection. The anaesthetic effect also allows confirmation that the lesion injected is responsible for the patient's symptoms. Injections into a tendon sheath follow the same principle, the distal joint being moved before injection to ensure the needle has not entered the tendon itself. Tendinitis affecting the rotator cuff is treated by injecting into the subacromial bursa, and bursitis at other sites may be similarly injected.

Resistant tenosynovitis, epicondylitis, and de Quervain's stenosing tenovaginitis may also be managed surgically. When formally studied, outcomes for surgery as a first-line treatment are no better than for injection.

Carpal tunnel syndrome

Among keyboard operators, splinting has been found to be effective to relieve work-induced symptoms. However, it is rarely curative. Corticosteroid injections are effective in 60–70 per cent of cases where an underlying cause is excluded. In a randomized controlled trial, 25 mg hydrocortisone was as effective as higher doses or as long-acting triamcinolone. The injection is usually directed under the flexor retinaculum on the ulnar side of the palmaris longus tendon, though a more proximal wrist injection technique has been described. Surgical decompression of the carpal tunnel is effective in over 90 per cent of cases, though it necessitates a prolonged recovery period.

Chronic upper limb pain

It is important to establish a positive diagnosis of chronic upper limb pain at an early stage (though it is a diagnosis of exclusion). The outcome is poorer when intervention is delayed, particularly if the patient has previously had one or more other upper limb disorders incorrectly diagnosed. The patient must be reassured there is no tissue damage. An explanation in terms of muscle strain and fatigue resulting in tightening of muscles and/or nerve compression (as appropriate to the individual's symptoms) may aid the patient's understanding, encouraging their participation in a rehabilitative programme.

A multidisciplinary team employing a biopsychological approach to treatment is ideal in the management of chronic upper limb pain.

The physician's main role is to establish the diagnosis, excluding contributory factors, and consider pharmacological interventions as appropriate. Tricyclic antidepressants (e.g. 10–50 mg amitriptyline, taken at about 6 p.m. to avoid morning drowsiness) are useful in relieving neuropathic pain and regaining a restorative sleep pattern. The more selective selective serotonin reuptake inhibitor (SSRI)-type anti-depressants are better tolerated but generally less effective in this setting. Anxiolytics or antispasmodic drugs (benzodiazepines are better than baclofen or methacarbamol) may be helpful if there is considerable muscle spasm inhibiting stretching and mobilization exercises. Generally, simple analgesics and nonsteroidal anti-inflammatory drugs (NSAIDs) are inappropriate in chronic upper limb pain.

The physiotherapist will direct a graduated exercise programme for the relevant muscles, developing aerobic fitness, muscle endurance and correcting imbalance between mobilizing and stabilizing groups of muscles. Acute, localized complaints may be treated with ice or with ultrasound (though objective evidence for these is limited).

Occupational therapists, particularly those with a specialist interest in work-related upper limb disorders, can offer expert advice on adaptations in the workplace, short-term use of splints, split keyboards, etc. For example, a volar splint (holding the wrist in mild extension), worn at night and selectively by day, is useful for localized symptoms in the wrist or for de Quervain's disease.

While evidence exists that adverse ergonomic factors play a part, the role of psychosocial factors in the causation of symptoms is more problematic. The involvement of a clinical psychologist may only be appropriate if the patient accepts that psychological factors are a significant component in their presentation.

Occupational health practitioners are an important part of the multidisciplinary team (often a nurse specialist in the workplace) though it is important to have the consent of the patient. None the less, the value of the preventive measures discussed above should be emphasized to the patient.

Rehabilitation and prevention

The rehabilitative and preventative aspects of a patient's care are critical to a successful return to work, irrespective of any other treatment used. The advice 'if it hurts, stop' runs contrary to all accepted principles of behavioural management of chronic pain and may lead to chronicity. Job rotation, rest breaks, and a graduated rehabilitation programme may be necessary.[19] Success depends upon informed assessment of risk, a sharing of information between medical personnel and employees, and the implementation by managers of risk-reduction measures. These include advice and training to ensure better working practices and suitable induction of new staff. Work with visual display units now falls under the Health and Safety Regulations of 1992, which are based on the premise that use of visual display units is associated with musculoskeletal effects, visual fatigue, and mental stress that can be helped by simple ergonomic principles.[20]

References

1. Cleland, L.G. (1987). RSI: a model of social iatrogenesis. *Med. J. Aust.* **147**, 236–237.
2. Urwin, M., Symmons, D., Allison, T. *et al.* (1998). Estimating the burden of musculoskeletal disorders in the community: the comparative prevalence of symptoms at different anatomical sites, and their relation to social deprivation. *Ann. Rheum. Dis.* **57**, 649–655.
3. Palmer, K., Coggon, D., and Cooper, C. (1998). Work related upper limb disorders: getting down to specifics. *Ann. Rheum. Dis.* **57**, 445–446.
4. Melhorn, J.M. (1998). Cumulative trauma disorders and repetitive strain injuries: the future. *Clin. Orthop.* **351**, 107–126.
5. Harrington, J.M., Carter, J.T., Birrell, L., and Gompertz, D. (1998). Surveillance case definitions for work related upper limb pain syndromes. *Occup. Environ. Med.* **55**, 264–271.
6. Palmer, K., Walker-Bone, K., Linaker, C., Kellingray, S., Reading, I., Coggon, D., and Cooper C. (2000). The Southampton examination schedule for the diagnosis of musculoskeletal disorders of the upper limb. *Ann. Rheum. Dis.* **59**, 5–11.
7. Hart, D.A., Archambault, J.M., Kydd, A., Reno, C., Frank, C.B., and Herzog, W. (1998). Gender and neurogenic variables in tendon biology and repetitive movement disorders. *Clin. Orthop.* **351**, 44–56.
8. Thomas, P.R. and Clarke, D. (1992). Vibration white finger and Dupuytren's contracture: are they related? *J. Soc. Occup. Med.* **42**, 155–158.
9. Liss, G. and Stock, S. (1996). Can Dupuytren's contracture be work-related? A review of the evidence. *Am. J. Ind. Med.* **29**, 521–532.
10. Dennett, X. and Fry, H.J.H. (1988). Overuse syndrome: a muscle biopsy study. *Lancet* **8591 i**, 905–908.
11. Hoppmann, R.A. and Patronne, N.A. (1989). A review of musculoskeletal problems in instrumental musicians. *Semin. Arthritis Rheum.* **19**, 117–126.
12. Pritchard, M.H., Pugh, N., Wright, I., and Brownlee, M. (1999). A vascular basis for repetitive strain injury. *Rheumatology* **38**, 636–639.
13. Sjøgaard, G. and Søgaard, K. (1998). Muscle injury in repetitive motion disorders. *Clin. Orth.* **351**, 21–31.
14. McKinnon, S.E. and Novak, C.B. (1997). Clinical perspectives: repetitive strain in the workplace. *J. Hand Surg. (Am.)* **22A**, 2–18.
15. Gerr, F. and Letz, R. (1992). Risk factors for carpal tunnel syndrome in industry: blaming the victim? *J. Occup. Med.* **34**, 1117–1119.
16. Viikari-Juntura, E. (1998). Risk factors for upper limb disorders. *Clin. Orthop.* **351**, 39–43.
17. Australian National Occupational Health and Safety Commission (1986). *Repetition strain injury (RSI): a report and model code of practice.* Australian Government Publishing Service, Canberra.
18. Sheon, R.P. with members of the Goff Group (1997). Repetitive strain injury: an overview of the problem. *Postgrad. Med.* **102**, 53–71.
19. Higgs, P., Young, V.L., Seaton, M., Edwards, D., and Feely, C. (1992). Upper extremity impairment in workers performing repetitive tasks. *Plast. Reconstr. Surg.* **90**, 614–620.
20. Health and Safety Executive (1992). *Health and safety (display screen equipment) regulations, 1992.* HMSO, London.
21. Coggon, D., Palmer, K.T., and Walker-Bone, K. (2000). Occupation and upper limb disorders. *Rheumatology* **39**, 1057–1059.
22. James, M. and Wynn-Parry, C.B. (1992). Performing arts medicine. *Br. J. Rheum.* **31**, 795.
23. Levenstein C. (1999). Economic losses from repetitive strain injuries. *Occup-Med.* **14**, 149–161.
24. Ramel, E. and Moritz, V. (1994). Self-reported musculoskeletal pain and discomfort in professional ballet dancers in Sweden. *Scand. J. Rehab. Med.* **26**, 11–16.
25. Yassi, A. (1997). Repetitive strain injuries. *Lancet* **349**, 943–947.

6.14 Hypermobility

Howard Bird

Definition of hypermobility

Articular hypermobility, perhaps better termed joint hyperlaxity, describes the possession by an individual of a joint or joints with a much wider range of movement than average. A single joint or many joints may be so affected. The term does not define aetiology since many factors contribute to a wide range of movement at a joint and several may contribute. The threshold at which the syndrome can be defined remains the subject of debate, not least because the range of movement at a given joint displays a Gaussian distribution in a population. The cut-off point above which generalized hypermobility is held to be present is therefore somewhat arbitrary. Hyperlaxity is not synonymous with reduced joint stiffness though rheologically this is often present. Neither does it equate with functional disability, though in many circumstances hyperlax joints do contribute to impairment of function and often produce symptoms of pain and sometimes, paradoxically, stiffness.

The most common variant, diagnosed on clinical grounds, is 'benign joint hypermobility syndrome' (BJHS), though hypermobility may also be a feature of rare inherited connective tissue disorders including Ehlers–Danlos syndrome (EDS), Marfan's syndrome, and osteogenesis imperfecta amongst others. These conditions account for only a very small proportion of examples encountered, though some consider there may be overlap between these discrete structural abnormalities of connective tissue, for which faulty genes are known or may be suspected, and the more benign variant (BJHS).

Acquired inflammatory disease may also promote joint hyperlaxity either by damage to collagen or by the stretching effect of an effusion and by the drugs used in the treatment of this (e.g. prednisolone and D-penicillamine), but this will not be considered further in this chapter.

Diagnostic criteria and standard scoring systems

The simple clinical scoring system in most common use is that proposed by Beighton *et al.* in 1973.[1] This evolved from a scoring system originally devised by Carter and Wilkinson in 1964,[2] which was subsequently subjected to serial amendments.[3, 4] The Beighton score is depicted in Table 1 (Figs 1 and 2).

The Beighton scoring system is simple, taking just a few seconds, hyperextension at the elbow and knee being measured with a simple angle goniometer or even by eye. The use of the little finger is preferred to the use of other fingers since the latter excludes too many persons. Although the inclusion of ankle movements has been suggested, they tend to show little variation between individuals in a

Table 1

1. Passive dorsiflexion of the little fingers beyond 90° (one point for each hand) – two points

2. Passive apposition of the thumbs to the flexor aspects of the forearm (one point for each thumb) – two points

3. Hyperextension of the elbows beyond 10° (one point for each elbow) – two points

4. Hyperextension of the knee beyond 10° (one point for each knee) – two points

5. Forward flexion of the trunk with knees fully extended so that palms of the hands rest flat on the floor – one point.

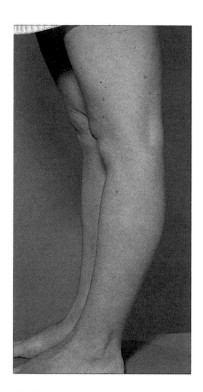

Fig. 1 Hyperextensible knee joints

normal population. It should be recalled that forward flexion of the trunk, a measure of composite joint movement, often segregates from the other four features in epidemiological studies. A study on 502 normal adult South African Blocks in which 94 per cent of males and 80 per cent of females achieved scores of 0, 1, or 2, is fairly typical of the sensitivity of this instrument.[1]

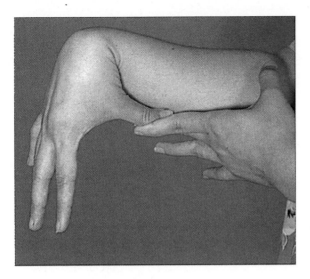

Fig. 2 Hyperextensible joints affecting the thumb with wrists.

An alternative scoring system from Contompasis,[5] described in detail by Poul and Fait,[6] is more complex, providing a maximum score of 72, but has not gained general acceptance. It is now only occasionally used,[7] mainly because it takes so long. It is hard to remember and describe and adds little to the simplified Beighton[1] scoring system.

More recent criteria for the definition of BJHS have been proposed by Mishra *et al.*[8]. Also simple, these diagnostic criteria incorporate extraarticular features characteristically associated with inherited joint hyperlaxity.

Comparison of alternative scoring systems

A seminal paper from Bulbena *et al.*[9] compared the Carter and Wilkinson 1964 scoring system with a new system popular in France[10] and found the 1964 version, even before its 1973 modification, was as effective as any. The 1973 modification remains the most satisfactory for simple use in general rheumatology clinics to alert suspicion to the possibility of joint hypermobility.

With increased attention to aetiology, however, the desirability of more sophisticated measurements, perhaps restricted to a single joint, became appreciated. A comprehensive account of the ranges of joint movement that can be measured throughout the body with simple goniometry is to be found in a booklet published by the American Academy of Orthopaedic Surgeons in 1965.[11] The sums of all the measured arcs of movement have been incorporated into a 'global index'[12] for comparison with simpler systems. In parallel, sophisticated mechanical devices have been invented to accurately measure serial change in the range of movement at a single joint. An example is the Leeds finger hyperextensometer[13] that is depicted in Fig. 3. A preset torque (in practice 2.6 kg cm^{-1}) is applied to the index finger of the hand, and the resulting angle of hyperextension recorded on a dial. This has proved accurate to one or two degrees and allowed the first demonstration of enhanced peripheral joint laxity prior to parturition in pregnant females,[14] probably attributable to circulating serum relaxin,[15] which combines with the weight of the gravid uterus to expand the pelvis prior to delivery.

A subsequent study of the hyperextensometer showed it conveyed more applied information at the joint measured, only partially

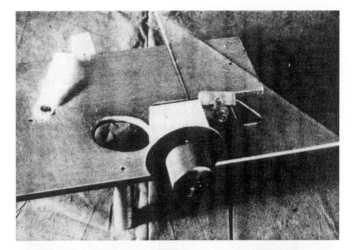

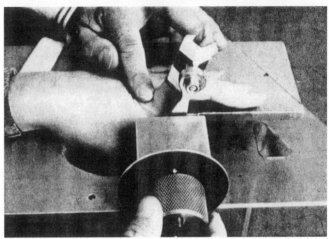

Fig. 3 A finger hyperextensometer for the quantification of joint laxity. The finger of the subject is hyperextended at the metacarpophalangeal joint by the application of a pre-set fixed torque. The resultant angle of hyperextension is read off on the dial.

correlating with the Beighton (1973) score. When correlations were sought between the ranges of movement at different joints in the same hyperlax individual, the greatest correlations were observed between joints of comparable anatomical structure (e.g. the shoulder correlating with the hip; the elbow correlating with the knee).

Epidemiology

The range of normal joint movement decreases rapidly throughout childhood and more slowly in adulthood. This has been confirmed in Edinburgh children,[16] a South African population,[1] and London children.[17] Joint laxity continues to diminish throughout adult life.[3]

The joints of females are invariably more lax than comparable joints in age-matched males,[18] although this has been disputed by some authors[17] and is not always seen in the spine. The concept of pauci-articular hypermobility, that is hypermobility restricted to just a small number of joints (and therefore by implication resulting from causes other than collagen structure) has been reviewed in detail by Larsson *et al.*[19]

(a)

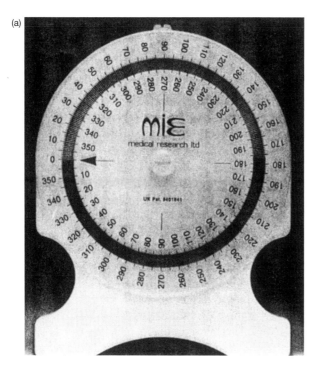

(b)

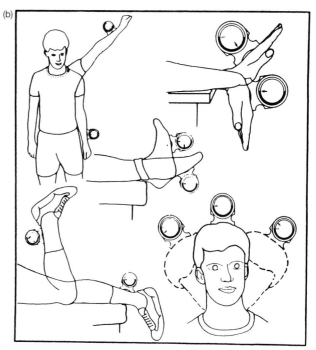

Fig. 4 (a) A clinical goniometer capable of measuring arcs of movement in any direction. Manufactured by MIE Medical Research Ltd, 6 Wortley Moor Road, Leeds LS12 4JF, UK. (b) The goniometer in use.

In the adult, joints in the dominant hand are invariably less lax (by a factor of some 10 per cent) compared to those in the non-dominant hand. This is normally attributed to the increased muscular tone in the forearm that develops with literacy.

The study of interethnic variation is in its infancy. Considering the thumb, Asian Indians show more hyperextension than Africans who in turn have more hyperextension than Europeans.[18] Similar results have been obtained by comparing the finger joints of these different racial groups in the same country (southern Africa).[20] Some races may be endowed with particular laxity. A recent study from Iraq suggests that this may be the case there.[21] Even Hippocrates drew attention to the remarkable joint laxity in Scythians, a race inhabiting the region a little to the north of Iraq in antiquity.

Regular training undoubtedly affects the range of movement, either due to alteration in muscle control or stretching of the joint capsule.[22] It is therefore important to specify whether an individual measured is 'warmed up' or participating in a physical training programme,[23] the increase in range of movement achieved by applying 'warm up' being substantial. Sophisticated studies in athletes have also demonstrated a diurnal variation in joint hypermobility, the effect most marked in late afternoon and least in the early morning, correlating well with and therefore probably partly attributable to diurnal variation in plasma cortisol.

The spine is a complex set of joints, capable of some compensation in the presence of local injury, so simple surface techniques that measure the range of the whole spine through goniometry only tell part of the picture.[24] Plumb-line techniques have been described but the hydrogoniometer (Fig. 4) is probably the simplest method of measurement both for the spine and for peripheral joints. For the spine it becomes important to specify the level at which the angle of movement is measured. More sophisticated techniques, including stereoradiography, vector stereography, and three-dimensional optical systems are available,[25] but may yet be superseded by systems such as the Polehemus Navigation Sciences 3 Space Isotrak system in specialist centres, a technique that has proved capable of confirming the diurnal variation in spinal movement throughout a 24-hour period.[26]

Aetiology

Seminal studies performed by Johns and Wright in 1962[27] sectioned various tissues in turn at the wrist joint of anaesthetized cats. An arthrographic technique quantified the extent to which each separate tissue contributed to the rheological phenomenon of stiffness. The joint capsule contributed 47 per cent, passive action of the muscles 41 per cent, the tendons 10 per cent, and the restraining action of the skin 2 per cent. However, this represents a single joint and rheology does not necessarily correlate with the range of joint movement.

Based upon epidemiological evidence it has been argued that three main determinants need to be considered in the pathogenesis of joint hyperlaxity:[28] bony surfaces; collagen; and neuromuscular control. In addition, the role of proprioception has recently also attracted attention.

Bony surfaces

The characteristics of joints vary considerably in the body from those that make up the vault of the skull, allowing no movement, to ball and socket joints such as the hip and shoulder, allowing maximum movement. Between these two extremes various adaptions have evolved to modify the range of movement. At the elbow there is bony locking to prevent hyperextension, though the increase in carrying angle in women allows for a greater degree of hyperextension at this joint than in males. At the ankle, lateral movement is restricted by bony prominences. The knee, a hinge joint, depends upon its ligaments for stability.

Local inherited bony modification may alter this. A shallow acetabulum, for example, contributes substantially to congenital dislocation of the hip,[29, 2] and there is a strong suspicion that this group, in whom hyperlaxity is often restricted to the hip and the shoulder, may be susceptible to premature osteoarthritis localized to those sites. Up to the age of epiphyseal fusion at puberty, however, the shape of the bone may be influenced to some extent by external forces in the form of vigorous training.

Collagen

There is substantial scope for variation between the amino acid content of the chains, the extent to which these are twisted (which also confers strength), and the extent to which these are further consolidated by disulfide bridges (the phenomenon that accounts for the increased stiffness in collagen with ageing). The density of packing of the collagen fibres within a tissue, perhaps ligament or tendon, may be influenced by stress but the majority of variation in collagen structure between individuals is inherited.

A characteristic of inherited collagen weakness as the main contributing factor is the widespread distribution of joint laxity, and such individuals score highly overall on the Beighton 1973 system, particularly at the fingers, thumb base, and knees.

Basic biomechanics have been performed on collagen,[17] mainly in the tails of rats. After an initial brief alignment of the force/extension curve, there follows an essential linear extension during which Hooke's law is obeyed. At a certain point, a failure of individual fibres occurs and the tendon ruptures. By contrast, elastin fibres can undergo appreciable extension under the action of relatively small forces, returning to their original dimension when the force is removed. Elastin accounts for the elasticity of the skin and a characteristic of joint hypermobility related to inherited collagen structure is that the skin is often elastic as well, sometimes bruising easily.

Neuromuscular control

The importance of neurological 'servo' mechanisms in allowing joint stability to be altered is well recognized by sporting coaches and forms the basis for the methods of proprioceptive neuromuscular facilitation that can enhance the range of joint movement in athletic training.[30, 31] Massage and warmth may also help,[32] and the enhanced range of movement achieved through yoga and other relaxation techniques attests to the importance of this. The integrity of the Golgi tendon organs and muscle spindles is thus important in determining the range of joint movement, the quality and nature of muscle fibres also contributing in terms of their physiological ability to stabilize the joint and their anatomical bulk, which might act to impede the range of movement by creating an obstructive muscular mass. The widespread joint laxity often seen in Down syndrome may be a manifestation of this phenomenon, perhaps partly inherited but also largely acquired.

Proprioception

Proprioception is the ability of the individual, albeit subconsciously, to detect the precise position of a joint at any one time.

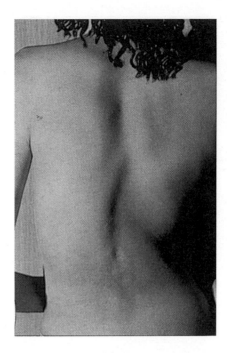

Fig. 5 A young woman with EDS VI having especially severe kyphoscoliosis and very obvious rib and chest deformities.

That joint laxity can lead to premature osteoarthritis in the accompaniment of neurological conditions as diverse as subacute combined degeneration of the cord, syringomyelia, and tabes dorsalis attests to the importance of adequate joint protection by the nervous system during normal life. Anecdotally, clinicians have felt for many years that 'joint instability' is more potent than 'joint hypermobility' alone in the pathogenesis of premature osteoarthritis. A slightly unstable, almost ataxic, gait is a characteristic of a proportion of patients with generalized hypermobility, and suspicion has recently concentrated on abnormal proprioception as a further contributing cause. This falls with age.[33] In animal experiments, low-threshold knee joint mechanoreceptors discharge maximally towards the extremes of the range of movement.[34] Powerful reflex effects on the limb muscles act to prevent hyperextension of a joint.[35] There is a correlation of abnormal proprioception acuity and joint hyperlaxity in the interphalangeal joint[36] and knee joint.[37] This research is in its infancy, not always adequately controlled, and further studies are needed to determine whether known non-weight-bearing joints that are lax with impaired proprioception are less susceptible to osteoarthritis than weight-bearing joints with impaired proprioception. Nevertheless, proprioception clearly needs to be considered in the list of causative factors.

Heritable hypermobility syndromes

The best known of these disorders is the EDS, (Fig. 5) characterized by the clinical triad of articular hypermobility, dermal hyperextensibility, and cutaneous scarring (Fig. 6).[38, 39] A recent reclassification has reduced the number of recognized variants from the 13 (that had replaced the original five) to six. This diversity provides an example of the way in which candidate genes are being increasingly recognized for

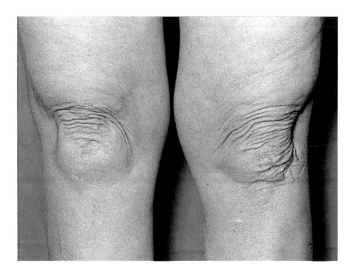

Fig. 6 Typical patellar scarring of EDS I. The velvety softness of the skin is also very apparent.

the relatively rare conditions. In the case of Marfan's syndrome, the fibrillin gene plays a role and the abnormality in osteogenesis imperfecta, which is also associated with joint hyperlaxity, is under active investigation.

Genetics

Clearly, any candidate genes identified for EDS, Marfan's syndrome, and osteogenesis imperfecta are not necessarily applicable to the BJHS, a condition segregated from the others by the lack of abnormal scar tissue, the lack of skin extensibility, and the lack of major skeletal deformity including kyphoscoliosis. Nevertheless, some have suggested that BJHS may be a mild form of such conditions, perhaps with incomplete penetration or perhaps ameliorated by hormonal influences. Of the different subgroups of EDS, the hypermobile variant (formerly EDS type III) was the candidate most likely to confuse. Benign hypermobile Marfanoid syndrome has also been described,[40] and in osteogenesis imperfecta joint laxity occasionally predominates over bony fracture.[41]

The possibility of a mutation in the genes encoding the chains for type V collagen (as in EDS types I and II), the genes for type I collagen and the procollagen N-proteinase (as in EDS type VII), or the fibrillin gene (as in Marfan-like syndromes) cannot be excluded. A comprehensive up-to-date review is available elsewhere.[42] Variation can occur at a multitude of sites, including the intracellular events in the biosynthesis of collagen and the extracellular events such as fibril assembly.

Although the protein polymer systems form the basis for the extracellular matrix of tendons, ligaments, and joint capsules, correct tissue function also depends on cell-mediated alignment of collagen fibrils and fibrillin microfibrils during the organization of the tissue. An increased understanding of the basic biology of tendons and ligaments, other than more general connective tissues, remains a prerequisite for the development of medical understanding of the genetic and acquired forms of joint hypermobility. Ultimately gene-specific treatment may follow but this still seems some way ahead.

Benign joint hypermobility syndrome

In many ways this is a diagnosis of exclusion. It implies individuals fulfilling diagnostic criteria, as specified above, in whom there is also no evidence of the more severe inherited disorders of connective tissue such as Ehlers–Danlos syndrome or Marfan's syndrome.

Prevalence

The true prevalence is unknown. Generalized ligamentous laxity, the prerequisite, is seen in perhaps 10 per cent of healthy individuals.[43] Pauci-articular hypermobility is even more prevalent. Amongst 660 North American students, 47 per cent of males and 78 per cent of females were identified as having at least one hypermobile joint.[44] Of 9275 patients attending a rheumatology clinic at Guy's Hospital, London in the 1980s, 2 per cent were diagnosed as suffering from BJHS.[45] There was a marked female preponderance in this series, as in most.

Articular features

Arthralgia and myalgia are common. The pathogenetic mechanism is obscure but unaccustomed physical exertion is a common predisposing factor. It has been postulated that there may be overstimulation of sensory nerve endings, poorly supported by defective collagen fibrils.[46] Changes in climate may contribute, particularly the onset of damp or cold weather. There may be a temporal relationship to menstruation (probably in the progestogen-dominated phase of the cycle) and progestogens and relaxin may account for the deterioration in symptoms during pregnancy. Physical activity may contribute.

Intriguingly, there appears to be a positive association between BJHS and epicondylitis and adhesive capsulitis. The reason for this is unclear, though the apparent association with nerve compression (e.g. carpal tunnel syndrome)[47] may be attributable to floppy tissues. There is more controversy over whether there is or is not an association with fibromyalgia as defined by the American College of Rheumatology (ACR) criteria.[48]

Chondromalacia patellae frequently occur and may be associated with genu recurvatum (hyperextensibility of the knee).[49]

If symptoms are present at a single joint there may be soft tissue swelling with an effusion and late chronic traumatic synovitis that can be identified by magnetic resonance imaging (MRI) scan. This may ultimately lead to the development of a popliteal (Baker's) cyst at the knee joint.

Joints sublux and dislocate easily, particularly the patella[50] and shoulder. Temporomandibular joint dysfunction, possibly through instability, is also associated.[51] Sometimes an anteromedial displacement of the disc occurs. This can be confirmed by MRI scan.

The association with premature osteoarthritis is more contentious. Scott *et al.*[52] compared joint mobility in a group of 50 consecutive patients aged 50 and over with symptomatic osteoarthritis with age- and sex-matched controls. There was a greater frequency of hypermobility amongst the individuals with osteoarthritis. A statistically significant association between joint hypermobility and osteoarthritis has also been established in a general rheumatology clinic ($p < 0.01$).[53] An Icelandic study[54] has shown that hypermobile patients were characterized more severely with thumb base osteoarthritis (though less severe osteoarthritis of the interphalangeal joints) whereas in non-hypermobile patients the converse was true.

Clearly, mechanical factors may be superimposed upon the genetic influence, for example, meniscoid tears (or even the old-fashioned operation of total meniscectomy, now largely superseded by partial meniscectomy, which leaves the rim of the meniscus intact with much less biomechanical insult).

In the spine, spondylolysis with or without isthmic spondylolisthesis is frequent in loose-jointed individuals.[55] The loose back syndrome[56] may be a milder variant. There is the anecdotal impression that these individuals are more susceptible to prolapsed intervertebral disc and radiological abnormalities of the spine, including scoliosis and transitional vertebrae at the lumbosacral junction, and partes interarticulares defects were found to be more common in a large radiological study.[57]

Bone fragility may occur in BJHS or may reflect overlap with osteogenesis imperfecta. Patients with BJHS may be more susceptible to stress fracture, though this is unusual and would normally prompt a consideration of diagnosis in case a more serious inherited abnormality had been missed. Whether prophylactic anti-osteoporotic therapy has any role in BJHS still has to be determined. At present, the decision should be guided by the results of a dual-energy X-ray absorptiometry (DEXA) scan when this is compared to that of age-matched non-hypermobile normals.

Extraarticular features

The skin is not infrequently thin and may be soft in texture. A significant correlation has been demonstrated between extensibility of the skin and joint hypermobility score.[8]

There is controversy about whether mitral valve prolapse occurs[58, 59] or is an artefact of the less strict criteria used before 1990.[8] In most series, aortic root dilatation, a feature of Marfan's syndrome, has not been seen in BJHS.

Some patients show eyelid abnormalities of which lid laxity is the most common. Occasionally, dislocation of the lenses means that this is more reminiscent of Marfan's syndrome.

Hernia occurs more frequently[60] as does rectal prolapse[61] and uterine prolapse.[62]

Spontaneous pneumothorax has long been recognized,[63] probably reflecting collagen fragility in the lung. A postal questionnaire survey has demonstrated an apparent increase in asthma, which is the subject of further investigation at present.[64]

Clinical features of associated disorders

EDS

Many of these overlap with BJHS but the spinal abnormalities, coupled with the lack of abnormalities in scar formation and/or the lack of aneurysm formation, allow the majority of cases to be separated.

Marfan's syndrome

This causes less confusion. Normally in Marfan's syndrome the long thin digits, the subluxation of the ocular lens, and the aortic and mitral valve disease provide confirmatory features.

Osteogenesis imperfecta

Classically, this is associated with bone fragility, blue sclerae, and wormian bones in the skull. Hypermobility of the digits is often seen and ligamentous laxity may play a part in the development of spinal abnormalities, which occur in a proportion of individuals. One rare form, the Bruck syndrome, is associated with articular rigidity rather than laxity.[65]

Differential diagnosis

The presence of appropriate diagnostic criteria, in particular with the demonstration of the joint hypermobility that forms an essential part of these, is normally enough to confirm an adequate clinical diagnosis. The situation is more complicated when the joint hypermobility is restricted to a small number of joints. Non-specific symptoms in the absence of demonstrable joint hypermobility would not normally be attributed to this diagnosis. The only major problem is therefore with rheumatic diseases that may mimic the condition in a patient who has borderline hypermobility, perhaps restricted to a small number of joints.

The principal causes for confusion are there.

1. *Fibromyalgia.* If the ACR diagnostic criteria are adhered to, there is normally no overlap between classic fibromyalgia and classic BJHS. The problem arises when localized joint hyperlaxity causes muscle pain that mimics the symptoms of fibromyalgia.

2. *Inflammatory polyarthritis.* If joint hyperlaxity is most pronounced at a small number of joints, a chronic traumatic synovitis may occur. This has been studied arthroscopically when it is sometimes associated with pyrophosphate deposition.[66] Classic inflammatory polyarthritis affects more joints and is associated with a greater degree of inflammation as judged by increased joint tenderness, a more angry effusion, and, at a later stage, X-ray change.

3. *Osteoarthritis.* Discussion continues on whether premature osteoarthritis is a natural result of BJHS. Sometimes osteoarthritis localized to a single joint causes laxity of the ligaments at that site by stretching.

4. *EDS.* The most likely overlap is the original type III, now defined as the hypermobile variant.

Investigation

With a clear-cut clinical diagnosis, investigation normally lacks relevance. If tiredness and myalgia predominate, it is judicious to arrange for a full blood count and full biochemical profile. Inflammatory arthritis is excluded by the presence of a normal C-reactive protein (CRP), viscosity, and/or erythrocyte sedimentation rate (ESR). Connective tissue disorders such as lupus are excluded by appropriate serology, as is rheumatoid arthritis, which also causes X-ray changes.

Affected joints, particularly if there is associated synovitis, may require imaging either by ultrasound or MRI scan or arthrography. Osteoarthritis may be present on X-ray at the worst affected joints.

Overall, investigation of the joints in hypermobile individuals adds little, except in injuries where associated pathologies are suspected.

Management

Rest

Particularly if symptoms are precipitated by acute soft tissue injury or strain, the hyperlax joint should be rested, if necessary with the use of a small local splint. Dynamic splinting may be helpful as the injury improves but widespread rest has less place in the management of BJHS. It is probably not appropriate to encourage children to rest their joints excessively if this restricts their activities.

Physiotherapy

There is some conflict of views here. Previously, gentle stretching was recommended but this only seems to suit a relatively small number of patients. Recent research has shown that exercise designed to strengthen the muscles around the most hyperlax joints not only reduces the range of movement but also relieves symptoms in the hyperlax joints. This would therefore now seem to be the approach of first choice, stretching perhaps being tried if stabilization of the joint proves ineffective. Massage and hydrotherapy may be helpful at the discretion of the physiotherapist.

Drug treatment

Analgesics will relieve pain. If paracetamol alone fails to help, the compound generic analgesics (co-proxamol, co-codamol, and co-dydramol, probably in that order) should be tried. More potent and expensive analgesics such as meptazinol and tramadol can be left in reserve.

Non-steroidal anti-inflammatory drugs (NSAIDs) may have a role, particularly if joints are inflamed as a result of trauma. Ibuprofen is probably the safest but naproxen, ketoprofen, diclofenac, and piroxicam, all provide generic alternatives that are inexpensive. A new range of selective COX-2 inhibitors has become available.

Topical applications may be helpful. These may be analgesics (e.g. felbinac gel) or NSAIDs (most of the generic preparations are available for topical application). Capsaicin, a counterirritant, may also have a role.

The role of steroid injections is more controversial. Steroids reduce the total amount of collagen and might be harmful but could be used judiciously in the case of persistent effusion.

Podiatry

Laxity of the ankle and foot region invariably leads to flattening of the longitudinal arch (pes planus). This may be accompanied by secondary pronation of the forefoot and, in severe cases, valgus deformity of the hindfoot. Appropriate orthoses are required to correct the biomechanical abnormality, relieving pain in the foot.[67]

Surgery

Where possible this should usually be avoided. Surgery is often technically more difficult because of fragility of tissues. Bleeding requires more precise control and may lead to the formation of a haematoma with a consequent greater risk of infection. Scarring can be unsightly. However, these problems are relatively insignificant compared to the general impression of a majority of hypermobile patients who have undergone surgery who invariably express disappointment with the results. By implication, biomechanics are already finely balanced and,

once altered, will not necessarily lead to better function unless the problem of recurrent dislocation was causing recurrent traumatic damage in its own right. Severe rupture of ligaments at the ankle or knee is probably best treated by open repair,[68] and persistent synovitis may be treated by synovectomy. A major problem, however, is delayed healing, particularly if there is laxity of the skin. Refractory trochanteric bursitis (often associated with a snapping hip in hyperlax individuals) may respond to partial excision of the iliotibial band.[69]

The main controversy is whether recurrent dislocation should be remedied by stabilizing surgery. The Trillat procedure for recurrent anterior shoulder dislocation, introduced in 1965, in which the coracoid process is osteotomized and tilted downward so that it serves as a bone block, has given excellent results in 73 per cent of patients.[70] Laser-assisted capsule shrinkage may play a role,[71] and this has sometimes been associated with arthroscopic replacement of the glenoid labrum reattachment in the treatment for chronic anterioinferior shoulder dislocation.[72] An arthroscopic multiple suture technique has been introduced for the treatment of recurrent posterior instability.[73]

In the hand and wrist, recurrent dislocation of the distal interphalangeal joint (Fig. 7) can be successfully treated by arthrodesis[74] and chronic subluxation of the dislocating inferior radioulnar joint may be treated with surgical reconstruction using the tendon of flexor carpi ulnaris.[75]

At the knee, the Krogius tenoplasty and pes anserinus transfer are probably not of value in hypermobile patients.[76, 77] Recurrent subluxation of the patella that fails to respond to conservative treatment (strengthening the quadriceps and vastus medialis and stretching the tight lateral structures) may be best treated by translocating the entire quadriceps and patella mechanism medially using the Insall procedure.[78]

For severe instability of the ankle, an operation passing the anterior part of the peroneus brevis tendon through the fibula and fastening it on to the talocalcaneum interosseum ligament may be performed.[79] An alternative procedure is the Brotstrom operation in which the torn ligament is reattached to the lateral malleolus or talus, depending on the site of the rupture.[80]

Instability of the talus has been successfully treated by a brace or reconstruction of the interosseous talocalcaneal ligament.[81]

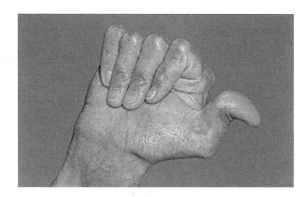

Fig. 7 Hyperextensible joints affecting the thumb with terminal phalanx with EDS IV.

Table 2

The Hypermobility Syndrome Association
PO BOX 1122
Nailsea, Bristol BS48 2YZ
Website: www.hypermobility.org

A support group, organized by people who are hypermobile themselves.
Please send a stamped, self-addressed envelope for more information.

Ehlers-Danlos Syndrome Support Group
PO BOX 335, Farnham,
Surrey GU10 1XJ
Website: www.ehlers-danlos.org

A support group which publishes a range of literature about this condition.
Please send a stamped, self-addressed envelope for more information.

Marfan Association UK
Rochester House, 5 Aldershot Road,
Fleet, Hants GU51 3NG
Website: www.marfan.org.uk

A support group which publishes a range of literature about this condition.
Please send a stamped, self-addressed envelope for more information.

Support and information

Patient self-help and support groups play an important role in providing information. The EDS Support Group has been conspicuously successful in printing a large number of pamphlets and handbooks about the condition. The addresses of the principal support groups are given in Table 2.

References

1. Beighton, P.H., Solomon, L., and Soskolne, C.L. (1973). Articular mobility in an African population. *Ann. Rheum. Dis.* **32**, 413–418.

2. Carter, C. and Wilkinson, J. (1964). Persistent joint laxity and congenital dislocation of the hip. *J. Bone Joint Surg. (Br.)* **46**, 40–45.

3. Kirk, J.A., Ansell, B.M., and Bywaters, E.G.L. (1967). The hypermobility syndrome. *Ann. Rheum. Dis.* **26**, 419–425.

4. Grahame, R. and Jenkins, J.M. (1972). Joint hypermobility—asset or liability. *Ann. Rheum. Dis.* **31**, 109–111.

5. McNerney, J.E. and Johnston, W.B. (1979). Generalised ligamentous laxity, hallux abducto valgus and the first metatarsocuneiform joint. *J. Am. Podiatr. Assoc.* **69**, 69–82.

6. Poul, J. and Fait, M. (1986). Genalisierte Bandalaxität bei Kindern. *Z. Orthop.* **124**, 336–339.

7. Morgan, A.W. and Bird, H.A. (1994). Conference report: special interest group for joint hypermobility. *Br. J. Rheumatol.* **33**, 1089–1091.

8. Mishra, M.B., Ryan, P., Atkinson, P., *et al.* (1996). Extra-articular features of benign joint hypermobility syndrome. *Br. J. Rheumatol.* **35**, 861–866.

9. Bulbena, A., Duro, J.C., Porta, M., Faus, S., Vallescar, R., and Martin-Santos, R. (1992). Clinical assessment of hypermobility of joints: assembling criteria. *J. Rheumatol.* **19**, 115–122.

10. Rotés, J. and Argany, A. (1957). La laxité articulaire considerée comme facteur des altérations de l'appareil locomoteur. *Rev. Rhum. Mal. Osteoartic.* **24**, 535–539.

11. American Academy of Orthopaedic Surgeons (1965). *Joint motion: method of measuring and recording.* Churchill Livingstone, Edinburgh.

12. Bird, H.A., Brodie, D.A., and Wright, V. (1979). Quantification of joint laxity. *Rheumatol. Rehabil.* **18**, 161–166.

13. Jobbins, B., Bird, H.A., and Wright, V. (1979). A joint hyperextensometer for the quantification of joint laxity. *Eng. Med.* **8**, 103–104.

14. Bird, H.A., Calguneri, M., and Wright, V. (1981). Changes in joint laxity occurring during pregnancy. *Ann. Rheum. Dis.* **40**, 209–212.

15. Maclennan, A.H., Green, R.C., Nicolson, R., and Bath, M. (1986). Serum relaxin and pelvic pain of pregnancy. *Lancet* **ii**, 243–245.

16. Wynne-Davis, R. (1970). Acetabular dysplasia and familial joint laxity: two aetiological factors in congenital dislocation of the hip. *J. Bone Joint Surg. (Br.)* **52**, 704–708.

17. Silverman, S., Constine, L., Harvey, W., and Grahame, R. (1975). Survey of joint mobility and *in vivo* skin elasticity in London schoolchildren. *Ann. Rheum. Dis.* **34**, 177–180.

18. Harris, H. and Joseph, J. (1949). Variation in extension of the metacarpophalangeal and interphalangeal joints of the thumb. *J. Bone Joint Surg. (Br.)* **31**, 547–549.

19. Larsson, L-G., Baum, J., and Mudholkar, G.S. (1987). Hypermobility: features and differential incidence between the sexes. *Arthritis Rheum.* **30**, 1426–1430.

20. Schweitzer, G. (1970). Laxity of metacarpophalangeal joints of the finger and interphalangeal joint of the thumb: a comparative interracial study. *S. Afr. Med. J.* **44**, 246–249.

21. Al-Rawi, Z.S., Al-Aszawi, A.J., and Al-Chalabi, T. (1985). Joint mobility among university students in Iraq. *Br. J. Rheumatol.* **24**, 326–331.

22. Atha, J. and Wheatley, D.W. (1976). The mobilising effects of treatment on hip flexion. *Br. J. Sports Med.* **10**, 22–25.

23. Barton, L., Bird, H.A., Lindsay, M., Newton, J., and Wright, V. (1995). The effect of different joint interventions on the range of movement at a joint. *J. Orthop. Rheumatol.* **8**, 87–92.

24. Hilton, R.C., Ball, J., and Benn, R.T. (1978). *In vitro* mobility of the lumbar spine. *Ann. Rheum. Dis.* **38**, 378–383.

25. Pearcy, M. (1986). Measurement of back and spinal mobility. *Clin. Biomech.* **1**, 44–51.

26. Russell, P., Weld, A., Pearcy, M.J., Hogg, R., and Unsworth, A. (1992). Variation in lumbar spine mobility measured over a 24-hour period. *Br. J. Rheumatol.* **31**, 329–332.

27. Johns, R.J. and Wright, V. (1962). Relative importance of various tissues in joint stiffness. *J. Appl. Physiol.* **17**, 824–828.

28. Bird, H.A. (1983). Joint and tissue laxity. In *Topical reviews of the rheumatic disorders*, Vol. 2 (ed. V. Wright), pp. 133–166. John Wright and Sons, Bristol.

29. Massie, W.K. and Howarth, M.B. (1951). Congenital dislocation of the hip. *J. Bone Joint Surg. (Am.)* **33**, 171–198.

30. Holt, L.E., Travis, T.M., and Okita, T. (1970). Comparative study of three stretching techniques. *Percept. Skills* **31**, 611–616.

31. Knott, M. and Voss, D.E. (1968). *Proprioceptive neuromuscular facilitation: patterns and techniques.* Harper and Rowe, New York.

32. Wiktorsson-Möller, M., Oberg, B., Aekstrand, J., and Gillguist, J. (1983). Effects of warming up, massage and stretching of range of motion and muscle strength in the lower extremity. *Am. J. Sports Med.* **11**, 249–252.

33. Ferrell, W.R., Crighton, A., and Sturrock, R.D. (1992). Position sense at the proximal interphalangeal joint is distorted in patients with rheumatoid arthritis of finger joints. *Expt. Physiol.* **77**, 675–680.

34. Ferrell, W.R. (1980). The adequacy of stretch receptors in the cat knee joint for signalling joint angle throughout a full range of movement. *J. Physiol.* **299**, 85–99.

35. Baxendale, R.H. and Ferrell, W.R. (1981). The effect of knee joint afferent discharge on transmission in flexion reflex pathways in decerebrate cats. *J. Physiol.* **315**, 231–242.

36. Malick, A.K., Ferrell, W.R., McDonald, A., and Sturrock, R.D. (1994). Impaired proprioceptive acuity at the proximal interphalangeal joint in patients with the hypermobility syndrome. *Br. J. Rheumatol.* **33**, 631–637.

37. Hall, M.G., Ferrell, W.R., Sturrock, R.D., Hamblen, D.L., and Baxendale, R.H. (1995). The effect of the hypermobility syndrome on knee joint proprioception. *Br. J. Rheumatol.* **34**, 121–125.

38. Ehlers, E. (1901). Cutis laxa, niegung zu Haemorrhagien in der Haut, Lockerung mehrer Artikulationen. *Derm. Z.* **8**, 173–175.

39. Danlos, M. (1908). Un cas de cutis laxa avec tumeurs par contusion chronique des coudes et des genoux (xanthome juvenile pseudodiabetique de MM Hallopeau et Mace de Lepinay). *Bull. Soc. Franc. Derm. Syph.* **19**, 70–72.

40. Viljoen, D. and Beighton, P. (1990). Marfan syndrome: a diagnostic dilemma. *Clin. Genet.* **37**, 417–422.

41. Weil, U.H. (1981). Osteogenesis imperfecta. *Clin. Orthop.* **159**, 6–10.

42. Kadler, K. and Wallis, G. (1999). The molecular basis of joint hypermobility. In *Hypermobility of joints*, 3rd edn (ed. P. Beighton, R. Grahame, and H. Bird), pp. 23–37. Springer-Verlag, London.

43. Birrell, F.N., Adebajo, A.O., Hazleman, B.L., and Silman, A.J. (1994). High prevalence of joint laxity in West Africans. *Br. J. Rheumatol.* **33**, 56–59.

44. Larrson, L.-G., Baum, J., and Mudholkar, G.S. (1987). Hypermobility: features and differential incidence between the sexes. *Arthritis Rheum.* **30**, 1426–1430.

45. Grahame, R. (1971). Clinical manifestations of the joint hypermobility syndrome. *Revmatologia (USSR)* **2**, 2024.

46. Child, A.H. (1986). Joint hypermobility syndrome: inherited disorder of collagen synthesis. *J. Rheumatol.* **13**, 239–242.

47. Francis, H., March, L.M., Terenty, T., and Webb, J. (1987). Benign joint hypermobility with neuropathies: (II) documentation and mechanism of tarsal tunnel syndrome. *J. Rheumatol.* **14**, 577–581.

48. Hudson, N., Starr, M.R., Esdaile, J.M., and Fitzcharles, M.-A. (1995). Diagnostic associations with hypermobility in rheumatology patients. *Br. J. Rheumatol.* **34**, 1157–1161.

49. Al-Rawi, Z. and Nessan, A.H. (1997). Joint hypermobility in patients with chondromalacia patellae. *Br. J. Rheumatol.* **36**, 1324–1327.

50. Runow, A. (1983). The dislocating patella. Etiology and prognosis in relation to joint laxity and anatomy of patella articulation. *Acta Orthop. Scand.* **202** (suppl.), 1–53.

51. Gage, J.P. (1985). Collagen biosynthesis related to temporomandibular joint clicking in childhood. *J. Prosthet. Dent.* **53**, 944–946.

52. Scott, D., Bird, H.A., and Wright, V. (1979). Joint laxity leading to osteoarthrosis. *Rheumatol. Rehabil.* **18**, 167–169.

53. Bridges, A.J., Smith, E., and Reid, J. (1992). Joint hypermobility in adults referred to rheumatology clinics. *Ann. Rheum. Dis.* **51**, 793–796.

54. Jonsson, J. and Valtysdottir, S.T. (1995). Hypermobility features in patients with hand osteoarthritis. *Osteoarthritis Cartilage* **3**, 1–5.

55. Morgan, A.W., Gibbon, W., and Bird, H.A. (1996). A controlled study of spinal laxity in subjects with joint hyperlaxity and Ehlers–Danlos syndrome [abstract]. *Br. J. Rheumatol.* **36** (Suppl. 1), 58.

56. Howes, R.J. and Isdale, I.C. (1971). The loose back: an unrecognised syndrome. *Rheumatol. Phys. Med.* **11**, 72–77.

57. Grahame, R., Edwards, J.C., Pitcher, D., Gabell, A., and Harvey, W. (1981). A clinical and echocardiographic study of patients with the hypermobility syndrome. *Ann. Rheum. Dis.* **40**, 541–546.

58. Propock, W.A. and Barlow, J.B. (1971). Aetiology and electrocardiographic features of the following posterior mitral leaflet syndrome: analysis of a further 130 patients with a later systolic murmur or non-ejection systolic click. *Am. J. Med.* **51**, 73–78.

59. Brown, O.R., Dermots, H., Kloster, J.E., Roberts, A., Menasche, V.D., and Beals, R.K. (1975). Aortic root dilatation and mitral valve prolapse in Marfan's syndrome. *Circulation* **52**, 651–657.

60. Wynne-Davies, R. (1971). Familial joint laxity. *Proc. R. Soc. Med.* **64**, 689–690.

61. Marshman, D., Percy, J., Fielding, I., and Delbridge, L. (1987). Rectal prolapse: relationship with joint mobility. *Aust. NZ J. Surg.* **57**, 827–829.

62. Al-Rawi, Z.S. and Al-Rawi, Z.T. (1982). Joint hypermobility in women with genital prolapse. *Lancet* i, 1439–1441.

63. Brear, S.G., Beton, D., Slaven, Y.M., and Honeybourne, D. (1984). Spontaneous pneumothoraces are associated with mitral valve prolapse. *Thorax* **39**, 219.

64. Morgan, A.W., Pearson, S.B., and Bird, H.A. (1996). Respiratory symptoms in Ehlers–Danlos syndrome and the benign joint hypermobility syndrome. *Arthritis Rheum.* **39**, S136.

65. Viljoen, D., Versfeld, G., and Beighton, P. (1989). Osteogenesis imperfecta with congenital joint contractures (Bruck syndrome). *Clin. Genet.* **36**, 122–126.

66. Bird, H.A., Tribe, C.R., and Bacon, P.A. (1978). Joint hypermobility leading to osteoarthritis and chondrocalcinosis. *Ann. Rheum. Dis.* **37**, 203–211.

67. Agnew, P. (1997). Evaluation of the child with ligamentous laxity. *Clin. Podiatr. Med. Surg.* **14**, 117–130.

68. Coughlin, L., Oliver, J., and Beretta, G. (1987). Knee bracing and anterolateral rotatory instability. *Am. J. Sports Med.* **15**, 161–163.

69. Zoltan, D.J., Clancy, W.G. Jr, and Keene, J.S. (1986). A new approach to snapping hip and refractory trochanteric bursitis in athletes. *Am. J. Sports Med.* **14**, 201–204.

70. Gerber, C., Terrier, F., and Ganz, R. (1988). The Trillat procedure for recurrent anterior instability of the shoulder. *J. Bone Joint Surg. (Br.)* **70**, 130–134.

71. Markel, M.D., Hayashi, K., Thabit, G., and Thielke, R.J. (1996). Changes in articular capsular tissue using holmium:YAG laser at non-ablative energy densities. Potential application in non-ablative stabilisation procedures. *Orthopade* **25**, 37–41.

72. Hardy, P., Thabit, G.S., Fanton, G.S., Blin, J.L., Lortat-Jacob, A., and Beniot, J. (1996). Arthroscopic management of recurrent anterior shoulder dislocation by combining a labrum suture with anter-inferior holmium: YAG laser capsular shrinkage. *Orthopade* **25**, 91–93.

73. McIntyre, L.J., Caspari, R.B., and Savoie, F.H. (1997). The arthroscopic treatment of posterior shoulder instability: two year results of a multiple suture technique. *Arthroscopy* **13**, 426–432.

74. Kornberg, M. and Aulicino, P.L. (1985). Hand and wrist joint problems in patients with Ehlers-Danlos syndrome. *J. Hand Surg. (Am.)* **10**, 193–196.

75. Tsai, T.-M. and Stilwell, J.R. (1984). Repair of lateral subluxation of inferior radio-ulnar joint using flexor carpi ulnaris tendon. *J. Hand Surg. (Br.)* **9**, 289–294.

76. Bauer, F.C.H., Wredmark, T., and Isberg, B. (1984). Krogius tenoplasty for recurrent dislocation of the patella. Failure associated with joint laxity. *Acta Orthop. Scand.* **55**, 267–269.

77. Hovelius, L., Westerlind, G., and Breggen, B. (1985). Pes anserinus transfer for unstable knee. *Acta Orthop. Scand.* **56**, 127–129.

78. Insall, J.N., Aglietti, P., and Tria, A.J. (1983). Patellar pain and incongruence. II: clinical application. *Clin. Res. Rel. Res.* **176**, 225–232.

79. Eyring, E.J. and Guthrie, W.D. (1986). A surgical approach to the problem of severe instability of the ankle. *Clin. Orthop.* **206**, 185–191.

80. Javors, J.R. and Violet, J.T. (1985). Correction of lateral instability of the ankle by use of the Brotstrom procedure. *Clin. Orthop.* **198**, 201–207.

81. Kato, T. (1995). The diagnosis and treatment of instability of the sub-talar joint. *J. Bone Joint Surg. (Br.)* **77**, 400–406.

6.15 Complex regional pain syndromes: definitions and pathogenesis

Tarnya Marshall, Carol Chong, Rajesh Munglani, and Adrian Crisp

The cardinal symptom of many soft tissue rheumatic disorders is pain. Patients may present in a number of settings, and the perception of the disorder, its diagnosis, and its management may vary accordingly. Often, the more complex the disorder the greater the number and diversity of treatment approaches. A good example of this is the patient with complex regional pain syndrome. Patients are commonly seen in the rheumatology and/or pain clinics and approaches taken in these settings have both similarities and differences. This is illustrated in Chapters 6.16 and 6.17.

Introduction

Complex regional pain syndrome type I (CRPS type I) is one of many terms used to describe the syndrome of pain and swelling, often with a history of a precipitating or inciting factor. It has been described in almost any region of the body, and may cause marked disability and morbidity. It is often poorly recognized, which may make treatment more challenging. The aetiology and pathophysiology remain unclear and, as a result, treatment is not tailored specifically to the pathological mechanism. Despite this, treatment may be successful and recovery full. The condition is recognized to be relapsing in some patients and involvement of a different site in the same individual at a later time point has also been described. Staging of the disease has been undertaken, but the natural history remains to be established.

Historical features and nomenclature

Historically, the first references to a condition of pain and swelling following an injury were in 1766, particularly with regard to the soft tissue changes that may be seen. Greater experience of the condition was achieved during the American Civil War, when a large number of limb gunshot wounds was seen.[1] Burning pain, then named 'causalgia', was described in detail in a patient with a thigh wound and direct nerve trauma. However, because of lack of recognition of the syndrome and also the severity of the pain experienced by soldiers with associated disability, the authorities were often reluctant during times of war—in particular during the American Civil War and the First World War—to believe their injured men, and dishonourable dismissal from the Army was not uncommon.

Sudeck reported the first radiological abnormalities in this condition in 1900, and described the different patterns of bone loss seen at different stages of the syndrome.[2] He was also the first clinician to describe the pseudo inflammatory component of CRPS type I. The term 'Sudeck–Leriche syndrome' was coined for painful posttraumatic osteoporosis following the description of bone rarefaction by the pathologist

Leriche.[3] In 1946 Evans coined the term reflex sympathetic dystrophy[4] because patients with this syndrome obtained relief with sympathetic blockade. Many other synonyms have been in use, with national variation in the preferred term. For example, the favoured French term is algodystrophy, whereas in English-speaking countries reflex sympathetic dystrophy (RSD) is the term of choice. The Germans most commonly use 'Sudeck's atrophy'. Some of the synonyms cover involvement of a specific region of the body, for example, shoulder–hand syndrome. Other terms, for example, algoneurodystrophy, attempt to encompass the presumed pathophysiology. Other terms, such as regional migratory osteoporosis and transient demineralization of the hip of pregnancy, are considered by some to concern separate entities, as the conditions are almost always self-limiting and appear to run a far more benign course.[5, 6] However, similarities do certainly exist, with pain and difficulty weight bearing usually the presenting features and with evidence of osteopenia on plain radiographs. The term CRPS has been introduced as many of the other terms imply a mechanism or pathology, or imply that the condition involves only one particular region of the body. The term RSD, although the favoured term in English-speaking countries, does imply that the syndrome is a reflex response to an inciting factor, that the sympathetic nervous system is the culprit in pathophysiological terms, and that dystrophic changes occur in all cases. Table 1 lists the various synonyms for CRPS.

In 1994, the term complex regional pain syndrome (CRPS) was introduced by a working group of the International Association for the Study of Pain (IASP).[7] In using the term CRPS, the word *complex* indicates how varied the presentation of this condition can be, not only between patients but also at different times in the same patient. *Regional* indicates the distribution of symptoms, which is typically non-dermatomal. *Pain* is usually disproportional to the precipitating

Table 1 Synonyms for complex regional pain syndrome

Causalgia
Acute bone atrophy
Posttraumatic osteoporosis
Shoulder–hand syndrome
Sudeck's acute inflammatory atrophy
Sudeck's disease
Sudeck–Leriche syndrome
Steinbrocker's syndrome
Postinfarct sclerodactyly
Idiopathic painful decalcification of the foot
Algoneurodystrophy
Posttraumatic sympathetic dystrophy
Transient osteoporosis
Regional migratory osteoporosis
Transient demineralization of the hip of pregnancy

events and *syndrome* describes the signs and symptoms that make up this clinical entity. Despite the introduction of the term CRPS 7 years ago, the terms reflex sympathetic dystrophy and causalgia are still commonly used in medicine.

The criteria set out by the IASP are listed below.

1. The presence of an initiating noxious event or a cause of immobilization.

2. Continuing pain, allodynia, or hyperalgesia in which the pain is disproportionate to any known inciting event.

3. Evidence at some time of oedema, changes in skin blood flow, or abnormal sudomotor activity in the region of pain (sign or symptom).

4. This diagnosis is excluded by the existence of other conditions that would otherwise account for the degree of pain and dysfunction.

Criteria number 1 is not necessary for diagnosis as 5–10 per cent of patients will not give this history. CRPS type I is defined as a pain syndrome that usually develops after an initiating noxious event, is not limited to the distribution of a single peripheral nerve, and is apparently disproportionate to the inciting event. CRPS type I encompasses RSD, algodystrophy, and all the other terms used. CRPS type I occurs much more commonly than CRPS type II.

The IASP criteria have been criticized for several reasons. First, they lack specificity. More importantly they are unable to predict the response of such a condition to various treatments nor the long-term prognosis for these patients. Modifications of these criteria have been proposed by other authors to include symptoms and signs in these categories: sensory; vasomotor; sudomotor/oedema; and motor/trophic.[4, 7] The inclusion of these signs and symptoms is particularly useful for research where more specific criteria are required.[8]

The involvement of the sympathetic nervous system is not constant in this syndrome and thus the word 'sympathetic' is not used in the definition. In patients with CRPS, there may be components of sympathetically maintained pain (SMP) or sympathetically independent pain (SIP). SMP is defined as pain that is maintained by sympathetic nervous system activity including circulating catecholamines. Sympathetic pain is now defined as a *symptom* and not a clinical entity.[9]

Further clinically relevant points are not included in the IASP definition. Involvement may be either unilateral or bilateral. Most commonly recognized is peripheral disease,[10] although CRPS type I may affect any region of the trunk or limbs. Case reports describe involvement of the spine and mandible. In the upper limb, reports of CRPS type I tend to involve the hand, although CRPS type I may affect a single digit alone, or indeed the distal extremity of a digit.[11] There is usually evidence of osteopenia on plain radiographs, and the pattern of this is helpful in making the diagnosis and staging the disease. Motor abnormalities have been reported, in particular, tremor, involuntary movement, and muscle spasm.[12] Contractures may occur in the later stages.

Other diagnostic criteria

To add further to the confusion relating to CRPS, three further sets of diagnostic criteria exist, adding to the lack of consistency in studies. The most recent and widely quoted diagnostic criteria are those of Kozin *et al.* described in 1981.[13] The criteria do not take investigations into account, but concentrate on clinical findings. However, as will be discussed, none of the investigations performed in patients

Table 2 Kozin's diagnostic criteria (reference 14)

Definite CRPS type I
Pain and tenderness in the distal extremity
Signs and/or symptoms of vasomotor instability
Swelling in the extremity
(Dystrophic changes usually present)

Probable CRPS type I
Pain and tenderness
and
Vasomotor instability
or
Swelling
(Dystrophic skin changes often present)

Possible CRPS type I
Vasomotor instability
or/and
Swelling
No pain, but mild to moderate tenderness may be present

Doubtful CRPS type I
Unexplained pain and tenderness in an extremity

with CRPS type I is infallible, and all have limited sensitivity and specificity. The criteria are outlined in Table 2.

Steinbrocker *et al.* outlined the stages of the disease,[15] and Doury *et al.* the radiographic abnormalities.[15] All criteria have disadvantages. The natural history of CRPS type I remains unclear and, because of this, Steinbrocker's criteria are of limited use. Doury's criteria assume that all cases of CRPS type I have radiographic abnormalities, which has not been established and may certainly be untrue in the early course of CRPS type I.

Epidemiology

Due to the varied nature and different regions of the body affected by CRPS type I, the true epidemiology remains unclear. The condition is recognized in children, who may have particularly marked vasomotor changes.[17–19] The epidemiology is more easily determined following an incident that is recognized to be associated with CRPS type I. It has been suggested that up to 5 per cent of all cases of limb trauma are complicated by CRPS type I.[20] Several studies of patients who sustained Colles' fracture describe the incidence of CRPS type I as a complication of fracture. Atkins *et al.*[21] found that 40 per cent of patients had evidence of CRPS type I 9 weeks after a Colles' fracture in a group of 60 patients. A larger study of 109 patients describe an incidence of 25 per cent at 9 weeks following Colles' fracture, although this had fallen to 16 per cent at a 6-month review.[22] An observational study of outcome at 10 years following Colles' fracture found that as many as 26 per cent of patients in a group of 55 patients had at least one feature of CRPS type I.[23] A smaller group of 36 patients underwent distal ulnar excision following wrist injury, with 86 per cent having a Colles' fracture, and one or more features of RSD were found in 60 per cent of patients at 6 years.[24]

CRPS type I has been described in other patients following fracture. This includes reports of anterior chest wall syndrome in patients following fracture of the clavicle.[25] In each case, patients described allodynia. Arthroscopic surgery has also been associated with CRPS type I.[26, 27] One paper reviewed the outcome of 63 different arthroscopic techniques and discovered that 2.3 per cent of all complications were due to CRPS type I.[28] This equates to a risk of one case following 2500 arthroscopies. Trauma to either the central or nervous system has been associated with the development of CRPS type I. In a prospective study of brain-injured patients, CRPS type I was found after an average of 4 months following injury.[29]

Of patients undergoing carpal tunnel release, 5 per cent have been described as developing CRPS type I.[30–32] CRPS type I is also described in patients who have carpal tunnel syndrome but who have not undergone decompressive surgery, although the incidence is low.[33]

Shoulder–hand syndrome occurs following myocardial infarction, and one series suggested an incidence of 5 per cent.[34] A similar incidence is seen following revascularization of a previously ischaemic periphery.

Aetiology

There is often a history of trauma, occasionally of such low significance that it may be overlooked by the patient. Symptoms may occur up to 6 months after injury.[35] Other triggering factors have been reported. Several drugs have been implicated, for example, phenobarbitone, phenytoin, isoniazid,[16] and the immunosuppressive agents cyclosporin[36] and tacrolimus.[37] Rapamycin is currently under investigation as an immunosuppressive agent administered after solid organ transplantation. A recent report associated this drug with bone pain, osteolysis on plain radiographs, and high uptake of tracer on isotope bone scanning. Resolution of symptoms occurred on withdrawal or reduction of rapamycin, or following administration of the bisphosphonate pamidronate.[38] Surgery or a neurological event have also been implicated, particularly with peripheral manifestations, and the incidence of CRPS type I following different surgical techniques is described above. Concurrent medical conditions may predispose to CRPS type I and diabetes mellitus, hyperthyroidism, hyperparathyroidism, and type 1V hyperlipidaemia have all been associated. Chronic pain in a poorly understood condition may cause depression and isolation and, although a higher rate of psychological abnormalities has been reported with CRPS type I, this appears to be little different from that in other patient groups who suffer chronic pain.[39, 40] There is evident localized bone loss that cannot be solely attributed to immobility. The pain is often most severe during stages 1 and 2 when the rate of bone loss is most rapid. Similarities exist between CRPS type I and Charcot's neurarthropathy of diabetes (Figs 1 and 2).

Pain occurs in each condition, although Charcot's joints are classically painless in the later stages. Histologically, there is bone loss with a normal underlying bone architecture in CRPS type I, with predominantly trabecular bone resorption,[41] whereas a destructive pattern of bone loss is seen in the Charcot's joint.

The Charcot's joint is typically hyperaemic whereas the limb involved by CRPS type I, especially in the later stages, is cooler. The pathogenesis of both conditions remains elusive, but a common pathway towards rapid bone loss does not seem unreasonable. A painful limb is not subjected to normal weight-bearing, and immobility must be considered as a mechanism of bone loss. This may be

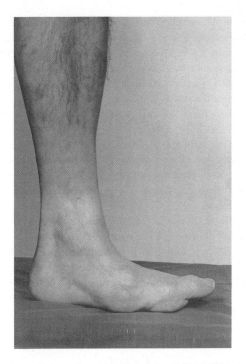

Fig. 1 Diabetic neurarthropathy commonly presents with swelling, warmth, and pain. Clinically, there may be evidence of a joint effusion. (Courtesy of Dr A. Marshall.)

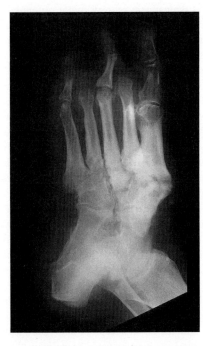

Fig. 2 Radiographically, diabetic neurarthropathy may reveal periosteal calcification, minimal subluxation, fracture, and fragmentation. The radiographic appearance of late disease, as demonstrated here, is that of a disordered joint. (Courtesy of Dr. A. Marshall.)

compared to the bone loss that occurs in the postoperative period, which is not associated with the severe burning pain that characterizes CRPS type I, and the rate of bone loss due to immobility does not match the speed of bone loss that must occur in CRPS type I to cause osteopenia on plain radiographs.[42]

Central and peripheral nervous system damage are also recognized as causes of CRPS type I. Trauma to the brain or spinal cord may predispose to CRPS type I,[29, 43, 44] with features of CRPS type I occurring as soon as 24 hours after surgery. In patients with myelopathy, CRPS type I is typically seen to develop 4–12 weeks following the injury or trauma.

Whether generalized osteopenia or osteoporosis is an independent risk factor for CRPS type I has yet to be resolved. One study of 19 patients indicated that lumbar bone density was lower than expected, although this was not a significant finding.[45] Individuals with lower than average bone density may therefore be at risk of developing CRPS type I following what would have otherwise been a relatively minor traumatic incident.

In patients with cancer, CRPS type I may occur as a result of a direct effect of metastatic tissue, or remotely from cancerous tissue. A case of CRPS type I in a patient with squamous carcinoma of the lung is described, in whom resolution of the symptoms of CRPS type I occurred following resection of the tumour.[46] CRPS type I occurring as a result of venepuncture or due to insertion of arteriovenous shunts is also reported. Cigarette smoking was considered a possible inciting factor for CRPS type I, although the evidence for this is slim.[47]

Pathogenesis of CRPS

The pathogenesis of CRPS is unclear and there is evidence for both central and peripheral mechanisms. This syndrome has many components such as sympathetic, sensory, motor, autonomic, inflammatory, and psychological. In any given patient some or all of these components may be present in varying degrees. Over time, the contribution of each component to the syndrome may change or vary, making research into its mechanisms difficult.

Proponents of peripheral mechanisms for CRPS have shown that these patients have increased extravasation of plasma proteins when cutaneous nerves are stimulated, leading to postulations that neuropeptides might impair blood flow and oxygen delivery.[48] These neuropeptides may cause increased skin temperature, increased hair and nail growth, and oedema in the acute phase.[49] Primary afferent nociceptors are not normally sensitive to catecholamines but become 'activated' in pathological conditions.

However, central mechanisms also contribute to CRPS. Schurmann and colleagues have used Doppler flowmetry to show that sympathetic nervous system disturbances are systemic and not restricted to the affected limb.[49] After nerve injury, there is a lot of 'cross-talk' that occurs between the sensory system and sympathetic system. These individual sensory nerve endings become very sensitive to mechanical and thermal influences, circulating catecholamines, and stimulation from postganglionic sympathetic neurons. The latter work via $\alpha 1$ and $\alpha 2$ adrenoreceptors and neuropeptide Y.[50, 51] This state of central sensitization could be maintained from persistent nociceptive input arising from ectopic activity in neuromas, ectopic activity in dorsal root ganglions, and sympathetic sensory fibre interaction from alpha adrenoceptors and neuropeptide Y receptor sensitivity in nociceptors.[52]

It is likely that CRPS involves both peripheral and central mechanisms. One postulated hypothesis is that an initial injury causes activation of nociceptors and results in signalling along pain pathways from the periphery to the spinal cord. Neuromodulation occurs in the spinal cord, which causes central pain signalling neurons (dorsal root ganglia) to

become sensitized. Animal experiments have shown postganglionic sympathetic fibres sprouting to form basket-like terminals with the dorsal root ganglia.[53] These sensitized dorsal root ganglia therefore respond to mechanical stimulation, seen clinically as allodynia.[54]

Although there is a lot of evidence for the effects of the sympathetic system on the somatosensory nerves, the sympathetic system itself may show decreased activity after nerve injury. Animal experiments show that there is atrophy of sympathetic cell bodies and fibres after a peripheral nerve lesion. This could account for the increase in skin temperature and increased sweating observed in the affected limb in the acute stages of CRPS. The initial impairment in sympathetic output could result in a 'denervation supersensitivity' of the blood supply to the affected limb in the more chronic phase of CRPS. Possible mechanisms for denervation supersensitivity include upregulation of postjunctional receptors or second messenger systems, decrease in neurotransmitter uptake, or an increase in neurotransmitter affinity for receptors. These findings could account for a 'cooler' limb that may become cooler when exposed to circulating cathecholamines or stress. Perhaps this explains the cold allodynia so frequently seen in sympathetically mediated pain.

Nevertheless, sympathetic overactivity has been traditionally considered to be the underlying mechanism. However, plasma concentrations of adrenaline, noradrenaline, and metabolites, which would be expected to be found in higher concentrations if sympathetic overactivity were present, are lower than in controls.[55] Attempts to quantify the sympathetic skin response have been statistically insignificant in comparison with attempts in control subjects.[56, 57] These findings, which refute the presence of sympathetic overactivity, are supported by Arnold et al.'s findings of altered sensitivity of adrenoceptors to sympathetic neurotransmitters in the veins from the affected areas in patients with CRPS type I.[58] The success of sympathetic blocks in the treatment of CRPS type I did add credibility to the hypothesis of sympathetic overactivity as the pathological mechanism in CRPS type I. However, two papers have described the powerful placebo effect of sympathetic blockade, and have demonstrated that neuropathic pain is not influenced significantly by placebo, alpha adrenergic agonist, or antagonist.[59, 60]

In support of the original description by Sudeck[21] of the pseudo-inflammatory nature of CRPS type I, patients with CRPS have an inflammatory component to their pain. The affected limb is often painful, oedematous, and red. Calcitonin-gene-related peptide (CRGP) and substance P are released from afferent nerve endings. CRGP causes vasodilatation and substance P induces the extravasation of plasma proteins. It is possible that these inflammatory changes could produce longer-term neural or vascular impairment.[61] Interestingly, Hannington-Kiff has reported successful use of intravenous guanethidine in patients with rheumatoid arthritis.[62] The role of inflammatory free radicals in CRPS type I is supported by two studies. In animal models, tert-butylhydroperoxide, a free radical donor, was administered intraarterially causing symptoms of acute CRPS, that is, an oedematous, painful warm extremity with impaired function.[63] In the second study, Zollinger and colleagues administered vitamin C, a free radical scavenger, prophylatically and showed that this decreased the incidence of CRPS after wrist fractures.[64]

Further studies have shown abnormalities of high-energy phosphate metabolism in muscle of affected areas in the patients with CRPS type I, perhaps providing an explanation as to why patients may have difficulty moving the muscles of the affected limb.[65]

In addition, reduced mitochondrial enzyme activity has been demonstrated, which results in reduced oxygenation within muscle, providing a further explanation for muscle dysfunction.[66]

Staging and progression

The natural history of CRPS type I is still unclear as it would appear that not all cases progress unremittingly and that resolution may occur during any stage. Some cases seem to respond rapidly to treatment while others may be resistant. Three stages are recognized, with clinical and radiographic features utilized in the staging (Table 3).[16, 67] Stage 1 is characterized by onset of pain, with swelling and oedema and evidence of patchy bone loss on plain radiographs. Stage 2 recognizes more established disease, with continuing pain, atrophy of the skin and tissues, and contracture of the joint. Diffuse bone loss is seen on plain radiographs. In stage 3 pain is less prominent and, as there is little active movement, pain is most marked during passive movement. Those patients who develop a trophic, cold limb may be less responsive to treatment and, the longer the duration of the disease, the less favourable the outcome. However, no studies have compared treatments or outcomes between the three stages. In some, the intractable pain is sufficient for amputation to be considered and undertaken. High recurrence of CRPS type I in the stump following amputation has, however, been described[68] and, unless the amputation is performed for reasons of ongoing severe infection, radical surgery is usually avoided. In others, there may be resolution of signs and symptoms, either spontaneously or following treatment.

Recurrence may occur subsequently at the original or at a completely separate anatomical site. Many studies that assess treatment of CRPS type I fail to use staging methods, and as a result the natural history and value of early treatment with regard to outcome remain to be clarified. The largest observational study to date describes the clinical features in 829 patients.[69] Progression from stage 1 to stage 3 was not confirmed, but patients could be divided into those with a warm limb and those with a cold limb. Although, in general, the longer the disease had been established the more likely the presence of a cold limb, 13 per cent of patients had a cold limb early in the disease and warm limbs were described in patients who had longstanding CRPS type I of many years duration.

Summary

CRPS is a clinical entity about which there has been much debate. The pathophysiology giving rise to such clinical symptoms may vary from patient to patient. This controversy over CRPS extends from its name,

Table 3 Stages of CRPS type I: Steinbrocker et al.'s criteria (reference 15)

Stage 1. Hypertrophic stage
Pain, oedema, swelling
Hyperhidrosis, warmth, redness

Stage 2. Atrophic stage
Pain, cyanosis, atrophic, cold skin
Reduced range of movement

Stage 3. Atrophic, cold skin
Reduced range of movement, less pain

symptoms and signs, pathophysiology, and methods of treatment. Until increased comprehension of CRPS is acquired, our treatment of this group of patients will inevitably be empirical and anecdotal in part.

References

1. **Mitchell, S.W., Morehouse, G.R., and Keen, W.W.** (1864). *Gunshot wounds and other injuries of nerves.* Lippincott, New York.
2. **Sudeck, P.** (1900). Uber die akute entzundliche Knochenatropie. *Arch. Klin. Chir.* **62**, 147–156.
3. **Leriche, R.** (1939). *Physiologie et pathologie du tissu osseux.* Masson, Paris.
4. **Bruehl, S.,** *et al.* (1999). External validation of IASP diagnostic criteria for complex regional pain syndrome and proposed research diagnostic criteria. *Pain* **81**, 147–154.
5. **Duncan, H., Frame, B., Frost, H.M., and Arnstein, R.** (1969). Regional migrating osteoporosis. *South. Med. J.* **62**, 41–44.
6. **Curtiss, P.H. and Kincaid, W.E.** (1959). Transitory demineralisation of the hip in pregnancy. A report of three cases. *J. Bone Joint Surg.* **41**, 1327–1332.
7. **Harden, R.N.** *et al.* (1999). Complex regional pain syndrome: are the IASP diagnostic criteria valid and sufficiently comprehensive? *Pain* **83**, 211–219.
8. **Birklein, F. and Handwerker, H.O.** (2001). Complex regional pain syndrome: how to resolve the complexity. *Pain* **94**, 1–6.
9. **Baron, R., Fields, H.L., Janig, W., Kitt, C., and Levine, J.D.** (2002). National Institutes of Health Workshop: reflex sympathetic dystrophy/complex regional pain syndromes—state-of-the-science. *Anesth. Analg.* **95** (6), 1812–1816.
10. **Seale, K.S.** (1989). Reflex sympathetic dystrophy of the lower extremity. *Clin. Orthop.* **243**, 50.
11. **Kline, S. and Holder, L.** (1993). Segmental reflex sympathetic dystrophy: clinical and scintigraphic criteria. *J. Hand Surg. Am.* **18**, 853–859.
12. **Veldman, P.H., Reynen, H.M., Arntz, I.E.** *et al.* (1993). Signs and symptoms of reflex sympathetic dystrophy; prospective study of 829 patients. *Lancet* **342** (8878), 1012–1016.
13. **Kozin, F., Ryan, L.M., Carerra, G.F., Soin, J., and Wortmann, R.L.** (1981). The reflex sympathetic dystrophy syndrome (RSDS) III. Scintigraphic studies, further evidence for the therapeutic efficacy of systemic corticosteroids, and proposed diagnostic criteria. *Am. J. Med.* **70**, 23–30.
14. **Kozin, F.** (1992). Reflex sympathetic dystrophy: a review. *Clin. Exp. Rheumatol.* **10**, 401–409.
15. **Steinbrocker, O., Spitzer, N., and Friedman, H.** (1948). The shoulder–hand syndrome in reflex dystrophy of the upper extremity. *Ann. Intern. Med.* **29**, 22–52.
16. **Doury, P., Dirheimer, Y., and Pattin, S.** (1981). *Algodystrophy: diagnosis and therapy of a frequent disease of the locomotor apparatus.* Springer-Verlag, Berlin.
17. **Wilder, R.T., Berde, C.B., Wolohan, M., Vieyra, M.A., Masek, B.J., and Micheli, L.J.** (1992). Reflex sympathetic disorder in children. *J. Bone Joint Surg. (Am.)* **74**, 910–919.
18. **Silber, T.J. and Majd, M.** (1988). Reflex sympathetic dystrophy syndrome in children and adolescents. *Am. J. Dis. Child.* **142**, 1328–1330.
19. **Coughlan, R.J., Kavanagh, R.T., and Hazleman, B.L.,** *et al.* (1995). The clinical features of algodystrophy in childhood. *J. Orthop. Rheumatol.* **8**, 146–150.
20. **Bronica, J.J.** (1979). Causalgia and other reflex sympathetic dystrophies. In *Advances in pain research and therapy*, p. 141. Raven Press; New York.
21. **Atkins, R.M., Duckworth, T., and Kanis, J.A.** (1989). Features of Algodystrophy after Colles' fracture. *J. Bone Joint Surg. (Br.)* **72**, 105–110
22. **Atkins, R.M., Duckworth, T., and Kanis, J.A.** (1989). Algodystrophy following Colles' fracture. *J. Hand Surg. (Br.)* **14**, 161–164.
23. **Field, J., Warwick, D., and Bannister, G.C.** (1992). Features of algodystrophy 10 years after Colles' fracture. *J. Hand Surg. (Br.)* **17**, 318–320.
24. **Field, J., Majkowski, R.J., and Leslie, I.J.** (1993). Poor results of Darrach's procedure after wrist injuries. *J. Bone Joint Surg. (Br.)* **75**, 53–57.

25. Ivey, M., Britt, M., and Johnson, R.V. (1991). Reflex sympathetic dystrophy after clavicle fracture: case report. *J. Trauma* **31**, 276–279.

26. Kim, H.J., Kozin, F., Johnson, R.J., and Hines, R. (1979). Reflex sympathetic dystrophy of the knee following meniscectomy. *Arthritis Rheum.* **22**, 177–181.

27. Waldman, S.D. and Waldman, K.A. (1992). Reflex sympathetic dystrophy of the knee following arthroscopic surgery: successful treatment with neural blockade utilising anaesthetics. *J. Pain Symtom Manag.* **7**, 243–245.

28. Small, N.C. (1993). Complications in arthroscopic surgery of the knee and shoulder. *Orthopaedics* **16**, 985–988.

29. Gellman, H., Keenan, M.A., Stone, L., Hardy, S.E., Waters, R.L., and Stewart, C. (1992). Reflex sympathetic dystrophy in brain-injured patients. *Pain* **51**, 307–311.

30. MacDonald, R.I., Lichtman, D.H., Hanlon, J.J., and Wilson, J.N. (1978). Complications of surgical release for carpal tunnel syndrome. *J. Hand Surg.* (*Am.*) **1**, 70–76.

31. Clayburgh, R.M., Breckenbaugh, R.D., and Dobyns, J.H. (1987). Carpal tunnel release in patients with diffuse peripheral neuropathy. *J. Hand Surg.* (*Am.*) **12**, 380–383.

32. Kushner, S.H., Brien, W.W., Johnson, D., and Gellman, H. (1991). Complications associated with carpal tunnel syndrome. *Orthop. Rev.* **20**, 346–352.

33. Fitzcharles, M.A. and Esdaile, J.M. (1990). Carpal tunnel syndrome complicated by reflex sympathetic dystrophy. *Br. J. Rheumatol.* **30**, 468–470.

34. Rosen, P.S. and Graham, W. (1957). The shoulder–hand syndrome: historical review with observations on 73 patients. *Can. Med. Assoc. J.* **77**, 86–91.

35. Levine, D.Z. (1991). Burning pain in an extremity: breaking the destructive cycle of reflex sympathetic dystrophy. *Postgrad. Med.* **90** (2), 175–185.

36. Munoz-Gomez, J., Collado, A., Gratacos, J., Campistol, J.M., Lomena, F., Llena, J., and Andreu, J. (1991). Reflex sympathetic dystrophy syndrome of the lower limbs in renal transplant patients treated with cyclosporin A. *Arthritis Rheum.* **34**, 625–630.

37. Villaverde, V., Cantalejo, M., Balsa, A., *et al.* (1999). Leg bone pain syndrome in a kidney transplant patient treated with tacrolimus (FK506). *Ann. Rheum. Dis.* **58**, 653–654.

38. Crosbie, O., Collier, J., Bateman, E. *et al.* A pilot study of Sirolimus (rapamycin) as primary immunosuppression following liver transplantation [abstract]. *Hepatology* **30**, 185.

39. Lynch, M.E. (1992). Psychological aspects of reflex sympathetic dystrophy: a review of the paediatric literature. *Pain* **49**, 337–347.

40. Ciccicone, D.S., Bandilla, E.B., and Wu, W.H. (1997). Psychological dysfunction in patients with reflex sympathetic dystrophy. *Pain* **71**, 323–333.

41. Bickerstaff, D.R., Charlesworth, D., and Kanis, J.A. (1993). Changes in cortical and trabecular bone in algodystrophy. *Br. J. Rheumatol.* **32**, 46–51.

42. del Puente, A., Pappone, N., Mandes, M.G., Mantova, D., Scarpa, R., and Oriente, P. (1996). Determinants of bone mineral density in immobilisation: a study on hemiplegic patients. *Osteoporosis Int.* **6**, 50–54.

43. Cremer, S.A., Maynard, F., and Davidoff, G. (1989). The reflex sympathetic dystrophy syndrome associated with traumatic myelopathy: a report of 5 cases. *Pain* **37**, 187–192.

44. Philip, P.A., Philip, M., and Monga, T.N. (1990). Reflex sympathetic dystrophy in central cord syndrome: case report and review of the literature. *Paraplegia* **28**, 48–54.

45. Cepollaro, C., Gonnelli, S., Pondrelli, C., Martini, S., Montagnani, A., Rossi, B., and Gennari, C. (1998). Usefulness of ultrasound in Sudeck's atrophy of the foot. *Calcif. Tissue Int.* **62**, 538–541.

46. Prowse, M., Higgs, C.M.B., Forrester-Wood, C., AND McHugh, N. (1989). Reflex sympathetic dystrophy associated with squamous cell carcinoma of the lung. *Ann. Rheum. Dis.* **48**, 339–344.

47. Parvelka, S., Fiallca, V., and Ernst, E. (1993). Reflex sympathetic dystrophy and cigarette smoking [letter]. *J. Hand Surg.* (*Am.*) **18**, 168.

48. Weber, N., *et al.* (2001). Facilitated neurogenic inflammation in complex regional pain syndrome. *Pain* **91**, 251–257.

49. Schurmann, M., Gradl, G., *et al.* (2000). Peripheral sympathetic function as a predictor of complex regional pain syndrome type 1 (CRPS 1) in patients with radial fracture. *Auton. Neurosci.* **86**, 127–134.

50. Tracey, D.J., *et al.* (1995). Peripheral hyperalgesia in experimental neuropathy: exacerbation by neuropeptide. *Brain Res.* **669**, 245–254.

51. Coughnon, N., *et al.* (1997). The therapeutic potential of NPY in central nervous system disorders with special reference to pain and sympathetically maintained pain. *Expert Opin. Invest. Drugs* **6**, 759–769.

52. Munglani, R., *et al.* (1998). Therapeutic potential of NPY. *Drugs* **52**, 371–389.

53. Chung, K., *et al.* (1997). Sprouting sympathetic fibers from synaptic varicosities in the dorsal root ganglion of the rat with neuropathic injury. *Brain Res.* **75**, 275–280.

54. Campbell, J.N. (1996). Complex regional pain syndrome and the sympathetic nervous system. In *Pain 1996 an updated review (refresher course syllabus)* (ed. J.N. Campbell). IASP Press, Seattle.

55. Drummond, P.D., Finch, P.M., and Smythe, G.A. (1991). Reflex sympathetic dystrophy: the significance of differing plasma catecholamine concentrations in affected and unaffected limbs. *Brain* **12**, 263–267.

56. Casale, R. and Elam, M. (1992). Normal sympathetic nerve activity in a reflex sympathetic dystrophy with marked skin vasoconstriction. *J. Auton. Nerv. Syst.* **41**, 215–219.

57. Clinchot, D.M. and Lorch, F. (1996). Sympathetic skin response in patients with reflex sympathetic dystrophy. *Am. J. Phys. Med. Rehabil.* **75**, 252–256.

58. Arnold, J., Teasell, R., Macleod, A., Brown, J., and Carruthers, G. (1993). Increased venous alpha-adrenoceptor responsiveness in patients with reflex sympathetic dystrophy. *Ann. Intern. Med.* **118**, 619–621.

59. Verdugo, R. and Ochoa, J. (1994). Sympathetically maintained pain. I. Phentolamine block questions the concept. *Neurology*, **44**, 1003–1010.

60. Verdugo, R., Campero, M., and Ochoa, J. (1994). Phentolamine sympathetic block in painful polyneuropathies. II. Further questioning of the concept of sympathetically maintained pain. *Neurology* **44**, 1010–1014.

61. Drummond, P.D. (2001). Mechanism of complex regional pain syndrome: no longer excessive sympathetic outflow? *Lancet*, **358**, 168–170.

62. Hannington-Kiff, J.G. (1994). Sympathetic nerve blocks in painful limb disorders. In *Textbook of pain*, 3rd edn. (ed. P.D. Wall and R. Melzack), pp 1035–1052. Churchill Livingstone, Edinburgh.

63. van-der-Laan, L., *et al.* (1998). Clinical signs and symptoms of acute reflex sympathetic dystrophy in one hindlimb of the rat, induced by infusion of a free-radical donor. *Acta Orthop. Belg.* **64**, 210–217.

64. Zollinger, P.E., *et al.* (1999). Effect of vitamin C on frequency of reflex sympathetic dystrophy in wrist fractures: a randomised trial. *Lancet* **354**, 2025–2028.

65. Heerschap, A., Hollander, J., Reynen, H., and Goris, R. (1993). Metabolic changes in RSD: a 31P NMR spectroscopy study. *Muscle Nerve* **16**, 367–373.

66. Tilman, P., Stadhouders, A., Jap, P., and Goris, R. (1990). Histopathologic findings in skeletal muscle tissue of patients suffering from reflex sympathetic dystrophy. *Micron Microscop. Acta* **21**, 271–272.

67. Steinbrocker, O. (1947). The shoulder–hand syndrome. Associated painful homolateral disability of the shoulder and hand with swelling and atrophy of the hand. *Am. J. Med.* **3**, 402–407.

68. Dielissen, P.W., Claasen, A.T., Veldman, P.H., and Goris, R.J. (1995). Amputation for reflex sympathetic dystrophy. *J. Bone Joint Surg.* (*Br.*) **77**, 270–273.

69. Veldman, P.H., Reynen, H.M., Arntz, I.E., and Goris, R.J. (1993). Signs and symptoms of reflex sympathetic dystrophy: prospective study of 829 patients. *Lancet* **342**, 1012–1016.

6.16 Complex regional pain syndromes in the rheumatology clinic

Tarnya Marshall and Adrian Crisp

Differential diagnosis

The differential diagnosis of complex regional pain syndrome (CRPS) type I is wide and includes almost any other cause of regional pain (Table 1). There may be a history of trauma, including surgery, preceding the onset of symptoms, and other causes of localized pain include fracture and ligamentous injury. In view of this, fracture should be considered as a differential diagnosis. However, the two may coexist, usually with CRPS type I developing as a complication of fracture but, if a fracture is present, this must be diagnosed so that correct management may be instituted. As CRPS type I often involves a joint, the diagnosis of septic arthritis and other causes of a monoarthritis should be considered. Vascular disease may also present as regional pain associated with colour change and, as a consequence, some patients with CRPS type I present initially to vascular surgeons. Later on in the disease, the diagnosis may be difficult to differentiate from a disuse syndrome, as pain is most marked during passive movement and the affected area may demonstrate contractures and appear cold and blue with muscle and soft tissue wasting.

Clinical evaluation

The history should establish the age and sex of the patient, duration of symptoms, and any preceding trauma (Table 2). The latter may be severe, such as in fractures. In the case of some patients, especially those with knee involvement, there may be a history of surgery, such as arthroscopy. The history of trauma need not be present and in some may be so mild that the patient feels it unworthy of mention. The degree of disability should also be established. Some individuals are unable to weight-bear for any length of time or have difficulty with personal care if an upper limb is involved. There may be a history of sensitivity of the affected region, so that the draught under a door or the light touch of a sheet may cause severe discomfort or pain. There

may be a history of colour change in the area, which may be particularly marked in the periphery. Past medical history should be noted in detail, as several conditions, particularly those of an endocrinological nature are associated with the development of CRPS type I. This is discussed further in the 'Aetiology' section in Chapter 6.15. Drug history may be relevant, and prescribed medication is increasingly being associated with the development of CRPS type I. A recent publication has raised the question of systemic osteoporosis, with lumbar spine involvement in particular, as an independent risk factor for CRPS type I. Although confirmation of this is awaited, it does raise the question of assessment of bone health and reduction of risk factors for osteoporosis as part of routine history taking in patients with CRPS type I.

Examination

A full medical examination should be performed, and a detailed regional examination to exclude other causes of regional pain (Table 2). In cases of CRPS type I, the affected area often relates to a joint. The clinical findings vary depending on the stage of the disease. During stage 1, there may be swelling and oedema, and discolouration. The vasomotor changes may be marked during the early stages and, as a result, the affected area may appear erythematous and warm or, indeed, cold and blue. The vasomotor disturbance may fluctuate and there may be no temperature difference or discolouration, even though the history may be suggestive of this. A variety of motor disturbances are reported, including incoordination, tremor, involuntary movements, muscle spasm, paresis, and pseudoparalysis. The largest

Table 1 Differential diagnosis

Septic arthritis
Inflammatory monoarthritis
Crystal arthropathy
Lymphoedema
Stress fracture
Osteonecrosis
Ischaemia
Soft tissue pathology
Diabetic neurarthropathy
Disuse syndrome

Table 2 Clinical evaluation

History
Trauma

Predisposing factors

Disability

Colour change

Sensitivity

Drug history

Examination
Skin and soft tissue changes, e.g. atrophy, colour change

Temperature in comparison with contralateral side

Hyperaesthesia

Motor abnormalities

Passive and active joint movements

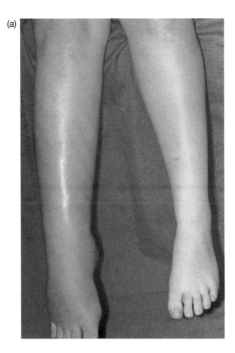
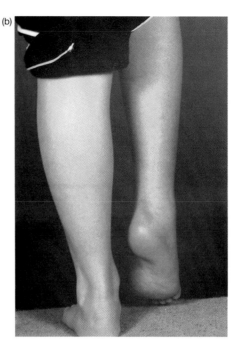

Fig. 1 The legs of a boy with CRPS type I affecting his right lower leg are seen. He is unable to bear-weight because of pain, and has atrophy of his left Achilles tendon. His leg demonstrates hyperaemia and swelling.

prospective, observational study described incoordination in as many as 54 per cent of their cohort of 829 patients, and tremor in 49 per cent.[1] Perhaps as a result of the clinically significant altered sympathetic nerve supply, increased hair and nail growth may be seen in up to 10 per cent of patients with early CRPS type I (see Fig. 1).[2]

Investigations

The diagnosis can often be made on clinical grounds alone. However, a range of diagnostic tools is available. Routine haematology and biochemistry are generally unhelpful and inflammatory markers are usually within normal limits. Bone-specific alkaline phosphatase may be marginally elevated in early disease, but this is not a consistent finding. Plain radiographs are more useful diagnostically and may show evidence of osteopenia in the affected area, indicating bone loss of at least 30 per cent (see Figs 2 and 3).

The pattern of bone loss depends on the stage of the syndrome, with patchy loss occurring early and diffuse loss seen in the later stages.[3–6] In order to show unilateral osteopenia, both the affected site and the non-affected ipsilateral site must be X-rayed simultaneously to standardize exposure of the X-ray. Generalized skeletal osteopenia may be obvious on a plain radiograph of any region of the body—another reason why the affected area should be compared with the ipsilateral side. The advantages of plain radiographs are that they may be obtained quickly and cheaply and are non-invasive. The dose of radiation is low, especially if a peripheral site is exposed to the radiation beam and no important organs are exposed. One drawback, however, is that bone loss of less than 30 per cent is not obvious on plain radiographs, and mild disease or early disease may be overlooked. No studies to date identify the rate of bone loss, or the optimum time to request plain radiographs.

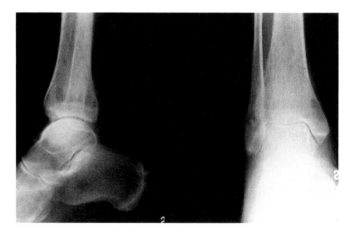

Fig. 2 The plain radiograph demonstrates diffuse osteopenia throughout the calcaneum in a patient with CRPS type I of the left foot.

Another diagnostic and validated method is *thermography* (Fig. 4). An infrared camera semiquantifies heat emission from the skin, by monitoring near-surface blood flow in the limbs, and vasomotor instability may therefore be monitored.[7–9] No radiation is involved, and the technique is non-invasive. Thermography cameras, however are not necessarily in general use.

Three-phase bone scintigraphy typically demonstrates increased local blood flow and increased soft tissue uptake immediately following administration of the radioactive isotope. Delayed images, at 3–4 hours, indicate increased uptake within the bone and, if these strict criteria are met, Mackinnon and Holder reported high sensitivity

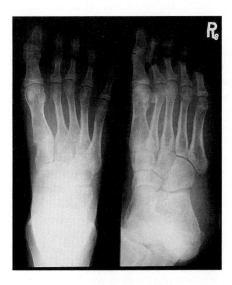

Fig. 3 In comparison with Fig. 2 of the previous section, this plain radiograph shows earlier CRPS and the pattern of ostopenia is more patchy.

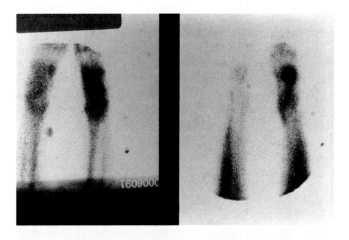

Fig. 5 Triple-phase isotope bone scan of a patient with early disease. Clinically, the right lower leg and foot is warm and erythematous and there is evidence of increased local blood flow on scan. At this stage in this disease, and with these scintigraphic findings, the diagnosis is undisputed (Courtesy of Professor M. Peters).

(a)

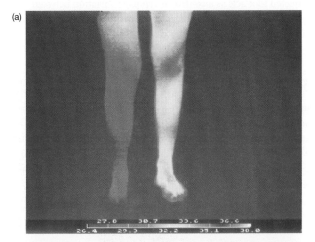

(b)

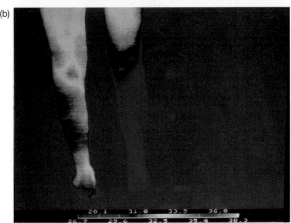

Fig. 4 (a and b) Thermography: the heat emission from a patient with CRPS type I affecting the right leg. On both the anterior and posterior views, the leg appears cooler than the normal unaffected side. The patient has either unstable vasomotor change (early disease), pictured while the leg is clinically cool, or has a permanently cold leg (established disease) (Courtesy of Dr B.L. Hazleman and Mrs M. Smith).

(96 per cent) and specificity (98 per cent) for this technique.[10] This has been challenged by other authors. Werner *et al.*[11] reported a sensitivity of only 50 per cent, with a higher specificity (92 per cent), whereas Pollock found high specificity and low sensitivity. The effect of sympathetic blockade on three-phase bone scintigraphy remains unanswered and, as Hoffman *et al.* demonstrated,[12] 7 of 15 patients with CRPS type I who later received an analgesic benefit from sympathetic blockade had normal isotope bone scintigraphy before the procedure was performed. No studies have assessed bone scintigraphy following sympathetic blockade. However, it would seem appropriate to perform bone scintigraphy before any treatment regimes are instigated. In children, decreased uptake is more commonly seen at the affected site.[13]

The changes seen in stage 3 disease are difficult to interpret and are often indistinguishable from a disuse syndrome. Five-stage bone scintigraphy has been used diagnostically, but appears to offer little further information, and is more work-intensive. Bone scintigraphy does carry a radioactive disadvantage and requires the intravenous administration of the radioactive isotope. If CRPS type I is suspected clinically, a three-phase scan must be discussed with the nuclear medicine physicians, as this is not routinely performed for other indications (Fig. 5).

More recently, *magnetic resonance imaging* (MRI) has been used with success and has the advantage of excluding other pathologies, for example, stress fracture.[14] The typical findings are those of bone oedema and soft tissue swelling on T2-weighted fat-suppressed sequences. MRI is not a useful technique at quantifying bone but may demonstrate changes in magnetic signal within the bone. A recent report described a high frequency of joint effusion on MRI in patients with CRPS type I and the authors have argued the importance of this as a diagnostic sign (Fig. 6).[15] MRI is a more expensive diagnostic technique than the other techniques used in the diagnosis of CRPS type I and, although no radiation is administered, some patients find the experience uncomfortable, claustrophobic, and noisy.

Vascular scintigraphy has been used with success in the diagnosis of CRPS type I. Human albumin-labelled technetium is administered to compare the haemodynamic flow patterns over a 20-minute period between the affected and non-affected sides. As with thermography and bone scintigraphy, the changes seen in stage 1 disease are markedly different to the changes seen in the later stages. A high flow pattern is seen in stage 1, representing vasodilatation and high blood flow, whereas a low flow pattern is seen in stages 2 and 3. This technique offers no benefit over other investigative techniques and is not used in routine clinical practice.

Histological studies, including synovial biopsies and studies of amputated limbs in cases of severe CRPS type I, have shown no consistent diagnostic features.[16] It may be argued that locally invasive techniques should be avoided unless there is a need to exclude other pathologies, because the diagnostic yield is low and the opportunity to exacerbate the disease could be great.

Ultrasound of the calcaneum is becoming increasing accepted in the assessment of bone density, although dual-energy X-ray absorptiometry (DEXA) remains the gold standard. A recent study has looked closely at the role of quantitative ultrasound of the calcaneum in patients with unilateral CRPS type I of the foot.[17] Two measurable quantities, namely, broadband ultrasound attenuation and 'stiffness' (a term used to quantify bone quality), were reduced but improved with calcitonin therapy and were associated with a reduction in reported pain levels. Ultrasound may therefore be more useful than DEXA in this group of patients, although other causes of unilateral bone loss are not excluded.[18] One of the difficulties in assessing the efficacy of treatments has been the lack of objective evidence and quantification of the response to treatment. Attempts have been made to quantify the sympathetic response,[19, 20] but this is unlikely to be very useful as CRPS type I is characterized by vasomotor instability. Bone loss appears to start early in the disease and patchy osteoporosis is evident in cases with a short history (Fig. 7). Quantification of this bone resorption may be an indirect measure of disease progression and resolution. In cases where there is unilateral involvement, the unaffected foot acts as a control as reported variation between two normal feet is minimal. Precision, determined by repeated measurements in normal subjects, is 0.9 per cent.[17]

Management

A variety of treatments have been used with anecdotal success and there is a great need for randomized controlled studies (Table 3). Physiotherapy remains the cornerstone of treatment and rehabilitation of the affected area starting with light touch and slowly moving on to passive, then active movements with weight-bearing exercises is often undervalued.

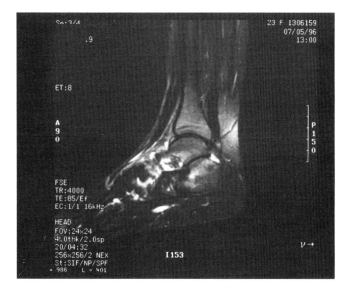

Fig. 6 T2-weighted image.

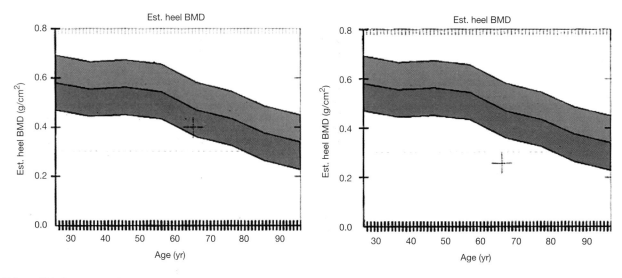

Fig. 7 (a and b) Quantitative ultrasound of both heels of a 62-year-old woman with generalized osteoporosis and CRPS type I of her right foot. There is lower attenuation in the affected foot than in her unaffected foot. The result in her normal foot is below average, perhaps a reflection of systemic osteopenia, which was diagnosed using bone densitometry.

Table 3 Management options

Physical therapy
Physiotherapy (exercise and hydrotherapy)
Occupational therapy
Transcutaneous nerve stimulation
Acupuncture
Hypnotherapy

Pharmacological therapies
Calcitonin
Bisphosphonates
Antineuralgic agents, e.g. gabapentin

Sympathetic blockade
Chemical
Surgical

Proprioceptive exercises are often built into the exercise programme, for example, swivel boards may be used in the treatment of lower limb CRPS type I, and may benefit those in whom proprioception is reduced.[21] Hydrotherapy is often of benefit, particularly in patients who are reluctant to weight-bear or to allow passive movement of their affected limb. Recent studies have assessed the role of physiotherapy in the treatment of early CRPS type I in adults favourably.[22, 23] The role of physiotherapy in late disease is less clear. One study assessing outcome in late disease noted a reduction in pain levels of 75 per cent in 70 per cent of patients undergoing physical therapy over a follow-up period varying between 10 and 36 months.[24] In children, physical therapy has been shown to be effective, often reducing the need for invasive measures.[25, 26] Some benefit has been described with acupuncture[27] and hypnotherapy.[28]

A multidisciplinary team approach is necessary in the treatment of patients with CRPS type I. Physiotherapists and occupational therapists have central roles. Drug therapy should be considered and pain specialists and psychologists should all have input. Many patients with chronic pain benefit from this approach.

Sympathetic blockade, induced by surgical or chemical methods, has been beneficial in reducing pain. Chemical blockade may be administered singly or repeatedly. The use of regional intravenous guanethidine, a favoured agent for this technique, is, however, no more effective than placebo.[29, 30] Sympathetic blockade is discussed in greater detail in Chapter 6.17. Historically, oral prednisolone was prescribed with little success, often in conjunction with calcium channel antagonists, to reduce the inflammatory response and to increase local blood flow.[31–33] The dose of prednisolone varies, although in one paper the prescription of high-dose prednisolone (60–80 mg) was tapered rapidly over 3–4 weeks.[32] Because prednisolone is recognized to cause bone loss and the efficacy of treatment was unproven, corticosteroids are no longer widely used. Gabapentin has been used to treat the pain of CRPS type I with anecdotal benefit,[34] although randomized controlled studies are required to evaluate this further.

Calcitonin and the bisphosphonates have also been used with some success. Both are established treatments for osteoporosis, Paget's disease, and hypercalcaemia of malignancy. Their use in CRPS type I where there is localized bone loss is reasonable. Calcitonin may be administered intranasally or subcutaneously, and there may be compliance implications particularly with patients who are required to self-administer subcutaneous injections daily. Side-effects include nausea, vomiting, facial flushing, and local skin reactions at the site of injection. Calcitonin is believed to have an analgesic as well as an antiresorptive effect.[35, 36] One study[37] found no benefit of intranasal calcitonin in comparison with placebo, although a weak statistical significance was achieved when comparing intranasal calcitonin and physiotherapy with physiotherapy alone.[38] Several papers report success with subcutaneous calcitonin in the management of CRPS type I,[39, 40] although only one was a randomized, controlled study. The length of treatment varies considerably, with some authors prescribing calcitonin for 4 weeks, while others prescribe it for up to 10 months.

The role of bisphophonates is being explored as a treatment for CRPS type I. Administration may be oral or intravenous, although there are no reports of oral bisphosphonate therapy in the treatment of CRPS type I. Intravenous pamidronate has an analgesic and perhaps therapeutic role in patients with metastatic bone disease.[41] The analgesic effect of bisphosphonates may have an important role in CRPS type I. Anecdotal pain relief was first described in a patient with CRPS type I in 1988.[42] No controlled trials exist to assess the effects of the bisphosphonates in CRPS type I, although analgesic and functional success is reported with both intravenous pamidronate[43–45] and intravenous alendronate.[46] The regimes are variable but bisphosphonate infusions were usually given over 3 consecutive days as tolerated in these studies. Each of these trials included small numbers of patients, and the period of follow-up was short. No studies attempted to administer a further dose of bisphosphonate at a later date if there had been a partial response, and the effect of repeated doses therefore remains to be clarified. Further randomized controlled studies to assess the efficacy of the bisphosphonates and calcitonin are required, as the evidence is conflicting[17, 39, 40] and long-term studies are lacking. Other bisphosphonates, such as clodronate, are also reported to have analgesic effects, although this has not been assessed in patients with CRPS type I.

Bisphosphonates are usually well tolerated and the gastrointestinal side-effects of oral bisphosphonates are often avoided with intravenous administration. Patients may also suffer symptoms of fever, myalgia, and flushes and hypersensitivity reactions. The mechanism for the analgesic properties of bisphosphonate drugs remains unclear.

Prostaglandin E2 and other nociceptive substances have been postulated.[47] Bisphosphonates have been shown to sensitize afferent nerve fibres. The neuropeptides and neuromodulators released from these nerve endings produce vasodilatory and inflammatory effects that may cause pain and perhaps trophic changes in soft tissues and bone.[48, 49]

Patients with CRPS type I may be considered malingerers by some as no pathophysiological or histological findings have been confirmed and in some cases there may be litigation and compensation cases pending. This is an attitude that other patient groups who suffer chronic pain may not invite. For example, patients with postherpetic neuralgia have a similar rate of depression, anxiety, and suicidal ideation.

Summary

Chronic regional pain syndrome type I remains a poorly understood condition, which may be associated with chronic pain and disability.

Although a number of aetiological factors have been associated with the development of the condition, the pathophysiology remains unclear. Despite the variety of diagnostic tests available, no particular test has shown high sensitivity and specificity during the early stages of the disease, partly because of the instability of the vasomotor changes. Treatments, which have been anecdotally reported as successful, have yet to be formally assessed in randomized, controlled trials with consistent, reproducible objective outcome measures. However, a multidisciplinary team approach early in the disease may be valuable in preventing long-term disability. Further research is required to establish the pathophysiology and tailor the most effective treatment plan accordingly.

References

1. Veldman, P.H., Reynen, H.M., Arntz, I.E., and Goris, R.J. (1993). Signs and symptoms of reflex sympathetic dystrophy: prospective study of 829 patients. *Lancet* **342**, 1012–1016.

2. Doury, P. (1988). Algodystrophy. Reflex sympathetic dystrophy syndrome. *Clin. Rheumatol.* **7**,173–180.

3. Steinbrocker, O. and Argyros, T.G. (1958). The shoulder-hand syndrome: present status as a diagnostic and therapeutic entity. *Med. Clin. N. Am.* **42**, 1533–1553.

4. Herrmann, L.G., Reineke, H.G., and Caldwell, J.A. (1942). Post traumatic painful osteoporosis: a clinical and roentgenological entity. *Am. J. Roentgenol.* **47**, 353–361.

5. Genant, H.K., Kozin, F., Bekerman, C., McCarty, D.J., and Sims, J. (1975). The reflex sympathetic dystrophy: a comprehensive analysis using fine-detail radiography, photon absorptiometry and bone and joint scintigraphy. *Radiology* **117**, 21–32.

6. Kozin, F., Genant, H.K., Bekerman, C., and McCarty, D.J. (1976). The reflex sympathy dystrophy syndrome II. Roentgenographic and scintigraphic evidence of bilaterality and of periarticular accentuation. *Am. J. Med.* **60**, 332–338.

7. Pachaczevsky, R. (1987). Thermography in post traumatic pain. *Am. J. Sports Med.* **15**, 243–250.

8. Karstetter, K.W. and Sherman, R.A. (1991). Use of thermography for initial detection of early reflex sympathetic dystrophy. *J. Am. Podiatr. Med. Assoc.* **81**, 198–205.

9. Bruehl, S., Lubenow, T.R., Nath, H., and Ivankovich, O. (1996). Validation of thermography in the diagnosis of reflex sympathetic dystrophy. *Clin. J. Pain* **12**, 316–325.

10. Mackinnonn, S.E. and Holder, L.E. (1984). The use of three-phase radionucleotide bone scanning in the diagnosis of reflex sympathetic dystrophy. *J. Hand Surg.* **9A**, 556–563.

11. Werner, R., Davidoff, G., Jackson, D., Cremer, S., Ventocilla, C., and Wolf, L. (1989). Factors affecting the sensitivity and specificity of the three phase technetium bone scan in the diagnosis of reflex sympathetic dystrophy syndrome in the upper extremity. *J. Hand Surg. (Am.)* **14**, 520–523.

12. Hoffman, J., Phillips, W., Blum, M., Barohn, R., Ramamurthy, S. (1993). Effect of sympathetic block demonstrated by triple phase bone scan. *J. Hand Surg. (Am.)* **18**, 860–864.

13. Goldsmith, D.P., Vivino, F.B., Eichenfield, A.H., Athreya, B.H., and Heyman, S. (1989). Nuclear imaging and clinical features of childhood reflex neurovascular dystrophy: comparison with adults. *Arthritis Rheum.* **32**, 480–485.

14. Schweitzer, M.E., Mandel, S., Schwartzman, R.J., Knobler, R.L., and Tahmoush, A.J. (1995). Reflex sympathetic dystrophy revisited: MR imaging before and after infusion of contrast material. *Radiology* **195**, 211–214.

15. Graif, M., Schweitzer, M.E., Marks, B., Matteucci, T., and Mandel, S. (1998). Synovial effusion in reflex sympathetic dystrophy: an additional sign for the diagnosis and staging. *Skeletal Radiol.* **27**, 262–265.

16. van der Laan, L., ter Laak, H.J., Gabreels-Festen, A., Gabreels, F., and Goris, R.J.A. (1998). Complex regional pain syndrome type 1: pathology of skeletal muscle and peripheral nerve. *Neurology* **51**, 20–25.

17. Cepollaro, C., Gonnelli, S., Pondrelli, C., Martini, S., Montagnani, A., Rossi, B., and Gennari, C. (1998). Usefulness of ultrasound in Sudeck's atrophy of the foot. *Calcif Tissue Int.* **62**, 538–541.

18. Prowse, M., Higgs, C.M.B., Forrester-Wood, C., and McHugh, N. (1989). Reflex sympathetic dystrophy associated with squamous cell carcinoma of the lung. *Ann. Rheum. Dis.* **48**, 339–344.

19. Casale, R. and Elam, M. (1992). Normal sympathetic nerve activity in a reflex sympathetic dystrophy with marked skin vasoconstriction. *J. Auton. Nerv. Syst.* **41**, 215–219.

20. Clinchot, D.M. and Lorch, F. (1996). Sympathetic skin response in patients with reflex sympathetic dystrophy. *Am. J. Phys. Med. Rehabil.* **75**, 252–256.

21. Veldman, P.H., Reynen, H.M., Arntz, I.E., *et al.* (1993). Signs and symptoms of reflex sympathetic dystrophy; prospective study of 829 patients. *Lancet* **342** (8878), 1012–1016.

22. Oerlemans, H.M., Goris, J.A., de Boo, T., and Oostendorp, R.A. (1999). Do physical therapy and occupational therapy reduce the impairment percentage in reflex sympathetic dystrophy? *Am. J. Phys. Med. Rehabil.* **78**, 533–539.

23. Oerlemans, H.M., Oostendorp, R.A., de Boo, T., van der Laan, L., Sevenson, J.L., and Goris, J.A. (2000). Adjuvant physical therapy versus occupational therapy in patients with reflex sympathetic dystrophy/complex regional pain syndrome type 1. *Arch. Phys. Med. Rehabil.* **81**, 49–56.

24. Robaina, F.J., Rodriquez, J.L., De Vera, J.A., Martin, M.A. (1989). Transcutaneous electrical nerve stimulation and spinal cord stimulation for pain relief in reflex sympathetic dystrophy. *Stereotact. Funct. Neurosurg.* **52**, 53–62.

25. Dietz, F.R., Mathews, K.D., and Montgomery, W.J. (1990). Reflex sympathetic dystrophy in children. *Clin. Orthop.* **258**, 225–231.

26. Wilder, R.T., Berde, C.B., Wolohan, M., Viegra, M.A., Masek, B.J., and Micheli, L.J. (1992). Reflex sympathetic dystrophy in children. *J. Bone Joint Surg. (Am.)* **74**, 910–919.

27. Fralka, V., Resch, K.L., Ritter-Dietrich, D., Alacamliogh, Y., Chen, O., Lechta, T., Kluger, R., and Ernst, F. (1993). Acupuncture for reflex sympathetic dystrophy. *Arch. Intern. Med.* **153**, 661–662.

28. Garner, M.J. (1992). Hypnotherapy for reflex sympathetic dystrophy. *Am. J. Clin. Hypn.* **34**, 227–232.

29. Jadad, A.R., Carroll, D., Glynn, C.J., and McQuay, H.J. (1995). Intravenous regional blockade for pain relief in reflex sympathetic dystrophy: a systematic review and a randomised, double-blind crossover study. *J. Pain Symptom Manage.* **10**, 13–20.

30. Ramamurthy, S., Hoffman, J., and the Guanethidine Study Group (1995). Intravenous regional guanethidine in the treatment of reflex sympathetic dystrophy/causalgia: a randomised, double blind study. *Anaesth. Analg.* **81**, 718–723.

31. Glick, E.N. (1973). Reflex sympathetic dystrophy (algoneurodystrophy). Results of treatment by corticosteroids. *Rheumatol. Rehabil.* **12**, 84.

32. Kozin, F., McCarty, D.J., Sims, J., and Gerant, H. (1976). The reflex sympathetic dystrophy syndrome. I. Clinical and histological studies. Evidence of bilaterality response to steroids, and articular involvement. *Am. J. Med.* **60**, 332–338.

33. Christensen, K., Jensen, E.M., and Noer, I. (1982). The reflex dystrophy syndrome. Response to treatment with systemic corticosteroids. *Acta Chir. Scand.* **148**, 653–655.

34. Mellick, G.A. and Mellick, L.B. (1997). Reflex sympathetic dystrophy treated with gabapentin. *Arch. Phys. Med. Rehabil.* **78**, 98–105.

35. Pecile, A., Ferri, S., Braga, P.C., and Olgiati, V.R. (1975). Effects of intracerebroventricular calcitonin in the conscious rabbit. *Experientia.* **31**, 332–333.

36. Fraioli, F., Fabbri, A., Gnessi, L., Moretti, C., Santora, C., and Felici, M. (1982). Subarachnoid injection of salmon calcitonin induces analgesia in man. *Eur. J. Pharmacol.* **78**, 381–382.

37. Bickerstaff, D.R. and Kanis, J.A. (1991). The use of nasal calcitonin in the treatment of posttraumatic algodystrophy. *Br. J. Rheumatol.* **30**, 291–294.

38. Gobelet, C., Walburger, M., and Meier, J.L. (1992). The effects of adding calcitonin to physical treatment on reflex sympathetic dystrophy. *Pain* **48**, 171–175.

39. Arlet, J. and Mazieres, B. (1997). Medical treatment of reflex sympathetic dystrophy. *Hand Clinics* **13**, 477–483.

40. Sawicki, A., Szulc, P., Subczk, T., Goliszewski, J., Garnier, P., and Labuszewski, R. (1992). Influence of calcitonin treatment on the osteocalcin concentration in the algodystrophy of bone. *Clin. Rheumatol.* **11**, 346–350.

41. Latreille, J., Conte, P.J., Mauriac, L., *et al.* (1994). Aredia infusions in breast cancer: a randomised phase III trial to assess delay in progression of bone metastases [abstract]. *Proc. Annu. Meet. Am. Soc. Clin. Oncol.* **13**, 78.

42. Devogelaer, J.P., Dall'Armellina, S., Huaux, J.P., and Nagant de Deuxchaisnes, C. (1988). Dramatic improvement of intractable reflex sympathetic dystrophy syndrome by intravenous infusions of the second generation bisphosphonate APD [abstract 213]. *J. Bone Miner. Res.* **3**, S122.

43. Rehman, M.T.A., Clayson, A.D., Marsh, D., Adams, J., Cantrill, J., and Anderson, D.C. (1992). Treatment of reflex sympathetic dystrophy with intravenous pamidronate [abstract]. *Bone* **13**, 116.

44. Maillefert, J.F., Chatard, C., Owen, S., Peere, T., Tavernier, C., and Tebib, J. (1995). Treatment of refractory reflex sympathetic dystrophy with pamidronate. *Ann. Rheum. Dis.* **54**, 687.

45. Cortet, B., Flipo, R.-M., Coquerrelle, P., Duquesnoy, B., and Delcambre, B. (1997). Treatment of severe, recalcitrant reflex sympathetic dystrophy: assessment of efficacy and safety of the second generation bisphosphonate pamidronate. *Clin. Rheumatol.* **16**, 51–56.

46. Adami, S., Fossaluzza, V., Gatti, D., Fracassi, E., and Braga, V. (1997). Bisphosphonate therapy of reflex sympathetic dystrophy syndrome. *Ann. Rheum. Dis.* **56**, 201–204.

47. Strang, P. (1996). Analgesic effect of bisphosphonates on bone pain in breast cancer patients. *Acta Oncol. Suppl.* **35**, 50–54.

48. Schott, G.D. (1995). An unsympathetic view of pain. *Lancet* **345**, 634–636.

49. Dray, A. (1996). Neurogenic mechanisms and neuropeptides in chronic pain. *Prog. Brain Res.* **110**, 85–94.

6.17 Complex regional pain syndrome (type I): the pain clinic perspective

Carol Chong and Rajesh Munglani

Patients with complex regional pain syndrome (type I) (CRPS) are often seen in the pain clinic, where the approach can differ from that in the rheumatology setting.

Additional investigations in the pain clinic

Investigations are not usually helpful but may help to exclude other conditions. There are no pathognomonic blood tests. In 40 per cent of patients, there is radiological evidence of bone demineralization of the periarticular area on plain X-ray films. These changes are seen after 4–8 weeks.[1]

A triple phase bone scan using radiolabelled technetium 99 can be used to evaluate blood flow to the effected limb. In early CRPS, there may be increased blood flow, whereas blood flow is decreased when the condition is in its later stages. There is often periarticular pooling in the late phase of this scan. The usefulness of this technique has been questioned.[1]

Magnetic resonance imaging (MRI) of the affected limb could show oedema in the muscle and periarticular connective tissue. An increased enhancement occurs after gadolinium and indicates increased vascular permeability. This is less dramatic than changes seen with arthritis or infections.[1]

A difference in temperature between affected and unaffected limbs of at least 1 °C is considered significant and thermography is used to establish this.

There are various other tests involving measurement of cutaneous blood flow with Doppler flowmetry and measuring skin conductivity or abnormalities of sweat secretion. However, these techniques are rarely used in clinical practice in the United Kingdom.

Diagnostic blocks

The use of sympathetic blockade allows us to see if there is a significant sympathetic component to the patient's pain. Sympathetically maintained pain (SMP) is diagnosed if at any stage of the pain history a placebo-controlled block of the sympathetic system causes relief of symptoms. This can be achieved in several ways.

Intravenous phentolamine test

An intravenous phentolamine test is a practical way of determining SMP as it is easy to perform and can be placebo-controlled. Phentolamine is an antagonist of $\alpha 1$ and $\alpha 2$ adrenoceptors that may be involved in SMP. Monitoring should include blood pressure and electrocardiography. An infusion containing phentolamine (0.5–1 mg/kg)

is administered via a peripheral vein in an unaffected extremity over a period of 20 minutes. The patient should experience significant levels of pain relief when compared to a placebo infusion. The possible side-effects related to this technique are hypotension, flushing, nasal congestion, and headaches. However, the advantages of performing this test include relative lack of invasiveness, minimal risk of discomfort, and placebo control. Further, analgesia obtained from local anaesthetic blockade of sensory nerves or systemic uptake can be ruled out.

Local anaesthetic diagnostic blockade

The sympathetic supply to the upper and lower limbs is carried in the stellate and lumbar sympathetic ganglia, respectively. Local anaesthetic can be placed on the stellate or lumbar sympathetic ganglia and these techniques will be briefly described below. We will not attempt a detailed description of these techniques as there are some excellent books on neural blockade available.[2, 3] However, the use of such blocks for diagnosis or treatment is controversial as local anaesthetic may spread inadvertently on to somatosensory nerves resulting in false-positives.[4–6] Verdugo and Ochoa have shown that their patients with CRPS were relieved of motor weakness and movement disorders when placebo nerve blockade was performed.[7]

There is also controversy as to the subjective evaluation of whether sympathicolysis has been achieved. Schurmann and colleagues[1] showed that 48 per cent of patients who had a temperature rise after stellate ganglion blockade had an undisturbed sympathetic nervous function when this was assessed with laser Doppler flowmetry.

Treatment

The treatment of CRPS involves treating all its components. This includes pharmacological manipulation, sympathetic blocks, neuromodulation, physiotherapy, behavioural therapy, and rehabilitation. However, there is lack of evidence to support most of these treatments as few randomized controlled trials have been performed.

Sympathetic blockade

Sympathetic blockade is achieved either by intravenous regional anaesthesia using a drug such as guanethidine or via injections of the appropriate ganglia. The interruption of the periarterial sympathetic supply for sympathetic pain was first described by Leriche.[8] Many authors have questioned the role of the sympathetic system in CRPS and several have dismissed the value of sympathectomy in these patients.[9–12] The sympathetic system interacts at many neuroanatomical levels with the patient's pain state and therefore patients will present with a range of pathophysiology that is dynamic and changeable. This could account for the varying response seen when sympathectomies are performed in CRPS.

Intravenous regional block

Hannington-Kiff [13] first described this technique, which is essentially a Bier's block using guanethidine. Guanethidine depletes nerve endings of noradrenaline and prevents its reuptake. It is not available for this use in the United States. Other drugs that have been used include bretylium, ketorolac, reserpine, phentolamine, and ketanserin. This technique has advantages in that it is technically easy to perform and can be done in an anticoagulated patient. A dose of guanethidine of 10–20 mg diluted in saline is administered intravenously (IV) in the affected limb. However this injection usually causes pain and it is common to administer this with lignocaine 10–20 mg. It is emphasized in the literature that a positive response to IV regional guanethidine (IVRG) is not diagnostic of CRPS. Possible complications include hypotension and neuropraxia from the cuff. The author (Munglani, unpublished observations) has seen one case of pulmonary embolism on deflation of a leg cuff. The benefit of IVRG is controversial. The duration of pain relief is said to increase with consecutive blocks,[14] and it is quite common to perform a 'series' of three guanethidine blocks over a fortnight.

Some authors have reported very good success with IV regional blockade (IVRB) using guanethidine.[15, 16] However, more recent randomized, controlled trials have failed to show any benefit in groups of patients though individual dramatic responses are common.[17, 18] This suggests either a placebo response, an effect from the inflated cuff, or our failure to understand the complex, dynamic nature of SMP in CRPS.

Sympathetic blocks

There are several ganglia where sympathetic blockade may be achieved. This is done pharmacologically by injecting these areas with local anaesthetic, local anaesthetic and steroid, or various neurolytic agents, the most common being phenol, glycerol, or alcohol. For further reading on neurolytic agents, see Myers.[19] Neurolytic agents may spread further than the intended area of block and carry the risk of permanent injury.

In recent years, the technique of radiofrequency denervation has also been used for ablating the sympathetic nervous system. This can be performed percutaneously and has the advantage of being more site-specific as very small lesions are made. On the other hand, open surgical ablation of the sympathetic nervous system goes back to Leriche's technique of stripping of perivascular sympathetic nerves.[4]

It is important to stress that all sympathetic blocks should be done in a closely monitored environment with full resuscitation facilities. The following are several areas of sympathetic blockade commonly performed.

Stellate ganglion block

The stellate ganglion receives sympathetic fibres from the head and neck that originate from the anterolateral horn of the spinal cord at T1–2. It also receives sympathetic fibres from the upper limbs that originate from T8–9. These fibres travel as white rami to join the sympathetic chain and synapse at the stellate, middle, or superior cervical ganglion. The stellate ganglion is approximately 2.5 cm long × 1 cm wide × 0.5 cm thick. It lies over the transverse processes of C7–T1.

There are several techniques to block the stellate ganglion and the reader is referred to the excellent texts mentioned above for further information. This block is usually performed under local anaesthetic with full monitoring and resuscitation facilities available. Stellate ganglion blockade is used in SMP of the upper limb or head and neck. Its side-effects include Horner's syndrome, nasal congestion, conjunctival injection, perforated trachea or oesophagus, nerve injury, and inadvertent vascular or intrathecal injections.

The success rate of stellate ganglion blockade in the hands of experienced operators is said to be only 75 per cent.[20] Forouszanfar and colleagues, in a recent retrospective analysis, have shown radiofrequency lesioning of the stellate ganglion to have the same efficacy as traditional methods of blockade.[21]

Lumbar sympathetic block

The lower limbs are innervated by preganglionic sympathetic fibres that arise from the anterolateral dorsal horn from T10 to L2–3. These travel through the white rami and sympathetic trunk to the sympathetic and sacral ganglia and then usually join the L1 to S3 spinal nerves by way of grey rami or form a diffuse plexus around the iliac arteries.

There are many techniques of lumbar sympathetic blockade and once again the reader is referred to the excellent books available. This block is usually carried out with image intensifier at L3, as a higher level carries more risk to the genitofemoral nerve, causing neuralgia. Successful diagnostic blockade using local anaesthetic is usually only followed by a 30 per cent success rate when the neurolytic block is done. The neurolytic blocks have a duration of action of 6–12 months. This high false-positive rate has been attributed to the local anaesthetic inadvertently blocking somatosensory nerves or from systemic absorption.[22]

Complications that may result include bleeding, perforation of abdominal viscera, hypotension, and inadvertent intravascular, intrathecal, or epidural injection.

Thoracic sympathetic block

This block may be indicated in some malignant pains with a strong component of SMP. One of the authors (R.M.) has had excellent results with T2 thoracic sympathetic blocks either with local anaesthetic or radiofrequency in the treatment of posttraumatic neck pain and upper arm symptoms with strong autonomic symptoms. Prithvi Raj et al. state that the incidence of pneumothorax is 4 per cent even in experienced hands.[3]

Coeliac plexus and splanchnic block

Although coeliac plexus blockade is usually performed for visceral abdominal pain, it is included here for completeness. SMP originating from the abdomen is rare. The coeliac plexus lies anterolateral to the aorta and receives sympathetic fibres from T5 to T12 that pass through the splanchnic nerves. All abdominal viscera except part of the transverse colon, descending colon, rectum, and pelvic viscera receive innervation from the coeliac plexus. Neurolytic coeliac plexus blocks usually last about 6–12 months before the nerves regenerate. This block carries risk of visceral injury, pneumothorax, haemorrhage, hypotension, impotence, and diarrhoea. Splanchnic nerve radiofrequency at T11 may offer an alternative way of producing similar results and one of the authors (R.M.) has seen good response for lower chest and upper abdominal myofascial pain syndromes with it.

Sphenopalatine ganglion block

This ganglion is located posterior to the middle turbinate and receives communications from the first and second division of the trigeminal nerve, facial nerve, and carotid plexus. There is a direct communication with the cervical sympathetic and parasympathetic fibres via the superficial petrosal nerve. It is possible to block this ganglia using topical cocaine or local anaesthesia as it lies in close proximity to the nasal mucosa. Alternatively, it can also be approached laterally using an image intensifier. A needle is passed under the zygoma lateral to the mandible to enter the sphenopalatine fossa. This ganglion can be blocked either with local anaesthetic or radiofrequency procedures. It is used for patients with cluster headaches, migraines, and Sluder's neuralgia. Adverse effects include epistaxis and numbness of the hard palate and teeth.

Ganglion of impar (Walther) block

This technique for the treatment of intractable neoplastic perineal pain of sympathetic origin was described by Plancarte and colleagues in 1996.[22] The ganglion of impar lies retroperitoneally at the level of the sacrococcygeal junction. It is possible to reach it through the sacrococcygeal membrane or with a bent needle around the coccyx.

Other interventions

There have been other interventions described for the treatment of CRPS. These include continuous infusions of local anaesthetic or opioids to the brachial or lumbar plexuses, spinal cord stimulators, and intrathecal therapies.

The use of continuous local anaesthetic[23] or low-dose morphine[24] for brachial plexus blockades has been reported but again raises the question as to whether these drugs have been deposited on somatosensory nerves or have systemic uptake. They are administered via a catheter in the brachial plexus and may be difficult to maintain in out-patients. The exact mechanism and site of action of drugs in this situation is not clear.

In randomized controlled trials, Kemler and colleagues found that spinal cord stimulation produced significant relief of pain in patients with chronic CRPS[25] but no clinically important improvement in functional ability. The same authors reported in another study that spinal cord stimulation in CRPS patients had no effect on pain thresholds for pressure, warmth, and cold.[26] This technique is invasive, expensive, and, even in experienced hands, has a 25 per cent complication rate.

Van Hilten et al.[27] conducted a randomized controlled cross-over trial using intrathecal baclofen in seven patients with generalized dystonia from CRPS. There was marked improvement in upper limb dystonia in six of these seven women after a single bolus dose but less improvement was seen with the lower limbs. Baclofen is an agonist of gamma aminobutyric acid B (GABA-B) and activation of these receptors results in presynaptic inhibition of sensory input to the motor neurons of the spinal cord. Implantable intrathecal pumps of baclofen are already used in multiple sclerosis.

Pharmacotherapy

The use of pharmacotherapy in CRPS is also an area that has not been subjected to many properly randomized, double-blind, controlled trials. It is common for patients to be on several drugs from different groups at the same time or for patients to have tried many groups of drugs in the past. The following are used in the management of CRPS.

Anti-depressants

The 'older' tricyclic antidepressants such as amitryptyline have been shown to be effective in the management of neuropathic pain,[28] but no studies have been done to evaluate the use of antidepressants in CRPS. These agents may be useful in patients with CRPS who experience burning or shooting pain. It is not known if these drugs exert their analgesic effect in the same way as their antidepressant effect, that is, to inhibit the reuptake of noradrenaline and serotinin. The doses required for analgesia are much less than those required to treat depression. Therefore it is important that these drugs be titrated to individual patient's requirements. The use of the 'newer' slow serotonin reuptake inhibitors (SSRIs) in CRPS has produced varying anecdotal reports of this group being beneficial[29] or disappointing.[30]

Anti-epileptics agents

There are no controlled studies evaluating the use of anti-epileptic agents in CRPS. However the use of gabapentin was first reported in reflex sympathetic dystrophy in 1995 by Mellick et al.[31] Its efficacy in neuropathic pain has been demonstrated in randomized controlled trials of diabetic neuropathy[32] and postherpetic neuralgia.[33] It may also be of benefit in patients with CRPS who have shooting, burning pain.

Nonsteroidal anti-inflammatory drugs (NSAIDs)

There is a rationale for using NSAID in the early stages of CRPS or in patients where there is a significant inflammatory component.[34] Harden advocated the use of ketoprofen and it has more antibradykinin and antiprostacyclin action in addition to the antiprostaglandin effect.[30]

Opioids

Stanton-Hicks and colleagues recommend a trial of opioids in the early stages of CRPS, preferably intravenously.[29] The use of opioids for non-malignant pain always raises concerns of dependence and abuse, especially when its efficacy in CRPS remains unproven.

(N-methyl-D-aspartate) NMDA antagonists

There have been reports suggesting that ketamine is useful in neuropathic pain[24] or chronic pain.[25] However, the use of ketamine or dextromethorphan in chronic pain syndromes seem to be limited by the high incidence of side-effects. This is so even when the drug is administered orally.

Capsaicin

Cheshire and Snyder reported the use of topical capsaicin in CRPS in 1990.[36] This agent is thought to act by depleting the nerve endings of substance P. A trial of capsaicin is suggested by Stanton-Hicks et al.[29] in patients with specific areas of hyperalgesia.

Calcitonin and bisphosphonates

The use of calcitonin in CRPS was described by Bickerstaff et al.[37] and Gobelet et al.[38] with varying success. Its mechanism of action in CRPS is unknown. There have been reports of success with the bisphosphonate clodronate which is administered intravenously. This randomized controlled trial showed that patients had less pain than those who received a placebo.[39] Adami and colleagues used IV alendronate versus placebo in 20 patients and found less pain and swelling in the treated group.[40] The mechanism of bisphosphonate action in analgesia is unknown but it is thought to prevent bone resorption. However, we know that less than half of patients with CRPS show radiological evidence of bone resorption.

Other agents used in the management of CRPS include corticosteroids, calcium channel antagonists, and alpha 2 agonists such as clonidine. The use of pamidronates is discussed in Chapter 6.16.

Physical therapies

A consensus meeting in 1998 recommended the use of physiotherapy and occupational therapy for functional restoration in a time-limited algorithm.[29] The use of medication and sympathetic blocks was only recommended if these therapies were unsuccessful after 3 weeks. Physiotherapy aims to improve mobility, function, prevent dependent oedema, and to encourage tactile input to the effected area. The techniques used include joint motion exercises, massage, and neuromuscular electrical stimulation (NMES).[41] The reader is referred to this consensus report,[29] the review by Harden,[30] and references 41–43 for more details on these aspects of CRPS management.

However, Bogduk stresses that very few of these methods have been subjected to randomized controlled trials.[44] Oerlemans et al. randomized 135 patients with upper limb reflex sympathetic dystrophy to receive physiotherapy, occupational therapy, or a control group.[45] They found no difference in impairment at 12 months between any of the three groups. The same authors have found no difference in pain between the three groups.[46]

Psychology

It is important that patients with CRPS receive psychological support as there is a high incidence of depression and anxiety in these patients.[46] Cognitive behavioural therapy is used and is said to be the most effective technique in these patients.[29]

Once again, there are no randomized controlled trials evaluating these therapies in this group of patients.

References

1. Schurmann, M., et al. (1994). Clinical and physiologic evaluation of stellate ganglion block for complex regional pain syndrome type 1. Clin. J. Pain 17 (1), 94–100.
2. Cousins, M.J. and Bridenbaugh, P.O. (1998). Neural blockade. Lippincott–Raven, Philadelphia.
3. Prithvi Raj, P., et al. (1996). Autonomic blocks. In Pain medicine (ed. P. Prithvi Raj), pp. 227–258. Mosby, St Louis.
4. Charlton, J.E. (1986). Current views on the use of nerve blocking in the relief of chronic pain. In The therapy of pain (ed. M. Swerdlow), pp. 133–164. MTP, Lancaster.
5. Hogan, Q.H. (1997). Neural blockade for diagnosis and prognosis. Anesthesiology 86, 216–214.
6. Stolker, R.J., et al. (1994). The management of chronic spinal pain by blockades: a review. Pain 58, 1–20.
7. Verdugo, R.J. and Ochoa, J.L. (2000). Abnormal movements in complex regional pain syndrome: assessment of their nature. Muscle Nerve 23, 198–205.
8. Leriche, R. (1916). De la causalgie envisagee comme une nevrite du sympathique ed des son traitment par la dendation et l'excision des plexus nerveux periarterials. Presse Medicale 24, 178–180.
9. Max, M.B., et al. (1999). Sympathetically maintained pain: has the emperor no clothes? Neurology 52, 905–907.
10. Schott, G.D. (1998). Interrupting the sympathetic outflow in causalgia and reflex sympathetic dystrophy: a futile procedure for many patients. Br. Med. J. 316, 792–793.
11. Verdugo, R.J., et al. (1994). Phentolamine sympathetic block in painful polyneuropathies. Further questioning of the concept of "sympathetically maintained pain". Neurology 44, 1010–1014.
12. Raja, S.N., et al. (1991). Systemic alpha-adrenergic blockade with phentolamine: a diagnostic test for sympathetically maintained pain. Anesthesiology 74, 691–698.
13. Hannington-Kiff, J.G. (1977). Relief of Sudeck's atrophy by regional intravenous guanethidine. Lancet 1, 1132–1133.
14. Lee, D.J. and Benzon, H.T. (1999). Anesthesiologic treatments for complex regional pain syndrome. In Essentials of pain medicine and regional anesthesia (ed. H.T. Benson and S.N. Raja). Churchill-Livingstone, Philadelphia.
15. Ramamurthy, S., Hoffman, J., and Guanethidine Study Group. (1995). Intravenous regional guanethidine in the treatment of reflex sympathetic dystrophy/causalgia: a randomised double blind study. Anaesth. Analg. 81, 718–723.
16. Wahren, L.K., et al. (1995). Effects of regional intravenous guanethidine in patients with neuralgias in the hand: a follow up study over a decade. Pain 62, 24–30.
17. Jadad, A.R., et al. (1995). Intravenous sympathetic blockade for pain relief in reflex sympathetic dystrophy: a review and a randomised double blind crossover study. J. Pain Symptom Manage. 10, 13–20.
18. Kaplan, R., et al. (1996). Intravenous guanethidine in patients with reflex sympathetic dystrophy. Acta Anaesthesiol. Scand. 40, 1216–1222.
19. Myers, R.M. (1998). Neuropathology of neurolytic agents. In Neural blockade in clinical anesthesia and management of pain, 3rd edn (ed. M.J. Cousins and P.O. Bridenbaugh). Lippincott-Raven, Philadelphia.
20. Stanton-Hicks, M., et al. (1996). Use of regional anaesthetics in the diagnosis of reflex sympathetic dystrophy and sympathetically maintained pain. In Reflex sympathetic dystrophy: a reappraisal (ed. W. Janig and M. Stanton-Hicks), pp. 217–237. IASP Press, Seattle.
21. Forouszanfar, T., et al. (2000). Radiofrequency lesions of the stellate ganglion in chronic pain syndromes: a retrospective analysis of clinical efficacy in 86 patients. Clin. J. Pain 16 (2), 164–168.
22. Plancarte, R., et al. (1996). Neurolytic blocks of the sympathetic axis. In Cancer pain (ed. R.B. Patt), pp. 377–426. Lippincott, Philadelphia.
23. Wang, L.K., et al. (2001). Axillary brachial plexus block with patient controlled analgesia for complex regional pain syndrome type 1: a case report. Reg. Anesth. Pain Med. 26, 68–71.
24. Azad, S.C. (2000). Continuous axillary brachial plexus analgesia with low dose morphine in patients with complex regional pain syndromes. Eur. J. Anaesthesiol. 17, 185–188.
25. Kemler, M.A., et al. (2000). A controlled trial of spinal cord stimulation in patients with chronic reflex sympathetic dystrophy. N. Engl. J. Med. 343, 618–624.
26. Kemler, M.A., et al. (2001). Impact of spinal cord stimulation on sensory characteristics in complex regional pain syndrome type 1: a randomised trial. Anesthesiology 95, 72–80.
27. Van Hilten, B.J., et al. (2000). Intrathecal baclofen for the treatment of dystonia in patients with reflex sympathetic dystrophy. N. Engl. J. Med. 343, 625–630.

28. McQuay, H.J., *et al.* (1996). A systematic review of antidepressants in neuropathic pain. *Pain* **68**, 217–227.

29. Stanton-Hicks, M., *et al.* (1998). Consensus report. Complex regional pain syndrome: guidelines for therapy. *Clin. J. Pain* **14**, 155–166.

30. Harden, R.N. (2001). Complex regional pain syndrome. *Br. J. Anaesth.* **87**, 99–106.

31. Mellick, G.A., Mellick, L.B., and Mellick, J.D. (1995). Gabapentin in the management of reflex sympathetic dystrophy. *J. Pain Symptom Manage.* **10**, 265–266.

32. Backonja, M., *et al.* (1998). Gabapentin for the symptomatic treatment of painful neuropathy in patients with diabetes mellitus. *J. Am. Med. Assoc.* **280**, 1831–1836.

33. Rowbotham, M., *et al.* (1998). Gabapentin for the treatment of postherpetic neuralgia: a randomised controlled trial. *J. Am. Med. Assoc.* **280**, 1837–1842.

34. Eide, P.K., *et al.* (1994). Relief of post-herpetic neuralgia with N-methyl-D-aspartic acid receptor antagonist ketamine: a double-blind, cross-over comparison with morphine and placebo. *Pain* **5**, 347–354.

35. Haines, D.R. and Gaines, S.P. (1999). N of 1 randomised controlled trials of oral ketamine in patients with chronic pain. *Pain* **83**, 283–287.

36. Cheshire, W.P. and Snyder, C.R. (1990). Treatment of reflex sympathetic dystrophy with topical capsaicin: a case report. *Pain* **42**, 307–311.

37. Bickerstaff, D.R., *et al.* (1991). The use of nasal calcitonin in the treatment of post-traumatic algodystrophy. *Br. J. Rheumatol.* **30**, 291–294.

38. Gobelet, C., *et al.* (1986). The effect of adding calcitonin to physical treatment on reflex sympathetic dystrophy syndrome. *Clin. Rheumatol.* **5**, 382–388.

39. Varenna, M., *et al.* (2000). Intravenous clodronate in the treatment of reflex sympathetic dystrophy syndrome. A randomised double blind, placebo, controlled study. *J. Rheumatol.* **27**, 1477–1483.

40. Adami, S., *et al.* (1997). Bisphosphonate therapy of reflex sympathetic dystrophy syndrome. *Ann. Rheum. Dis.* **56**, 201–204.

41. Hareau, J. (1996). What makes treatment for reflex sympathetic dystrophy successful? *J. Hand Ther.* **9**, 367–370.

42. Parsley, C. (1998). The progression of reflex sympathetic dystrophy and the implications for therapy. BAHT, 14–16.

43. Lampen-Smith, R.A. (1997). Complex regional pain syndrome 1 (RSD) and the physiotherapeutic intervention. *NZ J. Physiother.* **25**, 19–23.

44. Bogduk, N. (2001). Complex regional pain syndrome. *Curr. Opin. Anaesthesiol.* **14**, 541–546.

45. Oerlemans, M.H., *et al.* (1999). Do physical therapy and occupational therapy reduce the impairment percentage in reflex sympathetic dystrophy? *Am. J. Phys. Med. Rehabil.* **78**, 533–553.

46. Oerlemans, H.M., *et al.* (1999). Adjuvant physical therapy versus occupational therapy in patients with reflex sympathetic dystrophy/complex regional pain syndrome type 1. *Arch. Phys. Med. Rehabil.* **81**, 49–56.

47. Bruehl, S. and Carlson, C.R. (1992). Predisposing psychological factors in the development of reflex sympathetic dystrophy: a review of the empirical evidence. *Clin. J. Pain* **8**, 287–299.

Index